Handbook of
Depression in Children and Adolescents

Issues in Clinical Child Psychology

Series Editors: **Michael C. Roberts,** *University of Kansas–Lawrence, Kansas*
                    Lizette Peterson, *University of Missouri–Columbia, Missouri*

BEHAVIORAL ASPECTS OF PEDIATRIC BURNS
Edited by Kenneth J. Tarnowski

CHILDREN AND DISASTERS
Edited by Conway F. Saylor

HANDBOOK OF DEPRESSION IN CHILDREN AND
ADOLESCENTS
Edited by William M. Reynolds and Hugh F. Johnston

INTERNATIONAL HANDBOOK OF PHOBIC AND ANXIETY
DISORDERS IN CHILDREN AND ADOLESCENTS
Edited by Thomas H. Ollendick, Neville J. King, and William Yule

MENTAL HEALTH INTERVENTIONS WITH PRESCHOOL
CHILDREN
Robert D. Lyman and Toni L. Hembree-Kigin

A Continuation Order Plan is available for this series. A continuation order will bring
delivery of each new volume immediately upon publication. Volumes are billed only
upon actual shipment. For further information please contact the publisher.

Handbook of
Depression in Children and Adolescents

Edited by

William M. Reynolds

University of British Columbia
Vancouver, British Columbia, Canada

and

Hugh F. Johnston

University of Wisconsin
Madison, Wisconsin

Plenum Press • New York and London

Library of Congress Cataloging in Publication Data

On file

ISBN 0-306-44742-8

© 1994 Plenum Press, New York
A Division of Plenum Publishing Corporation
233 Spring Street, New York, N. Y. 10013

Printed in the United States of America

Contributors

Jessie C. Anderson, Division of Child and Adolescent Psychiatry, Children's Pavilion, Dunedin Hospital, Dunedin, New Zealand

William R. Beardslee, Judge Baker Children's Center, Department of Psychiatry, Harvard University Medical School, Boston, Massachusetts 02115

Jules R. Bemporad, Department of Psychiatry, The New York Hospital–Cornell Medical Center, White Plains, New York 10605

Lori Breedlove, Burrell Center, Springfield, Missouri 65804

Ronald T. Brown, Department of Psychiatry and Behavioral Sciences, Emory University School of Medicine, Atlanta, Georgia 30322

Dennis P. Cantwell, Department of Psychiatry and Biobehavioral Science, Neuro-psychiatric Institute, University of California at Los Angeles, Los Angeles, California 90024

Gabrielle A. Carlson, Division of Child and Adolescent Psychiatry, Department of Psychiatry and Behavioral Sciences, State University of New York at Stony Brook, Stony Brook, New York 11794-8790

Dante Cicchetti, Mt. Hope Family Center, University of Rochester, Rochester, New York 14608

Harvey F. Clarizio, Department of Counseling and Educational Psychology, Michigan State University, East Lansing, Michigan 48824-1034

Gregory N. Clarke, Division of Child Psychology, Oregon Health Sciences University, Portland, Oregon 97201

Bruce E. Compas, Department of Psychology, University of Vermont, Burlington, Vermont 05405-0134

Geraldine Downey, Department of Psychology, Columbia University, New York, New York 10027

Graham J. Emslie, Department of Psychiatry, University of Texas Southwestern Medical Center, and Children's Medical Center at Dallas, Dallas, Texas 75235-9070

Sydney Ey, Medical College of South Carolina, Charleston, South Carolina 29425

Scott Feldman, Department of Psychology, Columbia University, New York, New York 10027

Sarah Friedman, Department of Psychology, Columbia University, New York, New York 10027

J. Jay Fruehling, Child Psychopharmacology Information Center, Department of Psychiatry, University of Wisconsin, Madison, Wisconsin 53792

Kathryn E. Grant, Cook County Medical Center, Chicago, Illinois 60626

Kay Hodges, Department of Psychology, Eastern Michigan University, Ypsilanti, Michigan 48197

Hugh F. Johnston, Division of Child and Adolescent Psychiatry, Department of Psychiatry, University of Wisconsin Medical School, Madison, Wisconsin 53792

Javad H. Kashani, Department of Psychiatry, University of Missouri School of Medicine, Columbia, Missouri 65212

Nadine J. Kaslow, Department of Psychiatry and Behavioral Sciences, Emory University School of Medicine, Atlanta, Georgia 30322

Alan E. Kazdin, Department of Psychology, Yale University, New Haven, Connecticut 06520-8205

Betsy D. Kennard, Department of Psychiatry, University of Texas Southwestern Medical Center, and Children's Medical Center at Dallas, Dallas, Texas 75235-9070

Jananne Khuri, Department of Psychology, Columbia University, New York, New York 10027

Robert A. Kowatch, Department of Psychiatry, University of Texas Southwestern Medical Center, and Children's Medical Center at Dallas, Dallas, Texas 75235-9070

Cynthia Kurowski, Department of Educational Psychology, University of Texas, Austin, Texas 78712

Peter M. Lewinsohn, Oregon Research Institute, Eugene, Oregon 97403-1983

James J. Mazza, Department of Psychology, St. John's University, Jamaica, New York 11439

Rob McGee, Department of Preventive and Social Medicine, University of Otago Medical School, Dunedin, New Zealand

Laura L. Mee, Department of Psychiatry and Behavioral Sciences, Emory University School of Medicine, Atlanta, Georgia 30322

Hartmut B. Mokros, Rutgers University, New Brunswick, New Jersey 08903

Barry Nurcombe, Division of Child and Adolescent Psychiatry, Department of Psychiatry, Vanderbilt University School of Medicine, Nashville, Tennessee 37212

Elva O. Poznanski, Rush–Presbyterian–St. Luke's Medical Center, Chicago, Illinois 60612

Gary R. Racusin, Connecticut Mental Health Center, Yale University, New Haven, Connecticut 06516

William M. Reynolds, Psychoeducational Research and Training Centre, University of British Columbia, Vancouver, British Columbia V6T 1Z4, Canada

Fred A. Rogosch, Mt. Hope Family Center, University of Rochester, Rochester, New York 14608

Paul Rohde, Oregon Research Institute, Eugene, Oregon 97403-1983

Lawrence W. Rouse, Department of Educational Psychology, University of Texas, Austin, Texas 78712

Patrick Schloss, Assistant Vice President, Graduate Studies and Research, Bloomsburg University, Bloomsburg, Pennsylvania 17815

Holly Sher, Department of Special Education, University of Missouri, Columbia, Missouri 65211

Donald L. Sherak, Child and Adolescent Services, Taunton State Hospital, Taunton, Massachusetts 02780

Patricia L. Speier, Langley Porter Psychiatric Institute, University of California at San Francisco, San Francisco, California 94143-0984

Kevin D. Stark, Department of Educational Psychology, University of Texas, Austin, Texas 78712

Sheree L. Toth, Mt. Hope Family Center, University of Rochester, Rochester, New York 14608

Paul V. Trad, Department of Psychiatry, The New York Hospital–Cornell Medical Center, White Plains, New York, 10605

Warren A. Weinberg, Department of Neurology, University of Texas Southwestern Medical Center, and Children's Medical Center at Dallas, Dallas, Texas 75235-9070

Ingrid Wheelock, Judge Baker Children's Center, Department of Psychiatry, Harvard University Medical School, Boston, Massachusetts 02115

Lech Wisniewski, Department of Special Education, Eastern Michigan University, Ypsilanti, Michigan 48197

Preface

Anyone who has ever been close to a seriously depressed child has undoubtedly been affected by the youngster's vulnerability, misery, and pain. Indeed, it is much like caring for a child who is in physical pain. For the child in the depths of depression, no activity is fun, nothing can be enjoyed, and no one can provide enough consolation or comfort. At times, the youngster may cry or whimper. There may be fits of defiance or rage and sometimes withdrawal into a numb, sullen silence. A child in this state tries the patience of parents and siblings. Remedies of every sort are tried, including gifts, punishments, bribes, lectures, pleading, and a host of others. Such efforts occasionally provide temporary relief, but more often they seem to make matters worse. Commonly, there is an emotional wall of anger and frustration between a depressed child and other family members that may inevitably lead to further isolation and withdrawal. If too much time passes without their being helped, many depressed children and adolescents come to believe that suicide offers the only real relief for their pain.

Currently, there is a Depression Awareness Week that includes free screening at participating health and mental health settings around the United States and is designed to identify depression in adults, suggesting that society's awareness of depression and psychiatric disorders is focused to a large extent on adults. Although professionals acknowledge the existence of depression in children and adolescents, with epidemiological studies suggesting significant prevalence, the scope of the problem is still unrecognized by the general public. For children and adolescents, the school typically provides a natural setting for the identification of depression, with a number of schools already having adopted a screening model for this purpose. Sadly, too little is yet being done to identify and treat depressed children and adolescents.

Depression in children and adolescents is manifested by many of the same symptoms we find in depressed adults. Depression in the young may last for years with little respite or even relief from treatment. As this handbook illustrates, depression in young people represents a complex interplay of developmental, environmental, dynamic, interpersonal, cognitive, behavioral, and biological factors. The multitude and magnitude of these factors are well represented and presented.

The need for a comprehensive handbook on depression in children and adolescents became evident to one of the editors (WMR) several years ago when he was writing a chapter on depression for a book on internalizing disorders. After he had completed an initial 200-page draft of his chapter, it was clear that no chapter nor, realistically, no one single-authored book could do justice to the depth and breadth of understanding depression in children and adolescents. This handbook is the result of our perception that the scope of this disorder merits a broad and multidisciplinary approach. Toward this end, the book includes contributions by many of the leading experts on child and adolescent depression in the fields of psychology and psychiatry.

This book was written for professionals as well as graduate students with clinical and research interests in child and adolescent psychopathology in general, and in depression in young people in particular. We anticipate that the book will be particularly useful to psychologists, psychiatrists, social workers, pediatricians, counselors, nurses, and other mental health professionals. The chapters cover a range of disciplines and orientations to provide a balanced and comprehensive treatment of depression in children and adolescents.

The 25 chapters are organized in six parts. Part I, an introduction to depression in children and adolescents, consists of a brief introduction to the field, chapters on the description and epidemiology of depression in youngsters, phenomenology and treatment of bipolar disorder, and a thoughtful chapter on the validity of depression as a clinical disorder in young people. Part II describes a wide range of theories and models of depression, with specific attention to children and adolescents. This range is illustrated by chapters on dynamic theories, cognitive–behavioral models, developmental models, and neurobiological models. Part III focuses on classification, diagnosis, and assessment of depression in youngsters, with a chapter on systems of classification and diagnosis, and chapters on assessment by clinical interviews, self-report procedures, and assessment by significant others. The last chapter in this part discussed the important issue of variability in reports of child depression across informants. Part IV provides a comprehensive examination of treatment approaches for depression in children and adolescents, with chapters on the psychological treatment of children, the treatment of adolescents, family therapy, and a chapter on psychopharmacotherapy for depression in children and adolescents. Part V, which examines depression in special populations, includes chapters on depression in infants, children with medical illness, and youngsters in special education placements within school settings. Part VI provides coverage of a wide range of important topics, with chapters on children of parents with depressive disorders, maltreatment and depression in children, the effects of psychosocial stressors, suicide and suicidal behaviors in children and adolescents, and the nature of comorbidity of other disorders and depression in children and adolescents. Each chapter in this handbook provides a comprehensive examination of an important topic related to depression in young people. Readers will find a useful blend of theory, research, and clinical practice within the overall scope of the book.

This handbook is dedicated foremost to the millions of children and adolescents who suffer from depression and whose plight is the book's focus. Although by design the book is a compilation of current research and knowledge on depression in children and adolescents, we hope and anticipate that readers will go beyond the individual chapters and integrate this information into a comprehensive picture of our understanding of depression in young people.

We are grateful to many individuals who by direct or indirect means assisted us, provided comments, support, example, or by their writings and research enhanced our knowledge of depression in children and adolescents. Each of the editors has gained from interactions with colleagues at the University of Wisconsin–Madison. Among those who have helped both of us on our journey to this point, we wish to thank Dr. John H. Greist of the University of Wisconsin Medical School and Dean of the Foundation for Health, Research, and Education. Bill also thanks his friends and colleagues, Drs. Gloria Miller, Joe Czajka, Maribeth Gettinger, Allan Cohen, Bob Smith, Richard Rankin, Kevin Stark, Kevin Coats, James Mazza, Thomas Evert, and Gail Anderson, for their support, encouragement, and friendship over the years. In particular, he wishes to thank Dr. Norman Sundberg, friend and mentor for the past twenty years, for his support, friendship, and example. Hugh wishes to thank Drs. Bill Swift, Jack Westman, and Richard Anderson for years of thoughtful mentorship. Hugh also has a special thanks for Dr. Lorna Benjamin, who taught him the art of listening, and for J. Jay Fruehling, who has been incredibly helpful in too many ways to list. At Plenum, we were very fortunate to have the guidance, encouragement, and support of Mariclaire Cloutier with whom it was wonderful to work. We also wish to acknowledge the late Joachim Puig-Antich, M.D., who, by his exceptional work in the field, greatly enhanced our knowledge of depression in young people.

We are most grateful to the many authors who have contributed to this handbook and who by their contributions have helped us to illuminate the many facets of depression in young people. They represent the leading researchers and experts in the field of child and adolescent depression, and we are especially honored by their contributions and dedication to this book and, more important, by their enhancement of our understanding of depression in children and adolescents. We also received a great deal of support and encouragement from the contributors, who, as the handbook took shape, shared their enthusiasm and commitment to the project.

Both editors also wish to thank and acknowledge the indirect assistance provided by the many hundreds of children and adolescents we have seen in our research and clinical experience who have provided us with the insights and understanding of depression in young persons.

Finally, but most significantly, we wish to acknowledge the importance and support of our families. Bill is especially grateful to his family and wishes to thank his wife, Margaret, and his children, Annie and Sean, for their love, affection, and encouragement, and for their support during the many days and nights he spent cloistered with his PC. Bill also wishes to acknowledge his parents, Martha and Hugh, sister Judy, and brothers Dan and Bob and their families. Hugh wishes to thank his wife, Amy Rock, for her steady love, encouragement, support, affection, and patience with her "workaholic" spouse.

WILLIAM M. REYNOLDS
HUGH F. JOHNSTON

Contents

Part I. Introduction and General Issues

1. The Nature and Study of Depression in Children and Adolescents   3

   William M. Reynolds and Hugh F. Johnston

2. Phenomenology and Epidemiology of Mood Disorders in Children and
   Adolescents 19

   Elva O. Poznanski and Hartmut B. Mokros

3. Adolescent Bipolar Disorder: Phenomenology and Treatment Implications . . 41

   Gabrielle A. Carlson

4. The Validity of the Diagnosis of Major Depression in Childhood and
   Adolescence 61

   Barry Nurcombe

Part II. Theories and Models of Depression

5. Dynamic and Interpersonal Theories of Depression 81

   Jules R. Bemporad

6. Cognitive and Behavioral Correlates of Childhood Depression:
   A Developmental Perspective 97

   Nadine J. Kaslow, Ronald T. Brown, and Laura L. Mee

7. A Developmental Psychopathology Perspective on Depression in Children
   and Adolescents 123

   Dante Cicchetti, Fred A. Rogosch, and Sheree L. Toth

8. Neurobiological Aspects of Depression in Children and Adolescents 143

*Graham J. Emslie, Warren A. Weinberg, Betsy D. Kennard,
and Robert A. Kowatch*

Part III. Approaches to Assessment and Diagnosis

9. Classification and Diagnostic Criteria of Depression in Children and
Adolescents 169

Donald L. Sherak, Patricia L. Speier, and Dennis P. Cantwell

10. Evaluation of Depression in Children and Adolescents Using Diagnostic
Clinical Interviews 183

Kay Hodges

11. Assessment of Depression in Children and Adolescents by Self-Report
Questionnaires 209

William M. Reynolds

12. Assessment of Depression in Children and Adolescents by Parents, Teachers,
and Peers 235

Harvey F. Clarizio

13. Informant Variability in the Assessment of Childhood Depression 249

Alan E. Kazdin

Part IV. Treatment Approaches

14. Psychological Treatment Approaches for Depression in Children 275

Kevin D. Stark, Lawrence W. Rouse, and Cynthia Kurowski

15. Psychological Approaches to the Treatment of Depression in Adolescents ... 309

Peter M. Lewinsohn, Gregory N. Clarke, and Paul Rohde

16. Family Therapy for Depression in Young People 345

Nadine J. Kaslow and Gary R. Racusin

17. Pharmacotherapy for Depression in Children and Adolescents 365

Hugh F. Johnston and J. Jay Fruehling

Part V. Depression in Special Populations

18. Depression in Infants 401

   Paul V. Trad

19. Depression in Medically Ill Youngsters 427

   Javad H. Kashani and Lori Breedlove

20. Depression in Special Education Populations 445

   Patrick Schloss, Holly Sher, and Lech Wisniewski

Part VI. Selected Topics in the Study of Depression in Young People

21. Children of Parents with Affective Disorders: Empirical Findings and
   Clinical Implications 463

   William R. Beardslee and Ingrid Wheelock

22. Maltreatment and Childhood Depression 481

   Geraldine Downey, Scott Feldman, Jananne Khuri, and Sarah Friedman

23. Psychosocial Stress and Child and Adolescent Depression: Can We Be More
   Specific? 509

   Bruce E. Compas, Kathryn E. Grant, and Sydney Ey

24. Suicide and Suicidal Behaviors in Children and Adolescents 525

   William M. Reynolds and James J. Mazza

25. Comorbidity of Depression in Children and Adolescents 581

   Jessie C. Anderson and Rob McGee

   Index 603

I

INTRODUCTION AND GENERAL ISSUES

1

The Nature and Study of Depression in Children and Adolescents

William M. Reynolds and Hugh F. Johnston

Introduction

Depression is a serious mental health problem in children and adolescents. It has been estimated that nearly 1 of every 6 youngsters admitted to psychiatric hospitals in the United States had an intake diagnosis of a depressive disorder (Silver, 1988). Depression is also one of the most frequently found psychiatric disorders among suicidal children and adolescents [Reynolds and Mazza (Chapter 24)]. Over the past two decades, the study of depression in children and adolescents has become an area of extensive research in the fields of psychiatry, psychology, and related disciplines. The range of research domains, from neuroendocrinology to cognitive deficits, suggests an enormous interest on the part of professionals in the nature, evaluation, and treatment of depression in young people. What is most impressive is that the vast majority of research on depression in children and adolescents has been conducted since the mid-1970s. This delay in our focus on depression in young people may be in part a function of the long-term psychodynamic perspectives of depression as nonexistent in children or normative in adolescents. In particular, the notion or myth of adolescent turmoil overshadowed for many professionals the validity of depression as a form of psychopathology in this age group (Offer & Schonert-Reichl, 1992).

In this chapter, we will touch on a number of topics and issues related to our understanding of depression in children and adolescents. Rather than risk redundancy by delving deep into each topic, we instead seek to lay out a road map for the purpose of integrating and organizing the material that follows. It is our hope that this chapter will

William M. Reynolds • Psychoeducational Research and Training Centre, University of British Columbia, Vancouver, British Columbia V6T 1Z4, Canada.   **Hugh F. Johnston** • Division of Child and Adolescent Psychiatry, Department of Psychiatry, University of Wisconsin Medical School, Madison, WI 53792.

Handbook of Depression in Children and Adolescents, edited by William M. Reynolds and Hugh F. Johnston. Plenum Press, New York, 1994.

provide a larger view of the forest that will help and orient the reader as she or he explores the chapters that make up the trees of this text.

Depression in children and adolescents is generally considered to be an internalizing disorder (Reynolds, 1992a). Unlike externalizing problems and disorders—such as conduct disorder or attention-deficit hyperactivity disorder—that cause distress to others such as parents, peers, and teachers, depression has its primary impact on the child. The depressed youngster may cause very little consternation or discomfort to others, yet feel intense misery, demoralization, and distress. Many depressed children and adolescents do not come to the attention of teachers or parents, and if they do, referral for treatment appears to be relatively infrequent. This is not to say that some depressed youngsters do not have difficulties in school. Depressed youngsters tend not to be actively engaged in school learning, with consequent reductions in grades and other indicators of achievement (Cole, 1990; Kovacs & Goldston, 1991). Lowered school performance by depressed youngsters is consistent as an outcome of several symptoms of depressive disorders, including poor concentration and thinking ability, decreased productivity in school, fatigue, psychomotor retardation or agitation, and insomnia. A number of researchers have suggested a linkage between learning disabilities and depression in children and adolescents (Forness, 1988; Rourke, Young, & Leenaars, 1989; Weinberg & Emslie, 1988).

While depression is ultimately viewed as an internalizing disorder, it must be remembered that the initial clinical presentation of depressed children is protean. Some children withdraw in sadness, others lash out with formidable anger. Indeed, a strong predictor of having externalizing symptoms is the presence of internalizing symptoms, with many youngsters showing symptoms of both broad-bandwidth domains (Achenbach & McConaughy, 1992). Furthermore, depression in children has been closely associated with conduct disorders (Puig-Antich, 1982). At times, we have felt that the use of the term "depression" as a label for this disorder is misleading. Perhaps it might be better labeled "miserable mood disorder of childhood."

The current level of attention to depression in children and adolescents is well warranted, especially when we consider the results of epidemiological studies that suggest that as many as 5% of children and between 10% and 20% of adolescents from the general population have experienced a depressive disorder (Reynolds, 1992a, 1994). There also appears to be among young people a cohort trend for increasing rates of depression (Klerman, 1988; Klerman & Weissman, 1989). Thus, we may find greater numbers of depressed children and adolescents in the future. To compound the problem, most youngsters do not receive treatment, and there is some question as to the efficacy of contemporary treatments (Keller, Lavori, Beardslee, Wunder, & Ryan, 1991). In addition to the study of depression in children and adolescents, there has been strong research and clinical interest in depression in infants and preschool-age youngsters [e.g., Trad, 1986; Trad (Chapter 18)].

It is ironic that much of the modern research in childhood depression is modeled after similar work that has been conducted in adults. During the first 60 years of this century, it was widely accepted that depression in adults had its roots in early childhood experience (Freud, 1946) and that depression could not occur in the undeveloped psyche of the child (Mahler, 1961). We are only now at the threshold of realizing that this illness affects all age groups, albeit with important developmental differences.

The study of developmental psychopathology has assisted in our understanding of depression in children, with particular reference to research on attachment, maltreatment, temperament, and the development of the self [e.g., Cicchetti, Rogosch, and Toth (Chapter 7); Downey, Feldman, Khuri, and Friedman (Chapter 22)]. Developmental perspectives on the nature and ontogenesis of depression and depressive states in infants, children, and adolescents are not new, with the works of Spitz and Wolf (1946) and Bowlby (1973, 1980, 1982) providing an early developmental focus on depression in children. Renewed interest in the development of psychopathology in children emerged in the 1980s (e.g., Bowlby, 1988; Cicchetti & Olsen, 1990; Cicchetti & Schneider-Rosen, 1984; Cytryn, et al., 1984; Garber, 1984; Rutter, 1988). It is useful to note that developmental models of depression, and in particular separation–attachment models, have also been extensively investigated in nonhumans (e.g., Lewis, McKinney, Young, & Kraemer, 1976; Kraemer, Ebert, & McKinney, 1983; Mineka & Suomi, 1978; Suomi & Harlow, 1977).

Classification

The present state of the art in the classification of mood disorders is comparable to the classification of respiratory illness before the discovery of the microbe. In those early days of medicine, scholars made serious distinctions between wet cough and dry cough, green sputum and yellow sputum, cough with a fever and cough without a fever. Undoubtedly, learned discussions were held regarding the advantages, disadvantages, and nuances of various classification systems. In a similar way, we struggle mightily with our current objective–descriptive classifications of most psychiatric illness. These comments are not intended to diminish the importance of the laborious work that has given us our current diagnostic system. They do highlight, however, the critical need for greater understanding of the etiology and pathophysiology of depressive disorder. Ultimately, the greatest value of a classification system is its ability to suggest the most effective treatment. We now realize that knowing that a cough is caused by pneumococcus is far more important than knowing whether it is, say, a wet cough with yellow sputum.

There have been a number of perspectives and systems for the classification of depression in young people. In the early 1970s, Weinberg and colleagues (Ling, Oftedal, & Weinberg, 1970; Weinberg, Rutman, Sullivan, Penick, & Dietz, 1973) provided a set of criteria for the classification of depression in children that included the presence of both (1) dysphoric mood and self-deprecatory thoughts and (2) two or more of the following eight symptoms: sleep disturbance, change in school performance, aggressive behavior, diminished socialization, change in attitude toward school, somatic complaints, loss of usual energy, and unusual change in appetite or weight or both. According to Weinberg et al. (1973), symptoms of depression need to be present for more than 1 month and to be a change in the child's usual behavior. Other formulations that recognized the validity of depression in children include those of Connell (1972), Kuhn and Kuhn (1971), McConville, Boag, and Purohit (1973), and Poznanski and Zrull (1970). A number of other formulations specific to depression in infants, children, and adolescents have been presented (e.g., Cytryn & McKnew, 1972; Malmquist, 1971; Rie, 1966; Spitz & Wolf, 1946) and provide evidence of the broad interest in understanding depression in children and adolescents and precursors to contemporary perspectives. Although predicted for the most part on adult criteria, contemporary diagnostic criteria do identify "cases" of depression in young children, including those of preschool age (e.g., Kashani & Carlson, 1987; Kashani, Holcomb, & Orvaschel, 1986).

The most commonly used classification system for the clinical description of depressive disorders in North America is the *Diagnostic and Statistical Manual of Mental Disorders* (DSM), which, with the publication of the 3rd edition and its subsequent revision (DSM-III and DSM-III-R) (American Psychiatric Association, 1980, 1987), set the standard for the classification of depressive disorders in children and adolescents. DSM is currently in its 4th edition (DSM-IV), published by the American Psychiatric Association (1994). DSM-IV delineates a number of depressive disorders, including Major Depressive Disorder, which may be either a single episode or recurrent; Dysthymic Disorder; and Depressive Disorder Not Otherwise Specified (NOS). These latter disorders are consistent with the notion of unipolar depression. Also included under the general classification of mood disorders are Bipolar Disorders, which include Bipolar I Disorder, with the form of this disorder differentiated on the basis of whether the most recent episode was manic, hypomanic, depressed, mixed depression and mania, or currently manic with prior episodes of depression or hypomania; Bipolar II Disorder (recurrent major depression with hypomania); Cyclothymic Disorder; and Bipolar Disorder NOS. In addition, Mood Disorder Due to a General Medical Condition and Substance-Induced Mood Disorder are included under the classification of mood disorders along with Mood Disorder NOS. Although not included within the larger category of mood disorders, Adjustment Disorder with Depressed Mood is another DSM-IV disorder that is relevant for the study of depression in children and adolescents. Table 1 summarizes the primary disorders included in the DSM-IV category of mood disorders.

The current formulation of DSM continues to ignore, for the most part, the potential for developmental differences or features unique to depression in children. Furthermore, the heavy reliance on DSM criteria for identification of depressed youngsters may limit some avenues of research and clinical practice. For instance, Sherak, Speier, and Cantwell (Chapter 9) note that both DSM-III- and DSM-III-R-diagnosed depressed children do not respond to trials of antidepressants as do adults diagnosed with similar criteria. To judge the medications ineffectual with youngsters may be too limiting if we allow that groups of depressed youngsters who do not meet DSM criteria may nevertheless respond to antidepressant medications. This inconsistency and others in the current diagnostic formulation of depression in children and adolescents have led some investigators to question the existence of depression in youngsters as a clinical entity derived by adult criteria [Nurcombe (Chapter 4); Nurcombe et al., 1989].

Assessment

The study and our understanding of depression in children and adolescents have been greatly enhanced by the development of measures for the assessment and diagnosis of depression in young people. The two primary modes of assessment are by direct self-report [e.g., Reynolds (Chapter 11)] and structured and semistructured clinical interviews with youngsters and parents [e.g., Hodges (Chapter 10)]. In addition to these assessment methodologies, a multitude of sources, such as parents, teachers, and peers, have been

Table 1. Summary of Primary DSM-IV Mood Disorders

Depressive disorders	Bipolar disorders	Other disorders
Major Depression[a–c,f]	Bipolar Disorder I[d,e,g]:	Mood Disorder Due to Medical
Single Episode	Manic: Single; Most Recent	Condition
Recurrent[d,g]	Episode[c,f]	With Manic Features
Dysthymic Disorder[b]	Depressed: Most Recent Episode[a,b,f]	With Depressive Features
Depressive Disorder	Hypomanic: Most Recent Episode	With Major Depressive-Like Episode
NOS	Mixed: Most Recent Episode[a–c,f]	With Mixed Features
	Most Recent Episode Unspecified	Substance-Induced Mood Disorder
	Bipolar Disorder II:	With Manic Features
	Recurrent Major Depression with	With Depressive Features
	Hypomania[a–g]	With Mixed Features
	Cyclothymic Disorder	With Onset During Intoxication
	Bipolar Disorder Not Otherwise	With Onset During Withdrawal
	Specified	Mood Disorder Not Otherwise
		Specified

[a–g] May also include: [a] With Melancholic Features; [b] With Atypical Features; [c] With Catatonic Features; [d] With Seasonal Pattern; [e] With Rapid Cycling; [f] With Postpartum Onset; [g] With/Without Interepisode Recovery.

used to provide reports of children's depressive symptomatology [e.g., Clarizio (Chapter 12)]. When we examine the results of various sources of information using measures for the assessment of depression, we find significant disagreement between sources, such as between parent and child, child and peer, and so forth [Kazdin (Chapter 13)]. In the case of adolescents, parents generally report significantly fewer symptoms of depression than are reported by youngsters (Fleming, Boyle, & Offord, 1993; Verhulst & van der Ende, 1992). The issue of informant variability is an important consideration, since it will affect our interpretation of much of the research on the nature, etiology, classification, and treatment of depression in children.

A significant body of research on the assessment of depression in children and adolescents has been generated. Most of the research on depression and depressive symptomatology in children and adolescents has utilized self-report methods. Given the internalized nature of most depressive symptomatology and the subjective nature of the depressive experience, self-report measures appear to be a viable approach with young people (Reynolds, 1993). For the most part, the data suggest that children and adolescents are reliable reporters of their depressive symptoms (Reynolds, 1989; Reynolds & Graves, 1989; Shain, Naylor, & Alessi, 1990). Naturally, when we examine specific measures of depression, whether they are clinical interviews, self-report, peer report, or parent report, issues of reliability, validity, norms, and other salient psychometric as well as developmental aspects must be considered. Likewise, when we evaluate depression in children, an important consideration must be the evaluation of information from different sources. Explicating the relative level of a child's depression from conflicting sources of information is often a complex task that must consider multiple factors in deciding how we might differentially weight the information [Kazdin (Chapter 13)].

Epidemiology

The epidemiology of childhood depression is frightening because it informs us of the mass of untreated suffering in our society. Furthermore, the presence of a cohort effect suggests that the problem is worsening. Although at one level this possibility is disturbing, it is also intriguing. As a rule, very common illnesses or disorders exist for interesting reasons. For example, sickle cell anemia is the result of a genetic adaptation that provides some protection for carriers who live in areas where malaria is present. Given the high prevalence of mood disorders in children and adolescents, we must wonder whether there is a connection with some adaptive trait. It also seems conceivable that our modern existence has become such a poor fit with our evolved psychophysiology that mood disorders are inevitable.

The prevalence of depression in children and adolescents may be inferred from the results of several recent epidemiological studies of psychopathology and depression in children and adolescents. However, the extent to which young people experience depression is in large part a function of how we conceptualize depression, e.g., as syndrome, disorder, or cumulative severity of depressive symptomatology (Reynolds, 1994). Likewise, estimates of prevalence vary across studies as a function of prevalence time period (e.g., 1-month, 6-month, 12-month, lifetime). From the results of epidemiological studies (e.g., Fleming et al., 1993; Fleming, Offord, & Boyle, 1989; Garrison, Addy, Jackson, McKeown, & Waller, 1992; Kashani et al., 1987; Lewinsohn, Hops, Roberts, Seeley, & Andrews, 1993; Reinherz, Giaconia, Lefkowitz, Pakiz, & Frost, 1993), it is evident that the prevalence of depression follows a developmental trajectory in its prevalence among youngsters, with higher rates of depression, both point prevalence and lifetime prevalence, found in adolescents. Recent studies of adolescents (e.g., Garrison et al., 1992; Lewinsohn et al., 1993) suggest a lifetime prevalence of 15–20%. These data indicate that between 1 of 6 and 1 of 5 youngsters from the general population experience a DSM depressive disorder at some time in their childhood or adolescence. Thus, the results from epidemiological studies provide us with evidence that a very large number of youngsters experience a depressive episode of sufficient severity to warrant a diagnosis of major depression, dysthymic disorder, or bipolar disorder, although the latter disorder is relatively rare in children.

Comorbidity

A significant finding over the past decade has been the relatively high degree of comorbidity of depressive disorders and other internalizing and externalizing disorders in children and adolescents. The comorbidity of internalizing disorders and other psychopathology is an area of growing and critical research interest (Reynolds, 1992b). Research shows that a wide range of other psychiatric disorders are found among youngsters with depressive disorders, including anxiety disorders (Alessi, Robins, & Dilsaver, 1987; Keller et al., 1992; Kovacs, Gatsonis, Paulauskas, & Richards, 1989; Last, 1992; Last, Perrin, Hersen, & Kazdin, 1992), conduct problems (Alessi & Magen, 1988; Harrington, Fudge, Rutter, Pickles, & Hill, 1990, 1991; Kovacs, Paulauskas, Gatsonis, & Richards, 1988), attention-deficit disorder (J. C. Anderson, Williams, McGee, & Silva, 1987; Biederman & Steingard, 1989; Jensen, Burke, & Garfinkel, 1988), eating disorders (Alessi, Krahn, Brehm, & Wittekindt, 1989; Rastam, 1992; Smith & Steiner, 1992), and substance-abuse disorders (Bukstein, Glancy & Kaminer, 1992; Deykin, Levy, & Wells, 1987), among other disorders.

The study of comorbidity of depressive disorders and other psychopathology in youngsters is important for several reasons. The existence of comorbidity of depression and other psychopathology appears to increase the potential for long-term mental health problems (Harrington et al., 1990, 1991; Kovacs, 1985, 1989). Our understanding of subtypes or developmentally robust forms of depressive disorders is quite limited and basically a minimal revision of adult criteria. Subtypes of depressive disorders based on comorbidity or depression with significant features of other disorders may prove to be a clinically useful way of describing and understanding depression in young people. Understanding the relationship between comorbid disorders may help us in designing appropriate treatment modalities that systematically integrate treatment components that target unique and common aspects of the comorbid disorders. Anderson and McGee (Chapter 25) have examined comorbidity in a large cohort of youngsters with major depression followed longitudinally to provide an understanding of the course of such disorders and the implications of comorbidity as a function of whether the depression precedes or succeeds the comorbid condition.

Environmental Factors

Environmental factors are those stressors that initiate, interact with internal vulnerability and biological factors, maintain, or exacerbate depression in children and adolescents. The definition describes a very broad class of factors and includes familial, interpersonal, extrafamilial, catastrophic, and traumatic events and setting, as well as minor chronic stressors that we sometimes characterize as "hassles." These factors are those that typically produce stress in the individual. The delineation of these environmental stressors encompasses a wide range of domains, including family factors, such as parental psychopathology [Beardslee, Bemporad, Keller, & Klerman, 1983; Beardslee and Wheelock (Chapter 21); Downey & Coyne, 1990; Hammen, Burge, Burney, & Adrian, 1990; Rutter & Quinton, 1984], maltreatment [Downey et al. (Chapter 22); Kaufman, 1991], parent–child conflict (Asarnow, Carlson, & Guthrie, 1987; Cole & Rehm, 1986; Kashani, Burbach, & Rosenberg, 1988; Puig-Antich et al., 1993, 1985a), and marital separation and divorce (Forehand, McCombs, Long, Brody, & Fauber, 1988; Reynolds, 1985); peer difficulties (Puig-Antich et al., 1985b); Reynolds & Coats, 1982); catastrophic and traumatic events (Kinzie, Sack, Angell, Manson, & Rath, 1986; Saigh, 1992); and physical illness [Kaplan, Busner, Weinhold, & Lenon, 1987; Kashani and Breedlove (Chapter 19)]. Placement or status in a special class within the school environment [Dalley, Bolocofsky, Alcorn, & Baker, 1992; Reynolds & Miller, 1985; Schloss, Sher, and Wisniewski (Chapter 20)] is a source of distress and stress for youngsters that is meaningful in its potential contribution to depression and depressive states. Another environmental factor related to depression in youngsters is social support—more specifically, the lack of social support (e.g., G. K. Anderson & Reynolds, 1993; Hops, Lewinsohn, Andrews, & Roberts, 1990). Research also suggests that there are developmental as well as gender differences in youngsters' depression as a response to stress [G. K. Anderson & Reynolds, 1993; Compas, Grant and Ey (Chapter 23); Wagner & Compas, 1990].

Biological Factors

In research, clinical practice, and office and cocktail party conversation, we are drawn into the nature vs. nurture debate. Perhaps the most interesting theme in modern neuroscience is that nature shapes nurture and that nurture is a most powerful modifier of nature. The early work of Hubel and Weisel (1970) demonstrating that patching a kitten's eye causes drastic differences in the structure and function of the visual cortex is compelling evidence that developmental experiences can overwhelm the predestiny of neuronal tissues. Conversely, the developing child exerts profound influences on his or her caregivers, helping to *create* the environment in which he or she will develop. It seems likely to us that a most important piece of the puzzle will ultimately be the interaction of biology and experience.

Research on the biological bases and correlates of depression in children and adolescents is to a large extent driven by previous research with adults. Much of this research has focused on neurobiological abnormalities associated with depression in young people (e.g., Puig-Antich, 1986, 1987a,b; Puig-Antich et al., 1989). As noted by Emslie, Weinberg, Kennard, and Kowatch (Chapter 8), biological correlates assist us in understanding the physiology of depression as well as the potential for diagnosis via biological markers. Biological and genetic research on depressive disorders has depended to some extent on the differentiation of qualitative as well as quantitative subtypes or classes of depressive disorders. For example, research suggests a genetic contribution to the etiology of bipolar disorder. However, whether this contribution is a function of the qualitative difference of this disorder from other depressive disorders or the quantitative difference within a liability threshold model in which depressive disorders are distinguished by their symptom variability–severity along a continuum is a domain of discussion and investigation (e.g., McGuffin & Katz, 1986).

A major line of the research on the psychobiology of depression in youngsters as well as adults has focused on the relationship between the functioning of the hypothalamic–pituitary–adrenal axis and depression. Specific to the latter area of research has been the investigation of the dexamethasone suppression test (DST), a somewhat uneven biological marker for endogenous forms of major depression. A relatively large number of studies of the DST with depressed children and adolescents (Reynolds, 1985, 1992a) have indicated that there are youngsters who show abnormal DST results, although the data do not suggest a high level of sensitivity for major depression. Research on biological correlates of depression in children and adolescents has included the study of growth hormone secretion (Puig-Antich et al., 1984), sleep architecture (Emslie, Roffwarg, Rush, Weinberg, & Parkin-Feigenbaum, 1987), and natural-killer-cell activity associated with the functioning of the immune system (Shain et al., 1991), to name a few of the biological areas of research on correlates of depression in children and adolescents.

Psychotherapy

Although there is a large literature base on psychological treatments of childhood psychological disorders (e.g., Kazdin, 1990), there has been limited research on the use of psychotherapy for the treatment of depression in children and adolescents. The experimental-treatment research on psychotherapy for depression in children and adolescents published in North American and English language journals comprises fewer than a dozen studies (Butler, Miezitis, Friedman, & Cole, 1980; Fine, Forth, Gilbert, & Haley, 1991; Kahn, Kehle, Jenson, & Clark, 1990; Lewinsohn, Clarke, Hops, & Andrews, 1990; Liddle & Spence, 1990; Marcotte & Baron, 1993; Reynolds & Coats, 1986; Stark, Reynolds, & Kaslow, 1987). These studies, although few given the prevalence of depression in youngsters and in comparison to the number of treatment studies of depression in adults, provide strong evidence for the utility of psychologically based therapies for depression in young people.

A number of researchers have provided useful clinical guidelines for the application of cognitive–behavioral and interpersonal therapies for the treatment of depression in children and adolescents [Lewinsohn, Clarke, and Rohde (Chapter 15); Mufson, Moreau, Weissman, & Klerman, 1993; Stark, 1990; Stark, Rouse, and Kurowski (Chapter 14)]. The research to date, along with the structured treatment procedures developed by researchers, suggests that reasonably effective means are available for the treatment of many depressed youngsters. It is evident that much more research is necessary to ascertain which children and adolescents may best benefit from psychotherapy and whether forms of depression in youngsters are best treated by one therapy or another. Furthermore, there has not been a published study on the efficacy of combined psychotherapy and pharmacotherapy, nor has there been a comparison of these two procedures within a randomly assigned and controlled study. As Johnston and Fruehling (Chapter 19) note, antidepressant medication should not be considered the first line of treatment in children, a perspective that requires knowledge and availability of efficient psychotherapies. The effectiveness of these psychotherapies in comparison to medications is therefore an important research question, as is the question of whether treatment effectiveness is enhanced by the combination of these treatment approaches. Such research is of critical importance if we are to deal effectively with the multitude of youngsters with depressive disorders.

Pharmacotherapy

We need only read newspapers and magazines and watch television talk shows to realize that we are entering a brave new world of psychopharmacology. New agents are being developed and marketed at an unprecedented rate. Progress has been clear-cut, with many of the newer compounds having greater efficacy and fewer side effects. The ability of pharmacological agents in fine-tuning mood and cognitive states has been cause for rejoicing, caution, and, for some, alarm. We have grave concerns about the alacrity with which these compounds are given to children. This abandon is especially worrisome given the current regulatory and drug-marketing climate, which essentially discourages research about the effects these drugs have on children. Yet we also see the potential for relief of suffering.

The pharmacotherapy of depression in children and adolescents has generally been found to be less effective than the use of pharmacological agents with adults [Ambrosini, Bianchi, Rabinovich, & Elia, 1993; Johnston & Fruehling (Chapter 17); Strober, Lampert, Schmidt, & Morrell, 1993]. Yet, as is suggested by Johnston and Fruehling (Chapter 17), a substantial number of child psychiatrists utilize antidepressant medications to treat depression (as well as other psychiatric disorders) in children and adolescents, although such treatment is not without risk (e.g., Biederman, 1991; Riddle et al., 1991). The research on psychopharmacological interventions for depression in children and adolescents has focused on four classes of medications: tricyclic antidepressants (TCAs), monoamine oxidase inhibitors (MAOIs), the newer selective serotonin reuptake inhibitors (SSRIs), and lithium carbonate, which is generally used for the treatment of bipolar disorder. Of all medications used for the treatment of depression in children and adolescents, the most effective appears to be lithium use with bipolar-disordered youngsters, with reports of efficacy similar to that found with adults [Carlson (Chapter 3)]. There is also preliminary evidence for the efficacy of fluoxetine, an SSRI (e.g., Simeon, Dinicola, Ferguson, & Copping, 1990) that has generated some controversy (Riddle et al., 1989; Teicher, Glod, & Cole, 1990) and is contraindicated in combination with MAOIs (Ryan, 1992).

Major questions concerning the use of drugs for the treatment of depression in children and adolescents relate to specific guidelines for the selection, administration, monitoring, and combination of medications, as well as safety issues. A number of authors have addressed many of these issues [e.g., Johnston & Freuhling (Chapter 17); Petti, 1983; Rancurrello, 1996; Ryan, 1992], although the complexities and limited data supporting efficacy contribute to the need for caution in the prescription of antidepressant medications with young people.

Summary and Conclusions

The current state of our understanding of depression in children and adolescents suggests that depression in young people, as in adults, is a relatively common mental health problem that often presents itself along with other forms of psychopathology. The subjective misery experienced by the depressed youngster, as well as the interpersonal and social difficulties (Gotlib & Hammen, 1992), along with the potential for negative long-term outcome (Kovacs et al., 1984b; Kovacs, Feinberg, Crouse-Novak, Paulauskas, & Finkelstein, 1984a), suggest that the depression in many youngsters is relatively long-lasting even with treatment.

There are a number of factors that suggest that developmental factors are relevant to the nature and understanding of depression in young people. Bemporad (Chapter 5) suggests differences between children and adolescents as a function of dynamic stages of development, although the roles of trauma and maltreatment are clearly factors related to the etiology of depression in young people. Gender differences in the prevalence of depression tend to appear around puberty, when we find depressive symptomatology increasing in girls at a higher rate than in boys. These differences are manifested in the prevalence of depression as well as differential response to particular stressors and modifiers. In this manner, research should examine characteristics, correlations, and etiological bases and interactions separate for males and females.

It is encouraging to find the quality and extensive coverage of research on depression in children and adolescents that has been published over the past decade. We have learned a great deal about the nature, etiological factors, methods for reliable and valid assessment, psychological and pharmacological treatment approaches, and other aspects of depression in youngsters. By most standards, we still have a great deal to learn in all areas. The exponential growth of research in this broad field of inquiry suggests a tremendous

interest on the part of professionals in many mental-health-related disciplines. We anticipate that a similar level of interest and research will be evident over the next decade, with
the benefits of this attention accruing to children and adolescents who manifest a
propensity for depression.

References

Achenbach, T. M., & McConaughy, S. H. (1992). Taxonomy of internalizing disorders of childhood and
adolescence. In W. M. Reynolds (Ed.), *Internalizing disorders in children and adolescents* (pp.
19–60), New York: John Wiley.

Alessi, N. E., Krahn, D., Brehm, D., & Wittekindt, J. (1989). Prepubertal anorexia nervosa and major
depressive disorder. *Journal of the American Academy of Child and Adolescent Psychiatry, 28,*
380–384.

Alessi, N. E., & Magen, J. (1988). Comorbidity of other psychiatric disturbances in depressed psychiatrically
hospitalized children. *American Journal of Psychiatry, 145,* 1582–1584.

Alessi, N. E., Robbins, D. R., & Dilsaver, S. C. (1987). Panic and depressive disorders among psychiatrically
hospitalized adolescents. *Psychiatry Research, 20,* 275–283.

Ambrosini, P. J., Bianchi, M. D., Rabinovich, H., & Elia, J. (1993). Antidepressant treatments in children and
adolescents. I. Affective disorders. *Journal of the American Academy of Child and Adolescent
Psychiatry, 32,* 1–6.

American Psychiatric Association (1980). *Diagnostic and statistical manual of mental disorders,* 3rd ed.
Washington, DC: Author.

American Psychiatric Association (1987). *Diagnostic and statistical manual of mental disorders,* 3rd ed.,
revised. Washington, DC: Author

American Psychiatric Association (1994). *Diagnostic and statistical manual of mental disorders,* 4th ed.
Washington, DC: Author.

Anderson, G. K., & Reynolds, W. M. (1993). Models of stress, coping, and depression in adolescents: A path
analytic investigation. Unpublished manuscript.

Anderson, J. C., Williams, S., McGee, R., & Silva, P. A. (1987). DSM-III disorders in preadolescent children:
Prevalence in a large sample from the general population. *Archives of General Psychiatry, 44,* 69–76.

Asarnow, J. R., Carlson, G. A., & Guthrie, D. (1987). Coping strategies, self-perceptions, hopelessness, and
perceived family environments in depressed and suicidal children. *Journal of Consulting and
Clinical Psychology, 55,* 361–366.

Beardslee, W. R., Bemporad, J., Keller, M. B., & Klerman, G. L. (1983). Children of parents with major
affective disorder: A review. *American Journal of Psychiatry, 140,* 825–832.

Biederman, J. (1991). Sudden death in children treated with a tricyclic antidepressant. *Journal of the
American Academy of Child and Adolescent Psychiatry, 30,* 495–498.

Biederman, J., & Steingard, R. (1989). Attention-deficit hyperactivity disorder in adolescents. *Psychiatric
Annals, 19,* 587–596.

Bowlby, J. (1973). *Attachment and loss,* Vol. 2, *Separation, anxiety and anger.* New York: Basic Books.

Bowlby, J. (1980). *Attachment and loss,* Vol. 3, *Loss, sadness and depression.* New York: Basic Books.

Bowlby, J. (1982). *Attachment and loss,* Vol. 1, 2nd ed., *Attachment.* New York: Basic Books.

Bowlby, J. (1988). Developmental psychiatry comes of age. *American Journal of Psychiatry, 145,* 1–10.

Bukstein, O. G., Glancy, L. J., & Kaminer, Y. (1992). Pattern of affective comorbidity in a clinical population of
dually diagnosed adolescent substance abusers. *Journal of the American Academy of Child and
Adolescent Psychiatry, 31,* 1041–1045.

Butler, L., Miezitis, S., Friedman, R., & Cole, E. (1980). The effect of two school-based intervention programs
on depressive symptoms in preadolescents. *American Educational Research Journal, 17,* 111–119.

Cicchetti, D., & Olsen, K. (1990). The developmental psychopathology of child maltreatment. In M. Lewis &
S. M. Miller (Eds.), *Handbook of developmental psychopathology* (pp. 261–279). New York: Plenum
Press.

Cicchetti, D., & Schneider-Rosen, K. (1984). Toward a transactional model of childhood depression. In D.
Cicchetti & K. Schneider-Rosen (Eds.), *Childhood depression* (pp. 81–105). San Francisco: Jossey-
Bass.

Cole, D. A. (1990). Relation of social and academic competence to depressive symptoms in childhood.
Journal of Abnormal Psychology, 99, 181–190.

Cole, D. A., & Rehm, L. P. (1986). Family interaction patterns and childhood depression. *Journal of Abnormal Child Psychology, 14*, 297–314.

Connell, H. M. (1972). Depression in childhood. *Child Psychiatry and Human Development, 4*, 71–85.

Cytryn, L., & McKnew, D. H. (1972). Proposed classification of childhood. *American Journal of Psychiatry, 129*, 149–155.

Cytryn, L., McKnew, D. H., Zahn-Waxler, C., Radke-Yarrow, M., Gaensbauer, T. J., Harmon, R. J., & Lamour, M. (1984). A developmental view of affective disturbances in the children of affectively ill parents. *American Journal of Psychiatry, 141*, 219–222.

Dalley, M. B., Bolocofsky, D. N., Alcorn, M. B., & Baker, C. (1992). Depressive symptomatology, attributional style, dysfunctional attitude, and social competency in adolescents with and without learning disabilities. *School Psychology Review, 21*, 444–458.

Deykin, E. Y. Levy, J. C., & Wells, V. (1987). Adolescent depression, alcohol and drug abuse. *American Journal of Public Health, 77*, 178–182.

Downey, G., & Coyne, J. C. (1990). Children of depressed parents: An integrative review. *Psychological Bulletin, 108*, 50–76.

Emslie, G. J., Roffwarg, H. P., Rush, A. J., Weinberg, W. A., & Parkin-Feigenbaum, L. (1987). Sleep EEG findings in depressed children and adolescents. *American Journal of Psychiatry, 144*, 668–670.

Fine, S., Forth, A., Gilbert, M., & Haley, G. (1991). Group therapy for adolescent depressive disorder: A comparison of social skills and therapeutic support. *Journal of the American Academy of Child and Adolescent Psychiatry, 30*, 79–85.

Fleming, J. E., Boyle, M. H., & Offord, D. R. (1993). The outcome of adolescent depression in the Ontario child health study follow-up. *Journal of the American Academy of Child and Adolescent Psychiatry, 32*, 28–33.

Fleming, J. E., Offord, D. R., & Boyle, M. H. (1989). Prevalence of childhood and adolescent depression in the community: Ontario child health study. *British Journal of Psychiatry, 155*, 647–654.

Forehand, R., McCombs, A., Long, N., Brody, G., & Fauber, R. (1988). Early adolescent adjustment to recent parental divorce: The role of interparental conflict and adolescent sex as mediating variables. *Journal of Consulting and Clinical Psychology, 56*, 624–627.

Forness, S. R. (1988). School characteristics of children and adolescents with depression. *Monograph in Behavioral Disorders, 10*, 117–203.

Freud, S. (1946). Mourning and melancholia. In *Standard edition* (Vol. 14 (pp. 243–258). London: Hogarth Press (original published in 1917).

Garber, J. (1984). The developmental progression of depression in female children. In D. Cicchetti & K. Schneider-Rosen (Eds.), *Childhood depression* (pp. 29–58). San Francisco: Jossey-Bass.

Garrison, C. Z., Addy, C. L., Jackson, K. L., McKeown, R., & Waller, J. L. (1992). Major depressive disorder and dysthymia in young adolescents. *American Journal of Epidemiology, 135*, 792–802.

Gotlib, I. H., & Hammen, C. L. (1992). *Psychological aspects of depression: Toward a cognitive–interpersonal integration*. New York: John Wiley.

Hammen, C., Burge, D., Burney, E., & Adrian, C. (1990). Longitudinal study of diagnoses in children of women with unipolar and bipolar affective disorder. *Archives of General Psychiatry, 47*, 1112–1117.

Harrington, R., Fudge, H., Rutter, M., Pickles, A., & Hill, J. (1990). Adult outcomes of childhood and adolescent depression. I. Psychiatric status. *Archives of General Psychiatry, 47*, 465–473.

Harrington, R., Fudge, H., Rutter, M., Pickles, A., & Hill, J. (1991). Adult outcomes of childhood and adolescent depression. II. Links with antisocial disorders. *Journal of the American Academy of Child and Adolescent Psychiatry, 30*, 434–439.

Hops, H., Lowinsohn, P. M., Andrews, J. A., & Roberts, R. E. (1990). Psychosocial correlates of depressive symptomatology among high school students. *Journal of Clinical Child Psychology, 19*, 211–220.

Hubel, D. H., & Weisel, T. N. (1970). The period of susceptibility to the physiological effects of unilateral eye closure in kittens. *Journal of Physiology* (Lond.), *206*, 419–436.

Jensen, J. B., Burke, N., & Garfinkle, B. D. (1988). Depression and symptoms of attention deficit disorder with hyperactivity. *Journal of the American Academy of Child and Adolescent Psychiatry, 27*, 742–747.

Kahn, J. S., Kehle, T. J., Jenson, W. R., & Clark, E. (1990). Comparison of cognitive–behavioral, relaxation, and self-modeling interventions for depression among middle-school students. *School Psychology Review, 19*, 196–211.

Kaplan, S. L., Busner, J., Weinhold, C., & Lenon, P. (1987). Depressive symptoms in children and adolescents with cancer: A longitudinal study. *Journal of the American Academy of Child and Adolescent Psychiatry, 26*, 782–787.

Kashani, J. H., Burbach, D. J., & Rosenberg, T. K. (1988). Perception of family conflict resolution and depressive symptomatology in adolescents. *Journal of the American Academy of Child and Adolescent Psychiatry, 27*, 42–48.

Kashani, J. H., & Carlson, G. A. (1987). Seriously depressed preschoolers. *American Journal of Psychiatry, 144*, 348–350.

Kashani, J. H., Carlson, G. A., Beck, N. C., Hoeper, E. W., Corcoran, C. M., McAllister, J. A., Fallahi, C., Rosenberg, T. K., & Reid, J. C. (1987). Depression, depressive symptoms, and depressed mood among a community sample of adolescents. *American Journal of Psychiatry, 144*, 931–934.

Kashani, J. H., Holcomb, W. R., & Orvaschel, H. (1986). Depression and depressive symptoms in preschool children from the general population. *American Journal of Psychiatry, 143*, 1138–1143.

Kaufman, J. (1991). Depressive disorders in maltreated children. *Journal of the American Academy of Child and Adolescent Psychiatry, 30*, 257–265.

Kazdin, A. E. (1990). Psychotherapy for children and adolescents. *Annual Review of Psychology, 41*, 21–54.

Keller, M. B., Beardslee, W., Lavori, P. W., Wunder, J., Drs, D. L., & Samuelson, H. (1988). Course of major depression in non-referred adolescents: A retrospective study. *Journal of Affective Disorders, 15*, 235–243.

Keller, M. B., Lavori, P. W., Beardslee, W. R., Wunder, J., & Ryan, N. (1991). Depression in children and adolescents: New data on "undertreatment" and a literature review on the efficacy of available treatments. *Journal of Affective Disorders, 21*, 163–171.

Keller, M. B., Lavori, P. W., Wunder, J., Beardslee, W., Schwartz, C., & Roth, J. (1992). Chronic course of anxiety disorders in children and adolescents. *Journal of the American Academy of Child and Adolescent Psychiatry, 31*, 595–599.

Kinzie, J. D., Sack, W. H., Angell, R. H., Manson, S., & Rath, B. (1986). The psychiatric effects of massive trauma on Cambodian children. I. The children. *Journal of the American Academy of Child and Adolescent Psychiatry, 25*, 370–376.

Klerman, G. L. (1988). The current age of youthful melancholia: Evidence for increase in depression among adolescents and young adults. *British Journal of Psychiatry, 152*, 4–14.

Klerman, G. L., & Weissman, M. M. (1989). Increasing rates of depression. *Journal of American Medical Association, 261*, 2229–2235.

Kovacs, M. (1985). The natural history and course of depressive disorders in childhood. *Psychiatric Annals, 15*, 387–389.

Kovacs, M. (1989). Affective disorders in children and adolescents. *American Psychologist, 44*, 209–215.

Kovacs, M., Feinberg, T. L., Crouse-Novak, M., Paulauskas, S. L., & Finkelstein, R. (1984a). Depressive disorders in childhood. I. A longitudinal prospective study of characteristics and recovery. *Archives of General Psychiatry, 41*, 229–237.

Kovacs, M., Feinberg, T. L., Crouse-Novak, M., Paulauskas, S. L., Pollock, M., & Finkelstein, R. (1984b). Depressive disorders in childhood. II. A longitudinal study of the risk for a subsequent major depression. *Archives of General Psychiatry, 41*, 643–649.

Kovacs, M., Gatsonis, C., Paulauskas, S. L., & Richards, C. (1989). Depressive disorders in childhood. IV. A longitudinal study of comorbidity with and risk for anxiety disorders. *Archives of General Psychiatry, 46*, 776–782.

Kovacs, M., & Goldston, D. (1991). Cognitive and social cognitive development of depressed children and adolescents. *Journal of the American Academy of Child and Adolescent Psychiatry, 30*, 388–392.

Kovacs, M., Paulauskas, S. L., Gatsonis, C., & Richards, C. (1988). Depressive disorders in childhood. III. A longitudinal study of comorbidity with and risk for conduct disorders. *Journal of Affective Disorders, 15*, 205–217.

Kraemer, G. W., Ebert, M. H., & McKinney, W. T. (1983). Separation models and depression. In J. Angst (Ed.), *Origins of depression: Current concepts and approaches* (pp. 133–145). Berlin: Springer-Verlag.

Kuhn, V., & Kuhn, R. (1971). Drug therapy for depression in children: Indications and methods. In A. Annell (Ed.), *Depressive states in childhood and adolescence* (pp. 455–459). Stockholm: Almqvist & Wiksell.

Last, C. G. (1992). Anxiety disorders in childhood and adolescence. In W. M. Reynolds (Ed.), *Internalizing disorders in children and adolescents* (pp. 61–106). New York: John Wiley.

Last, C. G., Perrin, S., Hersen, M., & Kazdin, A. E. (1992). DSM-III-R anxiety disorders in children: Sociodemographic and clinical characteristics. *Journal of the American Academy of Child and Adolescent Psychiatry, 31*, 1070–1076.

Lewinsohn, P. M., Clarke, G. N., Hops, H., & Andrews, J. (1990). Cognitive–behavioral treatment for depressed adolescents. *Behavior Therapy, 21*, 385–401.

Lewinsohn, P. M., Hops, H., Roberts, R. E., Seeley, J. R., & Andrews, J. A. (1993). Adolescent psychopathology. I. Prevalence and incidence of depression and other DSM-III-R disorders in high school students. *Journal of Abnormal Psychology, 102*, 133–144.

Lewis, J. K., McKinney, W. T., Young, L. D., & Kraemer, G. W. (1976). Mother–infant separation in rhesus monkeys as a model of human depression: A reconsideration. *Archives of General Psychiatry, 33,* 699–705.

Liddle, B., & Spence, S. H. (1990). Cognitive–behaviour therapy with depressed primary school children: A cautionary note. *Behavioural Psychotherapy, 18,* 85–102.

Ling, W., Oftedal, G., & Weinberg, W. (1970). Depressive illness in childhood presenting as severe headache. *American Journal of Diseases in Children, 120,* 122–124.

Mahler, M. S. (1961). On sadness and grief in infancy and childhood. *Psychoanalytic Study of the Child, 16,* 332–351.

Malmquist, C. P. (1971). Depressions in childhood and adolescence. *New England Journal of Medicine, 284,* 887–893.

Marcotte, D., & Baron, P. (1993). L'efficacité d'une stratégie d'intervention emotivo-rationnelle auprès d'adolescents dépressifs du milieu scolaire. *Canadian Journal of Counseling, 27,* 77–92.

McConville, B. J., Boag, L. C., & Purohit, A. P. (1973). Three types of childhood depression. *Canadian Psychiatric Association Journal, 18,* 133–138.

McGuffin, P., & Katz, R. (1986). Nature, nurture and affective disorder. In J. F. W. Deakin (Ed.), *The biology of depression* (pp. 26–52). Washington, DC: American Psychiatric Press.

Mineka, S., & Suomi, S. J. (1978). Social separation in monkeys. *Psychological Bulletin, 85,* 1376–1400.

Mufson, L., Moreau, D., Weissman, M. M., & Klerman, G. L. (1993). *Interpersonal psychotherapy for depressed adolescents.* New York: Guilford Press.

Nurcombe, B., Seifer, R., Scioli, A., Tramontana, M. G., Grapentine, W. L., & Beauchesne, H. C. (1989). Is major depressive disorder in adolescence a distinct diagnostic entity? *Journal of the American Academy of Child and Adolescent Psychiatry, 28,* 333–342.

Offer, D., & Schonert-Reichl, K. A. (1992). Debunking the myths of adolescence: Findings from recent research. *Journal of the American Academy of Child and Adolescent Psychiatry, 31,* 1003–1014.

Petti, T. A. (1983). Imipramine in the treatment of depressed children. In D. P. Cantwell & G. A. Carlson (Eds.), *Affective disorders in childhood and adolescents—An update* (pp. 375–415). Jamaica, NY: Spectrum Publications.

Poznanski, E. O., & Zrull, J. P. (1970). Childhood depression: Clinical characteristics of overtly depressed children. *Archives of General Psychiatry, 23,* 8–15.

Puig-Antich, J. (1982). Major depression and conduct disorder in prepuberty. *Journal of the American Academy of Child Psychiatry, 21,* 118–128.

Puig-Antich, J. (1986). Psychobiological markers: Effects of age and puberty. In M. Rutter, C. E. Izard, & P. B. Read (Eds.), *Depression in young people: Developmental and clinical perspectives* (pp. 341–381). New York: Guilford Press.

Puig-Antich, J. (1987a). Affective disorders in children and adolescents: Diagnostic validity and psychobiology. In H. Y. Melzer (Ed.), *Psychopharmacology: The third generation of progress* (pp. 843–859). New York: Raven Press.

Puig-Antich, J. (1987b). Sleep and neuroendocrine correlates of affective illness in childhood and adolescence. *Journal of Adolescent Health Care, 8,* 505–529.

Puig-Antich, J., Dahl, R., Ryan, N., Novacenko, H., Goetz, D., Goetz, R. M., Twomey, J., & Klepper, T. (1989). Cortisol secretion in prepubertal children with major depressive disorder: Episode and recovery. *Archives of General Psychiatry, 46,* 801–809.

Puig-Antich, J., Kaufman, J., Ryan, N. D., Williamson, D. E., Dahl, R. E., Lukens, E., Todak, G., Ambrosini, P., Rabinovich, H., & Nelson, B. (1993). The psychosocial functioning and family environment of depressed adolescents. *Journal of the American Academy of Child and Adolescent Psychiatry, 32,* 244–253.

Puig-Antich, J., Lukens, E., Davies, M., Goetz, D., Brennan-Quattrock, J., & Todak, G. (1985a). Psychosocial functioning in prepubertal children with major depressive disorders. II. Interpersonal relationships after sustained recovery from affective episode. *Archives of General Psychiatry, 42,* 511–517.

Puig-Antich, J., Lukens, E., Davies, M., Goetz, D., Brennan-Quattrock, J., & Todak, G. (1985b). Psychosocial functioning in prepubertal children with major depressive disorders. I. Interpersonal relationships during the depressive episode. *Archives of General Psychiatry, 42,* 500–507.

Puig-Antich, J., Novacenko, H., Davies, M., Chambers, W. J., Tabrizi, M. A., Krawiec, V., Ambrosini, P. J., & Sachar, E. J. (1984). Growth hormone secretion in prepubertal major depressive children. I. Sleep related plasma concentrations during a depressive episode. *Archives of General Psychiatry, 41,* 455–460.

Rancurello, M. (1986). Antidepressants in children: Indications, benefits, and limitations. *American Journal of Psychotherapy, 40,* 377–392.

Rastam, M. (1992). Anorexia nervosa in 51 Swedish adolescents: Premorbid problems and comorbidity. *Journal of the American Academy of Child and Adolescent Psychiatry, 31,* 819–829.

Reinherz, H. Z., Giaconia, R. M., Lefkowitz, E. S., Pakiz, B., & Frost, A. K. (1993). Prevalence of psychiatric disorders in a community population of older adolescents. *Journal of the American Academy of Child and Adolescent Psychiatry, 32,* 369–377.

Reynolds, W. M. (1985).Depression in childhood and adolescence: Diagnosis, assessment, intervention strategies and research. In T. R. Kratochwill (Ed.), *Advances in school psychology,* Vol. 4 (pp. 133–189). Hillsdale, NJ: Erlbaum Associates.

Reynolds, W. M. (1989). Suicidal ideation and depression in adolescents: Assessment and research. In P. F. Lovibond & P. Wilson (Eds.), *Clinical and abnormal psychology* (pp. 125–135). Amsterdam: Elsevier.

Reynolds, W. M. (1992a). Depression in children and adolescents. In W. M. Reynolds (Ed.), *Internalizing disorders in children and adolescents* (pp. 149–254). New York: John Wiley.

Reynolds, W. M. (1992b). Internalizing disorders in children and adolescents: Issues and recommendations for further research. In W. M. Reynolds (Ed.), *Internalizing disorders in children and adolescents* (pp. 311–318). New York: John Wiley.

Reynolds, W . M. (1993). Self-report methods. In T. H. Ollendick & M. Hersen (Eds.), *Handbook of child and adolescent assessment* (pp. 98–123). New York: Plenum Press.

Reynolds, W. M. (1994). Depression in adolescents: Contemporary issues and perspectives. In T. H. Ollendick & R. J. Prinz (Eds.), *Advances in clinical child psychology,* Vol. 16 (pp. 261–316). New York: Plenum Press.

Reynolds, W. M., & Coats, K. I. (1982). Depression in adolescents: Incidence, depth and correlates. Paper presented at the 10th International Congress of the International Association for Child and Adolescent Psychiatry, Dublin, July 1982.

Reynolds, W. M., & Coats, K. I. (1986). A comparison of cognitive–behavioral therapy and relaxation training for the treatment of depression in adolescents. *Journal of Consulting and Clinical Psychology, 54,* 653–660.

Reynolds, W. M., & Graves, A. (1989). Reliability of children's reports of depressive symptomatology. *Journal of Abnormal Child Psychology, 17,* 647–655.

Reynolds, W. M., & Miller, K. L. (1985). Depression and learned helplessness in mentally retarded and nonretarded adolescents: An initial investigation. *Applied Research in Mental Retardation, 6,* 295–307.

Riddle, M. A., Brown, N., Dzubinski, D., Jetmalani, A. J., Law, Y., & Woolston, J. L. (1989). Fluoxetine overdose in an adolescent. *Journal of the American Academy of Child and Adolescent Psychiatry, 28,* 587–588.

Riddle, M. A., Nelson, J. C., Kleinman, C. S., Rasmusson, A., Leckman, J. F., King, R. A., & Cohen, D. J. (1991). Sudden death in children receiving Norpramin: A review of three reported cases and commentary. *Journal of the American Academy of Child and Adolescent Psychiatry, 30,* 104–108.

Rie, H. E. (1966). Depression in childhood: A survey of some pertinent contributions. *Journal of the American Academy of Child Psychiatry, 5,* 553–583.

Rourke, B. P., Young, G. C., & Leenaars, A. A. (1989). A childhood learning disability that predisposes those afflicted to adolescent and adult depression and suicide risk. *Journal of Learning Disabilities, 22,* 169–175.

Rutter, M. (1988). Epidemiological approaches to developmental psychopathology. *Archives of General Psychiatry, 45,* 486–495.

Rutter, M., & Quinton, D. (1984). Parental psychiatric disorder: Effects on children. *Psychological Medicine, 14,* 853–880.

Ryan, N. D. (1992). Pharmacological treatment of major depression. In M. Shafii & S. L. Shafii (Eds.), *Clinical guide to depression in children and adolescents* (pp. 219–232). Washington, DC: American Psychiatric Press.

Saigh, P. A. (1992). The behavioral treatment of child and adolescent posttraumatic stress disorder. *Advances in Behavior Research and Therapy, 14,* 247–275.

Shain, B. N., Kronfol, Z., Naylor, M., Goel, K., Evans, T., & Schaefer, S. (1991). Natural killer cell activity in adolescents with major depression. *Biological Psychiatry, 29,* 481–484.

Shain, B. N., Naylor, M., & Alessi, N. (1990). Comparison of self-rated and clinician-rated measures of depression in adolescents. *American Journal of Psychiatry, 147,* 793–795.

Silver, L. B. (1988). The scope of the problem in children and adolescents. In J. G. Looney (Ed.), *Chronic mental illness in children and adolescents* (pp. 39–51). Washington, DC: American Psychiatric Press.

Simeon, J., Dinicola, V. F., Ferguson, H. B., & Copping, W. (1990). Adolescent depression: A placebo-controlled fluoxetine treatment study and follow-up. *Progress in Neuropsychopharmacology and Biological Psychiatry, 14,* 791–795.

Smith, C., & Steiner, H. (1992). Psychopathology in anorexia nervosa and depression. *Journal of the American Academy of Child and Adolescent Psychiatry, 31*, 841–843.

Spitz, R. A., & Wolf, K. M. (1946). Anaclitic depression: An inquiry into the genesis of psychiatric conditions in early childhood. II. *Psychoanalytic Study of the Child, 2*, 313–347.

Stark, K. D. (1990). *Childhood depression: School-based intervention*. New York: Guilford Press.

Stark, K. D., Reynolds, W. M., & Kaslow, N. J. (1987). A comparison of the relative efficacy of self-control therapy and behavioral problem-solving therapy for depression in children. *Journal of Abnormal Child Psychology, 15*, 91–113.

Strober, M., Lampert, C., Schmidt, S., & Morrell, W. (1993). The course of major depressive disorder in adolescents. I. Recovery and risk of manic switching in a follow-up of psychotic and nonpsychotic subtypes. *Journal of the American Academy of Child and Adolescent Psychiatry, 32*, 34–42.

Suomi, S. J., & Harlow, H. F. (1977). Production and alleviation of depressive behaviors in monkeys. In J. D. Maser & M. E. P. Seligman (Eds.), *Psychopathology: Experimental methods* (pp. 131–173). San Francisco: W. H. Freeman.

Teicher, M. H., Glod, C., & Cole, J. O. (1990). Emergence of intense suicidal preoccupation during fluoxetine treatment. *American Journal of Psychiatry, 147*, 207–210.

Trad, P. V. (1986). *Infant depression: Paradigms and paradoxes*. New York: Springer-Verlag.

Verhulst, F. C., & van der Ende, J. (1992). Agreement between parents' reports and adolescents' self-reports of problem behavior. *Journal of Clinical Psychology and Psychiatry, 33*, 1011–1023.

Wagner, B. M., & Compas, B. E. (1990). Gender, instrumentality, and expressivity: Moderators of the relation between stress and psychological symptoms during adolescence. *American Journal of Community Psychology, 18*, 383–406.

Weinberg, W. A., & Emslie, G. J. (1988). Adolescents and school problems: Depression, suicide, and learning disorders. In A. R. Stiffman & R. A. Feldman (Eds.), *Advances in adolescent mental health: A research–practice annual*, Vol. 3, *Depression and suicide* (pp. 181–205). Greenwich, CT: JAI Press.

Weinberg, W. A., Rutman, J., Sullivan, L., Penick, E. C., & Dietz, S. G. (1973). Depression in children referred to an educational diagnostic center: Diagnosis and treatment. *Journal of Pediatrics, 83*, 1065–1072.

2

Phenomenology and Epidemiology of Mood Disorders in Children and Adolescents

Elva O. Poznanski and Hartmut B. Mokros

Until recently, researchers lacked standardized assessment instruments and formal criteria to use in making a mood disorder diagnosis in children and adolescents. These two methodological developments have been fundamental to making mood disorders in youth, particularly depression in childhood, one of the most active areas of research within child psychiatry (Mokros & Poznanski, 1992). Indeed, many review articles and several books devoted exclusively to childhood depression have now been published (e.g., Schulterbrand & Raskin, 1977; Cantwell & Carlson, 1983; Petti, 1983; Weller & Weller, 1984; Cicchetti & Schneider-Rosen, 1984; Rutter, Izard, & Read, 1986; Shafii & Shafii, 1992).

This chapter examines developments in this area of research, focusing specifically on the phenomenology and epidemiology of mood disorders in children and adolescents. It should be noted at the outset that this literature is skewed in two directions. First, the vast majority of extant research has investigated depression, with investigations of bipolar disorders in this age group being rare. Second, the research literature has focused largely on the study of prepubertal children, with research on adolescents relatively neglected. In the following discussion, this focus is revealed in the relatively greater emphasis given to depression in childhood than to other mood disorders and to the manifestation of mood disorders in adolescents.

Elva O. Poznanski • Rush—Presbyterian—St. Luke's Medical Center, Chicago, Illinois 60612. **Hartmut B. Mokros** • Rutgers University, New Brunswick, New Jersey 08903.

Handbook of Depression in Children and Adolescents, edited by William M. Reynolds and Hugh F. Johnston. Plenum Press, New York, 1994.

Elva O. Poznanski
and Hartmut B.
Mokros

Phenomenology of Mood Disorders in Youth

The notion that mood disorders, particularly depressive disorders, may manifest themselves in childhood and adolescence is now accepted. Yet this acceptance did not emerge until relatively recently. This section will first examine historical shifts in attitudes toward mood disorders in youth. This introduction is followed by a brief discussion of the range of evidence now available that has led to the current assumption of equivalence of mood disorders across the life span. Finally, this section discusses criteria currently in use in the diagnosis of mood disorders, criteria that identify the accepted current model of the phenomenology of these disorders in youth.

Historical Attitudes

Interest in depression in childhood dates back to the 1940s (Spitz, 1946) and the early 1950s (Depert, 1952). Resistance to the concept of clinical depression in childhood came both from the psychoanalytical school (Rie, 1966) and from those who argued that depressive symptoms represented transient experiences associated with normative development (Lefkowitz & Burton, 1978). That is to say, sadness as a *symptom* was viewed as part of everyday experience. But sadness as one of a number of co-occurring symptoms defining a depressive *syndrome*, a syndrome that might evidence a defined temporal course (i.e., *depressive disorder*), was viewed as exceedingly rare if not impossible in youth.

Yet clinical evidence indicated that dysphoria did indeed, and not uncommonly, seem to express itself as syndrome and disorder in children (Poznanski & Zrull, 1970; Poznanski, Krahenbuhl, & Zrull, 1976). Nevertheless, a prominent early formulation of childhood depression held that the expression of depression in children differed from its expression in adults in that the depressive affect was missing. Indeed, a description of a child's affect was missing in all mental status reports until very recently. Hence, the constructs of "masked depression" and "depressive equivalents" were introduced to cover this void (e.g., Cytryn & McKnew, 1974; Glaser, 1967), although such terms proved untenable over time for both clinical and research purposes (Carlson & Cantwell, 1980a).

A more moderate position assumed that depressive manifestations in childhood differ from those in adults and argued that adult-like depressive symptomatology was manifest by children, but that additional symptoms unique to children define the depressive syndrome (e.g., Frommer, 1968; Poznanski & Zrull, 1970). This position is still held to some extent by many clinicians and researchers (e.g., Ney, Colbert, Newman, & Young, 1986). Indeed, as will be discussed in the final section of this chapter, an increasingly influential research movement known as developmental psychopathology (e.g., Cicchetti & Schneider-Rosen, 1984; Kovacs, 1989; Rutter, 1986) has strongly argued, in opposition to the currently prevailing climate of opinion presented in the next section, in favor of such a position for the development of a phenomenology of mood disorders in youth.

At least two criteria systems tailored specifically to children, those of Poznanski (Poznanski, Mokros, Grossman, & Freeman, 1985) and Weinberg (Weinberg, Rutman, Sullivan, Penick, & Dietz, 1973) have been discussed in the literature, although neither of these systems considers the full range of mood disorders, concentrating instead on depression.

Assumption of Equivalence of the Phenomenology of Mood Disorders across the Life Span

The past decade has witnessed increased acceptance of the view that mood disorders experienced in youth are phenomenologically equivalent to the adult experience (e.g.,

Ambrosini & Puig-Antich, 1985). Support of this position comes from a variety of sources. First, symptom clusters, defined as a depressive syndrome, appear comparable between children and adults (e.g., Carlson & Kashani, 1988). Second, family history research indicates high levels of affective disturbance among relatives of children diagnosed with affective disorder (e.g., Dwyer & DeLong, 1987; Puig-Antich et al., 1989; Strober et al., 1988) and high risk for affective disorder among offspring of affectively disturbed parents (e.g., Beardslee, Bemporad, Keller, & Klerman, 1983), with the added finding that offspring of unipolars are more prone to unipolar disorders (Weissman et al., 1987) and offspring of bipolars are more prone to bipolar disorders (Klein, Depue, & Slater, 1985). Third, research on biological correlates has provided potential evidence for both state (Poznanski et al., 1982) and trait (Puig-Antich et al., 1984) markers of prepubertal major depressive disorder. Fourth, longitudinal study of prepubertal depressives indicates the presence of clearly defined temporal episodes (Kovacs, Feinberg, Crouse-Novak, Paulauskas, & Finkelstein, 1984a) as well as a longitudinal course marked by greatly increased risk for new episodes of illness once an initial episode has been experienced (Kovacs et al., 1984b; Poznanski et al., 1976).

These lines of evidence have led to the adoption of adult criteria, with minor modification, in the diagnostic evaluation of children and adolescents.

Phenomenology of Mood Disorders in Diagnostic Criteria: DSM-IV

Two adult diagnostic systems have most commonly been applied in research and clinical practice with children. These are the Research Diagnostic Criteria (RDC) (Spitzer, Endicott, & Robins, 1978) and the American Psychiatric Association's criteria contained in the *Diagnostic and Statistical Manual of Mental Disorders*, currently in its 4th edition (DSM-IV). Although differences exist between these systems in both the definitions of disorders and the subtypes of disorder considered, the overlap between them is great. While the RDC has been extensively used in research, particularly in pharmacological study of depression as in the studies of Puig-Antich and colleagues, DSM-IV has become the standard for clinical practice. For this reason, the discussion will focus on the phenomenology of mood disorders as they are defined in the most recently published revision of DSM, DSM-IV. We will describe the mood disorder criteria as they appear in DSM-IV and highlight those changes made since the DSM-III that have direct relevance to the phenomenology of mood disorders in children and adolescents. Two families of disorder, depressive and bipolar disorder, comprise these mood disorders.

Depressive Disorders. The discussion of depressive disorders will focus on the two major types—Major Depressive Disorder and Dysthymia (formerly known as Depressive Neurosis)—identified by DSM-IV. The discussion will trace the relationship between symptom and syndrome in the definition of these disorders.

Major Depressive Disorder. Consideration of a Major Depressive Disorder diagnosis requires evidence for a Major Depressive Episode. The depressive syndrome is defined by the clustering of at least five of nine symptoms within a 2-week period that marks a change from previous functioning. These five symptoms must include either (1) a depressed or irritable mood or (2) loss of interest and pleasure in usual activities as *essential symptoms* (Poznanski et al., 1985) if the diagnosis is to be considered. The remaining symptoms, or *qualifying symptoms* (Poznanski et al., 1985), necessary to define the presence of a depressive syndrome include appetite disturbance, sleep disturbance, psychomotor agitation or retardation, loss of energy, feelings of worthlessness or inappropriate guilt, diminished ability to think or concentrate, and recurrent thoughts of death or suicide.

Once evidence for a depressive syndrome has been established, it is further necessary to rule out (1) concomitant organic factors that may have caused or maintained the syndrome, (2) the manifestation of the syndrome as a product of a normal bereavement process, (3) the presence of delusions or hallucinations in the absence of mood symptoms, and (4) evidence for underlying thought disorders.

These criteria for major depressive episodes include notable changes from DSM-III that are of particular relevance in application to children. DSM-III contained several symptom qualifications that applied only to children under 6 and required one less associated symptom in this age group. The hypoactivity substitution for psychomotor retardation was dropped from DSM-III-R, as was the reduction in the number of associated symptoms required for diagnosis of children under 6. DSM-III-R dropped an age qualification for these symptoms, thus applying symptoms by observation across all ages. This practice, a common one in child psychiatry, has now expanded for use in adult psychiatry!

In addition, numerous changes have been made in criteria included for the melancholic subtype, such as the incorporation of prior good response to somatic antidepressant therapy as a criterion. This criterion, in particular, has limited relevance for child and adolescent work because of poor response of these age groups to antidepressant medication, an issue discussed in detail below.

Once evidence for a major depressive episode has been established, a major depressive disorder diagnosis is defined either as a *single episode*, if the patient's history reveals no evidence for any prior episodes, or as *recurrent* if such evidence is obtained.

Dysthymia. Whereas major depressive episodes describe episodic mood disturbances, Dysthymia represents a milder although chronic course. A depressed or irritable mood prominent and present most days over at least 1 year defines the essential symptom for Dysthymia. In addition, at least two of six qualifying symptoms must cluster with the essential symptom. These symptoms include appetite disturbance, sleep disturbance, low energy, low self-esteem, poor concentration, and feelings of hopelessness. In addition: (1) Remission of this symptom presentation cannot have extended for more than 2 months during the episode and there can be (2) no evidence of major depression during the episode, (3) no evidence in the history of manic or hypomanic disorder, (4) no underlying thought disorder, and (5) no organic basis for the symptom presentation can be established.

Although the boundaries between dysthymia and major depression are particularly unclear in children and adolescents, the work of Kovacs et al. (1984a) has established that the distinction can be made and, indeed, that it is not uncommon to identify children with double depressions in which a major depressive episode is superimposed on preexisting dysthymia.

Bipolar Disorders. The two major types of bipolar disorders identified by DSM-IV—Bipolar Disorder and Cyclothymia—provide the focus of the following discussion. Specifically, the discussion first examines symptoms that constitute a manic syndrome and then examines the relationship of this manic syndrome to other mood impairment symptoms requiring consideration in defining a bipolar disorder.

Bipolar Disorder. Consideration of a Bipolar Disorder diagnosis requires evidence for a manic episode. The essential symptom of the disorder is a notable period of abnormally and persistently elevated, expansive, or irritable mood. Unlike the criteria for a Major Depressive Episode, the duration of this disturbance of mood is not specifically defined. In addition to evidence of an essential symptom, three of seven (four if evidence of the essential symptom is irritability) qualifying symptoms must also be present. These symptoms include grandiosity, decreased need for sleep, increased talkativeness, flight of ideas, ease of distractibility, increased goal-directed activity, and excessive and counter-productive involvement in pleasurable activities. A manic episode is said to be present if in addition this disturbance of mood results in marked impairment in usual functioning.

As with the depressive disorders, the manic syndrome may be diagnosed as a manic episode only if there is additionally (1) no evidence of delusions or hallucinations over a 2-week period in the absence of the mood disturbance, (2) no evidence of underlying thought disorder, and (3) no evidence of an organic basis for the mood disturbance.

A current episode of a manic episode or a history of a manic episode provides the basis for diagnosing a bipolar disorder. The bipolar disorder is diagnosed as *mixed type* if both manic and major depressive episodes show a recurrent pattern of cycling within the same time frame, as *manic type* if only a manic episode is present, or as *depressed type* if the history reveals evidence of a manic episode but the current mood disturbance is a major depressive episode.

These criteria for manic episode and bipolar disorder have been largely unchanged since DSM-III.

Cyclothymia.   Cyclothymia refers to chronic mood disturbance of at least 1 year's duration during which numerous periods of depressed mood and hypomanic episodes are experienced. Hypomanic episodes are defined as identical to the criteria for manic episodes shown in Table 3, with the exception that marked impairment in social and occupational functioning is not required for hypomanic episodes. In order to entertain a Cyclothymia diagnosis for the period of mood disturbance, (1) hypomanic and depressive symptoms cannot have been absent for more than 1 month, (2) there is no evidence of major depressive or manic episode, (3) there is no evidence of underlying thought disorder, and (4) there is no evidence of organic involvement.

The criteria for hypomanic episodes were more clearly defined in DSM-III-R than in its predecessor. These changes are of particular relevance for the diagnosis of mood disorder in adolescents. DSM-III merely defined hypomania as a clinical syndrome similar to, but less severe than, mania. The inclusion of evidence of a hypomanic episode in making a cyclothymia diagnosis also represents a shift in DSM-III-R. Thus, the DSM-III-R and DSM-IV criteria are more stringent in defining the manic component of cyclothymia, while the depressive component is more easily met. Whereas DSM-III required that at least three associated symptoms accompany a depressed mood or loss of interest or pleasure, DSM-III-R specified only that a period of depressed mood or loss of interest or pleasure that does not meet full symptom criteria for a major depressive episode need be present.

Summary

The DSM-IV criteria reviewed above represent the current working model of the phenomenology of mood disorders. Acceptance of these criteria as defining phenomenology implicitly involves acceptance of the position that mood disorders are phenomenologically equivalent across the life span. Potential difficulties with making such an assumption will be considered following a review of the epidemiological literature offered in the next section.

Epidemiology of Mood Disorders in Youth

Numerous studies in the recent literature provide data about the prevalence of dysphoric mood and depressive disorder in children and adolescence. In contrast, epidemiological study of bipolar disorder has been negligible, reflecting, in part, the rarity of the disorder within this age group as well as the difficulty of establishing the diagnosis in children and adolescents. We will therefore focus primarily on the epidemiology of depression and conclude with a brief summary of research on child and adolescent bipolar disorder.

Epidemiology of Depression and Depressive Disorders

Prevalence rates of depression in children have ranged from 0.14% (Rutter, Tizard, & Whitmore, 1970) to over 60% (Brumbach, Jackoway, & Weinberg, 1980). Factors that account for this variability include differences in populations studied (e.g., normal vs. clinical), methods of assessment (e.g., self-report or questionnaire vs. clinical interview), definitions of depression (i.e., symptom, syndrome, or disorder), and methods for defining evidence of depression (e.g., cutoff scores on self-reports vs. diagnostic criteria).

Although considerable variability in prevalence rates has been reported, several notable findings have emerged. First, both dysphoric mood and depressive disorder appear to increase in youth, with the lowest rates in the preschool years and the highest rates in adolescence. Second, although depression is identifiable before puberty, the incidence of depression increases dramatically after puberty. Third, the pattern of depression found in adults, with significantly more females depressed than males, does not appear until adolescence. Fourth, comparison of research that has employed comparable methodology indicates that variability in identified prevalence rates is much less than is often suggested. Finally, although the frequency with which various symptoms of depression are reported differs across age groups, Carlson and Kashani (1988) note that the basic phenomenology of depression does not differ between children across ages (i.e., preschool, prepubertal, adolescents) or between children and adults.

Our review of this literature will be divided into three parts according to age groupings investigated: preschool-age children, prepubertal children, and adolescents. Within each age group, the results are discussed separately for clinical and nonclinical samples. Although we will review both studies that define depression on the basis of diagnostic assessment and criteria and studies that define depression on the basis of self-report or questionnaire cutoff data, discussion of studies of clinical samples will be confined to those employing diagnostic assessments and criteria. Our aim here is to identify factors that account for differences in prevalence rates, difficulties in interpreting the available data, conclusions that may be drawn, and questions left unanswered.

Depression and Depressive Disorder in Preschool-Age Children.
Nonclinical Populations.   To date, two studies have been reported that provide data about depressive disorder in "normal" preschool-age children. Kashani and Ray (1983) surveyed the parents of 241 preschoolers, via questionnaire, and found no evidence of depressive disorder within this sample. Indeed, only 1 child (0.4%) was reported as sad, with this child also reported as experiencing suicidal ideation. Although the results of this study would suggest that depression is exceedingly rare among preschool children, the fact that information was obtained from only a single informant responding on a single questionnaire limits the conclusions that may be drawn.

A more recent study (Kashani, Holcomb, & Orvaschel, 1986) of 109 nursery school children between the ages of 2.5 and 6 years that employed multiple measures obtained from combined parent and teacher ratings identified 9 children (8.3%) as possible major depressive or dysthymic disorders. However, psychiatric interviews with these 9 children identified only 1 child (0.9%) who met DSM-III criteria for major depressive disorder. Nevertheless, these data do suggest that depressive symptoms are not as rare in this age group as suggested by the earlier study (Kashani & Ray, 1983) and, moreover, confirm that a diagnosis of depression may be made in this age group.

Clinical Populations. Several studies have reported prevalence data for one clinical population of preschool-age children. Kashani, Ray, and Carlson (1984) report that 4% (2 boys and 2 girls) of 100 consecutive referrals to a child development unit met diagnostic criteria for depression. The diagnoses included 1 definite major depressive disorder and 1 definite and 2 probable dysthymic disorders. In a later report, Kashani, Carlson, Horwitz, and Reid (1985) reported that 17% of these 100 children were identified as predominantly dysphoric by their parents and that all symptoms associated with the diagnosis of depression were more severe among the dysphoric than among the nondysphoric children. Significantly, of the dysphoric children, 82% lived in a household with at least one biological parent absent, compared to 55% of the nondysphoric group.

A more recent publication, based on evaluations of 1000 preschoolers from the same setting (Kashani & Carlson, 1987), identified 9 children (0.9%) as major depressive disorders according to DSM-III *adult* criteria. All the depressed children came from a "broken home," as compared to 33% of 18 controls drawn from among the nondepressed children. In addition, all the depressed children had been abused or severely neglected, in comparison to 22% of the control group. Hence, environmental factors are clearly associated with depression in this age group, raising the issue that depression in young children may be more easily related to psychosocial factors and hence possibly more "reactive" than the adult counterpart.

Depression and Depressive Disorder in School-Age Children

Nonclinical Populations. Two studies have reported prevalence estimates of depression for a single school-age cohort all born the same year in the same hospital in Dunedin, New Zealand. The initial report (Kashani et al., 1983), which provides data for these children at age 9 years, found a current point prevalence of 1.8% for major depression and past prevalence of 1.1%. The second study, of 792 of these children at age 11 years (Anderson, Williams, McGee, & Silva, 1987), reports 1-year prevalence estimates for all DSM-III psychiatric diagnoses. Psychiatric diagnoses were identified for 17.6% of the children studied, with depression diagnoses (i.e., major depression and dysthymia) accounting for 10% of all primary psychiatric diagnoses, thus establishing a 1-year depression prevalence of 1.8%. Thus, these two studies established identical prevalence estimates (1.8%) of depression for this sample at two different time points.

Rates of disorder from studies that have assessed depressive symptomatology exclusively, through interview, self-report or peer nomination, have reported slightly higher but also fairly consistent prevalence rates. Poznanski et al. (1984) interviewed children from one elementary school and found 5.4% qualified for a major depression diagnosis. Using a self-report measure of depression, Strauss, Forehand, Frame, and Smith (1984) identified a 6.3% prevalence rate on the basis of a Children's Depression Inventory cutoff score. Finally, Lefkowitz and Tesiny (1985), in a study of 3020 children using the Peer Nomination Inventory of Depression, established a prevalence rate on the basis of peer nomination of 5.2%. The similarity of rates obtained through these three different methods of assessment raises the interesting research question as to the actual overlap of children identified as depressed by all three methods.

The studies reviewed also reveal some interesting findings about epidemiological patterns. For example, prepubertal depressive disorders are more common among boys than among girls, a pattern contrary to that found in adults (Rutter, 1986). Anderson et al. (1987) report that in their study, the sex ratio for depression was 5.4:1, male/female, compared to a ratio for all diagnoses of 1.7:1, male/female. However, when studies using severity measures of depression were examined, depression scores were found to be higher for females than for males, although the differences were not significant (Lefkowitz & Tesiny, 1985; Poznanski et al., 1984).

It has commonly been assumed that rates of depression are higher among socioeconomically disadvantaged classes of society. No convincing evidence has been presented to support this assumption.

Finally, no convincing evidence has emerged to suggest that the prevalence of depression increases with age within the school-age years. Although our data in general indicate that depressive symptomatology is less common among 6- to 7-year-olds than among older children, some depression-associated symptoms are in fact more common among these younger than among older children. Clearly, further research on developmental factors in the epidemiology of prepubertal depression is needed.

Thus, full diagnostic assessments have identified roughly 2% of prepubertal school-age children as depressed, while measures that assess only depression have identified between 5.2% and 6.3% using three distinctly differing methods of assessment (i.e., clinician rating, self-report, and peer nomination).

Clinical Populations.   A number of studies have provided reports of the prevalence of depression among clinical populations. We will review prevalence data for two populations: children hospitalized in psychiatric units and children assessed for learning disabilities. Although depression prevalence data have been reported for other clinical populations such as residential schools (Handford, Mattison, Humphrey, & McLaughlin, 1986), these studies have not employed formal criteria to diagnose depression, relying instead on self-report measures.

Prevalence rates of psychiatric diagnoses among prepubertal psychiatric patients indicate that depressive disorders accompanied by impairment in functioning severe enough to require hospitalization are common in this age range. Petti (1978) reported that 59% of psychiatric inpatients were depressed according to modified Weinberg criteria. Depression prevalence rates reported in studies employing DSM-III criteria have been much lower. Using DSM-III criteria, Carlson and Cantwell (1980b) report depression in 28% of 102 children; Ney et al. (1986), in 20% of 282 children; Alessi and Magen (1988), in 16% of 160 children; and Kashani, Cantwell, Shekim, and Reid (1982), in 13% of 100 children.

Research on the association between depression and learning disabilities represents a growing research area (e.g., Hunt & Cohen, 1984; Mokros, Poznanski, & Merrick, 1989). This interest has been spurred by the clinical observation that learning disabilities are quite common among depressed children. Kashani et al. (1982) reported that learning difficulties were significantly more common among depressed (62%) than among nondepressed (22%) children in their inpatient study. Brumbach et al. (1980) reported that 62% of 100 prepubertal children referred to an educational diagnostic center met Weinberg diagnostic criteria for depression. This rate would presumably have been much lower if DSM-III criteria had been applied. Although this study suggests a very high rate of depression in children referred for evaluation of learning disabilities, the fact that these workers did not systematically assess psychiatric diagnoses other than depression is a serious shortcoming. Moreover, no formal criteria for learning disabilities (i.e., DSM-III specific developmental disorders) were applied.

Conflicting results have also been reported. Baker and Cantwell (1987) studied the risk for DSM-III psychiatric disorder in 300 children (all under age 16) referred for speech and language disorders. Although psychiatric diagnoses were common (44%) at initial referral, only 2% of the children were diagnosed as mood disorders. Similarly, at a 5-year follow-up, 60% of the children received a psychiatric diagnosis, with only 5% diagnosed as mood disorders. Hence, the prevalence rate for mood disorder is comparable to that in nonclinical populations. Factors that might account for the wide discrepancy among these studies are unclear. The lack of an elevated prevalence of depressive disorders in the Baker and Cantwell (1987) study argues against a common hypothesis that the frustration created by learning difficulties encourages the development of reactive depression (Livingston, 1985). Further investigation of this hypothesis is clearly warranted, however, since it offers a mechanism for understanding the emergence and persistence of reactive depressions in childhood.

Depression and Depressive Disorder in Adolescents

Nonclinical Populations.   Two recent studies have employed structured interviews to identify the prevalence of depressive disorders in adolescents according to DSM-III criteria. Deykin, Levy, and Wells (1987) used the Diagnostic Interview Schedule (Robins, Helzer, Crougham, & Ratcliff, 1981) to study the relation of depression, alcohol, and drug abuse in 424 college students between the ages of 16 and 19 years, of whom 94% were between the ages of 18 and 19 years. They found a lifetime prevalence of 6.8% for major depressive disorder. However, since neither an estimate of current point prevalence nor complete age of depression onset data were reported, it is difficult to compare this result with the prior work. It would be important in future research to identify the extent of convergence between the age of onset for first depression obtained from a lifetime prevalence study with available point-prevalence studies across age groups.

For a younger age group (14–16 years), Kashani et al. (1987) report a current point prevalence of 4.7% for major depressive disorder and 3.3% for dysthymic disorder based on interviews with 150 adolescents and their parents according to a modified version of the Diagnostic Interview for Children and Adolescents (DICA). These data indicate a 4-fold jump (8.0% vs. 1.9%) in the prevalence of affective disorders among 14- to 16-year-olds when compared to data from 11-year-olds reported in the Anderson et al. (1987) and Kashani et al. (1983) studies.

Several aspects of the methodology and results of the Kashani et al. (1987) study merit further consideration. In addition to the presence of DSM-III symptom criteria, they required evidence of significant dysfunction as well as clinical judgment that the adolescent needed treatment before they made a depression diagnosis. No comparable criteria have been included in other studies. When the dysfunction and treatment criteria were dropped, an additional 22% of subjects were found to meet criteria for major depression or dysthymia. Kashani et al. (1987) also report that additional psychiatric diagnoses were high across all subjects studied, with all (100%) of the depressed children qualifying for an additional DSM-III diagnosis and 26% of the 77 children with no symptom of dysphoria meeting criteria for DSM-III diagnoses. The high rate of unqualified depressive disorders (30%) together with the high prevalence of at least one other psychiatric diagnosis (42%) suggests either that the sensitivity of the clinical raters was inordinately elevated in identifying symptomatology in this study or that DSM-III criteria, as assessed by the DICA, are overly liberal in identifying disorder in community studies.

Most reported research of depression prevalence in normal adolescents has relied on self-report instruments. In the largest study to date, Kandel and Davies (1982) had 8206 14- to 18-year-olds complete a brief self-report depression inventory, derived from the Symptom Checklist—90. They report that 18% of these subjects were "highly depressed."

A number of studies have used the Beck Depression Inventory (BDI) to assess depression. Albert and Beck (1975) studied 63 7th and 8th graders (ages 11–15 years) using a shortened (13-item) form of the BDI. They found that 33.3% of subjects were moderately depressed (scores of 8 and above) and 3.2% severely depressed. Among studies that have used the complete 21-item BDI, Teri (1982) reports moderate depression for 27% and severe depression for 5% of 568 14- to 17-year-olds; Reynolds (1983), moderate and severe depression for 18% of 2875 13- to 18-year-olds; and Kaplan, Hong, and Weinhold (1984), moderate depression for 7.3% and severe depression for an additional 1.3% of 385 11- to 18-year-olds. Thus, across these four BDI studies, rates of at least moderate depression ranged from 8.6% to 36.5%.

Epidemiological studies have also provided information about mood regulation in adolescence. Kandel and Davies (1982) found that adolescents were significantly higher in self-ratings of dysphoria than a matched sample of parents. For example, when asked, "During the past year how often were you troubled by feeling unhappy, sad or depressed?," 19.7% of adolescents reported that they were much bothered, compared to 6.5% of their parents so reporting. Similar evidence has been discussed by Csikszentmihalyi and Larson (1984). They report significantly greater variability in adolescent ratings of moods when compared to adults, indicating that normal adolescents expressed a greater range and frequency of both highs and lows than their adult counterparts. Thus, whereas Offer and colleagues (Offer, 1969; Offer, Ostrov, & Howard, 1981) argued that traditional attitudes exaggerated the stressful character of adolescence, the studies discussed above suggest that the image Offer provides may have swung our view of adolescence too far in the opposite direction.

The most robust sociodemographic correlate of depression identified in these studies is evidence for greater rates of depression among females than among males, a pattern like that seen in adults. Kashani et al. (1987) found that among depressed subjects, girls outnumbered boys 5:1. Kandel and Davies (1982) and Reynolds (1983) also report significant sex differences, as does Teri (1982). However, Albert and Beck (1975) and Kaplan et al. (1984) found no sex difference. Their samples, however, included a sizeable number of prepubertal children. Since it is assumed that hormonal changes at puberty may well be related to the flip-flop in the sex ratio of depression, then mixing samples with prepubertal and pubertal children would militate against finding sex differences. Nevertheless, when the prepubertal and adolescent data are combined, there is a clear emergence of higher rates of mood disorder among females in adolescence.

As with studies of prepuberal children, most studies of adolescents have failed to identify sociodemographic differences in depression on such variables as race, religion, socioeconomic status, and parental education.

Again, as with prepubertal studies, those studies that have included a sufficiently large age range to allow for meaningful assessment have failed to identify any age trends in terms of prevalence or correlates of depression.

Clinical Populations. Prevalence rates in clinical samples of adolescents are similar to those found for prepubertal psychiatric inpatients. For example, Robbins, Alessi, Cook, Poznanski, and Yanchysyn (1982) reported a 27% and Strober, Green, and Carlson (1981) an 18.7% rate of depressive disorder among adolescents in an inpatient psychiatric setting. Thus, although the prevalence of depressive disorder appears to show a dramatic increase in the normal population at puberty, the proportion of prepubertal and adolescent children seen in psychiatric settings diagnosed as depressed does not appear to rise appreciably.

Summary. Several points are of interest in summarizing across age groups. First, children as young as 2.5 years have now been successfully assessed using adult diagnostic criteria. Second, a clear age trend is evident in the prevalence of depression. Before the age of 6, the disorder is extremely rare even in individuals assumed to be at high risk. This rarity does not extend to the school-age years. Diagnostic studies that ruled out other psychiatric disorders have established a roughly 2% prevalence rate for major depressive disorders, while studies that assessed only the depressive syndrome report a depression prevalence rate between 5.2% and 6.3%. Among adolescents, there is a dramatic increase in reported depression as determined both diagnostically and through self-report measures. Although there clearly appear to be differences in the rates of expression of depressive disorders and depressive symptomatology across the three age ranges reviewed, no evidence emerged to suggest age trends within these age groupings. The fact that several study samples included subjects selected from a wide range of ages within both prepubertal and adolescent studies would suggest that this lack of evidence is not a sampling artifact.

Putting these two contradictory age-related findings together suggests a third major point, namely, that shifts in prevalence of depression are not specifically age-related at all, but are instead related to accelerated biological maturation at puberty. Several findings support this hypothesis (i.e., the rapid increase in both suicide attempts and completions, and the emergence of bipolar disorder following puberty, all of which are exceedingly rare in the prepubertal years). Whether biological factors may account for the equally dramatic jump in depression among school-age as compared to preschool children is less clear. More likely, such factors as the greater self-awareness of school-age children, the cognitive capacity to conceptualize, and the verbal ability to report symptoms, along with the increased performance and social pressures they experience, account for this jump in depression.

The fourth point of interest is the lack of clear sex difference and possibly greater propensity for depression among males prior to puberty, with a clearly greater propensity for depression among females after puberty.

Not apparent from the studies reviewed is whether there has been an increase in the rate of depression diagnosis over time (i.e., cohort effects). Many studies reviewed mask the possibility of secular trends in depression. There is convincing evidence now available that a real, 3-fold, increase in adolescent suicide has occurred over the past 20 years, an increase not attributable to greater sensitivity in case identification (Shaffer & Fisher, 1981). Given the assumed link between suicidal behavior and affective disorder, one might assume that there has also been an increase in depression among youth. Klerman (1988) reports data to suggest that the age of onset of depression and the prevalence of depression among adolescents are greater among the postwar baby boom generation than among prior generations. However, it is difficult to identify direct evidence in support of such a hypothesis because of diagnostic confusion and incompleteness of records. Indeed, evidence in support of such a hypothesis may merely reflect greater reporting of depression as assessment instruments and diagnostic criteria have become increasingly standardized and accepted.

Epidemiology of Mania and Bipolar Disorders

Manic–depressive illness or bipolar disorder is much rarer in the general population than major depressive disorders, with lifetime prevalence estimates of 0.4–1.2% according to DSM-III-R. On the basis of retrospective study of adult bipolars, onset during adolescence is not uncommon and appears to increase during the adolescent years (Carlson, 1983), although estimates of the rate of bipolar onset prior to age 18 have all been under 30% (Strober et al., 1988). Moreover, the appearance of bipolar illness before puberty appears to be extremely rare if adult criteria are used. In an early review of the literature, Anthony and Scott (1960) identified only three children described in the literature, all age 11 years, who met their quite stringent criteria for manic–depressive psychosis. The review of the literature by Carlson (1983) identified 14 cases described in the literature (including those identified by Anthony and Scott), with 8 of these having onsets under the age of 9 and 6 an onset between the ages of 9 and 12 years. Several additional case reports of prepubertal bipolar illness have been reported since (e.g., Reiss, 1985; Sylvester, Burke, McCauley, & Clark, 1984), with one study reporting a case of hypomania in a 4-year-old (Poznanski, Israel, & Grossman, 1984). To date, no large-scale clinical studies have been reported. An additional problem exists for the epidemiological study of bipolar illness in children in that the diagnosis is quite difficult to make in this age group (Carlson, 1983).

Given the low base rate of the disorder, true epidemiological study of bipolar disorder would require study of very large samples in order to establish prevalence estimates. An alternative approach is at-risk study.

In adolescence, bipolar disorder is easier to identify, although some diagnostic confusion remains. For example, Carlson and Strober (1978), in their classic study, reevaluated the diagnostic records of six early adolescents initially diagnosed as schizophrenic and found that all were best diagnosed as manic–depressive. Recent epidemiological study (Carlson & Kashani, 1988) reveals that mania symptoms occur more frequently in adolescents than previously recognized. Of 150 randomly selected 14- to 16-year olds, 20 endorsed four or more manic items on the DICA.

Unanswered Issues in the Current Understanding of the Phenomenology of Mood Disorders in Youth

Overview

We began this chapter by noting that an important historical change in attitude toward the understanding of mood disorders in children and adolescents has occurred during the past several decades. This change involved a move from denial that these disorders occurred at all in childhood to the assumption that childhood and adult expressions of mood disturbance referenced the same disorder. Along with this shift came the development of standardized methods of assessment and diagnostic criteria that facilitated empirical research. Although these measures represent an important first step, it would be highly premature to regard methods of assessment as complete or to assume that future diagnostic criteria will not need revision.

Research has certainly substantiated that children may be directly assessed for depression and that depressed children can yield a phenomenological profile similar to that of depressed adults. Epidemiological research indicates that cases of depression may be identified in the community and that there are noteworthy shifts in the prevalence of depression, with greater prevalence in the adolescent years.

To this point, we have left unchallenged the assumption that child and adult mood disorders are equivalent. It is our contention that this assumption, i.e., that mood disorders in childhood represent the same entities as their adult counterparts, is still not resolved. Although many similarities have been identified, tantalizing differences also exist.

Studies that have specifically compared clinical phenomenology of major depressive disorders across broad age groups (Kovacs & Gatsonis, 1989; Mitchell, McCauley, Burke, & Moos, 1988; Ryan et al., 1987) and studies of changes in social–cognitive correlates of childhood depression have reported few developmental differences. However, since these studies have employed the known adult phenomenology as the starting point for their investigations, it may be argued that they have thereby restricted the type of phenomenological profile that may emerge for youth.

Specific findings within the literature also raise questions. For example, if there is continuity of disorders, then what is the significance of the negligible expression of mania in prepubertal children? What is the significance of the common presence of high levels of comorbidity among mood-disordered youth? And what are the implications of the related observation that psychosocial impairments commonly do not abate following remission of the affective symptomatology? Finally, why is there a lack of crisp response to antidepressants among depressed children and adolescents? All these questions may be viewed as challenges to the assumption of equivalence of mood disorders across the life span. In the remainder of this chapter, we will examine some of these concerns in more detail.

An important critique of the equivalence assumption, known as developmental psychopathology (Rutter & Garmezy, 1983), has charged that developmental considerations have been ignored in the evolution of the phenomenology of mood disorders in youth (Cicchetti & Schneider-Rosen, 1984, 1986; Rutter et al., 1986). Researchers in this tradition would argue that models of pathology have not been adequately linked to the emerging understanding of normative development and have thereby missed how processes of biological maturation and psychosocial development may mediate expressions of disorder. Additionally, they argue that demands of assessment procedures are insensitive in varying degrees to the cognitive and social facilities of children. Finally, developmental psychopathology suggests that in identifying a mood disorder as a child's problem, there is a tendency in both diagnosis and remediation not to appreciate the broader developmental system within which the mood disorder is situated and the impact that both the disorder and its remediation have on other areas of functioning in the child's development.

For these reasons, some researchers in this tradition have suggested that taxonomic classifications should be derived empirically rather than rationally (Achenbach & Edelbrock, 1984). For example, Achenbach and Edelbrock (1984) suggest that disorders of childhood are better thought of in terms of "broad-band" (e.g., "externalizing" and "internalizing") rather than "narrow-band" disorders such as depression.

The Issue of Comorbidity

Rutter (1986) notes that the relationship between diagnostic entities and the extent of concurrence or overlap between diagnoses has received insufficient attention. Study of collateral diagnosis is important for gauging the clarity of boundaries between disorders and for determining whether the identification of overlapping diagnoses proves useful for the description of groups at risk. This study is particularly important for research on depression, since many of the symptoms of depression, including dysphoria, may well constitute symptoms of primarily nonaffective syndromes.

Extent of Comorbidity. Additional psychiatric disorders have been found to commonly accompany depressions in childhood. For example, in an epidemiological study of 792 11-year-olds (Anderson et al., 1987), 11 (79%) of 14 children diagnosed as depressed received an additional psychiatric diagnosis. In contrast, of 125 children with nonaffective diagnoses, only 27% received an additional psychiatric diagnosis. Of those 11 depressed children who received an additional diagnosis, 8 received concurrent attention-deficit disorder, anxious/phobic disorder, and conduct disorder/oppositional disorder diagnoses, 2 anxious/phobic and conduct oppositional disorder diagnoses, and 1 conduct/oppositional disorder. Thus, anxiety disorders were identified in 10 of the 14 depressed children, conduct disorders in 11 of the 14, and attention-deficit disorder in 8 of the 14. Additionally, 3 children were found to also suffer from dysthymic disorder.

Kashani et al. (1987) report similarly high levels of comorbidity in their community study of adolescent depression. All 12 depressed children in their study had at least one additional diagnosis, with anxiety disorder in 75%, oppositional disorder in 50%, conduct disorder in 33%, alcohol abuse in 25%, and drug abuse in 25%. In addition, single cases of mania, attention-deficit disorder, and enuresis were also identified. Of the 12 depressions, 7 were major depressions, and all of these also had a coexisting dysthymia. Thus, comorbidity is extremely common among both prepubertal and adolescent depressed children identified in the community.

High rates of comorbidity have also been identified in clinically based studies of depressed children, although the rates of diagnoses have shown greater variability than in the two community studies reviewed above. This variation may reflect the greater diagnostic precision made possible in the clinical situation, where assessments are not confined to one-time interviews. Thus, Marriage, Fine, Moretti, and Haley (1986) found that among 60 children referred for depression, 33 were diagnosed with affective disorders. Of these, 33% were pure major depressive disorders and 33% pure dysthymic disorders. The remaining third had concurrent conduct disorders, with 10 of these 11 meeting criteria for dysthymic disorders. Identification of this high percentage of pure depressive disorders (67%) and the lack of additional diagnoses other than conduct disorder is the exception rather than the rule in clinical research studies.

Kovacs et al. (1984a) found that 79% of subjects with a major depressive disorder had other Axis I diagnoses. The most common were dysthymic disorder (38%), anxiety disorder (33%), and conduct disorder (7%). Of subjects with a dysthymic disorder, 93% had other Axis I diagnoses, with a superimposed major depressive disorder most common (57%), followed by anxiety disorder (36%), attention-deficit disorder (14%), and conduct disorder (11%). The presence of either, any, or specific concurrent diagnoses failed to show a difference in the duration of the depressive episode (Kovacs et al., 1984a) and neither increased nor decreased the probability of the recurrence of a depressive episode (Kovacs et al., 1984b). However, the small sample sizes in this research limit the confidence that may be placed in these later findings.

Mitchell et al. (1988) also report high rates of comorbidity in their study of the phenomenology of depression in children and adolescents. Coexisting disorder was identified in 89% of the prepubertal children and 86% of the adolescents in their study. No differences were identified between children and adolescents in the prevalence of coexisting disorders, although conduct disorders, which were equally common in children (16%) and adolescents (14%), did show differences between age groups according to the child's gender. Conduct disorders were found only among prepubertal males (26%), whereas they were roughly equally common among adolescent males (10%) and females (17%). By far the most commonly identified coexisting diagnoses were anxiety disorders, and these were found to be related to higher depression-severity scores.

Consistent with epidemiological studies, these clinical studies all found high rates of comorbidity among depressed children. However, these studies do not indicate whether these high rates of comorbidity are in fact specific to depression. One recent clinical study that has made such a comparison found, in contrast to epidemiological findings, that the extent of psychiatric comorbidity in depressed children did not differ from that in children with other psychiatric diagnoses (Alessi & Magen, 1988).

Anxiety Disorder and Mood Disorders.   Several studies have specifically investigated the relationship between anxiety and mood disorders. For example, Puig-Antich and Rabinovich (1985) report that most of the depressed children in their study presented with anxiety symptoms. However, anxiety symptoms were no more prevalent in a depressed group of 80 children compared with a psychiatric nondepressed group of 43 children. In assessing family history data, they found no difference in the expression of major depressive disorder or mania among nondepressed children with a diagnosis of separation anxiety compared with children diagnosed with major depressive disorder. The presence of anxiety disorder in a depressed child does not result in differential prediction of treatment response to imipramine nor a psychobiological profile (e.g., sleep architecture) that is different from a child without anxiety disorder. Mood disorders among parents may predispose children to separation anxiety disorder, which may itself be a precursor to depressive disorder.

Hershberg, Carlson, Cantwell, and Strober (1982) also report on the relation between anxiety and depression for a sample of 102 psychiatrically ill children and adolescents. They found high levels of anxiety among the depressed children in this sample, a pattern that is similar to what has been reported for adult depressives. In contrast, low levels of depression were found among the anxiety-disordered children in the sample. (Of note, anxiety disorders showed less similarity to adult anxiety disorders than did depressive disorders.) Evidence for depressive disorders among relatives was comparable in both groups; however, only anxiety disorders had a family history of anxiety disorder and only depressed had family history of bipolar illness and schizoaffective illness.

Substance Abuse and Mood Disorders.   An issue of particular interest in adolescence is the relation of alcohol and drug use with depression. Deykin et al. (1987) studied the interrelation of these factors and found that both alcohol and substance abuse were associated with major depressive disorder, with alcohol abuse specific to major depressive disorder but substance abuse related to other psychiatric disorders as well. When these disorders overlapped, the onset of major depressive disorder almost always preceded that of alcohol and substance abuse. Hence, alcohol and substance abuse may initially represent efforts at self-medication. A similar conclusion has been offered by Paton, Kessler, and Kandel (1977), who studied the relation between depressive mood and illegal drug use. Two findings stand out. First, depressed mood was found to be an important predictor of illicit drug use, other than marijuana use, among adolescents who had already experimented with marijuana. Second, in longitudinal study, these workers found a decrease in depressed mood over time among depressed users who continued drug use and an increase in depressed mood among the depressed users who stopped using drugs. As with the Deykin study, this study also suggests the possibility that drug abuse is at first an attempt at self-medication to relieve depressive states. Clearly, longitudinal research of depressed children is warranted to ascertain the vulnerability of these children to other disorders, particularly alcohol and substance abuse.

Summary.   The issue of comorbidity represents a central theoretical concern for defining the phenomenology of mood disorders, particularly depression, in youth. Puig-Antich et al. (1989) note that "the search for 'pure' (i.e., noncomorbid) forms of very early onset of affective illness may be a futile undertaking, as comorbidity may be an intrinsic characteristic of children with major affective illness and their families." While this may be so, this position retains the assumption that affective or mood disorders in youth are at their core phenomenologically equivalent to adult disorders. It is possible that high rates of comorbidity seriously compromise this assumption. Thus, it would seem necessary for research to forswear the assumption of equivalence and to provide clarification of the general nosology of childhood psychopathology, through studies of longitudinal course and of differential risks associated with such pathology, as well as study of treatment-response patterns.

Psychopharmacological Treatment

Successful pharmacological management of affectively disordered adults has represented one of the more notable accomplishments of modern psychiatry. The assumed similarity in the phenomenology of mood disorders across the life span has led to the increased adoption of pharmacological treatment strategies in children and adolescents, including the antidepressants, lithium carbonate, and monoamine oxidase inhibitors. Interestingly, relative to children, psychopharmacological research on adolescents has been particularly neglected (Campbell & Spencer, 1988). This section examines the efficacy of antidepressant treatment of depressed children and adolescents as a further issue of relevance for defining the phenomenology of mood disorders in youth.

Elva O. Poznanski
and Hartmut B.
Mokros

Clinical Efficacy of Antidepressant Medication. The clinical efficacy of anti-depressants in the treatment of depressed children and adolescents has been reported anecdotally in case reports, and in open trials (e.g., Brumbach, Schmidt-Dietz, & Weinberg, 1977). The strongest substantiation of clinical efficacy has come from studies of dose/plasma levels in prepubertal children, with the most favorable treatment outcomes occurring when dose/plasma levels fell in the same therapeutic range as reported for adults (e.g., Geller, Cooper, Chestnut, Anker, & Schulter, 1986; Preskorn, Weller, & Weller, 1982; Preskorn, Weller, Weller, & Glotzbach, 1983; Puig-Antich et al., 1987). For adolescents, however, Ryan et al. (1986) found no relation between drug plasma level and clinical response.

In contrast, data from controlled double-blind studies have been inconclusive for both children and adolescents. Whereas a small sample study (Preskorn, Weller, Hughes, Weller, & Bolte, 1987) found imipramine to be effective in the treatment of children with major affective disorder, two other small sample studies, one of children (Kashani, Shekim, & Reid, 1984) and one of adolescents (Kramer & Fieguine, 1981), showed no benefits of treatment. In the largest controlled study reported to date of the clinical efficacy of antidepressant treatment of prepubertal children, Puig-Antich et al. (1987) report no difference between actively treated and control groups. Positive response was seen in 56% of the imipramine-treated children and in 68% of the control subjects! Finally, the most methodologically sophisticated double-blind placebo-controlled study to date, which included a fixed plasma level and placebo washout period in the design, failed to establish any difference between active and placebo response (Geller, Cooper, McCombs, Graham, & Wells, 1989).

Summary. Psychopharmacological interventions with children and adolescents lack convincing evidence of the same effectiveness as reported in adults. The failure to obtain evidence for the clinical efficacy of antidepressants brings further into question the assumption of equivalence of mood disorders across the life span. Even successes in open trials raise questions. For example, Puig-Antich et al. (1985a,b) have demonstrated that children whose affective symptoms improve with antidepressant treatment nevertheless continue to experience impaired psychosocial functioning. This finding clearly suggests broadening the conceptualization of the phenomenology of mood disorders as currently described by DSM-IV.

Conclusions

Childhood mood disorders are now recognized as valid clinical entities. Although the clinical pattern presents many parallels to adult mood disorders, with some children showing the anlage of adult mood disorders, the clinical picture is not as well defined and shows clear differences from adults. In bipolar disorders, the illness shifts from vague clinical presentation prepubertally to more psychotic, more visible manic episodes after puberty. Depression in children is less severe prepubertally than in adolescence, and psychosocial factors are more easily identified.

Two issues, treatment response and psychiatric comorbidity, underscore the differences between childhood and adult mood disorders. Given the many clinical similarities between children and adults, the lack of response of prepubertal children to antidepressants is troubling. Too little is known about adolescents to comment. Whether in children this is due to difference in disease state or a different biological mechanism in young organisms is unknown. The issue of comorbidity is a difficult one and will not likely be resolved by research on depression alone. To some extent, comorbidity is a reflection of the general fuzziness of diagnostic nomenclature in children—an area that has vastly improved over the last two decades but is still more difficult than in adult nosology.

The etiology of these disorders has been only partly explored, with both biological and psychosocial factors uncovered. The typical clinical case is rarely definable in terms of either biological or psychosocial etiology. Thus, treatment often involves the introduction of multimodal approaches. Future studies of childhood and adolescent mood disorders need to further study the etiology of these disorders, clarify initial patterns in childhood, explore protective environments, study the forms of impact on development, and define guidelines for diagnosis and treatment.

The search for appropriate treatment strategies should also be broadened to consider a much-neglected topic, namely, the potential long-term side effects of treatment. This is particularly important in the use of psychopharmacological agents with children. Although acute biological side effects are well known, the possibility of delayed effects has been largely unexplored. A neglected concern is the potential impact of medication on cortical and cognitive development and, experientially, of bypassing normal development. For example, lithium has been felt to be a benign drug with minor side effects. Yet Carlson, Rapport, and Kelly (1992) recently reported effects of cognitive dulling during lithium therapy measured in terms of a lowered performance on a computerized paired-associate learning task and a computerized performance task. Studies of such effects for other psychopharmacological agents ought to be encouraged.

The fact that depressed children can be diagnosed using adult criteria does not really address the issue of whether they are the same entities in children and adults and also whether adult criteria are sufficiently defined for the diagnosis of children. In the future, we need to focus both on the effect of development on depression and on the effect of depression on development.

References

Achenbach, T. M., & Edelbrock, C. (1984). Psychopathology of childhood. *Annual Review of Psychology*, *35*, 227–256.

Albert, N., & Beck, A. T. (1975). Incidence of depression in early adolescence: A preliminary study. *Journal of Youth and Adolescence*, *4*, 301–307.

Alessi, N. E., & Magen, J. (1988). Comorbidity of other psychiatric disturbances in depressed psychiatrically hospitalized children. *American Journal of Psychiatry*, *145*, 1582–1584.

Ambrosini, P. J., & Puig-Antich, J. (1985). Major depression in children and adolescents. In D. Shaffer, A. A. Ehrhardt, & L. L. Greenhill (Eds.), *The clinical guide to child psychiatry* (pp. 182–191). New York: Free Press.

Anderson, J. C. Williams, S., McGee, R., & Silva, P. A. (1987). DSM-III disorders in preadolescent children. *Archives of General Psychiatry*, *44*, 69–76.

Anthony, J., & Scott, P. (1960). Manic depressive psychosis in childhood. *Journal of Child Psychology and Psychiatry and Allied Disciplines*, *1*, 52–72.

Baker, L., & Cantwell, D. P. (1987). A prospective psychiatric follow-up of children with speech/language disorders. *Journal of the American Academy of Child Psychiatry*, *26*, 546–553.

Beardslee, W. R., Bemporad, J., Keller, M., & Klerman, G. L. (1983). Children of parents with major affective disorder: A review. *American Journal of Psychiatry*, *7*, 825–832.

Brumbach, R. A., Jackoway, M. K., & Weinberg, W. A. (1980). Relationship of intelligence to childhood depression in children referred to an educational diagnostic center. *Perceptual and Motor Skills*, *50*, 11–17.

Brumbach, R. A., Schmidt-Dietz, S. G., & Weinberg, W. A. (1977). Depression in children referred to an educational diagnostic center: Diagnosis and treatment and analysis of criteria and literature review. *Diseases of the Nervous System*, *38*, 529–535.

Campbell, M., & Spencer, E. K. (1988). Psychopharmacology in child and adolescent psychiatry: A review of the past five years. *Journal of the American Academy of Child Psychiatry*, *27*, 269–279.

Cantwell, D. P., & Carlson, G. A. (Eds.) (1983). *Affective disorders in childhood and adolescence—An update.* New York: Spectrum Publications.

Carlson, G. A. (1983). Bipolar affective disorders in childhood and adolescence. In D. P. Cantwell & G. A. Carlson (Eds.), *Affective disorders in childhood and adolescence—An update* (pp. 61–84). New York: Spectrum Publications.

Carlson, G. A., & Cantwell, D. P. (1980a). Unmasking masked depression in children and adolescents *American Journal of Psychiatry, 137,* 445–449.

Carlson, G. A., & Cantwell, D. P. (1980b). A survey of depressive symptoms, syndrome and disorder in a child psychiatric population. *Journal of Child Psychology and Psychiatry and Allied Disciplines, 21,* 19–24.

Carlson, G. A., & Kashani, J. H. (1988). Manic symptoms in a nonreferred adolescent population. *Journal of Affective Disorders, 15,* 219–226.

Carlson, G. A., & Strober, M. (1978). Affective disorder in adolescence: Issues in misdiagnosis. *Journal of Clinical Psychiatry, 39(59),* 63–66.

Carlson, G. A., Rapport, M. D., & Kelly, K. L. (1992). The effects of methylphenidate and lithium on attention and activity level. *Journal of the American Academy of Child and Adolescent Psychiatry, 31,* 262–268.

Cicchetti, D., & Schneider-Rosen, K. (Eds.) (1984). *Bringing child development to child depression: New directions for child development,* No. 26. San Francisco: Jossey-Bass.

Cicchetti, D., & Schneider-Rosen, K. (1986). An organizational approach to childhood depression. In M. Rutter, C. E., Izard, & P. E. Read (Eds.), *Depression in young people* (pp. 71–134). New York: Guilford Press.

Csikszentmihalyi, M., & Larson, R. (1984). *Being adolescent: Conflict and growth in the teenage years.* New York: Basic Books.

Cytryn, L., & McKnew, D. H. (1974). Factors influencing the changing clinical expression of the depressive process in children. *American Journal of Psychiatry, 131,* 879–881.

Depert, J. L. (1952). Suicide and depression in children. *Nervous Child, 9,* 378–389.

Deykin, E. Y., Levy, J. C., & Wells, V. (1987). Adolescent depression, alcohol and drug abuse. *American Journal of Public Health, 77,* 178–182.

Dwyer, J. T., & DeLong, G. R. (1987). A family history of twenty probands with childhood manic–depressive illness. *Journal of the American Academy of Child Psychiatry, 26,* 176–180.

Frommer, E. (1968). Depressive illness in childhood. *British Journal of Psychiatry, 2,* 117–123.

Geller, B., Cooper, T. B., Chestnut, E. C., Anker, J. A., & Schulter, M. D. (1986). Preliminary data on the relationship between nortriptyline plasma level and response in depressed children. *American Journal of Psychiatry, 143,* 1283–1286.

Geller, B., Cooper, T. B., McCombs, H. G., Graham, D., & Wells, J. (1989). Double-blind placebo-controlled study of nortriptyline in depressed children using a "fixed plasma level" design. *Psychopharmacology Bulletin, 25,* 101–108.

Glaser, K. (1967). Masked depression in children and adolescents. *American Journal of Psychotherapy, 21,* 565–574.

Handford, H. A., Mattison, R., Humphrey, F. J., & McLaughlin, R. E. (1986). Depressive syndrome in children entering a residential school subsequent to parent death, divorce or separation. *Journal of the American Academy of Child Psychiatry, 25,* 409–414.

Hershberg, S. G., Carlson, G. A., Cantwell, D. P., & Strober, M. (1982). Anxiety and depressive disorders in psychiatrically disturbed children. *Journal of Clinical Psychiatry, 43,* 358–361.

Hunt, R. D., & Cohen, D. J. (1984). Psychiatric aspects of learning difficulties. *Pediatric Clinics of North America, 31,* 471–497.

Kandel, D. B., & Davies, M. (1982). Epidemiology of depressive mood in adolescence. *Archives of General Psychiatry, 39,* 1205–1212.

Kaplan, S. L., Hong, G. K., & Weinhold, C. (1984). Epidemiology of depressive symptomatology in adolescents. *Journal of the American Academy of Child Psychiatry, 23,* 91–98.

Kashani, J. H., Cantwell, D. P., Shekim, W. O., & Reid, J. C. (1982). Major depressive disorder in children admitted to an inpatient community mental health center. *American Journal of Psychiatry, 139,* 671–672.

Kashani, J. H., & Carlson, G. A. (1987). Seriously depressed preschoolers. *American Journal of Psychiatry, 144,* 348–350.

Kashani, J. H., Carlson, G. A., Beck, N. C., et al. (1987). Depression, depressive symptoms, and depressed mood among a community sample of adolescents. *American Journal of Psychiatry, 144,* 931–934.

Kashani, J. H., Carlson, G. A., Horwitz, E., & Reid, J. (1985). Dysphoric mood in young children referred to a child development unit. *Child Psychiatry and Human Development, 15,* 234–242.

Kashani, J. H., Holcomb, W. R., & Orvaschel, H. (1986). Depression and depressive symptoms in preschool children from the general population. *American Journal of Psychiatry*, *143*, 1138–1143.

Kashani, J., McGee, R. O., Clarkson, S. E., et al. (1983). Depression in a sample of 9-year-old children. *Archives of General Psychiatry*, *40*, 1217–1223.

Kashani, J. H., & Ray, J. S. (1983). Depressive related symptoms among preschool-age children in a child development unit. *Child Psychiatry and Human Development*, *13*, 233–238.

Kashani, J. H., Ray, J. S., & Carlson, G. A. (1984). Depression and depressive-like states in preschool-age children in a child development unit. *American Journal of Psychiatry*, *141*, 1397–1402.

Kashani, J. H., Shekim, W. O., & Reid, J. C. (1984). Amitriptyline in children with major depressive disorder: A double-blind crossover study. *Journal of the American Academy of Child Psychiatry*, *23*, 348–351.

Klein, D. N., Depue, R. A., & Slater, J. F. (1985). Cyclothymia in the adolescent offspring of parents with bipolar affective disorder. *Journal of Abnormal Psychology*, *94*, 115–127.

Klerman, J. (1988). The current age of youthful melancholia: Evidence for increase in depression among adolescents and young adults. *British Journal of Psychiatry*, *152*, 4–14.

Kovacs, M. (1989). Affective disorders in children and adolescents. *American Psychologist*, *44*, 209–215.

Kovacs, M., Feinberg, T. L., Crouse-Novak, M. A., Paulauskas, S. A., & Finkelstein, R. (1984a). Depressive disorders in childhood. I. A longitudinal prospective study of characteristics and recovery. *Archives of General Psychiatry*, *41*, 229–237.

Kovacs, M., Feinberg, T. L., Crouse-Novak, M. A., Paulauskas, S. A., Pollock, M., & Finkelstein, R. (1984b). Depressive disorders in childhood. II. A longitudinal study of the risk for a subsequent major depression. *Archives of General Psychiatry*, *41*, 229–237.

Kovacs, M., & Gatsonis, C. (1989). Stability and change in childhood-onset depressive disorders: Longitudinal course as a diagnostic validator. In L. Robins, J. L. Fleiss, & J. Barrett (Eds.), *The validation of psychiatric disorders* (pp. 57–75). New York: Raven Press.

Kovacs, M., Paulauskas, S., Gatsonis, C., & Richards, C. (1988). Depressive disorders in childhood. III. A longitudinal study of comorbidity with and risk for conduct disorders. *Journal of Affective Disorders*, *15*, 205–217.

Kramer, A. D., & Feiguine, R. J. (1981). Clinical effects of amitriptyline in adolescent depression. *Journal of the American Academy of Child Psychiatry*, *20*, 636–644.

Lefkowitz, M. M., & Burton, N. (1978). Childhood depression: A critique of the concept. *Psychological Bulletin*, *85*, 716–726.

Lefkowitz, M. M., & Tesiny, E. P. (1985). Depression in children: Prevalence and correlates. *Journal of Consulting and Clinical Psychology*, *53*, 647–656.

Livingston, R. (1985). Depressive illness and learning difficulties, research needs and practical implications. *Journal of Learning Disabilities*, *18*, 518–520.

Marriage, K., Fine, S., Moretti, M., & Haley, G. (1986). Relationship between depression and conduct disorder in children and adolescents. *Journal of the American Academy of Child Psychiatry*, *25*, 687–691.

Mitchell, J., McCauley, E., Burke, P. M., & Moss, S. J. (1988). Phenomenology of depression in children and adolescents. *Journal of the American Academy of Child Psychiatry*, *27*, 12–20.

Mokros, H. B., & Poznanski, E. O. (1992). Standardized approaches to the clinical assessment of depression in children and adolescents. In M. Shafii & S. Shafii (Eds.), *Clinical guide to depression in children and adolescents*. Washington, DC: American Psychiatric Press (in press).

Mokros, H. B., Poznanski, E., & Merrick, W. A. (1989). Depression and learning disabilities in children: A test of an hypothesis. *Journal of Learning Disabilities*, *22*, 230–233, 244.

Ney, P., Colbert, P., Newman, B., & Young, J. (1986). Aggressive behavior and learning difficulties as symptoms of depression in children. *Child Psychiatry and Human Development*, *17*, 3–14.

Offer, D. (1969). *The psychological world of the teenager*. New York: Basic Books.

Offer, D., Ostrov, E., & Howard, K. (1981). *The adolescent: A psychological self-portrait*. New York: Basic Books.

Paton, S., Kessler, R., & Kandel, D. (1977). Depressive mood and adolescent illegal drug use: A longitudinal analysis. *Journal of Genetic Psychology*, *131*, 267–289.

Petti, T. A. (1978). Depression in hospitalized child psychiatry patients: Approaches to measuring depression. *Journal of the American Academy of Child Psychiatry*, *17*, 49–59.

Petti, T. A. (1983). *Childhood depression*. New York: Haworth Press.

Poznanski, E. O., Carroll, B. J., Banegas, M. C., Cook, S. C., & Grossman, J. A. (1982). The dexamethasone suppression test in prepubertal depressed children. *American Journal of Psychiatry*, *139*, 321–324.

Poznanski, E. O., Grossman, J., Mokros, H. B., Buchsbaum, Y., Freeman, L., & Spiegelman, L. (1984).

Depressive symptomatology in an urban elementary school. Paper presented at the 137th Annual Meeting of the American Psychiatric Association, Los Angeles.

Poznanski, E. O., Israel, M. C., & Grossman, J. (1984). Hypomania in a four-year-old. *Journal of the American Academy of Child Psychiatry, 23*, 105–110.

Poznanski, E. O., Krahenbuhl, V., & Zrull, J. P. (1976). Childhood depression: A longitudinal perspective. *Journal of the American Academy of Child Psychiatry, 15*, 491–501.

Poznanski, E. O., Mokros, H. B., Grossman, J., & Freeman, L. (1985). Diagnostic criteria in childhood depression. *American Journal of Psychiatry, 142*, 1168–1173.

Poznanski, E. O., & Zrull, J. P. (1970). Childhood depression: Clinical characteristics of overtly depressed children. *Archives of General Psychiatry, 23*, 8–15.

Preskorn, S. H., Weller, E. B., Hughes, C. W., Weller, R. A., & Bolte, K. (1987). Depression in prepubertal children: Dexamethasone nonsuppression predicts differential response to imipramine vs. placebo. *Psychopharmacology Bulletin, 23*, 128–133.

Preskorn, S. R., Weller, E. B., & Weller, R. A. (1982). Depression in children: Relationship between plasma imipramine levels and response. *Journal of Clinical Psychiatry, 43*, 450–453.

Preskorn, S. R., Weller, E. B., Weller, R. A., & Glotzbach, E. (1983). Plasma levels of imipramine and adverse effects in children. *American Journal of Psychiatry, 140*, 1332–1335.

Puig-Antich, J., Goetz, D., Davies, M., et al. (1989). A controlled family history study of prepubertal major depressive disorder. *Archives of General Psychiatry, 46*, 406–418.

Puig-Antich, J., Lukens, E., Davies, M., Goetz, D., Brennan-Quattrock, J., & Todak, G. (1985a). Psychosocial functioning in prepubertal major depressive disorders I. *Archives of General Psychiatry, 42*, 500–507.

Puig-Antich, J., Lukens, E., Davies, M., Goetz, D., Brennan-Quattrock, J., & Todak, G. (1985b). Psychosocial functioning in prepubertal major depressive disorders II. *Archives of General Psychiatry, 42*, 511–517.

Puig-Antich, J., Novacenko, H., Davies, M., Chambers, W. J., Tabrizi, M. A., Krawiec, V., Ambrosini, P., & Sachar, E. J. (1984). Growth hormone secretion in prepubertal children with major affective disorders. I. Final report on response to insulin-induced hypoglycemia during a depressive episode. *Archives of General Psychiatry, 41*, 455–460.

Puig-Antich, J., Perel, J. M., Lupatkin, W., et al. (1987). Imipramine in prepubertal major depressive disorders. *Archives of General Psychiatry, 44*, 81–89.

Puig-Antich, J., & Rabinovich, H. (1985). Relationship between affective and anxiety disorders in childhood. In R. Gittelman (Ed.), *Anxiety disorders of childhood* (pp. 136–156). New York: Guilford Press.

Reiss, A. L. (1985). Developmental manifestations in a boy with prepubertal bipolar disorder. *Journal of Clinical Psychiatry, 46*, 441–443.

Reynolds, W. M. (1983). Depression in adolescents: Measurement, epidemiology, and correlates. Paper presented at the annual meeting of the National Association of School Psychologists, Detroit.

Rie, H. E. (1966). Depression in childhood: A survey of some pertinent contributions. *Journal of the American Academy of Child Psychiatry, 5*, 553–583.

Robins, D. R., Alessi, N. E., Cook, S. C., Poznanski, E. O., & Yanchysyn, G. W. (1982). The use of the Research Diagnostic Criteria for depression in adolescent psychiatric inpatients. *Journal of the American Academy of Child Psychiatry, 21*, 251–255.

Robins, L. N., Helzer, J. E., Croughan, J., & Ratcliff, K. S. (1981). National Institute of Mental Health Diagnostic Interview Schedule: Its history, characteristics, and validity. *Archives of General Psychiatry, 38*, 381–389.

Rutter, M. (1986). Depressive feelings, cognitions, and disorders: A research postscript. In M. Rutter, C. E. Izard, & P. E. Read (Eds.), *Depression in young people* (pp. 491–519). New York: Guilford Press.

Rutter, M., & Garmezy, N. (1983). Developmental psychopathology. In P. H. Mussen (Ed.), *Handbook of child psychology*, E. M. Hetherington (Ed.), Vol. IV, *Socialization, personality and social development* (pp. 775–911). New York: John Wiley.

Rutter, M., Izard, C. E., & Read, P. E. (Eds.) (1986). *Depression in young people.* New York: Guilford Press.

Rutter, M., Tizard, J., & Whitmore, K. (1970). *Education, health, and behaviour.* London: Longman.

Ryan, N. D., & Puig-Antich, J. (1987). Pharmacological treatment of adolescent psychiatric disorders. *Journal of Adolescent Health Care, 8*, 137–142.

Ryan, N. D., Puig-Antich, J., Ambrosini, P., et al. (1987). The clinical picture of major depression in children and adolescents. *Archives of General Psychiatry, 44*, 854–861.

Ryan, N. D., Puig-Antich, J., Cooper, T., et al. (1986). Imipramine in adolescent major depression: Plasma level and clinical response. *Acta Psychiatrica Scandinavica, 73*, 275–288.

Schulterbrand, J. G., & Raskin, A. (Eds.) (1977). *Depression in childhood: Diagnosis, treatment and conceptual models.* New York: Raven Press.

Shaffer, D., & Fisher, P. (1981). The epidemiology of suicide in children and young adolescents. *Journal of the American Academy of Child Psychiatry, 20*, 545–561.

Shafii, M., & Shafii, S. L. (Eds.). (1992). *Clinical guide to depression in children and adolescents.* Washington, DC: American Psychiatric Press.

Spitz, R. (1946). Anaclitic depression. *The Psychoanalytic Study of the Child, 2,* 313–342.

Spitzer, R. L., Endicott, J., & Robins, E. (1978). Research diagnostic criteria: Rationale and reliability. *Archives of General Psychiatry, 35,* 773–782.

Strauss, C. C., Forehand, R., Frame, C., & Smith, K. (1984). Characteristics of children with extreme scores on the children's depression inventory. *Journal of Child Clinical Psychology, 13,* 227–231.

Strober, M., Green, J., & Carlson, G. (1981). Reliability of psychiatric diagnosis in hospitalized adolescents. *Archives of General Psychiatry, 38,* 141–145.

Strober, M., Morrell, W., Burroughs, J., Lampert, C., Danforth, H., & Freeman, R. (1988). A family study of bipolar I disorder in adolescence: Early-onset of symptoms linked to increased familial loading and lithium resistance. *Journal of Affective Disorders, 15,* 255–268.

Sylvester, C. E., Burke, P. M., McCauley, E. A., & Clark, C. J. (1984). Manic psychosis in childhood. *Journal of Nervous and Mental Disease, 172,* 12–15.

Teri, L. (1982). The use of the Beck Depression Inventory with adolescents. *Journal of Abnormal Child Psychology, 10,* 277–284.

Weinberg, W. A., Rutman, J., Sullivan, L., Penick, E. C., & Dietz, S. G. (1973). Depression in children referred to an educational diagnostic center: Diagnosis and treatment. *Behavioral Pediatrics, 83,* 1065–1072.

Weissman, M. M., Gammon, G. D., John, K., et al. (1987). Children of depressed parents: Increased psychopathology and early onset of major depression. *Archives of General Psychiatry, 44,* 847–853.

Weller, E. B., & Weller, R. A. (Eds.) (1984). *Current perspectives on major depressive disorders in children.* Washington, DC: American Psychiatric Press.

3

Adolescent Bipolar Disorder

Phenomenology and Treatment Implications

Gabrielle A. Carlson

Introduction

Manic–Depressive Illness, or Bipolar Disorder as it has been designated since DSM-III (American Psychiatric Association, 1980), has captured the interest of clinicians and nonclinicians virtually since the beginning of recorded history. It is at once fascinating and almost inconceivable that an illness could render its sufferer so maniacal one moment, so depressed and immobile the next, and so absolutely normal the third. While its recurrent nature and protean manifestations were recognized intermittently over the centuries, Kraepelin (1921) was the first person to systematically and prospectively study hundreds of people afflicted in such a way that patterns could be observed in terms of symptom cluster, periodicity, and mood oscillation. Although replicated, the many individual and committee hours spent on the task have not significantly improved on his work.

Despite the mention by Kraepelin (1921) of a 6-year-old manic–depressive child, and an onset of disorder in many by late adolescence, it took several decades for interest in juvenile manic–depression to surface. A volume of *The Nervous Child* published in 1952 was first devoted to the subject of juvenile manic–depressive psychosis, and some of the definitional issues presented reflect some of the same diagnostic uncertainties still extant. The next noteworthy advance was a paper by Anthony and Scott (1960) that helped clarify two important definitions. First, these workers emphasized the importance of distinguishing between children and adolescents; second, they required the diagnosis to contain both poles of the disorder, mania and depression. This was at a time when manic–depression was defined by recurrence of depression but not necessarily by both mania and depression. Juvenile manic–depression was still considered a rarity, however. It took the promulgation of antidepressant and mood-stabilizing medication to stimulate a real interest in the disorder. At that point, it became more than an academic exercise to correctly classify

Gabrielle A. Carlson • Division of Child and Adolescent Psychiatry, Department of Psychiatry and Behavioral Sciences, State University of New York at Stony Brook, Stony Brook, NY 11794-8790.

Handbook of Depression in Children and Adolescents, edited by William M. Reynolds and Hugh F. Johnston. Plenum Press, New York, 1994.

psychiatric disorders in young people. Even so, there remained a prevailing notion that manic–depressive psychosis/illness was very rare in childhood.

Part of the reason for the alleged rarity had to do with whether, by "childhood," one meant young children or adolescents. Anecdotal reports of "children" with manic–depression increased with the chronological age of the child, but until Anthony and Scott (1960) wrote their important review, the age boundary was blurred. Another misconception had to do with the term "psychosis." The endogenous (i.e., without obvious cause), episodic, often psychotic dimensions of manic–depression *without ultimate deterioration* were part of the concept "manic–depressive psychosis." According to Kraepelin (1921) and his successors for the next several decades, it was not necessary to have a manic episode to be manic–depressive. As Goodwin and Jamison (1990) point out, it was *endogenous* depressions that Leonhard in 1957 divided into "unipolar" and "bipolar" subtypes. This was subsequently confirmed by both Angst and Perris in 1966, using family history information to determine that the presence or absence of mania may make a difference in the person's overall illness course. It was thus *endogenous* depressions that were felt to be very uncommon in children and even adolescents (for further discussion, see Carlson and Garber, 1986). This point has been lost in the gentrification of manic–depressive insanity to manic–depressive illness to affective disorder with unipolar and bipolar subtypes to mood disorder.

The usual explanation given for the lack of recognition of juvenile bipolar disorder has been that clinicians were blinded by the prevailing psychoanalytical conceptualization that children (including adolescents) have insufficiently developed superegos. That is, the hostility and rage directed against internalized objects that have disappointed or abandoned the subject do not yet produce guilt and resultant depression and its defense, mania. It is hard to believe that this view, relatively esoteric and idiosyncratic (to the United States), should account for a *worldwide* dearth of interest in and identification of juvenile manic–depression for so many years. Differences between diagnostic practices in the United States and Great Britain, for instance, that produced such differences in diagnosis of schizophrenia and manic–depression (Cooper et al., 1972) do not help us with the underidentification of juvenile manic–depression. The European depression literature, less influenced by psychoanalytical and Meyerian tradition that supposedly led us astray for so long, does not report vastly different numbers of juvenile manic–depressives.

Carlson and Strober (1978, 1979) have reported elsewhere that a number of biases keep clinicians from recognizing the implications of their patients' symptoms and behavior. First, it is easy to attribute low spells and high spells to the behavioral vicissitudes of adolescence or to the numerous psychosocial changes they may be experiencing. Thus, in mild cases, adjustment disorders are frequently diagnosed. In extreme cases, where the adolescent is raving and psychotic, schizophrenia has been the diagnosis most frequently made. These diagnostic problems will be discussed at greater length later in this chapter. However, it is curious that there has been a bias against recognizing a disorder that has, in many cases, an *onset in adolescence.*

In reality, the inconsistency between the fact that bipolar disorder has its onset in adolescence and that bipolar disorder was considered almost nonexistent in adolescents, may have to do with the time lag between symptom onset and an episode of severity sufficient to require treatment. In data derived from studies of the Old Order Amish, Blumenthal, Egeland, Sharpe, Nee, and Endicott (1987) report that the *median* age of onset for Bipolar I patients varied by 11 years from first noticeable symptoms (age 14.7) to first hospitalization (age 25.8), with age at both first Research Diagnostic Criteria (RDC) major affective disorder and first treatment being about age 22. McGlashan (1988) reports similar findings in adolescent-onset mania. There were about 5 years between first symptoms (*mean* age 16 ± 3) and first hospitalization (*mean* age 21 ± 6); the time span between first symptoms and first hospitalization in adult-onset patients, interestingly, was less (*mean* ages 30 ± 9 and 32 ± 10, respectively). Note that the use of means rather than medians captures the fact that the long age of risk artificially inflates means compared to medians. This strongly suggests that (1) *fully symptomatic* bipolar disorder may be less common in adolescence and (2) the time span to full symptoms in early-onset patients is longer than for adults. The latter interpretation is further supported by data that reveal shortening of cycle length (i.e., time between episodes) with increasing age and age of onset (see the review in Goodwin & Jamison, 1990, p. 135). Although data from Carlson, Davenport, and Jamison (1977) and from McGlashan (1988) do not find significant differences in outcome between adolescent- and adult-onset bipolar patients, onset in both studies was symptom, not treatment, onset. A question of particular interest is the prognostic significance of becoming *treatably psychiatrically ill and hospitalized* (i.e., variables usually measured in studies) with bipolar depression or mania early. Additionally worth knowing is whether and under what circumstances these fully symptomatic adolescents have had a prepubertal prodrome because of the long onset time as opposed to an unusually short cycle or time to full episode. Whereas the original observation was that manic–depression was rare in childhood and adolescence, the answer may simply be that, like many other illnesses, it takes a while to get going and reach its fully recognized state. Juvenile bipolar disorder was understudied because adult psychiatric institutions and studies rarely include patients below age 18 and virtually never include those below age 15. Adolescents with endogenous/psychotic disorders occurring below age 15 were and are sufficiently uncommon to require a concerted effort to obtain adequate samples to study.

Bipolar Disorder—Clinical Aspects

Classic bipolar disorder is not difficult for the clinician to recognize, but diagnostic acumen is important in less fully developed cases and in atypical cases, i.e., the ones most likely to occur in young people. Clinicians working only with children and young adolescents, who have not had fairly extensive exposure to "classic" phenomenology, are at a disadvantage in diagnosing the disorder. The reason is both that they have had limited experience with classic cases and that they are forced to deal with more complicated, developmentally confounded, early cases. Their adult-oriented colleagues cannot help much because their grounding in development and psychopathology in children is also lacking. Although the DSM criteria help to operationalize the clinical picture, they do not begin to substitute for seeing patients with the disorder. Since we did not evolve a clinical picture of juvenile bipolar disorder from hundreds of cases followed longitudinally as Kraepelin and his contemporaries did, we are forced to apply adult criteria to identify youngsters who have disorders similar to those of adults. Unfortunately, we are at risk of developing the ludicrous situation of having increasing numbers of children "meeting criteria" out of the context from which the criteria were developed.

Age of Onset

As mentioned above, there is a considerable discrepancy between the age of onset of first affective symptoms and the age of onset of either first treatment or first psychiatric hospitalization. When the latter is the criterion, the mean age of onset for bipolar disorder is about age 28; the median age is lower, however, and probably the more important number. The reason for the difference, as mentioned earlier, is that the age of risk to development of the disorder continues into senescence and thus raises the mean age. The older literature, as cited by Angst (1988), reports percentage onsets under age 20 in a similar range [Mendel (1881), 19%; Kraepelin (1921), 33%; Wertham (1919), 20%]. This has been substantiated in recent literature [e.g., Baron et al., 1983, 11%; Loranger and Levine (1978), 20%; Joyce (1984), 42%). Akiskal, Djenderedjian, Rosenthal, and Khani (1977) reported that 60% of cyclothymes had their onset by age 25. What is particularly relevant to youth, however, is that there are strong correlates with family history. Thus, both Angst (1988) and Weissman, Warner, Wickramaratne, and Prusoff (1988) found that those with early-onset major depressive and bipolar disorder had family members with early onset. Similarly, Strober et al. (1988) found the highest rates of positive family histories in adolescent bipolars with prepubertal psychopathology.

Type of Onset and Change of Diagnosis

What is the prognostic significance of the type of onset, manic or depressive, in bipolar disorder? When a young person presents with a first episode of obvious mania, it is highly likely that further episodes will follow. Though it is difficult to predict time to recurrence, the course of bipolar disorder is quite certain. More problematic is the young person who presents with a depressive episode. Depending on the age of the patient, the number of episodes already experienced, and the length of follow-up, the diagnosis will change fro unipolar to bipolar in between 4% and 33% of cases (Angst, 1988). In adolescents, the rate of diagnostic change is about 20% over about a 4-year period (Akiskal et al., 1985a; Strober and Carlson, 1982; Strober, Lampert, Schmidt, & Morrell, 1993). There is some suggestion that this rate may hold for older preadolescents as well (Kovacs and Gatsonis, 1989; Asarnow, personal communication, April 17, 1991).

Since, in childhood and adolescence, one is invariably dealing with first onset, accurate prediction of a bipolar course when a young person appears with a serious depression is difficult. Strober and Carlson (1982) originally reported that the best predictors to bipolar course in hospitalized adolescents with major depression were acute onset, hypomanic response to an antidepressant medication, strong family history of major depression/bipolar disorder, and *psychotic symptoms* (see Table 1). Strober et al. (1993) have recently replicated these findings insofar as 28% of adolescents with psychotic depressions went on to have subsequent manic episodes and none of the nonpsychotic

Table 1. Significant Schedule for Affective Disorders and Schizophrenia Intake Ratings of Depression in Bipolar and Nonbipolar Adolescents[a]

Item (range)	Bipolar ($N = 12$) Mean (SD)	Nonbipolar ($N = 48$) Mean (SD)	t	p
Duration of onset (1 = acute; 9 = insidious)	4.94 (0.81)	6.02 (0.96)	3.60	0.001
Depressed mood (1–7)	5.94 (1.02)	5.08 (1.13)	2.38	0.02
Self-reproach (1–6)	4.98 (0.99)	4.18 (1.13)	2.22	0.05
Suicidal tendencies (1–7)	3.69 (0.91)	4.37 (0.96)	2.27	0.05
Weight gain (1–6)	1.24 (0.46)	1.77 (0.79)	2.21	0.05
Bodily concerns (1–6)	4.18 (0.94)	3.24 (1.06)	2.85	0.01
Diminished concentration (1–6)	4.67 (0.76)	3.98 (0.88)	2.46	0.02
Irritability (1–6)	3.37 (0.92)	4.12 (1.12)	2.34	0.05
Retardation (1–6)	4.44 (0.80)	3.29 (1.11)	3.23	0.01
Self-pity (1–6)	2.21 (0.72)	2.78 (0.79)	2.37	0.02
Demandingness (1–6)	1.86 (0.67)	2.55 (0.78)	2.87	0.01
Psychosis present: delusions or hallucinations (%)	75%	6%	Fisher's exact test	0.000

[a]From Strober and Carlson (1982).

depressives did. Of additional import is that studies of patients with *first episodes* of psychosis in young people report similar findings. For instance, Brockington, Helzer, Hillier, and Francis (1982), in a study of hospitalized psychotic patients, found that 6 of 11 patients with mood-congruent psychotic symptoms during their depressive episodes went on to have a manic–depressive course during a 6-year follow-up. This finding was not true of those with mood-incongruent psychotic symptoms. However, in the Vancouver, British Columbia, study of first episodes of psychosis, Beiser, Iacono, and Erickson (1989) found that DSM-III diagnosis of major depression predicted a 14% bipolar switch by 9 months and a 20% bipolar switch by 18 months. [This risk for "switching" into mania may occur differentially in younger age samples with first episodes. In a 1-year follow-up of 92 psychotically depressed adults with a mean age at interview of 42, only 3% became manic according to Johnson, Horvath, and Weissman (1991).] Beiser and colleagues make the point that *the temporal precedence of affective psychopathology to psychotic symptoms was a better predictor of bipolar and affective course than mood congruence of symptoms.* In other words, if there are clear depressive symptoms before the onset of psychosis, the prognostic significance for an affective-disorder course is greater than the level or severity of either affective or psychotic symptoms during the nadir of the episode. This is essentially the same observation made by Carlson and Goodwin (1973) in reporting the sequence of manic symptoms and psychosis during a manic episode. The diagnostic confusion with schizophrenia will be discussed in another part of this chapter.

Duration of Episodes

Most studies of episode length have compared unipolar with bipolar depressions. One must turn to the older literature to discern the natural duration of episodes not complicated by treatment. Basically, bipolar episodes are shorter, averaging between 4 and 6 months untreated. There is wide variability, however. As cited by Angst (1988), Huhn and Pauly found 75% of adolescents to have recovered by 6 months. Data from Strober's sample of hospitalized depressed adolescents specifically selected to have uncomplicated, primary affective disorder by RDC criteria suggest that the duration of adolescent depressive episodes may be longer than that of adult episodes (Strober et al., 1994). His findings were compared with those from the National Institute of Mental Health Collaborative depression study (Keller, Shapiro, Lavori, & Wolfe, 1982), which admittedly had a more heterogeneous population of depressed adults. However, for adolescents, the 3- to 4-month (16-week) recovery rate (from time of hospital admission) was 17%, the 6-month (28-week) recovery rate was 62%, and the 1-year recovery rate was 81%. These rates compared with 63%, 69%, and 74% for adults, respectively. Thus, ultimate recovery rates were the same, but it took adolescents longer to get there. There was no significant difference in episode duration in Strober's psychotic (and thus more likely bipolar) depressives. What is more discouraging about these findings is that Strober's sample was a treated sample; nonetheless, episode duration was similar to that of untreated depressed samples.

Recovery Rates and Cycle Length

When Kraepelin (1921) originally wrote that manic–depressive psychosis had a good prognosis for recovery (in contrast to dementia praecox), he was addressing recovery from an episode rather than remaining symptom-free forever. In fact, recovery from a first episode of bipolar disorder is remarkably high, though, as noted above, it may not occur quickly. Kraepelin reports of patients remaining severely manic or depressed for decades and then spontaneously remitting. Of relevance to the study of adolescent-onset bipolar disorder is the observation that cycle lengths decrease with time. Thus, the average time between the start of the first episode and the start of the second is about 5 years. This time shortens with subsequent episodes and is shorter in patients with a later age of onset (for a review, see Goodwin & Jamison, 1990). On the other hand, in any given patient, there appears to be considerable consistency of episode length from episode to episode (Angst, 1988).

With regard to recovery, there is a distinction between symptomatic recovery and social recovery, rates of the former being higher than rates of the latter. Reviewing a large number of long-term follow-up studies, Goodwin and Jamison (1990, pp. 149–150) found that approximately 60% of patients ultimately show a return to premorbid levels of functioning. This return may not be immediately apparent and improves with time after symptomatic recovery, as it takes time to recover from the consequences of an episode. If one defines chronicity as continuous criteria for an episode for 2 years or more, rates of between 10% and 25% are generally given. "Recovery," defined as 5 years without symptoms, is also low, however (23%), attesting to the number of recurrences of the disorder. Over the shorter term, many patients suffer high rates of enduring symptoms (Harrow, Goldberg, Grossman, & Meltzer, 1990). It is difficult to make an intelligent statement about the number of episodes likely to occur over a person's lifetime, since data addressing this question depend on how long a follow-up has been executed. In those studies in which follow-up exceeds 25 years, single episodes are rare (0–8%), 10–30% of patients will escape with 2 or 3 episodes, 25–50% of patients will have 7 or more episodes (Goodwin & Jamison, 1990, p. 133).

There have been a number of longitudinal follow-up studies of early-onset bipolar patients (Annesley, 1961; Carlson et al., 1977; Landolt, 1957; McGlashan, 1988; Olsen, 1961; Welner, Welner, & Fishman, 1979; Werry, McClellan, & Chard, 1991). Only three (Carlson et al., 1977; Coryell and Norten, 1980; McGlashan, 1988) directly compared findings to adults in the same sample. Coryell and Norten (1980) found that over 8.4 years, adolescent bipolars spent 12.6% of time in hospital compared to adults 9.4%. Carlson et al. (1977) reported that of the 28 adolescent-onset patients studied, 60% had good social outcomes (though they might have had recurrences) and had a mean episode frequency per year of 0.38. This finding was not different from that for those patients with onsets over age 45. The findings of McGlashan (1988) were similar. In general, these studies conclude that bipolar disorder is not benign, but that *symptom* onset prior to adulthood does not necessarily doom the patient to a worse outcome. Factors associated with a worse outcome have more to do with poor intermorbid functioning. Such poor functioning may occur because of either personality disorder (Kutcher, Marton, & Korenblum, 1990) or co-occurring psychiatric disorders such as substance abuse (Black, Winokur, Bell, Nasrallah, & Hulbert, 1988).

Clinical Picture

Although the phenomenology of depression and the current state of its nosology have been discussed elsewhere in this volume, there are certain symptoms, somewhat more typical of bipolar depressions, that deserve emphasis. First, although depressed mood is the sine qua non of depressive disorders, patients with bipolar depressions do not always describe or even recognize themselves as depressed. In that respect, the DSM-III criterion of dysphoria is more accurate. Those afflicted feel indescribably dreadful. However, they feel that *depression* is something one feels about a circumstance and that it is in a somewhat normal realm of experience. They do not necessarily liken their incomprehensible mood to anything anyone has ever experienced. This completely apathetic state and dulling of all feelings is what is mistaken for a "flat" affect and is sometimes confused with schizophrenia. DSM-III (American Psychiatric Association, 1980) tried to capture this experience in its melancholic descriptor, "distinct quality of depressed mood i.e. different from the feeling following the death of a loved one." DSM-III-R (American Psychiatric

Association, 1987) replaced this criterion with "lack of reactivity to usually pleasurable stimuli." While this mood state is not invariably present in bipolar depressions, its appearance is more common to bipolar than to unipolar depressions.

Other symptoms and behaviors consistent with a slowed, vegetative state are seen in bipolar depressions, too. Slowed mentation impairs the ability to concentrate and, in some cases, appears as a foggy, confused state. In the elderly, it contributes to a diagnostic confusion with dementia. In adolescents, this symptom is responsible for precipitous drops in grades in previously good students and for sudden antisocial cutting of classes because the work is so hopelessly impossible to concentrate on and execute. Slowed physical behavior manifests itself in hypersomnia (including napping), slowed, monotonous speech, lack of spontaneous speech, and long latencies of response.

Psychotic symptoms (hallucinations and delusions) are not infrequent in bipolar depressions. For instance, Winokur, Clayton, and Reich (1969) reported that 33% of depressed bipolar patients had delusions; 6% had auditory hallucinations. The prognostic significance of psychotic symptom content (mood congruency), intensity, and relationship to affective symptoms is unresolved. DSM-IV draft (American Psychiatric Association, 1991) states that

> the presence of psychotic symptoms predicts severity but is not synonymous with it. Psychotic depression predicts a relatively poor prognosis compared with nonpsychotic depression, including more chronicity, hospitalization, episodes, impairment and perhaps suicide risk. . . . Individuals diagnosed with psychotic mood disorder [this includes manic episodes] are more likely to develop psychotic symptoms during recurrences and often maintain the particular content of their delusions across episodes.

This issue is particularly salient in adolescents with depressive episodes, since they have a much higher frequency of psychotic symptoms. For instance, Carlson and Strober (1979) found that 66% of bipolar depressed adolescents had delusions and 50% had hallucinations. Rosen, Rosenthal, Van Dusen, Dunner, and Fieve (1983) found that 62% of 13 adolescent-onset bipolar patients had three or more psychotic symptoms "sometime in the course of their illness" (it was not clear in the study report whether the symptoms were manic or depressed). This is in contrast to patients over age 30, with 28% having three or more psychotic symptoms, and over age 40, who, when they had psychotic symptoms, had only one or two. As mentioned earlier, Strober et al. (1993) describe the 2-year course of 58 depressed (by RDC criteria) (Spitzer, Endicott, & Robins, 1978) hospitalized adolescents of whom 18 (31%) were psychotic. A comparison with the nonpsychotic depressives revealed significantly greater severity, and more psychosocial impairment at 6 months but not by 24 months (by which time 89% had recovered and 90% of the nonpsychotic depressives had recovered). Of the 18, 5 (27.7%) had "switched" polarity (none of the nonpsychotics "switched"). Of these, 5 became manic on the heels of their depressive episode, and 3 developed a manic or hypomanic episode after recovery from the index depression. Given the consistency of this finding with other reports of first episodes of psychosis (see above), the implications of psychotic symptoms during initial depressive episodes of younger patients, and especially early-onset patients, may therefore be somewhat different from those for older patients.

Mania

Duration

Keeping in mind that mania usually occurs in episodes, and therefore has an onset and offset, in its fully developed state it is clearly different from the patient's usual state of being.

Between DSM-III, -III-R, and -IV, there have been alterations in duration needed to qualify for an "episode." While 7 days is the DSM-III criterion, there is nothing sacred about 1 week, and it defies common sense not to "count" an otherwise clear episode that, for some reason, lasts only 6 days. Not specifying duration, however, has artificially increased the rates of mania to the point of unbelievability. Thus, using information from a structured-interview assessment of nonpsychiatrically referred 14- to 16-year-olds, Carlson and Kashani (1988) found that 13% of the sample endorsed enough "manic symptoms" to meet criteria for mania if duration was not clearly defined. Classically, manic episodes last several weeks to several months. The histories described by patients with fully developed bipolar disorder, however, indicate that early in their course, there were brief (days) episodes of mania or hypomania. Drug-induced manic and hypomanic episodes are often brief as well. The diagnostic significance of these episodes, however, is much clearer retrospectively than they are prospectively.

Clinical Picture

While an acute manic episode is unmistakable, the boundaries between optimistic or emotionally labile temperament and mild mania (hypomania) and severe, psychotic, disorganized mania and schizophrenia are fuzzier (Carlson, 1984, 1990). Carlson and Goodwin (1973) conceptualized mania as having "stages": In Stage I (hypomania), characteristic symptoms are present, but impairment is equivocal or mild; in Stage II, mania is clearly symptomatic and incapacitating; Stage III is characterized by a severe, psychotic, sometimes dysphoric state. In each state, the various components of mood, cognition, and activity level increase in velocity. While one can often delineate "stages," the boundaries between them, again, are nebulous. One can occasionally state a precise day on which an episode began or ended; more often, however, one knows only that it was not present before or after a particular time frame. Most important is the distinction between manic symptoms and the person's premorbid personality. As noted in DSM-IV, "the episode is associated with an unequivocal change in functioning that is uncharacteristic of the person when not depressed." For people with a normally tempestuous life-style, or in adolescents with a preexisting externalizing disorder, the identification of an episode becomes very difficult.

Symptoms. While severity of disorder is problematic in distinguishing mania at both ends of the severity range, developmental issues pose an additional confound in making a diagnosis of hypomania and mania. Elation, euphoria, and a sense of beatific well-being are the mood states associated with mania. This feeling is quickly reduced to anger and hostility, however, when the person is impeded. Many patients have depressive feelings simultaneously such that they are easily reduced to tears or, in more serious mania, are clearly quite dysphoric and frightened at times. The statements and metaphors used to describe the feeling of being high are important, as is the person's ready wit and convivial merriment. True elation, however, appears to be particularly uncommon in young children, though in recent years people have tried to squeeze the silly, disinhibited behavior of some hyperactive children under this criterion. The uncharacteristicness of the behavior and feeling may prove most helpful. Thus, a psychiatrically hospitalized, prepubertal, 12-year-old boy who had suffered many hardships and was chronically depressed became hypomanic on fluoxetine. As his hypomania was unfolding, he developed a perpetually silly grin and made statements such as these: "I know I don't have a family or a place to live but I suddenly feel like all that doesn't matter anymore. I feel like all my troubles are gone; it doesn't make sense 'cause none of that stuff has changed." "I should feel bad because I lost my weekend pass but I feel really great!" Not surprisingly, the significance of those remarks was not recognized at the time. After several days of escalating behavior fulfilling all the criteria for a full manic episode, and after the fluoxetine was discontinued, the youngster became euthymic (i.e., no longer depressed). He recognized that his total lack of concern for his future was an alien, albeit enjoyable feeling for him. He no longer felt either hopeless or euphoric. While many children deny their problems, it was the patient's change in attitude both from depression to mania and from mania to euthymia that was most revealing here.

A second critical feature of mania is the vastly increased energy level with which it is suffused. Thoughts, words, and actions are in fast motion. Although DSM-III and -III-R have replaced "increase in activity" with "increase in goal-directed activity," this author doubts that anyone can measure the "goal-directedness" of activity. Moreover, in the years prior to somatic treatment, it is unlikely that patients who died from manic exhaustion were particularly goal-directed. Whether, in fact, excessive activity is goal-directed or not may be an important distinction between hypomania, where the person is still in some degree of control, and mania, where he or she no longer is. The only redeeming value in the change may be that it should distinguish the hyperactivity of children with attention-deficit hyperactivity disorder (ADHD), in which tasks are never completed. However, the *episodic nature* of the hyperactivity is probably a more reliable distinction between mania or hypomania and ADHD than are levels of goal-directedness.

Racing thoughts, flight of ideas, and increased verbal production with puns, word plays, and incessant speech are also characteristics of mania. Overtalkativeness, however, is a not infrequent complaint from parents about their behavior-disordered child and can be seen in both chronically anxious children and children with ADHD. In fact, we have observed verbal children with pervasive developmental disorders to have a push of speech and incessant perseveration on certain topics (idiosyncratic to the particular child) that is as compelling as that seen in mania. On the other hand, this problem, too, is relatively chronic, and follow-up so far has not revealed a bipolar outcome.

Thought content is striking in mania. What is not usually emphasized is that this often reflects and magnifies the person's premorbid conflicts, life-style, preoccupations, and other concerns. Thus, literary people are more likely than truck drivers to feel that they are writing the world's greatest novel. Those with strong religious backgrounds are more likely to hear from God than are atheists. It is interesting that grandiosity, which in true mania can become psychotic, with the person hearing voices and having visions to confirm his or her special place in the world schema, is uncommon in young children and begins to appear around age 9 or 10 (Carlson, 1983). There may be some confusion, however, with childhood denial of weakness and impotence. Ask any 6-year-old what he would do with a "robber" who came into his room at night, and you will usually hear how he will beat the "bad guy" up and throw him down the stairs. No amount of reasoning seems to change the conviction that the child is strong and capable enough to overcome the aggressive adult adversary as easily as the "good guys" seen on TV. Similarly, children who threaten to run away after they feel they have been wronged will talk with great bravado about how they can live without adult supervision. They are certainly "grandiose," but it is not considered deviant developmentally.

Another manic symptom that may have different implications in children is hypersexuality. Postpubertal adolescents and adults may become uncharacteristically preoccupied with sexual themes or become involved sexually with people in ways that are different from their usual behavior. Children, especially those who have been abused, neglected, or are chronically disinhibited in a variety of ways, are frequently called sexually provocative. They may display themselves, be disrespectful of other people's physical boundaries, or masturbate publicly. Since the behavior may occur intermittently, especially when the child is upset or frustrated, it can be described as episodic.

Since sexually provocative children are frequently also irritable, impulsive, explosive, and hyperactive, it is not surprising that they are being diagnosed as manic with increasing frequency. As will be described shortly, studies of lithium responsiveness in such children have been discouraging, and even a recent study of such children who had parents with major depression or bipolar disorder showed an unimpressive response (Carlson, Rapport, Kelly, & Pataki, 1992a,b).

One boundary problem that occurs in young people, then, is between behavior disorders (which obviously include the spectrum of ADHD, conduct disorder, and opposi- tional defiant disorder) and mania/hypomania. This is not simply a problem of one diagnosis or the other. There are a considerable number of anecdotal reports (e.g., Davis, 1979; Dyson & Barcai, 1970; Weinberg & Brumback, 1976; White & O'Shanick, 1977) and systematic studies that describe bipolar patients with a prior history of hyperactivity or conduct disorder or both (for reviews, see Carlson, 1983, 1984; Casat, 1982; also Akiskal et al., 1985a; Endicott et al., 1985; Koehler-Troy, Strober, & Malenbaum, 1986; Reiss, 1985). In addition, several studies have found a particularly high rate of affected relatives in people with early-onset bipolar disorder (Rice et al., 1987; Smeraldi, Gasperini, Macciardi, Bussoleni, & Morabito, 1983). Strober et al. (1988) additionally reported that adolescent bipolar patients with prepubertal histories of behavior disorder had even higher rates of affected relatives than adolescent-onset bipolars without prepubertal psychopathology (44.1% vs. 23.5% for affective disorder by RDC criteria; 29.4% vs. 8.6% bipolar disorder). In all these case histories, a positive lithium response or a positive family history of bipolar disorder or both were used to confirm the relationship.

Studies of children at risk for bipolar disorder by virtue of being offspring of bipolar parents reveal a wide range of psychopathology that includes substantial numbers of children with behavior disorders (e.g., Decina et al., 1983; Gershon et al., 1985; Mayo, O'Connell & O'Brien, 1979). Interestingly, a reexamination of data from the Stony Brook High-Risk Project (Weintraub, 1987) on offspring (ages 7–15) of a bipolar parent revealed the following: (1) The bipolar risk group ($N = 114$) compared to a normal control group ($N = 108$) showed significantly more conduct problems (27% vs. 16%) and attention- deficit problems (30% vs. 16%). (2) Of the bipolar risk group diagnosed with affective disorder at young-adult follow-up ($N = 110$ with an attrition rate of 17.9%), 33.3% had exhibited childhood conduct problems and 45.5% had exhibited childhood attention problems. These rates were significantly higher than those in young "at-risk" adults who remained diagnosis-free, who had rates of 11.5% for conduct problems and 18.8% for attention problems (Carlson and Weintraub, 1993). What complicates the interpretation of these findings is the high rate of comorbidity in parents, the impact of assortative mating, and the fact that there were also high rates of substance abuse among the young adults with affective disorders. It is thus unclear whether the childhood attentional/behavioral prob- lems represent an affective disorder prodrome, a substance-abuse prodrome, or non- specific other psychopathology resulting from living with mentally ill parents. What is unequivocal, however, is that diagnosis-free young adults who are through the age of risk for early-onset bipolar disorder had psychopathologically unremarkable childhoods. Sys- tematic studies of hyperactive children examining the possibility that they are "masked manics" have not supported the hypothesis that a relationship exists between ADHD and bipolarity. Were there a relationship, one might anticipate that there would be significant numbers of bipolar relatives in families of hyperactive children, that some hyperactive children would respond dramatically to lithium, or that longitudinal follow-up would reveal manic–depressive outcomes. However, neither family studies (Biederman et al., 1986; Cantwell, 1972; Lahey et al., 1988; Morrison & Stewart, 1971; Stewart, DeBlois, & Cummings, 1980), treatment studies (Whitehead & Clark, 1970; Greenhill, Reider, Wender, Buchsbaum, & Zahn, 1973), nor follow-up studies of hyperactive children into adulthood (Gittelman, Mannuzza, Shenker, & Bonagura, 1985; Weiss, Hechtman, & Lily, 1986) have confirmed a relationship.

Some authors claim that the earliest prodromes of bipolar disorder are manifest in a "variant" syndrome (Davis, 1979) that is distinguished from nonaffective behavior disorder by the presence of "affective storms," i.e., overreactive, explosive anger and aggression or severe emotional lability, extroversion, and expansiveness (e.g., Decina et al., 1983; Feinstein, Feldman-Rotman, & Woolsey, 1982; Kestenbaum, 1979). While this pattern may be found retrospectively in early histories of some confirmed bipolars, systematic, long-term follow-up of such youngsters, defining the syndrome in a reliable way, has not been done. Recently, Carlson et al. (1992a) treated 11 children who fit a pattern of hyperactivity, explosive anger, and poor response to stimulants. In 4 children treated in an open trial with lithium, there was a positive response. However, in 7 cases prospectively selected for bipolar symptoms, affective storms, and a positive family history of affective disorder, a double-blind trial of lithium produced only modest results. Response was most obvious by 8 weeks and was not reversed by return to placebo medication. The authors felt that the response did not appear to be a robust confirmation of acute manic tendencies and may have represented a more nonspecific, antiaggressive response.

In summary, there appears to be some relationship between prepubertal behavior disorder and some cases of early-onset bipolar disorder. Whether the behavior disorder represents a prodrome or subsyndromal mania, or is simply a nonspecific response to the considerable family psychopathology in which it generally occurs, remains to be clarified (for further discussion, see Carlson, 1990). It is safe to say, however, that the information is less useful prospectively in predicting bipolarity than we might have hoped.

Psychotic Mania.   If there is diagnostic confusion between hyperactivity or emotional lability and hypomania on the less severe pole of the manic spectrum, there is serious diagnostic confusion between psychotic mania and schizophrenia on the severe end of the spectrum. In 1973, Carlson and Goodwin (1973) reacquainted psychiatry with the fact that mania could appear very psychotic and disorganized, usually at the peak of the illness (Stage III), during which time it could be easily confused with schizophrenia. Carlson and Strober (1978, 1979) describe how easily psychotic adolescents with bipolar disorder were misdiagnosed with schizophrenia. Since then, a number of people have confirmed this observation (Hassanyeh & Davison 1980; Ballenger, Reus, & Post, 1982; Joyce, 1984; Rosen et al., 1983; Werry et al., 1991). It must be emphasized that the level of psychosis observed in young people sometimes goes beyond what has always been recognized as the mood-compatible hallucinations and delusions of a manic episode.

The following is a quote from the description by Kraepelin (1921, p. 73) of delirious mania:

> Mood during this delirium is very changing, sometimes anxiously despairing ("thoughts of death"), timid and lachrymose, distracted, sometimes unrestrainedly merry, erotic or ecstatic, sometimes irritable or unsympathetic and indifferent. At the beginning the patients frequently display the signs of senseless raving mania; dance about, perform peculiar movements, shake their head, throw the bedclothes Pell-Mell, are destructive, pass their motions under them, smear everything, make impulsive attempts at suicide, take off their clothes.
>
> The patients do not trouble themselves at all about their surroundings; they do not listen, they give no information, obey no requests, are resistive, strike out. Their linguistic utterances alternate between inarticulate sounds, praying, abusing, entreating, stammering, disconnected talk, in which clang associations, senseless rhyming, diversion by external impressions, persistence of individual phrases, are recognized.

It is no wonder that confusion with schizophrenia occurs. What is interesting is that it occurs so selectively in young people. While this confusion occurs with symptoms of psychotic depressions as well, mania is especially troublesome. Joyce (1984) found that

72% of young manics (onset prior to age 20) vs. 24% of manics with onsets after age 30 were initially judged to be schizophrenic. Werry et al. (1991) followed up 61 young people who had been psychiatrically hospitalized with initial diagnoses of schizophrenia, schizophreniform psychosis, bipolar, schizoaffective disorder, or psychotic depression. Although all the young people with follow-up diagnoses of schizophrenia had been given that diagnosis initially, over half of those with bipolar diagnoses at follow-up had initially been mislabeled as schizophrenic.

The confusion occurs in part because, for reasons that are as yet unknown, young people seem to have more psychotic symptoms than their older counterparts (Ballenger et al., 1982; Rosen et al., 1983). It also occurs because, although bipolar disorder has a young age of onset, schizophrenia has a younger age of onset and is more likely to come to psychiatric attention earlier with psychotic symptoms. An examination of age of onset of DSM-III-diagnosed people with first episodes of psychosis (Iacono and Beiser, 1989) revealed that 43% of schizophrenics were between the ages of 16 and 20, in contrast to 26% with bipolar disorder. Over the next 5 years, the rates of onset were similar (30% and 32%, respectively). The tendency for schizophreniform psychosis, which also predominated between ages 16 and 25 (45% before age 20, 36% between 21 and 25), to evolve into schizophrenia (58%) was much greater than for affective disorder (18.3%).

There are few studies examining the diagnostic stability of psychosis (Horgan, 1981; Parker, O'Donnell, & Walter, 1985), and the study of Werry et al. (1991) is the only one that examines the question in adolescents using modern criteria and long-term follow-up. They found that only 57% of bipolars and 63% of schizophrenics are diagnosed accurately at first hospitalization (all the youth ultimately diagnosed with either schizophrenia or bipolar disorder originally received those diagnoses, however). If these observations are typical, one must conclude that a very open mind must be kept at a first episode of psychosis in adolescence that is not obviously manic or depressive. At this time, the diagnostic pendulum may be swinging too far in the direction of overdiagnosing bipolar disorder, and it should be kept in mind that there is still better than an even chance that a youngster who looks schizophrenic in fact is.

Are there any ways of increasing diagnostic accuracy? The best predictors of a bipolar outcome appear to be acute onset, good premorbid functioning, unequivocal affective symptoms that clearly precede the psychosis (it seems to be the case, if one reads the schizo-affective literature correctly, that a less successful predictor of outcome is the prominence of affective symptoms or which specific psychotic symptoms prevail), and a positive family history of episodic affective disorder. Predictors of a chronic psychotic outcome include poor premorbid functioning with such personality variables as extreme introversion, asociality and aggression, attentional and information-processing abnormalities, neurodevelopmental problems and low IQ (Eggers, 1978, 1989; McGlashan, 1988; Nuechterlein, 1986; Hellgren, Gillberg, Enerskog, 1987), and possibly a family history of schizophrenia (Gottesman and Shields, 1976).

Clinical Picture in Prepubertal Children. Because of the phenomenological overlap between behavior disorders and affective disorders in this younger age group, the *differential diagnostic issues* are different (Carlson, 1990). In addition, the *phenomenology* of the disorder in young children may also be different. In an examination of 14 published cases reports of children under age 12 with bipolar disorder, Carlson (1983) found that there were clear symptom changes between those under age 9 and those age 9 and over. Specifically, the youngest children had episodes that were difficult to delineate, usually because they were superimposed on organic problems or other psychopathology. Psychomotor retardation in thought, speech, and motor activity was not reported in the youngest children. With regard to mood, true euphoria was not reported in younger children, and irritability and dysphoria seemed to be as prominent in mania as elevated mood. Convincing delusions (those that were clear breaks from reality and were not simply age-appropriate) were also absent. As has been the case with adolescents, there may be a number of cases that have been misdiagnosed (Weller, Weller, Tucker, & Fristad, 1986). On the other hand, unlike the situation with adolescents, where the literature abounds with follow-up studies pointing out the error of our ways in misdiagnosing psychotic young people, that is not the case with "misdiagnosed" behavior disorders. In fact, as mentioned earlier, quite the contrary is true. Whether the report of 14 psychotic manics admitted to a prepubertal children's psychiatric unit over a 6-month period (Varanka, Weller, Weller, & Fristad, 1988) represents true mania, misdiagnosed phenocopy, or a combination awaits validating abilities we currently lack.

Clinical Picture in Mental Retardation.   People with mental retardation develop both depressive and bipolar disorders (for reviews, see Carlson, 1979; Sovner & Hurley, 1983). The clinical picture they present is instructive in disentangling the interaction between age and so-called "cognitive immaturity" (Carlson, 1979, 1980). In general, the activity level and vegetative symptoms seen in postpubertal mentally retarded people regardless of IQ are comparable to those seen in uncomplicated postpubertal or adult bipolar disorder. The impact of IQ, not surprisingly, is more in keeping with language-based symptoms (Carlson, 1979). An inspection of several proposed mania criteria interpretations for the severely mentally retarded population include the following (Sovner & Hurley 1982): *generalized, undirected hyperactivity* (increase in goal-directed activity), *flight of ideas, not as clever, perseveration, disjointed thoughts* (increased rate of speech/racing thoughts); *concrete delusions, grandiosity may center around mastery of daily living skills* (inflated self-esteem). For depression, *disruptive behavior seen most at bedtime or observed sleep monitoring* (insomnia/hypersomnia); *decreased energy and slowed movements* (fatigue, psychomotor retardation); *decrease in IQ on retesting, change in attention span while performing usual activities* (decreased concentration) (Sovner & Hurley, 1982). What is most critical in this population, of course, is an information source who has observed the patient closely over a long period of time so that episodic changes in behavior can be described. What complicates assessment is both that institutional care may not provide such a source and that the not infrequent changes in structure and staff result in considerable behavioral disorganization with such patients and must be factored into understanding "episodes."

In summary, three major variables seem to impact on the phenomenology of bipolar depression and mania: the patient's current age (young child, adolescent, adult), whether the episode is early in the course of the disorder (episodic course not yet clear, symptoms not yet fully expressed), and the person's salient premorbid "trait" characteristics (IQ, other psychopathology, personality attributes).

Treatment

That pharmacotherapy has revolutionized the acute and prophylactic treatment of bipolar disorder is incontrovertible. A summary of placebo-controlled studies with adults yields an overall success rate in acute treatment of mania as follows: with lithium, about 78% (Tyrer, 1985); with neuroleptics, about 30–50% (Tyrer, 1985); with carbamazepine, about 71% (Goodwin & Jamison, 1990, p. 621); and with valproic acid (though the numbers of patients are considerably fewer), 53–64% (Freeman, Clothier, Pazzaglia, Lesem, & Swann, 1992; Pope, McElroy, Keck, & Hudson, 1991). With respect to prevention of relapse, in follow-ups that range from about 5 months to several years (i.e., not very long-term), placebo-controlled studies show that those on placebo have a high likelihood of relapse (81%) and those on lithium a 34% rate of relapse (Goodwin & Jamison, 1990,

p. 688). A report using survival analysis of 14 studies of lithium discontinuation reveals that 50% of those who stopped lithium have relapsed by 5 months, with mania likely to occur much sooner (2.7 months) than depression (14 months); relapse rates of 72% and 84% occurred by 1 and 2 years, respectively (Suppes, Baldessarini, Faedda, & Tohen, 1991). In other words, not only has no cure been effected, but also there is the implicit suggestion that the patient is vulnerable to a vastly shortened cycle length on medication discontinuation. Whether this decrease persists or reflects only an increased vulnerability immediately after withdrawal, which can be mitigated by more gradual withdrawal, remains to be seen.

Hidden within the optimistic numbers of response to treatment and prophylaxis is also a wide range of variability, in terms of both the kinds of patients who achieve therapeutic response and the kind of responses they obtain. Where acute and prophylactic treatment has been most successful, it has aborted the current episode and attenuated future episodes so that they appear to be fewer, more widely spaced, and milder in symptomatology.

While a closer scrutiny of responders vs. nonresponders produces no conclusive predictors, there are several observations that might have bearing on young people. Patients with mixed episodes/dysphoric mania (Post et al., 1989; Prien, Himmelhoch, & Kupfer, 1988), those with interepisode comorbidity (Black et al., 1988; Himmelhoch, Mulla, Neil, Detre, & Kupfer, 1976), and rapid cyclers (Prien, Caffey, & Klett, 1974) have the poorest acute and prophylactic response to lithium, and there is some suggestion that anticonvulsant mood stabilizers (carbamazepine and valproic acid) may prove more effective (Freeman et al., 1992; Post et al., 1989).

Demonstrations of medication efficacy for bipolar disorder in children and adolescents have been much more scarce, reflecting in part the observation that adolescents hospitalized with and treated for bipolar disorder, compared to adults, are relatively uncommon in one institution. Until the situation is rectified with systematic, placebo-controlled studies, we are left to interpolate information from the adult literature and the limited information that exists on adolescents.

A review of anecdotal reports on the subject of lithium treatment of juvenile bipolar disorder (Annell, 1969; Campbell, Green, & Deutsch, 1985; Carlson & Strober, 1978; DeLong & Aldershof, 1987; Hassanyeh & Davison, 1980; Horowitz, 1977; van Krevelen & van Voorst, 1959; Youngerman & Canino, 1978) suggests a range of responses similar to that found in adults. There are no placebo-controlled studies to confirm that, however. Furthermore, there is only one study of the effects of lithium prophylaxis (Strober, Morrell, Lampert, & Burroughs, 1990). In this undertaking, 37 adolescents were followed over 18 months in a naturalistic, prospective design. Of the 13 who discontinued medication (on their own), 92% relapsed; of the 24 who were compliant with medication, 37% relapsed. These data are thus similar to reports of adults with more systematic lithium discontinuation.

Reports addressing treatment-response variability in adolescents are consistent with the adult literature. Thus, adolescents with preadolescent and probably comorbid behavior disorder or personality disorders or both (Himmelhoch & Garfinkel, 1986; Kutcher et al., 1990; Strober et al., 1988) had much poorer responses to lithium acutely than their bipolar peers without these attributes. Although rapid cycling is more likely a phenomenon of older people, one report of 4 cases of early-onset rapid cycling described only a 50% response rate to lithium (Jones & Berney, 1987), consistent with the less complete response described in adults. Finally, when bipolar disorder occurs in mentally retarded people, mood stabilizers appear to ameliorate mood disorder in some cases (e.g., McLaughlin, 1987; Steingard & Biederman, 1987).

The question of efficacy in schizoaffective states largely depends on the definition of schizoaffective. It would appear that as long as "schizoaffective" is defined only on the basis of what may be psychosis severity (i.e., mood incongruence) during an episode (and the evidence of intermorbid functioning is similar to that seen in bipolar disorder, i.e., without psychosis), treatment and prophylaxis response is similar to that in bipolar disorder (Bouman, Niemantsverdriet-van Kampen, Ormel, & Slooff, 1986). Data would suggest that "schizomanic" disorder is very similar to bipolar disorder; however, "schizodepressive" (i.e., nonbipolar) disorder is more similar to schizophrenia (Brockington, Wainwright, & Kendall, 1980). The implications for adolescents, of course, are that young-onset patients appear to be the most psychotic and the most likely to be defined as schizoaffective. Whether there are diagnostic and treatment implications for later-onset "schizoaffective disorder" is as yet unknown.

What treatment implications can be drawn from the foregoing discussion? With regard to fully established, unequivocal adolescent bipolar disorder, while there are no definitive studies, there are, as yet, no data to suggest that the presence of adolescence per se should change treatment recommendations for either acute or prophylactic medication. Questions somewhat particular to adolescent-onset bipolar disorder are: (1) how aggressively to pursue antimanic therapy in clinical situations where the diagnosis is unclear, (2) whether drug holidays should be undertaken if a person has had only one episode of mania, and (3) whether early treatment with prophylactic medication in a confirmed bipolar or one at risk merely postpones the inevitable or improves the course of the disorder.

There are no definitive answers to these questions. In the case of an acute psychosis that is clearly neither manic nor depressive, even though the odds slightly favor a schizophrenic course, a trial of mood-stabilizing medication (lithium or an anticonvulsant) should be considered. At some point, however, the question of whether this medication is adding anything to the patient's treatment must be asked. If withdrawal of neuroleptic exacerbates the patient's psychosis, but gradual withdrawal of mood stabilizer (with maintenance at very low blood levels) does not change the clinical picture with maintenance neuroleptic, perhaps the additional drug should be withdrawn. Weight gain poses a significant compliance deterrent, especially to appearance-conscious adolescents, and prolonged combined therapy should be avoided where possible.

Another therapeutic dilemma is posed by emotionally labile young people who may or may not have cyclothymia. On one hand, there is clear evidence of a relationship between true subsyndromal affective disorder and ultimate emergence of major affective disorder (Akiskal et al., 1985a; Depue et al., 1981), suggesting that prophylactic treatment might be helpful. On the other hand, in a population not "at risk" for a bipolar outcome, the prognostic significance is less clear. For example, young adults with a DSM-I disorder, "emotionally unstable character disorder," seemed, in an open trial, to respond favorably to lithium. Follow-up subsequently determined that their condition dissipated with further maturity, rather than blossoming into bipolar disorder (Rifkin, Quitkin, Carillo, Blumberg, & Klein, 1972; Rifkin, Levitan, Galweski, & Klein, 1972,b). There have been efforts to reconcile the relationship between subsyndromal mood disorder and borderline personality disorder as well (Akiskal, Yerevanian, Davis, King, & Lemmi, 1985b; McGlashan, 1983). Whether or not such young people should be tried on mood-stabilizing drugs, at this point, must be decided on a case-by-case basis. There is no wholesale evidence that positive response is probable, however, and the clinician must not be deluded, nor delude the patient, about the experimental nature of such a trial. Clear determination of efficacy is necessary before committing the adolescent to a long-term treatment.

Finally, the question of drug holidays needs reconsideration in light not only of the evidence of very high rates of mania recurrence after lithium discontinuation (Suppes et al., 1991), but also that the patient might become resistant to treatment with a drug to which he or she formerly responded (R. D. Post, as quoted in the *Psychiatric Times*, July 1991). In the case of adolescents and their families who are terrified about what appears to be a lifetime disorder with a lifetime commitment to medication, the possibility of a drug holiday still seems worthy of consideration. Subsequent course (i.e., how symptom-free), and evaluation of degree of remission compared to premorbid state, degree of compliance, level of support system, and other factors, will influence the decision. If discontinuation is decided on, current recommendations are that it be done very gradually over several weeks to a month.

In conclusion, there is considerable circumstantial evidence that juvenile bipolar disorder simply represents the youngest onset of a disorder with a long age range of risk. A number of pathoplastic modifications are conferred by age, biology, and beginning (vs. fully developed) disorder. There is some evidence that age of onset is decreasing in bipolar disorder (Gershon, Hamovit, Guroff, & Nurmberger, 1987), which, if true, increases the importance of our understanding the implications of this disorder in young people and will provide us the opportunity of studying it further.

References

Akiskal, H. S., Downs, J., Jordan, P., Watson, S., Daugherty, D., & Pruitt, D. B. (1985a). Affective disorders in referred children and younger siblings of manic depressives. *Archives of General Psychiatry, 42*, 996–1004.

Akiskal, H. S., Djenderedjian, A. H., Rosenthal, R. H., & Khani, M. (1977). Cyclothymic disorder: Validating criteria for inclusion in the bipolar affective group. *American Journal of Psychiatry, 134*, 1227–1233.

Akiskal, H. S., Yerevanian, B. L., Davis, G. C., King, D., & Lemmi, H. (1985b). The nosologic status of borderline personality: Clinical and polysomnographic study. *American Journal of Psychiatry, 142*, 192–198.

American Psychiatric Association (1980). *Diagnostic and statistical manual of mental disorders*, 3rd ed. Washington, DC: Author.

American Psychiatric Association (1987). *Diagnostic and statistical manual of mental disorders*, 3rd ed., revised. Washington, DC: Author.

American Psychiatric Association (1994). *Diagnostic and statistical manual of mental disorders*, 4th ed. Washington, DC: Author.

Angst, J. (1988). Clinical course of affective disorders. In T. Helgason & R. J. Daly (Eds.), *Depressive illness: Prediction of course and outcome* (pp. 1–48). New York: Springer-Verlag.

Annell, A. L. (1969). Lithium in the treatment of children and adolescents. *Acta Psychiatrica Scandinavica Supplementum, 207*, 19–33.

Annesley, P. T. (1961). Psychiatric illness in adolescence: Presentation and prognosis. *Journal of Mental Science, 107*, 268–278.

Anthony, E. J., & Scott, P. (1960). Manic depressive psychosis in childhood. *Journal of Child Psychology and Psychiatry, 1*, 53–72.

Ballenger, J. C., Reus, V. I., & Post, R. M. (1982). The "atypical" presentation of adolescent mania. *American Journal of Psychiatry, 139*, 602–606.

Baron M., Risch N., & Mendlewicz J. (1983). Age at onset in bipolar-related major affective illness: Clinical and genetic implications. *Journal of Psychiatric Research, 17*, 5–18.

Beiser, M., Iacono, W. G., & Erikson, D. (1989). Temporal stability in the major mental disorders. In L. N. Robins & J. E. Barret (Eds.), *The validity of psychiatric diagnoses* (pp. 77–97). New York: Raven Press.

Biederman, J., Munir, K., Knee, D., Habelov, W., Armentano, M., Autor, S., Hoge, S. K., & Waternaux, C. (1986). A family study of patients with attention deficit disorder and normal controls. *Journal of Psychiatric Research, 20*, 263–274.

Black, D. W., Winokur, G., Bell, S., Nasrallah, A., & Hulbert, J. (1988). Complicated mania—Comorbidity and immediate outcome in the treatment of mania. *Archives of General Psychiatry, 45*, 232–236.

Blumenthal, R. L., Egeland, J. A., Sharpe, L., Nee, J., & Endicott, J. (1987). Age onset in bipolar and unipolar illness with and without delusions and hallucinations. *Comprehensive Psychiatry, 28*, 547–554.

Bouman, T. K., Niemantsverdriet-van Kampen, J. G., Ormel, J., & Slooff, C. J. (1986). The effectiveness of lithium prophylaxis in bipolar and unipolar depressions and schizo-affective disorders. *Journal of Affective Disorders, 11*, 275–280.

Brockington, I. F., Helzer, J. F., Hillier, V. F., & Francis, A. F. (1982). Definitions of depression: Concordance and prediction of outcome. *American Journal of Psychiatry, 139*, 1022–1027.

Brockington, I. F., Wainwright, S., & Kendall, R. E. (1980). Manic patients with schizophrenic or paranoid symptoms. *Psychological Medicine, 10,* 73–83.

Campbell, M., Green, W. H., & Deutsch, S. I. (1985). *Child and adolescent psychopharmacology.* Beverly Hills: Sage Publications.

Cantwell, D. P. (1972). Psychiatric illness in the families of hyperactive children. *Archives of General Psychiatry, 27,* 414–417.

Carlson, G. A. (1979). Affective psychoses in mental retardates. *Psychiatric Clinics of North America, 2,* 499–510.

Carlson, G. A. (1980). *Manic–depressive illness and cognitive immaturity.* New York: Spectrum Publications.

Carlson, G. A. (1983). Bipolar affective disorders in childhood and adolescence. IN D. P. Cantwell & G. A. Carlson (Eds.), *Affective disorders in childhood and adolescence—An update* (pp. 61–84). New York: Spectrum Publications.

Carlson, G. A. (1984). Issues of classification in childhood bipolar disorder. *Psychiatric Developments, 4,* 273–285.

Carlson, G. A. (1990). Annotation: Child and adolescent mania—Diagnostic considerations. *Journal of Child Psychology and Psychiatry, 31,* 331–341.

Carlson, G. A., Davenport, Y. B., & Jamison, K. (1977). A comparison of outcome in adolescent and late onset bipolar manic depressive illness. *American Journal of Psychiatry, 134,* 919–922.

Carlson, G. A., & Garber, J. (1986). Developmental issues in the classification of depressive disorders in children. In M. Rutter, C. E. Izard, & P. B. Read (Eds.), *Depression in children: Developmental perspective.* (pp. 399–434). New York: Guilford Press.

Carlson, G. A., & Goodwin, F. K. (1973). The stages of mania. *Archives of General Psychiatry, 134,* 919–922.

Carlson, G. A., & Kashani, J. H. (1988). Manic symptoms in non-referred adolescent population. *Journal of Affective Disorders, 15,* 219–226.

Carlson, G. A., Rapport, M. D., Kelly, K. L., & Pataki, C. S. (1992a). Lithium and methylphenidate in children. *Journal of the American Academy of Child and Adolescent Psychiatry, 31,* 262–270.

Carlson, G. A., Rapport, M. D., Pataki, C. S., & Kelly, K. L. (1992b). Lithium in hospitalized children at 4 and 8 weeks: Mood, behavior, and cognitive effects. *Journal of Psychology and Psychiatry, 33,* 411–425.

Carlson, G. A., & Strober, M. (1978). Manic depressive illness in early adolescence: A study of clinical and diagnostic characteristics in six cases. *Journal of the American Academy of Child Psychiatry, 17,* 138–153.

Carlson, G. A., & Strober, M. (1979). Affective disorders in adolescence. *Psychiatric Clinics of North America, 2,* 511–525.

Carlson, G. A., & Weintraub, S. (1993). Childhood behavior problems and bipolar disorder—relationship or coincidence? *Journal of Affective Disorders, 28,* 143–154.

Casat, C. D. (1982). The under- and over-diagnosis of mania in children and adolescents. *Comprehensive Psychiatry, 23,* 552–559.

Cooper, J. E., Kendell, R. E., Gurland, B. J., Sharpe, L., Copeland, J. R. M., & Simon, R. (1972). *Psychiatric diagnosis in New York and London: A comparative study of mental hospital admissions. Maudsley Monograph No. 20.* London: Oxford University Press.

Coryell, W., & Norten, S. G. (1980). Mania during adolescence. *Journal of Nervous and Mental Disease, 168,* 611–613.

Davis, R. E. (1979). Manic depressive variant syndrome of childhood: A preliminary report. *American Journal of Psychiatry, 136,* 702–706.

Decina, P., Kestenbaum, C. J., Farber, S., Kron, L., Gargan, M., Sackheim, H. A., & Fieve, R. R. (1983). Clinical and psychological assessment of children of bipolar probands. *American Journal of Psychiatry, 140,* 545–553.

DeLong, G. R., & Aldershof, A. L. (1987). Long-term experience with lithium treatment in childhood: Correlation with clinical diagnoses. *Journal of the American Academy of Child and Adolescent Psychiatry, 26,* 389–394.

Depue, R. A., Slater, J. F., Wolfstetter-Kausch, H., Klein, D., Goplerud, E., & Farr, D. (1981). A behavioral paradigm for identifying persons at risk for bipolar depressive disorder: A conceptual framework and five validation studies. *Journal of Abnormal Psychology, 90,* 381–437.

Dyson, W. L., & Barcai, A. (1970). Treatment of children of lithium responding parents. *Current Therapy Research, 12,* 286–290.

Eggers, C. (1978). Course and prognosis of childhood schizophrenia. *Journal of Autism and Childhood Schizophrenia, 8,* 21–36.

Eggers, C. (1989). Schizo-affective psychoses in childhood: A follow-up study. *Journal of Autism and Developmental Disorders, 19,* 327–342.

Endicott, J., Nee, J., Andreasen, N., Clayton, P., Keller, M., & Coryell, W. (1985). Bipolar II: Combine or keep separate? *Journal of Affective Disorders, 8*, 17–28.

Feinstein, S. C., Feldman-Rotman, S., & Woolsey, A. B. (1982). *Diagnostic aspects of manic–depressive illness in children and adolescents.* Stratton, NY: Thieme.

Freeman, T. W., Clothier, J. L., Pazzaglia, P., Lesem, M. D., & Swann, A. C. (1992). A double-blind comparison of valproate and lithium in the treatment of acute mania. *American Journal of Psychiatry, 149*, 108–111.

Gershon, E. S., Hamovit, J. H., Guroff, J. J., & Nurnberger, J. I. (1987). Birth-cohort changes in manic and depressive disorders in relatives of bipolar and schizoaffective patients. *Archives of General Psychiatry, 44*, 314–319.

Gershon, E. S., McKnew, D., Cytryn, L., Hamovit, J., Schreiber, J., Hibbs, E., & Pellegrini, D. (1985). Diagnoses in school-age children of bipolar affective disorder patients and normal controls. *Journal of Affective Disorders, 8*, 283–291.

Gittelman, R., Mannuzza, S., Shenker, R., & Bonagura, N. (1985). Hyperactive boys almost grown up. I. Psychiatric status. *Archives of General Psychiatry, 42*, 937–947.

Goodwin, F. K., & Jamison, K. R. (1990). *Manic depressive illness.* New York: Oxford University Press.

Gottesman, I. I., & Shields, J. (1976). A critical review of recent adoption, twin and family studies of schizophrenia: Behavior genetics perspectives. *Schizophrenia Bulletin, 2*, 360–401.

Greenhill, L. L., Reider, R. O., Wender, P. H., Buchsbaum, H., & Zahn, P. (1973). Lithium carbonate treatment of hyperactive children. *Archives of General Psychiatry, 28*, 636–640.

Harrow, M., Goldberg, J. F., Grossman, C. A., & Meltzer, H. Y. (1990). Outcome in manic disorders: A naturalistic follow-up study. *Archives of General Psychiatry, 47*, 665–671.

Hassanyeh, F., & Davison, K. (1980). Bipolar affective psychosis with onset before age 16: Report of 10 cases. *British Journal of Psychiatry, 137*, 530–539.

Hellgren, L., Gillberg, C., & Enerskog, I. (1987). Antecedents of adolescent psychoses: A population-base study of school health problems in children who develop psychosis in adolescence. *Journal of the American Academy of Child and Adolescent Psychiatry, 26*, 351–355.

Himmelhoch, J. M., & Garfinkel, M. E. (1986). Sources of lithium resistance in mixed mania. *Psychopharmacology Bulletin, 22*, 613–620.

Himmelhoch, J. M., Mulla, D., Neil, J. F., Detre, T. P., Kupfer, D. J. (1976). Incidence and significance of mixed affective states in a bipolar population. *Archives of General Psychiatry, 33*, 1062–1066.

Horgon, D. (1981). Change in diagnosis to manic–depressive illness. *Psychological Medicine, 11*, 517–523.

Horowitz, H. A. (1977). Lithium and the treatment of adolescent manic depressive illness. *Diseases of the Nervous System, 6*, 480–483.

Iacono, W. G., & Beiser, M. (1989). *The emergence of a new discipline: Rochester symposium on developmental psychopathology.* Hillsdale, NJ: Erlbaum Associates.

Johnson, J., Horvath, E., & Weissman, M. M. (1991). The validity of major depression with psychotic features based on a community sample. *Archives of General Psychiatry, 48*, 1075–1981.

Jones, P. M., & Berney, T. P. (1987). Early onset rapid cycling bipolar affective disorder. *Journal of Child Psychology and Psychiatry, 28*, 731–738.

Joyce, P. R. (1984). Age onset in bipolar affective disorder and misdiagnosis as schizophrenia. *Psychological Medicine, 14*, 145–149.

Keller, M. B., Shapiro, R. W., Lavori, P. W., & Wolfe, N. (1982). Recovery in major depressive disorder: Analysis with life table and regression models. *Archives of General Psychiatry, 39*, 905–910.

Kestenbaum, C. J. (1979). Children at risk for manic–depressive illness: Possible predictors. *American Journal of Psychiatry, 136*, 1206–1208.

Koehler-Troy, C., Strober, M., & Malenbaum, R. (1986). Methylphenidate-induced mania in a prepubertal child: A case report. *Journal of Clinical Psychiatry, 47*, 566–567.

Kovacs, M., & Gatsonis, C. (1989). Stability and change in childhood-onset depressive disorders: Longitudinal course as a diagnostic validator. In L. N. Robins & J. E. Barrett (Eds.), *The validity of psychiatric diagnosis* (pp. 57–73). New York: Raven Press.

Kraepelin, E. (1921). *Manic depressive insanity and paranoia.* Livingstone: Edinburgh.

Kutcher, S. P. Marton, P., & Korenblum, M. (1990). Adolescent bipolar illness and personality disorder. *Journal of the American Academy of Child and Adolescent Psychiatry, 29*, 355–358.

Landolt, A. D. (1957). Follow-up studies on circular manic depressive reactions occurring in the young. *Bulletin of the New York Academy of Medicine, 33*, 65–73.

Loranger, A. P. W., & Levine, P. M. (1978). Age of onset of bipolar affective illness. *Archives of General Psychiatry, 35*, 1345–1348.

Mayo, J. A., O'Connell, R. A., & O'Brien, J. D. (1979). Families of manic–depressive patients: Effect of treatment. *American Journal of Psychiatry, 136*, 1535–1539.

McGlashan, T. H. (1983). The borderline syndrome. II. Is it a variant of schizophrenia or affective disorder? *Archives of General Psychiatry, 40,* 1319–1323.

McGlashan, T. H. (1988). Adolescent versus adult onset of mania. *American Journal of Psychiatry, 145,* 221–224.

McLaughlin, M. (1987). Bipolar affective disorder in Down's syndrome. *British Journal of Psychiatry, 151,* 116–117.

Morrison, J. R., & Stewart, M. A. (1971). A family study of the hyperactive child syndrome. *Biological Psychiatry, 3,* 189–195.

Neuchterlein, K. (1986). Childhood precursors of adult schizophrenia. *Journal of Child Psychology and Psychiatry, 27,* 133–144.

Olsen, T. (1961). Follow-up study of manic–depressive patients whose first attack occurred before the age of 19. *Acta Psychiatrica Scandinavica Supplementum, 162,* 45–51.

Parker, G., O'Donnell, M., & Walter, S. (1985). Changes in the diagnoses of functional psychoses associated with the introduction of lithium. *British Journal of Psychiatry, 146,* 377–382.

Pope, H. G., Jr., McElroy, S. L., Keck, P. E., Jr., & Hudson, J. L. (1991). Valproate in the study of acute mania: A placebo controlled study. *Archives of General Psychiatry, 48,* 62–68.

Post, R. M., Rubinow, D. R., Uhde, T. W., Roy-Byrne, P., Linnoila, M., Rosoff, A., & Cowdry, R. (1989). Dysphoric mania: Clinical and biologic correlates. *Archives of General Psychiatry, 46,* 353–358.

Prien, R. F., Caffey, E. M., Jr., & Klett, J. (1974). Factors associated with the treatment success in lithium carbonate prophylaxis: Report to the Veterans Administration and National Institute of Mental Health Collaborative Study Group. *Archives of General Psychiatry, 31,* 189–192.

Prien, R. F., Himmelhoch, J. H., & Kupfer, D. J. (1988). Treatment of mixed mania. *Journal of Affective Disorders, 15,* 9–15.

Rice, J., Reich, T., Andreasen, N. C., Endicott, J., Van Eerdewegh, M., Fishman, R., Hirschfeld, R. M. A., & Klerman, G. L. (1987). The familial transmission of bipolar illness. *Archives of General Psychiatry, 44,* 441–450.

Reiss, A. L. (1985). Developmental manifestations in a boy with prepubertal bipolar disorder. *Journal of Clinical Psychiatry, 41,* 441–443.

Rifkin, A., Levitan, S. J., Galweski, J., & Klein, D. F. (1972a). Emotionally unstable character disorder—A follow-up study. 1. Description of patients and outcome. *Biological Psychiatry, 4,* 65–79.

Rifkin, A., Levitan, S. J., Galweski, J., & Klein, D. F. (1972b). Emotionally unstable character disorder—a follow-up study. II. Prediction of outcome. *Biological Psychiatry, 4,* 81–88.

Rifkin, A., Quitkin, F., Carillo, C., Blumberg, A. G., & Klein, D. F. (1972). Lithium carbonate in emotionally unstable character disorder. *Archives of General Psychiatry, 27,* 519–523.

Rosen, L. N., Rosenthal, N. E., Van Dusen, P. H., Dunner, D. L., & Fieve, R. R. (1983). Age at onset and number of psychotic symptoms in bipolar I and schizoaffective disorder. *American Journal of Psychiatry, 140,* 1523–1524.

Smeraldi, G., Gasperini, M., Macciardi, F., Bussoleni, C., & Morabito, A. (1983). Factors affecting the distribution of age of onset in affective parents. *Journal of Psychiatric Research, 17,* 309–317.

Sovner, R., & Hurley, A. D. (1982). Diagnosing depression in the mentally retarded: Diagnosing mania in the mentally retarded. *Psychiatric Aspects of Mental Retardation Newsletter, 1,* 1–12.

Sovner, R., & Hurley, A. D. (1983). Do the mentally retarded suffer from affective illness? *Archives of General Psychiatry, 40,* 61–67.

Spitzer, R. L., Endicott, J., & Robins, E. (1978). *Research Diagnostic Criteria.* New York: New York State Psychiatric Institute.

Steingard, R., & Biederman, J. (1987). Case report: Lithium responsive manic-like symptoms in two individuals with autism and mental retardation. *Journal of the American Academy of Child and Adolescent Psychiatry, 26,* 932–935.

Stewart, M. D., DeBlois, S., & Cummings, C. (1980). Psychiatric disorder in the parents of hyperactive boys and those with conduct disorder. *Journal of Child Psychology and Psychiatry, 21,* 283–292.

Strober, M., & Carlson, G. A. (1982). Bipolar illness in adolescents with major depression: Clinical, genetic and psychopharmacologic predictors. *Archives of General Psychiatry, 39,* 549–555.

Strober, M., Lampert, C., Schmidt, S., & Morrell, W. (1993). The course of major depressive disorder in adolescents: Recovery and risk of manic switching in a 24–month prospective, naturalistic follow-up of psychotic and non-psychotic subtypes. *Journal of the American Academy of Child and Adolescent Psychiatry, 32,* 34–42.

Strober, M., Morrell, N., Lampert, C., & Burroughs, J. (1990). Lithium carbonate in prophylactic treatment of bipolar I illness in adolescents: A naturalistic study. *American Journal of Psychiatry, 147,* 457–461.

Strober, M., Morrell, W., Burroughs, J., Lampert, C., Danforth, H., & Freeman, R. (1988). A family study of bipolar I disorder in adolescence. *Journal of Affective Disorders, 15,* 255–268.

Suppes, T., Baldessarini, R. J., Faedda, G. L., & Tohen, M. (1991). Risk of recurrence following discontinuation of lithium treatment in bipolar disorder. *Archives of General Psychiatry, 48,* 1082–1088.

Tyrer, S. P. (1985). Lithium in the treatment of mania. *Journal of Affective Disorders, 8,* 251–157.

van Krevelen, D., & van Voorst, J. (1959). Lithium in the treatment of a cryptogenic psychosis of a juvenile. *Acta Paedopsychiatrica, 26,* 148–152.

Varanka, T. M., Weller, E. B., Weller, K. A., & Fristad, M. A. (1988). Lithium treatment of psychotic features in prepubertal children. *American Journal of Psychiatry, 145,* 1557–1559.

Weinberg, W. A., & Brumback, R. A. (1976). Mania in childhood: Case studies and literature review. *American Journal of Diseases of Childhood, 130,* 380–385.

Weintraub, S. (1987). Risk factors in schizophrenia: The Stony Brook High-Risk Project. *Schizophrenia Bulletin, 13,* 439–450.

Weiss, G., Hechtman, L. T., & Lily, R. (1986). *Hyperactive children grown up—Empirical findings and theoretical considerations.* New York: Guilford Press.

Weissmann, M. M., Warner, V., Wickramaratne, P., & Prusoff, B. A. (1988). Early onset major depression in parents and their children. *Journal of Affective Disorders, 15,* 269–277.

Weller, R. A., Weller, E. B., Tucker, S. G., & Fristad, M. A. (1986). Mania in prepubertal children: Has it been underdiagnosed? *Journal of Affective Disorders, 11,* 151–154.

Welner, A., Welner, Z., & Fishman, R. (1979). Psychiatric adolescent inpatients 8 to 10 year follow up. *Archives of General Psychiatry, 36,* 698–700.

Werry, J. S., McClellan, J. M., & Chard, L. (1991). Childhood and adolescent schizophrenic, bipolar and schizoaffective disorders: A clinical and outcome study. *Journal of the American Academy of Child and Adolescent Psychiatry, 30,* 457–465.

Wertham, F. I. (1929). A group of benign psychoses: Prolonged manic excitements with a statistical study of age, duration, and frequency in 2000 manic attacks. *American Journal of Psychiatry, 9,* 17–28.

White, J. H., & O'Shanick, G. (1977). Juvenile manic–depressive illness. *American Journal of Psychiatry, 134,* 1035–1036.

Whitehead, P. L., & Clark. L. D. (1970). Effect of lithium carbonate, placebo, and thioridazine on hyperactive children. *American Journal of Psychiatry, 127,* 824–825.

Winokur, G., Clayton, P. J., & Reich, T. (1969). *Manic depressive illness.* St. Louis: C. V. Mosby.

Youngerman, J., & Canino, I. (1978). Lithium carbonate use in children and adolescents: A survey of the literature. *Archives of General Psychiatry, 35,* 216–224.

4

The Validity of the Diagnosis of Major Depression in Childhood and Adolescence

Barry Nurcombe

Introduction

This chapter concerns the question of whether, in children and adolescents, major depression can be discriminated from other forms of misery. Beginning with a description of the historical evolution of the question, it sets out the criteria by which a categorical depressive disorder could be validated and analyzes the empirical evidence for and against the hypothesis that there is indeed a distinct depressive disorder in childhood and adolescence. The chapter ends with a consideration of "dysthymia," a classificatory wasteland into which many problems have been dumped

The question is more than mere nit-picking or personal taste. The empirical evidence, as will be shown, supports the contention that in most patients, depression is dimensional. There is, however, good evidence supporting the validity, in adults, of a categorically distinct depressive disorder (known as "major depression," "endogenous depression," or "melancholia"). Dimensional psychopathology is the outcome of phenotypic heterogeneity, polygenic inheritance, or a multifactorial mix of genes, temperament, and experience. On the other hand, the categorical distinctness of a syndrome represents a prima facie case for a pathochemical, pathophysiological, or histopathological etiology. We will return to this point later, pausing first to make subtle distinctions between the terms *symptom*, *syndrome*, *disorder*, and *disease*.

Discussions concerning the affective phenomena of depression are hampered by semantic confusion. The term "depression" can be interpreted in several ways:

Barry Nurcombe • Division of Child and Adolescent Psychiatry, Department of Psychiatry, Vanderbilt University School of Medicine, Nashville, Tennessee 37212.
Handbook of Depression in Children and Adolescents, edited by William M. Reynolds and Hugh F. Johnston. Plenum Press, New York, 1994.

1. As a momentary *affect* ("I felt depressed when you said that").
2. As a prevailing *mood* ("He looked depressed yesterday").
3. As a reference to a *psychodynamic constellation*, a complex of conscious and unconscious ideas and feelings related to actual or symbolic loss ("He has unresolved depression following the loss of his mother").
4. As a *syndrome*, it refers to a concurrent set of symptoms and signs dominated by depressive mood.
5. As a *disorder*, "depression" refers to a depressive syndrome that is categorically distinct.
6. As a hypothetical *disease*, it refers to a depressive disorder linked to a specific genetic, pathochemical, pathophysiological, or structural abnormality.

Can a distinct depressive disorder be identified from a larger population of patients with a depressive syndrome? If so, can the disorder be associated with biological dysfunction? As previously noted, the validation of a categorical disorder is a first step toward uncovering a biomedical etiology.

According to Kendell (1976), categories "carve nature at the joints." Categorical distinctness indicates a natural boundary or "point of rarity" between the disorder in question and other syndromes or disorders. In regard to the distinction between major depression and dysthymia, patients with features of both syndromes should be fewer than those with either condition. In other words, the blacks and the whites should exceed the grays.

Categorical Depression in Descriptive Psychiatry

By the turn of the century, Bonhoeffer (1910) had distinguished exogenous psychoses—those caused by physical disease—from endogenous psychoses. Endogenous psychoses were thought to arise from inner ("autochthonous") sources and to be linked to innate defects (Morel, 1857) or constitutional predispositions (Moebius, 1893). In 1896, Kraepelin (1896) divided endogenous psychoses into manic–depressive insanity and dementia praecox. Within the former, he grouped mania, depression, and mixed states. Subsequently, British psychiatrists (e.g., Gillespie, 1929) distinguished neurotic (or reactive) depression from endogenous depression, the latter being thought to arise from inner dysfunction, the former from life stress. Endogenous depression was characterized by a subjectively distinct kind of misery, diurnal variation, psychomotor retardation, disturbance of appetitive functions, and mood-congruent hallucinations and delusions. The more severe forms of endogenous depression were known as "melancholia," characterized, in accordance with the patient's psychomotor activity, as "agitated" or "retarded." In DSM-III-R (American Psychiatric Association, 1987), "endogenous depression" is known as Major Depression. Reactive Depression has been renamed Dysthymia, a term borrowed from Kahlbaum (1863).

During the 1960s, bipolar manic–depressive disorder was separated from other types of affective disorder. The concept of bipolarity was borrowed from Leonhard (1957). The term "unipolar depression" is currently used to contrast with "bipolar depression," an episode of depression occurring in a cyclical bipolar disorder. Gershon, Bunney, and Leckman (1976) have distinguished Bipolar I disorder (with manic and depressive episodes) from Bipolar II disorder (which has hypomanic and depressive episodes).

During and after the 1930s, a vigorous debate arose, one side (associated with Lewis, 1934) contending that reactive and endogenous depression formed a continuum differing only in severity, the other side (e.g., Kiloh & Garside, 1963) asserting that the two conditions were categorically distinct. Following World War II, the debate was fought out in a series of factor–analytical studies of depressed patients. Kendell and Gourlay (1970) found evidence for a dimensional model, whereas Kiloh and Garside (1963) and Kiloh, Andrews, Neilson, and Bianchi (1972) repeatedly extracted a factor contrasting "endogenous" with "neurotic" depression. Subsequent cluster analyses of mixed samples (e.g., Everitt, Gourlay, & Kendell, 1971; Grove et al., 1987; Matussek, Soldner, & Nagel, 1982; Paykel, 1971; Pilowsky, Levine, & Bolton, 1969) have consistently identified a distinct endogenous group. On the other hand, reactive depression has repeatedly decomposed into heterogeneity and may be no more than a diagnostic artifact (Kiloh & Garside, 1977). Others have suggested that the "neurotic" pole of the aforementioned "endogenous– neurotic" factor is a mix of anxiety and coping style rather than "neurotic depression" per se (Mullaney, 1984; Parker et al., 1990).

The Concept of Depression in Child Psychiatry

Psychoanalysis fostered the concept that children could become depressed. Working from observations made during play therapy, Melanie Klein (1948, 1949) theorized that normal infants pass through a depressive stage. From a different perspective, Freud and Burlingham (1944) noted the depressive responses of evacuated children who had been separated from their mothers during the London blitz. The work of Klein and Freud foreshadowed that of Spitz and Wolf (1946) on anaclitic depression and hospitalism and evolved into the theories of Bowlby (1952, 1969, 1973, 1980) concerning attachment, separation, and loss.

On the other hand, although many European psychiatrists (e.g., Kuhn, 1963) diagnosed depression in children, psychoanalysts (e.g., Finch, 1960; Rie, 1966; Rochlin, 1959) were of the opinion that prior to adolescence, children lack the superego development required to manifest a true melancholia. If pathological guilt were to be regarded as the cardinal feature of melancholia, the psychoanalytic viewpoint was undoubtedly true; however, pessimism and low self-esteem are commonly manifest by depressed children and may be the preadolescent counterpart of depression.

The issue was reopened in the 1960s when several authors (e.g., Toolan, 1962; Glasser, 1967; Malmquist, 1971) suggested that oppositional behavior, conduct problems, poor school performance, and somatic symptoms could, in some cases, represent "depressive equivalents" or the manifestations of "masked depression." Pathological guilt was displaced as the essential ingredient of childhood depression. Subsequently, stimulated by advances in biological psychiatry, several authors designed rating scales and structured interviews that adapted adult criteria to the diagnosis of childhood depression (e.g., Ling, Oftedal, & Weinberg, 1970; Weinberg, Rutman, Sullivan, Penick, & Deitz, 1973; Cytryn & McKnew, 1972; Poznanski & Zrull, 1970; Kovacs, 1982, 1985; Puig-Antich & Chambers, 1978; Herjanic & Campbell, 1977; Hodges, Klein, Stern, Cytryn, & McKnew, 1982; Costello, Edelbrock, Kalas, Kessler, & Klaric, 1982). In a landmark study, Carlson and Cantwell (1980) found that depressive mood and vegetative signs were prevalent among depressed children—in other words, that depressive phenomenology could be unmasked by systematic interviewing. These findings were corroborated by Cytryn, McKnew, and Bunney (1980), Carlson and Kashani (1988), and Ryan et al. (1987). As a result, the only concession made to childhood depression in DSM-IV (American Psychiatric Association, 1994) criteria is to substitute irritability for depression and reduce the time requirement for dysthymia from 2 years to 1 year.

During the past decade, research into childhood depression has burgeoned, particularly with regard to its epidemiology (e.g., Kashani & Simonds, 1979; Kashani et al., 1983) and biochemistry (Puig-Antich, 1986). Major depression and dysthymia are frequently diagnosed, and antidepressant medication is freely prescribed.

Despite the convictions of many clinicians, the empirical evidence for major depression is incomplete. Studies that apply adult depressive criteria to children and adolescents introduce potential fallacies. Many disturbed children are polysymptomatic; rating scales and interviews designed with preconceptions about the symptomatic structure of a depressive disorder could isolate a spurious syndrome from a larger set of nonspecific clinical phenomena. Clinicians affected by confirmatory bias may unwittingly suggest symptoms to their interviewees or encourage them to endorse marginal complaints, whereas "halo" effects will incline interviewers to detect the remaining criteria for a favorite syndrome after the cardinal features have been identified. In this way, square pegs are jammed into round pigeonholes. Furthermore, as Kovacs (1986) has described, metacognitive immaturity prevents children from exhibiting the introspective, self-monitoring thought required to report accurately on their subjectivity. These problems are magnified when an emotionally disturbed child, removed from a disruptive home and placed in unfamiliar surroundings, is confronted by a curious stranger who launches into an interminable and apparently irrelevant interrogation.

Validating Criteria

How, then, can a disorder be validated? Taken together, the following criteria support the hypothesis that a particular syndrome is categorically distinct:

1. *Natural history*: Patients with the syndrome have a predictable onset, course, and outcome.
2. *Psychobiological markers*: The syndrome is associated with abnormalities of pathophysiology, pathochemistry, or structure.
3. *Genetic studies*: Pedigree, twin, adoption, and chromosomal studies support a genetic etiology.
4. *Response to treatment*: Patients with the hypothetical disorder should respond predictably to treatment aimed at etiology.
5. *Construct validity*: Using multivariate analysis, the clinical syndrome on which the disorder is based should be both empirically isolable and capable of identifying a distinct cluster of patients from a larger population. The patients thus categorized should exhibit the natural history, markers, genetic features, and response to treatment described above.

Let us apply these criteria to the concept of a categorical unipolar major depression in adulthood.

Natural History

Unipolar depression usually begins in middle age (Perris, 1966). Patients, on average, have three to five episodes (Perris, 1966). The first episode usually has a precipitant stressor, but subsequent episodes are less likely to (Zis & Goodwin, 1979). Episodes in later life are more severe (Cutler & Post, 1982). Untreated episodes usually last 7–14 months (Perris, 1966). Before the introduction of electroconvulsive therapy, the suicide rate was 15–30% (Tsuang, 1978). Dysthymia, which is almost certainly heterogeneous, has no such historical clarity.

Psychobiological Markers

Gold, Goodwin, and Chrousos (1988a,b) have reviewed research into the markers of depression. The most consistent finding is hypercortisolism not suppressed by dexamethasone and without the diurnal rhythmicity manifest by normal adults. Less consistent findings concern diminished somatostatin and arginine vasopressin, a blunted response of growth hormone to clonidine or insulin-induced hypoglycemia, and an attenuated response of thyroid-stimulating hormone to thyrotropin-releasing hormone. It is postulated that melancholia is a chronic, generalized stress response that has escaped counterregulation by glucocorticords.

Major depression is associated with an alteration of circadian rhythm, as well as polysomnographic evidence of shortened REM latency, redistribution of REM sleep to early in the period of sleeping, prolonged sleep latency, wakefulness, decreased arousal threshold, and early morning waking (Wehr & Goodwin, 1981).

Genetic Studies

Affective illness congregates in the family trees of unipolar depressives (Rice & McGuffin, 1986). Gershon, Bunney, and Leckman (1976) and Bertelsen, Hawald, and Hauge (1977) found that about 50% of monozygotic twins were concordant for unipolar depression compared to about 25% of dizygotic twins. No convincing evidence has been gathered of a genetic difference between unipolar depression and dysthymia. Most of the research on gene loci has concerned bipolar disorder and will not be summarized here.

Response to Treatment

Somatic therapies are required to relieve melancholia. Akiskal (1986) summarizes numerous controlled studies as follows: Electroconvulsive therapy aborts about 90% of melancholic episodes, heterocyclic antidepressants about 70%.

Construct Validity

Empirical evidence for the categorically distinct nature of major depression has accrued gradually during the last 30 years. Several statistical techniques have been employed to investigate this matter (Trull, Widiger, & Guthrie, 1990): principal component analysis (PCA), cluster analysis, bimodality analysis, admixture analysis, and latent class analysis. Up to this time, the first three of these techniques have been the most often applied in construct validity studies.

PCA validates a factorial syndrome, but it is not helpful in determining whether the syndrome is categorically distinctive, since all subjects score on all the factors derived. It serves best to isolate syndrome factors that can then be used as the basis for cluster or bimodality analysis.

Cluster analysis sorts out homogeneous subgroups on the basis of a measure of similarity such as a factor score. However, it is uncertain which of the numerous techniques of cluster analysis should be employed, nor is it clear how to determine the correct number of clusters. Grove and Andreason (1986) and Meehl (1979) suggest that cluster analysis should be used for hypothesis-testing rather than exploration.

Bimodality analysis (e.g., Hasselblad, 1966; Lord, 1958; Wainer, 1978) tests for a gap or gaps in the distribution of scores on a factor. However, bimodality emerges only if there is little overlap between two distributions, and Grayson (1987) asserts that in some circumstances, bimodality can be exhibited by dimensional variables.

Admixture analysis examines the distribution of canonical coefficient scores derived from discriminant function analysis in order to determine whether a distribution is best explained by one or more components. However, discriminant function analysis requires a prior diagnostic categorization, thus potentially introducing a circular logic.

Maximum covariance analysis (Meehl, 1973), a form of latent class analysis, utilizes the concept that the covariance between two signs of a latent class variable will be minimized in homogeneous groups and maximized in mixed groups.

As already discussed, numerous factor-analytical and cluster-analytical studies of mixed adult depressive populations have isolated a depressive syndrome within which a distinctive group of depressed patients have congregated.

Validating Major Depression in Children and Adolescents

Natural History

Zeitlin (1972, 1985) compared three groups: people who had been treated at the Maudsley Hospital both as children and as adults, patients who had been treated only as children, and a sample treated only as adults. Of those depressed adults who had been treated as children, few had had depressive conditions when younger. Of those children regarded as depressed, few were subsequently diagnosed as depressed in adulthood. However, among a small subsample who were depressed on both occasions, there was a clear continuity in the clinical picture. Rutter (1986) noted that this study does not clarify whether depressive disorder should be diagnosed regardless of its associated symptomatology or whether depression is best considered a response to stress rather than an illness. To complicate matters, one might add that either explanation could be valid, depending on the child in question.

Kovacs, Feinberg, Crouse-Novak, Paulauskas, and Finkelstein (1984a) and Kovacs et al. (1984b) conducted a 5-year follow-up of children diagnosed as having major depression, dysthymia, and adjustment disorder with depressed mood. Children with major depression and adjustment disorder recovered more quickly than those with dysthymia. Subsequent major depression occurred in 70% of those who had had major depression or dysthymia when younger, and was virtually restricted to them. Garber, Kriss, Cock, and Lindholm (1988) found that 100% of a sample of depressed adolescent inpatients had a recurrence of depression over the next 8 years. Kovacs et al. (1984b) found that 70% of child and adolescent major depressives had had a further major depression within 5 years.

Harrington, Fudge, Rutter, Pickles, and Hill (1990) located from existing psychiatric records 80 child and adolescent depressives and 80 matched controls. Subjects were located an average of 18 years after initial contact, using evaluators blind to the original diagnosis. Among the index group, there was a 58% incidence at follow-up of adult depression of any type and a 35% incidence of major depression. Compared to the controls, the depressed group, as adults, were 5 times more likely to exhibit any form of depression and 7 times more likely to suffer from major depression. It should be noted that the majority of the youthful depressives who exhibited major depression in adulthood were adolescent at the time of initial diagnosis.

Treatment Response

Despite the enthusiasm with which antidepressant drugs are prescribed today, there have been only four controlled studies of their efficacy in children and adolescents. Puig-Antich et al. (1987) and Geller, Cooper, McCombs, Graham, and Wells (1989) found that imipramine and nortriptyline failed to surpass placebo in the treatment of prepubertal major depression, while Kramer and Feiguine (1981) and Geller (1989) found amitriptyline and nortriptyline no better than placebo in the treatment of adolescent depression. Thus far, no controlled study of antidepressant medication has demonstrated a significant experimental effect.

Puig-Antich et al. (1981, 1984) found that, compared to dysthymic and nondepressed controls, a small group of prepubertal children with major depression secreted less growth hormone in response to insulin-induced hypoglycemia and more growth hormone while asleep. In prepubertal major depressives, no evidence has been found for a blunting of the response of thyroid-stimulating hormone to thyrotropin-releasing hormone (Wagner, Saeed, Skyiepal, & Meyer, 1991). Cavallo, Hejazi, Richard, and Meyer (1987) found lower nocturnal plasma levels of melatonin in a small sample of major depressive children compared to short-statured controls. After promising earlier studies (Puig-Antich et al., 1979; Puig-Antich, 1983), Puig-Antich et al. (1989a) and Doherty et al. (1986) found no evidence of hypercortisolism when children with major depression were compared with nonaffective psychiatric controls. However, Weller et al. (1985) found evidence for hypercortisolism in a sample of hospitalized prepubertal major depressives. Studies of dexamethasone suppression in childhood depression have been reviewed by Casat, Arana, and Powell (1989). The results have been contradictory; the specificity of the test has been questioned, and the sensitivity has varied between 40% and 60%.

Puig-Antich et al. (1982) and Young, Knowles, MacLean, Boag, and McConville (1982) found that the polysomnographic records of prepubertal major depressives did not reveal the decreased REM latency, decreased slow wave sleep, increased REM density, decreased sleep efficiency, or abnormal REM distribution that characterize adult depressives and that the sleep architecture of depressed children did not differ from that of normal children. Lahmeyer, Poznanski, and Beller (1983) and Goetz et al. (1987) found changes in the sleep patterns of depressed adolescents, but their results were not consistent. A recent study by Emslie, Rush, Weinberg, Rintelmann, and Roffwarg (1990), comparing prepubertal major depressives to normal controls, has detected longer sleep latency, shorter REM latency, more individual short REM latency intervals, and a greater amount of REM sleep.

In summary, psychobiological studies of childhood and adolescent depression have yielded inconsistent findings. However, because too little is known concerning the effect of normal developmental neuroendocrine changes on the functions in question, these studies should be regarded as preliminary.

Genetic Studies

Puig-Antich et al. (1989b) conducted a controlled study of the family history of prepubertal major depressives, nonaffective psychiatric controls, and normals. Compared with major depression in later life, the diagnosis of major depression before 20 years of age was associated with an increased rate of major depression in first-degree relatives. Depressive children had significant higher rates of major depression, alcoholism, and other diagnoses in first-degree and second-degree relatives. Puig-Antich has suggested that familial alcoholism potentiates prepubertal depression in genetically vulnerable children, that the search for a "pure" major depression in childhood might be futile, and that major depression allied to conduct disorder might be a nongenetic phenocopy of major depression. No twin or adoption studies have been undertaken with prepubertal or adolescent depressives.

Construct Validity

The multivariate analyses of child and adolescent symptomatology have been discussed by Achenbach and Edelbrock (1978), Dreger (1982), and Quay (1986). Quay reviewed 61 factor analyses of behavior ratings, case history studies, peer ratings, and self-reports in samples of both sexes from 3 to 18 years of age, derived from school, special classes, delinquency institutions, clinics, and hospitals. The most common factors isolated corresponded to *undersocialized aggression, socialized conduct problems, attention-deficit, mixed dysphoria, schizoid withdrawal,* and *social ineptness.* The typical elements of the mixed dysphoria factor were as follows: anxious, shy, depressed, sensitive, feeling worthless, self-conscious, lacking in confidence, confused, weepy, aloof, and worrying. This factor appears to be an amalgam of emotionality, sadness, and shyness.

Working from a large outpatient sample, Achenbach and Edelbrock (1983) isolated a mixed *depressed–withdrawal–delinquent* factor for adolescent girls, but no depressive factor for adolescent boys. The following "depressive" factor was isolated from prepubertal boys: feeling worthless, guilty, needing to be perfect, feeling unloved, worrying, depressed, fearing own impulses, suicidal talk, and lonely. This factor is similar to the mixed dysphoria factor already described.

Lessing, Williams, and Revelle (1981) isolated a depressive syndrome by cluster-analyzing parents', teachers', and clinicians' ratings of a predominantly outpatient sample. Ryan et al. (1987) factor-analyzed Kiddie Schedule for Affective Disorders and Schizophrenia (K-SADS) (Chambers et al., 1985) data elicited from prepubertal and adolescent patients attending an affective disorders clinic. The following factors were isolated: *depressed–anhedonia; negative cognition–suicide; anxious–insomniac–somatizing; appetite–weight;* and *irritable–agitated–antisocial.* The first factor was composed of the following items: anhedonia, fatigue, psychomotor retardation, withdrawal, depressed mood, hypersomnia, anorexia, decreased weight, and diurnal mood change.

In a principal-components analysis of K-SADS data derived from 95 children (aged 9–16 years) and their parents referred to a depression clinic, Kolvin et al. (1991) extracted four factors: *endogenous depression, negative cognition, anxiety,* and *anger–agitation.* These factors are consistent with those isolated by Ryan et al. (1987). Subsequent cluster analysis identified three broad clusters: *negative cognition, endogenous depression,* and a mixed *conduct problems–neurosis* group. There was reasonable consistency between these clusters and clinical diagnosis. The "endogenous depression" factor derived from children was composed of the following items: anhedonia, withdrawal, dysphoric mood, loss of appetite, loss of energy, irritability, and somatic complaints.

Kolvin et al. (1991) suggest that "comorbidity" explains the lack of concordance between clinical and empirical diagnosis that has been noted in some studies (e.g., Nurcombe et al., 1990). However, Achenbach (1991) suggests that apparent comorbidity may arise as an artifact of diagnostic models that impute false boundaries between dimensionally continuous syndromes. In some cases, apparent comorbidity might stem from a higher-order pattern of concurrent problems reflecting a single diagnostic grouping, rather than the overlap between two separate disorders.

In two related studies, Nurcombe et al. (1989) and Seifer, Nurcombe, Scioli, and Grapentine (1989) employed multivariate techniques in order to search for a depressive factor among adolescent and child outpatient and inpatient samples. In doing so, they adapted the following ground rules from Ni Bhrolchain (1979);

1. Multivariate analysis should be used deductively, not to generate hypotheses.
2. A hypothesis having been stated, every attempt should be made to maximize the chance of finding the reverse.
3. The data should be elicited by or from people with no preconception about the hypothesis. Omnibus instruments should be used in order to avoid the kind of circular logic that many structured interviews entail.
4. Principal-components analysis is best used to identify syndromes. Cluster analysis lends itself to the isolation of categorical subgroups.
5. Syndromal factors and categorical clusters should be isolated from current symp-

tomatology and mental status. Clusters can then be validated by associating them with other features such as family history, outcome, psychobiological characteristics, and response to treatment.

6. The results of one cluster analysis should be checked with a second clustering technique.

Data for the Nurcombe–Seifer analyses were derived from parental Child Behavior Checklists (CBCLs) on 126 adolescent outpatients, 216 adolescent inpatients, 193 child outpatients, and 91 child inpatients. Principal-components analysis of adolescent outpatients did not identify a convincing depressive factor. However, the analysis of adolescent inpatients yielded three factors: *conduct problems*, *depression*, and *social ineptness*. The depression factor was not bimodal in distribution. Table 1 lists the items that loaded most heavily on the depression factor.

Two separate hierarchical cluster analysis were then performed on Z-scaled factor scores. Both analyses isolated a depression cluster containing 11–15% of the sample. The cluster was validated against Minnesota Multiphasic Personality Inventory and Children's Depression Inventory scores, but not against clinical diagnosis, suggesting a trend toward an overdiagnosis of depressive disorder by hospital clinicians.

A similar multivariate analysis of 284 6- to 12-year-old inpatients and outpatients extracted only a weak depressive component (see Table 2). Two separate cluster analyses failed to isolate a depressive category. There was no evidence of bimodality in the prepubertal depressive factor.

Using an expanded data set of 1345 child and adolescent outpatients and inpatients from multiple rural and urban sites, Weiss and Nurcombe (1992) undertook a complex multivariate analysis of CBCL data. Only adolescent inpatients yielded a convincing depression factor (attempts suicide, fears school, fears own impulses, has to be perfect, feels unloved, feels persecuted, feels worthless, likes to be alone, anxious, guilty, self-conscious, shy, moody, sulks, talks of suicide, insomniac, anergic, sad, withdrawn, worrying). Despite two cluster analyses and one latent class analysis, no convincing depressive cluster was isolated.

In summary, there have been many factor-analytical studies of child and adolescent psychopathology, but few have identified a convincing depressive factor. In most instances, depressive phenomena are commingled with emotionality and social ineptitude. However, since most of these studies were of outpatients, pure depression may have been too uncommon to be detected. Several recent studies—two of children and adolescents in a mood disorders clinic and two of hospitalized adolescents—have identified cleaner depressive factors. Only two studies (Kolvin et al., 1991; Nurcombe et al., 1989) have identified a categorically distinct depression cluster; however, few cluster analyses have been attempted in children and adolescents.

Table 1. Depression Factor Items and Factor Loadings Derived from Adolescent Inpatients[a]

Item	Loading	Item	Loading
1. Threatens suicide	(0.58)	7. Shy	(0.52)
2. Depressed	(0.57)	8. Overtired	(0.52)
3. Worrying	(0.57)	9. Nightmares	(0.51)
4. Anxious	(0.54)	10. Fears doing bad	(0.51)
5. Feels worthless	(0.54)	11. Underactive	(0.51)
6. Trouble sleeping	(0.53)		

[a]From Nurcombe et al. (1989).

Discussion

The concept of major depression in adulthood is supported by studies of its natural history and response to treatment. It is associated with changes in neuroendocrine function and disruption of circadian rhythms. The diagnosis is further supported by family aggregation and twin studies. Multivariate analyses of mixed data sets have repeatedly identified a factor that polarizes endogenous depression and neurosis and have isolated a cluster of patients consistent with a categorical major depression. Dysthymia, on the other hand, decomposes, on analysis, into a mixture of temporary reactions to life stress, grief reactions, chronic personality traits, coping style, and the residua of major depression. It is probably a diagnostic artifact.

Contemporary enthusiasm for the diagnosis of major depression in childhood has come almost entirely from the application of adult criteria and techniques. However, it is unlikely that the phenomenology of childhood depression is completely isomorphic with that in adults. Furthermore, children—especially emotionally disturbed children—lack the metacognitive competency required to report their own psychopathology with accuracy.

Three studies have demonstrated a continuity of depressive syndromes between childhood, adolescence, and adulthood. Some depressed children appear to grow up to become major depressives in adolescence or adulthood. These three studies represent the most impressive support for the validity of the diagnosis. However, there are numerous problems. The suicide rate is markedly higher in adolescents than in children and has increased in the last 20 years. Among children, male depressives are twice as prevalent as female, the reverse of the sex ratio in adolescence. Furthermore, in children and adolescents, major depression and dysthymia are entangled with aggressivity, antisocial behavior, anxiety, and substance abuse more frequently than is the case with adults (Puig-Antich, 1987).

The diagnosis of depression in childhood and adolescence has not been supported by the efficacy of antidepressant therapy, and the psychobiological evidence in favor of this diagnosis is patchy. However, it is fair to say that all the evidence is not yet available. The failure to find consistent pharmacological or psychobiological support for the validity of the diagnosis could be explained by small sample size, instrument insensitivity, faulty original case selection, the rarity of major depression, or, finally, the invalidity of the diagnosis.

One family pedigree study has found an aggregation of major depression, alcoholism, and other psychiatric disorders among the relatives of depressed children. As with the comorbidity question, the relationship between childhood depression and parental alcoholism, depression, and mental illness is probably complex. It is unlikely to be solely hereditary in nature.

Table 2. Depression Factor Items and Factor Loadings Derived from Child Inpatients and Outpatients[a]

Item	Loading	Item	Loading
1. Worrying	(0.61)	6. Fears doing bad	(0.51)
2. Must be perfect	(0.57)	7. Nightmares	(0.50)
3. Feels worthless	(0.57)	8. Suicidal ideation	(0.46)
4. Too guilty	(0.57)	9. Anxious	(0.46)
5. Depressed	(0.54)	10. Self-conscious	(0.40)

[a]From Seifer et al. (1989).

Construct-validity analyses have offered inconsistent support for the existence of a depressive syndrome. In most studies, depression emerges as part of an impure dysphoria factor, along with anxiety and social ineptitude or withdrawal. However, recent research has isolated an acceptable depressive syndrome from hospitalized or mood-disordered patients, possibly because these samples contained more severe or developed cases. In one study, a categorical depressive cluster was found in adolescent inpatients, but not in either adolescent outpatients or a mixed sample of prepubertal children. Among adolescents, there is some empirical evidence for the existence of a small group of patients who have a categorical depression and a larger group whose depression is dimensional and nonspecific in nature.

A Speculative Conclusion

Without question, many children and adolescents suffer from emotional problems in which sadness is a prominent feature. It is still unclear, however, whether a true categorical depressive disorder can be isolated, linked to a predictable genetic background, psychobiology, and natural history, and associated with a specific etiology and treatment. To pursue these ends, we require high-risk longitudinal studies (e.g., of the progeny of high-risk pedigrees) utilizing a variety of methods for gathering phenomenological data and combining descriptive psychiatry with studies of the attitudes of high-risk children to themselves, their social environments, and their futures. At the same time, the search for family aggregations, psychobiological markers, and effective treatments should continue. How can developmental psychopathology contribute to this enterprise?

The panoramic developmental theories of Freud and Piaget are in decline. Contemporary developmental researchers shuttle to and fro between their data and parsimonious constructs derived from information-processing, social learning, and ethological theories. Up to now, they have had little contact with descriptive psychiatrists and biological researchers, who hunt for needles of melancholia in the haystack of dysthymia. How can the two groups communicate?

Sroufe and Rutter (1984), Santostefano (1978), and Cicchetti and Schneider-Rosen (1986) suggest that behavior can be interpreted only within a total psychosocial and developmental context; for example, the misery of bereavement may have a different significance from sadness following punishment. Later experience does not have a random effect on individuals; it is assimilated in accordance with temperament, previous experience, and previously learned coping techniques. Development is not linear. It results from the incorporation, reorganization, and subordination of old and new elements, proceeding from global, inflexible, fragmentary origins toward increasingly specific, flexible, and hierarchically organized ends. There is no need to postulate fixation or regression as the basis of psychopathology. Disturbed behavior results from a failure to reorganize and subordinate anachronisms that continue to operate in an inflexible, fragmentary, and ultimately maladaptive manner.

The attachment system is a particularly promising field of research. Activated by the threat of danger, attachment entails behavior that is later incorporated within and subordinated to the emerging systems of social affiliation, mating, and parenting. The link between early attachment experience and later behavior is conceivably via internal representations or "working models" of the self-in-relation-to-significant-others (Bowlby, 1969; Bretherton, 1985). Theoretically, then, disruption in early attachment could be linked to later depressive psychopathology via global, inflexible, poorly organized, unintegrated, and dysfunctional self–other representations (Cicchetti & Schneider-Rosen, 1986; Cummings & Cicchetti, 1990).

A number of questions spring to mind:

1. What is the influence of heredity in predisposing individuals to later depressive conditions? Does it operate by making some individuals more vulnerable to attachment disruption or to subsequent risk factors? Does it limit or define the coping techniques available? Does it render biochemically predisposed individuals more likely to tip over from misery into melancholia?

2. If attachment disruption is a significant antecedent stress, does it act in an undifferentiated manner, or do such perturbations as parental depression, separation, bereavement, abandonment, rejection, or abuse have differential effects?

3. If the effects of different types of attachment disruption are differentiated, can they be related to definable types of pathology in self–other representations? For example, does a mixture of parental coercion, inconsistency, and neglect predispose children to conduct problems? What are its inner representations? Do such representations engender hostile, provocative transactions with others, leading to self-fulfilling prophecies of failure, disappointment, rejection, and self-hatred?

4. Can a depressive precursor condition be identified (cf. Cicchetti & Aber, 1986)? Is it homotypic or heterotypic with later depression? Does it evolve into depression through invariant stages, with definable turning points?

5. If a precursor–outcome evolution can be delineated, what are the environmental, psychological, and biological factors that propel individuals toward a depressive outcome? What protects them from moving in that direction?

6. Can protracted dysthymia tip over into a neuroendocrinologically decompensated melancholia? If so, what are the hereditary, biological, or psychosocial factors that push individuals over the melancholic edge? At what age is such a decompensation possible?

7. How does helplessness relate to hopelessness? Why do some individuals give up hope, and how does their doing so affect the neuroendocrine system?

These questions suggest a complex linkage between genetic predisposition, attachment disruption, representational pathology, dysfunctional social interaction, precursor states, risk/protective factors, "dysthymia," and melancholic neuroendocrine decompensation (cf. Cicchetti & Aber, 1986). Naive? Certainly. But a potentially useful scaffolding for research design.

ACKNOWLEDGMENTS. The author would like to express his appreciation to Drs. Thomas Ban, Judy Garber, Peter Loosen, Bahr Weiss, Robert Begtrup, and Dante Cicchetti for their help in the preparation of this chapter.

References

Achenbach, T. M. (1991). "Comorbidity" in child and adolescent psychiatry: Categorical and quantitative perspectives. *Journal of Child & Adolescent Psychopharmacology, 1,* 271–278.

Achenbach, T. M., & Edelbrock, C. S. (1978). The classification of childhood psychopathology: A review and analysis of empirical efforts. *Psychological Bulletin, 85,* 1275–1301.

Achenbach, T. M., & Edelbrock, C. S. (1983). *Manual for the Child Behavioral Checklist and revised Child Behavioral Profile.* Burlington, VT: Queen City Printers.

Akiskal, H. S. (1986). The clinical management of affective disorders. In J. E. Helzer & S. B. Guze (Eds.), *Psychiatry,* Vol. 2, *Psychoses, affective disorders and dementia* (pp. 119–146). New York: Basic Books.

American Psychiatric Association (1994). *Diagnostic and statistical manual of mental disorders,* 4th ed. Washington, DC: Author.

Bertelsen, A., Hawald, B., & Hauge, M. A. (1977). A Danish twin study of manic–depressive disorders. *British Journal of Psychiatry, 130,* 330–351.

Bonhoeffer, K. (1910). *Die symptomatischen Psychosen.* Leipzig: Deuticke.

Bowlby, J. (1952). *Maternal care and mental health.* Geneva: World Health Organization.

Bowlby, J. (1969). *Attachment and loss*, Vol. 1, *Attachment*. New York: Basic Books.

Bowlby, J. (1973). *Attachment and loss*, Vol. 2, *Separation, anxiety and anger*. New York: Basic Books.

Bowlby, J. (1980). *Attachment and loss*, Vol. 3, *Loss, sadness, and depression*. New York: Basic Books.

Bretherton, I. (1985). Attachment theory: Retrospect and prospect. In I. Bretherton & E. Waters (Eds.), *Growing points of attachment theory and research* (pp. 3–38). Monograph of the Society for Research in Child Development, Vol. 50, Whole Numbers 1–2.

Carlson, G. A., & Cantwell, D. P. (1980). Unmasking masked depression in children and adolescents. *American Journal of Psychiatry, 137*, 445–449.

Carlson, G. A., & Kashani, J. H. (1988). Phenomenology of major depression from childhood through adulthood: Analysis of three studies. *American Journal of Psychiatry, 1245*, 1222–1225.

Casat, C. D., Arana, G. W., & Powell, K. (1989). The DST in children and adolescents with major depressive disorders. *American Journal of Psychiatry, 146*, 503–507.

Cavallo, A., Hejazi, M. S., Richard, G. E., & Meyer, W. J. (1987). Melatonin circadian rhythm in childhood depression. *Journal of the American Academy of Child and Adolescent Psychiatry, 26*, 395–399.

Chambers, W., Puig-Antich, J., Hirsch, M., Paes, P., Ambrosini, P. J., Tabrizi, M. A., & Davies, M. (1985). The assessment of affective disorders in children and adolescents by semi-structured interview: Test-retest reliability of the K-SADSA-P. *Archives of General Psychiatry, 42*, 696–702.

Cicchetti, D., & Aber, J. L. (1986). Early precursors of later depression: An organizational perspective. In L. Lipsett & C. Rovee-Collier (Eds.), *Advances in infancy*, Vol. 4 (pp. 87–137). Norwood, NJ: Ablex.

Cicchetti, D., & Schneider-Rosen, K. (1986). An organizational approach to childhood depression. In M. Rutter, C. E. Izard, & P. B. Read (Eds.), *Depression in young people: Clinical and developmental perspectives* (pp. 71–134). New York: Guilford Press.

Costello, A. J., Edelbrock, C., Kalas, R., Kessler, M. D., & Klaric, S. H. (1982). The NIMH Diagnostic Interview Schedule for Children (DISC). Unpublished interview schedule. Pittsburgh: Department of Psychiatry, University of Pittsburgh.

Cummings, E. M., & Cicchetti, D. (1990). Toward a transactional model of relations between attachment and depression. In M. Greenberg, D. Cicchetti, & E. M. Cummings (Eds.), *Attachment in the preschool years* (pp. 339–372). Chicago: University of Chicago Press.

Cutler, N. R., & Post, R. M. (1982). Life course of illness in untreated manic–depressive illness. *Comprehensive Psychiatry, 23*, 101–115.

Cytryn, L., & McKnew, D. H. (1972). Proposed classification of childhood depression. *American Journal of Psychiatry, 129*, 149–155.

Cytryn, L., McKnew, D. H., & Bunney, W. E. (1980). Diagnosis of depression in children: A reassessment. *American Journal of Psychiatry, 137*, 22–25.

Doherty, M. B., Mandansky, D., Kraft, J., Carter-Ake, L. L., Rosenthal, P. A., & Coughlin, B. F. (1986). Cortisol dynamics and test performance of dexamethasone suppression test in 97 psychiatrically hospitalized children aged 3–16 years. *Journal of the American Academy of Child and Adolescent Psychiatry, 25*, 400–408.

Dreger, R. M. (1982). The classification of children and their emotional problems: An overview. II. *Clinical Psychology Review, 2*, 349–385.

Emslie, G. J., Rush, A. J., Weinberg, W. A., Rintelmann, J. W., & Roffwarg, H. P. (1990). Children with major depression show rapid eye movement latencies. *Archives of General Psychiatry, 47*, 119–124.

Everitt, B. S., Gourlay, A. J., & Kendell, R. E. (1971). An attempt at validation of traditional psychiatric syndromes by cluster analysis. *British Journal of Psychiatry, 119*, 399–412.

Finch, S. M. (1960). *Fundamentals of child psychiatry*. New York: Norton.

Freud, A., & Burlingham, D. (1944). *Infants without families*. New York: International Universities Press.

Garber, J., Kriss, M. R., Cock, M., & Lindholm, L. (1988). Recurrent depression in adolescents: A follow-up study. *Journal of the American Academy of Child and Adolescent Psychiatry, 27*, 49–54.

Geller, B. (1989). A double-blind placebo-controlled study of nortriptyline in adolescents with major depression. Paper presented at the annual meeting of the New Clinical Drug Evaluation Unit, National Institute of Mental Health, Washington, DC.

Geller, B., Cooper, T. B., McCombs, H. G., Graham, D., & Wells, J. (1989). Double-blind placebo-controlled study of nortriptyline in depressed children using a "fixed plasma level" design. *Psychopharmacology Bulletin, 25*, 101–108.

Gershon, E., Bunney, W., & Leckman, J. (1976). The inheritance of affective disorders: A review of data and hypotheses. *Behavioral Genetics, 6*, 227–261.

Gillespie, R. D. (1929). The clinical differentiation of types of depression. *Guy's Hospital Report, 2*, 306–344.

Glasser, K. (1967). Masked depression in children and adolescents. *American Journal of Psychotherapy, 21*, 565–574.

Goetz, R. R., Puig-Antich, J., Ryan, N., Rabinovich, H., Ambrosini, P. J., Nelson, B., & Krawiec, V. (1987). Electroencephalographic sleep of adolescents with major depression and normal controls. *Archives of General Psychiatry, 46,* 61–68.

Gold, P. W., Goodwin, F. K., & Chrousos, G. P. (1988a). Clinical and biochemical manifestations of depression. I. Relation to the neurobiology of stress. *New England Journal of Medicine, 319,* 348–353.

Gold, P. W., Goodwin, F. K., & Chrousos, G. P. (1988b). Clinical and biochemical manifestations of depression. II. Relation to the neurobiology of stress. *New England Journal of Medicine, 319,* 413–420.

Grayson, D. (1987). Assessment of evidence for a categorical view of schizophrenia. *Archives of General Psychiatry, 43,* 712–713.

Grove, W. M., & Andreasen, N. C. (1986). Multivariate statistical analysis in psychopathology. In T. Million & G. L. Klerman (Eds.), *Contemporary directions in psychopathology: Toward the DSM-IV* (pp. 347–362). New York: Guilford Press.

Grove, W. M., Andreason, N. C., Young, M., Endicott, J., Keller, M. B., Hirschfeld, R. M. A., & Reich, T. (1987). Isolation and characterization of a nuclear depressive syndrome. *Psychological Medicine, 17,* 471–484.

Harrington, R., Fudge, H., Rutter, M., Pickles, A., & Hill, J. (1990). Adult outcomes of childhood and adolescent depressions. I. Psychiatric status. *Archives of General Psychiatry, 47,* 465–473.

Hasselblad, V. (1966). Estimation of parameters for a mixture of normal distributions. *Technometrics, 8,* 431–444.

Herjanic, B., & Campbell, W. (1977). Differentiating psychiatrically disturbed children on the basis of a structured interview. *Journal of Abnormal Child Psychiatry, 5,* 127–134.

Hodges, K., Klein, J., Stern, L., Cytryn, L., & McKnew, D. (1982). The development of a child assessment interview for research and clinical use. *Journal of Abnormal Child Psychiatry, 10,* 173–189.

Kahlbaum, K. (1863). *Die Gruppierung der psychischen Krankheiten und die Enteilung der Seelenstörungen.* Danzig: Kaufman.

Kashani, J. H., McGee, R. D., Clarkson, S. E., Anderson, J. C., Walton, L. E., William, S., Silver, P. A., Robins, A. J., Cytryn, L., & McKnew, D. H. (1983). Depression in a sample of nine-year-old children: Prevalence and associated characteristics. *Archives of General Psychiatry, 40,* 1217–1227.

Kashani, J. H., & Simonds, J. F. (1979). The incidence of depression in children. *American Journal of Psychiatry, 136,* 1203–1205.

Kendell, R. E. (1976). *The role of diagnosis in psychiatry.* Oxford: Blackwell.

Kendell, R. E., & Gourlay, J. (1970). The clinical distinction between psychotic and neurotic depressions. *British Journal of Psychiatry, 117,* 257–266.

Kiloh, L. G., Andrews, G., Neilson, M., & Bianchi, G. N. (1972). The relationship of the syndromes called endogenous and neurotic depression. *British Journal of Psychiatry, 121,* 183–196.

Kiloh, L. G., & Garside, R. F. (1963). The independence of neurotic depression and endogenous depression. *British Journal of Psychiatry, 109,* 451–463.

Kiloh, L. G., & Garside, R. F. (1977). Depression: A multivariate study of Sir Aubrey Lewis' data on melancholia. *Australian and New Zealand Journal of Psychiatry, 11,* 149–156.

Klein, M. (1948). *Contributions to psychoanalysis 1921–1945.* London: Hogarth.

Klein, M. (1949). *The psychoanalysis of children.* London: Hogarth.

Kolvin, I., Barrett, M. L., Bhate, S. R., Berney, T. P., Famnyiwa, O. O., Fundudis, T., & Tyrer, S. (1991). The Newcastle child depression project: Diagnosis and classification of depression. *British Journal of Psychiatry, 159 (Supplement 11),* 9–21.

Kovacs, M. (1982). The Interview Schedule for Children (ISC). Unpublished manuscript. Pittsburgh: Department of Psychiatry, University of Pittsburgh.

Kovacs, M. (1985). The children's depression inventory. *Psychopharmacology Bulletin, 21,* 995–998.

Kovacs, M. (1986). A developmental perspective on methods and measures in the assessment of depressive disorders: The clinical interview. In M. Rutter, C. E. Izard, & P. B. Read (Eds.), *Depression in young people: Developmental and clinical perspectives* (pp. 435–462). New York: Guilford Press.

Kovacs, M., Feinberg, T. L., Crouse-Novak, M. A., Paulausaks, S. L., & Finkelstein, R. (1984a). Depressive disorders in childhood, I. A longitudinal prospective study of characteristics and recovery. *Archives of General Psychiatry, 41,* 229–237.

Kovacs, M., Feinberg, T. L., Crouse-Novak, M. A., Paulauskas, S. L., Pollack, M., & Finkelstein, R. (1984b). Depressive disorders in childhood. II. A longitudinal study of the risk for a subsequent major depression. *Archives of General Psychiatry, 41,* 643–649.

Kraepelin, E. (1896). *Lehrbuch der Psychiatrie,* 5th ed. Leipzig: Barth.

Kramer, A. D., & Feiguine, R. J. (1981). Clinical effects of amitriptyline in adolescent depression: A pilot study. *Journal of the American Academy of Child and Adolescent Psychiatry, 20,* 636–644.

Kuhn, R. (1963). Über kindlichen Depressionen und ihre Behandlung. *Schweizer Medizinische Wochenschrift*, *93*, 86–90.

Lahmeyer, H. W., Poznanski, E. O., & Beller, S. N. (1983). EEG sleep in depressed adolescents. *American Journal of Psychiatry*, *140*, 1150–1153.

Leonhard, K. (1957). *Aufteilung der endogenen Psychosen*. Berlin: Akademie-Verlag.

Lessing, E. E., Williams, V., & Revelle, W. (1981). Parallel forms of the IJR behavior checklist for parents, teachers, and clinicians. *Journal of Consulting and Clinical Psychology*, *49*, 34–50.

Lewis, A. J. (1934). Melancholia: A clinical survey of depressive states. *Journal of Mental Science*, *80*, 277–378.

Ling, W., Oftedal, G., & Weinberg, W. (1970). Depressive illness in children presenting as severe headaches. *American Journal of Diseases of Children*, *120*, 122–128.

Lord, F. M. (1958). *Multimodal score distributions on the Myers–Briggs Type Indicator—I* (ETS RM 58-8). Princeton, NJ: Education Testing Service.

Malmquist, C. P. (1971). Depressions in childhood and adolescence. *New England Journal of Medicine*, *284*, 887–893.

Matussek, P., Soldner, M. L., & Nagel, D. (1982). Neurotic depression: Result of cluster analyses. *Journal of Nervous and Mental Disease*, *170*, 588–597.

McConville, B. J., Boag, L. C., & Purohit, A. P. (1973). Three types of childhood depression. *Canadian Psychiatric Association Journal*, *18*, 133–138.

Meehl, P. E. (1973). MAXCOV-HITMAX: A taxonomic search for loose genetic syndromes. In *Psychodiagnosis: Selected papers* (pp. 200–224). Minneapolis: University of Minnesota Press.

Meehl, P. E. (1979). A funny thing happened to us on the way to latent entities. *Journal of Personality Assessment*, *43*, 563–581.

Moebius, J. P. (1893). *Abriss der Lehre von den Nervenkrankheiten*. Leipzig: Deuticke.

Morel, B. A. (1857). *Trité des dégénérescences physiques, intellectuelles et morales de l'espèce humaine*. Paris: Balliere.

Mullaney, J. A. (1984). The relationship between anxiety and depression: A review of some principal component analytic studies. *Journal of Affective Disorders*, *7*, 139–148.

Ni Bhrolchain, M. (1979). Psychotic and neurotic depression. I. Some points of method. *British Journal of Psychiatry*, *134*, 87–93.

Nurcombe, B., Seifer, R., Scioli, A., Tramontana, M. G., Grapentine, W. L., & Beauchesne, H. C. (1989). Is major depressive disorder in adolescence a distinct diagnostic entity? *Journal of the American Academy of Child and Adolescent Psychiatry*, *28*, 333–342.

Parker, G., Hadzi-Pavlovic, D., Boyce, P., Wilhelm, K., Brodaty, H., Mitchell, P., Hickie, I., & Eyers, K. (1990). *British Journal of Psychiatry*, *157*, 55–65.

Paykel, E. S. (1971). Classification of depressed patients: A cluster analysis derived grouping. *British Journal of Psychiatry*, *118*, 275–288.

Perris, C. (1966). A study of bipolar (manic–depressive) and unipolar recurrent depressive psychoses. *Acta Psychiatrica Scandinavica*, *194*(supplement), 1–189.

Pilowsky, I., Levine, S., & Boulton, D. M. (1969). The classification of depression by numerical taxonomy. *British Journal of Psychiatry*, *115*, 937–945.

Poznanski, E., & Zrull, J. (1970). Child depression: Clinical characteristics of overtly depressed children. *Archives of General Psychiatry*, *23*, 8–15.

Puig-Antich, J. (1983). Neuroendocrine and sleep correlates of prepubertal major depressive disorder: Current status of the evidence. In D. P. Cantwell & G. A. Carlson (Eds.), *Affective disorders in childhood and adolescence—An update* (pp. 211–228). New York: Spectrum Publications.

Puig-Antich, J. (1986). Psychobiological markers: Effects of age and puberty. In M. Rutter, C. E. Izard, & P. B. Read (Eds.), *Depression in young people: Developmental and clinical perspectives* (pp. 341–382). New York: Guilford Press.

Puig-Antich, J. (1987). Affective disorders in children and adolescents: Diagnostic validity and psychobiology. In H. Y. Meltzer (Ed.), *Psychopharmacology: The third generation of progress* (pp. 843–860). New York: Raven Press.

Puig-Antich, J., & Chambers, W. (1978). The Schedule for Affective Disorders and Schizophrenia for School-Aged Children. Unpublished interview schedule. New York: New York State Psychiatry Institute.

Puig-Antich, J., Chambers, W., Halpern, F., Hanlon, C., & Sachar, E. J. (1979). Cortisol hypersecretion in prepubertal depressive illness: A preliminary report. *Psychoneuroendocrinology*, *4*, 191–197.

Puig-Antich, J., Dahl, R., Ryan, N., Novacenko, H., Goetz, D., Goetz, R., Toomey, J., & Kleper, T. (1989a). Cortisol secretion in prepubertal children with major depressive disorder. *Archives of General Psychiatry*, *46*, 801–809.

Puig-Antich, J., Goetz, D., Davies, M., Kaplan, T., Davies, S., Ostrow, L., Asnis, L., Toomey, J., Iyengar, S., & Ryan, N. (1989b). A controlled family history study of prepubertal major depressive disorder. *Archives of General Psychiatry, 46,* 406–418.

Puig-Antich, J., Goetz, R., Hanlon, C., Tabrizi, M. A., Davies, M., & Weitzman, E. (1982). Sleep architecture and REM sleep measures in prepubertal major depressives during an episode. *Archives of General Psychiatry, 39,* 932–939.

Puig-Antich, J., Novacenko, H., Davies, M., Chambers, W. J., Tabrizi, M. A., Krawiec, V., Ambrosini, P. J., & Sachar, E. J. (1984). Growth hormone secretion in prepubertal major depressive children. I. Sleep-related plasma concentrations during a depressive episode. *Archives of General Psychiatry, 41,* 455–460.

Puig-Antich, J., Perel, J. M., Lupatkin, W., Chambers, W. J., Tabrizi, M. A., King, J., Goetz, R., Davies, M., & Stiller, R. L. (1987). Imipramine in prepubertal major depressive disorders. *Archives of General Psychiatry, 44,* 81–89.

Puig-Antich, J., Tabrizi, M. A., Davies, M., Chambers, W., Halpern, F., & Sachar, E. J. (1981). Prepubertal endogenous major depressives hyposecrete growth hormone in response to insulin-induced hypoglycemia. *Journal of Biological Psychiatry, 16,* 801–818.

Quay, H. C. (1986). Classification. In H. C. Quay & J. S. Werry, *Psychopathological disorders of childhood,* 3rd ed. (pp. 1–34). New York: John Wiley.

Rice, J. P., & McGuffin, P. (1986). Genetic etiology of schizophrenia and affective disorders. In J. E. Helzer & S. B. Guze (Eds.), *Psychiatry,* Vol. II, *Psychoses, affective disorders and dementia* (pp. 147–170). New York: Basic Books.

Rie, H. E. (1966). Depression in childhood: A survey of some pertinent contributions. *Journal of the American Academy of Child Psychiatry, 5,* 653–685.

Rochlin, G. (1959). The loss complex. *Journal of the American Psychoanalytic Association, 7,* 299–316.

Rutter, M. (1986). The developmental psychopathology of depression. In M. Rutter, C. E. Izard, & P. B. Read (Eds.), *Depression in young people: Developmental and clinical perspectives* (pp. 3–32). New York: Guilford Press.

Ryan, N. D., Puig-Antich, J., Ambrosini, P., Rabinovich, H., Robinson, D., Neilson, B., Iyenhar, S., & Toomey, J. (1987). The clinical picture of major depression in children and adolescents. *Archives of General Psychiatry, 44,* 854–861.

Santostefano, S. (1978). *A biodevelopmental approach to clinical child psychology.* New York: John Wiley.

Seifer, R., Nurcombe, B., Scioli, A., & Grapentine, W. L. (1989). Is major depressive disorder in childhood a distinct diagnostic entity? *Journal of the American Academy of Child and Adolescent Psychiatry, 28,* 935–941.

Spitz, R. A., & Wolf, K. M. (1946). Anaclitic depression: An inquiry into the genesis of psychiatric conditions in early childhood. *Psychoanalytic Study of the Child, 2,* 313–342.

Sroufe, L. A., & Rutter, M. (1984). The domain of developmental psychopathology. *Child Development, 55,* 17–29.

Toolan, J. M. (1962). Depression in children and adolescence. *American Journal of Orthopsychiatry, 32,* 404–414.

Trull, T. J., Widiger, T. A., & Guthrie, P. (1990). Categorical versus dimensional status of borderline personality disorder. *Journal of Abnormal Psychology, 99,* 40–48.

Tsuang, M. T. (1978). Suicide in schizophrenics, manics, depressives, and surgical controls: A comparison with general population suicide mortality. *Archives of General Psychiatry, 135,* 153–155.

Wagner, K. D., Saeed, M. A., Skyiepal, B., & Meyer, W. J. (1991). Thyrotrophin and growth hormone responses to TRH stimulation are normal in 6–12 year-old children with major depression. *Journal of Child & Adolescent Psychopharmacology, 1,* 199–206.

Wainer, H. (1978). Gapping. *Psychometrika, 43,* 203–212.

Wehr, T. A., & Goodwin, F. K. (1981). Biological rhythms and psychiatry. In S. H. Arieti & K. H. Brodie (Eds.), *The American handbook of psychiatry,* Vol. VII, 2nd ed. (pp. 46–74). New York: Basic Books.

Weinberg, W. A., Rutman, J., Sullivan, L., Penick, E. C., & Deitz, S. G. (1973). Depression in children referred to an educational diagnostic center: Diagnosis and treatment. *Behavioral Pediatrics, 83,* 1065–1072.

Weiss, B., & Nurcombe, B. (1992). Age, clinical severity, and the differentiation of depressive symptomatology: A test of the orthogenetic hypothesis. *Development and Psychopathology, 4,* 115–126.

Weller, E. B., Weller, R. A., Fristad, M. A., Preskorn, S. H., & Teare, M. (1985). The dexamethasone suppression test in prepubertal depressed children. *Journal of Clinical Psychiatry, 46,* 511–513.

Young, W., Knowles, J. B., MacLean, A. W., Boag, L., & McConville, B. J. (1982). The sleep of childhood depressives: Comparison with age-matched controls. *Biological Psychiatry, 17,* 1163–1168.

Zeitlin, H. (1972). A study of patients who attended the children's department and later the adults' department of the same psychiatric hospital. Unpublished M.Phil. dissertation. London: University of London.

Zeitlin, H. (1985). *The natural history of psychiatric disorder in children*. Institute of Psychiatry, Maudsley Monograph. London: Oxford University Press.

Zis, A. P., & Goodwin, F. K. (1979). Major affective disorders as a recurrent illness: A critical review. *Archives of General Psychiatry, 36*, 835–839.

II
THEORIES AND MODELS
OF DEPRESSION

5

Dynamic and Interpersonal Theories of Depression

Jules R. Bemporad

Introduction

In contrast to the wealth of literature on psychodynamic and interpersonal theories of depression in adults, there is a paucity of contributions examining these aspects of depression in adolescents, and particularly in children. This relative neglect of psychodynamic approaches to juvenile depression may seem surprising, since some of the major psychoanalytic theorists of depression, such as those of Freud and Abraham, specifically implicated childhood events in the etiology of adult mood disorders. Freud suggested the loss of a love object or the love of that object in early childhood as predisposing to adult melancholia, if a substitute object could not be found. Abraham went so far as to postulate the existence of a childhood episode of depression, termed "primal parathymia," secondary to a disappointment in the child's relationship with his or her mother in the history of adult depressives. Later psychoanalytic authors such as Rado and Jacobson continued to consider adult depression as the result of childhood experiences that were devoid of adequate care or love, often casting the adult experience as a reliving of the childhood disillusionment with needed others and the frustration of not receiving the required nurturance from parental figures.

Even more surprising, given the theoretical reliance on an earlier depressive episode as a precursor to the adult disorder, was the uniform belief that true depression could not occur in childhood. The reasons for this prevailing opinion were that children had not as yet formed a true superego or an appropriate self-representation, both of which were held to be crucial to the intrapsychic creation of the experience of depression. In actuality, this distinction was intended to separate the melancholic disorder of adults, which was noted for its marked self-recriminations and low self-regard, from the transient dysphoric moods of children. Therefore, when the classic psychoanalytic formulations of depression,

Jules R. Bemporad • Department of Psychiatry, The New York Hospital–Cornell Medical Center, White Plains, New York 10605.
Handbook of Depression in Children and Adolescents, edited by William M. Reynolds and Hugh F. Johnston. Plenum Press, New York, 1994.

such as anger turned against the self or as the realization of a great disparity between the ego ideal and the true self, were applied to children, the theories simply did not readily fit either the clinical picture of depression or existing knowledge of the developmental capabilities of children. As Rie (1966) concluded in an early review of childhood depression, the developmental lack of a future orientation in children precluded their succumbing to hopelessness in the face of frustration; therefore, adult forms of depression could not be experienced or expressed by children. The major difficulty seemed to be that the psychodynamic models used to explain some, and usually severe, forms of adult depression were inapplicable to the immature psychic structure of children.

A possible theoretical avenue toward resolution appeared in the 1950s and 1960s with a newer and more simplified formulation of depression. In 1953, Bibring (1953) proposed a novel psychodynamic explanation of adult depression, devoid of the prior metapsychological constraints and assumptions, that could find applications to individuals of all ages. Bibring proposed that depression was the emotional counterpart of a perceived helplessness of the ego to obtain needed narcissistic supplies from the environment. When an individual was deprived of some crucial area of gratification or meaning, and was helpless to restore whatever was lost, he or she experienced a sense of ego helplessness, together with the affect of depression and a breakdown of the usual mechanisms for maintaining self-esteem. This narcissistic blow could result from the acknowledgment that some lofty aspiration for success or power was doomed to failure, or that the individual would never achieve some cherished state of self, or that one's need to be loved by an important other would remain unfulfilled. Different deprivations would affect different individuals in different ways, depending on each individual's particular need and the relationship of that need to the establishment of self-esteem. Depression, for Bibring, had a common core: the loss of self-esteem secondary to the painful awareness that one is helpless to fulfill highly important narcissistic needs. The degree to which one succumbs to helplessness may depend on one's prior history, one's ability to substitute other sources of psychic gratification, as well as external factors. Similarly, some individuals may "complicate" this basic depressive mechanism by self-reproaches or self-accusations, while others may try to defend against this painful state through denial, escape into action, or substance abuse. The key feature of Bibring's innovative approach is that by reducing the cause of depression to helplessness in the face of narcissistic deprivation, he made it theoretically possible for this affect and its concomitant clinical disorder to be applied theoretically to children and adolescents, as well as adults.

A decade after Bibring's contribution, Sandler and Joffee (1965) enlarged on Bibring's formulation and specifically utilized this newer model in the understanding of childhood depression. These authors described depression as a basic psychobiological affective reaction that arises automatically whenever an individual has lost a prior sense of well-being. Like anxiety, another fundamental negative affect, depression is seen as becoming abnormal when it persists for an undue length of time or when the child is unable to adapt to it appropriately. Sandler and Joffee agree with Bibring that the essence of depression is the feeling of having lost, or being unable to attain, something that is essential to narcissistic integrity and that coupled with this feeling is the sense of being helpless and being unable to remedy the loss. This painful state results whenever a necessary structure for maintaining a sense of well-being is lost, be it through the absence of a loved one, the frustration of some aspiration, or the curtailment of some meaningful function or activity. It is when the individual sees him or herself as helpless, impotent, and resigned in the face of deprivation that depression is experienced. However, not all individuals who experience depressed affect, as most people do at one time or another, go on to develop a clinical disorder. Most can overcome their plight through a variety of health-promoting or adaptive maneuvers, while others succumb to increasing melancholia, which further hampers return to normal functioning and feeling. The latter individuals who cannot deal successfully with the initial and normal psychobiological affective reaction collapse into the clinical disorder. Sandler and Joffee found that these more vulnerable individuals have failed to properly individuate and move beyond their early attachment to parental figures or that they hold unrealistic expectations of themselves. These authors present a two-stage model of depression in which the first step represents a ubiquitous, automatic affective reaction that is rooted in our neurobiology, while the second step represents a pathological failure to deal with the initial affective reaction. The vulnerability responsible for the progression to the second stage resides in a developmental failure to achieve autonomy and reality orientation in terms of relationships and expectations.

Sandler and Joffee's significant contribution—which formulated a practical theoretical psychodynamic model for, as well as delineated a clinical description of, childhood depression—has had relatively little impact on the current study of this disorder in a pediatric patient population. One possible reason for this neglect may be attributable to the particular time at which their article appeared. In the late 1960s, there was still a fairly uniform opinion among psychoanalysts that children could not suffer from depression because of their immature psychic structure. At that time, true depression was conceptualized as severe melancholia with predominant manifestation of self-reproaches, which were believed to display the basic mechanism of anger turned against the self. Milder depressions that did not present with blatant self-recrimination but still displayed lowered self-esteem were interpreted as due to a felt disparity between the real self and the ego ideal, a comparison beyond the psychic abilities of children.

However, just as newer theoretical approaches (such as Bibring's formulations) that were less encumbered by metapsychological presuppositions were starting to make some inroads in analytical circles, the remarkable success of monamine oxidase inhibitors (MAOIs), and, later, of tricyclic compounds, in ameliorating many symptoms of depression initiated a revolution of the manner in which this disorder was conceptualized. Many practitioners revised their ideas of the etiology of depression from being based on childhood maltreatment or loss (which was carried forward in the psyche to adult life) to one of biochemical imbalance resulting from a genetic defect. The triggering role of a precipitant was still accepted in the production of a clinical depressive episode, but the individual vulnerability to decompensation was thought to reside in the activation of a physiological defect rather than in a reliving of a childhood trauma.

This transformation in the interpretation of depressive phenomena mirrored a more universal paradigm shift from a Freudian interpretive model to a Kraepelinian empirical, descriptive approach to illness that allegedly shunned any theoretical bias. Therefore, psychiatric conditions, depression included, were reexamined in terms of strict phenomenology or presenting symptoms without assumptions as to a meaningful connection between symptoms or the supposed psychological purpose of certain symptoms. Disorders were accepted as they presented and were described in objective detail in order to permit uniformity in diagnosis with an absolute minimum of subjective interpretation.

The past few decades have witnessed a virtual explosion of research on depressive disorders from an empirical framework. There have been innumerable studies on the epidemiology of depression in order to assess its true prevalence in the population and natural clinical course, on the family medical histories of depressed individuals in the search for patterns of inheritance, on "biological markers" that could point the way to the genetic locus of a depressogenic defect by revealing a linkage to known inherited characteristics, and on biochemical processes of the nervous system usually involving neurotransmitters and their receptors.

The study of psychopathology was dominated by this "medical model" of psychiatric disorder when clinicians and researchers began to turn their attention to depressive states in children and adolescence. It is not surprising that the majority of investigations into pediatric mood disorders have reflected the current psychiatric zeitgeist and have focused on descriptive or organic aspects of these conditions. In contrast, studies looking at psychosocial factors have been few and far between, although such studies have begun to appear in recent years (see below). Throughout this shift from a psychodynamic "understanding" to a genetic "explanation" of depressive disorders in childhood, another area of disagreement has centered on the effect of a child's developmental progress on the experience and manifestation of mood disorders. It has been argued that depression, as an organic illness, has a uniform mode of expression with minimal modification regardless of age, so that diagnostic criteria for adults can be applied readily to children. Others have proposed that depression, as a psychological phenomenon, should vary in its presentation in keeping with the relative degree of overall development.

The foregoing introduction should make clear that there remain a good many unresolved issues regarding the etiology of depression as it occurs in individuals of all ages. This chapter will present those studies that consider depression as a psychological reaction to major disappointments or losses or to a chronically frustrating environment in which basic emotional needs remain frustrated. This literature will be reviewed in a developmental framework, assuming that the phenomenon of depression is modified in parallel to the increased cognitive and social capacities of the developing child.

Descriptions of Depressive States

One of the earliest clinical studies in the child psychiatry literature described the occurrence of depression-like states in infancy. In this pioneer paper, Spitz (1946) recorded the reactions of 6-month old infants after abrupt separation from their mothers. These children were described as sad, listless, weepy, and withdrawn. They also exhibited little spontaneous movement, slow reactivity to stimuli, and appetite and sleep disturbances. Spitz concluded that this reaction to separation was an infantile mood disorder, which he called "anaclitic depression," emphasizing its age-appropriate dependent qualities. The setting for Spitz's observation was a prison in which female inmates were allowed to keep their infants until the infants reached 6 months of age, at which time they were removed to a special nursery that, while apparently sanitary and medically adequate, offered minimal human contact or care. It may be of interest that in keeping with the prevalent theory of the day, Spitz attempted to explain the infants' depressive response on the basis of aggression turned against the self. He argued that these children were deprived of an external (maternal) object to absorb their innate aggressive drive and were prevented from other possible release by reduced mobility, so that they had to turn their hostility onto themselves. Others have interpreted Spitz's observations differently, stressing the children's sudden loss of the physical warmth, emotional caring, and cognitive stimulation that had been supplied by the now-absent mother and the lack of appropriate substitution following separation.

The key role of attachment and the pathological effects of separation in infancy were further elaborated by Bowlby (1960), who described a sequential process of stages of separation observed in young children. The first stage is that of protest, in which the infant is very upset and possibly attempts to summon the mother by screaming, crying, or thrashing about. If the mother does not return, the infant demonstrates the stage of despair, with silent crying, sad faces, and social withdrawal. If reunion has still not occurred, the child moves on to the state of defense or detachment, during which he or she seems to deny the separation and will relate to new adults in a friendly manner. In fact, during this last stage, the infant may ignore the mother if she reappears. Bowlby did not consider any of these stages as equal to depression, as a clinical entity, but described the stages as a universal reaction to separation. In contrast to Spitz and other psychoanalysts of his time, Bowlby (1973) conceived of the infant's attachment to the mother from an ethological point of view, stressing innate behavior sequences on the part of both mother and child that initiate and strengthen an emotional bond that forms independently of any postulated oral gratification.

It may therefore not be surprising to find that the Bowlby sequence of protest–despair–detachment has been observed among higher subhuman primates who were separated from their mothers, or from peers when raised in a group living situation (McKinney, 1988). After an initial phase of postseparation protest, infant monkeys demonstrate less physical activity, a lack of interest in their environment, decreased socialization, reduced food and water consumption, and a variety of sleep disorders. These symptoms mirror many of those found in melancholic forms of adult depression and may point to a primal, evolutionary model of all later affective disorders. The finding that drugs that increase norepinephrine levels reduce the severity of the symptoms in monkeys, while drugs that reduce the levels of this neurotransmitter exacerbate the reaction, also points to a common physiological basis for depressive affect in monkeys, infants, and adults.

However, despite these intriguing points of convergence, the phenomenon resulting from separation demonstrated by simian or human infants cannot be equated with true clinical depression. This reaction represents an innate and age-appropriate reaction to separation in an immature organism that is time-limited and, from an ethological standpoint, may serve the function of eliciting nurturance from other adult caretakers, thereby ensuring the survival of the orphaned young in a social group. This reaction does resemble depression physiologically, at least in terms of drug response, but is more like adult mourning than melancholia in most other respects.

Clayton, Herjanic, Murphy, and Woodruff (1974) compared the symptom picture of acutely bereaved and of severely depressed individuals and found important differences. The bereaved group manifested less lowered self-esteem, fewer self-recriminations, less suicidal ideation, and less psychomotor retardation. The depressed group expressed many more feelings of hopelessness and worthlessness as well as a greater loss of interest in social activities and relationships. Perhaps the interesting difference between the two groups was that the bereaved group experienced their anguish as a normal continuation of their usual psychic life, while the depressed group experienced their dysphoria as an abnormal state that was discontinuous with their usual sense of self and included a qualitative change in their relationship to their surroundings. Therefore, adult bereavement was seen as an understandable response to a major external loss that was accepted by the bereaved as an extension of their normal identity and (in time) resolved spontaneously. In these characteristics, mourning resembles those depression-like syndromes of infancy more than does adult clinical depression. At present, the infant's reaction to separation appears to be a prototype of later affective disorders and may exemplify the evolutionary and physiological foundation for adult depression but is not equal to it.

Early Childhood

Although there are some theoretical attempts to account for a possible psychodynamic structure of depression in early childhood, actual documentation of true affective disorders existing during this developmental stage is most infrequent. Poznanski and Zrull (1970) looked for evidence of depression in the charts of children who attended a psychiatric clinic for a 5-year period. Of 1788 clinic records reviewed, they could find only 1 of a child under age 5 whose symptoms were suggestive of a depressive disorder. Similar results were reported by Kashani, Ray, and Carlson (1986) in their evaluation of 100 consecutive preschoolers referred to a child development unit. Only 1 child, who was beyond the age of 6, met DSM-III criteria for major depression, and only 1 other child, also 6 years of age, could be diagnosed as suffering from a dysthymic disorder. These children, as well as 2 others, both age 4, who displayed partial dysthymic disorders, revealed other difficulties, in addition to having been raised in very disturbed home environments. Of the 4 children, 2 responded rapidly to intervention, while 1 was lost to follow-up and the other continued to be symptomatic 1 year later, but may not have received treatment. Therefore, there is some question whether these dysphoric states of young children are truly depressive disorders, in the sense of an actual illness, or whether they represent understandable reactions to a chronically frustrating environment colored by the relative immaturity of the individual.

The reactive nature of these conditions may be observed in most cases when the children return rapidly to normal functioning when the source of their distress is removed or when they are placed in situations that offer proper emotional care and stimulation. This timely recovery leads one to ask whether anything internal in the child's psyche had been altered greatly, since there may be little evidence of the prior dysphoria. No one would doubt that young children display depressive affects, but there is reason to doubt whether this mood carries with it an alteration of self-evaluations or of negative occurrence in the future.

For example, a young child [who has been reported previously (Bemporad, 1982)] was admitted to a psychiatric unit because of chronic dysphoria and suicidal threats. This girl was being raised by her great grandmother, who resented the child and felt her to be an unfair burden. The great grandmother gave the child adequate housing and nutrition, but very little in terms of emotional care. She would often leave the child at home alone at night while she went drinking with friends and would return home intoxicated, where-upon she would degrade the child, telling her how much she resented having to take care of her. On the unit, this girl quickly became cheerful and responded well to the support given to her from staff. In her doll play, she re-created her home situation by having a child doll being rebuked by a mother doll. When asked why the child doll was being scolded, the child replied that the doll had been "bad." When asked what she meant by "being bad," the child replied that she was being scolded. This circular logic was appropriate for her maturational stage, which according to Piaget (1952) is characterized by a "moral realism" indicating that actions are judged by their consequences rather than their intent. It became clear that this girl was reacting to a painful and frustrating emotional environment, but that this experience had not, as yet, affected her view of herself or of others. She was responding to her environment and was not able to reach conclusions that went beyond her immediate experience.

McConville, Boag, and Purohit (1973) also found that the expression of depressive affect varies with developmental level. In a study of 75 depressed children, they found that children of the ages between 6 and 8 manifested an almost pure state of sadness without accompanying cognitive aspects such as loss of self-esteem or guilt that typified the depressive experience of older children. Therefore, depression in young children may be qualitatively different from that in the older child, reflecting an immaturity of cognitive and social development.

As for the role of current frustration or disappointment as a prime factor in producing depressive responses in children who appear more able to rebound than do adults when put in better situations, Kazdin, Moser, Colbus, and Bell (1985) addressed this question in a study of the relationship of physical abuse and depression in a group of 79 inpatients, ages 6–13. They found a higher rate of depression among abused than among nonabused children, but only in those children who were still suffering abuse. Children with a history of past abuse scored similarly to nonabused children on measures of depression and hopelessness, but did show significantly lowered self-esteem. It is not stated whether this difference was more marked in the older children in their sample. These findings suggest that depression in younger children is not a truly self-perpetuating illness based on relatively fixed, conscious or unconscious, pessimistic evaluations of the self and others, and support the view that it is merely a situation-bound reaction.

Ultimately, the question whether transient, externally evoked episodes of dysphoria represent a depressive disorder depends on how this illness is defined. Rather than arbitrarily putting limits on the definition of depression, it might be more heuristic to conceive of depressive phenomena as varying in complexity in parallel with the overall development of the child. As Anthony (1975b) has cogently argued, depression may be best characterized as undergoing development in parallel with the child's development in symbolism, representation, language, and logical operations. For younger children, this response appears to be a rather uncomplicated reaction to continued deprivation of emotional care from parents or to an uncompensated loss of a former love object.

Middle and Late Childhood

Piaget (1952) describes the child's entry into the stage of concrete operations as the supremacy of thought over appearance. This developmental achievement entails the formation of specific schemata, or organizational concepts, through which experience is judged and interpreted. The child no longer reacts to his immediate perceptual world, but evaluates his experience according to cognitive filters. At this stage of development, the child begins to look for reasons behind events in the early attempt to make some logical sense out of the world around him or her and no longer accepts reality as a given. One of the ramifications of this transformation is that the older child responds less directly to unpleasantness in his environment and more to feelings of disappointment from within. For example, McConville et al. (1973) found that depressed children of ages 8–10 expressed a sense of low self-esteem that had been absent in the manifestations of the dysphoria of younger children.

The older child may still react with depressive affect to a situation of loss or deprivation, but in addition to an expression of direct frustration may give reasons for the unfortunate turn of events. The child may believe that he or she deserved their misfortune because of some prior misdeed or because of some alleged imperfection in himself or herself. This inner-generated dysphoria results from judgments that remain stable over time and therefore do not respond readily to alterations in the environment. Similarly, the dysphoria will be more generalized, affecting school performance or relationship with peers, in addition to behavior at home. Therefore, this is the age when depressive reactions become more stable and prolonged, even after a change in circumstances. Some researchers, such as Kovacs and Beck (1977) and Puig-Antich (1982), have decided to investigate only older children in their studies of depression, perhaps considering the dysphoria of younger children as too unstable or as too difficult to diagnose with certainty.

Most descriptions of depression in this older age group report cognitive components in addition to a dysphoric mood. Kazdin et al. (1985) found a high degree of hopelessness and low self-esteem in depressed children who were physically abused. Similarly, Kaufman (1991) reports a high prevalence of depression among a sample of 56 maltreated children (mean age 9 years, 7 months). Those maltreated who were depressed were found to be older, to have evidence of more severe physical abuse, and to have experienced more emotional deprivation, greater out-of-home placements, and fewer sources of social support. The depressed children also showed significant differences in cognitive style, attributing the outcome of positive events to external, unstable, and specific causes and attributing the outcome of negative events to internal, stable, and global qualities. This last finding, in particular, demonstrated the beginning of a mode of thought that may perpetuate the depressive reaction and underlie such associated depressive symptoms as low self-esteem or hopelessness. Kaufman (1991, p. 264) concludes that "it is not just what happens to children, but how they make sense of events that happen to them that determines their likelihood for developing a depressive disorder."

Therefore, the depressive reactions of the older child may be considered of a different magnitude and quality than those of younger children. The child is now responding to internal judgments rather than simply reacting to environmental circumstances. However, this self-generated nature of depressive reactions should not be allowed to negate the powerful influences of external events. The child reacts differently, but is still immersed in a depriving, maltreating environment. The lack of emotional warmth in the families of depressed children, the repeated separations, and the inappropriate burdens placed on these children have been noticed even by researchers who were primarily interested in biological aspects of the disorder. Puig-Antich et al. (1985) found that their sample of 52 depressed children showed greater problems in familial relationships than did neurotic or normal controls. The depressed children were more impaired in verbal and affective communication skills and were more rejected by their mothers. They were also more involved in parental conflicts, had more troubled sibling relationships, and were teased more by peers. These psychosocial difficulties were still manifest after the acute depressive episode had resolved and seemed to constitute long-standing problems of interpersonal relationships.

Difficulties in relationships had also been found in a group of older children by Poznanski and Zrull (1970) in one of the first reported clinical series on childhood depression. The 14 children described were uniformly withdrawn, often failing to make eye contact with the research interviewers. These children were also self-derogatory, feared failure, anticipated unfair treatment, and exhibited destructive and aggressive behavior. It is of interest that the depressive disorders were not immediately reactive to the loss of a loved person or a new situation, but rather appeared as part of an ongoing process in the emotional life of the child. The parents of the depressed children were often depressed themselves, but also critical of and emotionally detached from the index children. This sample of depressed children was reevaluated in adolescence (Poznanski, Krakenbuhl, & Zrull, 1976), when it was found that half were still depressed. In this subsample, the parental rejection and criticism had continued.

A sample of 12 depressed youngsters, ages 7–17, reported by Bemporad and Lee (1984) showed personality characteristics and familial relationships remarkably similar to those found by Poznanski and Zrull. All the 12 children had been under considerable emotional stress for some time, and when a precipitant could be identified, it appeared to be but the last in a series of frustrations or losses. The mothers of the depressed children gave evidence of chronic depression together with other forms of psychopathology. The fathers, when present in the household, were also depressed. The parents often used the index children as scapegoats for their own misfortunes and frequently were openly critical and rejecting. Additional characteristics found by Bemporad and Lee were that the depressed children were burdened by responsibilities beyond their years and that their behavior was strictly controlled by the parent. In contrast to nondepressed controls, the children were very involved in parental problems and appeared exploited by the parents for support and counsel. They seemed to have limited extrafamilial relationships and few independent interests to compensate for the difficulties experienced within the household. These children described a mode of familial relationship that is similar to the "affectionless control" found by Parker (1981) in his studies of childhood memories of adult depressives.

These studies characterize the depressed older child as having evolved a very low sense of self-worth secondary to chronic criticism from parents, as demonstrating social isolation and a lack of compensatory relationships due to familial control or restrictiveness, and as having assumed inappropriate emotional burdens of discontented parents and dysfunctional families. As with younger depressed children, chronic rejection by parents and their lack of warmth or empathic understanding seem to play an important role in the development of the disorder. At this stage of development, however, the child has created an intrapsychic self-image that reflects his or her prior upbringing. The child now fears failure, anticipates maltreatment, has stifled normal strivings toward autonomy or mastery, and has developed an adherence to the strict behavior demands of the parents, in direct relation either to them or to their internalized intrapsychic representations.

Adolescence

With the child's passage into adolescence, the potential for experiencing depressive feelings and true depressive illness greatly increases. In an epidemiological study of psychiatric disorders among 2000 children on the Isle of Wight, Rutter (1986) found only 3 cases of depression at age 10 but 35 cases at ages 14–15. Similarly, Kashani, Rosenberg, and Reid (1989) found the prevalence of depression in a community sample to be 4 times greater at age 17 than at ages 8 and 12. The reasons for this marked increase in affective disturbance following puberty may derive partially from external social expectations at this time of life and partially from internal maturational changes that transform the manner in which the self and the environment are phenomenologically apprehended.

In Western culture, the passage into adolescence involves the psychological abandonment of the family unit and the establishment of a new network of relationships and roles in society. The established and reliable modes of receiving affirmations of one's worth from family members or familiar teachers and friends may no longer be effective as the youngster is faced with expectations of autonomy, new forms of relational behavior toward peers and adults, and greater demands in terms of work or academic performance. These pressures for more adult-like behavior are experienced at a time when major internal changes are also occurring. The youngster achieves biological maturity and begins to experience sexual feelings and longings. While much has been made of the disruptive effects of puberty on the psychic equilibrium of the child, secondary sexual characteristics may pose a greater threat to one's self-esteem than lustful urges, particularly in the modern context of our more permissive age. Secondary sexual characteristics are especially problematic to the adolescent because these characteristics take on a public quality. The bodily transformations that accompany puberty can be seen by others and can therefore be judged by them. These physiological changes (or their retardation) may be perceived as attracting admiration (or ridicule) from others and thereby greatly influence a teenager's opinion of himself or herself. The advent of procreative capacity also brings with it the possibility of a new level of intimacy in relationships that can magnify fears of rejection, exploitation, or responsibility. Therefore, the biological maturation of the reproductive system causes immense alterations in the adolescent's psychological and social life, not only in terms of sexual feelings but also in causing marked changes in one's body and in creating a demand for new codes of interpersonal behavior.

Equally if not more radical inner changes occur in the adolescent's cognitive capacities. As is well known, this is the time that true abstract thought becomes possible, and this new potential has important ramifications in how the individual conceives of himself or herself. Piaget (1952) describes these new abilities in thought as allowing for the conceptualization of the hypothetical as well as for the actual, while simultaneously rendering a more realistic account of the world. The adolescent is now able to project the self into the future, so as to connect present actions with long-range consequences. However, while the youngster has the understanding that some present occurrence will affect his or her later life, the adolescent lacks the backlog of life experience to moderate his or her predictions. Therefore, failing an exam precludes forever the possibility of some cherished profession or being turned down for a date means certain isolation for all eternity. Everyday occurrences are automatically but erroneously generalized, with a magnification of importance and affective response. The expansion of cognitive abilities also prevents the adolescent from utilizing childhood denial to obliterate or nullify the painful affects that are part of a truthful acceptance of one's limitations. Easson (1977,

p. 262) has described this process as a time when "the dreams, hopes, fantasies, and fears all meet reality," which normally and naturally brings on a state of sadness and mourning.

The coincidence of these major internal transformations with the social expectations of greater emancipation, self-regulation, and responsibility helps to explain the ubiquity of mood swings during adolescence. Happily, while profound, these mood swings are short-lived as the adolescent rebounds between despair and euphoria. A recent study by Csikszentmihalyi and Larson (1984), in which adolescents reported their activities, thoughts, and feelings at random intervals, indicated that they were less stable in terms of a continuous baseline of feeling than are adults. The adolescents were more likely to experience a euphoria during which they perceived the world as perfect, and utter despair secondary to unexpected events. These extremes passed rapidly and alternated with each other, in contrast to the more constant mood state of adults.

Among psychoanalysts, Jacobson (1961) has interpreted these adolescent mood swings as manifesting the pressures of the id and superego at different times on an ego that is weakened by the pressure for adaptive challenges. She views these emotional highs and lows as a necessary part of the transition from childhood to adult life during which a new sense of self is gradually created. Along the way, the individual may be under the sway of a replenished id, and so act out impulses without restraint, or of a still tyrannical superego, causing a massive sense of shame and guilt. With increasing experience, the ego gains greater mastery over its environment and can better deal with these intrapsychic pressures. Therefore, most if not all adolescents can be expected to go through transient dysphoric states as they establish reliable avenues of esteem and worth to replace those childhood sources of narcissistic supplies that have been relinquished.

These passing interludes of dysphoria, while at times filled with an anxious sense of urgency for relief or with the darkest existential despair, should not be taken as true depressive disorders (although these disorders should not be simply ignored either). As mentioned above, such states have a relatively benign course and transpire on their own as the individual discovers new sources of esteem or realigns his or her goals as part of the gradual acceptance of oneself that defines the growth to the maturity of adult status. However, true depressive disorders do occur as well and at times may be difficult to distinguish from the more frequent transient mood states. Anthony (1975a) has noted this difficulty in assessment, recommending a careful consideration of the patient's past history as a possible aid to diagnosis. Anthony argues that youngsters with true depressive disorders will have demonstrated prior difficulties, leaving them more vulnerable to the usual emotional blows encountered in vicissitudes of everyday adolescent life. Anthony further suggests that these more serious depressions often occur after minimal provocation, while the transient depressive reactions are in response to a major environmental precipitant. These clinical observations imply that true and severe depressive disorders during adolescence occur in those individuals who are especially vulnerable on the bases of a poor premorbid level of adaptation and of a weakened psychological state that can be disrupted by minor losses or disappointments. These more impaired individuals do not recover rapidly and, if untreated, may go on to develop chronic and severe affective disorders. In such cases, the loss of a relationship, social status, or anticipated achievement that previously protected the individual against a dreaded, and not uncommonly hated, sense of self leaves the individual with decreased ability to regain an adequate sense of worth (Bemporad 1988). Deprived of narcissistic supplies on which an inordinate amount of self-worth depended, the youngster is crippled by his or her own psychological limitations from instituting new activities that might compensate for his or her deprivation. The individual collapses psychologically when deprived of the narcissistic props that had previously maintained a fragile sense of self-regard.

These more severe depressive episodes take on two major clinical and psycho-dynamic forms, which Anthony has described as relating to different developmental stages.

The earlier, preoedipal type, which corresponds in adults to the anaclitic type of Blatt (1974) or the self-claiming type of Arieti (1962), is characterized by a continuing symbiotic tie to a mother figure. The second, more oedipal type, which corresponds in adults to the introjective type of Blatt (1974) and the self-blaming type of Arieti (1962) is associated with a great deal of guilt stemming from a severe superego.

These two clinical types also may be considered in terms of their ability to master the psychological requirements of adolescence. The "preoedipal" or "anaclitic" form of depression seems to typify those youngsters whose prior development has not prepared them sufficiently to deal with the demands of life outside the family orbit. These adolescents appear to have failed in the developmental tasks of latency, if one assumes those tasks to include the de-idealization of the parents and a shift of psychological interest to peers and extrafamilial adults, the derivation of mastery and enjoyment through autonomous activities, and a sense of connectedness to one's society. The adolescents prone to anaclitic depression continue to rely excessively on their nuclear families for comfort or esteem and are not comfortable in the culture of their peers. They are simply not ready for the biological and cognitive changes that are transpiring in their bodies and minds. Nor are they prepared to meet the new expectations for self-reliance or the choices that are inherent in the greater autonomy offered to adolescents. This developmental stasis is usually the result of subtle sabotaging, by the parents, of the youngsters' budding drive toward freedom and extrafamilial allegiances during late childhood. Often, the families are quite dysfunctional, and the child is so involved in the parental arguments or turmoil that he or she is cheated of the opportunity to progress normally through latency and establish a solid psychological foothold outside the family orbit. These youngsters are overwhelmed at having to act on their own, at having to make their own decisions, and at existing without the familiar structure of their home environment. In addition to depressed mood, they exhibit anxiety, bewilderment, and shame as they perceive that they are not up to the demands that constantly confront the self. These youngsters may be drawn to becoming members of cults or fall prey to a charismatic leader in their search for a parental substitute who can structure their lives and relieve them of the burden of individuation.

The introjective form of depression occurs in adolescents who are able to separate from home and function independently but who carry unrealistic aspirations or restrictions within their psyches. These unconscious systems of shoulds were gradually internalized during childhood and by adolescence have become an inherent stable part of the estimation of oneself. These youngsters are threatened by the freedom allowed them as they encounter a peer group or school society whose values are quite different from their own. They are equally disturbed by the cognitive changes that permit them to question familial prohibitions and standards and by the normal erotic desires that accompany puberty. They find it difficult to reconcile their nascent impulses and thoughts with the social role and modes of conduct that were reinforced during childhood. More often, these youngsters cannot tolerate the reevaluation of their abilities that is forced on them as they strive for greater achievement against stiffer competition. A not atypical circumstance for this form of depression occurs when a youngster had performed so well as to be admitted to a prestigious university or prep school, or chosen as a member of a top-ranked athletic team, only to find that he or she no longer stands out since his new school or teammates are equal, if not superior, in their ability.

These youngsters find they cannot live up to their internalized standards, and this realization leads to a pervasive sense of failure and a loss of interest in most activities. This form of depression usually presents with guilt, inhibition, anhedonia, and, not uncommonly, suicidal ideation. Hendin (1975) described this type of individual in his study of college students who had attempted suicide. He found that his subjects were still tied to their parents in an emotional knot that precluded any pleasure or freedom. They had to continue to live out the parental dictates in terms of moral conduct or personal achievement. When confronted with a more relaxed, hedonistic, and liberated life-style, they found themselves in an escapable dilemma: To join in with their peers meant to suffer the guilt of betraying their family values, yet to continue to live out their internalized prohibitions now meant to live a barren, inauthentic existence. According to Hendin, suicide became a means of escape from this conflict.

These two forms of depression share an inability to transcend a childhood sense of self so as to master the new and complex developmental tasks of adolescence. This older sense of self cannot adapt to the changes that occur in the individual's mind and body or to those that transpire in his or her environment. In this sense, adolescent depression is not dissimilar from adult mood disorders in being caused by atavistic remnants of childhood that no longer apply to one's stage of development.

Conclusion

In the foregoing presentation, the formulation of depression by Bibring (1953) as resulting from the uncompensated deprivation of narcissistic needs has been applied to the sequence of developmental stages. The source of narcissistic gratification varies with the differing psychological maturation of the child throughout ontogeny. During infancy, the mother satisfies most, if not all, of the child's needs for security, bodily comfort, and emotional communication. Her loss deprives the infant of a whole host of necessary gratifications and results in the lack of crucial stimulation and protection required for normal growth. The young child reacts with almost a pure feeling state of sadness to chronic maltreatment or disapproval from parental figures. At this stage, the child reacts directly to his or her environment, so that the dysphoric response is in direct relationship to environmental circumstances. As the child matures, the environment still impacts greatly on his or her psychic life, but more as the result of inner cognitive conclusions by the child than as an immediate response to the situation at hand.

Therefore, in the older child, inability to meet parental expectations, negative appraisals by others, or failure of some valued aspiration can elicit a more persistent state of depression that includes cognitive elements such as low self-esteem in addition to alterations in mood. Finally, adolescence puts its own distinctive stamp on the precipitation and manifestation of depressive states. At this developmental stage, the prime causes of depression are a self-perceived failure to live up to one's aspiration for autonomy, achievement, or particular codes of conduct. By now, the values of the past have been internalized, resulting in the failure to meet developmental tasks being experienced as a failure to meet one's own standards. This sequence of symptoms, psychodynamics, and precipitants of depression at the various steps in development is presented in Table 1. At the extreme right are listed stages of ego development, corresponding to each form of depression, as distilled by Loevinger (1976) from the literature on ego psychology. Therefore, each developmental form of depression may be seen in the context of the overall normal development of the child.

While the delineation of stage-specific reactions may be helpful in organizing the conceptualization of depression as dependent for its characteristic on the maturational level of the child, such a delineation must ultimately be considered a distortion. Development is a fluid process that is not readily captured by static pictures of stable stages. The attempt to ascribe causes for child psychopathology to one event at one specific stage rather than to the long-term sequelae of that event throughout the maturational years is usually incorrect and misleading. This is certainly the case for depressive disorders that result from prolonged deprivations and maltreatment that are gradually integrated in the child's psychological development.

This role of chronicity of traumata for later pathogenicity has been portrayed

Table 1. Symptoms and Causes of Depression at Various Stages of Development

Developmental stage	Symptoms	Major psychodynamics	Type of dysphoria	Loevinger ego development stages
Infancy	Withdrawal after crying and protest	Loss of stimulation, security, and well-being supplied by the mother	Deprivation of needed stimulation	Presocial, symbiotic
Early childhood	Inhibition, clinging behavior	Disapproval by parents	Inhibition of gratification of emerging sense of will	Impulsive, self-protective, fear of being caught, externalizing blame, opportunistic
Middle childhood	Sadness as automatically responsive to the immediate situation	Rejection by parents, loss of gratifying activities (i.e., chronic illness)	Sadness, unsustained crying directly related to frustrating or depriving situation	Conformist: conformity to external rules, shame and guilt for breaking rules, superficial niceness
Late childhood	Depression with low self-esteem	Unable to meet parental ideal, unable to sustain threat to parental relationship	Depression with a cognitive component in terms of affect resulting from deduction about circumstances	Conscientious: conformist, differentiation of norms and goals, awareness of self in relation to group, helping
Adolescence	Depression with exaggerated urgency, time distortion, and impulsivity	Unable to fulfill internalized parental ideal, unable to separate from family	Accentuation of depression by cognitive distortions about the finality of events	Conscientious: self-evaluated standards, guilt for consequences, long-term goals and ideals

Source: Reprinted by permission from *Psychiatry* 1982: *The American Psychiatric Association Annual Review*, Vol. 1, edited by L. Grinspoon. Copyright 1982 American Psychiatric Press. Originally adapted from J. Loevinger, 1976, *Ego development*. San Francisco: Jossey-Bass.

admirably by Brown, Harris, and Bifulco (1986) in their studies on the relationship of childhood loss to adult depression. They studied a group of women who had all lost their mothers (through death or other separation) in childhood, but only half of whom had suffered a depressive episode. It was found that the postloss lives of those women who had become depressed differed markedly from those of depression-free individuals. Those women who later became depressed described their having been sent away to institutions or to unwelcoming relatives after maternal separation. These environments were so devoid of care that these women sought to escape their circumstances through marriage precipitated by early pregnancy. As a result, they often found themselves, as young adults, locked in an unhappy marriage with an unsuitable spouse, burdened by numerous young children at home, and unable to procure employment due to their failure to obtain vocational training or an adequate education. In contrast, the nondepressed women were largely able to remain at home following maternal loss and did not find themselves in situations of emotional deprivation that prompted escape by early motherhood and marriage. These women were able to finish school, find more suitable spouses, and experience parenthood at a more judicious age. Therefore, the depressed group may have become vulnerable to affective disorders by becoming trapped by a combination of external limitations on a satisfying way of life. While these real-life obstacles undoubtedly played a part in pathogenesis, they do not describe the internal attitudes and self-perceptions of the two groups of women. Those with postloss lack of care experiences developed a sense of hopelessness early in their lives. They felt themselves to be burdens to others and failed to solidify stable esteem-building resources. These personality characteristics enhanced their later vulnerability to succumb to depression following provocation.

One salient contribution of this work is that depression results from chronic emotional maltreatment that affects the individual's inner life and external circumstances. This formulation is most applicable to those depressions of childhood in which the individual is faced with a chronic deprivation of urgently needed warmth, concern, or approval and is deprived by circumstances he or she cannot control of the benefit of compensatory experiences. As the child matures, he or she will eventually adapt to such situations by lowered self-regard, a pervasive sense of hopelessness, and an inability to maintain self-worth separate from external sources, resulting in a greater vulnerability to, if not a chronic state of, depression.

References

Anthony, E. J. (1975a). Two contrasting types of adolescent depression and their treatment. In E. J. Anthony & T. Benedek (Eds.), *Depression and human existence* (pp. 445–460). Boston: Little, Brown.

Anthony, E. J. (1975b). Childhood depression. In E. J. Anthony & T. Benedek (Eds.), *Depression and human existence* (pp. 231–277). Boston: Little, Brown.

Arieti, S. (1962). The psychotherapeutic approach to depression. *American Journal of Psychotherapy, 16,* 397–406.

Bemporad, J. R. (1982). Childhood depression from a developmental perspective. In L. Grinspoon (Ed.), *Annual review of psychiatry,* Vol. 1 (pp. 272–280). Washington, DC: American Psychiatric Press.

Bemporad, J. R. (1988). Psychodynamic treatment of depressed adolescents. *Journal of Clinical Psychiatry, 49(Supplement),* 26–31.

Bemporad, J. R., & Lee, K. W. (1984). Developmental and psychodynamic aspects of childhood depression. *Child Psychiatry and Human Development, 14,* 145–157.

Bibring, E. (1953). The mechanism of depression. In P. Greenacre (Ed.), *Affective disorders* (pp. 13–48). New York: International Universities Press.

Blatt, S. J. (1974). Levels of object representation in anaclitic and introjective depression. *Psychoanalytic Study of the Child, 29,* 107–158.

Bowlby, J. (1958). *Attachment and Loss, Vol. 2, Anxiety and Anger.* London: Hogarth.

Bowlby, J. (1960). Grief and mourning in infancy and early childhood. *Psychoanalytic Study of the Child*, *15*, 9–52.

Brown, G., Harris, T., & Bifulco, A. (1986). Long-term effects of early loss of parent. In M. Rutter, C. Izard, & P. Read (Eds.), *Depression in young people* (pp. 251–296). New York: Guilford Press.

Clayton, P. J., & Merjanic, & Murphy, G. R. (1979). Mourning and depression: Their similarities and differences. *Canadian Journal of Psychiatry*, *19*, 309–312.

Csikszentmihalyi, M., & Larson, R. (1984). *Being adolescent*. New York: Basic Books.

Easson, W. H. (1977). Depression in adolescence. In S. C. Feinstein & P. Giovacchini (Eds.), *Adolescent psychiatry*, Vol. 5 (pp. 257–275). New York: Aronson.

Hendin, H. (1975). Growing up dead: Student suicide. *American Journal of Psychotherapy*, *29*, 327–338.

Jacobson, E. (1961). Adolescent moods and the remodeling of psychic structures in adolescence. *Psychoanalytic Study of the Child*, *16*, 164–183.

Kashani, J. H., Ray, J. S., & Carlson, G. A. (1986). Depression and depressive-like states in preschool age children in a child development unit. *American Journal of Psychiatry*, *141*, 1397–1402.

Kashani, J. H., Rosenberg, T. K., & Reid, J. C. (1989). Developmental perspectives in child and adolescent depressive symptoms in a community sample. *American Journal of Psychiatry*, *146*, 871–876.

Kaufman, J. (1991). Depressive disorders in maltreated children. *Journal of the American Academy of Child and Adolescent Psychiatry*, *30*, 257–265.

Kazdin, A., Moser, J., Colbus, D., & Bell, R. (1985). Depressive symptoms among physically abused and psychiatrically disturbed children. *Journal of Abnormal Psychology*, *94*, 298–307.

Kovacs, M., & Beck, A. T. (1977). An empirical–clinical approach toward a definition of childhood depression. In J. G. Schulterbrandt & A. Raskin (Eds.), *Depression in childhood* (pp. 1–26). New York: Raven Press.

Loevinger, J. (1976). *Ego development*. San Francisco: Jossey-Bass.

McConville, B., Boag, L., & Purohit, A. (1973). Three types of childhood depression. *Canadian Psychiatric Association Journal*, *18*, 133–138.

McKinney, W. (1988). Animal models for depression. In A. Georgotas & R. Cancro (Eds.), *Depression and mania* (pp. 181–196). New York: Elsevier.

Parker G. (1981). Parental reports of depressives. *Journal of Affective Disorders*, *3*, 131–140.

Piaget, J. (1952). *The origins of intelligence in childhood*. New York: International Universities Press.

Poznanski, E. O., Krahenbuhl, V., & Zrull, P. (1976). Childhood depression: A longitudinal perspective. *Journal of the American Academy of Child Psychiatry*, *15*, 491–501.

Poznanski, E. O., & Zrull, P. (1970). Childhood depression. *Archives of General Psychiatry*, *239*, 8–15.

Puig-Antich, J. (1982). Psychobiological correlates of major depressive disorder in children and adolescents. In L. Grinspoon (Ed.), *Annual review of psychiatry*, Vol. 1 (pp. 288–296). Washington, DC: American Psychiatric Press.

Puig-Antich, J., Lukens, E., Davies, M., Goetz, D., Brennan-Quattrock, J., & Todak, G. (1985). Psychosocial functioning in prepubertal major depressive disorders. *Archives of General Psychiatry*, *42*, 500–507, 511–517.

Rie, H. E. (1966). Depression in childhood: A survey of some pertinent contributions. *Journal of the American Academy of Child Psychiatry*, *5*, 653–685.

Rutter, M. (1986). The developmental psychopathology of depression. In M. Rutter, C. E. Izard, & P. B. Read (Eds.), *Depression in young people* (pp. 3–32). New York: Guilford Press.

Sandler, J., & Jaffee, N. G. (1965). Notes on childhood depression. *International Journal of Psychoanalysis*, *46*, 88–96.

Spitz, R. (1946). Anaclitic depression. *Psychoanalytic Study of the Child*, *5*, 113–117.

6

Cognitive and Behavioral Correlates of Childhood Depression

A Developmental Perspective

Nadine J. Kaslow, Ronald T. Brown, and Laura L. Mee

Cognitive–behavioral models have received widespread attention pertaining to the etiology, symptom display, and treatment of depressed children and adolescents. This chapter addresses the myriad cognitive–behavioral perspectives relevant to depression in youth. This work is integrated with principles from developmental psychology. A developmental perspective for conceptualizing the cognitive and behavioral functioning of children necessitates understanding children as organisms who are different from adults rather than deficient relative to adults, and viewing children's behavior in the context in which it is embedded. The incorporation of notions from developmental psychology within a cognitive–behavioral framework enhances our understanding of the development of competencies and deficits as manifested in depressed youth of different ages.

This chapter begins with a discussion of the major cognitive and behavioral theories of adult depression that during the past decade have been applied to the study of children. The most influential cognitive and behavioral theories of depression are the social-skills and activity-level perspective of Lewinsohn (1974), the cognitive model of Beck (1967, 1976), the twice-revised learned-helplessness theory (Seligman, 1975; Abramson, Seligman, & Teasdale, 1978; Abramson, Metalsky, & Alloy, 1989), and the self-control model of Rehm (1977). The discussion of these models is followed by a comprehensive review of the research in the childhood depression literature relevant to key cognitive and behavioral variables. To aid in understanding these research findings within a developmental framework, a brief overview of pertinent developmental literature is presented.

Nadine J. Kaslow, Ronald T. Brown, and Laura L. Mee • Department of Psychiatry and Behavioral Sciences, Emory University School of Medicine, Atlanta, Georgia 30322.

Handbook of Depression in Children and Adolescents, edited by William M. Reynolds and Hugh F. Johnston. Plenum Press, New York, 1994.

We concur with developmental psychopathologists who assert that children from diverse familial and cultural environments, with varying biological endowments, manifest depressive symptoms in age-appropriate ways (Cicchetti & Schneider-Rosen, 1986). This approach highlights the interplay among advances and lags in cognitive, social, emotional, and neurobiological systems for the developing child. The developmental psychopathology model describes the link among attachments with caretakers, negative cognitive schemata, difficulties with the modulation of negative affect, and the development of depressive symptoms (Cicchetti & Schneider-Rosen, 1986; P. M. Cole & Kaslow, 1988; Kaslow, Celano, & McCarthy, 1994). We deem such a model useful in conceptualizing the interaction between the depressed youth and the environment and the individual competencies and environmental resources associated with resiliency in overcoming depression. Given that other chapters in this handbook devote their attention to developmental psychopathology, affect regulation, and interpersonal processes, the primary aim of this chapter is to focus on cognitive and behavioral processes associated with childhood depression. It is recognized, however, that these constructs are embedded in the broader framework of developmental psychopathology (Lewis & Miller, 1990).

Cognitive–Behavioral Models of Depression

Behavioral Model

The social-skills and activity-level model of Lewinsohn (1974) has its origins in operant psychology. According to this perspective, depressed persons receive insufficient positive reinforcement from significant others due to the depressives' inadequate social skills for eliciting positive interpersonal responses. These social-skill deficits are viewed as causative in eliciting a depressogenic pattern of reinforcement. Depressed individuals are often less adept at reinforcing others, further diminishing the rate of reciprocal social reinforcement. Further, depressed individuals engage in too few activities and have difficulties experiencing activities as pleasurable. This low activity level combined with difficulty in experiencing pleasure without inhibitory anxiety exacerbates one's depressive state.

Cognitive Model

The cognitive model of Beck (1967, 1976) posits the existence of schemata through which individuals filter and interpret their experience. These schemata are influenced by the person's developmental history prior to the onset of psychological stress. Individuals prone to depression develop distorting negative schemata that often remain latent until activated by stressful situations. When activated, the negative cognitive triad is evident. This cognitive triad is characterized by a negative view of the self, the world, and the future. The negative view of the self is manifested in low self-esteem, a negative self-evaluation, increased self-criticism, and an underestimation of one's abilities. A negative view of the world is evidenced in a depressed individual's propensity to provide negatively biased explanations for situations that he or she encounters and for world events. A negative view of the future is associated with the development of hopelessness, a negative expectation for the future. According to Beck, depressed individuals also evidence cognitive distortions that are systematic errors in reasoning. These dysfunctional beliefs, attitudes, and assumptions are internal regulators of behavior as they override common sense and realistic responses. The systematic cognitive errors associated with depression include arbitrary influence, selective abstraction, personalization, and absolutistic, dichotomous thinking. It is important to note that there is research suggesting that individuals in whom depression is diagnosed may not actually distort information, but rather may perceive reality in a more realistic, albeit depressing, manner (Alloy & Abramson, 1979; Coyne & Gotlib, 1983). As Alloy and Abramson (1979) have noted, depressives may be "sadder but wiser."

Learned-Helplessness Model

In 1975, Seligman (1975) proposed the original learned-helpless model based on empirical investigations with laboratory animals and work with depressed patients. According to the original learned-helplessness model, individuals become helpless and depressed when they perceive events in their environment as uncontrollable and when they hold a belief in response–outcome independence. Simply stated, learned helplessness occurs when one "gives up" because one believes that one's behavior cannot influence the environment. When an individual learns that outcomes are uncontrollable, he or she becomes depressed, exhibits diminished self-esteem, and evidences cognitive and motivational deficits that impair problem-solving abilities.

After several years of empirical investigations with humans (for a review, see Garber & Seligman, 1980), the model was revised and the attributional reformulation of learned helplessness was proposed (Abramson et al., 1978). Central to this model is the construct of attributions or explanatory style. Explanatory style, the manner in which a person explains the causes of positive and negative events, is the cognitive process by which learned helplessness is modulated. According to this model, the causal attributions people make for life events, particularly negative life events, and the degree of importance attached to them contribute to the development of expectations of hopelessness and depressive symptoms. Individuals whose explanatory style is characterized by internal, stable, and global attributions for negative outcomes are at greater risk for developing depressive symptoms in response to negative events. These individuals are likely to blame themselves for the negative event (internal) and to view the cause of the event as stable over time (stable) and generalizable across situations (global). The opposite style, external–unstable–specific attributions for positive events, is also characteristic of the depressive's cognitions.

More recently, the learned-helplessness model has been revised further and presented as the hopelessness theory of depression (Abramson et al., 1989). In this revision, the diathesis–stress component of the theory is underscored. Specifically, attributional style (the diathesis) serves as a mediator between perceived negative life events (stress) and depression. Explanatory style is considered a distal contributory cause, and the hopelessness belief is the proximal, sufficient cause of a depression.

Self-Control Model

The self-control model of depression of Rehm (1977) is derived from the more general self-control theory of Kanfer (1970) that described the adaptive processes of self-monitoring, self-evaluation, and self-reinforcement. Depressed individuals are believed to have deficits in one or more specific self-control behaviors. In terms of self-monitoring, depressives selectively attend to negative events to the exclusion of positive events, and they frequently monitor immediate as opposed to delayed consequences of behavior. Deficits in self-evaluation refer to the setting of overly stringent self-evaluative criteria and the failure to make adaptive causal attributions. Depressives' deficits in self-reinforcement are their tendency to provide insufficient contingent positive self-reinforcement and excessive self-punishment.

Summary of Cognitive–Behavioral Models

Despite their unique characteristics, there is considerable overlap among the theories reviewed above. Central constructs among the theories include: contingency reinforcement (social skills, activity level), information-processing (self-schemata, cognitive distortions), view of self (self-evaluation, perceived competence), hopelessness, learned helplessness (instrumental responding, locus of control, attributional style), and self-control. Rehm (1988) asserted that these constructs can be viewed collectively as ways in which individuals process their experience to draw inferences and judgments, which are then used as a basis for problem-solving and decisions regarding future actions. The following section will provide a review of the literature pertaining to the relevance of each of these constructs to the expression of depression in children and adolescents.

Cognitive–Behavioral Models and Depression in Children and Adolescents

Contingent Reinforcement: Social Skills and Activity Level

Children are social beings from birth onward (Stern, 1985). Their social behavior is a reflection of their inherent temperament, the social behavior modeled by their caretakers, the responses they receive for their social interactions from significant others, and the socialization influences on the developmental course of their affective expression (Garber & Kashani, 1991; Lewis & Saarni, 1985; Thomas & Chess, 1977). Children whose individual characteristics and interpersonal environment enable them to achieve normal social development evidence competent interpersonal responding (Dodge, 1986), the capacity for perspective-taking, and empathy for other's affective experiences (Selman, 1980).

There are few empirical studies specifically addressing social skills in depressed youth. However, it has been found that parent- and self-reported social-skills deficits are significantly related to youths' current levels of depression and predictive of future levels of depressive symptomatology (Wierzbicki & McCabe, 1988). This finding provides some evidence for Lewinsohn's social-skills deficit model of depression in children.

The model proposed by Lewinsohn postulates that one manifestation of social-skills deficits is decreased pleasant-activity level. Although depressed adolescents do not report engaging in fewer pleasant activities than nondepressed adolescents, adolescents who rate themselves as depressed endorse engaging in more unpleasant activities (Carey, Kelley, Buss, & Scott, 1986). In a study that examined the daily states and time-use patterns of youths, no differences were found between youths high and low on a self-report measure of depressive symptoms in terms of any daily activities, with the exception of sports (Larson, Rafaelli, Richards, Ham, & Jewell, 1990). This study is of particular importance due to the ecological validity of the methodology employed.

Given the paucity of research pertaining to social skills and activity level, the literature regarding the interpersonal functioning of depressed children and adolescents merits attention. Depressed youths display deficits in social functioning with their parents, siblings, and peers (Altmann & Gotlib, 1988; Blechman, McEnroe, Carella, & Audette, 1986; John, Gammon, Prusoff, & Warner, 1987; Kazdin, Esveldt-Dawson, Sherick, & Colbus, 1985; Puig-Antich et al., 1985a; Sacco & Graves, 1984). These findings have been replicated when the reports of the child's depression status are derived from the child or from peer nominations (Blechman et al., 1986). Moreover, children with concurrent depressive and externalizing disorders (e.g., conduct, attention-deficit disorders) are more rejected and manifest less socially competent behavior than do inpatient youths diagnosed with depression only (Asarnow, 1988).

Compared to their nondepressed counterparts, depressed elementary school children are rated by peers and adults as less likeable and attractive, as emitting fewer positive behaviors, and as being in greater need of psychotherapy (Mullins, Peterson, Wonderlich, & Reaven, 1986; Peterson, Mullins, & Ridley-Johnson, 1985). Depressed youths experience others as less friendly, often report wanting to be alone, and spend less time in public places and more time in their bedrooms (Larson et al., 1990). Depressed males spend less time with their peers than do nondepressed males, suggesting that social isolation may be more characteristic of boys than of girls with depression (Larson et al., 1990). Interestingly, depressed youths who have interpersonal deficits are less satisfied with their performance and perceive themselves as less socially competent (e.g., Altmann & Gotlib, 1988; Fauber, Forehand, Long, Burke, & Faust, 1987; Faust, Baum & Forehand, 1985; Sacco & Graves, 1984). In fact, some of these interpersonal deficits persist even on remission from a depressive episode (Puig-Antich et al., 1985b).

Social problem-solving skills are potential mediators of psychopathology. Despite findings of social problem-solving deficits in depressed adults and interpersonal difficulties in depressed youths, there is little evidence for a relationship between depression and interpersonal problem-solving abilities in children and adolescents (Joffe, Dobson, Fine, Marriage, & Haley, 1990; Mullins, Siegel, & Hodges, 1985; Rotheram-Borus, Trautman, Dopkins, & Shrout, 1990; Siegel & Griffin, 1984). It appears that deficits in problem-solving skills are primarily characteristic of suicidal youngsters (Rotherman-Borus et al., 1990) and youngsters with externalizing disorders (Joffe et al., 1990).

Future research devoted to the specific nature and course of depressed children's interpersonal interactions with peers, family, and authority figures is warranted. Given that impairments in interpersonal functioning appear ubiquitous in youths who evidence a range of emotional and behavioral disorders, Kovacs (1989) has called for an examination of the unique characteristics of the social skills of depressed children. It may be particularly fruitful for this work to focus on interpersonal communications via-à-vis affective states. Given that depression may reflect a failure to utilize adaptive cognitive, behavioral, and interpersonal strategies in modulating sad affect (P. M. Cole & Kaslow, 1988; Garber & Kashani, 1991), it behooves future investigators to examine these children's ability to gain awareness about their own affective states, recognize emotions in others, and develop an understanding of the interpersonal consequences of their own emotional behavior (Fuchs & Thelen, 1988). Research with normally developing children has begun to assess empirically the development of awareness of others' affective states as well as awareness of one's own affective state, with a particular focus on sadness (Glasberg & Aboud, 1981) and rejection (Barden, Garber, Leiman, Ford, & Masters, 1985). Similar paradigms may be used to study emotional awareness of self and others in clinically depressed children. Additionally, there is a need for future research that examines from a developmental perspective depressed children's interpersonal competence as reflected in their social information-processing and their capacity to empathize with other's affective states.

Information-Processing

Self-Schema. Information-processing theory underscores the importance of the self-as-schema model. The self-schema has been defined as the body of knowledge stored in long-term memory that facilitates and biases the encoding and recall of personally relevant information. Research with depressed adults reveals self-schemata that contain primarily negative content. It has been suggested that the activation of these negative self-schemata and associated dysfunctional attitudes are underlying vulnerabilities that if triggered will activate depressive cognitive sets leading to the emergence of the affective, motivational, and vegetative symptoms of depression.

Data from developmental psychology reveal that the capacity to encode with respect to the self increases with age, with this capacity emerging during the elementary school years. The solidification of this cognitive capacity occurs at the commencement of adolescence. Thus, children as young as 8 years of age can differentiate judgments regarding their own characteristics. These self-descriptions can be stored in memory in a fashion consistent with organized schemata. Children of elementary school age evidence superior recall of self-descriptive adjectives when utilizing self-reference instructions as opposed to semantic or structural orienting instructions.

Only recently have researchers utilized information-processing paradigms to test the self-schema model of depression in children. Hammen and Zupan (1984) compared, on an incidental recall task of self-descriptive traits, normal schoolchildren who scored high on the Children's Depression Inventory (CDI) with those who scored low on the CDI. As predicted, children who scored low on the CDI (nondepressed) recalled more positive self-descriptive traits, but not negative ones. Thus, they exhibited mood-congruent, content-specific recall. Rather than recalling more negative self-descriptive traits than structurally encoded traits as was predicted, the high scorers on the CDI (depressed) recalled approximately equal numbers of negative and positive self-referential traits. Hammen and Zupan propose two explanations for their findings. First, it may be that the high scorers on the CDI did not have a sufficient depressive history to develop a consistent negative-content self-schema. Alternatively, the children in the study, while high scorers on the CDI, may not have been clinically depressed or sufficiently depressed to evidence the mood-congruent, content-specific recall effects.

Utilizing a methodology in which schoolchildren high or low on self-reported depressive symptoms were compared on recall of words from a word-association task, Whitman and Leitenberg (1990) found that compared to nondepressed children, children with depressive symptoms were less accurate in their recall of words previously answered correctly and remembered fewer of their own correct responses. Additionally, these depressed children performed more poorly than their nondepressed counterparts when asked to recall the correct answers. Despite these between-group differences, the two groups of children did not differ on their recall of previously incorrect words.

Two related studies, also conducted by Hammen and colleagues, deserve mention. These studies compared the self-schemata of children at high risk for depression on the basis of having a depressed mother with those of children at relatively low risk for depression. In testing the cognitive vulnerability hypothesis, Zupan, Hammen, and Jaenicke (1987) found that 60% of the children of depressed mothers had a history of recent or current mood disorder. Although the depressed youth who had depressed mothers recalled more of the negative self-referent words than structurally encoded words in one study (Zupan et al., 1987), these findings were not replicated in another study (Jaenicke et al., 1987). In both studies, however, the depressed children failed to demonstrate the predicted effect for positive self-descriptive adjectives. Neither positive nor negative self-schemata were correlated with the duration of the children's depressive episodes or with the history of prior depressions (Zupan et al., 1987). Further, the low-risk children manifested stronger positive self-schemata in both studies (Jaenicke et al., 1987; Zupan et al., 1987). The results of these studies suggest that maternal factors may contribute to the development of self-schemata. Specifically, maternal depression, high levels of stress, and criticism of the child are associated with the development of a less positive self-schema in children (Jaenicke et al., 1987).

Taken together, these studies provide only minimal support for the notion that depressed children have a less positive self-schema or a more negative self-schema than do nondepressed youth. More data need to be gathered before the applicability of negative self-schema to depressed children can be ascertained. The specificity regarding the relationship between negative self-schema and depression in children has not been addressed. Thus, it is unclear whether or not the aforementioned findings are pertinent to troubled children in general or unique to depressed youth. Additionally, it remains to be demonstrated whether or not the results obtained thus far are indicative of impairments in the encoding process, the retrieval process, or both. Further, there is minimal information regarding the effects of age and gender on the information-processing strategies of depressed youths.

Cognitive Distortions. Cognitive distortions, misperceptions through which individuals process incoming information regarding themselves, the environment, and their future (Ingram & Kendall, 1987), are based on previous experiences. Negative cognitive distortions, the tendency to misconstrue information in a manner consistent with a negative view of the self, the world, and the future, play a central role in the development and maintenance of depression (Beck, 1967). Empirical investigations with adults have yielded findings consistent with the postulations formulated by Beck's cognitive theory. These studies have revealed that depressed adults report significantly more negatively distorted cognitions on self-report measures than do their nondepressed counterparts.

The burgeoning research examining cognitive distortions in children has yielded similar findings. Haley, Fine, Marriage, Moretti, and Freeman (1985) conducted a study to determine the relationship between cognitive distortion and depression in a sample of inpatient and outpatient children and adolescents, 8–16 years of age. To assess cognitive distortions, the investigators developed the Cognitive Bias Questionnaire for Children (CBQC). Children who self-reported depression or received a psychiatric diagnosis of depression, or both, endorsed more depressed–distorted cognitions than did the youth with nonaffective disorders. The presence of depressed–distorted cognitions was associated with the youths' severity of depression and discriminated between children with and without a primary mood disorder.

Leitenberg, Yost, and Carroll-Wilson (1986) developed the Children's Negative Cognitive Error Questionnaire (CNCEQ), which measures the following negative cognitive errors derived from Beck's cognitive theory of depression: overgeneralizing predictions of negative outcomes, catastrophizing the consequences of negative events, incorrectly taking personal responsibility for negative outcomes, and selectively attending to negative features of an event. Using the CNCEQ, Leitenberg et al. (1986) found that normally developing children did not report elevations on the aforementioned negative cognitive errors. However, compared to their nondepressed, nonanxious, and high-self-esteem counterparts, children who self-reported high levels of depressive and anxious symptoms and low self-esteem endorsed significantly more negative cognitive errors, particularly overgeneralization. These relationships emerged when children from extreme groups on the distribution of depression scores in a large sample were compared.

Robins and Hinkley (1989) administered a series of questionnaires assessing cognitive constructs, including the CNCEQ, to normal elementary-school-age children. Similar to the findings of Leitenberg et al. (1986), Robins and Hinkley (1989) found that children who self-reported elevations on the Depression Self-Rating Scale revealed more negative cognitive errors only on questions addressing interpersonal issues. The utilization of a normal sample, coupled with the relatively small sample size, limits the conclusions that may be drawn from this study. Kazdin (1990) assessed spontaneous negative self-statements and intrusive cognitions associated with depression utilizing the Automatic Thoughts Questionnaire (ATQ) developed for children. The findings that emerged supported the convergent validity of the measure and associated construct. Specifically, children who scored high on the ATQ evidenced greater symptoms of depression, more helplessness, lower self-esteem, and an external locus of control.

Kendall, Stark, and Adam (1990) reported data from a series of three studies that examined whether or not depressed children evidenced cognitive distortions as noted above or whether or not these distortions reflected underlying deficits in information-processing. The findings supported the notion that depressed children evidence cognitive distortions, particularly pertaining to self-evaluative information. In other words, compared to teachers' observations, depressed children reported themselves more negatively. However, on more neutral tasks that tap non-personally relevant and non-affectively charged information (Matching Familiar Figures Test), depressed children did not evidence impairments. The findings were interpreted as supporting a cognitive-distortion hypothesis and as contradictory of a cognitive-deficiency model.

Research efforts will need to focus on clarifying the specific nature of cognitive distortions in depressed youngsters as they relate to personal vs. nonpersonal material and affectively laden vs. affectively neutral information. Particular attention needs to be paid to the development of cognitive distortions in normally developing and depressed children, so that critical periods may be identified to determine at which time these cognitions develop. Further, the specificity of the cognitive distortions of depressed children vs. those of children who manifest other forms of psychopathology needs to be determined.

View of Self

Self-Esteem. Negative self-evaluation is conceptualized as a central factor in the development and maintenance of depression according to cognitive–behavioral (e.g., Beck, 1967; Rehm, 1977) and psychodynamic theories (e.g., Arieti & Bemporad, 1978; Bibring, 1953; Freud, 1957). Writers assert that depressed individuals experience feelings of inadequacy, inferiority, worthlessness, and incompetence. Throughout development, an individual constructs a self-concept defined as a personal perspective on one's thoughts, feelings, and behaviors. One's self-concept is continually reformulated as one is exposed to new information in the environment (Harter, 1990). One particularly relevant component of self-concept is self-esteem, a construct that refers to judgments we make about our self-worth (Harter, 1990). As children mature, their self-evaluations become more differentiated and less global (Harter, 1994). Both longitudinal and cross-sectional findings indicate that one's overall self-concept as well as one's estimation of social and physical self-worth increase with age, except in early elementary school and during the transition to junior high school. A strong relationship exists between children's self-evaluations and their performance (Harter, 1990).

Developmental research reveals that by elementary school, children are capable of self-reflection and self-evaluation. In fact, even preschoolers make self-evaluations, albeit in absolute and unqualified terms (McCandless & Evans, 1973). Elementary schoolchildren use increased internal descriptors of themselves and demonstrate the capacity to evaluate themselves on the basis of identity as well as their actions. They also begin to evaluate themselves in comparison to others, rather than in absolute terms. Additionally, they make a transition from action-based to competency-based conceptions of the self. These changes in cognitive processes may be prerequisites for making self-evaluations (Cicchetti & Schnieder-Rosen, 1986), including negative self-evaluations associated with depressive schemata.

The bulk of the empirical work examining self-esteem in depressed youths has utilized self-report inventories. The primary inventories used include the Coopersmith Self-Esteem Inventory (CSEI) (Coopersmith, 1967), the Self-Perception Profile for Children (Harter, 1982), the Piers–Harris Children's Self-Concept Scale (Piers & Harris, 1969), and the Offer Self-Image Questionnaire (OSIQ) (Offer, Ostrov, & Howard, 1981). These scales assess the child's self-evaluation in global terms and in specific domains of functioning, notably academic, social, physical, and athletic (Harter, 1982).

Children who are depressed report lower self-esteem than do nondepressed children, and there is considerable correlational evidence revealing a moderate relationship between children's self-reports of depressive symptoms and self-esteem. In samples of nonclinic elementary school children, depressive symptoms as measured by the CDI significantly correlate in the negative direction with self-reports of self-esteem on the Piers–Harris (e.g., Saylor, Finch, Spirito, & Bennett, 1984b; Strauss, Forehand, Frame, & Smith, 1984; Ward, Friedlander, & Silverman, 1987; Windle et al., 1986) and the CSEI (Kaslow, Rehm, & Siegel, 1984). Altmann and Gotlib (1988) reported that children with high scores on both the CDI and the Peer Nomination Inventory of Depression (PNID) (Lefkowitz & Tesiny, 1980) endorsed less overall competence on the Self-Perception Profile for Children. They indicated particularly low self-esteem in the following domains: scholastic competence, athletic competence, physical appearance, and conduct. Despite the strong correlations between self-reported depression and self-esteem, the association between peer-rated depression and self-esteem is minimal (Lefkowitz & Tesiny, 1980; Saylor, Finch, Baskin, Furey, & Kelly, 1984a).

In nonclinic samples of adolescents, Fauber et al. (1987) examined the relationship between CDI scores and self-esteem (social and cognitive competence) as measured by the Perceived Competence Scale for Children completed by the adolescents, parents, and teachers. Findings were that depression scores were significantly and negatively related to self-competency ratings. In a related vein, the only adolescent variable that was found to be predictive of depression was negative self-evaluation (Simons & Miller, 1987). Body image has been found to be a particularly important predictor of depression in adolescents and young adults (Noles, Cash & Winstead, 1985; Teri, 1982). It appears that body image is a critically important aspect of self-esteem in this age group, and it functions as both an antecedent and a strong correlate of depressive symptoms in adolescents (Allgood-Merten, Lewinsohn, & Hops, 1990).

Self-esteem has also been examined in clinically depressed children and adolescents. Similar to findings with nonclinic samples, these studies have found evidence that depressed children exhibit low self-esteem (Asarnow & Pates, 1988; Asarnow, Carlson, & Guthrie, 1987; McCauley, Mitchell, Burke, & Moss, 1988). Children whose depressive episodes have remitted have higher self-esteem than do children who are in a depressive episode (Asarnow & Bates, 1988; McCauley et al., 1988), suggesting that low self-esteem is state-dependent rather than reflective of an underlying trait. However, the literature reveals a lack of specificity in the association between depression and low self-esteem. Specifically, studies of clinic samples revealed that the depressed children with lower self-esteem frequently had comorbid psychiatric disorders including conduct, attention, and anxiety disorders (Asarnow & Bates, 1988; Asarnow et al., 1987; McCauley et al., 1988). Additionally, low self-esteem is related to cognitive measures of inattention and impulsivity, as well as depression, in nonclinic children (McGee, Anderson, Williams, & Silva, 1986). Although the bulk of the literature has revealed a strong correlation between depression and low self-esteem, not all studies have confirmed this relationship (Kazdin, Colbus, & Rodgers, 1986a; Kazdin, French, Unis, Esveldt-Dawson, & Sherick, 1983).

A number of gender differences regarding the relationship between depression and self-esteem have been found. In a sample of normally developing elementary school-children, Altmann and Gotlib (1988) found a gender–depression interaction indicating that the depressed girls felt more positively about their social competence and conduct than did the depressed boys. In adolescence, females not only reported more depressive symptoms than did their male counterparts, but also endorsed lower self-esteem and a more negative body image (Allgood-Merten et al., 1990).

Finally, self-concept has been enhanced via cognitive–behavioral interventions with depressed children. Stark, Reynolds, and Kaslow (1987) found that although depressed children who received either self-control therapy or behavioral problem-solving therapy demonstrated significant amelioration of their depressive symptoms as compared to children in the wait-list control condition, only children receiving the self-control therapy showed an improvement in self-concept. Reynolds and Coats (1986) found that depressed adolescents who received either a cognitive–behavioral therapy intervention or relaxation training evidenced significant improvements in self-concept that were not found in children in the wait-list control condition. Similar findings were found with early adolescent subjects, as those depressed children who received cognitive–behavioral therapy, relaxation training, and self-modeling interventions evidenced a significant decrease in depression and an increase in self-esteem as compared to those children assigned to the wait-list control condition (Kahn, Kehle, Jenson, & Clarke, 1990).

The accumulating body of data suggests avenues worthy of future investigation. The first of these is a determination of whether or not low self-esteem and depression represent a unitary construct or whether or not they occur independently. In other words, it is unclear whether or not there are children or adolescents who meet diagnostic criteria for depression but do not manifest low self-esteem. In a related vein, it is unclear whether or not there are components of cognitive–behavioral interventions for depressed children that are efficacious specifically in enhancing self-esteem. A second area awaiting investigation relates to a more detailed examination of the specificity of low self-esteem to depression in children. Finally, given the data that self-esteem concerns regarding body image are salient for adolescents, particularly females, it behooves researchers to focus attention on specific vulnerable content areas associated with low self-esteem at varying ages and across genders.

Perceived Competence. It is important to ascertain whether or not the low self-esteem characteristic of depressed youngsters reflects an accurate perception of their competence or is indicative of a negative distortion in self-perception. There is considerable evidence to suggest that depressed youngsters actually have impaired cognitive functioning (e.g., Fauber et al., 1987; Hodges & Plow, 1990; Kaslow et al., 1984; Lefkowitz, & Tesiny, 1980; Seagull & Weinshank, 1984; Tesiny, Lefkowitz, & Gordon, 1980) and social functioning (e.g., Altmann & Gotlib, 1988; Fauber et al., 1987; Faust et al., 1985; Jacobsen, Lahey, & Strauss, 1983; Lefkowitz & Tesiny, 1980; Puig-Antich et al., 1985a,b; Slotkin, Forehand, Fauber, McCombs, & Long, 1988). Doubly incompetent children, that is, those with both academic and social difficulties, evidence the highest level of depressive symptoms (Blechman et al., 1986; D. A. Cole, 1990). However, Saylor et al. (1984a,b) have presented contradictory findings that suggest that not all depressed children evidence impaired competence.

There are relatively scant data addressing subjective vs. objective indices of competence within a given sample of depressed children. While some research reveals that self-reported depression is correlated significantly with objective indices of cognitive functioning (Fauber et al., 1987; Worchel, Little, & Alcala, 1990), the data are far from conclusive. Some studies have found that depressed youths rate themselves more negatively than nondepressed youths despite comparable task performance (Meyer, Dyck, & Petrinack, 1989; McGee et al., 1986; Worchel et al., 1990). Additionally, the tendency to underestimate academic competence is significantly related to academic performance (D. A. Cole, 1990).

To clarify the contradictory findings that have emerged regarding depressed youths' perceptions of their own competence, more systematic studies need to be undertaken to identify relevant domains of functioning that may be impaired in depressed youths at various stages of development and across gender. Given the heterogeneity in actual levels of competence among depressed youths, the varying courses of the depressive disorder based on the number and nature of domains of functioning that are impaired deserve careful study. Finally, more attention needs to be paid to the accuracy of depressed youths' perceptions of their own competency. In other words, it is unclear whether or not their perceptions are distorted or whether or not these perceptions reflect accurate estimations of their abilities.

Hopelessness, negative expectancies for the future, is a central characteristic of depression in adults (Beck, 1967) and a key predictor of adult suicide (Beck, Steer, Kovacs, & Garrison, 1985). A number of authors have challenged children's capacity to become hopeless, given their limited temporal perspective and lack of a future orientation (Bemporad & Wilson, 1978). Siomopoulos and Inamdar (1979) have argued that it is not until adolescence that youths have sufficient cognitive–affective development and the concept of time to become hopeless, and thus they assert that it is not until adolescence that individuals present a clinical picture of depression similar to that of adults. However, as reviewed by Rehm and Carter (1990), research conducted within the rubric of developmental psychology reveals that by the time children attain stable concrete operational thinking, they are able to conceptualize the interval between events (temporal duration) and the succession of events (temporal sequence), constructs associated with a future perspective. This capacity to conceptualize time is a prerequisite to children's having negative expectations about the future or becoming hopeless. It is interesting to note that in a sample of 8-, 12-, and 17-year-olds, there was no evidence for developmental differences between children, preadolescents, and adolescents in their self-reports of hopelessness (Kashani, Reid, & Rosenberg, 1989).

Investigators have begun to examine the construct of hopelessness in childhood, primarily utilizing the Hopelessness Scale for Children (HSC) (Kazdin et al., 1983). In the majority of studies, children with high scores (more pessimistic) on the HSC have been found to be at greater risk for low self-esteem, depression, suicide, and a range of psychopathology (Asarnow & Bates, 1988; Asarnow et al., 1987; Kashani et al., 1989; Kazdin et al., 1983; Kazdin, Rodgers, & Colbus, 1986b; McCauley et al., 1988). However, not all studies have confirmed this association (Simons & Miller, 1987). In addition to having overall negative expectations about their future, depressed youths are also pessimistic with regard to specific outcomes (e.g., employment) and possibilities for success (Feather, 1983). Additionally, children who self-report high levels of hopelessness evidence deficits in social behavior (Kazdin et al., 1986). Further, high scorers on the HSC have been found to make internal, stable, global attributions for negative events (Spirito, Williams, Stark, & Hart, 1988). In addition to the positive correlation between hopelessness and depression, there is a strong relationship between hopelessness and suicidal ideation and behavior. There is some indication that the association between hopelessness and suicidality is stronger (Kazdin et al., 1983). However, when level of depression is controlled, the relationship between hopelessness and suicidal behavior diminishes (Asarnow et al., 1987).

There is some debate over the specificity of the construct of hopelessness to depression in youths. McCauley et al. (1988) found that only youths in a depressive episode obtained elevated scores on the HSC. Similar elevations were not found for youths whose depression had remitted or for youths with other psychiatric difficulties. Asarnow and Bates (1988) reported similar findings with an inpatient sample. These findings suggest that hopelessness is not an enduring trait, but rather a statelike phenomenon that dissipates once a depressive episode has remitted. Furthermore, Benfield, Palmer, Pfefferbaum, and Stowe (1988) noted few differences in self-reported levels of hopelessness between an inpatient sample of youths diagnosed with major depression or dysthymic disorder and a nondepressed inpatient control group. Additionally, no between-group differences were found on self-reported depression or life stress.

There continues to be debate in the literature regarding the applicability of hopelessness cognitions to depression in youngsters based on their level of cognitive development. Thus, it is crucial for future research endeavors to provide both longitudinal and cross-sectional data regarding the manifestation of hopelessness in depressed youths as it interacts with various stages of cognitive and social–emotional development. Additionally, more research on the relationship between hopelessness, depression, and suicidal behavior in children and adolescents should be conducted to elucidate the complex interaction between these constructs.

Learned Helplessness

Instrumental Responding.   Shortly after birth, children begin to engage in activities that increase competence and mastery. By preschool, children are capable of making attributions for their successes and failures. The development of these causal attributions affects children's expectations regarding the impact of their behavior on future outcomes. These expectancies in turn influence the extent to which children are motivated to persist in associated situations in the future. Infants and preschoolers typically develop unsophisticated explanations for their successes and failures that enable them to continue to engage in mastery-oriented behaviors.

By elementary school, children develop conceptualizations regarding the causes of their successes and failures based on a wider array of information and their capacity to differentiate the attributional variables of ability and effort. Those children who experience themselves as efficacious in controlling their environment develop mastery-oriented attributions that facilitate their sustaining motivation and thus lead to adaptive instrumental responding. Conversely, those children who believe that failure is insurmountable and success unattainable develop a helpless stance that leads to decreased persistence and an associated deterioration of performance (learned helplessness) (Dweck & Leggett, 1988). These children evidence deficits in instrumental responding.

Children thus develop either mastery-oriented or helpless attributions and associated styles of instrumental responding. These attributions are derived utilizing information that children glean from the environment regarding how capable they are based on their actual performance, how well their performance compares to that of peers, and the reinforcement that they receive from adults in their environment (namely, parents and teachers). Interestingly, gender differences have emerged to suggest that normally developing girls are more likely than their male peers to exhibit the helpless pattern of attributions, low expectancies for success, and an associated decline in performance (Dweck & Leggett, 1988). Some have argued that the development of this response repertoire sets the stage for elevated rates of depression and associated learned-helplessness behaviors in adult women vs. men (Nolen-Hoeksema, 1990).

There are few studies that have addressed the motivational deficit of helplessness hypothesized as central to depression (Kaslow, Tanenbaum, Abramson, Peterson, & Seligman, 1983; Schwartz, Friedman, Lindsay, & Narrol, 1982). These investigations have found that children who score high on the CDI have impaired performance on higher-order cognitive tasks such as block design on the Wechsler Intelligence Scale for Children-Revised (WISC-R), solving anagrams, and performance on the Matching Familiar Figures Test, a cognitive measure of reflection–impulsivity. Additionally, children diagnosed as depressed have lower performance on arithmetic achievement than on verbal tasks (Hodges & Plow, 1990), a finding consistent with the learned-helplessness literature (Dweck & Licht, 1980). These authors interpreted their findings as supportive of deficits in instrumental responding in depressed children. The methodological limitations of these studies have precluded direct examination of instrumental responding in these children.

In a more methodologically sophisticated experiment examining cognitions and behavior associated with learned helplessness in children with high and low scores on the CDI, no relationship was found between depressive symptoms and a behavioral measure of learned helplessness (Bodiford, Eisenstadt, Johnson, & Bradlyn, 1988). These researchers interpreted their findings to suggest that children with depressive symptoms may not demonstrate the hypothesized behavioral and motivational deficits associated with learned helpless. However, they note that problems with the behavioral task utilized limit the conclusions that may be gleaned from this investigation. Finally, Nolen-Hoeksema, Girgus, and Seligman (1986) examined explanatory style, academic achievement, and teachers' ratings of mastery-oriented and learned-helplessness behaviors in the classroom. Findings were that helplessness in the classroom, poorer school achievement, and depressive symptoms were significantly intercorrelated. Future research should be directed toward a more in-depth examination of the actual instrumental responding behavior of depressed youngsters.

Locus of Control. Another aspect of the learned-helplessness model relates to individuals' perception of control. As a trait, locus of control refers to a generalized belief in one's ability to affect the environment so as to maximize rewards and minimize negative outcomes. On the basis of research with adults, it has been argued that depressed youngsters perceive a lack of control over important events in their environment. Experiences with prior uncontrollable outcomes and the consequent expectation that future events would be uncontrollable have been linked to serious cognitive and motivational deficits and dysphoric affect.

Social-cognition research reveals that the differentiation between internal and external locus of control is blurred in preschoolers' explanatory schemata. These relatively undifferentiated inferential reasoning processes lead preschoolers to incorrect conclusions about causality (Sedlak & Kurtz, 1981). By the time children enter elementary school, they develop more stylized patterns for assessing the locus of control. With age, a child's locus of control becomes more internal and less external (Nowicki & Duke, 1974).

There are a few studies that assess directly the association between depression in children, locus of control, and perception of controllability. In an early study, Moyal (1977) found that children's scores on the Nowicki–Strickland Children's Locus of Control Scale (Nowicki & Strickland, 1973) were significantly correlated with depressive symptoms in a manner suggesting that children who reported depressive symptoms also endorsed a more external locus of control. Additionally, those children with an external locus of control had lower self-esteem and were more likely to choose helpless, self-blaming, or externalized blaming responses on the Moyal–Miezitis Stimulus Appraisal Scale. Consistent with these findings, other researchers have found that higher levels of depression are associated with a more external locus of control in children (Butler, Miezitis, Friedman, & Cole, 1980; Lefkowitz, Tesiny & Gordon, 1980; McCauley, et al., 1988; Mullins, et al., 1985; Tesiny et al., 1980) and adolescents (Siegel & Griffin, 1984). Additionally, children who endorsed high levels of depressive symptoms and an external locus of control evidenced deficits in school achievement (Tesiny et al., 1980).When social-class variables are considered, the joint effects of low family income and an external locus of control are associated with the highest levels of depression (Lefkowitz et al., 1988). In two of the aforementioned studies (Mullins et al., 1985; Siegel & Griffin, 1984), scores on the Nowicki–Strickland were found to account for nearly a third of the variance in predicting depression in relation to other variables.

Weisz and colleagues (Weisz et al., 1989; Weisz, Weiss, Wasserman, & Rintoul, 1987) have utilized a two-dimensional model of control cognitions to examine beliefs about the contingencies of outcomes (outcome contingency) and beliefs about one's competence to perform outcome-relevant behavior (personal competence). In a series of thoughtfully conceptualized and well-designed studies, Weisz and colleagues examined control-related beliefs and cognitions in clinic-referred and inpatient children and adolescents. For clinic-referred youths (Weisz et al., 1987) who endorsed high levels of depression on the CDI, low levels of perceived personal competence were also found. However, outcome contingency beliefs were not associated with CDI scores. Similar findings were reported by Weisz et al. (1989) in their work with inpatient samples. These studies suggest that depressive symptoms in youths are associated more closely to "personal helplessness" in the form of perceived incompetence and contingency uncertainty than to universal helplessness as reflected in perceived noncontingency.

Attributional Style. The attributional reformulation of the learned-helplessness model retains an emphasis on perceived control (Abramson et al., 1978). These authors argued that it is not uncontrollability per se, but the nature of attributions an individual makes regarding life events and perceived noncontingency between actions and outcomes, that determine whether or not the person becomes depressed and the specific characteristics of the resultant depression (Abramson et al., 1978). In the revised model, the perception that an important event is uncontrollable remained an important component in the event–attribution–depression sequence. More recently, however, the construct of uncontrollability has diminished in its centrality to the theory and has been replaced by an emphasis on the attributions that individuals offer for either negative or positive events.

There are four dimensions of attributional style relevant to depressive cognitions: controllability, internality, stability, and globality. The dimension of controllability was described above, and as noted, a belief that important events are beyond one's control is associated with feelings of depression. Internal causation refers to causes located within the person (e.g., intelligence, interpersonal skills), whereas external causation refers to causes external to the person (e.g., fate, behavior of others, external circumstances). Individuals who make internal attributions for negative events (i.e., those who blame themselves for bad events) are likely to experience dysphoric affect, and these attributions to internal causes are presumed to underlie the self-esteem deficits that accompany depression. Those persons who make global attributions for negative events and thus view the causes of these events as generalizable across situations are likely to develop depressions that influence all areas of their lives. Finally, the use of stable attributions for negative events implies that the individual believes that the cause of the event is relatively enduring over time and thus is likely to develop a sense of hopelessness about the future and a chronic depression. Research with depressed adults reveals that these individuals exhibit more internal, stable, and global attributions for failure and external, unstable, and specific attributions for success relative to nondepressives (Peterson & Seligman, 1984).

There has been considerable research pertaining to the development of attributions in children and adolescents. The genesis of attributions may be found in infancy when mastery is attained as a result of an infant's actions. By preschool, children are able to make attributions about their successes and failures. They are more likely to attribute greater motivation to individuals who are externally induced to perform and greater effort to more competent people, and tend not to differentiate luck from skill. These attributional patterns in turn affect children's expectancies of success and failure. As children proceed through elementary school and high school, their attributional patterns are marked by an increased consistency in their understanding of events and future outcomes, greater capacity to integrate past events with present situations, and a more realistic assessment of the control that they have over their own behavior and events in the environment.

The primary measure utilized in the assessment of children's attributional styles is the Children's Attributional Style Questionnaire (CASQ) (Seligman et al., 1984). This measure has also been referred to in the literature as the KASTAN Children's Attributional Style Questionnaire. The original CASQ consisted of 48 items; the recently revised measure includes 24 items. The CASQ includes forced-choice items, each of which consists of a situation (e.g., "You get good grades") and two possible attributions to explain why the situation occurred (e.g., "I am a hard worker" vs. "Schoolwork is simple"). Half of the situations represent positive (good) outcomes; half represent negative (bad) outcomes. Three dimensions of attributional style (internality, globality, stability) are assessed. Two composite scores are derived: a positive composite and a negative composite. The lower the positive and the higher the negative composite scores, the more depressive the attributional style as conceptualized by the revised learned-helplessness theory of depression (Abramson et al., 1978). An overall composite score can be obtained by subtracting the composite score for negative events from the composite score for positive events. The lower this composite score, the more depressive the attributional style.

In the initial study examining the development of the CASQ and the relationship between scores on the CASQ and CDI scores, Seligman et al. (1984) found that in 8- to 13-year-old elementary school children, those children who attributed negative events to internal, stable, and global causes were more likely to report depressive symptoms than were children who attributed these events to external, unstable, and specific causes. Additionally, children who attributed positive events to external, unstable, and specific causes were more likely to endorse high levels of depressive symptoms on the CDI than were youths who attributed these events to internal, stable, and global causes. Seligman and Peterson (1986) examined these findings in more detail and found that children who scored low on depression were less likely than children with high scores on the CDI to explain positive and negative events evenhandedly. Nondepressed children who make internal, stable, and global attributions for success, while making asymmetrical, external, unstable, and specific attributions for failure, may have a lopsided attributional style in which they have optimistic distortions. Although this style may be less accurate than that of depressed children, it may be important for sustaining hope.

Several others authors have also found that nonclinic children who score high on the CDI make more internal, stable, and global attributions for failure and more external, unstable, and specific attributions for success than do low scorers (Blumberg & Izard, 1985; Bodiford et al., 1988; Kaslow et al., 1984; Nolen-Hoeksema et al., 1986; Robins & Hinkley, 1989; Saylor et al., 1984b). These differences in attributional styles are not due to self-report confounds such as social desirability or to personal and demographic variables including intellectual level, achievement, socioeconomic status, race, or gender (Bodiford et al., 1988). However, there are data that suggest that when psychological variables (e.g., stress, affective state) and other explanatory variables (e.g., socioeconomic status, school, or employment problems) are also considered, the contribution of attributional style in predicting depression decreases (Blumberg & Izard, 1985; Hammen, Adrian, & Hiroto, 1988; Robins & Hinkley, 1989; Siegel & Griffin, 1984; Simons & Miller, 1987). Thus, future studies should examine other potential mediating factors between attribution and depression.

A maladaptive attributional style also characterizes inpatient and outpatient youths who meet criteria for depression (Asarnow & Bates, 1988; Benfield et al., 1988; Curry & Craighead, 1990; Kaslow, Rehm, Pollack, & Siegel, 1988; McCauley et al., 1988; Saylor et al., 1984). There is evidence for the specificity of this maladaptive attributional style to depression (Benfield et al., 1988; Kaslow et al., 1988; McCauley et al., 1988). However, studies with psychiatric populations of children generally indicate a weaker relationship between a self-deprecatory attributional style and depression than is found in nonclinic samples (e.g., Kaslow et al., 1988). In these psychiatric samples, between-group differences in attributions for positive events are more pronounced than those for negative life events (Benfield et al., 1988; Curry & Craighead, 1990). These maladaptive cognitive patterns appear to be characteristic of many depressed youths (55%), but not all, suggesting a heterogeneity of cognitive patterns in these children (Asarnow & Bates, 1988).

Depressed children have been found to endorse a more maladaptive attributional style when compared both to youths who had a prior episode of depression but were not currently depressed and to nondepressed psychiatric controls (Asarnow & Bates, 1988; McCauley et al., 1988). In one study, these group differences were accounted for by attributions for positive but not negative events (McCauley et al., 1988). Of further interest is the finding that the association between attributional patterns and level of depression differs between depressed and nondepressed psychiatric samples (Benfield et al., 1988; Hammen et al., 1988). Finally, the attributional styles of suicidal youths have been examined. Suicidal youths as a group have not been found to evidence a maladaptive attributional style, yet those suicidal youths who are also depressed possess the attributional style characteristic of depressed youths (e.g., Rotheram-Borus et al., 1990). Although the aforementioned studies suggest a relationship between depressive symptoms and disorders and attributional styles measured by the CASQ, the specific nature of this relationship is not consistent across studies. This inconsistency may be attributable to the psychometric limitations of the CASQ, the variable nature of the populations studied, and the heterogeneity of depressive disorders manifested in children and adolescents.

A few studies have evaluated attributional correlates of depressive symptoms in children using other measures. Using the Cognitive Process Inventory for Children, a series of vignettes followed by questions designed to tap aspirations, expectations, and attributions, children classified as depressed attributed positive events to external causes and negative events to internal causes more than nondepressed children (Leon, Kendall, & Garber, 1980). Siegel and Griffin (1984) found that adolescents who endorsed high levels of depressive symptoms on the Beck Depression Inventory also evidenced a maladaptive attributional style on the Attributional Style Scale for Adolescents (ASSA), a modification of the Attributional Style Questionnaire (ASQ) for adults (Seligman, Abramson, Semmel, & von Baeyer, 1979). In this study, a positive correlation was found between level of depression and a tendency to attribute outcomes to internal, stable, and global causes; this correlation becomes stronger when attributions are weighted by the subjective significance of the event (Siegel & Griffin, 1984).

Meyer et al. (1989) examined causal explanations for performance on solvable and unsolvable problems using two attribution wheels. Children were asked to evaluate the relative importance of ability, effort, task difficulty, and luck in enhancing or impeding their performance. The results revealed partial support for the reformulated model of learned helplessness, particularly the personal-helplessness component of the theory. Specifically, children who endorsed high levels of depressive symptoms emphasized ability factors as causally related to their failures, whereas low scorers focused on factors other than ability. However, depressed children did not externalize their successes relative to nondepressed children, and nondepressed children did not externalize their failures more than their depressed counterparts. Further, both groups emphasized effort, a controllable factor, as causal of their successes (Meyer et al., 1989). In a related study, however, Ward et al. (1987) found no significant differences in causal attributions for success or failure on an anagram task between children rated as depressed and nondepressed by their peers.

Bodiford et al. (1988) also examined the relationship between attributions and actual task performance. Data from this study indicated that helpless behavior on a block design task was not associated with a helpless attributional style, although attributional style in this study was found to be associated with depression. These results suggest the need to examine further the nature of the correspondence between attributional style and actual performance.

Brown and Siegel (1988) conducted a study that examined the role of perceived control in the attributions that adolescents made for negative life events and their association to depression. In their prospective study of stress and adaptive functioning in adolescence, Brown and Siegel (1988) found that internal, stable, and global attributions for negative events attributed to uncontrollable causes were associated with increased levels of depression, whereas internal, global attributions for negative events attributed to controllable causes were found to be inversely related to increases in depression levels.

In both nonclinic and clinic samples, using a variety of measures of attributional styles, researchers have begun to examine developmental and gender differences in the association between attributional style and depression. Some studies have found developmental changes in attributional style (McCauley et al., 1988; Nolen-Hoeksema et al., 1986; Robins & Hinkley, 1989), but contradictory evidence has also been presented (Kaslow et al., 1984). Additionally, while some researchers have found differential attributional patterns between boys and girls (Blumberg & Izard, 1985), other investigators have found no gender differences (Robins & Hinkley, 1989). The limited available data and the contradictory findings support the need for further research in this area.

A few studies have examined attributional styles longitudinally. Composite attributional styles appear relatively stable over time. An internal, stable, and global way of construing the causes of negative events has been found to be predictive of depressive symptoms in children up to 1 year later, with initial level of depression partialed out (Nolen-Hoeksema et al., 1986; Seligman et al., 1984). Additionally, maladaptive explanatory styles appear to make a unique contribution in predicting future depression, and the association appears not to be merely reflective of explanatory style being a symptom of depression or to the influence of earlier depressive symptoms on explanatory style (Nolen-Hoeksema et al., 1986). Further, children who evidence a maladaptive explanatory style have been found to be more prone to experience depressive symptoms during the subsequent year (Nolen-Hoeksema et al., 1986). These findings suggest that this maladaptive attributional style may be one risk factor for depression. In a related vein, there is some evidence that depressive symptoms predict explanatory style at future times (Nolen-Hoeksema et al., 1986). However, there are data that suggest that in children with depressed mothers, neither attributional style alone nor its interaction with stress significantly predicted the development of depressive symptoms, but was associated with the development of nondepressive disorders (Hammen et al., 1988).

Attributional style has also been assessed as it relates to constructs associated with depression in children and has been found to correlate with school achievement and behavior (Nolen-Hoeksema et al., 1986). Specifically, children with a maladaptive attributional style demonstrate impairments in achievement according to standardized achievement scores. These children were also rated by teachers as evidencing more helpless and fewer mastery behaviors in the classroom (Nolen-Hoeksema et al., 1986). However, Bodiford et al. (1988) found no relationship between self-reports of attributional style on the CASQ and helplessness behaviors exhibited on a task (Dweck & Repucci, 1973) designed to assess children's responses to academic failure. Measures of attributional patterns have been found to be correlated significantly with measures of self-perception in inpatient youths; this association is not accounted for by level of depression (Asarnow & Bates, 1988). These findings suggest that analysis of attributional patterns may be important for the development of children's self-perceptions. Adolescent suicide attempters who reported high levels of hopelessness on the HSC also reported depressive attributions for both negative and positive events (Spirito et al., 1988).

One particularly noteworthy finding is that in early adolescence, maladaptive attributional styles are associated with less secure attachment to parents, although not to peers (Armsden, McCauley, Greenberg, Burke, & Mitchell, 1990). The association between security of parental attachment, attributional style, and depressive disorders suggests that depressogenic cognitive schemata may promote the link between depression and insecure attachments. Alternatively, the endorsement of less secure parental attachment by depressed adolescents may reflect their cognitive distortions rather than be indicative of actual impairments in the attachments.

The attributional reformulation of the learned-helplessness theory is a diathesis–stress model. Thus, it is important to examine the data pertaining to the interaction between negative life events and attributional style. There is some research to suggest that the combination of negative life events and a maladaptive attributional style increases a child's vulnerability to depression. However, findings regarding this association are inconsistent (Nolen-Hoeksema et al., 1986).

Some researchers have examined the origins of attributional style. These investigations have studied the association between the attributional style of children and their parents in order to ascertain whether or not children learn their attributional style from their parents. Seligman et al. (1984) found that nonclinic children's style of explaining the causes of negative events and their depressive symptoms converged with their mothers' explanatory style for events in their lives. However, a relationship between children's and fathers' attributional style was not found. Kaslow et al. (1988) examined the attributional styles of depressed clinic, nondepressed clinic, and normal children and both their mothers and fathers. Contrary to the study of Seligman et al. (1984), no relationship was found between the attributional style of children and their parents.

Several authors have underscored the value of attribution retraining for depressed children (Kaslow & Rehm, 1991; Nolen-Hoeksema et al., 1986). Potentially applicable programs have been described for depressed adults (Seligman, 1981) and helpless children (Dweck, 1975). Although no studies have examined directly the efficacy of attribution retraining for depressed children, a multidimensional treatment program has been shown to have positive effects in modifying attributional styles in both depressed and non-depressed psychiatric inpatients (Benfield et al., 1988).

To more fully test the validity of the attributionally reformulated theory of learned helplessness, future studies must utilize a longitudinal perspective in examining the diathesis–stress model. This research will entail developmentally oriented studies of depressive disorders, explanatory style, and life events. The association between attributional patterns and actual behavior deserves additional study. Further, the association between attributional theory and emotional expression should be studied in depressed children, and these youths' understanding of the implications of causal attributions for emotional experiences should be compared to that of their nondepressed counterparts (Stipek & DeCotis, 1988). More comprehensive investigations regarding how children learn attributions should include study of the reciprocal influences of parental cognitive processes and psychopathology, family interaction patterns, and cognitive processes and depression in the child.

Self-Control

During the past decade, increased attention has been paid to children's developing understanding of essential strategies for self-control and self-regulation. According to Vygotsky (1978), children initially learn self-regulatory strategies from watching their caretakers and more capable peers and from being the recipient of their parents' verbal guiding efforts to help them regulate their own actions and emotions. Vygotsky theorized that it was through this social guidance that children would begin to internalize verbal strategies that they could then utilize (in the form of internal monologue) to guide their own behavior (Berk, 1989). The balance between children's capacity for independent functioning and their reliance on significant others for regulation of their behavior varies markedly with the task in question. In preschool, children use their overt verbalizations to guide their behaviors. As children mature, their speech is used increasingly to regulate and guide their behavior, thought processes, and affective expression. This speech eventually becomes the silent, internal dialogue that enables each individual to develop self-control strategies for self-monitoring, self-evaluation, and self-reinforcement (Berk, 1989).

There is an accumulating body of data examining self-control deficits in depressed children. Given that Rehm's self-control model incorporates tenets of the cognitive theory of depression, the learned-helplessness model and its attributional reformulation, and a social-skills perspective, much of the relevant data is reviewed in prior sections of this chapter. Only findings not covered elsewhere will be reviewed in this section.

In a sample of children of elementary and junior high school age, depressed children had lower expectations for task performance, set more stringent standards for poor scores but not good scores, and evaluated their performance more negatively (Kaslow et al., 1984). Despite similar performance between depressed and nondepressed youths, depressed youths provided lower evaluations of their performance (Meyer et al., 1989). Additionally, depressed children punished themselves significantly more than did nondepressed children, although no between-group differences were found for reward and depressed youths were more likely to recommend the use of punishment than reward as compared to their nondepressed peers. Females punished themselves significantly more than males, regardless of depression status (Kaslow et al., 1984). Similarly, in a sample of both clinic and nonclinic controls, depressed clinic children reported more overall self-control difficulties as measured by the Usually That's Me self-control measure (Humphrey, 1982) than did the nondepressed clinic children and the normal controls.

Cognitive–behavioral models suggest that a child's depression may occur as a result of a parent's modeling of depressive behaviors and cognitions or because the child's parents engage in faulty monitoring, evaluation, attribution, or reinforcement. To ascertain the relationship between cognitive factors in parents and depression and cognitive factors in children, both parents and children completed measures of depression and self-control behaviors. Kaslow et al. (1988) found no differences in the self-control styles of parents of depressed clinic, nondepressed clinic, and normal controls. Additionally, no relationship was found between the self-control behavior of children and their parents. These parents were also evaluated on rates of and criteria for reinforcement. Findings were that mothers of depressed clinic and nonclinic children both set very high criteria for providing their children with rewards when compared to mothers of clinic/nondepressed children (D. A. Cole & Rehm, 1986). No differences in father ratings were obtained.

Future research endeavors should include behavioral observations of depressed children's interactions with their caretakers, with a focus on the self-control strategies that caretakers utilize, the caretakers' efforts to help the child regulate himself or herself, and caretakers' responses to children's efforts at self-regulation. Additionally, with older children, the relationship between self-reported monitoring, evaluation, and reinforcement, the actual enactments of these processes, and associated behavioral responding deserve attention.

Summary and Conclusions

This chapter has delineated the myriad cognitive and behavioral impairments associated with depression in school-age children and adolescents. Taken together, research reveals that depressed children differ from their nondepressed counterparts in the following cognitive and behavioral processes: contingent reinforcement, information-processing, view of self, hopelessness, learned helplessness, and self-control. Depressed children have impaired interpersonal functioning with parents, siblings, peers, and teachers, and these impairments tend to persist even on recovery from the depressive episode. Unlike the situation with regard to adults, there is insufficient evidence regarding differential participation by depressed and nondepressed youngsters in pleasurable and unpleasurable activities. Similarly, it remains unclear whether or not depressed children manifest self-schemata different from those of their nondepressed counterparts.

Consistent with the adult literature, which suggests that depressed individuals report significantly more negatively distorted cognitions on self-report measures, depressed children evidence similar cognitive distortions. Depressed youths have low self-esteem that appears to reflect only in part actual impairments in competencies in social and academic domains. Youths who are depressed typically feel hopeless about their future, and high levels of hopelessness are a risk factor for suicidal behavior. There are some data suggesting that deficits in instrumental responding and associated feelings of learned helplessness are characteristic of children who report high levels of depressive symptoms.

The large body of research addressing attributional patterns in depressed youths has led to contradictory findings. However, the bulk of this work reveals that compared to their nondepressed counterparts, depressed youngsters evidence a more internal, stable, and global attributional pattern for negative events and a more external, unstable, and specific attributional style for positive events. Finally, depressed children appear to have deficits in self-monitoring, self-evaluation, and self-reinforcement.

While the evidence for cognitive and behavioral deficits in depressed children and adolescents is quite compelling, and cognitive–behavioral interventions have been found efficacious in ameliorating depressive symptoms in youngsters, a focus only on these processes is insufficient. Rather, a more comprehensive model for understanding impairments in functioning and for developing effective treatment strategies must take into account the child's level of cognitive, social, and emotional development. Additionally, given that depression in children generally emerges within an interpersonal context, it is essential that considerable attention be paid to the interpersonal environment in which depressive cognitions and behaviors are learned, manifested, and perpetuated. Finally, given that depression in children reflects a failure to regulate negative affect due to children's lack of adaptive cognitive, behavioral, and interpersonal strategies for affect regulation, treatment efforts should be devoted to assisting children in developing age-appropriate cognitive and behavioral techniques for affect regulation. These interventions need to be sensitive to the children's development, existing cognitive schemata, and strengths and resources. Additionally, these interventions should include family involvement in order to enable the families to utilize more adaptive cognitive and behavioral processes in regulating both their own and their children's thoughts, feelings, and behaviors. Family involvement is particularly relevant because children's development is embedded within the family context.

References

Abramson, L. Y., Metalsky, G. I., & Alloy, L. B. (1989). Hopelessness depression: A theory-based subtype of depression. *Psychological Bulletin, 96,* 358–372.

Abramson, L. Y., Seligman, M. E. P., & Teasdale, J. (1978). Learned helplessness in humans: Critique and reformulation. *Journal of Abnormal Psychology, 87,* 49–74.

Allgood-Merten, B., Lewinsohn, P. M., & Hops, H. (1990). Sex differences and adolescent depression. *Journal of Abnormal Psychology, 99,* 55–63.

Alloy, L. B., & Abramson, L. Y. (1979). Judgement of contingency in depressed and nondepressed students: Sadder but wiser? *Journal of Experimental Psychology General, 108,* 441–485.

Altmann, E. O., & Gotlib, I. H. (1988). The social behavior of depressed children: An observational study. *Journal of Abnormal Child Psychology, 16,* 29–44.

Arieti, S., & Bemporad, J. (1978). *Severe and mild depression: The psychotherapeutic approach.* New York: Basic Books.

Armsden, G. C., McCauley, E., Greenberg, M. T., Burke, P. M., & Mitchell, J. R. (1990). Parent and peer attachment in early adolescent depression. *Journal of Abnormal Child Psychology, 18,* 683–697.

Asarnow, J. R. (1988). Peer status and social competence in child psychiatric inpatients: A comparison of children with depressive, externalizing, and concurrent depressive and externalizing disorders. *Journal of Abnormal Child Psychiatry, 16,* 151–162.

Asarnow, J. R., & Bates, S. (1988). Depression in child psychiatric inpatients: Cognitive and attributional patterns. *Journal of Abnormal Child Psychology, 16,* 601–615.

Asarnow, J. R., Carlson, G. A., & Guthrie, D. (1987). Coping strategies, self-perceptions, hopelessness, and perceived family environments in depressed and suicidal children. *Journal of Consulting and Clinical Psychology, 55,* 361–366.

Barden, R. C., Garber, J., Leiman, B., Ford, M. E., & Masters, J. C. (1985). Factors governing the effective remediation of negative affect and its cognitive and behavioral consequences. *Journal of Personality and Social Psychology, 49*, 1040–1053.

Beck, A. T. (1967). *Depression: Clinical, experimental and theoretical aspects*. New York: Hoeber.

Beck, A. T. (1976). *Cognitive therapy and emotional disorders*. New York: International Universities Press.

Beck, A. T., Steer, R. A., Kovacs, M., & Garrison, B. (1985). Hopelessness and eventual suicide: A 10-year perspective study of patients hospitalized with suicidal ideation. *American Journal of Psychiatry, 142*, 559–563.

Bemporad, J. R., & Wilson, A. (1978). A developmental approach to depression in childhood and adolescence. *Journal of the American Academy of Psychoanalysis, 6*, 325–352.

Benfield, C. Y., Palmer, D. J., Pfefferbaum, B., & Stowe, M. L. (1988). A comparison of depressed and nondepressed disturbed children on measures of attributional styles, hopelessness, life stress and temperament. *Journal of Abnormal Child Psychology, 16*, 397–410.

Berk, L. E. (1989). *Child development*. Boston: Allyn & Bacon

Bibring, E. (1953). The mechanism of depression. In P. Greenacre (Ed.), *Affective disorders* (pp. 13–48). New York: International Universities Press.

Blechman, E. A., McEnroe, M. J., Carella, E. T., & Audette, D. P. (1986). Childhood competence and depression. *Journal of Abnormal Psychology, 95*, 223–227.

Blumberg, S. H., & Izard, C. E. (1985). Affective and cognitive characteristics of depression in 10- and 11-year old children. *Journal of Personality and Social Psychology, 49*, 194–202.

Bodiford, C. A., Eisenstadt, T. H., Johnson, J. H., & Bradlyn, A. S. (1988). Comparison of learned helpless cognitions and behavior in children with high and low scores on the Children's Depression Inventory. *Journal of Clinical Child Psychology, 17*, 152–158.

Brown, J. D., & Siegel, J. M. (1988). Attributions for negative life events and depression: The role of perceived control. *Journal of Personality and Social Psychology, 54*, 316–322.

Butler, L., Miezitis, S., Friedman, R., & Cole, E. (1980). The effect of two school-based intervention programs on depressive symptoms in preadolescents. *American Educational Research Journal, 17*, 111–119.

Carey, M. P., Kelley, M. L., Buss, R. R., & Scott, W. O. (1986). Relationship of activity to depression in adolescents: Development of the adolescent activities checklist. *Journal of Consulting and Clinical Psychology, 54*, 320–322.

Cicchetti, D., & Schneider-Rosen, K. (1986). An organizational approach to childhood depression. In M. Rutter, C. E. Izard, and P. B. Read (Eds.), *Depression in young people: Developmental and clinical perspectives* (pp. 71–135). New York: Guilford Press.

Cole, D. A. (1990). Relation of social and academic competence to depressive symptoms in childhood. *Journal of Abnormal Psychology, 99*, 422–429.

Cole, D. A., & Rehm, L. P. (1986). Family interaction patterns and childhood depression. *Journal of Abnormal Child Psychology, 14*, 297–314.

Cole, P. M., & Kaslow, N. J. (1988). Interactional and cognitive strategies for affect regulation: A developmental perspective on childhood depression. In L. B. Alloy (Ed.), *Cognitive processes in depression* (pp. 310–343). New York: Guilford Press.

Coopersmith, S. (1967). *The antecedents of self-esteem*. San Francisco: Freeman.

Coyne, J. C., & Gotlib, I. H. (1983). The role of cognition in depression: A critical appraisal. *Psychological Bulletin, 94*, 472–505.

Curry, J. F., & Craighead, W. E. (1990). Attributional style in clinically depressed and conduct disordered adolescents. *Journal of Consulting and Clinical Psychology, 58*, 109–115.

Dodge, K. A. (1986). A social information processing model of social competence in children. In M. Perlmutter (Ed.), *Minnesota symposia on child psychology*, Vol. 18 (pp. 77–125). Hillsdale, NJ: Erlbaum.

Dweck, C. S. (1975). The role of expectations and attributions in the alleviation of learned helplessness. *Journal of Personality and Social Psychology, 31*, 674–685.

Dweck, C. S., & Leggett, E. L. (1988). A social–cognitive approach to motivation and personality. *Psychological Review, 95*, 256–273.

Dweck, C. S., & Licht, B. G. (1980). Learned helplessness and intellectual achievement. In J. Garber and M. E. P. Seligman (Eds.), *Human helplessness: Theory and applications* (pp. 197–221). New York: Academic Press.

Dweck, C. S., & Repucci, N. D. (1973). Learned helplessness and reinforcement responsibility in children. *Journal of Personality and Social Psychology, 25*, 109–116.

Fauber, R., Forehand, R., Long, N., Burke, M., & Faust, J. (1987). The relationship of young adolescent Children's Depression Inventory (CDI) scores to their social and cognitive functioning. *Journal of Psychopathology and Behavioral Assessment, 9*, 161–172.

Faust, J., Baum, C. G., & Forehand, R. (1985). An examination of the association between social relationships and depression in early adolescence. *Journal of Applied Developmental Psychology, 6,* 291–297.

Feather, N. J. (1983). Causal attributions and beliefs about work and unemployment among adolescents in state and independent secondary schools. *Australian Journal of Psychology, 35,* 211–232.

Freud, S. (1957). Mourning and melancholia. In *Standard edition,* Vol. 14 (pp. 243–258). London: Hogarth Press (originally published in 1917).

Fuchs, D., & Thelen, M. H. (1988). Children's expected interpersonal consequences of communicating their affective state and reported likelihood of expression. *Child Development, 59,* 1314–1322.

Garber, J., & Kashani, J. H. (1991). Development of the symptom of depression. In M. Lewis (Ed.), *Child and adolescent psychiatry: A comprehensive textbook* (pp. 293–310). Baltimore: Williams & Wilkins.

Garber, J., & Seligman, M. E. P. (Eds.) (1980). *Human helplessness: Theory and applications.* New York: Academic Press.

Glasberg, R., & Aboud, F. E. (1981). A development perspective on the study of depression: Children's evaluative reactions to sadness. *Developmental Psychology, 17,* 195–202.

Haley, G. M. T., Fine, S., Marriage, K., Moretti, M. M. & Freedman, R. J. (1985). Cognitive bias and depression in psychiatrically disturbed children and adolescents. *Journal of Consulting and Clinical Psychology, 53,* 535–537.

Hammen, C., Adrian, C., & Hiroto, D. (1988). A longitudinal test of the attributional vulnerability model in children at risk for depression. *British Journal of Clinical Psychology, 27,* 37–46.

Hammen, C., & Zupan, B. A. (1984). Self-schemas, depression, and the processing of personal information in children. *Journal of Experimental Child Psychology, 37,* 598–608.

Harter, S. (1982). The perceived competence scale for children. *Child Development, 53,* 87–97.

Harter, S. (1990). Causes, correlates and the functional role of global self-worth: A life-span perspective. In R. Sternberg and J. Kolligian (Eds.), *Competence considered* (pp. 67–97). New Haven: Yale University Press.

Hodges, K., & Plow, J. (1990). Intellectual ability and achievement in psychiatrically hospitalized children with conduct, anxiety, and affective disorders. *Journal of Consulting and Clinical Psychology, 58,* 589–595.

Humphrey, L. L. (1982). Children's and teachers' perspectives on children's self-control: The development of two rating scales. *Journal of Consulting and Clinical Psychology, 50,* 624–633.

Ingram, R. E., & Kendall, P. C. (1987). The cognitive side of anxiety. *Cognitive Therapy and Research, 11,* 523–536.

Jacobsen, R. H., Lahey, B. B., & Strauss, C. C. (1983). Correlates of depressed mood in normal children. *Journal of Abnormal Child Psychology, 11,* 29–40.

Jaenicke, C., Hammen, G., Zupan, B., Hiroto, D., Gordon, D., Adrian, C., & Burge, D. (1987). Cognitive vulnerability in children at risk for depression. *Journal of Abnormal Child Psychology, 15,* 559–572.

Joffe, R. D., Dobson, K. S., Fine, S., Marriage, K., & Haley, G. (1990). Social problem-solving in depressed, conduct-disordered, and normal adolescents. *Journal of Abnormal Child Psychology, 18,* 565–575.

John, K., Gammon, D., Prusoff, B., & Warner, V. (1987). The Social Adjustment Inventory for Children and Adolescents (SAICA): Testing a new semi-structured interview. *Journal of the American Academy of Child and Adolescent Psychiatry, 26,* 898–911.

Kahn, J. S., Kehle, T. J., Jenson, W. R., & Clarke, E. (1990). Comparison of cognitive–behavioral, relaxation, and self-modeling intervention for depression among middle-school students. *School Psychology Review, 19,* 195–210.

Kanfer, F. H. (1970). Self-monitoring: Methodological limitations and clinical applications. *Journal of Consulting and Clinical Psychology, 35,* 148–152.

Kashani, J. H., Reid, J. C., & Rosenberg, T. K. (1989). Levels of hopelessness in children and adolescents: A developmental perspective. *Journal of Consulting and Clinical Psychology, 57,* 496–499.

Kaslow, N. J., Celano, M. P., & McCarthy, S. M. (1994). Cognitive–behavioral perspectives on childhood depression: A developmental and contextual model. In V. B. Van Hasselt and M. Hersen (Eds.), *Handbook of behavior therapy and pharmacotherapy with children: A comparative analysis* (pp. 235–252). Boston: Allyn & Bacon.

Kaslow, N. J., & Rehm, L. P. (1991). Childhood depression. In R. Morris and T. R. Kratochwill (Eds.), *The practice of child therapy,* 2nd ed. (pp. 43–75). New York: Pergamon Press.

Kaslow, N. J., Rehm, L. P., Pollack, S. L., & Siegel, A. W. (1988). Attributional style and self-control behavior in depressed and nondepressed children and their parents. *Journal of Abnormal Child Psychology, 16,* 163–175.

Kaslow, N. J., Rehm, L. P., & Siegel, A. W. (1984). Social cognitive and cognitive correlates of depression in children. *Journal of Abnormal Child Psychology, 12,* 605–620.

Kaslow, N. J., Tanenbaum, R. L., Abramson, L. Y., Peterson, C., & Seligman, M. E. P. (1983). Problem-solving deficits and depressive symptoms among children. *Journal of Abnormal Child Psychology, 11,* 497–502.

Kazdin, A. E. (1990). Evaluation of the Automatic Thoughts Questionnaire: Negative cognitive processes and depression among children. *Psychological Assessment: A Journal of Consulting and Clinical Psychology, 2,* 73–79.

Kazdin, A. E., Colbus, D., & Rodgers, A. (1986). Assessment of depression and diagnosis of depressive disorder among psychiatrically disturbed children. *Journal of Abnormal Child Psychology, 14,* 499–515.

Kazdin, A. E., Esveldt-Dawson, K., Sherick, R. B., & Colbus, D. (1985). Assessment of overt behavior and childhood depression among psychiatrically disturbed children. *Journal of Consulting and Clinical Psychology, 53,* 201–210.

Kazdin, A. E., French, N. H., Unis, A. S., Esveldt-Dawson, K., & Sherick, R. B. (1983). Hopelessness, depression, and suicidal intent among psychiatrically disturbed inpatient children. *Journal of Consulting and Clinical Psychology, 51,* 504–510.

Kazdin, A. E., Rodgers, A., & Colbus, D. (1986b). The Hopelessness Scale for Children: Psychometric characteristics and concurrent validity. *Journal of Consulting and Clinical Psychology, 54,* 241–245.

Kendall, P. C., Stark, K. D., & Adam, T. (1990). Cognitive deficit or cognitive distortion in childhood depression. *Journal of Abnormal Child Psychology, 18,* 255–270.

Kovacs, M. (1989). Affective disorders in children and adolescents. *American Psychologist, 44,* 209–215.

Larson, R. W., Raffaelli, M., Richards, M. H., Ham, M., & Jewell, L. (1990). Ecology of depression in late childhood and early adolescence: A profile of daily states and activities. *Journal of Abnormal Psychology, 99,* 92–102.

Lefkowitz, M. M., Tesiny, E. P., & Gordon, N. H. (1980). Childhood depression, family income, and locus of control. *The Journal of Nervous and Mental Disease, 168,* 732–735.

Lefkowitz, M. M., & Testiny, E. P. (1980). Assessment of childhood depression. *Journal of Clinical and Consulting Psychology, 48,* 43–50.

Leitenberg, H., Yost, L. W., & Carroll-Wilson, M. (1986). Negative cognitive errors in children: Questionnaire development, normative data, and comparisons between children with and without self-reported symptoms of depression, low self-esteem, and evaluation anxiety. *Journal of Consulting and Clinical Psychology, 54,* 528–536.

Leon, G. R., Kendall, P. C., & Garber, J. (1980). Depression in children: Parent, teacher, and child perspectives. *Journal of Abnormal Child Psychology, 8,* 221–235.

Lewinsohn, P. M. (1974). A behavioral approach to depression. In R. M. Friedman and M. M. Katz (Eds.), *The psychology of depression: Contemporary theory and research* (pp. 157–185). New York: John Wiley.

Lewis, M., & Miller, S. M. (Eds.), (1990). *Handbook of developmental psychopathology.* New York: Plenum Press.

Lewis, M., & Saarni, C. (1985). *The socialization of emotions.* New York: Plenum Press.

McCandless, B. R., & Evans, E. D. (1973). *Children and youth psychosocial development.* Hinsdale, IL: Dryden Press.

McCauley, E., Mitchell, J. R., Burke, P., & Moss, S. (1988). Cognitive attributes of depression in children and adolescents. *Journal of Consulting and Clinical Psychology, 56,* 903–908.

McGee, R., Anderson, J., Williams, S., & Silva, P. A. (1986). Cognitive correlates of depressive symptoms in 11-year old children. *Journal of Abnormal Child Psychology, 14,* 517–524.

Meyer, N. E., Dyck, D. G., & Petrinack, R. J. (1989). Cognitive appraisal and attributional correlates of depressive symptoms in children. *Journal of Abnormal Child Psychology, 17,* 325–336.

Moyal, B. R. (1977). Locus of control, self-esteem, stimulus appraisal, and depressive symptoms in children. *Journal of Consulting and Clinical Psychology, 45,* 951–952.

Mullins, L. L., Peterson, L., Wonderlich, S. A., & Reaven, N. M. (1986). The influence of depressive symptomatology in children on the social responses and perception of adults. *Journal of Clinical Child Psychology, 15,* 233–240.

Mullins, L. L., Siegel, L. J., & Hodges, K. (1985). Cognitive problem-solving and life event correlates of depressive symptoms in children. *Journal of Abnormal Child Psychology, 13,* 305–314.

Nolen-Hoeksema, S. (1990). *Sex differences in depression.* Stanford: Stanford University Press.

Nolen-Hoeksema, S., Girgus, J. S., & Seligman, M. E. P. (1986). Learned helplessness in children: A longitudinal study of depression, achievement, and explanatory style. *Journal of Personality and Social Psychology, 51,* 435–442.

Noles, S. W., Cash, T. F., & Winstead, B. A. (1985). Body image, physical attractiveness, and depression. *Journal of Consulting and Clinical Psychology, 53,* 89–94.

Nowicki, S., & Duke, M. (1974). A preschool and primary inter–external control scale. *Developmental Psychology, 10*, 874–880.

Nowicki, S., & Strickland, B. (1973). A locus of control scale for children. *Journal of Consulting and Clinical Psychology, 40*, 148–154.

Offer, D., Ostrov, E., & Howard, K. I. (1981). *The adolescent: A psychological self-portrait.* New York: Basic Books.

Peterson, C., & Seligman, M. E. P. (1984). Causal explanations as a factor for depression: Theory and evidence. *Psychological Review, 91*, 347–374.

Peterson, L., Mullins, L. L., & Ridley-Johnson, R. (1985). Childhood depression: Peer reactions to depression and life stress. *Journal of Abnormal Child Psychology, 13*, 597–609.

Piers, E. V., & Harris, D. B. (1969). *The Piers–Harris Children's Self Concept Scale.* Nashville, TN: Counselor Recordings and Tests.

Puig-Antich, J., Lukens, E., Davies, M., Goetz, D., Brennan-Quattrock, J., & Todak, G. (1985a). Psychosocial functioning in prepubertal major depressive disorder I: Interpersonal relationships during the depressive episode. *Archives of General Psychiatry, 42*, 511–517.

Puig-Antich, J., Lukens, E., Davies, M., Goetz, D.,Brennan-Quattrock, J., & Todak, G. (1985b). Psychosocial functioning in prepubertal major depressive disorders II: Interpersonal relationships after sustained recovery from affective episode. *Archives of General Psychiatry, 42*, 511–517.

Rehm, L. P. (1977). A self-control model of depression. *Behavior Therapy, 8*, 787–804.

Rehm, L. P. (1988). Self-management and cognitive processes in depression. In L. B. Alloy (Ed.), *Cognitive processes in depression* (pp. 143–176). New York: Guilford Press.

Rehm, L. P. (in press). Psychotherapies for depression. In K. Schlesinger and B. Bloom (Eds.), *Proceedings of the first Boulder symposium on clinical psychology: Depression.* New York: Erlbaum.

Rehm, L. P. & Carter, A. S. (1990). Cognitive components of depression. In M. Lewis and S. M. Miller (Eds.), *Handbook of developmental psychopathology* (pp. 342–351). New York: Plenum Press.

Reynolds, W. M., & Coats, K. I. (1986). A comparison of cognitive–behavioral therapy and relaxation training for the treatment of depression in adolescents. *Journal of Consulting and Clinical Psychology, 54*, 653–660.

Robins, C. J., & Hinkley, K. (1989). Social–cognitive processing and depressive symptoms in children: A comparison of measures. *Journal of Abnormal Child Psychology, 17*, 29–36.

Rotheram-Borus, M. J., Trautman, P. D., Dopkins, S. C., & Shrout, P. E. (1990). Cognitive style and pleasant activities among female adolescent suicide attempters. *Journal of Consulting and Clinical Psychology, 58*, 554–561.

Sacco, W. P., & Graves, D. J. (1984). Childhood depression, interpersonal problem-solving, and self-ratings of performance. *Journal of Clinical Child Psychology, 13*, 10–15.

Saylor, C. F., Finch, A. J., Baskin, C. H., Furey, W., & Kelly, M. M. (1984a). Construct validity for measures of childhood depression: Application of multitrait–multimethod methodology. *Journal of Consulting and Clinical Psychology, 52*, 977–985.

Saylor, C. F., Finch, A. J., Spirito, A., & Bennett, B. (1984b). The Children's Depression Inventory: A systematic evaluation of psychometric properties. *Journal of Consulting and Clinical Psychology, 52*, 955–967.

Schwartz, M., Friedman, R., Lindsay, P., & Narrol, H. (1982). The relationship between conceptual tempo and depression in children. *Journal of Consulting and Clinical Psychology, 50*, 488–490.

Seagull, E. A. W., & Weinsbank, A. B. (1984). Childhood depression in a selected group of low-achieving seventh-graders. *Journal of Clinical Child Psychology, 13*, 134–140.

Sedlack, A. J., & Kurtz, S. T. (1981). A review of children's use of causal inference principles. *Child Development, 52*, 759–784.

Seligman, M. E. P. (1975). *Helplessness: On depression, development and death.* San Francisco: W. H. Freeman.

Seligman, M. E. P. (1981). A learned helplessness point of view. In L. P. Rehm (Ed.), *Behavior therapy for depression* (pp. 123–141). New York: Academic Press.

Seligman, M. E. P., Abramson, L. Y., Semmel, A., & von Baeyer, C. (1979). Depressive attributional style. *Journal of Abnormal Psychology, 88*, 242–247.

Seligman, M. E. P., & Peterson, C. (1986). A learned helplessness perspective on childhood depression: Theory and research. In M. Rutter, C. E. Izard, & P. B. Read (Eds.), *Depression in young people: Developmental and clinical perspectives* (pp. 223–249). New York: Guilford Press.

Seligman, M. E. P., Peterson, C., Kaslow, N. J., Tanenbaum, R. L., Alloy, L. B., & Abramson, L. Y. (1984). Attributional styles and depressive symptoms among children. *Journal of Abnormal Psychology, 93*, 235–238.

Selman, R. L. (1980). *The growth of interpersonal understandings.* New York: Academic Press.

Siegel, L. J., & Griffin, N. J. (1984). Correlates of depressive symptoms in adolescents. *Journal of Youth and Adolescence, 13,* 475–487.

Simons, R. L., & Miller, M. G. (1987). Adolescent depression: Assessing the impact of negative cognitions and socioenvironmental problems. *Social Work, July–August,* 326–330.

Siomopoulos, G., & Inamdar, S.C. (1979). Developmental aspects of hopelessness. *Adolescence, 14,* 233–239.

Slotkin, J., Forehand, R., Fauber, R., McComb, A., & Long, N. (1988). Parent-completed and adolescent-completed CDIs: Relationship to adolescent social and cognitive functioning. *Journal of Abnormal Child Psychology, 16,* 207–217.

Spirito, A., Williams, C. A., Stark, L. J., & Hart, K. J. (1988). The Hopelessness Scale for Children: Psychometric properties with normal and emotionally disturbed children. *Journal of Abnormal Child Psychology, 16,* 445–458.

Stark, K. D., Reynolds, W. M., & Kaslow, N. J. (1987). A comparison of the relative efficacy of self-control therapy and a behavioral problem-solving therapy for depression in children. *Journal of Abnormal Child Psychology, 15,* 91–113.

Stern, D. N. (1985). *The interpersonal world of the infant: A view from psychoanalysis and developmental psychology.* New York: Basic Books.

Stipek, D. J., & DeCotis, K. M. (1988). Children's understanding of the implications of causal attributions for emotional experiences. *Child Development, 59,* 1601–1616.

Strauss, C. C., Forehand, R., Frame, C., & Smith, K. (1984). Characteristics of children with extreme scores on the Children's Depression Inventory. *Journal of Clinical Child Psychology, 13,* 227–231.

Tesiny, E. P., Lefkowitz, M. M., & Gordon, N. H. (1980). Childhood depression, locus of control, and school achievement. *Journal of Educational Psychology, 12,* 506–510.

Thomas, A., & Chess, S. (1977). *Temperament and development.* New York: Brunner/Mazel.

Vygotsky, L. S. (1978). Internalization of higher psychological functions. In M. Cole, V. John-Steiner, S. Schribner, & E. Souberman (Eds.), *Mind in society: The development of higher psychological processes* (pp. 52–57). Cambridge, MA: Harvard University Press.

Ward, L. G., Friedlander, M. L., & Silverman, W. K. (1987). Children's depressive symptoms, negative self-statements, and causal attributions for success and failure. *Cognitive Therapy and Research, 11,* 215–227.

Weisz, J. R., Stevens, J. S., Curry, J. F., Cohen, R., Craighead, E., Burligame, W. V., Smith, A., Weiss, B., & Parmelee, D. X. (1989). Control-related cognitions and depression among inpatient children and adolescents. *Journal of the American Academy of Child and Adolescent Psychiatry, 28,* 358–363.

Weisz, J. R., Weiss, B., Wasserman, A. A., & Rintoui, B. (1987). Control-related beliefs and depression among clinic-referred children and adolescents. *Journal of Abnormal Psychology, 96,* 58–63.

Whitman, P. B., & Leitenberg, H. (1990). Negatively biased recall in children with self-report symptoms of depression. *Journal of Abnormal Child Psychology, 18,* 15–27.

Wierzbicki, M., & McCabe, M. (1988). Social skills and subsequent depressive symptomatology in children. *Journal of Clinical Child Psychiatry, 17,* 203–208.

Windle, M., Hooker, K., Lenerz, K., East, P. L., Lerner, J. V., & Lerner, R. M. (1986). Temperament, perceived competence and depression in early and late adolescents. *Developmental Psychology, 22,* 384–392.

Worchel, F., Little, V., & Alcala, J. (1990). Self-perceptions of depressed children on tasks of cognitive abilities. *Journal of School Psychology, 28,* 97–104.

Zupan, B. A., Hammen, C., & Jaenicke, C. (1987). The effects of current mood and prior depressive history on self-schematic processing in children. *Journal of Experimental Child Psychology, 43,* 144–158.

7

A Developmental Psychopathology Perspective on Depression in Children and Adolescents

Dante Cicchetti, Fred A. Rogosch, and Sheree L. Toth

The study of depression in children and adolescents has gone through a series of contradictory formulations as theorists have attempted to understand this complex form of disorder in youngsters. Conceptualizations have ranged from the belief that depression in children was impossible due to the immaturity of ego development prior to adolescence and the concomitant inability to experience guilt (Rie, 1966) to the belief that depression in children is prevalent and may be manifested in a variety of symptoms quite divergent from those evidenced in adulthood, i.e., depressive equivalents (Cytryn & McKnew, 1972; Glaser, 1967) to the assertion that symptoms indicating depression are the same across the age span from childhood to adulthood (American Psychiatric Association, 1987; Kashani et al., 1981; Puig-Antich, 1980). Such divergence in thinking indicates that the topic of depression in childhood and adolescence is an area of active and significant theoretical and empirical inquiry.

While it is at present generally accepted that children do experience depressive feelings and disorders, there are many disparate views about the origins of depression and subsequent approaches to intervention and prevention. Many such explanations of depression in children represent downward extensions of theory and empirical findings from the study of depression in adulthood. These explanations include, for example, depression as (1) a response to stress or negative life events, (2) a consequence of distortions in cognitions or attributional style, (3) a result of learned helplessness arising from reinforcement contingencies in the environment, (4) the result of interpersonal skill deficits or lack

Dante Cicchetti, Fred A. Rogosch, and Sheree L. Toth • Mt. Hope Family Center, University of Rochester, Rochester, New York 14608.

Handbook of Depression in Children and Adolescents, edited by William M. Reynolds and Hugh F. Johnston. Plenum Press, New York, 1994.

of social support, (5) an outgrowth of early unresolved loss or separation experiences, and (6) a genetically inherited disorder resulting in neurophysiological anomalies (see Rutter, Izard, & Read, 1986). Of course, additional conceptualizations could be added to this list. Although work such as this has provided a substantial contribution to beginning phases of inquiry into understanding child and adolescent depression, these accounts typically do not adequately consider the incomplete and evolving biological, affective, cognitive, social, representational, and social–cognitive capacities of the child. As a result, the disparate theoretical formulations can be vague regarding the processes or mechanisms by which the depressed outcomes are actually achieved by children, given the limitations imposed by their developmental level.

Developmental psychopathology is a newly emerging discipline (Cicchetti, 1984a,b, 1989; Cicchetti & Toth, 1991; Rutter, 1986; Sroufe & Rutter, 1984) that seeks to unify, within a developmental, life-span framework, the many contributions to the study of depression emanating from multiple fields of inquiry, including psychiatry, psychology, neuroscience, sociology, cultural anthropology, epidemiology, biostatistics, and psychometrics. Achenbach (1990) has described developmental psychopathology as a macroparadigm rather than a unitary theory. As such, developmental psychopathology represents a movement toward understanding psychopathology and its causes, determinants, course, sequelae, and treatment by integrating knowledge from multiple disciplines within a developmental framework. The undergirding developmental orientation forces theorists and researchers to begin to ask new questions about the phenomena they study. For example, it becomes necessary to move beyond identifying features that distinguish depressed and nondepressed children (e.g., attributional distortions, affect dysregulation) to articulating how such differences have evolved developmentally.

What Is Developmental?

Though the term would seem straightforward, understanding what "developmental" signifies often results in confusion and conflicting views. It is frequently presumed that any study involving children represents a "developmental" investigation. However, it is certainly possible to study children from a nondevelopmental perspective. Age, in and of itself, does not necessarily signify that a developmental process has been specified (Rutter, 1989).

Developmental psychopathology is concerned not only with children but also with individuals across the life span. The developmental approach is charged with two interrelated goals. First, the developmental perspective seeks to examine the specific evolving capacities that are characteristic of individuals at varying developmental stages across the life span. This examination requires formulating questions about a phenomenon in terms of what capacities are inherent in an individual during a particular developmental stage and how a given process or mechanism becomes manifested in view of the individual's developmental capacities and attainments. For example, the cognitive capacities from toddler to third grader to adolescent are progressively more advanced. As a result, meanings attributed to events and cognitive capacities for dealing with experiences are vastly different. Thus, to truly understand a phenomenon, it is necessary to consider developmental variations in cognitive capacities in order to ascertain how a hypothesized outcome is realized at different ages.

Second, a developmental analysis seeks to examine the prior sequence of adaptations in development that contribute to an outcome in a particular developmental period. This examination requires that the current status of a child's functioning be examined in the context of how that status was attained across the course of development. Such a life-course view seeks to move beyond the proximal causes of current outcomes to examine the developmental progression of distal sources of influence that have eventuated in current outcomes.

In keeping with these goals, Hammen (1992) has offered an exemplary developmental analysis of major contributors to depression in adults. Historically, factors such as biased cognitive appraisals, life stress, and interpersonal difficulties have each been examined extensively in regard to their effects on depressive outcomes. Hammen, however, has begun to ask the developmental questions of how individual differences in these proximal areas of influence evolved. Her analysis places the sources of current depression as originating in the stream of developmental process. The conceptualization of these constructs within a developmental perspective provides a richer, more in-depth understanding of the origins of depression and the processes that contribute to its continuation.

A Developmental Psychopathology Perspective

A concentration on the interface between normal and abnormal development is central to the developmental psychopathology perspective. This being the case, developmental psychopathology is interested not only in how knowledge from the study of normal development can inform the study of psychopathology, but also in how the study of psychopathology can inform the understanding of normal development (Cicchetti, 1989, 1990c). Thus, the application of knowledge of normal biological, affective, cognitive, and interpersonal development to the understanding of depression results in an articulation of how components of individual functioning in depressed children contribute to their symptomatic presentation. In turn, the study of aberrations in biological, affective, cognitive, and interpersonal capacities in depressed children assists in the provision of a more complete understanding of how these domains function in the normal course of development. The study of abnormal and the study of normal are intimately intertwined. For example, an understanding of the ramifications of a secure attachment relationship are best understood by contrasting children with secure and insecure attachments (Sroufe, 1990). Knowledge of the unfolding complications and difficulties that children with insecure attachments experience contributes to the understanding of how secure attachment relationships function to promote an adaptive course of development. It is through this dialectic that knowledge advances in the study of both normal and abnormal development.

In essence, developmental psychopathology is not primarily the study of disorders. That is not to say that the field does not seek to make a contribution to understanding psychopathology, including depression. However, the central focus of developmental psychopathology involves the elucidation of developmental processes and how they function as indicated and elaborated by the examination of extremes in developmental outcome.

Radke-Yarrow and Zahn-Waxler (1990) have highlighted how this approach contrasts with that of developmental psychology, which seeks to examine the central tendency of groups and uniformities and constancies in developmental progression. Extreme deviations from the mean in distributions are often viewed by developmental psychologists as problematic outliers that are best disregarded or that require adjustments to be made via statistical transformation to bring their scores closer to the mean. In contrast, the developmental psychopathologist is keenly interested in these extremes in their own right. Such extremes contribute substantial diversity to the possible outcomes in development, thereby enhancing our understanding of developmental processes. In addition to an interest in extremes in the distribution (i.e., children with disorders), the developmental psychopathologist also is interested in variations in the continuum between the mean and the extremes. These variations may represent individuals who are currently not divergent enough to be considered disordered but who may progress to further extremes as development continues. Such individuals may be vulnerable to developing future disordered outcomes. Therefore, tracking the ontogenetic course of these children is likely to broaden the complexity of understanding of developmental processes.

Diversity in process and outcome are hallmarks of the developmental psychopathology perspective. It is expected that there are multiple contributors to depressive outcomes in any individual, that the contributors vary between individuals with a depressive outcome, that there is heterogeneity among depressed children in the features of their depressive disturbance, and that there are numerous pathways to any depressive outcome. The principles of equifinality and multifinality derived from general systems theory are relevant in this regard (von Bertalanffy, 1968). Equifinality refers to the observation that a diversity of paths may lead to the same outcome. As such, a variety of developmental progressions may eventuate in depression, rather than positing a singular primary pathway to disorder. In contrast, multifinality suggests that any one component may function differently depending on the organization of the system in which it operates. Thus, for example, loss of a major attachment figure in childhood will result in numerous outcomes for children depending on the context of their environment and their individual competencies and coping capacities. Depression may be one such outcome in, for example, a child who already had insecure representational working models of attachment figures and of the self and who faces extremes of additional stress in conjunction with minimal support or nurturance from caregivers.

Given the diversity in process and outcome apparent in development, it should not be surprising that a developmental psychopathology approach to depression does not have a simple, unitary etiological explanation. The occurrence of depression during the life course likely results from a multiplicity of pathways in different individuals. Although commonalities in pathways in different clusters of depressed children may be delineated, it is also possible that depression is not the only outcome associated with each pathway. Further work exploring the developmental trajectories leading to depressive outcomes may delineate pathways that are depression-specific in some individuals. There are also likely to be, however, generic pathways that contribute to a range of dysfunctions and disorders (e.g., anxiety disorders, substance abuse, personality disorders), of which depression may be one. Thus, the study of depression needs to be part of a larger body of inquiry into the developmental patterns that promote adjustment difficulties and psychopathology.

The Organizational Approach

Drawing from the structuralist or organismic theory of development (Werner, 1948), the organizational approach to development (Cicchetti, 1990c; Cicchetti & Schneider-Rosen, 1986; Cicchetti & Sroufe, 1978; Sroufe & Waters, 1976) offers developmental psychopathology a powerful theoretical framework for conceptualizing the intricacies of the life-span perspective on psychopathology more generally and on depression more specifically. The organizational approach focuses on the quality of integration both within and between behavioral and biological systems of the individual. This focus on variations in the quality of integration provides the building blocks on which the developmental psychopathologist characterizes developmental status. Further, the organizational approach specifies how development proceeds. Development occurs as a progression of qualitative reorganizations within and among the biological, affective, cognitive, representational, and social systems proceeding through differentiation and subsequent hierarchical integration (Werner, 1948). The orthogenetic principle specifies that the developing individual moves from a state of relatively diffuse, undifferentiated organization to states of greater articulation and complexity by differentiation and consolidation of the separate systems, followed by hierarchical integration within and between systems. Initially, separate systems within the infant are relatively undifferentiated, but through development, the cognitive, affective, social, representational, and biological systems increasingly become more distinct or differentiated, and repeated hierarchical integrations among these systems lead to increasingly complex levels of organization.

At each juncture of reorganization in development, the concept of hierarchic motility specifies that prior developmental structures are incorporated into later ones by means of hierarchic integration. In this way, early experience and its effects on the organization of the individual are carried forward within the individual's organization of systems rather than having reorganizations override previous organizations. As a result, hierarchic motility suggests that previous areas of vulnerability or strength within the organizational structure may remain present although not prominent in the current organizational structure. Nevertheless, the presence of prior structures within the current organization allows for possible future access by way of regressive activation of those previous structures in times of stress or crisis. Thus, a behavioral or symptomatic presentation of a depressed individual may appear discrepant with recently evidenced adaptation, but in effect indicate the activation of prior maladaptive structures that were retained in the organizational structure through hierarchical integration.

Each state of development confronts the child with new challenges to which the individual must adapt. At each stage, successful adaptation or competence is signified by an adaptive integration within and among the emotional, cognitive, social, representational, and biological domains, as the child masters current developmental challenges. Waters and Sroufe (1983) view competence as the ability to use both internal and external resources to attain a successful adaptation. Because earlier structures of the child's organization are incorporated into later structures in the successive process of hierarchical integration, early competence tends to promote later competence. A child who has adaptively met the developmental challenges of a particular stage will be better equipped to meet successive new challenges in development. This is not to say that early adaptation ensures successful later adaptation, because major changes or stresses in the internal and external environment may tax subsequent adaptational capacities. However, early competence does provide a more optimal organization of behavioral and biological systems, thus offering, in a probabilistic manner, the greatest likelihood that adaptive resources are available to encounter and cope with new developmental demands.

In contrast, incompetence in development is fostered by difficulties or maladaptive efforts to resolve the challenges of a developmental period. Inadequate resolution of developmental challenges may result in a developmental lag or delay in, for example, one of the behavioral systems such as the emotional system. As a result, less than adequate integration within that domain will occur, and that poor intradomain integration will compromise adaptive interdomain integration as hierarchical integration proceeds. Thus, incompetence in development may be viewed as a problematic integration or lack of successful integration between domains or as an integration of pathological structures. Over time, difficulty in the organization of one behavioral system may tend to promote difficulty in the way in which other systems are organized as hierarchical integration between the separate systems occurs. The organization of the individual may then appear to consist of an integration of poorly integrated component systems. As the converse of the effects of early competence, early incompetence will tend to promote later incompetence because the child arrives at successive developmental stages with less than optimal resources available for responding to the challenges of that period. Again, this progression is not inevitable but probabilistic. Changes in the internal and external environment may lead to improvements in the ability to grapple with developmental challenges, resulting in a redirection in the developmental course.

The concept of "polarities of orthogenesis" (Kaplan, 1966) is useful in broadening the scope of understanding of variations in developmental adaptation and vulnerability to depression. The first polarity, rigid vs. flexible, involves the ability to use assimilation and accommodation (Piaget, 1952) to adapt to environmental challenges. The rigid individual is limited in this ability, whereas the flexible individual is not. The second polarity, labile vs. stable, involves the degree to which integrity is maintained in the process of achieving new adaptations. The labile individual undergoes extreme changes in psychological structure in response to minor environmental variation, whereas the stable individual maintains integrity and employs balanced and orderly strategies for adapting to environmental fluctuation. When manifested in the psychological structure, rigidity and lability in response to adaptational demands result in distress and mental pain for the individual. Structural rigidity and lability contribute to a child's experiencing anger and frustration as well as a loss of self-esteem and a sense of inability when met with environmental demands to which he or she struggles to adapt. As a result, feelings of helplessness and hopelessness, hallmarks of depressive experience, may be engendered.

Given the importance of a life-span view of developmental processes and an interest in delineating how prior development influences later development, a major issue in developmental psychopathology involves how continuity in the quality of adaptation across developmental time is determined. Sroufe (1979) has articulated the concept of coherence in the organization of behaviors in successive developmental periods as a means of identifying continuity in adaptation despite changing behavioral presentations of the developing individual. Crucial to this concept is a recognition that the same behaviors in different developmental periods may represent quite different levels of adaptation. Behaviors that indicate competence within a developmental period may indicate incompetence when evidenced within subsequent developmental periods. Normative behaviors early in development may indicate maladaptation when exhibited later in development. Thus, the manifestation of competence in different developmental periods is rarely indicated by isomorphism in behavioral presentation. Homotypic continuity is likely to be an unusual occurrence, particularly early in development.

An illustration of different behaviors representing continuity of adaptation (i.e., heterotypic continuity) is provided by Sroufe, Fox, and Pancake (1983) in discussing attachment and dependency. The surface interpretation of behaviors of infants in the Strange Situation, an experimental paradigm devised to assess parent–child attachment relations (Ainsworth & Wittig, 1969), might suggest that those who typically exhibit little distress on separation from their mothers and little affective response when reunited (Type A or anxious/avoidant classification) are exhibiting early signs of independence and autonomy. In contrast, infants who may exhibit distress and crying when separated and who eagerly approach and seek comfort from their mothers when reunited (subgroups of the Type B or secure attachment classification) might be considered to exhibit high dependence on their mothers. However, the organization of behaviors in the securely attached children is regarded as indicating a secure attachment to the caregiver, a more developmentally competent attainment, whereas the anxious/avoidant children's behavior is regarded as signifying anxiety and insecurity in the attachment relationship. Later in development, it is the anxious/avoidant group of children who exhibit helplessness and dependency, while those in the securely attached group are more likely to be autonomous and independent.

This example illustrates that if isomorphism in behaviors were to be the standard for judging continuity in development, the prior descriptions would suggest developmental discontinuity. However, when examined in the context of the coherence of the organization of behaviors across time, the presence of phenotypically different behaviors at different time points suggests continuity in the quality of adaptation, i.e., heterotypic continuity, rather than discontinuity. The underlying meaning of behaviors rather than the behaviors themselves is perpetuated across development. At the level of meaning in the preceding example, the securely attached children's behaviors on separation and reunion indicate trust in the mother's supportive presence and expectations of being comforted when distressed. This confidence in the ability to rely on the mother is internalized, resulting in more self-confident and autonomous behavior later in development. In contrast, the anxious/avoidant infant's behavior indicates doubts of the mother's availability to provide comfort and a restriction in affect to avoid unpredictable behavior from the mother. Later in development, the child has internalized this sense of doubt and uncertainty, exhibiting dependent and helpless behaviors.

Zahn-Waxler and Kochanska (1990) provide another example of behavior that might appear developmentally appropriate if the underlying organization and meaning of the behavior are not considered. Zahn-Waxler and Kochanska examined the development of guilt feelings in the children of depressed and nondepressed mothers. Although there were increases with age for all children in the guilt feelings they experienced, the underlying motives and functions of the guilt feelings varied for the children of depressed and nondepressed mothers. For the children of depressed mothers, guilt feelings were more frequently associated with primitive reasoning and irrationality, whereas the guilt feelings of children with nondepressed mothers were shown to function more adaptively. Thus, behaviors that might phenotypically appear appropriate and developmentally expected may be considered to be problematic when the context in which those behaviors occur is considered. The molar organization and meanings of behavior and the coherence of themes underlying the molecular behavioral presentation are likely to be more informative with respect to continuities in development. Transformations in the behavioral presentation may occur despite continuity in the coherence of the underlying organization of behavior.

In the course of development, there may be prototypic organizations of behavioral systems that have the potential for transformation into a spectrum of depressive presentations. There may be numerous forms of such depressotypic organizations that, depending on the course of subsequent experiences in development, may eventuate in depression or other forms of psychopathology or, in the event of corrective experiences, adaptive outcomes (Cicchetti, 1990b). What may be important is that early forms of incompetent organization of behavioral systems may not phenotypically resemble later depression, although a coherence in molar organization between a prior prototype and later depression may be discerned. For example, difficulty in managing anger may be an early prototypic feature with linkages to later depression. Difficulty in anger regulation through development may become integrated with changes in cognition and interpersonal relations that may eventually result in a depressive presentation. Alternatively, problems in regulating anger, given disparate developmental experiences, might eventuate in a different form of disorder, i.e., antisocial personality, or comorbidity of disorders, i.e., depression and antisocial personality. Nevertheless, for some individuals, there may be continuity between early difficulties in affect regulation and later depression, although the phenotypic behavioral presentation, poor early anger control vs. later dysphoria and chronic sadness, might appear discontinuous.

In view of the multiplicity of pathways that may eventuate in depressive disorders, various forms of depressotypic organizations should be anticipated. An example of a fairly typical outcome can be drawn from the attributional-theory literature. Within the cognitive domain, the child has developed a negative attributional style, blaming the self for negative occurrences and brushing off successes as a result of luck. There is a feeling of hopelessness about the future and a belief that the individual is unable to alter the situation. Emotionally, the child has low self-esteem and feelings of worthlessness and guilt. Sadness and dejection are frequently experienced in response to minor difficulties. There is little capacity to enjoy daily experiences. Socially, the child has poor relationships with family members and peers and does not expect others to desire contact with him or her.

Withdrawal from relationships has contributed to poor interpersonal skills. Biologically, a genetic propensity toward irritability exacerbates social encounters. In summary, this prototypic depressotypic organization suggests an integration of maladaptive features across the different behavioral and biological systems. Difficulties may arise in one component system and subsequently, through hierarchic integration, affect other behavioral systems. Such a depressotypic organization will have high potential for transforming into a depressive disorder given further experiences in development. This likelihood increases even more when one realizes that the child's cognitive schemata and inner mental representations will perpetuate involvement in situations that confirm prior experiences and a negative self-view.

Stage-Salient Developmental Issues

The evolution of such an organization may be seen as occurring through development as a child passes through stages in which new forms of adaptation are required. In each stage of development, there are specific issues that confront the child for the first time and require the child to garner and expand available resources in attempts to master new challenges. As stage-salient issues emerge in development, not only must they be negotiated at the time, but also adaptation requires a reintegration of prior stage-salient issues with the issue confronted in the current developmental period. Each stage-salient issue, thematically, becomes a lifelong feature of importance for adaptation. However, successful resolution of stage-salient tasks does not inoculate the individual against future difficulties. Likewise, unsuccessful resolution does not doom the individual to future dysfunction. Individuals continue to be affected by new experiences and changing conditions throughout their lives, and changes in the course of adaptation remain possible. The quality of resolution of stage-salient issues, however, does tend to constrain and canalize developmental pathways, making change less likely (Sroufe, 1989).

The initial developmental task occurring within the first 3 months of live is the achievement of homeostatic regulation. This includes the establishment of basic cycles and rhythms of sleep–wakefulness and feeding–elimination. During this period, the infant establishes a reliable signaling system that helps him or her achieve balance in inner state and external stimulation. A predictable, protective, engaging environment assists the infant in achieving regulation, whereas a chaotic, arbitrary, and hypo-/hyperstimulating environment contributes to difficulty in resolution of this task.

In the subsequent 4- to 6-month period, the infant develops a capacity for greater sustained attention to the environment. Infants begin to shift from primarily reflexive response to endogenous stimulations to contingent responses to exogenous environmental stimulation. Through this greater responsivity to the environment, the infant also differentiates various forms of affect expression and the intensity of these affects increases. Infants exhibit laughter in response to pleasurable stimulations, as well as frustration and rage when expected needs are not met. Maternal sensitivity and the infant's ability to elicit a maternal response promote successful negotiation of this issue, resulting in affective responsiveness and appropriate modulation. Difficulty in negotiation results in regulatory problems, with frequent irritability and difficulty in calming, affecting the ongoing quality of interactions with caregivers. Excessive irritability and difficulty in being soothed, both associated with failure on early stage-salient issues, may suggest early signs of affect dysregulation that may portend vulnerability to later affect-regulatory problems and depression.

The development of attachment relationships occurs between 6 and 12 months. The successful resolution of this task results in a secure attachment relationship with the primary caregiver, marked by increased attention and attunement to interpersonal inter-actions. Dyadic interactions are marked by synchrony, relatedness, resiliency to stress, and affective interchange. In contrast, insecure attachment relationships are characterized by fear and wariness, and the infant experiences considerable anxiety and uncertainty in the relationship with the caregiver. This negative resolution of attachment formation may suggest later difficulty in expecting comfort and support from others, thereby creating a sense of helplessness in one's ability to attain needed nurturance. This helplessness, in turn, may be linked to later depressive experience.

Subsequently, the growing infant is faced with the development of an autonomous self in the 18- to 36-month period. The infant must move out from the attachment relationship to explore the environment. The infant begins to understand the self as a separate and independent entity that has an effect on the environment and others. Self-regulation becomes increasingly important and is channeled through developing delay of gratification and frustration tolerance. Children also begin to have affective responses to self-recognition, experiencing themselves positively or negatively and evaluating them-selves in qualitative terms. As language and representational skills develop, the child's representations of self become increasingly complex and are integrated with affective reactions to the self. Negative representations of the self and associated affects are internalized by children who unsuccessfully resolve this task. Impoverished self-esteem and negative views about one's capabilities may create a sense of helplessness, again suggestive of future liability for depression.

Establishing peer relationships is the major developmental issue of the 36- to 60-month period. During this period, children develop an awareness of social roles and relationships and develop early emotional bonds with peers. Role-taking, empathy, and prosocial behavior become important features of interacting with agemates. Poor resolu-tion of this developmental task includes avoidance of peers or difficulty in establishing harmonious peer interactions and early friendships. This difficulty in peer engagement further suggests alienation in the interpersonal sphere that may relate to limitations in the ability to use interpersonal relations as a coping resource, thereby creating further vulnerability to depression.

The 6- to 12-year-period is marked by the need to adapt to school and participate in an organized environment of peers and nonfamilial adults. Feelings of agency, volition, and mastery become salient achievements. Children begin to assume responsibilities and accomplish tasks independently. They become increasingly aware of internal psychologi-cal processes and experiences of multiple emotions and their expression. Children having difficulty adapting to school derive a diminished sense of personal efficacy and belonging-ness. Such doubts about one's competence may increasingly set the stage for depressive ruminations about one's failures and inadequacies.

In the adolescent period, individuals must adapt to the physical changes inherent in puberty, forming relationships with opposite-sex peers, and establishing a sense of personal identity and uniqueness from one's family. Difficulty in resolving the developmen-tal tasks of this period are marked by problems and conflicts in negotiating being separate and unique as an individual while still maintaining harmonious relations with family. Difficulties in successfully resolving these additional issues of interpersonal and intraper-sonal adaptation further limit and restrict interpersonal and internal resources available to cope with stress, contributing to greater vulnerability to depression.

Thus, difficulties associated with failure on each stage-salient issue can be seen as resulting in an increased vulnerability to depression. Although intervening variables certainly may modify this course, the child who does not successfully resolve these developmentally salient issues clearly is at risk for the emergence of an affective disorder (Cicchetti, Toth, & Bush, 1988).

A Transactional Approach to Depression

Much of our discussion to this point has focused on the organization of developmental processes occurring within the developing child. Our attention shifts now to examining the means by which individual differences in developmental outcomes are conceptualized. A transactional model of development as originally articulated by Sameroff and Chandler (1975) provides the framework for a developmental perspective on how internal and external sources of influence are coordinated to shape the organizational structure of individuals along alternate pathways over the course of development. From the transactional perspective, reductionistic attempts to discern unitary, main-effect causes of depression (or other developmental outcomes) are inadequate. It is unlikely that a single cause of depression, in either the biological or the environmental sphere, will be found. Such an approach denies the complexity of development and the mutually influencing nature of constitutional, psychological, environmental, and sociological determinants over time. Further, the transactional conceptualization also moves beyond the mere interaction of factors in determining pathological outcomes. Thus, traditional diathesis–stress models (Gottesman & Shields, 1972) suggest that biological vulnerabilities to psychopathology are realized only under certain environmental conditions. Of course, it need not be the case that only biological agents cause disorder when moderated by environmental agents; environmental agents may also be considered causal factors in producing disorder given certain biological conditions. Nevertheless, interactive models remain essentially cross-sectional in nature. They posit a critical juncture between factors at a point in time rather than considering the successive ongoing transformations across domains that occur through the course of development.

The transactional model specifies that the interrelationships between the organization of developmental domains (biological, emotional, cognitive, interpersonal) and the environment (familial, social, community) are in a progressive exchange of mutual influence. Not only is the child influenced by environmental inputs resulting in transformation and reorganization, but also the environment is influenced by and responds to characteristics of the child. At successive points in development, the organizational structure of both the child and the environment are in a state of bidirectional influence. For example, early temperamental differences in children are transformed into a range of attachment organizations in response to variations in responding from caregivers. Subsequently, there are also likely to be alterations within caregivers as they respond to new variations in behavioral presentations of the child. Qualities of both the child and the environment are being mutually influenced as each evolves. These transactions of bidirectional influence will generate variations in the quality of the organization of their different biological and behavioral systems. At subsequent points in development, variations in the organization of the child, i.e., competent vs. incompetent, will alter the manner in which the child is able to respond to new experiences, positive or negative, and the pathways toward adaptation or maladaption that unfold.

The study of risk, vulnerability, and protective factors as they relate to the development of psychopathology has been an area of active inquiry consistent with transactional concepts of development (Rolf, Masten, Cicchetti, Nuechterlein, & Weintraub, 1990). In keeping with our developmental formulation, it is likely that a multitude of rather general factors across the broad domains of biology, psychology, and sociology will be at least indirectly related to depressive outcomes, because they represent the gamut of potential determinants of individual adaptation. A comprehensive articulation of the processes and mechanisms that have promoted or inhibited the development of competence over the course of development and, in particular, have resulted in a depressotypic organization of the individual may be more important than specific predictors of the immediate or proximal onset of depressive disorder. This approach is important because numerous characteristics related to depression, e.g., distorted attributional style, interpersonal relationship difficulties, feelings of helplessness and hopelessness, low self-esteem, and so on, are inevitably arrived at developmentally, and they will function as vulnerability factors for depression, in and of themselves.

Vulnerability factors are typically regarded as enduring or long-standing life circumstances or conditions that promote maladaptation. Major domains of influence on the child, including external (familial, social–environmental) and internal (biological, psychological), may serve as sources of vulnerability as they detract from the achievement of successful adaptation and competence. For example, parental psychopathology, parental drug abuse and alcoholism, marital conflict, divorce, child maltreatment, parental hostility, and lack of parental nurturance have all been shown to have detrimental effects on the developing child and his or her striving for adaptation. Similarly, factors such as low socioeconomic status, unsupportive social and familial networks, inadequate schools, high crime, and frequent hassles in daily living create stressful conditions that aggravate coping and detract from competent development. Biologically, a genetic predisposition to depression, biogenic amine anomalies, temperamental difficultness, and hyperreactive physiological responses to stress are among those issues that represent long-standing conditions that are likely to complicate the ease with which competent developmental achievements are attained. Through development, these vulnerability factors transact with the evolving organization of behavioral systems of the individual child to detract from the attainment of competence and may promote a depressotypic organization across the emotional, cognitive, social, representational, and biological systems.

In contrast, there are also enduring protective factors that promote competent adaptation in the child. Many of these, within the familial, social–environmental, and biological domains, are the polar opposites of the vulnerability factors listed above. For example, they would include parental mental health, harmonious marital relations, effective parenting, warmth and nurturance, adequate income levels, supportive social and familial networks, good schools, low crime, and no genetic predisposition for depression. These features are likely to enhance rather than hinder development.

In addition to these enduring competence-detracting and competence-promoting factors, there also exist transient influences that, though temporary in duration, may have a critical positive or negative impact, depending on the timing of such events or transitions in circumstances and the pertinent developmental issues for the child at the time. Further, the potency of specific risk and protective factors in influencing development will vary as a result of the developmental period in which they occur; a specific factor may be more influential in one developmental period as compared to another. For any individual child, the specific enduring features encountered, both vulnerability-producing and protective, will vary and exist within a dynamic balance. There will be greater likelihood of the development of incompetence and a depressotypic organization for those children for whom vulnerability and risk factors outweigh the protective and buffering influences (Cicchetti & Schneider-Rosen, 1984, 1986; Cummings & Cicchetti, 1990). There will be a potential for depressive disorders to emerge in those individuals in whom a depressotypic organization has evolved transactionally through development and whose coping capacities and protective resources are no longer effective in counteracting long-standing vulnerabilities and current stressors or acute risk factors.

Rutter (1990) has cautioned that risk, vulnerability, and protective factors are not variables causing pathological outcomes per se, but rather that they are indicators of more complex processes and mechanisms that impact on individual adaptation. Specifying the process or mechanism involved is essential. In our conceptualization, these factors are expected to operate chiefly by the significance they have in promoting or detracting from the development of competence at progressive stages of development and the consequent likelihood of an emerging depressotypic organization. Parental death per se does not cause depressive disorder, but in some children it may contribute to a sequence of negative transformations in the psychological and biological subsystems over the course of development. These changes, in turn, may result in the emergence of a depressotypic organization and a strong potential for depressive outcomes.

It should also be noted that the manner in which vulnerability, risk, and protective mechanisms exert their effects is likely to vary depending on the developmental period in which they occur. Some factors may have a much stronger influence at one developmental period as compared to another. High blood lead levels, for example, are likely to be far more detrimental early in development. Additionally, the same factor may function differently depending on the context in which it occurs. A parent losing a job may have varying degrees of impact on children depending on the socioeconomic conditions of the family. Thus, it is important to evaluate the effect of risk and protective processes on the basis of both the developmental and the social environmental context in which they occur.

An Illustration of a Developmental Psychopathology Analysis

We return now to examine in more detail two early stage-salient issues, attachment and the development of the self and autonomy, which emerge and become central life-span areas of personality organization with particular relevance for the study of depression. Attachment theory as originally formulated by Bowlby (1969, 1973, 1980, 1982) has placed central importance on the early propensity of humans to form and maintain strong affectional bonds. This need is seen as evolutionarily critical in that the human requires a lengthy span of development in which reliance on adults for care is essential for survival. Threats to the affectional bond via separation from or loss of the attachment figure arouse separation anxiety that is linked to survival concerns. Prolonged separation or actual loss results in mourning, with its affective, cognitive, social, and biological components. If mourning is unresolved, then the individual may be vulnerable to depression at subsequent points in the life span when loss-related events occur and feelings of separation anxiety and helplessness are reactivated.

Beyond the typically rare event of actual loss, infants experience a range of variations in the quality of the caregiving environment. Using the Strange Situation experimental paradigm (Ainsworth & Wittig, 1969), attachment-theory researchers have delineated patterns of individual differences in behaviors exhibited by infants in negotiating their relationships with their primary caregivers. These attachment organizations vary in the extent to which "felt security" is experienced by the infant in the relationship with the caregiver and how affect is regulated. Secure infants evidence trust in the caregiver and use her as a secure base from which to move out and explore the environment. They are assured that they can rely on the caregiver for emotional refueling when separation anxiety is aroused. In contrast, different types of insecure patterns have been articulated. The behaviors of these insecure infants indicate that modulation of separation anxiety is a more difficult task in that "felt security" is not readily experienced in the attachment relationship, and the infants must utilize alternate strategies for affect regulation. These strategies range from avoidance of the caregiver to angry resistance and protestations with the caregiver to more recently ascertained atypicalities and irregularities in behavior (e.g., appearing dazed, remaining still, freezing, and being otherwise apprehensive in the caregiver's presence).

Common to the various types of insecure attachment relationships are patterns of maternal insensitivity and unresponsiveness or psychological unavailability that disrupt the infant's ability to experience felt security in the relationship and lead to difficulties in regulating the relationship and, more generally, the arousal of separation anxiety and affect (Cicchetti, Ganiban, & Barnett, 1991; Cummings & Cicchetti, 1990). Noncontingency of maternal caregiving has been linked to insecure attachment relationships (Ainsworth, Blehar, Waters, & Wall, 1978), and this early pattern of caregiving may suggest early precursors to the development of learned helplessness (Abramson, Seligman, & Teasdale, 1978).

The various patterns of insecure attachment organization are important to our understanding of depression in that they represent early forms of aberrant organization of the biological, affective, cognitive, representational, and social behavioral systems with potential implications for an evolving depressotypic organization. With continuing development, the attachment relationship becomes increasingly complex as the infant begins to internalize features of the relationship. These internalized features have been labeled as representational models of the attachment figure and of the self and are conceptualized as cognitive and affective reconstructions of aspects of the attachment relationship experienced by the infant.

Different evolving memory systems contribute to the structure of the representational models. Crittenden (Crittenden, 1990; Crittenden, Partridge, & Claussen, 1991) has discussed a type of memory system, procedural memory, thought to develop in the sensorimotor period, in which information about relationships is encoded, retrieved, and expressed in the form of patterns of behavior. Bowlby (1980), applying the work of Tulving (1985, 1989) to attachment, has discussed two other memory systems, semantic and episodic. The semantic memory system stores and retrieves information in the form of generalizations about relationships. In contrast, the episodic memory system involves autobiographical information about events or episodes and actions of the self and others as well as associated affects at the time of specific events. The character of the different memory systems comprising the internal representational model is not necessarily consistent across the memory systems, and the ease of access between systems may be variable.

Bretherton (1990) has discussed the function of the representational models as useful in guiding interpersonal behavior on the basis of expectations of the behaviors of self and others and anticipated outcomes derived from prior experience. The representational models are thus economical in that they allow for choosing alternate strategies for interpersonal behavior on the basis of successes and failures in prior encounters. Thus, the child comes to use representational models, which operate outside conscious awareness, to interpret experiences and guide the course of interactions. As a result, a degree of stability in the features of representational models may be maintained, as experiences may be interpreted differentially in efforts to emphasize consistency with the existing models, and the types of interactions engaged in may be selected or avoided on the basis of anticipated outcomes. Through this process, representational models may contribute to the child's exerting an effect on shaping his or her environment.

Representational models are open to revision, however, if experiences continually contradict the model. Alternatively, continuity in the quality of attachment relationship experiences will contribute to consolidation and unification of the representations in the models across memory systems.

It is important to keep in mind that children typically develop attachments to more than their primary caregiver. Although primacy may be given to the representations associated with the primary caregiver, usually the mother, other representations of the father, for example, likely also develop. These representations may be largely consistent in quality and character with the internal representations of the mother and self in relation to the mother if the child experiences similar relationships with both parents. However, some children may experience quite discrepant relationships with their parents. For example, a child may have a positive relationship with the mother and a negative relationship with the father. How this inconsistency is processed by the child and how it affects internal representational models is uncertain (Bretherton, 1985). Children may derive separate models of other and self consistent with the different caregiver relationships they experience. Alternatively, a general representational model may develop based on the relationship with the primary attachment figure. Aspects of experience with the other attachment figure may be hierarchically integrated within this more general model and accessed later in development if experiences are consistent with qualitative features that were previously incorporated, though dormant.

For the child whose attachment figure does not provide a sense of felt security and ready affect modulation or soothing, an insecure representational model evolves from abstractions of encounters with the caregiver in which the child feels unloved, uncared for, unresponded to, and even threatened. Representations abstracted from such experiences influence expectations of the attachment figure and of others in close and intimate relationships. As development unfolds, the dyadic regulation of affect within the attachment relationship progressively shifts to regulation that is increasingly managed by the child. Thus, dyadic regulation increasingly becomes self-regulation (Sroufe, 1990). Similarly, the representations of the quality of the attachment relationship and its capacity and effectiveness to regulate affect and provide comfort and soothing become extended to representations of the self and its ability to regulate affective experience. For the child with an insecure representational model of the attachment figure and affect regulation within this relationship, corresponding representations of the self in the attachment relationship evolve. The self comes to be viewed as unlovable, unworthy, and rejected. Schneider-Rosen and Cicchetti (1984) have shown that infants who are insecurely attached are delayed in the emergence of visual self-recognition, suggesting some deviation in the process of self-development that has its roots in insecure attachment relationships.

For the child who develops an insecure representational model of the self and others based on experiences in the attachment relationship, we see what may be regarded as the germinal signs of a depressotypic organization with interpersonal, affective, and cognitive components. Qualitative aspects of an evolving self are carried forward from the attachment relationship, in addition to representations of the attachment relationship. Cicchetti and Schneider-Rosen (1986) have extended this analysis to later points in development to examine how affective components of the self that are relevant to depression, i.e., self esteem, are intertwined with growing cognitive components of the self, i.e., self-cognitions, self-schemata, and self-understanding (Damon & Hart, 1982, 1988). In doing so, Cicchetti and Schneider-Rosen provide a developmental framework for understanding how cognitive distortions and learned helplessness, considered to be prominent etiological factors in depression, may have been acquired through the course of development (see also Hammen, 1992).

In order to convey conceptual clarity, it is important to define different cognitive and affective components of the self that evolve developmentally. *Self-understanding* is a cognitive construction regarding oneself; it is the person's self-representation that has roots in the early evolving self-representations of the internal models of the attachment relationship. *Self-esteem* (and the loss of self-esteem), a central component of many theories of depression (Abramson et al., 1978; Beck, 1967; Bibring, 1953), is the affective component of the self; it is positively or negatively valenced in accord with how the self is represented. A *self-cognition* represents a particular usage of the cognitive structure in regard to the self. *Self-schemata* are structuralized representations of the self that result from repeated self-cognitions and accompanying affect over time. Self-schemata are hierarchically organized sets of self-cognitions with similar content. Self-schemata take on an enduring character over time, becoming the core structure of how the self is understood.

Self-cognitions are characterized by both content and style. Content refers to those aspects of the self that are being represented; style refers to the particular manner or process by which a person derives a specific thought about the self. In contrast, self-esteem is an affect that is dimensional in nature, varying from positive to negative. Negative or low self-esteem found in the intense dysphoria of depression may contrast with normal sadness not only quantitatively in its intensity but also qualitatively by way of different cognitive processes or styles that compose the self-cognitions. Self-cognitions and self-esteem are likely to influence each other reciprocally. Negative self-cognitions engender consistent associated affect or low self-esteem. In turn, low self-esteem as an affective state is likely to be accompanied by further self-cognitions that are negative in content. A negative cycle between affect and cognition, i.e., self-esteem and self-cognitions, is likely to perpetuate depressive experience.

Following Damon and Hart (1982, 1988), four characteristics of the self can be represented: material characteristics (e.g., possessions, physical characteristics), active characteristics (e.g., activities and skills), social characteristics (e.g., roles, relationships), and psychological characteristics (e.g., thoughts, emotions, personality processes). These domains may receive different emphasis in the self-representations of different individuals. More important, there is a distinctive developmental aspect to the complexity of these domains. A number of self- and person-perception researchers (Livesly & Bromley, 1973; Secord & Peevers, 1974; Selman, 1980) have noted a significant transition in the 7- to 8-year-old age range in how self-cognitions are constructed. This age shift corresponds to the cognitive transition from preoperational to operational thinking in the nonsocial arena and is associated with other transitions in social- and self-cognitions. Prior to the shift, children tend to view themselves in concrete, physical terms, such as physical appearance, possessions, games they like to play, and where they go to school (i.e., in terms of materialistic and active characteristics). Following the cognitive shift, children increasingly begin to abstract qualitative features from their experience and to view themselves in psychological terms, such as personal characteristics and traits, that are enduring over time.

Other important cognitive shifts also occur during this transition period. Children move from viewing themselves in relation to absolute standards to engaging in more social comparison, contrasting themselves with others. Children also shift from thinking of themselves in terms of their usual actions or habits to evaluating their competencies and skills in various areas. These shifts from physical to psychological, from absolute standards to comparative evaluations, and from habit-based to competency-based self-cognitions have implications for depression. Before the shift, there is likely to be some degree of variability in the affective valence of self-cognitions, e.g., whether children like their hairstyle or the friends they sit with at lunch. However, these self-cognitions relate to features that are subject to change and are specific and concrete, and associated affects are likely to be context-specific and transient. However, after the shift, as children become more abstract and form generalizations across situations and time, they begin to evaluate themselves in psychological, comparative, and competency-based terms. As a result, their cognitive capacities allow for self-cognitions to become more personal, global, and stable. These generalized self-evaluations will be accompanied by congruent affect regarding the self. For children making negative self-evaluations, there will be a trend to greater stability in associated negative affect regarding the self, or low self-esteem. Consequently, after the shift, there may be a greater tendency for negative self-cognitions to generate and perpetuate low self-esteem and dysphoria, contributing to depressive outcomes. Thus, advancing capacities for self-understanding may have negative consequences for children who are at risk for depression.

The features of self-cognitions made possible after the cognitive transition are relevant for understanding developmental aspects of the reformulated learned-helplessness theory of depression (Abramson et al., 1978). In this conceptualization, learned helplessness is conceptualized as a result of an individual's perception of noncontingency between responses and resulting rewards and punishments. This noncontingency is attributed on the basis of perceptions of failures that are a result of personal traits or characteristics, but not characteristics that apply universally. Further, the personal failings are viewed as global rather than situation-specific, and they are considered to be stable rather than transient, and thus are expected to endure over time. These attributions of personal, global, and stable features, used to explain noncontingency, are attributions that become possible after the previously discussed cognitive transition. Thus, attainments in normal cognitive development may serve as preconditions for generating self- cognitions that may contribute to depression via attributions of noncontingency.

More broadly, the character of self-cognitions attainable after the cognitive transition is likely to contribute to more ingrained self-schemata, and these internal structural representations, when negative, may be seen as contributing to the likelihood of depressive outcomes. Beck's cognitive theory of depression (Beck, 1967) centers around a cognitive triad of attributions, including negative cognitions about the self, about the world, and about the future. Again, these types of attributions become possible when children are able to form cognitions about the self and others that are psychological rather than physical, stable and enduring rather than unstable and changing, and global rather than specific.

Although advances in cognitive development appear to provide the conditions under which certain forms of negative self-cognitions may be linked to depressive outcomes, these advances do not explain why come children and not others going through these universal transitions become depressed. We believe that the balance of risk and protective factors as previously discussed will affect the affective valence of the types of self-cognitions made. More important, the representational models of self and others, derived from early experiences in the attachment relationship and elaborated through ongoing experience, are believed to contribute to the pathways taken in conjunction with advances in cognitive capacities. That is, insecure representational models that comprise part of a depressotypic organization of behavioral systems will contribute to cognitive advances being used to confirm and elaborate negative self-schemata, thereby increasing the risk for depressive outcomes (see Cummings & Cicchetti, 1990).

Conclusions and Future Directions

The developmental psychopathology approach to understanding depressive disorders in children and adolescents represents a comprehensive undertaking that seeks to unify contributions from multiple fields of inquiry into an integrated whole (cf. Cicchetti, 1990). Because current adaptation is viewed as a product of both current circumstances and conditions and prior experiences and adaptations (Sroufe, Egeland, & Kreutzer, 1990), depression is best understood in terms of current risk and protective factors within the context of prior developmental experiences that have been hierarchically integrated into the individual's organization of biological and behavioral systems. Understanding the developmental pathways between successive prior adaptations and current functioning (biological, cognitive, affective, representational, and interpersonal) is central to the developmental psychopathology approach.

We have seen that an appreciation for the developmental perspective holds promise for expanding and unifying various theoretical models of depression within a developmental framework. The developmental psychopathology approach allows for new questions to be addressed, moving beyond description of differences inherent among depressed individuals to exploring how such differences evolved. The multiplicity of pathways resulting from any one developmental experience and contributing to depressive disorders directs us toward studying the interface between normal and psychopathological development. Developmental psychopathology draws attention to both the similarities and the differences among normal and psychopathological conditions. As a result, we are able to distinguish the specific pathways leading to various psychopathologies (e.g., depression) as well as to understand the commonalities underlying both normal and psychopathological functioning. Through this integrated developmental approach, informed direction is given to efforts to prevent depressive disorders as well as to the provision of intervention for those who are already experiencing depression.

Because developmental psychopathology is a newly emerging discipline, there is much to be accomplished in advancing a developmental understanding of depression. The burgeoning literature emanating from attachment theory on internal representational processes is likely to prove fruitful in providing increased depth to our understanding of how organizations of affective, cognitive, representational, and interpersonal experiences are carried forward developmentally and affect the course of adaptation and the evolution of depressive disorders. Future research will benefit from increased attention to the interface between the psychological and biological domains. How, for example, might insecure internal representational models affect neurophysiological functioning, and how might genetic heritage alter tendencies for certain forms of representational processes to occur? Future research also should provide more detail regarding the differential strength of various risk and protective factors in development and how these vary during different developmental periods. Greater attention to the types and variety of precursor depressotypic organizations and how risk and protective factors influence these organizations also will be important. In summary, the developmental psychopathology perspective not only adds considerable but necessary complexity to the understanding of depressive disorders, but also provides a rich groundwork for exploring the development of depressive conditions.

ACKNOWLEDGMENT.   We acknowledge the support of the Prevention Research Branch of the National Institute of Mental Health (Grant MH45027).

References

Abramson, L. Y., Seligman, M. E. P., & Teasdale, J. D., (1978). Learned helplessness in humans: Critique and reformulation. *Journal of Abnormal Psychology, 87,* 49–74.

Achenbach, T. (1990). What is "developmental" about developmental psychopathology? In J. Rolf, A. Masten, D. Cicchetti, K. Nuechterlein, S. Weintraub (Eds.), *Risk and protective factors in the development of psychopathology* (pp. 29–48). New York: Cambridge University Press.

Ainsworth, M. D. S., Blehar, M. C., Waters, E., & Wall, S. (1978). *Patterns of attachment: A psychological study of the Strange Situation.* Hillsdale, NJ: Erlbaum Associates.

Ainsworth, M. D. S., & Wittig, B. A. (1969). Attachment and exploratory behavior of one year olds in a strange situation. In B. M. Foss (Ed.), *Determinants of infant behavior,* Vol. 4 (pp. 113–136). New York: John Wiley.

American Psychiatric Association (1987). *Diagnostic and statistical manual of mental disorders,* 3rd ed., revised. Washington, DC: Author.

Beck, A. T. (1967). *Depression: Causes and treatment.* Philadelphia: University of Pennsylvania Press.

Bibring, E. (1953). The mechanism of depression. In P. Greenacre (Ed.), *Affective disorders* (pp. 13–48). New York: International Universities Press.

Bowlby, J. (1969). *Attachment and loss,* Vol. 1, *Attachment.* New York: Basic Books.

Bowlby, J. (1973). *Attachment and loss,* Vol. 2, *Separation.* New York: Basic Books.

Bowlby, J. (1980). *Attachment and loss,* Vol. 3, *Loss.* New York: Basic Books.

Bowlby, J. (1982). *Attachment and loss,* Vol. 1, 2nd ed., *Attachment.* New York: Basic Books.

Bretherton, I. (1985). Attachment theory: Retrospect and prospect. In I. Bretherton & E. Waters (Eds.), Growing points of attachment theory and research (pp. 3–35). *Monographs of the Society for Research in Child Development, 50* ([1–2 (Serial No. 209)].

Bretherton, I. (1990). Open communication and internal working models: Their role in the development of attachment relationships. In R. A. Thompson (Ed.), *Nebraska symposium on motivation,* Vol. 36, *Socioemotional development* (pp. 57–113). Lincoln: University of Nebraska Press.

Cicchetti, D. (Ed.). (1984a). *Developmental psychopathology.* Chicago: University of Chicago Press.

Cicchetti, D. (1984b). The emergence of developmental psychopathology. *Child Development, 55,* 1–7.

Cicchetti, D. (Ed.). (1989). *Rochester symposium on developmental psychopathology,* Vol. 1, *The emergence of a discipline.* Hillsdale, NJ: Erlbaum Associates.

Cicchetti, D. (1990a). An historical perspective on the discipline of developmental psychopathology. In J. Rolf, A. Masten, D. Cicchetti, K. Nuechterlein, & S. Weintraub (Eds.), *Risk and protective factors in the development of psychopathology* (pp. 2–28). New York: Cambridge University Press.

Cicchetti, D. (1990b). Developmental psychopathology and the prevention of serious mental disorders: Overdue detente and illustrations through the affective disorders. In P. Muehrer (Ed.), *Conceptual research models for prevention of mental disorders* (pp. 215–254). Rockville, MD: National Institute of Mental Health.

Cicchetti, D. (1990c). The organization and coherence of socioemotional, cognitive, and representational development: Illustrations through a developmental psychopathology perspective on Down syndrome and child maltreatment. In R. A. Thompson (Ed.), *Nebraska symposium on motivation,* Vol. 36, *Socioemotional development* (pp. 259–366). Lincoln: University of Nebraska Press.

Cicchetti, D., Ganiban, J., & Barnett, D. (1991). Contributions from the study of high risk populations to understanding the development of emotion regulation. In J. Garber & K. Dodge (Eds.), *The development of emotion regulation* (pp. 15–48). New York: Cambridge University Press.

Cicchetti, D., & Schneider-Rosen, K. (1984). Toward a developmental model of the depressive disorders. *New Directions for Child Development, 26,* 5–27.

Cicchetti, D., & Schneider-Rosen, K. (1986). An organizational approach to childhood depression. In M. Rutter, C. Izard, & P. Read (Eds.), *Depression in young people: Developmental and clinical perspectives* (pp. 71–134). New York: Guilford Press.

Cicchetti, D., & Sroufe, L. A. (1978). An organizational view of affect: Illustration from the study of Down's syndrome infants. In M. Lewis & L. Rosenblum (Eds.), *The development of affect* (pp. 309–350). New York: Plenum Press.

Cicchetti, D., & Toth, S. L. (1991). The making of a developmental psychopathologist. In J. H. Cantor, C. C. Spiker, & L. H. Lipsitt (Eds.), *Child behavior and development: Training for diversity* (pp. 34–72). Norwood, NJ: Ablex Publishing.

Cicchetti, D., Toth, S. L., & Bush, M. (1988). Developmental psychopathology and incompetence in childhood: Suggestions for intervention. In B. Lahey & A. Kazdin (Eds.), *Advances in clinical child psychology* (pp. 1–71). New York: Plenum Press.

Crittenden, P. M. (1990). Internal representational models of attachment relationships. *Infant Mental Health Journal, 11,* 259–277.

Crittenden, P. M., Partridge, M. F., & Claussen, A. H. (1991). Family patterns of relationship in normative and dysfunctional families. *Development and Psychopathology, 3,* 491–512.

Cummings, E. M., & Cicchetti, D. (1990). Toward a transactional model of relations between attachment and depression. In M. T. Greenberg, D. Cicchetti, & E. M. Cummings (Eds.), *Attachment during the preschool years* (pp. 339–372). Chicago: University of Chicago Press.

Cytryn, L., & McKnew, D. H., Jr. (1972). Proposed classification of childhood depression. *American Journal of Psychiatry, 129,* 149–155.

Damon, W., & Hart, D. (1982). The development of self-understanding from infancy through adolescence. *Child Development, 53,* 841–864.

Damon, W., & Hart, D. (1988). *Self-understanding in childhood and adolescence.* New York: Cambridge University Press.

Glaser, K. (1967). Masked depression in children and adolescents. *American Journal of Psychotherapy, 21,* 565–574.

Gottesman, I., & Shields, J. (1972). *Schizophrenia and genetics: A twin study vantage point.* New York: Academic Press.

Hammen, C. (1992). Cognitive, life stress, and interpersonal approaches to a developmental psychopathology model of depression. *Development and Psychopathology, 4,* 191–208.

Kaplan, B. (1966). The study of language in psychiatry: The comparative developmental approach and its application to symbolization and language in psychopathology. In S. Arieti (Ed.), *American handbook of psychiatry,* Vol. 1 (pp. 659–688). New York: Basic Books.

Kashani, J. H., Husain, A., Shekim, W. O., Hodges, K. K., Cytryn, L., & McKnew, D. H. (1981). Current perspectives on childhood depression: An overview. *American Journal of Psychiatry, 138,* 143–153.

Lively, W. J., & Bromley, D. B. (1973). *Person perception in childhood and adolescence.* New York: John Wiley.

Piaget, J. (1952). *The origins of intelligence.* New York: Norton.

Puig-Antich, J. (1980). Affective disorders in childhood: A review and perspective. *Psychiatric Clinics of North America, 3,* 403–424.

Radke-Yarrow, M., & Zahn-Waxler, C. (1990). Research on children of affectively ill parents: Some considerations for theory and research on normal development. *Development and Psychopathology, 2*, 349–366.

Rie, H. E. (1966). Depression in childhood: A survey of some pertinent contributions. *Journal of the American Academy of Child Psychiatry, 5*, 653–685.

Rolf, J., Masten, A., Cicchetti, D., Nuechterlein, K., & Weintraub, S. (Eds.) (1990). *Risk and protective factors in the development of psychopathology.* New York: Cambridge University Press.

Rutter, M. (1986). Child psychiatry: The interface between clinical and developmental research. *Psychological Medicine, 16*, 151–160.

Rutter, M. (1989). Age as an ambiguous variable in developmental research: Some epidemiological considerations from developmental psychopathology. *International Journal of Behavioral Development, 12*, 486–500.

Rutter, M. (1990). Psychosocial resilience and protective mechanisms. In J. Rolf, A. Masten, D. Cicchetti, K. Nuechterlein, & S. Weintraub (Eds.), *Risk and protective factors in the development of psychopathology* (pp. 181–214). New York: Cambridge University Press.

Rutter, M., Izard, C., & Read, P. (Eds.) (1986). *Depression in young people: Developmental and clinical perspectives.* New York: Guilford Press.

Sameroff, A. J., & Chandler, M. J. (1975). Reproductive risk and the continuum of caretaking casualty. In F. D. Horowitz (Ed.), *Review of child development research*, Vol. 4 (pp. 187–244). Chicago: University of Chicago Press.

Schneider-Rosen, K., & Cicchetti, D. (1984). The relationship between affect and cognition in maltreated infants: Quality of attachment and the development of visual self-recognition. *Child Development, 55*, 648–658.

Secord, P., & Peevers, B. (1974). The development and attribution of person concepts. In T. Mischel (Ed.), *Understanding other persons.* Oxford: Blackwell Scientific.

Selman, R. (1980). *The growth of interpersonal understanding.* New York: Academic Press.

Sroufe, L. A. (1979). The coherence of individual development. *American Psychologist, 34*, 834–841.

Sroufe, L. A. (1989). Pathways to adaptation and maladaptation: Psychopathology as developmental deviation. *Rochester symposium on developmental psychopathology*, Vol. 1, *The emergence of a discipline* (pp. 13–40). Hillsdale, NJ: Erlbaum Associates.

Sroufe, L. A. (1990). Considering normal and abnormal together: The essence of developmental psychopathology. *Development and Psychopathology, 2*, 335–347.

Sroufe, L. A., Egeland, B., & Kreutzer, T. (1990). The fate of early experience following development change: Longitudinal approaches to individual adaptation in childhood. *Child Development, 61*, 1363–1373.

Sroufe, L. A., Fox, N., & Pancake, V. (1983). Attachment and dependency in developmental perspective. *Child Development, 54*, 1615–1627.

Sroufe, L. A., & Rutter, M. (1984). The domain of developmental psychopathology. *Child Development, 55*, 17–29.

Sroufe, L. A., & Waters, E. (1976). The ontogenesis of smiling and laughter: A perspective on the organization of development in infancy. *Psychological Review, 83*, 173–189.

Tulving, E. (1985). How many memory systems are there? *American Psychologist, 40*, 385–398.

Tulving, E. (1989). Remembering and knowing the past. *American Scientist, 77*, 361–367.

Waters, E., & Sroufe, L. A. (1983). Competence as a developmental construct. *Developmental Review, 3*, 79–97.

Werner, H. (1948). *Comparative psychology of mental development.* New York: International Universities Press.

Zahn-Waxler, C., & Kochanska, G. (1990). The origins of guilt. In R. A. Thompson (Ed.), *Nebraska symposium on motivation*, Vol. 36, *Socioemotional development* (pp. 183–258). Lincoln: University of Nebraska Press.

8

Neurobiological Aspects of Depression in Children and Adolescents

Graham J. Emslie, Warren A. Weinberg, Betsy D. Kennard, and Robert A. Kowatch

Introduction

Research on neurobiological correlates of depression in children and adolescents is at an exciting stage but lags substantially behind work in adults. Most of the areas studied have been chosen because of positive findings in adults. The positive side of this selective process is that many unproductive avenues of research are avoided by child researchers. However, assessing biological correlates of depression requires substantial normative data that are not readily available in child and adolescent populations, controlling for age, gender, and developmental stage.

The purpose of this chapter is to review studies available on neurobiological correlates that have at least some data available in the child and adolescent depressed population. The areas covered are neurology, neuropsychology, neuroimaging, neurochemistry, neuroendocrine, and polysomnographic findings. This chapter will focus on abnormalities associated with depression. Theories of the biochemical basis for depression have been discussed elsewhere and will be addressed only where appropriate. In some of these areas, e.g., neuroimaging, few data are available at this time in children and adolescents, but the areas hold significant promise. Extensive review of the available adult data will not be undertaken, but salient data from adults will be reviewed.

Identifying biological correlates of depression is important for several reasons

Graham J. Emslie, Betsy D. Kennard, and Robert A. Kowatch • Department of Psychiatry, University of Texas Southwestern Medical Center, and Children's Medical Center at Dallas, Dallas, Texas 75235-9070. **Warren A. Weinberg** • Department of Neurology, University of Texas Southwestern Medical Center, and Children's Medical Center at Dallas, Dallas, Texas 75235-9070.

Handbook of Depression in Children and Adolescents, edited by William M. Reynolds and Hugh F. Johnston. Plenum Press, New York, 1994.

(Table 1). Despite often initial enthusiasm and later disappointment, there is significant interest in identifying a marker for depression that would assist in diagnosis. Clearly, such a marker would be invaluable in populations at each end of the age spectrum where diagnosis becomes increasingly difficult. Biological correlates may identify more homogeneous subgroups for future study.

Although the identification of biological correlates that are specific and sensitive for depression is important, other uses of biological correlates cannot be ignored. It may be that one correlate is not a good diagnostic marker but may be useful in other areas. There is evidence that neurobiological markers can be useful in predicting response to acute treatment (Rush et al., 1989) and prediction of relapse or recurrence (Giles, Jarrett, Roffwarg, & Rush, 1987). This area of research will become increasingly important with clear definitions of what constitutes remission, relapse, and recurrence (Frank et al., 1991) and how these definitions can be applied to the course of childhood depression. Examples of neurobiological correlates being used to predict outcome can include many different areas. Dexamethasone nonsuppressors appear less likely to respond to placebo or psychosocial treatment alone (Brown, Dornseif, & Wernicke, 1988; Preskorn, Weller, Hughes, Weller, & Bolte, 1987; Robbins, Alessi, & Colfer, 1989). Certain soft neurological signs improve with remission (Brumback, 1988). Depressed adults with shortened REM latency appear more likely to respond to medication and more likely to relapse once treatment is discontinued (Giles et al., 1987; Rush et al., 1989). Abnormalities in neuropsychological testing and negative cognitions improve with treatment (Kennard, Nici, Emslie, & Weinberg, 1987; Kennard et al., 1991; Tems, 1989). These are all possible areas in which a neurobiological variable could assist in treatment and outcome.

A third area of importance in the identification of neurobiological abnormalities is in the area of family and genetic studies. Biological variables are often identified as state or trait variables. A state variable is present only when the individual is depressed and reverts to normal in a recovered state. Presumably, it was normal prior to the episode of depression. A trait variable presents theoretically from an early age and identifies an individual who is at risk for having depression. It has been suggested that shortened REM latency may have both a trait and a state component (Kupfer & Ehlers, 1989); i.e., it is abnormal prior to the episode and the difference increases during the episode. Clearly, it is difficult to identify individuals who are going to become depressed prior to their first episode, and so most variables investigated as possible trait variables are studied as to their stability into remission. At present, it is not possible to distinguish between a true trait variable and a "scar" variable, i.e., a more permanent change that arises as a result of a depressive episode. However, it becomes increasingly important to study children, with their shorter life history, not only because of the morbidity associated with the disorder in children themselves, but also to develop clues to what is central to the disorder and not a result of years of illness. A developmental perspective is central to research in childhood depression. Certain abnormalities may not show themselves in childhood because of developmental differences between adults and children.

Finally, biological correlates are important in increasing our understanding of the

---

Table 1. Utility of Biological Correlates of Affective Disorder

1. Diagnosis
2. Prediction of acute treatment response
3. Prediction of prognosis and recurrence
4. Understanding of basic pathophysiology
5. Genetic and family studies

---

basic pathophysiology of the disease. Neurological findings of subtle signs indicating left-sided weakness during a depressed state (Brumback, 1988; Freeman, Galaburda, Cabal, & Geschwind, 1985) are supported by decreased cerebral blood flow on the right (Ross & Rush, 1981). However, these findings are contradicted by other studies including studies of stroke victims (Robinson & Starkstein, 1990). Studies of the neuroendocrine system, e.g., growth hormone, were initially thought to be ways to assess central β-adrenergic neuron functioning, but now the control appears more complex than first believed. Numerous examples exist as to how further understanding of neurobiological findings may elucidate the common cause of these findings and the abnormality causing depression.

Neurobiological correlates tend to fall into two major groups: assessment of baseline functioning and of response to various challenges. To assess baseline functioning, groups of depressed and nondepressed subjects are compared in terms of, for example, 24-hour cortisol secretion. A challenge test stresses the system to enhance the possibilities of differences being identified. The best known of these is the dexamethasone suppression test (DST). Utilizing challenge tests developed with adults presents difficulties in defining an equivalent challenge for children of differing developmental stages.

The following sections will attempt to address some of the aforementioned issues in two general areas: structural abnormalities and functional abnormalities. Structural abnormalities include findings in neurology, neuropsychology, and neuroimaging. These disciplines attempt to identify localized deficits associated with depression, within and across cerebral hemispheres. Functional abnormalities include findings in neurochemistry, neuroendocrine systems, and polysomnography. These delineations may be arbitrary, as an understanding of depression requires the integration of findings in all these areas.

Structural Abnormalities

Neurology: Neurological Observations

Neuroanatomically, emotion is associated with the limbic system, which consists of a number of structures, including the amygdala, hippocampus, and cingulate gyrus. These structures connect to the hypothalamus and thalamus (diencephalon), which are also involved with emotion (Mesulam, 1985). The hypothalamus may be responsible for the primitive states and drives of appetite, thirst, sex, and fight or flight. The hypothalamus also receives input from the frontal lobes and the temporal–parietal cortex.

The cerebral cortex seems to modulate primitive functions and generate emotional expression (Bear, 1983; Heilman, Bowers, & Valenstein, 1983). Frontal lobe functions include volition, intention, and abiding by social rules. The temporal–parietal cortical functions include regulation of mood and affect, obsessions and compulsions, emotional qualities of social communication, and oral and written language. It remains to be determined whether or not observable emotion is primarily a function of the gray matter of cerebral cortex, limbic structures, or diencephalon, or of their interactions.

The lateralization of functions to either cerebral hemisphere is important in understanding the neuroanatomy of emotion. Both hemispheres are involved in expression of emotion (mood and affect), but debate continues about specific lateralization to the left or right hemisphere. The right hemisphere is involved in processing stimuli and producing responses that involve the comprehension of emotionality, while the left hemisphere is more analytical in its processing, focusing on the content or literal interpretation of stimuli (Bear, 1983; Flor-Henry, 1979; Geschwind & Galaburda, 1985; Kolb & Whishaw, 1980; Ross, 1981). The right hemisphere is probably responsible for the prosody or emotional tone of communication and language, the comprehension of nonverbal social cues, and subtle social nuances including wit and humor. The left hemisphere is primarily involved in the analytical processing of emotion, interpreting mood states from the content of speech, and assuming mood and affect from learned behaviors.

Neurological disease is often associated with psychiatric disturbance. Heilman et al. (1983) presented data and reviewed previous research that demonstrates the high prevalence of emotional disorders in adults with neurological disease. This prevalence has been demonstrated in children and adolescents by the Isle of Wight study (Rutter, Graham, & Yule, 1970). The prevalence of psychiatric disorders was 6.7% in the whole population, 11% in the nonneurological physically disabled children, and 34% in those with neurological findings. Similarly, Cantwell and Baker (1980) noted a high prevalence of psychiatric problems in children with neurodevelopmental problems.

Specific to depression, Flor-Henry (1979) sparked much interest in the relationship between disorders of mood and affect and right hemisphere dysfunction in adults by suggesting that depression was related to dysfunction of the "nondominant" (predominantly right) hemisphere. This has been partially supported by evidence of decreased cerebral blood flow on the right in depressed adults (Ross & Rush, 1981). Others, however, have found only global cortical blood flow reduction (Sackeim et al., 1990).

Extensive research has been conducted in adult patients following stroke, and depressive symptoms appear more common in left-side strokes. However, in the studies of depression in stroke patients, the question of whether the symptomatology represents a hypoactivity of the diseased brain or relative hyperactivity of the nonaffected hemisphere is a subject of debate and controversy (Lenhart & Katlin, 1986; Starkstein & Robinson, 1986). There are both intra- and interhemispheric considerations. One theory is that the observable behaviors are released by removal of a controlling influence or removal of the opposing behavior. Another consideration is that the two hemispheres are homologously paired. A disease in one part of the brain may promote the homologous (contralateral) part to act abnormally. This abnormal action in the contralateral side could be an overexpression or an absence of expression.

Neurological findings in depressed individuals without fundamental neurological disease have been reported. Focal neurological findings associated with depression include left-side hemiparesis in adults and children with major depressive disorders (Brumback, 1988; Freeman et al., 1985). Brumback, Staton, and Wilson (1980) reported on two depressed, learning-disabled children who evidenced signs of left hemiparesis and in whom treatment with a tricyclic antidepressant resulted in the disappearance of the focal neurological signs.

Important relationships between brain functions and behavior and disturbances of mood and affect are demonstrated by the Klein–Levin syndrome (Koerber et al., 1984; Waller, Jarriel, Erman, & Emslie, 1984). The Klein–Levin syndrome is an incapacitating disorder manifested by hypersomnolence, polyphagia, hypersexuality, and the feeling of dissociation. Interestingly, the patient described by Waller et al. (1984), on subsequent follow-up, developed discrete episodes of recurrent major depression and one episode of mania. This syndrome illustrates the relationship between the limbic system, right and left cerebral hemispheres, and affective disorders.

In summary, there is a body of data with adult stroke patients suggesting that depression results from destruction of left frontal–temporal lobes. However, others have reported left limb hemisyndrome in both adults and children manifesting major depressive disorder. The reported cases suggest resolution of the left hemiparesis with remission of the depression.

Neuropsychological Findings

Studies of normal populations in respect to brain function and mood have contributed much to the way we understand these relationships in the abnormal population. Overall studies of normal populations suggest an asymmetry of the brain in the interpretation and expression of emotions as found by observing human responses to specific stimuli. In general, these studies involve the selective presentation of stimuli to one hemisphere through the use of dichotic listening techniques (Haggard & Parkinson, 1971; Safer & Leventhal, 1977), split-field movies (Dimond & Farrington, 1977), tachistoscopically presented stimuli (Ley & Bryden, 1979; Suberi & McKeever, 1977), and electrophysiological studies (Davidson & Tomarken, 1989). The majority of these studies point to the conclusion that the hemispheres differ in function in the processing of emotion, with the left hemisphere primarily involved in analyzing information for content and the right hemisphere processing the emotional nature of the stimulus. Additionally, the hemispheres differ in their emotional interpretation of the environment, with the anterior part of the right hemisphere comparatively more activated when the emotional stimulus is negative than when the stimulus is positive (Davidson & Tomarken, 1989).

Neuropsychological studies of adults with major depressive disorder have found evidence for cognitive impairment in this population when compared with controls (Newman & Sweet, 1986). However, evidence for specific neuropsychological subtypes of impairment or for associating degree of impairment with severity of illness has been inconsistent (Newman & Sweet, 1986; Newman & Silverstein, 1987; Silverstein, Strauss, & Fogg, 1990).

Fromm and Schopflocher (1984) and Gray, Dean, D'Amato, and Rattan (1987), using neuropsychological measures, found a significant relationship between affective illness and right cerebral hemisphere impairment in an adult psychiatric population. Furthermore, Fromm and Schopflocher (1984) demonstrated improvement after treatment in those abilities that were most impaired.

Several studies have reported cognitive deficits associated with affective illness in children. Kaslow, Rehm, and Siegel (1984) reported a relationship between increased scores on the Children's Depression Inventory (CDI) (Kovacs, 1981) and poorer performance on the Block Design, Coding and Digit Span subtests of the Wechsler Intelligence Scale for Children—Revised (WISC-R). Other studies have reported similar associations between performance on the WISC-R performance subtests or similar nonverbal measures and self-report measures of depression (Blumberg & Izard, 1985; Brumback, 1988; Brumback et al., 1980; Brumback, Staton, & Wilson, 1984; Kaslow, Tanenbaum, Abramson, Peterson, & Seligman, 1983; Kron et al., 1982; Mullins, Siegel, & Hodges, 1985). While findings of poorer performance on nonverbal intellectual measures have been interpreted as representing right hemisphere dysfunction, others have suggested that these results reflect general problems with attention and concentration and slower speed on timed measures due to psychomotor retardation (Tramonta & Hooper, 1989). Conversely, attention, concentration, and psychomotor activity may be right brain functions (Heilman et al., 1983; Heilman, Watson, & Valenstein, 1985).

There have been a few studies that have sought to determine whether lateralization patterns of deficits similar to those reported in adults can be demonstrated in children with affective disorders. Kennard et al. (1987) performed neuropsychological evaluations on a group of child and adolescent inpatients with major depressive disorder. A pattern of weaker cognitive abilities emerged in higher-level cognitive functioning that included lower functioning in problem-solving, abstract reasoning, and attention and concentration. There was no evidence for consistent lateralization of deficits. Wilson and Staton (1984) reported cognitive improvements on neuropsychological measures following treatment for depression in 75 children. Whether their reported changes actually reflect improved functioning of the right hemisphere is uncertain, as many of their measures were non-lateralizing and the test–retest interval was short, confounding the results with practice effects.

A significant deficiency in the literature exists in regard to the impact of affective illness on the developing brain. Specifically, there are few longitudinal studies that examine relationships between depressive disorder and the development of cognitive abilities, social competence, and long-term academic achievement. Recently, Kovacs (1989) suggested that cognitive development is delayed and there is an interference with the acquisition of verbal abilities.

In a recent study, Kennard et al. (1991) attempted to address the issue of whether the cognitive deficits identified in children with major depression are state-related (directly associated with the presence of illness) or trait-related (stable over time). In their study, 37 psychiatric inpatients with a consensus diagnosis (based on structured interview and self- and parent-report measures) of major depressive disorder (MDD) were evaluated at admission and follow-up (average 30 months postadmission) on neuropsychological and depression measures. On admission, subjects evidenced mild impairment on cognitive measures. On follow-up, subjects improved significantly on measures of depression, but demonstrated no change on intellectual and academic measures and little significant change on neuropsychological measures. Poorer performance on measures of attention and flexibility of thought were associated with a greater percentage of time spent in a depressive episode. These data suggest that underlying cognitive dysfunction demonstrated by depressed patients is unaffected by their change in affective status. These results suggest that cognitive measures at time of diagnosis may be useful in determining prognosis.

In summary, there is increasing interest in the neuropsychological study of affective disorders in children and adolescents. However, comparison of different studies is complicated by whether or not neuropsychological testing vs. general measures of intelligence are used. Additionally, some studies rely on child self-report questionnaires for indication of depression, whereas others require the presence of full syndrome diagnostic criteria as determined by clinical interviews. These different methods have led to different study populations and results (Kazdin, 1989). More longitudinal studies are needed to address the impact of MDD on the development of cognitive, social, and academic abilities in these children.

Brain Imaging

Current radiological brain-imaging techniques available to study psychiatric disorders may be broadly divided into two groups: those techniques that image the *structure* of the central nervous system, computed tomography (CT) and magnetic resonance imaging (MRI), and those techniques that image the *function* of the central nervous system, positron emission tomography (PET), single-photon emission computed tomography (SPECT), and magnetic resonance spectroscopy (MRS). Figure 1 illustrates this division.

Structural Brain-Imaging Techniques. CT was first introduced in 1973 and utilizes standard X rays transmitted at many angles through the subject's brain. Radiation sensors detect X rays that have been transmitted through the head and attentuated by the various tissues. These data are collected and analyzed by a computer through a series of back-projection algorithms to provide a reconstructed set of images in the transverse plane. The advantages of CT are that it is widely available, can visualize bony structures as well as brain tissue, and is well understood and relatively economical. The disadvantages of CT are its poor contrast between gray and white matter, its use of ionizing radiation, possible allergic reactions to contrast material when used, its limitation to the transverse plane for imaging, and the problem of bony artifacts obscuring tissue in the posterior fossa.

MRI is based on the fact that certain species of atomic nuclei found in brain tissues behave as magnetic dipoles. Normally, these dipoles are randomly oriented, but when exposed to a strong external magnetic field, they will align and produce a measurable magnetic field. MRI then applies a high-strength radiofrequency signal that disturbs this bipolar alignment of the dipoles. When this radiofrequency signal is turned off, the MRI detectors measure the intensity of the electrical energy emitted as the atoms return to their magnetically imposed internal bipolar arrangement. Hydrogen nuclei (protons) are abundant in biological tissue and are the atomic species generally utilized for the creation of magnetic resonance images. MRI has the advantages of: no ionizing radiation like CT; superior gray–white matter delineation; the ability to image in three anatomical planes—transverse, coronal, and sagittal; high sensitivity for white matter lesions; no bone artifact in the posterior fossa, and no requirement for contrast material. Disadvantages of MRI are that it is less widely available and more expensive than CT and is limited by conditions that affect magnetic fields, e.g., aneurysm clips, pacemakers.

Hendren, Hodde-Vargas, Vargas, Orrison, and Dell (1991) used MRI to study a group of 37 psychiatric inpatients between the ages of 5 and 14 years, and 14 of these subjects were reported to have abnormal MRIs. Of these children, 2 were diagnosed to have a major depressive disorder by DSM-III-R criteria and reported to have abnormal MRIs. The first was a 13-year-old male whose MRI showed asymmetrical lateral ventricles, with the right ventricle greater than the left ventricle. The second subject was a 12-year-old male whose MRI showed a small area of abnormal signal intensity in the area of the left anterior basal ganglia or medial temporal lobe. Surprisingly, this is the only study that has been reported in which MRI was used to study children with major depression.

Functional Brain-Imaging Techniques. SPECT is a powerful, noninvasive method of determining regional cerebral blood flow. Normally, there is a tight coupling between cerebral blood flow, glucose metabolism, and neuronal activity in the brain. In practice, SPECT is a two-stage process. During the first stage of the procedure, the subject is injected or inhales a radioactively labeled compound. During a high-resolution SPECT scan, a radioactive element, such as technetium, is bound to a neutral, lipid-soluble agent, D,L-hexamethylpropylene amine oxime (HMPAO), and this compound is administered intravenously to the patient. This compound flows rapidly into the subject's brain with arterial circulation and is trapped in the brain within 30 seconds of the initial injection, thus producing a "snapshot" of brain activity at the time of injection. The second stage of this procedure occurs when the subject undergoes imaging by lying within a group of gamma ray detectors arrayed around the subject's head. For several hours, the bound technetium emits gamma rays that are detected by the gamma cameras.

Advantages of SPECT imaging are that it is widely available in most hospital nuclear

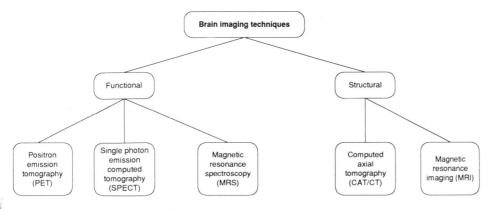

Figure 1. Brain-imaging techniques.

medicine departments, the radioisotopes that are used do not require a cyclotron for their production and thus are easily available, it is now possible to achieve spatial resolutions of 8 mm and resolutions of 2–3 mm are expected to be achieved in the near future, quantitative methods are available for measuring blood flow, and it is possible to study specific neurotransmitter receptors (e.g., muscarinic, dopaminergic, adrenergic, and opiate receptors). Disadvantages of SPECT include extracranial contamination from background radiation, its inability to measure glucose metabolic rates, and our lack of both clinical and research experience using SPECT.

Using the xenon inhalation method of SPECT imaging, Devous (1988) found significantly lower regional cerebral blood flow (rCBF) rates in the right temporal and parietal areas among adult patients with unipolar major depression relative to normal controls. Bipolar depressed patients in this same study were found to have higher rCBF rates in the left parietal and temporal lobes. Sackeim et al. (1990) reported their results of a study that compared the brain blood flow patterns of a group of 41 depressed adults vs. 40 matched controls. The depressed subjects were found to have a global deficit of CBF as well as specific deficits in selective frontal, central, superior temporal, and anterior parietal regions. They postulated that the blood flow deficits in these areas reflected dysfunction in the parallel distributed cortical network involving frontal and temporoparietal polymodal association areas. These polymodal association areas are thought to be directly involved in the mood changes seen in depressed patients (Tucker, 1988). Although there have been no functional brain-imaging studies of depressive illness in children or adolescents, one group in the Netherlands, Lou, Henriksen, Bruhn, and Psych (1984) used SPECT to study children with attention-deficit disorder. Using the xenon inhalation method of SPECT, they found reduced perfusion in the neostriatal and frontal cortex areas and a relative increase in flow in the primary sensory areas. This flow pattern was reversed by treatment with methylphenidate.

During PET, a cyclotron is used to produce short-lived isotopes of carbon, nitrogen, oxygen, or fluorine. These isotopes are then combined with a compound of interest and injected intravenously into the subject. The injected tracer will yield a positron that will collide with an electron and produce two photons that travel in exactly opposite directions. A detector "coincidence circuit" will recognize this simultaneous ionization and create an image from these events by filtered back-projection methods. The advantages of PET are that many specific receptors may be imaged, as well as rCBF and glucose metabolism. Disadvantages of PET scanning are that it is expensive and requires a cyclotron, which makes its availability to clinicians and researchers very limited. Since SPECT and PET are frequently confused, Table 2 contrasts these two imaging techniques.

A French group studied the resting-state cerebral metabolic rate of glucose using PET in 10 severely depressed adults and found significant hypofrontality and whole-cortex hypometabolism in the depressed state (Martinot et al., 1990). Zametkin et al. (1991) reported on a PET study that compared the cerebral glucose metabolism of a group of

Table 2. Comparison of Single-Photon Emission Computed Tomography (SPECT) and Positron Emission Tomography (PET)

Features	SPECT	PET
Radiation	Single photon (gamma ray)	Positron $\longrightarrow$ 2 photons
Images	rCBF and some receptors	rCBF, metabolism, and many receptors
Cost	$500.00	$1700.00
Availability	Wide (most nuclear medicine departments)	Limited (requires a cyclotron)

hyperactive adolescents vs. a group of normal controls and found significant reductions of glucose metabolism in 6 of 60 specific brain regions that were studied.

Magnetic resonance spectroscopy (MRS) is the newest imaging technique available to psychiatric researchers. MRS is capable of determining small variations in the resonant frequencies of different tissue compounds. A display of the magnetic resonance spectrum as a function of frequency shows the different chemical forms of an element forming peaks at characteristic positions. MRS can be used to study fats, membrane lipid metabolism, high-energy phosphate metabolism, glycogen, some neurotransmitters, amino acids, the citric acid cycle, lithium, and fluorinated compounds (Guze, 1991). The advantages of MRS are that it does not expose subjects to ionizing radiation and has no known side effects.Disadvantages of MRS are its limited spatial resolution, a 30- to 40-minute scan time, and a limited knowledge base in its use. There have been no studies of mood disorders using MRS in either adults or children, but because of its ability to study biochemical processes in vivo, it would seem an ideal technique with which to study these disorders.

In summary, despite the advances being made using various neuroimaging techniques in adult mood disorders, there is a dearth of research into child and adolescent mood disorders using these techniques. All the child psychiatric studies to date using the structural imaging techniques of MRI or CT have limited their studies to autism, attention-deficit hyperactivity disorder, or learning disabled children, in whom it was felt there would be a higher likelihood of finding "structural" abnormalities. A recent review article published by Kupperman, Gaffney, Hamdan-Allen, Preston, and Venkatesh (1990) entitled "Neuroimaging In Child Psychiatry" did not find any studies that utilized any brain-imaging technique, either structural or functional, to study children or adolescents with a mood disorder of any type. The future holds great promise for the use of these techniques to better understand the neurobiology of child and adolescent mood disorders.

Functional Abnormalities

Neurochemistry of Depression

Neurotransmitters (acetylcholine, monoamines, amino acids, neuropeptides, and other peptides and substances) are associated with emotion and fluctuations of mood and affect. At least 50 different substances have some or some combination of inhibitory, excitatory, or neuromodulatory effects on brain neurons. Currently, [5-hydroxytryptamine (5-HT)], serotonin, norepinephrine, and acetylcholine (ACh) are clearly implicated in the pathophysiology of affective illness (Coyle, 1987; Gold, Goodwin, & Chrousos, 1988; Willner, 1985; Zubenko, Moossy, & Kopp, 1990).

Study of neurotransmitters in depression accelerated with the observation that patients treated with reserpine, an antihypertensive drug, often develop severe depression. The mechanism of action of reserpine is to deplete catecholamines (noradrenaline, dopamine, and 5-HT). These data and others have led to the bioamine hypothesis for depression. The bioamine hypothesis has been further elaborated by the identification of the mode of action of known antidepressant drugs, e.g., monoamine oxidase inhibitors (MAOIs), tricyclic antidepressants (TCAs), and other serotonin and norepinephrine agonists.

Norepinephrine (Noradrenaline). Norepinephrine cells originate primarily from the locus ceruleus in the midpons. The noradrenergic system has connections to the hypothalamus, hippocampus, and throughout the cerebral cortex. Norepinephrine is synthesized from tyrosine intraneuronally, with the conversion of tyrosine to dopa by tyrosine hydroxylase being a rate-limiting step. Dopa is converted to dopamine by dopa decarboxylase, and dopamine is converted to norepinephrine by dopamine (β-hydroxylase (DBH). Norepinephrine and noradrenergic receptors have been extensively studied in adults with depression (Bunney & Davis, 1965; Golden & Potter, 1986; Schatzberg et al., 1982). Cerebrospinal fluid (CSF) concentrations of norepinephrine, 3-methoxy-4-hydroxyphenylglycol (MHPG), and DBH have not been clearly different in patients with depression. However, Maas, Fawcett, and Dekirmenjian (1968) reported decreased urinary excretion of MHPG in subjects in the bipolar depressed phase. Antidepressants cause down-regulation of post-synaptic β-receptors. Clonidine, a presynaptic α_2-receptor agonist, inhibits norepinephrine release in cerebral cortex. Clonidine also stimulates growth hormone (GH) release, apparently through postsynaptic α_2-receptors. A blunting of this response is seen in both adult and childhood depressives (Checkley, Slade, & Shur, 1981), as will be discussed later. While norepinephrine seems strongly associated with mood disorders, the exact mechanisms are unclear. Few data on child and adolescent depression are currently available.

Serotonin. 5-HT (serotonin) cells originate primarily in the raphe nuclei of the anterior midbrain. The serotonergic neurons provide innervation to the hypothalamus, forebrain, limbic system, and entire cortex and nuclei of the reticular system. The serotonergic neurons are involved in regulation of sleep, temperature, pain sensitivity, appetite, neuroendocrine secretions, and mood. 5-HT is synthesized from tryptophan. Tryptophan is converted to 5-hydroxytriptophan (5-HTP) by tryptophan hydroxylase, and the 5-HTP is decarboxylated to 5-HT. Tryptophan hydroxylase rarely becomes saturated, and as it is the rate-limiting step, the availability of tryptophan becomes an important factor in 5-HT synthesis.

Studies of serotonin in adult depressives are extensive (Agren, 1980; Glennon, 1987; Prange, Wilson, Lynn, Alltop, & Stikeleather, 1974; Van Praag, 1977). Studies measuring baseline CSF 5-hydroxyindole acetic acid (5-HIAA) are equivocal. The most comprehensive studies suggest a subgroup (30–40%) of depressives with low CSF 5-HIAA. Some studies suggest that this subgroup may show more aggression, anxiety, impulsivity, and suicidality. Positive pharmacological challenge tests in adults have included a blunting of prolactin response to tryptophan, fenfluramine, and chlorimipramine (Heninger, Chaney, & Sternberg, 1984). Again, few specific data are available in children and adolescents, though Birmaher et al. (1989) have presented data on 5-HTP challenge tests in children with MDD and normal controls. No difference was noted between the groups, but the study did raise methodological issues over appropriate dosage and timing of the challenge test.

Acetylcholine. Cholinergic neurons (ACh) originate primarily from the nucleus basalis of Meynert and other nuclear groups comprising the substantia innominata with radiations to the hypothalamus, hippocampus, and cerebral cortex. ACh is synthesized from choline via acetyltransferase; unlike other neurotransmitters, ACh has no system for synaptic reuptake.

In adults, there are data to support a "cholinergic–adrenergic balance" hypothesis of mood disorders (Janowsky, El-Yousef, Davis, & Sekerke, 1972) in which mood state is defined by interaction between central noradrenergic and cholinergic activity. Depression is associated with relative cholinergic predominance, whereas mania entails a relative adrenergic predominance. This hypothesis arises from many different indirect observations. Antiadrenergic depression-inducing drugs such as reserpine also have central and peripheral cholinomimetic actions. Most antidepressants have anticholinergic properties. The most direct evidence of ACh involvement came in the 1950s and 1960s from the study of people accidentally poisoned by insecticides that were cholinesterase inhibitors (Bowers, Goodman, & Sim, 1964; Gershon & Shaw, 1961). With regard to challenge tests, affectively ill subjects have a greater prolactin, cortisol, ACTH, and β-endorphin response to physostigmine (Janowsky, El-Yousef, Davis, & Sekerke, 1973; Risch, Cohen, Janowsky, Dalin, & Murphy, 1980), suggesting an overly active cholinergic system. In adults (Sitaram, Gillin, & Bunney, 1984), the cholinergic REM induction test (CRIT) involves intravenous injection of a centrally active muscarinic agent, arecoline, following the end of the first REM period. This procedure induces a quicker onset of the second REM period in unipolar and bipolar depressed patients, suggesting an increased cholinergic sensitivity. Cholinergic abnormalities have been studied in adolescents with major depression by McCracken, Poland, and Tondo (1991) using scopolamine. The adolescents showed an exaggerated response to scopolamine similar to that of their adult depressives.

While the "cholinergic–adrenergic balance" hypothesis of mood disorders does not account for all findings, it sets an important precedent in attempting to integrate the roles of more than one neurotransmitter.

Other Neurotransmitters and Neuromodulators. Many other neurotransmitters and neuromodulators are being investigated with regard to their importance in the understanding and treatment of mood disorders. Dopaminergic neurons originate from the substantia nigra, with major projections to the corpus striatum. Other groups of dopaminergic cells project to the limbic system, frontal cortex, and hypothalamic–pituitary axis. There is evidence that dopaminergic neurons play a role in motor functions, anger, arousal, thought disturbance, and possibly mood (Randrup et al., 1975). γ-Aminobutyric acid (GABA) (an inhibitory transmitter) has been found to be associated with affective disorders (Petty & Schlesser, 1981). GABA has been found to be low in plasma of patients with mood disorders, with primary or secondary unipolar depression and bipolar disorder, both manic and depressed phase (Petty & Sherman, 1982). There is also some suggestion that low plasma GABA may represent a fairly stable traitlike marker for mood disorders (Petty & Sherman, 1984).

In addition to GABA, there has been increasing interest in endogenous opiates, e.g., β-endorphin. The endorphins are intrinsic neuropeptides that stimulate opiate receptors and have analgesic and rewarding properties. Limited evidence is currently available as to whether changes or abnormalities in endorphins, or their impact on mood, are specifically related to affective disorders (Pickar et al., 1982).

In summary, the area of research in neurotransmitters, neuromodulators, and receptors is extensive in adult affective disorders, but limited in child and adolescent disorders. However, understanding of neurochemistry underlies all areas of investigation into the biology of depression. Little is known in humans about the relative rates of development of different neurotransmitter systems, an issue of unique importance to child psychiatry.

Neuroendocrine Abnormalities

Cortisol. Initially, clinicians noted a relationship between endocrinopathies and affective disturbance, and recent development of neuroendocrine assays and specific provocative tests has identified dysfunctions in the hypothalamic–pituitary–adrenal (HPA) axis, the hypothalamic–pituitary–thyroid (HPT) axis, and the hypothalamic–pituitary–growth hormone (HPGH) axis. The HPA axis has been the most thoroughly studied. Increased cortisol and corticosterone production that returns to near normal with clinical recovery from depression was noted initially (Gibbons, 1964, 1966). The data to date support the hypothesis of an overactivity in the HPA axis central regulatory mechanism in depression. Though the neurochemical basis for HPA axis overactivity in depression remains to be clarified, this hyperactivity is thought to be the result of the suprahypophyseal CNS dysfunction that causes depression. The neuroregulatory control of the

HPA axis at the level of the hypothalamus is thought to involve noradrenaline (NA) and dopamine (DA) as inhibitory neurotransmitters and ACh, 5H-T, and GABA as excitory neurotransmitters (Carroll and Mendels, 1976).

Carroll (1982) recognized that the HPA axis overactivity in depression was less pronounced than in Cushing's disease, and he developed the diagnostic use of the DST in major depression—particularly endogenous or melancholic depression. Reports in studies of adults (Carroll, Curtis, & Mendels, 1976; Carroll, Greden, & Feinberg, 1981; Rush, Giles, Roffwarg, & Parker, 1982) have suggested that the DST can usefully differentiate endogenous (melancholic) from nonendogenous (nonmelancholic) depressions and from normal controls. In addition, the DST may be a laboratory index of recovery (Albala & Greden, 1980; Angst, 1980; Goldberg, 1980; McLeod, 1972; Schlesser & Rush, 1981) or an indicator for early relapse, hospitalization, or suicide (Carroll et al., 1981; Coryell & Schlesser, 1981; Greden et al., 1980).

The information available in children and adolescents has been reviewed (Casat & Powell, 1988). Poznanski, Carroll, Banegas, Cook, and Grossman (1982) reported on the DST in prepubertal children using a 0.5 mg dexamethasone dose. They found that of 9 children diagnosed as having MDD, 5 showed nonsuppression, whereas in a group of 9 children with other diagnoses, only 1 showed nonsuppression; i.e., the sensitivity and specificity are similar to those in adults. Extein, Rosenberg, Pottash, and Gold (1982) and Robbins, Alessi, Yanchyshyn, and Colfer (1982) reported similar findings with a 1 mg dexamethasone dose in adolescents.

Doherty et al. (1986) reported that 15 (44%) of 34 patients aged 3–16 with MDD evidenced DST nonsuppression with a 1 mg dexamethasone dose compared to 1 (3%) of 34 nondepressed subjects. Emslie, Weinberg, Rush, Weissenburger, and Parkin-Feigenbaum (1987), in a sample of 94 child and adolescent inpatients, demonstrated that the incidence of DST nonsuppression in patients with major depression was 55% compared to 11% of those with no affective disorders. Depressive symptoms of decreased school performance and somatic complaints differentiated suppressors from nonsuppressors.

Growth Hormone. Secretion of GH from the anterior pituitary is stimulated by GH-releasing factor (GHRF) from the hypothalamus (Block et al., 1983). GHRF release is in turn stimulated by α-noradrenergic, dopaminergic, and serotonergic neuronal input (Mendelson, Jacobs, Sitaram, Wyatt, & Gilin, 1978). A variety of GH abnormalities have been found in adults with major depression, both during the episode of depression and during clinical remission. During an episode of major depression, adults demonstrate a reduction of GH secretion during the first 3 hours of sleep, and this abnormality persists during clinical remission of the depressive episode (Jarrett, Miewald, & Kupfer, 1990). Adults with MDD also show a reduction of GH secretion to a variety of pharmacological challenges, including insulin-induced hypoglycemia, clonidine, desmethylimipramine, and zimelidine (Risch & Judd, 1987). This "blunting" of the GH response to these pharmacological agents persists despite clinical remission of the depressive episode and may represent a "trait" marker for major depression in adults (Risch & Judd, 1987).

In contrast to depressed adults, prepubertal children during an episode of major depression were found by Puig-Antich et al. (1984a) to have increased levels of GH secretion during sleep. When restudied in a fully recovered state and off all medications, this hypersecretion of nocturnal GH was found to persist (Puig-Antich et al., 1984b). This hypersecretion of GH both during the episode of major depression and during recovery may represent a "trait" marker for major depression in prepuberty. Kutcher et al. (1991) studied nocturnal GH secretion in 12 adolescents with major depression and also found significant nocturnal hypersecretion of GH during the episode.

The strategy of various pharmacological challenges to the GH system that has been

2used to study adults has also proven useful in studying children and adolescents. A study by Puig-Antich et al. (1984c,d) found that prepubertal children with endogenous depression have significant hyposecretion of GH in response to insulin during the depressive episode and continue to show this same abnormality when drug-free and during recovery from their depressive episode. Jensen and Garfinkel (1990) studied the GH response to both L-dopa and clonidine and found that the 6 prepubertal boys in their sample hyposecreted GH in response to both these agents, whereas the 8 pubertal boys did not show differences in GH response to these agents. An intriguing study by Ryan et al. (1988) found that depressed adolescents secreted significantly less GH in response to intramuscular desmethylimipramine (DMI) than normal controls and that increasing suicidality on the Kiddie Schedule for Affective Disorders and Schizophrenia—Parent version rating scale was associated with significantly less secretion of GH in response to DMI.

Thyroid-Axis Abnormalities. Thyrotropin-releasing hormone (TRH) is produced by the hypophysiotropic neurons in the median eminence of the hypothalamus. TRH is secreted into the portal-venous system of the pituitary and stimulates synthesis and release of thyroid-stimulating hormone (TSH). TSH stimulates the thyroid gland to produce and secrete triiodothyronine (T_3) and thyroxine (T_4). These thyroid hormones produce negative feedback at the level of the pituitary and hypothalamus. The neurochemical control mechanisms for TRH is not fully understood, but involves both noradrenalin (stimulatory) and 5-HT (inhibitory). In adults, a blunted TSH response to TRH has been reported to occur in 30–40% of depressed subjects (Prange, Wilson, Lora, Alltop, & Breese, 1972; Rush et al., 1983; Targum, Byrnes, & Sullivan, 1982). Blunted TSH response has also been reported in alcoholics, bulimics, and schizophrenics (Baumgartner, Graf, Kurten, & Meinhold, 1988; Dackis, Bailey, Stuckey, & Extein, Pottash, Gold, 1985; Gwirtsman, Roy-Byrne, Yager, & Gemer, 1983; Loosen, Prange, & Wilson, 1979).

Studies of the thyroid axis in children and adolescents are few. Kutcher et al. (1991) reported on nocturnal secretory patterns of TSH in adolescent inpatients with major depression and controls. Nocturnal TSH values significantly differentiated the two groups at 1:00 A.M., but there was no significant difference in total amount of TSH secreted. Several studies of TSH response to TRH have been reported. Khan (1988) studied 100 inpatient adolescents with varied diagnoses and noted TSH blunting in 36% of depressed subjects and 43% with substance-abuse disorders. Brambilla, Musetti, Tacchini, Fontanillas, and Guareschi-Cazullo (1989) did not find blunting in 8 children and adolescents with dysthymia as compared with a matched normal control group. Garcia et al. (1991) used two doses of TRH, 2 mg/kg and 7 mg/kg, and compared 30 depressed subjects and 16 nondepressed psychiatric controls and found no difference in TSH response in the two groups adjusting for age. They did note a linear increase in TSH response with age, particularly in girls. They suggest that males may have a lower response of TSH to TRH in part due to an androgen blunting effect and because of their lower levels of estrogens.

At this time, the TRH stimulation test appears of limited clinical diagnostic utility due to low sensitivity and specificity. In addition, a study in adults (Baumgartner et al., 1988) suggests that it is not useful in predicting relapse.

In summary, neuroendocrine studies continue to be exciting areas of investigation. Currently, in the child and adolescent population, the study of GH regulation has significant promise. Neuroendocrine studies in children and adolescents pose problems unique to this age group. The rapid hormonal changes of puberty and individual variability make it hard to interpret both positive and negative results. Challenge tests, e.g., DST, TRH stimulation test, clonidine challenge, tend to be hard to interpret because of uncertainty about current dosage to allow comparison with adult studies. As yet, there is only limited clinical application for the large body of neuroendocrine research in mood disorders. The significance of neuroendocrine abnormalities to our understanding of the pathophysiology or etiology of depressive disorders remains uncertain. However, the increasing ability to detect and interpret neuroendocrine findings in all ages brings closer an understanding of the underlying neurobiology of depression.

Polysomnography

Disturbances in sleep, e.g., falling asleep, early morning awakening, and excessive sleepiness, have all been associated clinically with depression. Additionally, a substantial body of research in adults, utilizing direct laboratory recording of sleep, has identified abnormalities relatively unique to depression. In parallel, while sleep is a complex function, its basic mechanisms are beginning to be understood. In polysomnographic (PSG) recording of sleep, the subject's characteristic patterns of electroencephalogram (EEG), electromyogram (EMG), and electrooculogram (EOG) are used to stage sleep by standard scoring criteria (Rechtschaffen & Kales, 1968). Sleep is divided into stages 1, 2, 3, 4, which together constitute non–rapid eye movement (NREM) sleep, and rapid eye movement (REM) sleep. Stage 1 is a brief transition phase marking a change from awake state to sleep as indicated by EEG activity. Stage 2 is characterized by K-complexes and sleep spindles on the EEG. Stages 3 and 4 (delta or slow-wave sleep) are characterized by a predominance of low-frequency delta waves. REM sleep is identified by desynchronization of the EEG with rapid conjugate eye movements and muscular hypotonia. The approximate amount of time spent in each stage of sleep is: stage 1, 5–10%; stage 2, 45–55%; stages 3 and 4, 10–20%; and stage REM, 20–25%. The standard night of laboratory recording consists of four to five cycles of NREM/REM sleep. In the course of the night, there are decreasing amounts of stages 3 and 4 while REM sleep increases.

In adult depressives, the following have consistently been found: (1) sleep continuity disturbances, such as delayed sleep onset and decreased sleep efficiency (sleep efficiency is the proportion of the sleep recording period spent asleep, usually expressed as a percentage); (2) reduced delta (slow-wave) sleep; (3) increased REM density (i.e., the amount of REM activity during REM sleep); and (4) shortened REM latency (time from sleep onset to the first REM period) (Feinberg, Gillin,Carroll, Greden, & Zis, 1982; Gillin et al., 1984; Kupfer & Foster, 1972; Kupfer, Foster, Coble, McPartland, & Ulrich, 1978; Kupfer et al., 1985; Rush et al., 1982).

Diagnostically, these abnormalities are found more consistently in endogenous than in nonendogenous adult depressives. In a study by Rush et al. (1982), an REM latency threshold of less than 60.0 minutes distinguished melancholic from nonmelancholic depressed outpatients with a high diagnostic confidence (83%). In adults, studies have been completed comparing the sleep findings in depression with those in schizophrenia (Ganguli, Reynolds, & Rupfer, 1987), generalized anxiety disorder (Reynolds, Shaw, Newton, Coble, & Kupfer, 1983), and dementia (Reynolds et al., 1985). Generally, it appears that shortened REM latency is relatively specific for affective disorders. The sleep EEG may also provide important information about treatment selection and prediction of response in depressed patients. In one study of 34 medication-free patients with primary endogenous depression, EEG-monitored sleep criteria proved more significant than clinical status alone in predicting response to amitriptyline. Difficulty in sleep onset and a prolongation of REM latency following a single 50 mg dose of amitriptyline were the two variables that contributed to the prediction (Kupfer et al., 1981). Similar results have been found by Rush et al. (1989).

There is a growing body of evidence to suggest that reduced REM latency and perhaps other sleep abnormalities noted during the symptomatic episode of depression may persist into clinical remission, since most studies to date show that the sleep abnormalities tend to remain unchanged up to 2 years following remission (Rush et al., 1986). These initial findings suggest that sleep EEG abnormalities are probably more traitlike than statelike. To answer the question of whether sleep EEG features are simply residual scars of prior episodes of depression or are predictive of vulnerability even prior to the first episode will require family studies with longitudinal follow-up of these high-risk individuals.

In early studies of children with major depression, Puig-Antich et al. (1982) found no differences in the sleep EEG of depressed prepubertal children and normal controls. However, when the depressed children were studied during remission, REM latencies were significantly reduced when compared to controls (Puig-Antich et al., 1983). Recently, we reported on children of ages 8–13 with major depression and normal children (Emslie, Rush, Weinberg, Rintelmann, & Roffwarg, 1990). We compared 25 prepubertal children (mean age 11.5 years) with major depression to 20 age-matched normal controls. In the depressed group, REM latency was significantly shorter and total REM time and REM percentage of total sleep were significantly higher. NREM sleep stages were not significantly different between groups. When an REM latency threshold of less than 75 minutes was chosen, 17 (68%) of 25 depressed subjects compared to only 2 (13%) of 15 normal controls had at least one night of reduced REM latency.

Previously published data in adolescents have also been mixed. Lahmeyer, Poznanski, and Bellur (1983) found a significantly shorter REM latency and increased REM density in 13 depressed adolescents, both inpatients and outpatients, as compared to age-matched controls. Sleep-recording time was held constant for all subjects. Goetz et al. (1987) found sleep continuity disturbances in 48 depressed adolescents (mainly outpatients) as compared to 40 normal adolescent controls, but no differences in REM sleep measurements. Dahl et al. (1990) recently reported sleep parameter differences in 27 adolescents with MDD compared to 30 normal controls. In this study of a mixed population of inpatients and outpatients, suicidal MDD patients tended to have a shorter REM latency. The authors suggested that the differences in the data from different studies of adolescents may be accounted for by patient status (i.e., inpatient vs. outpatient), suicidality, or endogenicity. Because suicidal patients constituted most of the inpatients and endogenous patients in the group, it was not possible to separate the factors. Two recent studies of inpatient adolescents with major depression report significantly shortened REM latency in depressed adolescents as compared to normal controls (Emslie, Roffwarg, Rush, & Weinberg, 1991; Kutcher et al., 1991). Currently, it is unclear whether this apparent difference between inpatients and outpatients is a function of severity or type of illness or a result of methodological differences. Inpatients' sleep patterns are more easily stabilized prior to the time spent in the sleep laboratory as compared to depressed outpatients, possibly decreasing the artifact of irregular sleep patterns prior to the nights recorded.

In summary, depressed children and adolescents show less sleep continuity and NREM sleep differences compared to controls than do adults. As with adults, however, children show evidence of increased REM pressure early in the night. These findings suggest that of the several major sleep EEG abnormalities found in depressed adults, REM sleep changes are the most robust and earliest to manifest themselves.

Conclusion

This chapter highlights areas of research on neurobiological correlates in both adults and children. While not exhaustive, it does emphasize the breadth of information known and identifies areas in which substantial work is needed. While discussions of receptors and neurotransmitters at times may appear far removed from clinical care, these connections are gradually being made.

In the areas of neurological findings, the data from the studies of neurologically intact depressed individuals suggest that depression is evidenced by dysfunction of the right cerebral hemisphere. The data from stroke research, however, suggest more depression in left hemisphere strokes. This laterality may represent destruction of a tonic influence of mood from left to right brain. An interesting area of clinical importance for further research in behavioral neurology is the association of depression and learning disabilities. It is evident that depression, learning disabilities, and doing poorly in school are commonly associated (Livingston, 1985; Weinberg & Emslie, 1988; Weinberg & Rehmet, 1983; Weinberg, Rutman, Sullivan, Penick, & Dietz, 1973). Right hemisphere learning disabilities are being increasingly reported and are often associated with depressive symptomatology (Delong, 1978; Delong & Dwyer, 1988; Rourke, Young, & Leenaars, 1989; Voeller, 1986; Weinberg & McLean, 1986). The interaction between learning disabilities and depression requires further study.

In neuropsychological studies of depression, distinctions have to be made between studies conducted with subjects with depressive symptoms and those who meet criteria for major depression. Neuropsychological data of particular importance to children will be those assessing whether having chronic depression can lead to permanent structural or behavioral changes.

It is hoped that future research will be aided by neuroimaging studies. The pace of development of new technologies is outstanding. The development of scanning techniques that can picture brain function as well as structure with increasingly high resolution in an exciting development. Again, the lack of normative data on the developing brain limits our understanding at this time. The recent development of magnetic resonance spectroscopy, which does not require radiation exposure, will increase the availability of these studies in this age group.

The developments in the understanding of the neurochemistry of depression have direct clinical relevance, particularly to pharmacological treatment. Psychopharmacological research in children and adolescents is limited and results of treatment studies equivocal. Therefore, a greater understanding of the development of neurotransmitters and receptors, especially through puberty, becomes increasingly important. As research continues, it is clear that a neurochemistry model for depression will be more complex than originally believed and will involve the interaction of many neurotransmitters and their receptors.

Neuroendocrine studies of depression continue to be important areas of investigation, particularly cortisol and growth hormone studies. The identification of state or trait markers for depression will allow a more specific selection of high-risk populations to examine risk and protective factors, both biological and environmental, in susceptible individuals.

The study of sleep provides a window into the brain's physiological functioning. Sleep is a complex process that is beginning to be understood. The developmental norms are already available across the life span, making it easier to identify disorders. To date, results in depressed children and adolescents appear to show that inpatient subjects are more likely to show abnormal sleep, i.e., shorter REM latency, than outpatient depressives. This difference may be a function of severity or a methodological issue. It is possible that it takes the structure of an inpatient setting to stabilize sleep to bring out the sleep abnormalities in depressed children that are obscured in outpatients. Carefully controlled outpatient studies are needed to answer these questions.

In conclusion, the study of neurobiological correlates of depression requires substantial interaction between clinicians and basic neuroscience researchers. Study of children and adolescents is essential to an understanding of the developmental neurobiology of depression. It can be expected that further research in child and adolescent depression will assist understanding not just in this age group but in all age groups.

Agren, H. (1980). Symptom patterns in unipolar and bipolar depression correlating with monoamine metabolites in cerebrospinal fluid. I. General patterns. *Psychiatry Research, 3,* 211–223.

Albala, A. A., & Greden, J. F. (1980). Serial dexamethasone suppression tests (DST) in affective disorders. *American Journal of Psychiatry, 137,* 383.

Angst, J. (1980). Zur aetiologic und nosologic endogene depressiven Psychosen. *Monographs in Neurological Psychiatry, 112,* 1–18.

Baumgartner, A., Graf, K. J., Kurten, I., & Meinhold, H. (1988). The hypothalamic–pituitary thyroid axis in psychiatric patients and healthy subjects: Parts 1–4. *Psychiatry Research, 24,* 271–332.

Bear, D. M. (1983). Hemispheric specialization and neurology of emotion. *Archives of Neurology, 40,* 195–202.

Birmaher, B., Puig-Antich, K., Ryan, N., Dahl, R., Meyer, V., Thomas, C., Coleman, C., Brent, D., & Perel, J. (1989). 5HTP challenge test in children with major depressive disorder. *Scientific Proceedings of the Annual Meeting of the American Academy of Child and Adolescent Psychiatry, 5,* 48 (abstract).

Block, B., Brazeau, P., Ling, N., Bohlen, P., Esch, E., Wehrenberg, W. B., Benoit, R., Bloom, F., & Guillemin, R. (1983). Immunohistochemical detection of growth hormone–releasing factor in brain. *Nature, 301,* 607–608.

Blumberg, S. H., & Izard, C. E. (1985). Affective and cognitive characteristics of depression in 10- and 11-year-old children. *Journal of Personality and Social Psychology, 49,* 194–202.

Bowers, M. B., Goodman, E., & Sim, V. M. (1964). Some behavioral changes in man following anticholinesterase administration. *Journal of Nervous and Mental Disease, 138,* 383–389.

Brambilla, F., Musetti, C., Tacchini, C., Fontanillas, J., & Guareschi-Cazullo, A. (1989). Neuroendocrine investigation in children and adolescents with dysthymic disorders: The DST, TRN and clonidine tests. *Journal of Affective Disorders, 35,* 1231–1238.

Brown, W. A., Doinseif, B. E., & Wernicke, J. F. (1988). Placebo response in depression: A search for predictors. *Psychiatry Research, 26,* 259–264.

Brumback, R. A. (1988). Childhood depression and medically treatable learning disability. In D. L. Molfese & S. J. Segalowitz (Eds.), *Brain lateralization in children* (pp. 463–505). New York: Guilford Press.

Brumback, R. A., Staton, R. D., & Wilson, H. (1980). Neuropsychological study of children during and after remission of endogenous depressive episodes. *Perceptual and Motor Skills, 50,* 1163–1167.

Brumback, R. A., Staton, R. D., & Wilson, H. (1984). Right cerebral hemisphere dysfunction. *Archives of General Neurology, 41,* 248–249.

Bunney, W. E., Jr., & Davis, J. M. (1965). Norepinephrine in depressive reactions: A review. *Archives of General Psychiatry, 13,* 483–494.

Cantwell, D., & Baker, L. (1980). Academic failures in children with communication disorders. *Journal of the American Academy of Child Psychiatry, 19,* 579–591.

Carroll, B. J. (1982). The dexamethasone suppression test for melancholia. *British Journal of Psychiatry, 140,* 292–304.

Carroll, B. J., Curtis, G. C., & Mendels, J. (1976). Neuroendocrine regulation in depression. II. Discrimination of depressed from nondepressed patients. *Archives of General Psychiatry, 33,* 1051–1058.

Carroll, B. J., Greden, J. F., & Feinberg, M. (1981). Suicide, neuroendocrine dysfunction and CSF 5-HIAA concentrations in depression. In B. Angrast (Ed.), *Recent advances in neuropsychopharmacology: Advances in the biosciences,* Vol. 31 (pp. 301–313). New York: Pergamon Press.

Carroll, B. J., & Mendels, J. (1976). Neuroendocrine regulations in affective disorders. In E. J. Scahar (Ed.), *Hormones, behavior and psychopathology* (pp. 193–224). New York: Raven Press.

Casat, C., & Powell, K. (1988). Utility of the dexamethasone suppression test in children and adolescents with major depressive disorder. *Journal of Clinical Psychiatry, 49,* 390–393.

Checkley, S. A., Slade, A. P., & Shur, E. (1981). Growth hormone and other responses to clonidine in patients with endogenous depression. *British Journal of Psychiatry, 138,* 51–55.

Coryell, W., & Schlesser, M. A. (1981). Suicide and the dexamethasone suppression test in unipolar depression. *American Journal of Psychiatry, 138,* 1120–1121.

Coyle, J. T. (1987). Biochemical development of the brain: Neurotransmitters and child psychiatry. In C. Popper (Ed.), *Psychiatric pharmacosciences of children and adolescents.* Washington, DC: American Psychiatric Press.

Dackis, C. A., Bailey, I., Pottash, A. L., Stuckey, R. F., Extein, I. L., & Gold, M. S. (1985). Specificity of the DST and the TRH test for major depression in alcoholics. *American Journal of Psychiatry, 141,* 680–683.

Dahl, R. E., Puig-Antich, J., Ryan, N. D., Nelson, B., Dachille, S., Cunningham, S. L., Trubrick, L., & Klepper, T. P. (1990). EEG sleep in adolescents with major depression: The role of suicidality and inpatient status. *Journal of Affective Disorders, 19,* 63–75.

Davidson, R. J., & Tomarken, A. J. (1989). Laterality and emotion: An electrophysiological approach. In F. Boller & J. Grafman (Eds.), *Handbook of neuropsychology*, Vol. 3 (pp. 419–441). Amsterdam: Elsevier.

Delong, G. R. (1978). Lithium carbonate treatment of select behavior disorders in children suggesting manic–depressive illness. *Journal of Pediatrics, 93*, 689–694.

Delong, G. R., & Dwyer, J. T. (1988). Correlation of family history with specific autistic subgroups: Asperger's syndrome and bipolar affective disease. *Journal of Autism and Developmental Disorders, 18*, 593–600.

Devous, M. D., Sr. (1988). Imaging brain function by single-photon emission computed tomography. In N. C. Andreason (Ed.), *Brain imaging: Applications in psychiatry* (pp. 147–234). American Psychiatric Press.

Dimond, S. J., & Farrington, J. (1977). Emotional response to films shown to the right or left hemisphere of the brain measured by the heart rate. *Acta Psychologia, 41*, 255–260.

Doherty, M. B., Madansky, D., Kraft, J., Carter-Ake, L. L., Rosenthal, P. A., & Coughlin, B. F. (1986). Cortisol dynamics and test performance of the dexamethasone suppression test in 97 psychiatrically hospitalized children aged 3–16 years. *Journal of the American Academy of Child Psychiatry, 25*, 400–408.

Emslie, G. J., Roffwarg, H. P., Rush, A. J., & Weinberg, W. A. (1991). Sleep polysomnography in depressed adolescents. Paper presented at the Annual Meeting of the American Psychiatric Association, New Orleans.

Emslie, G. J., Rush, A. J., Weinberg, W. A., Rintelmann, J. W., & Roffwarg, H. P. (1990). Children with major depression show reduced rapid eye movement latencies. *Archives of General Psychiatry, 47*, 119–124.

Emslie, G. J., Weinberg, W. A., Rush, A. J., Weissenburger, J., & Parkin-Feigenbaum, L. (1987). Depression and dexamethasone suppression testing in children and adolescents. *Journal of Child Neurology, 2*, 31–37.

Extein, I., Rosenberg, G., Pottash, A., & Gold, M. (1982). The dexamethasone suppression test in depressed adolescents. *American Journal of Psychiatry, 139*, 1617–1619.

Feinberg, M., Gillin, J. C., Carroll, B. J., Greden, J. F., & Zis, A. P. (1982). EEG studies of sleep in the diagnosis of depression. *Biological Psychiatry, 17*, 305–316.

Flor-Henry, P. (1979). On certain aspects of the localization of the cerebral systems regulating and determining emotion. *Biological Psychiatry, 14*, 677–698.

Frank, E., Prien, R. F., Jarrett, R. B., Keller, M. B., Kupfer, D. J., Lavori, P. W., Rush, A. J., & Weissman, M. M. (1991). Conceptualization and rationale for consensus definitions of terms in major depressive disorder. *Archives of General Psychiatry, 48*, 851–855.

Freeman, R. L., Galaburda, A. M., Cabal, R. D., & Geschwind, N. (1985). The neurology of depression: Cognitive and behavioral deficits with focal findings in depression and resolution after electroconvulsive therapy. *Archives of Neurology, 42*, 289–291.

Fromm, D., & Schopflocher, D. (1984). Neuropsychological test performance in depressed patients before and after drug therapy. *Biological Psychiatry, 19*, 55–72.

Ganguli, R., Reynolds, C. F., III., & Kupfer, D. J. (1987). Electroencephalographic sleep in young, never-medicated schizophrenics: A comparison with delusional and nondelusional depressives and with healthy controls. *Archives of General psychiatry, 44*, 36–44.

Garcia, M. R., Ryan, N. D., Rabinovitch, H., Ambrosini, P., Twomey, J., Iyengar, S., Novacenko, H., Nelson, B., & Puig-Antich, J. (1991). Thyroid stimulating hormone response to thyrotropin in prepubertal depression. *Journal of the American Academy of Child and Adolescent Psychiatry, 30(3)*, 398–406.

Gershon, S., & Shaw, F. H. (1961). Psychiatric sequelae of chronic exposure to organophosphorus insecticides. *Lancet, 1*, 1371–1374.

Geschwind, N., & Galaburda, A. M. (1985). Cerebral lateralization: Biological mechanisms, associations, and pathology, a hypothesis and a program for research. *Archives of Neurology, 42*, 428–459, 521–522, 634–654.

Gibbons, J. L. (1964). Cortisol secretion rate in depressive illness. *Archives of General Psychiatry, 10*, 572–575.

Gibbons, J. L. (1966). The secretion rate of corticosterone in depressive illness. *Journal of Psychosomatic Research, 10*, 263–266.

Giles, D. E., Jarrett, R. B., Roffwarg, H. P., & Rush, A. J. (1987). Reduced rapid eye movement latency: A predictor of recurrence in depression. *Neuropsychopharmacology, 1*, 33–39.

Gillin, J. C., Sitaram, N., Wehr, T., Duncan, W., Post, R., Murphy, D. L., Mendelson, W. B., Wyatt, R. J., & Bunney, W. E. (1984). Sleep and affective illness. In R. M. Post & J. C. Ballenger (Eds.), *Neurobiology of mood disorders* (pp. 157–189). Baltimore: Williams & Wilkins.

Glennon, R. A. (1987). Central serotonin receptors as targets for drug research. *Journal of Medicinal Chemistry, 30*, 1–12.

Goetz, R. R., Puig-Antich, J., Ryan, N., Rabinovich, H., Ambrosini, P. J., Nelson, B., & Krawiec, V. (1987). Electroencephalographic sleep of adolescents with major depression and normal controls. *Archives of General Psychiatry, 44,* 61–68.

Gold, P. W., Goodwin, F. K., & Chrousos, G. P. (1988). Clinical and biochemical manifestations of depression: Relation to the neurobiology of stress. *New England Journal of Medicine, 319,* 348–353, 413–420.

Goldberg, I. K. (1980). Dexamethasone suppression tests in depression and response to treatment. *Lancet, 2,* 92.

Golden, R. M., & Potter, W. Z. (1986). Neurochemical and neuroendocrine dysregulation in affective disorders. *Psychiatric Clinics of North America, 9,* 313–327.

Gray, J. W., Dean, R. S., D'Amato, R. C., & Rattan, G. (1987). Differential diagnosis of primary affective depression using the Halstead–Reitan Neuropsychological Battery. *International Journal of Neuroscience, 35,* 43–49.

Greden, J. F., Albala, A. A., Haskett, R. F., James, N. M., Goodman, L., Steiner, M., & Carroll, B. J. (1980). Normalization of dexamethasone suppression test: A laboratory index of recovery from endogenous depression. *Biological Psychiatry, 15,* 449–459.

Guze, B. H. (1991). Magnetic resonance spectroscopy: A technique for functional brain imaging. *Archives of General Psychiatry, 48,* 572–574.

Gwirtsman, H. E., Roy-Byrne, P., Yager, J., & Gerner, R. H. (1983). Neuroendocrine abnormalities in bulimia. *American Journal of Psychiatry, 140,* 559–563.

Haggard, M. P., & Parkinson, A. M. (1971). Stimulus and task factors as determinants of ear advantages. *Quarterly Journal of Experimental Psychology, 23,* 168–177.

Heilman, K. M., Bowers, D., & Valenstein, E. (1983). Emotional disorders associated with neurological diseases. In K. M. Heilman & E. Valenstein (Eds.), *Neuropsychology* (pp. 377–402). New York: Oxford University Press.

Heilman, K. M., Watson, R. T., Valenstein, E. (1985). Neglect and related disorders. In K. M. Heilman & E. Valenstein (Eds.), *Clinical neuropsychology* (pp. 234–294). New York: Oxford University Press.

Hendren, R. L., Hodde-Vargas, J. E., Vargas, L. A., Orrison, W. W., & Dell, L. (1991). Magnetic resonance imaging of severely disturbed children—A preliminary study. *Journal of the American Academy of Child and Adolescent Psychiatry, 30(3),* 466–470.

Heninger, G. R., Charney, D. S., & Sternberg, D. E. (1984). Serotonergic function in depression: Prolactin response to intravenous tryptophan in depressed patients and healthy subjects. *Archives of General Psychiatry, 41,* 398–402.

Janowsky, D. S., El-Yousef, M. K., Davis, J., & Sekerke, H. J. (1972). A cholinergic–adrenergic hypothesis of mania and depression. *Lancet, 2,* 6732–6735.

Janowsky, D. S., El-Yousef, M. K., Davis, J. M., & Sekerke, H. J. (1973). Antagonistic effects of physostigmine and methylphenidate in man. *American Journal of Psychiatry, 130,* 1370–1376.

Jarrett, D. B., Miewald, J. M., & Kupfer, D. J. (1990). Recurrent depression is associated with a persistent reduction in sleep-related growth hormone reduction. *Archives of General Psychiatry, 47,* 113–118.

Jensen, J. B., & Garfinkel, B. D. (1990). Growth hormone dysregulation in children with major depression. *Journal of the American Academy of Child and Adolescent Psychiatry, 29(2),* 295–301.

Kaslow, N. J., Rehm, L. P., & Siegel, A. W. (1984). Social–cognitive and cognitive correlates of depression in children. *Journal of Abnormal Child Psychology, 12,* 605–620.

Kaslow, N. J., Tanenbaum, R. L., Abramson, L. Y., Peterson, C., & Seligman, M. E. P. (1983). Problem-solving deficits and depressive symptoms among children. *Journal of Abnormal Child Psychology, 11,* 497–502.

Kazdin, A. E. (1989). Identifying depression in children: A comparison of alternative selection criteria. *Journal of Abnormal Child Psychology, 17,* 437–454.

Kennard, B. D., Bass, C., Emslie, G. J., Weinberg, W. A., Nici, J., Guillion, C., & Rintelmann, J. (1991). Stability of cognitive deficits in children with MDD: A follow-up study. Paper presented at the Annual Meeting of the American Psychological Association, San Francisco, 1991.

Kennard, B. D., Nici, J., Emslie, G. J., & Weinberg, W. A. (1987). Neuropsychological and physiological measures in children with major depressive disorder. Paper presented at the Annual Meeting of the American Psychological Association, New York.

Khan, A. (1988). Sensitivity and specificity of TRH stimulation test in depressed and non-depressed adolescents. *Psychiatry Research, 25,* 11–17.

Koerber, R. K., Torkelson, R., Haven, G., Donaldson, J., Cohen, S. M., Case, M. (1984). Increased cerebrospinal fluid 5-hydroxytryptamine and 5-hydroxyindoleacetic acid in Klein–Levin syndrome. *Neurology, 34,* 1597–1600.

Kolb, B., & Whishaw, I. Q. (1980). *Fundamentals of human neuropsychology.* San Francisco: W. H. Freeman.

Kovacs, M. (1981). Rating scale to assess depression in school-aged children. *Acta Paedopsychiatrica, 46,* 303–315.

Kovacs, M. (1989). Affective disorders in children and adolescents. *American Psychologist, 44,* 209–215.

Kron, L., Decina, P., Kestenbaum, C. J., Farber, S., Gargan, M., & Fieve, R. (1982). The offspring of bipolar manic–depressives: Clinical features. *Adolescent Psychiatry, 10,* 273–298.

Kupfer, D. J., & Ehlers, C. L. (1989). Two roads to rapid eye movement latency. *Archives of General Psychiatry, 46,* 945–948.

Kupfer, D. J., & Foster, F. G. (1972). Interval between onset of sleep and rapid eye movement sleep as an indicator of depression. *Lancet, 11,* 684–686.

Kupfer, D. J., Foster, F. G., Coble, P. A., McPartland, R. J., & Ulrich, R. F. (1978). The application of EEG sleep for the differential diagnosis of affective disorders. *American Journal of Psychiatry, 135,* 69–74.

Kupfer, D. J., Spiker, D. G., Coble, P. A., Neil, J. F., Ulrich, R., & Shaw, D. H. (1981). Sleep and treatment prediction in endogenous depression. *American Journal of Psychiatry, 138,* 429–434.

Kupfer, D. J., Ulrich, R. F., Coble, P. A., Jarrett, D. B., Grochocinski, V. J., Doman, J., Matthews, G., & Borbely, A. (1985). Electroencephalographic sleep of young depressives. *Archives of General Psychiatry, 42,* 806–810.

Kupperman, S., Gaffney, G. R., Hamdan-Allen, G., Preston, D. F., and Venkatesh, L. (1990). Special article: Neuroimaging in child psychiatry. *Journal of the American Academy of Child and Adolescent Psychiatry, 29(2),* 159–172.

Kutcher, S., Malkin, D., Silverberg, J., Marton, P., Williamson, P., Malkin, A., Szalai, J., & Katic, M. (1991). Nocturnal cortisol, thyroid stimulating hormone, and growth hormone secretory profiles in depressed adolescents. *Journal of the American Academy of Child and Adolescent Psychiatry, 30(3),* 407–414.

Lahmeyer, H. W., Poznanski, E. O., & Bellur, S. N. (1983). Sleep in depressed adolescents. *American Journal of Psychiatry, 140,* 1150–1153.

Lenhart, R. E., & Katlin, E. S. (1986). Psychophysiological evidence for cerebral laterality effects in a high risk sample of students with subsyndromal bipolar depressive disorder. *American Journal of Psychiatry, 143,* 602–607.

Ley, R. G., & Bryden, M. P. (1979). Hemispheric differences in processing emotions and faces. *Brain and Language, 7,* 127–138.

Livingston, R. (1985). Depressive illness and learning difficulties: Research needs and practical implications. *Journal of Learning Disabilities, 18,* 518–520.

Loosen, P. T., Prange, A. J., & Wilson, I. C. (1979). TRH (protirelin) in depressed alcoholic men. *Archives of General Psychiatry, 36,* 540–547.

Lou, H. C., Henriksen, L., Bruhn, P., & Psych, C. (1984). Focal cerebral hypoperfusion in children with dysphasia and/or attention deficit disorder. *Archives of Neurology, 41,* 825–829.

Maas, J. W., Fawcett, J., & Dekirmenjian, H. (1968). 3-Methoxy-4-hydroxyphenylglycol (MHPG) excretion in depressed states: A pilot study. *Archives of General Psychiatry, 19,* 129–134.

Martinot, J. L., Hardy, P., Feline, A., Huret, J. D., Mazoyer, B., Attar-Levy, D., Pappata, S., & Syrota, A. (1990). Left prefrontal glucose hypometabolism in the depressed state: A confirmation. *American Journal of Psychiatry, 147(10),* 1313–1317.

McCracken, J., Poland, R., & Tondo, L. (1991). Differential effects of cholinergic blockage in adolescent major depression. *Scientific Proceedings of the Annual Meeting, American Academy of Child and Adolescent Psychiatry, 7,* 45 (abstract).

McLeod, W. R. (1972). Poor response to antidepressants and dexamethasone non-suppression. In B. M. Davies, B. J. Carroll, & R. M. Mowbray (Eds.), *Depressive illness: Some research studies* (pp. 202–206). Springfield, IL: Charles C. Thomas.

Mendelson, W. B., Jacobs, L. S., Sitaram, N., Wyatt, R. J., & Gilin, J. C. (1978). Methoscopolamine inhibition of sleep related growth hormone secretion. *Journal of Clinical Investigation, 61,* 1683–1690.

Mesulam, M. M. (1985). *Principles of behavioral neurology.* Philadelphia: Davis.

Mullins, L. J., Siegel, L. J., & Hodges, K. (1985). Cognitive problem-solving and life event correlates of depressive symptoms in children. *Journal of Abnormal Child Psychology, 13,* 305–314.

Newman, P. J., & Silverstein, M. L. (1987). Neuropsychological test performance among major clinical subtypes of depression. *Archives of Clinical Neuropsychology, 2,* 115–125.

Newman, P. J., & Sweet, J. J. (1986). The effects of clinical depression on the Luria–Nebraska Neuropsychological Battery. *International Journal of Clinical Neuropsychology, 8,* 109–114.

Petty, F., & Schlesser, M. A. (1981). Plasma GABA in affective illness: A preliminary investigation. *Journal of Affective Disorders, 3,* 339–343.

Petty, F., & Sherman, A. D. (1982). Plasma GABA: A blood test for bipolar affective disorder trait? *Research Communications in Psychology, Psychiatry and Behavior, 7,* 431–440.

Petty, F., & Sherman, A. D. (1984). Plasma GABA levels in psychiatric illness. *Journal of Affective Disorders*, *6*, 131–138.

Pickar, D., Extein, I., Gold, P. W., Naber, D., Summers, F. S., & Goodwin, F. K. (1982). Endorphins in affective disorders. In N. S. Shah & A. G. Donald (Eds.), *Endorphins and opiate antagonists in psychiatric illness* (pp. 375–397). New York: Plenum Press.

Poznanski, E. O., Carroll, V. J., Banegas, M. E., Cook, S. C., & Grossman, J. A. (1982). The dexamethasone suppression test in prepubertal depressed children. *American Journal of Psychiatry*, *139*, 321–324.

Prange, A. J., Jr., Wilson, I. C., Lora, P. P., Alltop, L. B., & Breese, G.R. (1972). Effects of thyrotropin releasing hormone in depression. *Lancet*, *2*, 999–1002.

Prange, A. J., Jr., Wilson, I. C., Lynn, C. W., Alltop, L. B., & Stikeleather, R. A. (1974). L-Tryptophan in mania: Contribution to a permissive hypothesis of affective disorders. *Archives of General Psychiatry*, *30*, 56–62.

Preskorn, S. H., Weller, E. B., Hughes, C. W., Weller, R. A., & Bolte, K. (1987). Depression in prepubertal children: Dexamethasone nonsuppression predicts differential response to imipramine vs. placebo. *Psychopharmacology Bulletin*, *23*, 128–133.

Puig-Antich, J., Goetz, R., Davies, M., Fein, M., Hanlon, C., Chambers, W. J., Tabrizi, M. A., Sachar, E. J., & Weitzman, E. D. (1948a). Growth hormone secretion in prepubertal children with major depression: Sleep-related plasma concentrations during a depressive episode. *Archives of General Psychiatry*, *41*, 463–466.

Puig-Antich, J., Goetz, R., Davies, M., Tabrizi, M. A., Novacenko, H., Hanlon, C., Chambers, W. J., Sachar, E. J., & Weitzman, E. D. (1984b). Growth hormone secretion in prepubertal children with major depression: Sleep-related plasma concentrations in a drug-free, fully recovered state. *Archives of General Psychiatry*, *41*, 479–483.

Puig-Antich, J., Goetz, R., Hanlon, C., Davies, M., Thompson, J., Chambers, W. J., Tabrizi, M. A., & Weitzman, E. D. (1982). Sleep architecture and REM sleep measures in prepubertal children with major depression: A controlled study. *Archives of General Psychiatry*, *39*, 932–939.

Puig-Antich, J., Goetz, R., Hanlon, C., Tabrizi, M. A., Davies, M., & Weitzman, E. D. (1983). Sleep architecture and REM sleep measures in prepubertal major depressives: Studies during recovery from the depressive episode in a drug-free state. *Archives of General Psychiatry*, *40*, 187–192.

Puig-Antich, J., Novacenko, H., Davies, M., Chambers, W. J., Tabrizi, M. A., Krawiec, V., Ambrosini, P. J., & Sachar, E. J. (1984c). Growth hormone secretion in pre-pubertal children with major depression. I. Final report on response to insulin-induced hypoglycemia during a depressive episode. *Archives of General Psychiatry*, *41*, 455–460.

Puig-Antich, J., Novacenko, H., Davies, M., Tabrizi, M. A., Ambrosini, P., Goetz, R., Bianca, J., Goetz, D., & Sachar, E. J. (1984d). Growth hormone secretion in pre-pubertal children with major depression. I. Response to insulin-induced hypoglycemia and after recovery from a depressive episode and in a drug-free state. *Archives of General Psychiatry*, *41*, 471–475.

Quattrocchi, M. M., Walker, A. M., Golden, C. J., & Fix, A. J. (1986). Regional cerebral blood flow and neuropsychological functioning among adolescent psychiatric inpatients. *Hillside Journal of Clinical Psychiatry*, *8*, 174–182.

Randrup, A., Munkvad, J., Fog, R., Gerlach, J., Molander, L., Kjellberg, B., & Scheel-Kruger, J. (1975). Mania, depression, and brain dopamine. In W. Essman & L. Valzelli (Eds.), *Current developments in psychopharmacology*, Vol. 2, New York: Spectrum.

Rechtschaffen, A., & Kales, A. (Eds.), (1968). *A manual of standardized terminology, techniques and scoring system for sleep stages of human subjects*. National Institute of Health Publication 204. Washington, DC: U.S. Government Printing Office.

Reynolds, C. F., III, Kupfer, D. J., Taska, L. S., Hoch, C. C., Spiker, D. G., Sewitch, D. E., Zimmer, B., Marin, R. S., Nelson, J. P., Martin, D., & Morycz, R. (1985). EEG sleep in elderly depressed, demented, and healthy subjects. *Biological Psychiatry*, *20*, 431–442.

Reynolds, C. F., III, Shaw, D. H., Newton, T. F., Coble, P. A., & Kupfer, D. J. (1983). EEG sleep in outpatients with generalized anxiety: A preliminary comparison with depressed outpatients. *Psychiatry Research*, *8*, 81–89.

Risch, S. C., Cohen, R. M., Janowsky, D. S., Dalin, N. H., & Murphy, D. L. (1980). Mood and behavioral effects of physostigmine on humans are accompanied by elevations in plasma beta-endorphin and cortisol. *Science*, *209*(4464), 1545–1546.

Risch, S. C., & Judd, L. L. (1987). Provocative challenges of growth hormone and prolactin secretion in schizophrenic and affective disorders. In C. B. Nemeroff & P. B. Loosen (Eds.), *The handbook of clinical psychoneuroendocrinology* (pp. 36–368). New York: Guilford Press.

Robbins, D. R., Alessi, N. E., & Colfer, M. V. (1989). Treatment of adolescents with major depression:

Implications of the DST and the melancholic clinical subtype. *Journal of Affective Disorders, 17,* 99–104.

Robbins, D. R., Alessi, N. E., Yanchyshyn, G. W., & Colfer, M. V. (1982). Preliminary report on the dexamethasone suppression test in adolescents. *American Journal of Psychiatry, 139,* 942–943.

Robinson, R. G., & Starkstein, S. E. (1990). Current research in affective disorders following stroke. *Journal of Neuropsychiatry and Clinical Neurosciences, 2,* 1–14.

Ross, E. D. (1981). The aprosodias: Functional–anatomic organization of the affective components of language in the right hemisphere. *Archives of Neurology, 36,* 144–148.

Ross, E. D., & Rush, A. J. (1981). Diagnosis and neuroanatomical correlates of depression in brain-damaged patients. *Archives of General Psychiatry, 38,* 1344–1354.

Rourke, B. P., Young, G. C., & Leenaars, A. A. (1989). A childhood learning disability that predisposes those afflicted to adolescent and adult depression and suicide risk. *Journal of Learning Disabilities, 22,* 169–175.

Rush, A. J., Erman, M. K., Giles, D. E., Schlesser, M. A., Carpenter, G., Vasavada, N., & Roffwarg, H. P. (1986). Polysomnographic findings in recently drug-free and clinically remitted depressed patients. *Archives of General Psychiatry, 43,* 878–884.

Rush, A. J., Giles, D. E., Jarrett, R. B., Feldman-Koffler, F., Debus, J. R., Weissenburger, J., Orsulak, P. J., & Roffwarg, H. P. (1989). Reduced REM latency predicts response to tricyclic medication in depressed outpatients. *Biological Psychiatry, 26,* 61–72.

Rush, A. J., Giles, D. E., Roffwarg, H. P., & Parker, R. C. (1982). Sleep EEG and dexamethasone suppression test findings in outpatients with unipolar and major depressive disorders. *Biological Psychiatry, 17,* 327–341.

Rush, A. J., Schlesser, M. A., Roffwarg, H. P., Giles, D. E., Orsulak, P. J., & Fairchild, C. J. (1983). Relationships among the TRH, REM latency and dexamethasone suppression tests: Preliminary findings. *Journal of Clinical Psychiatry, 44,* 23–29.

Rutter, M., Graham, P., & Yule, W. (1970). A neuropsychiatric study in childhood. *Clinics in Developmental Medicine.* No. 35–36. London: Spastics Society/Heinemann Medical.

Ryan, N. D., Puig-Antich, J., Rabinovich, H., Ambrosini, P. J., Robinson, D., Nelson, B., & Novacenko, H. (1988). Growth hormone response to desmethylimipramine in depressed and suicidal adolescents. *Journal of Affective Disorders, 15,* 323–337.

Sackeim, H. A., Prohovnik, I., Moeller, J. R., Brown, R. P., Apter, S., Prudic, J., Devanand, D. P., & Mukherjee, S. (1990). Regional cerebral blood flow in mood disorders. *Archives of General Psychiatry, 47,* 60–70.

Safer, M. A., & Leventhal, H. (1977). Ear differences in evaluating emotional tone of voice and verbal content. *Journal of Experimental Psychology, Human Perceptions and Performance, 3,* 75–82.

Schatzberg, A., Orsulak, P., Rosenbaum, A., Maruta, T., Kruger, E., Cole, J., & Schildkraut, J. (1982). Toward a biochemical classification of depressive disorders. V. Heterogeneity of unipolar depression. *American Journal of Psychiatry, 139,* 471–475.

Schlesser, M. A., & Rush, A. J. (1981). Serial changes in hypothalamic–pituitary adrenal axis activity among depressed patients receiving ECT. Read before the Society of Biological Psychiatry, New Orleans.

Silverstein, M. L., Strauss, B. S., & Fogg, L. (1990). A cluster analysis approach for deriving neuropsychologically-based subtypes of psychiatric disorders. *International Journal of Clinical Neuropsychology, 12,* 7–13.

Sitaram, N., Gillin, J. C., & Bunney, W. E., Jr. (1984). Cholinergic and catecholamine receptor sensitivity in affective illness: Strategy and theory. In R. M. Post & J. C. Ballenger (Eds.), *Neurobiology of mood disorders* (pp. 629–651). Baltimore: Williams & Wilkins.

Starkstein, S.E., & Robinson, R. C. (1986). Cerebral lateralization in depression. *American Journal of Psychiatry, 143,* 1631.

Suberi, M., & McKeever, W. F. (1977). Differential right hemispheric memory storage of emotional and non-emotional faces. *Neuropsychologia, 15,* 757–768.

Targum, S., Byrnes, S., & Sullivan, A. (1982). The TRH stimulation test in subtypes of unipolar depression. *Journal of Affective Disorders, 4,* 29–34.

Tems, C. L. C. (1989). Cognitive patterns in depressed and nondepressed children and adolescents. Doctoral dissertation. Dallas: University of Texas Southwestern Medical Center.

Tramontana, M. G., & Hooper, S. R. (1989). Neuropsychology of child psychopathology. In C. R. Reynolds & E. Fletcher-Janzen (Eds.), *Handbook of clinical child neuropsychology* (pp. 87–106). New York: Plenum Press.

Tucker, D. M. (1988). Neuropsychological mechanisms of affective self-regulation. In M. Kinsbourne (Ed.), *Cerebral hemisphere function in depression* (pp. 1–22). Washington, DC: American Psychiatric Press.

Van Praag, H. M. (1977). *Depression and schizophrenia: A contribution on their chemical pathologies.* New York: Spectrum Publications.

Voeller, K. (1986). Right-hemisphere deficit syndrome in children. *American Journal of Psychiatry, 143*, 1004–1009.

Voeller, K. K. S., & Heilman, K. M. (1987). Attention deficit disorder: A neglect syndrome in children? *Neurology, 37(Supplement 1)*, 221.

Waller, D. A., Jarriel, S., Erman, M., & Emslie, G. J. (1984). Recognizing and managing the adolescent with Klein–Levin syndrome. *Journal of Adolescent Health Care, 5*, 139–141.

Weinberg, W. A., & Emslie, G. J. (1988). Adolescents and school problems: Depression, suicide, and learning disorders. In R. A. Feldman & A. R. Stiffman (Eds.), *Advances in adolescent mental health*, Vol. 3, *Depression and suicide* (pp. 191–205). Greenwich, CT: JAI Press.

Weinberg, W. A., & McLean, A. (1986). A diagnostic approach to developmental specific learning disorders. *Journal of Child Neurology, 1*, 158–172.

Weinberg, W. A., & Rehmet, A. (1983). Childhood affective disorder and school problems. In D. P. Cantwell & G. A. Carlson (Eds.), *Affective disorders in childhood and adolescence: An update* (pp. 109–128). Jamaica, NY: Spectrum Publications.

Weinberg, W. A., Rutman, J., Sullivan, L., Penick, E. C., & Dietz, S. G. (1973). Depression in children referred to an educational diagnostic center: Diagnosis and treatment. *Journal of Pediatrics, 83*, 1065–1072.

Willner, P. (1985). *Depression: A psychobiological synthesis*. New York: John Wiley.

Wilson, H., & Staton, R. D. (1984). Neuropsychological changes in children associated with tricyclic antidepressant therapy. *International Journal of Neuroscience, 24*, 307–312.

Zametkin, A., Liebenauer, L., Fitzgerald, G., Minkunas, D., Herskovitch, P., Yamada, E., & Cohen, R. (1991). Brain metabolism in truly normal teenagers: Feasibility and comparison to hyperactives. *Scientific Proceedings of the Annual Meeting of the American Academy of Child and Adolescent Psychiatry, 7*, 50.

Zubenko, G. S., Moossy, J., & Kopp, U. (1990). Neurochemical correlates of major depression in primary dementia. *Archives of Neurology, 47*, 209–214.

III

APPROACHES TO ASSESSMENT AND DIAGNOSIS

9

Classification and Diagnostic Criteria of Depression in Children and Adolescents

Donald L. Sherak, Patricia L. Speier, and Dennis P. Cantwell

Diagnostic categories are the defining terminology for the study, classification, and treatment of psychiatric disorders. Each diagnostic term implies a coherent subset of symptoms from a larger possible grouping. A diagnosis also carries inherent implications regarding the disorder's possible etiology, natural history, and treatment response. Diagnostic classification systems are essential for scientific study of disease and for accurate communication between clinicians. Such systems allow clinicians to move beyond the anecdotal and case-report approach.

There have been historical objections to the process of psychiatric classification. Some have seen little point in making distinctions between disorders (Szurek & Berlin, 1956) or have argued that a psychiatric diagnosis was only "justifactory rhetoric" without meaning that led to unproven treatments (Szasz, 1978). Some were afraid that classification would obscure individual differences and prevent a detailed understanding of the disorders (Huschka, 1941). Szasz (1961) has further argued that the label, like the messenger, was to blame for the stigma experienced by those with the disorder. Most of these criticisms were leveled when psychiatric diagnosis was less precise (pre-DSM-III) and had not been as thoroughly validated and treatment options were both less specific and more limited.

Controversies in the diagnosis and classification of mental disorders have their roots in the philosophical underpinnings of Western thought. On one hand, the Platonic school holds that diseases express themselves in "ideal" forms that are distinct and different. This

Donald L. Sherak • Child and Adolescent Services, Taunton State Hospital, Taunton, Massachusetts 02780. **Patricia L. Speier** • Langley Porter Psychiatric Institute, University of California at San Francisco, San Francisco, California 94143-0984. **Dennis P. Cantwell** • Department of Psychiatry and Behavioral Science, Neuropsychiatric Institute, University of California at Los Angeles, Los Angeles, California 90024.

Handbook of Depression in Children and Adolescents, edited by William M. Reynolds and Hugh F. Johnston. Plenum Press, New York, 1994.

idea is the forerunner of the typological approach of Kraepelin (1915) and points toward the categorical foundations of DSM-III and onward. Kraepelin, working in the 19th-century European scientific tradition, took extensive clinical histories and made incisive, detailed records of signs and symptoms. He them grouped cases by similar orientation and defined syndromes or symptom complexes. Kraepelin observed a category of disease he termed "illogical psychoses." He separated clinical presentations into those that had a tendency toward deterioration and those that did not. This later group he termed the "manic–depressive psychoses," and this grouping is the forerunner of the contemporary mood-disorders class. In later revisions, he separated neurotic and reactive disorders under a general heading of manic–depressive psychoses. In pursuing a medical model, Kraepelin sought to uncover an etiology for each syndrome.

On the other hand, Hippocrates taught that disease was less an entity than a process, with symptoms emerging over time. Disease was an outgrowth of premorbid characteristics. Each case was unique. This was a forerunner of the dimensional approach and, to a lesser extent, the application of the multiaxial format instituted with DSM-III.

Robins (1976) takes a synthesizing approach to these antithetical positions. The categorical approach can be seen as the essential tool of a young science seeking to establish an intellectual beachhead. Fundamental aspects of a syndrome are laid down (Feighner et al., 1972), and the etiology, course, and treatment of the syndrome are investigated. Later, when more data have been gathered, the diagnostic boundaries are extended and refined. Variants and attenuated forms are elucidated.

The dimensional approach, when taken alone, has the risk of presenting a diagnosis that has blurred boundaries or that is an overly inclusive picture. When seeking the boundary between normalcy and clinically significant symptoms, the dimensional system faces some of the same difficulties as the categorical—what is the threshold for a treatable condition and how should borderline conditions be handled?

Much of the child work on dimensional analysis has been carried out by Achenbach (Achenbach, 1982; Achenbach & Edelbrock, 1978, 1981), who found that syndromes derived from multivariate analysis could be classified as broad-band (analogous to DSM categories). But, some DSM-III categories lacked empirical counterparts and, conversely, some empirical categories did not have DSM-III categorical correlates. The empirical approach has particular strengths—all classifications share a common derivation and treatment responses are easily measurable. However, the dimensional approach has some drawbacks—patients are limited to one diagnosis and the categories are not uniformly intuitive and not necessarily clinically relevant.

Utility of Diagnostic Systems

In assessing the utility of a diagnostic classification, one must consider the reliability, validity, feasibility, and coverage of the classification system. Reliability is the degree to which clinicians using the system would agree with one another on the diagnoses of a series of patients. Statistical methods can be used to compute the interrater reliability, or degree of agreement between diagnoses. Reliability of systems of classification will vary according to three factors: (1) the information provided (the information variance), (2) the way in which information is interpreted (the observation variance), and (3) how criteria are used to summarize the data collected (the criterion variance) (Cantwell, 1975). A categorical classification system, such as DSM, can never have the reliability of a dimensional system (such as Achenbach's), which is inextricably tied to specific assessment measures and therefore has less room for interrater disagreement. Starting with DSM-III, each revision has tried to incorporate research data to strengthen these measures.

Validity is the degree to which a measure gives an indication of a particular quality it claims to measure (American Psychiatric Association, 1975). In regard to diagnostic categories, it refers to the extent to which that system can be used to accurately communicate about and comprehend what is described (Spitzer & Williams, 1980). Four types of validity can be examined to assess the utility of a diagnostic system's categorization: *Face validity* is the correspondence of categories with clinical judgment and intuition. In the case of childhood depression, face validity has been more difficult to attain, since children can present depressive symptoms differently at different developmental stages. *Descriptive validity* refers to the uniqueness of each diagnostic category and is particularly difficult to attain in diagnostic categories for children. Because children have a more limited expression of symptoms compared to adults, there is greater diagnostic overlap. Also, certain diagnoses predispose to the development of other conditions, resulting in high rates of comorbid diagnoses. The higher the rate of comorbidity, the more problematic descriptive validity becomes. In general, however, the descriptive validity of mood disorders has been strengthened by studies showing strong family aggregation of mood disorders and other psychiatric disorders of probands of children with mood disorders. However, this approach does not address the issue of genetic or environmental etiology. For clinicians who generally use this diagnosis prognostically, *predictive validity* is the most important. Predictive validity refers to the usefulness of a diagnosis in predicting natural course and potential treatment outcome. *Construct validity* refers to the extent to which the classification supports a theory of the disorder's etiology and process. DSM, since it is descriptive and tries to be free of theoretical orientation, is less weighted toward a high constructive validity. As research into the etiology of mood disorders continues, however, construct validity should improve as theory and categorization more closely correspond.

Instead of examining diagnoses in light of these four types of validity, Klerman, Hirschfeld, and Andreason (1987) suggested that measures of internal and external validity should be strongly weighed when constructing a diagnostic classification. *Internal validity* is determined by the consistency of symptoms comprising the essential diagnostic criteria of the disorder and is usually arrived at statistically. *External validity* looks at whether disorders with different clinical presentations had differences other than their defining criteria. Klerman et al. (1987) describe six external validating criteria: (1) epidemiological factors (i.e., incidence, prevalence, life expectancy, morbidity), (2) family aggregation studies looking for patterns of psychopathology in families of probands with different mood disorders, (3) laboratory tests of biological markers, (4) psychosocial factors (such as early childhood experiences or personality traits), (5) studies of natural history, and (6) studies looking at response to treatment (Klerman et al., 1987). The external validating criteria for mood disorders in children have been discussed by Cantwell (1975), who notes that supporting data include natural history studies and studies of treatment response.

DSM-IV and ICD-10 have both attempted to draw on a wider database, seeking greater external validation for each diagnostic criterion. Although there is still some categorical disagreement between the two systems, this effort toward bridging the "criterion gap" should increase the international database validity across studies and improve communication and collaboration in the study of many psychiatric disorders, including mood disorders. Robins and Guze (1970) have outlined a five-stage scheme for validation of psychiatric disorders: clinical description, delimitation from other disorders, laboratory studies, family studies, and follow-up studies. Cantwell (1975) has argued for expansion of this scheme into a six-stage scheme: (1) overall clinical picture, including essential and associated features as well as exclusionary criteria; (2) physical and neurological features; (3) laboratory studies; (4) family aggregation studies; (5) follow-up studies; and (6) treatment studies. Cantwell's model is based on the premise that psychiatric disorders of children and adolescents are probably of multifactorial etiology and each diagnostic category may therefore contain etiologically distinct subgroups.

Long-term prospective studies of children diagnosed as having mood disorders will be needed to clearly determine potential adult-outcome diagnostic categories, and a careful initial delineation of associated features may help in delineating etiologies of subgroups. Treatment studies are of lesser utility in validating diagnostic criteria, both because a variety of psychopharmacological agents may be given for treatment of mood disorders and because of the lack of diagnostic specificity of many target symptoms. In the case of mood disorders, another confounding variable is the less robust response to antidepressants in children and adolescents.

Another criterion of importance to any diagnostic classification system is feasibility—the extent to which the system can be used successfully by the clinicians for whom it is designed. A system that is feasible must have clear, unambiguous instructions for use, must utilize routinely available information, and, for research purposes, should be in a form convenient to statistical manipulation (Rutter & Gould, 1985). By making the essential features for depression the same for both children and adults and allowing substitutions only for associated features, the developers of DSM-IV have sought to attain better feasibility for the diagnostic categories. This may be at the expense, however, of greater internal validity of age clusters within the categories.

The widespread use of DSM-III-R in many communities worldwide, especially those with significant cultural differences from North America (Africa, Asia, and South America), speaks to the high feasibility of using DSM as a classification system (Spitzer, Williams, & Skodol, 1983). Little is known, however, regarding the validity of these diagnostic categories in such different cultural contexts, and it may be premature to assume that this classification system can maintain its utility across cultural barriers without modification.

Coverage is a final important factor in assessing the utility of a diagnostic system. Coverage can be defined as the degree to which such a system can provide valid diagnostic categories for all patients (Spitzer & Williams, 1980). The coverage of a system is inversely proportional to the percentage of patients who have undiagnosed mental disorders. Increasing the number of disorders and broadening diagnostic criteria improve coverage, but also usually result in lowering reliability and external validity in the system and at least some of its categories.

The continued separation of the section of DSM-IV of disorders "Usually First Evident in Childhood and Adolescence" creates some potential problems concerning coverage. Many disorders, mood disorders being a primary example, first present in childhood or adolescence, yet are not found under this heading. Therefore, Major Depression, Bipolar Disorder, or other mood disorders may not be adequately considered in the differential diagnoses for children or adolescents, particularly by clinicians unfamiliar with these age groups. On the other hand, the mention of some age-specific differences in symptom criteria (e.g., the substitution, in children, of failure to make expected weight gain for weight loss in adults) acknowledges the possibility of developmentally different presentations. The inclusion of these substitute criteria may serve to broaden the coverage of these diagnostic categories.

Early Classifications

The first formal organization of psychiatric diagnoses in the United States, the *Diagnostic and Statistical Manual of Mental Disorders* (American Psychiatric Association, 1952), only made reference to childhood in four categories: chronic brain syndromes associated with birth trauma, schizophrenic reaction, childhood type, adjustment reaction of infancy, childhood and adolescence, and the specific symptom reactions (such as enuresis and somnambulism). DSM lacked strict operational criteria and was not uniformly phenomenological in approach. Partly in repsonse to this, over two dozen child and adolescent classification systems came into use. The Group for the Advancement of Psychiatry

Committee on Child Psychiatry made the reference to these in their 1966 classification system. The GAP system divided psychopathology into ten major groupings that stressed developmental level and psychodynamic factors. Categories ranged from mild ("healthy responses") to severe and enduring ("brain syndromes" and "mental retardation").

DSM-II (American Psychiatric Association, 1968) acknowledged for the first time the possibility of multiple concurrent diagnoses as well as a range in the severity of symptoms and the significance of acute vs. chronic conditions. A new section, "Behavioral Disorders of Childhood and Adolescence," was established to identify conditions more severe than situational disturbances and less severe than the neuroses and psychoses. These conditions included the hyperkinetic, withdrawing, overanxious, runaway, unsocialized aggressive, and group delinquent reactions of childhood and adolescence, as well as "other."

DSM-III (American Psychiatric Association, 1980), seeking greater organizational cohesion, moved the section for disorders "First Evident in Childhood and Adolescence" to the front of the volume. The section now contained over 40 disorders. However, the division made in this section was far from absolute. Some childhood disorders may not present for treatment until adulthood. Conversely many other diagnoses—psychotic disorders, mood disorders, dissociative disorders, adjustment disorders—frequently first begin prior to adulthood. This variable emergence can lead to a bias of underdiagnosing the childhood presentations of disorders not contained within this section. The dilemma of establishing some reasonable grouping raises the the issue of whether these disorders exist on a continuum or have fully separate child and adult presentations.

Prior to the work of Weinberg, Rutman, Sullivan, Penick, and Dietz (1973), there already was movement away from the strict psychoanalytical thinking that denied the possibility of the existence of a disease entity of depression in children. Clinicians knew empirically that children and adolescents experienced depressive phenomena. However, psychoanalysis had presented a hermetic system; children, by definition, lacked a developed superego. Because of this lack, they were not capable of negative introjects. And if this was a precondition of depression, children, by definition, could not be depressed.

Early attempts to define the reality of depressive disorders did not move to include children in adult categories, but worked from the premise that childhood depression was a condition inherently different from adult depression. Using terminology and concepts still grounded in psychoanalytical thinking, Frommer (1968) postulated three subtypes: enuretic depressives, pure depressives, and phobic depressives. She compared these types to each other and to a group of neurotic children suffering from a range of emotional disorders but not exhibiting significant depressive symptoms. The subtypes were compared in terms of such external validating criteria as natural history, family history, and therapeutic response. However, while these subtypes were presented as phenomenological entities, there was no presentation of essential inclusion criteria for making the diagnosis of depression or assignment to a subgroup. Also, no indication was presented that there was any statistically significant difference between the subgroups.

The "Childhood Depressive Phenomena: Tentative Classification" of Malmquist (1971) is also from this period. Malmquist used children's developmental level and disease etiology as criteria for grouping symptoms. He organized his observations into the following categories: (1) associated with organic disease states, (2) deprivation syndromes, (3) syndromes associated with difficulties in individualization, (4) latency types (including depressive equivalent), and (5) adolescent types, which included reaction to loss and "schizophrenias with prominent affective components."

About that time, McConville, Boag, and Purohit (1973) organized their clinical findings into three prepubertal categories and proposed etiologies to accompany each. The "affectual" subtype was more common in children aged 6–8 and was characterized by sadness, helplessness, and hopelessness. A negative self-esteem subtype, more common after the age of 8, was characterized by "thought feelings" relating to depression that

McConville thought developed out of the child's fixed ideas relating to negative self-esteem. The negative self-esteem was thought to be caused by multiple losses, such as multiple foster home placements. A third, rarer group, the "guilt" subtype, was more common in children aged 11 and older. The predominant feature here was depressive cognitions—these children felt that they were bad or should be killed. The underlying etiology was felt to be the punitive superego.

Modern Criteria

In 1972, the first modern criteria for adult depressive disorder were developed at Washington University. The "Feighner criteria" (Feighner et al., 1972) had four major criteria that were essential for diagnosis: (1) the presence of dysphoric mood (including depressed, sad, discouraged, despondent, or irritable; (2) a minimum of five of the following: poor appetite and weight loss, sleep difficulty—insomnia or hypersomnia, loss of energy, psychomotor agitation or retardation, loss of interest in usual activities including sex, feelings of self-reproach or guilt, a diminished ability to think or concentrate, and recurrent thoughts of death or suicide; (3) symptoms present for at least 1 month with no preexisting contributing psychiatric or medical condition; and (4) patients with severe distortions of perception or thinking as a primary manifestation of the disorder are excluded.

In a paper that was among the first to attempt to demonstrate a positive treatment response to antidepressants in children, Weinberg et al. (1973) set out a list of ten symptoms of childhood depression. At that time, this paper was controversial enough to carry a warning from the editor explaining that he felt it "necessary to stress extreme *caution* (1) in identifying any child as having a depressive illness and (2) in prescribing any medication for such a disorder." In Weinberg's system, dysphoric mood and self-deprecatory ideation were essential features, and two of eight additional criteria were necessary. Anhedonia was not considered as a separate category, but was subsumed under "changes in attitude toward school." Suicidal ideation and feelings of guilt were not separate categories, but were subsumed together, along with persecutory beliefs, under self-deprecatory ideation. Psychomotor retardation was not listed. However, changes in school performance, diminished socialization, and somatic complaints were essential categories. These categories were modified by Poznanski, Cook, and Carroll (1979), who included nonverbal dysphoria and social withdrawal in the essential criteria, but did not list psychomotor agitation or appetite disturbance as diagnostic symptoms.

Weinberg et al. (1973) had developed specific diagnostic criteria for children that deviated from the eventual DSM-III criteria: Weinberg required that children exhibit *both* depressed mood *and* low self-esteem. In contrast, DSM-III required *either* dysphoric mood *or* loss of pleasure in usual activities. Weinberg also required only two of the second grouping of symptoms. In this group, two are directly geared to academics—change in school performance and change in attitude toward school. Aggressive behavior is allowed as a counterpart to adult irritability and agitation. Somatic complaints, included here, are also a non-DSM-III criterion.

Poznanski, Cook, Carroll, and Corzo (1983) compared the Research Diagnostic Criteria (RDC) (Spitzer, Endicott, & Robins, 1978) and the DSM-III, Poznanski et al. (1979), and Weinberg et al. (1973) criteria in the diagnosis of depression in an outpatient population. All four criterion sets shared the verbal expression of dysphoric mood as an essential symptom. The systems had three associated features in common: sleep disturbance, excessive fatigue, and cognitive impairment. The RDC and Poznanski criteria required five associated features for a definite diagnosis of depression. DSM-III required four and the Weinberg criteria, the least stringent, stipulated only two. However, Poznanski et al. (1983) found an 86% agreement across the board for these systems in the determination of children as depressed or not depressed. Most of the disagreement was based on essential features. Over half the variance between the four systems was accounted for by two symptoms: (1) the clinician's rating of dysphoria based on the child's nonverbal expressions (a Poznanski and Weinberg criterion) and to a lesser extent (2) pervasive anhedonia (a DSM-III and RDC criterion). Pervasive anhedonia was found to have low sensitivity but diagnostic specificity approaching 100%. On the other hand, lowered self-esteem, found in all systems but the Weinberg, had high sensitivity but low specificity.

When Poznanski et al. (1983) compared the RDC (Feighner et al., 1972) and the DSM-III, Weinberg, and their own diagnostic criteria, they found a consensus among all four sets of criteria for the symptoms of sleep disturbance, fatigue, and cognitive impairment. However, there was disagreement as to whether dysphoric mood should be rated by clinician observation or by the child's or parents' reports.

DSM-III sought to establish broad usefulness in diagnosis and research through the implementation of an approach that was both atheoretical and categorical and placed within a multiaxial framework. The diagnoses are mostly descriptive of data directly observed (or reported by parents). Except in the cases of organic disorders, the classifications are, in most cases, free of etiological inferences. DSM-III also introduced the multiaxial format. The five axes give a more complex picture of the patient and have shown themselves to contribute to greater reliability and a more thorough diagnostic picture (Russell, Cantwell, Mattison, & Will, 1979). Axis II was reserved for developmental and personality disorders. The separate categorization of the learning and language disorders serves to highlight the interrelationship between these conditions and Axis I disorders. Impairments in these areas contribute to the component symptoms of such disorders as attention-deficit disorder, conduct disorder, and depression (Baker and Cantwell, 1989; Kashani, Strober, Rosenberg, & Reid, 1988).

In the revision of DSM-III, mental retardation, specific developmental, and pervasive developmental disorders were all joined on Axis II with the understanding that these disorders share common features of "generally having an onset in childhood or adolescence and usually persisting in a stable form without periods of remission or exacerbation into adult life" (American Psychiatric Association, 1987, p. 410). Additional Axis II changes included the division of developmental language disorder into expressive and receptive forms. The developmental expressive writing disorder was also new.

In DSM-IV (American Psychiatric Association, 1994), learning disorders, motor skills disorders, communications disorders and pervasive developmental disorders have been moved to Axis I. Axis II is reserved solely for Mental Retardation, Personality Disorders and subthreshold maladaptive personality features. Axis III continues to be reserved for general medical conditions that may be relevant to the understanding or prognosis of the individual's mental condition. Appendix G, a new addition, contains the ICD-9-CM codes for selected medical conditions and medication-induced disorders. In DSM-III-R, Axis IV was a rating scale for severity of chronic and acute stressors. In DSM-IV, Axis IV has become a checklist for specifying problems, in particular domains of life such as primary support group, housing, and access to health care services. Axis V continues as the Global Assessment of Functioning, but is now configured with examples over a span from 1 to 100.

Changes between DSM-III and DSM-III-R reconfigured inclusion criteria for some diagnoses to produce significant redefinition of case prevalence. DSM-III-R presented criteria that are operationally more stringent for dysthymia. For example, Lahey et al. (1990) applied both sets of criteria to a large group of latency-age outpatients and found that DSM-III-R dysthymia was over one third less prevalent than the DSM-III diagnosis.

The developers of DSM-III debated as to whether depression in adults and children should share the same essential features. In the finished document, there are allowances for substitutions only in some of the associated features. DSM-III accepted either dysphoric mood or loss of interest or pleasure in usual activities and four of a menu of eight symptoms including the two not shared by the Weinberg criteria—feeling of self reproach or guilt and recurrent thought of death or suicide. The DSM-III criteria for depression are more restrictive than the Weinberg criteria. Children meeting the DSM-III criteria had higher Childhood Depression Inventory scores than those fulfilling Weinberg criteria. The DSM-III criteria also appear to select cases in which there is a discrete onset (Carlson & Cantwell, 1982).

There is now widespread acceptance that mood disorders of childhood and adulthood present essentially as phenomenologically equivalent. Four lines of evidence support this view: (1) The equivalence between symptom clusters of adults and children (Carlson & Kashani, 1988). (2) Strong family history for affective disturbances in affectively disturbed children (Strober et al., 1988), as well as the increased vulnerability to the disorder for children with affectively disturbed parents (Beardslee, Bemporad, Keller & Klerman, 1983). Moreover, there is often specificity of transmission, with children of parents with unipolar disorder being more prone to unipolar affective disorder (Weissman, Gammon, & John, 1987) and offspring of parents with bipolar disorders being more prone to bipolar disorders. (3) The identification of biological correlates of both state markers (Poznanski et al., 1983) and trait markers (Puig-Antich et al., 1984) of prepubertal major depressive disorder. (4) Longitudinal studies that identify temporal episodes (Kovacs, Feinberg, Crouse-Novak, Paulauskas, & Finkelstein, 1984a) as well as an increased risk over time for the two episodes (Kovacs et al., 1984b; Poznanski, Krahenbuhl, & Zrull, 1976).

The presumption of diagnostic equivalence draws some attention away from the consideration of developmental nuances. Questions of biological maturation—including everything from neuroreceptor response capacity to cognitive development—may play important roles in both the etiology and the treatment response of mood disorders. Starting with DSM-III-R, greater attention has been paid to the existence of underlying states. DSM-III made no distinction between primary and secondary disorders. By the criteria of DSM-III-R, a primary mood disturbance is one that has emerged in the absence of any preexisting medical or psychiatric disorder. Secondary here defines the temporal relationship, not the causal connection. A depressive episode that emerges secondary to an ongoing medical disorder might be classified as a DSM-III-R organic affective syndrome. However, if the preexisting condition is an Axis I disorder such as conduct disorder or attention-deficit disorder, both are listed on Axis I, simply indicating that both are present at the same time of diagnosis.

Carlson and Cantwell have systematically studied the primary–secondary dichotomy in children and adolescents (Carlson and Cantwell, 1979, 1980a,b; Cantwell and Carlson, 1983). Although there were no significant differences in core depressive symptomatology, other symptoms such as aggressive behavior, noncompliance, hyperactivity, and somatic complaints were more common in children with secondary depression. This finding is not surprising, because these differences often reflected the comorbid psychiatric diagnoses of the subjects. There was a difference in family history in that many more children with a secondary depression had families with depressive spectrum disorders (according to Winokur's terminology) than did those children who had a primary depression.

The secondary depressed children tended to be more chronically ill, and at follow-up, which was conducted informally 5 years after they were initially seen, many of the primary depressives had remitted with regard to depressive symptomatology. The depressive symptoms of many of the secondary depressives had remitted as well. On the other hand, the secondary depressives continued to manifest signs of their primary psychiatric disturbance.

DSM-III-R represented a move toward a more unitary and more restrictive set of criteria for depressive disorders. In DSM-III, children under 6 required one fewer associated symptom. Also, hypoactivity could substitute for psychomotor retardation. In DSM-III-R, a full set of the symptoms associated with adult criteria is required to establish the diagnosis. Melancholic subtype included a pharmacological marker as a criterion—good prior response to antidepressant medication. Such criterion may prove to be a source of diagnostic difficulty, as they do not acknowledge the empirical data indicating that children and adolescents are historically less robust responders to antidepressant medications. This criterion also ignores the larger question of developmental neurobiology—in terms of disease pathology as well as capacity for pharmacological response.

DSM-III-R (American Psychiatric Association, 1987) and DSM-IV, as first presented in the *Options Book* (American Psychiatric Association, 1991), continued to refine criteria set forth in DSM-III—that children and adolescents be given any diagnosis if they meet the adult diagnostic criteria and do not fulfill exclusionary criteria. There are no diagnostic boundaries separating children and adolescents from adults. This approach represents an outgrowth of the decision by the Task Force on Nomenclature and Statistics for DSM-III to not list separate inclusion criteria for affective disorders in children and adolescents. DSM-III-R is explicit in telling the clinician how to proceed, stating that the *"essential features"* of mood disorders are the same in children and adolescents and in adults and that if the symptoms meet DSM criteria, the diagnosis should be assigned, regardless of age, with the caveat that "age specific *associated* features are included in the text" (American Psychiatric Association, 1987).

When DSM-III was being formulated, there was still controversy regarding the presence of clinical depression in children and, if it existed, whether or not it was fundamentally different from depression in adults (Spitzer & Wilson, 1976, p. 455). The existence of depressive states in children is no longer in question. The earlier debate reflected a paradigm shift away from a model based on psychodynamic theory to an empirically based phenomenological approach. In reality, this diagnosis continues to function as a compromise. In the DSM-III criteria, children over 6 years of age could be diagnosed by adult inclusion criteria. However, for children under 6 years old, dysphoric mood might have to be inferred by a persistently sad facial expression. This necessity is consistent with the finding of Carlson and Kashani (1988) that depressed preschoolers exhibited a depressed appearance, low self-esteem, somatic complaints, and hallucinations more than any other age group. In addition, children under 6 years of age were required to have three of the following four symptoms: poor appetite, sleeping problems, psychomotor agitation or retardation, and a loss of interest in or pleasure from visual interactions.

DSM-III established that a failure to make expected weight gains could serve as equivalent to adult-criteria depression with a seasonal pattern. The criteria for dysthymia were made more stringent, excluding cases that begin only after an initial major depressive episode. Primary-type specification, as opposed to secondary-type specification, was given to distinguish those cases that developed either prior to or in the absence of another chronic Axis I disorder. A determination of age of onset (early or late) was also given because evidence from field trials suggested that early onset characterizes a more homogeneous group.

Experience and feedback have helped framers of the DSM system to further clarify their mission, reemphasizing the limitations of the categorical approach. By viewing the categories as diagnostic prototypes, one can accept heterogeneity of class, recognize that individual cases fulfill criteria to greater or lesser degree, and allow for the validation of boundary preservation. This increase in the use of polythetic sets of criteria is reflected in increasingly complex diagnostic schemata.

In the 1980s, the United States Alcohol, Drug and Mental Health Administration and the World Health Organization collaborated in reviewing existing worldwide psychiatric diagnoses and classification. Out of this effort, new instruments for epidemiological assessment were developed for multicenter research studies. Clinicians and researchers from several disciplines and a wide range of perspectives developed a proposed classification system that was then field-tested in 10 languages that encompass most of the world's peoples. Data collected from this testing led to the expansion from 300 to the 1000 diagnostic categories of the *International Classification of Disease* and the elaboration of a multiaxial coding system similar to that of DSM-III.

International Classification of Disease—10

The *International Classification of Disease* (ICD) was created under the auspices of the World Health Organization (WHO) and has been accepted by most countries as the diagnostic guidelines for clinical settings. ICD-10, the latest revision, is being used to provide statistical data. In the ICD-10 system, diseases are typically organized along either etiological, situational, or body topographic lines. While one of the stated objectives of the DSM-IV Task Force was to conform to ICD-10, there is still significant divergence. For example, ICD-10 defines a "Mild Depressive Episode" that requires at least two of the following symptoms: depressed mood, marked loss of interest or pleasure in activities, and decreased energy or increased fatiguability. The additional seven from which two must be selected conform to the DSM criteria for depression with the addition of "loss of confidence and self-esteem" as a separate category. For this diagnosis, symptoms cannot be graded as "intense," but the cutoff is not clear. In addition, ICD-10 allows for a distinction between disorders with and without somatic symptoms. A "moderate" episode requires an additional symptom from the second menu of eight. Three of the symptoms must be present to a "marked degree." An alternative is to have seven symptoms overall, present to mild or moderate degree.

In contrast, for the "severe" episode, the additional criterion is that at least two of the symptoms must be of "severe" intensity and the rest must be "marked." The "severe" category can be with or without psychotic symptoms and then can be mood-congruent or -incongruent. A similar configuration exists for Recurrent Depressive Disorder—episodes can be "mild," "moderate," or "severe." "Severe" episodes can be with or without psychotic symptoms.

Akiskal (1985) has suggested that different thresholds might be appropriate criteria in different contexts. The broader Research Diagnostic Criteria (RDC) (dysphoric mood plus four symptoms for 1 week) may be appropriate for epidemiological studies. More restrictive criteria, such as those of Feighner et al. (1972)—dysphoric mood plus 4 weeks of five symptoms—may give more weight to genetic studies. The DSM-IV criteria with their interim 2-week threshold may represent a reasonable intermediate position for a treating clinician.

Akiskal (1985) has proposed sharpening the boundaries between the mood disorder and other mood-dominated states, including variants and subtypes. For example, "the blues" and major depression could be differentiated by the pharmacological response to the former and also by examining personal and family history of bipolarity or cyclicity, in addition to the degree of functional incapacitation.

Diagnostic and Statistical Manual of Mental Disorders, Fourth Edition

The Task Force on DSM-IV was appointed in 1988 to make revisions that would coincide with the publication of ICD-10 by the World Health Organization in 1993. Efforts were made to draw on the widest pool of data and an international group of experts. The Task Force had set a much higher threshold for revisions than was used in the past. To the extent possible, the focus was on empirical documentation.

For DSM-IV, disorders continue to be organized by one of three principles: (1) phenomenological similarity, such as all mood or anxiety disorders; (2) etiology, such as all substance-use or adjustment disorders; and (3) age of onset, such as disruptive behavior disorders. This arrangement continues to move rapidly over considerations relating to the onset of disorders such as mood disorders prior to adulthood and a presentation that, because of developmental differences, cannot fully conform to adult criteria.

Many additions were considered for the DSM-IV. However, most were relegated to Appendix B: Criteria Sets and Axes Provided for Further Study, because the Task Force had determined that there was an insufficient basis to include them as official categories. However, by publishing them, the Task force has sought to spur research that will test their utility and aid in further refinement of the categories.

The changes made in the depressive disorders in DSM-IV are mostly clarifications. While the nine symptoms listed in criterion A remained unchanged, Major Depressive Episode is now further defined by three additional criteria. Criterion C emphasizes that the symptoms must represent a clinically significant situation and criterion E has been added to clarify the relationship between depression and bereavement, with the latter diagnosis reserved for conditions lasting less than two months that do not cause functional impairment. Criterion B states explicitly that when the symptoms also meet the criteria for a Mixed Episode, that condition takes precedence, Also, DSM-IV states that the mood disorder must meet full criteria continuously for at least two years; a two month hiatus is no longer permitted.

The basic 5-digit codes for Major Depression are the same. However, specifiers have been modified. The melancholic features specifier is similar to the DSM-III criteria, but now requires, as criteria set A, either loss of pleasure or lack of reactivity to pleasurable stimuli, whereas the DSM-III required both. The DSM-III-R criteria for a prior depressive episode or the lack of a prior personality disturbance have been dropped. There are two new group B criteria: excessive guilt and distinctly depressed mood. While the DSM-IV specifier for Melancholic type no longer contains the criterion of prior good response to specific and adequate somatic antidepressant therapy, this does not imply that the DSM is moving away from the use of neurobiological markers. While eliminated from the criteria, medication response is discussed in the text as dexamethasone nonsuppression, reduced REM latency, and abnormal tyramine challenge test, among other "frequently associated . . . laboratory findings."

The seasonal pattern specifier is now to be applied only to depressive episodes. The 60-day window for symptoms has been eliminated and the relationship between seasonal and nonseasonal episodes shows further modifications, including the requirement of a two-year period of two seasonal episodes with no nonseasonal episodes.

Additional specifiers have been added—with catatonic features, with atypical features, with postpartum onset, and with rapid cycling. These reflect current understanding of clinical presentation as well as possible criteria that may imply differential treatment and prognosis. Longitudinal course specifiers have been added to focus on the prior pattern of recovery.

The categories of Substance-Induced Mood Disorder and Mood Disorder due to a General Medical Condition have been moved into the Mood Disorders section to facilitate differential diagnosis.

Changes in the DSM-IV criteria for Dysthymic Disorder reflect the overall conceptual thrust of this new edition. The importance of the clinical impact of the Symptom presentation is highlighted. The distinction made in DSM-III-R between primary secondary type was found to be not clinically valid and these subtypes have been eliminated.

Several other mood disorder categories were strongly considered for inclusion in DSM-IV, but the Task Force deemed it premature to make these official categories. These are all included in Appendix B: Criteria Sets and Axes Provided for Further Study. These include an alternate criteria set B for Dysthymic Disorder which does not refer to appetite and sleep but instead focuses on social withdrawal, anhedonia, brooding about the past, and excessive anger.

Minor Depressive Disorder refers to episodes that lack the full complement of criteria symptoms and may be less clinically significant. Other diagnoses include Recurrent Brief Depressive Disorder, which falls short of the two-week duration requirement for Major Depressive Episode, Mixed Anxiety-Depressive Disorder, and Depressive Personality Disorder. Premenstrual Dysphoric Disorder extends considerations first undertaken in Appendix A of DSM-III-R. Postpsychotic Depressive Disorder of Schizophrenia further refines the relationshp between mood disorders an dpsychosis.

Summary and Conclusions

From DSM-I through DSM-IV, many different classification schemes have been proposed. DSM-I and DSM-II were very rudimentary. DSM-III was the first "official" classification scheme to fully spell out criteria for various subtypes of mood disorders. This tradition has been carried on to DSM-III-R and DSM-IV. ICD-10 now has specific criteria in its research criteria. Along the way, a number of unofficial classification schemes, such as the Feighner criteria and the Research Diagnostic Criteria, have been developed on the basis of research data or clinical experience with adult populations or both. While the DSM's have stated that the criteria, at least in their core symptom pattern for mood disorders, are the same across the age span, there have been several attempts to develop more developmentally oriented classification schemes. However, none of them has achieved the kind of utility that has been reached by the DSM, RDC, and Feighner-type classification schemes.

For example, Weinberg attempted to modify the Feighner criteria slightly for use with children and adolescents. Carlson and Cantwell showed that the Weinberg criteria diagnosed a much wider group of children with mood disorders than did the DSM-III criteria. It remains to be seen whether the DSM-III-R and the DSM-IV criteria have the same utility in diagnosing mood disorders in children and adolescents as they do in adults. The DSM-III and -III-R criteria seem to identify a group of children and adolescents who do not have the same degree of response to tricyclic antidepressants as adult patients identified by the same criteria.

The answer to the question of whether natural history without treatment, family history, biological correlates, and other factors will be similar in children and adolescents with DSM-IV criteria awaits further research. Nevertheless, the use with children and adolescents of unmodified adult criteria, such as the RDC and the DSM-III criteria, has spurred research on mood disorders in children and adolescents that has reached a level far beyond what it had been prior to the onset of these classification schemes. Future research with existing adult-based criteria will help identify developmental changes that might need to be made on the basis of developmental state and age of the child or adolescent.

References

Achenbach, T. (1982). *Developmental psychopathology*, 2nd ed. New York: John Wiley.

Achenbach, T., & Edelbrock, C. S. (1978). The classification of child psychopathology: A review and analysis of empirical efforts. *Psychological Bulletin, 85*, 1275–1301.

Achenbach, T., & Edelbrock, C. S. (1981). Behavioral problems and competencies reported by parents of normal and disturbed children aged four through sixteen. *Monograph of Social Research and Childhood Development, 46* (Serial No. 188).

Akiskal, H. S. (1985). The boundaries of affective disorders: Implications for defining temperamental variants, atypical subtypes and schizoaffective disorder. For the Committee to Evaluate DSM-III. Washington, DC: American Psychiatric Association.

American Psychiatric Association (1952). *Diagnostic and statistical manual of mental disorders*, 1st ed. Washington, DC: Author.

American Psychiatric Association (1968). *Diagnostic and statistical manual of mental disorders*, 2nd ed. Washington, DC: Author.

American Psychiatric Association (1975). *A psychiatric glossary*, 4th ed. Washington, DC: Author.

American Psychiatric Association (1980). *Diagnostic and statistical manual of mental disorders*, 3rd ed. Washington, DC: Author.

American Psychiatric Association (1987). *Diagnostic and statistical manual of mental disorders*, 3rd ed., revised. Washington, DC: Author.

American Psychiatric Association (1991). Task Force on DSM-IV. *DSM options book*. Washington, DC: APA (September 1, 1991).

American Psychiatric Association (1994). *Diagnostic and statistical manual of mental disorders*, 4th ed. Washington, DC: Author.

Baker, L., & Cantwell, D. (1990). Association between emotional/behavioral disorders and learning disorders in a sample of speech/language impaired children. *Advances in Learning and Behavior Disorders*, 6, 27–46.

Beardslee, W. R., Bemporad, J., Keller, M. B., & Klerman, G. L. (1983). Children of parents with major affective disorder: A review. *American Journal of Psychiatry*, 140, 825–831.

Cantwell, D. P. (1975). A model for the investigation of psychiatric disorders of childhood: Its application in genetic studies of the hyperkinetic syndrome. In A. J. Anthony (Ed.), *Explorations in child psychiatry* (pp. 67–79). New York: Plenum Press.

Cantwell, D. P. (1985). Depressive disorders in children. *Psychiatric Clinics of North America*, 8, 779–792.

Cantwell, D. P., & Carlson, G. A. (1983). Issues in classification. In D. P. Cantwell & G. A. Carlson (Eds.), *Affective disorders in childhood and adolescence: An update.* (pp. 19–38). New York: Spectrum Publications.

Carlson, G. A., & Cantwell, D. P. (1979). A survey of depressive symptoms in a child and adolescent population. *Journal of the American Academy of Child Psychiatry*, 18, 587–599.

Carlson, G. A., & Cantwell, D. P. (1980a). A survey of depressive symptoms, syndrome, and disorder in a child psychiatric population. *Journal of Child Psychology and Psychiatry*, 21, 19–25.

Carlson, G. A., & Cantwell, D. P. (1980b). Unmasking masked depression in children and adolescents. *American Journal of Psychiatry*, 137, 445–449.

Carlson, G., & Cantwell, D. (1982). Diagnosis of childhood depression: A comparison of the Weinberg and DSM-III criteria. *Journal of the American Academy of Child Psychiatry*, 21, 247–250.

Carlson, G. A., & Kashani, J. H. (1988). Phenomenology of major depression from childhood through adulthood: Analysis of three studies. *American Journal of Psychiatry*, 145, 1222–1225.

Chambers, W. J., Puig-Antich, J., Hirsch, M., Paez, P., Ambrosini, P. J., Tambrizi, M. A., & Davies, M. (1985). The assessment of affective disorders in children and adolescents by semistructured interview: Test–retest reliability of the Schedule for Affective Disorders and Schizophrenia for School-Age Children, Present Episode version. *Archives of General Psychiatry*, 42, 696–702.

Feighner, J. P., Robins, E., Guze, S. B., Woodruff, R., Winokur, G., & Munoz, R. (1972). Diagnostic criteria for use in psychiatric research. *Archives of General Psychiatry*, 26, 57–63.

Frommer, E. A. (1968). Depressive illness in childhood. In A. Coppens & A. Walk (Eds.), *Recent developments in affective disorders* (pp. 117–136). Ashford, Kent: Headley Brothers.

Huschka, M. (1941). Psychopathological disorders in the mother. *Journal of Nervous and Mental Disease*, 94, 76–83.

Kashani, J. H., Strober, M., Rosenberg, T. K., & Reid, J. C. (1988). Correlates of psychopathology in adolescents. *Psychiatry Research*, 26, 141–148.

Klerman, G. L., Hirschfeld, R. M. A., & Andreasen, N. C. (1987). Major depression and related affective disorders. In G. L. Tischler (Ed.), *Diagnosis and classification in psychiatry: A critical appraisal of DSM-III* (pp. 3–31). New York: Cambridge University Press.

Kovacs, M., Feinberg, T. L., Crouse-Novak, M. A., Paulauskas, S. L., & Finkelstein, R. (1984a). Depressive disorders in childhood. I. A longitudinal prospective study of characteristics and recovery. *Archives of General Psychiatry*, 41, 229–237.

Kovacs, M., Feinberg, T. L., Crouse-Novack, M. A., Paulauskas, S. L., Pollack, M., & Finkelstein, R. (1984b). Depressive disorders in childhood. II. A longitudinal study of the risk for a subsequent major depression. *Archives of General Psychiatry*, 41, 643–649.

Kraepelin, E. (1915). *Compendium der Psychiatrie*. Leipzig: Abel.

Lahey, B., Loeber, R., Stouthamer-Loeber, M., Christ, M., Green, S., Russo, M., Frick, P., & Dulcan, M. (1990). Comparison of DSM-III and DSM-III-R diagnoses for prepubertal children: Changes in prevalence and validity. *Journal of the American Academy of Child and Adolescent Psychiatry, 29*, 620–626.

Malmquist, C. P. (19717). Depression in childhood and adolescence. *New England Journal of Medicine, 284*, 887–892, 955–961.

McConville, B. J., Boag, L. C., & Purohit, A. D. (1973). Three types of childhood depression. *Canadian Journal of Psychiatry, 18*, 133–138.

Poznanski, E., Cook, S., & Carroll, B. (1979). A depression rating scale for children. *Pediatrics, 64*, 442–450.

Poznanski, E. O., Cook, S. C., Carroll, B. J., & Corzo, H. (1983). Use of the Children's Depression Rating Scale in an inpatient psychiatric population. *Journal of Clinical Psychiatry, 44*, 200–203.

Poznanski, E. O., Krahenbuhl, V., & Zrull, J. P. (1976). Childhood depression: A longitudinal perspective. *Journal of the American Academy of Child Psychiatry, 15*, 491–501.

Puig-Antich, J., Novacenko, H., Davies, M., Chambers, W. J., Tabrizi, M. A., Krawiec, V., Ambrosini, P. J., & Sacher, E. J. (1984). Growth hormone secretion in prepubertal children with major depression, I. Final report on response. *Archives of General Psychiatry, 41*, 455–460.

Robins, E. (1976). Categories versus dimensions in psychiatric classification. *Psychiatric Annals, 6*, 39–55.

Robins, E., & Guze, S. B. (1970). Establishment of diagnostic validity and psychiatric illness: Its application to schizophrenia. *American Journal of Psychiatry*, 983–987.

Russell, A. T., Cantwell, D. P., Mattison, R., & Will, L. (1979). A comparison of DSM-II and DSM-III in the diagnosis of childhood psychiatric disorders. III. Multiaxial features. *Archives of General Psychiatry, 36*, 1223–1226.

Rutter, M., & Gould, M. (1985). Classification. In M. Rutter & I. Hersov (Eds.), *Child and adolescent psychiatry: Modern approaches*, 2nd ed. (pp. 304–324). Boston: Blackwell Scientific.

Spitzer, R. L., Endicott, J., & Robins, E. (1978). *Research diagnostic criteria for a selected group of functional disorders*, 3rd ed. New York: New York State Psychiatric Institute.

Spitzer, R. L., & Williams, J. B. W. (1980). Classification of mental disorders and DSM-III. In H. Kaplan, A. M. Freedman, & B. J. Sadock (Eds.), *Comprehensive textbook of psychiatry*, 4th ed. (pp. 591–613). Baltimore: Williams & Wilkins.

Spitzer, R. L., Williams, J. B.W., & Skodol, A. E. (1983). *International perspectives on DSM-III*. Washington, DC: American Psychiatric Press.

Spitzer, R. L., & Wilson, P. T. (1976). Nosology and the official psychiatric nomenclature. In A. M. Freedman, H. I. Kaplan, & B. J. Sadock (Eds.), *Comprehensive textbook of psychiatry*. Baltimore: Williams & Wilkins.

Szasz, T. (1961). *The myth of mental illness*. New York: Harper & Row.

Szasz, T. (1978). *The myth of psychotherapy: Mental healing as religion, rhetoric, and repression*. New York: Doubleday.

Szurek, S. A., & Berlin, I. N. (1956). Elements of psychotherapeutics with a schizophrenic child and his parents. *Psychiatry, 19*, 1–9.

Weinberg, W. A., Rutman, J., Sullivan, L., Penick, E. C., & Dietz, S. G. (1973). Depression in children referred to an educational diagnostic center: Diagnosis and treatment. *Behavioral Pediatrics, 83*, 1065–1072.

Weissman, M. M., Gammon, D., & John, K. (1987). Children of depressed parents: Increased psychopathology and early onset of major depression. *Archives of General Psychiatry, 44*, 847–853.

10

Evaluation of Depression in Children and Adolescents Using Diagnostic Clinical Interviews

Kay Hodges

This chapter will describe five of the most widely used diagnostic interviews and present psychometric data relevant to depression. In addition, a clinician-rated scale that is widely used in depression research—i.e., the Children's Depression Rating Scale (CDRS) (Poznanski, Cook, & Carroll, 1979)—will be reviewed because it is often used in conjunction with these structured interviews.

For most research purposes, a diagnostic interview is used, although frequently other instruments are employed as well. The standardization of the questions posed to the child and of the response items coded by the interviewer reduces information and criterion variance (Spitzer, Endicott, & Robins, 1975). Criterion variance should also be lessened across studies to the extent that each of the interviews attempts to use the criteria established by the most recent edition of the *Diagnostic and Statistical Manual of Mental Disorders*, e.g., DSM-III-R (American Psychiatric Association, 1987).

There is a growing consensus that interviews are preferred over symptom checklists and self-report questionnaires when clinical depression is of interest. In their review of the adult literature, Coyne and Downey (1991) demonstrate that the findings on the relationship between depression and social factors differ, depending on whether the specific study used interview-based diagnoses or a self-report depression questionnaire to assess depression. They conclude that the studies utilizing questionnaires probably reflect on the social correlates of distress, not depression.

Within the child literature, there is evidence that the sensitivity of questionnaires, such as the Children's Depression Inventory (CDI) (Kovacs, 1981) and the depression

Kay Hodges • Department of Psychology, Eastern Michigan University, Ypsilanti, Michigan 48197.

Handbook of Depression in Children and Adolescents, edited by William M. Reynolds and Hugh F. Johnston. Plenum Press, New York, 1994.

scale of the Child Behavior Checklist (CBCL) (Achenbach & Edelbrock, 1983), is too low for diagnostic purposes, such as differentiating depressed children from those with other psychiatric illnesses (e.g., Asarnow & Carlson, 1985; Hodges, 1990b; Kronenberg, Blumensohn, & Apter, 1988).

Additionally, interviews have the advantage of assessing for other diagnoses, which is important given the high rate of comorbidity observed for depression in children (Puig-Antich et al., 1989). The generalization of prognostic indicators, including expected outcome of specific treatments, may vary depending on co-occurring disorders. Thus, although these interviews are costly and labor-intensive, they will probably continue to be required assessment components.

Overview of the Interviews

There are five interviews that have had sufficient longevity to generate psychometric data relevant to depression. Three may be best described as standardized "clinical" interviews, in that they permit variations in the interview questions as needed to obtain a valid assessment of the child. The authors of these interviews state a preference for using clinicians as interviewers. These interviews are: the Child Assessment Schedule (CAS) (Hodges & Fitch, 1979), the Interview Schedule for Children (ISC) (Kovacs, 1983), and the Schedule for Affective Disorders and Schizophrenia in School-Age Children (K-SADS) (Puig-Antich & Chambers, 1978). Two other interviews are meant to be administered in a highly structured manner, with little variation in question presentation. As a result, lay interviewers, rather than professionals, can be easily used. These two interviews are the Diagnostic Interview for Children and Adolescents (DICA) (Herjanic, Herjanic, Brown, & Wheatt, 1975) and the Diagnostic Interview Schedule for Children (DISC) (Costello, Edelbrock, Dulcan, Kalas, & Klaric, 1984). Each of these five interviews generates the major diagnoses observed in children and adolescents, and in the past the interview items in each have been modified as the diagnostic criteria are revised. Each interview has a parallel version for parents, to inquire about the child's symptoms.

In the discussion that follows, the interviews are reviewed (in alphabetical order), with an emphasis on reliability and validity data for depression. Major depressive disorder (MDD) and dysthymic disorder (DD) are differentiated if separate data are available. After the interview is briefly described, psychometric data are presented separately on the use of the interview to determine the presence or absence of depression (i.e., diagnosis) and the use of depression symptom scales that can be derived from the interview (i.e., symptom scales).[1] Since parents are known to be more reliable reporters (e.g., Edelbrock, Costello, Dulcan, Kalas, & Conover, 1985), diagnoses based on both child and parent interviews are distinguished from those that are based on child interview only.

Unfortunately, there is no "gold standard" to which to compare the interviews' performance for the purposes of validity. Previously, it was hoped that parental report could serve as a gold standard. However, poor concordance has been consistently demonstrated between child report and that of other informants, including parents, clinicians, and teachers, across a variety of instruments (Achenbach, McConaughy, & Howell, 1987). At best, moderate concordance between parent and child would be anticipated across the interviews. Thus, following a precedent set by Edelbrock and Costello (1988), concordance between parent and child will be conceptualized as interinformant reliability.

---

[1]This chapter was written in early 1992. Thus, the review of the literature does not include work published since then or information on DSM-IV versions of any interviews.

For the reliability studies, the review will be restricted to (1) interrater studies that also included a test–retest component, (2) interinformant studies in which different interviewers were used to interview the informants, and (3) internal consistency studies.

The validity data for each interview are organized into the following categories: (1) relationship to other measures, (2) comparison to alternatively derived diagnoses, (3) comparisons among contrast groups, (4) developmental trends, (5) intervention studies, and (6) course of illness (i.e., follow-up studies). Inter-interview concordance studies are presented in the discussion of the first interview reviewed. Prevalence studies are not included, nor are studies testing specific hypotheses about correlates of depression, since there are no established results to which to compare the interviews.

The statistic typically used in determining diagnostic concordance is the kappa statistic (κ) (Bartko & Carpenter, 1976). In this review, the guidelines suggested in Fleiss (1981) will be used (i.e., excellent agreement beyond chance indicated by κ greater than 0.75; good, by κ between 0.59 and 0.75; fair, by κ between 0.40 and 0.58; and poor, by κ equal to or less than 0.40). Because κ is affected by base rates of the disorder, caution should be exercised in comparing values across studies (Robins, 1985). Agreement for continuous scores (i.e., scales) is quantified by the Pearson correlation (r) or Intraclass Correlation Coefficient (ICC). For test–retest and internal consistency data, a correlation of 0.70 or above is considered satisfactory.

Caution should be exercised in directly comparing findings across studies because of the varying conditions under which studies are conducted. Various factors that probably affect degree of diagnostic agreement are discussed in Cohen, O'Connor, Lewis, Velez, and Malachowski (1987) and Hodges and Zeman (1993).

Child Assessment Schedule

There are three versions of the CAS, which reflect the evolution of the interview. The original CAS, dated 1978, is the least structured and is useful for younger children (5–7 years old). The second version, with the last modification dated 1986, was primarily developed for children of ages 7–12 and was updated for DSM-III-R. A third version, dated 1990, is appropriate for adolescents and for use by highly trained lay interviewers. Throughout these versions, the core items of the interview have remained the same.

The CAS is thematically organized around 11 topic areas: (1) school; (2) friends; (3) activities and hobbies; (4) family; (5) fears; (6) worries, and anxieties; (7) self-image; (8) mood; (9) physical complaints; (10) expression of anger; and (11) reality-testing symptomatology. Diagnostically related items are embedded within these content areas. Approximately one half of the CAS items are diagnostically related, with the remainder inquiring about the child's problems or conflicts in everyday functioning (e.g., at school, with friends, within the family). The CAS resembles a traditional clinically oriented interview in that the interviewer strives to get an understanding of the child's symptoms, his functioning, the context in which he lives, and his insights and concerns about himself and his environment. The relationship between the content scales and the diagnostic items is outlined in Hodges and Saunders (1989).

There are four sections to the interview: content area questions (i.e., questions for the child and response items to score), onset and duration questions, interviewer observational judgments, and interviewer comments about the interview process. Quantitative scale scores are generated for (1) the total interview, (2) each diagnostically related symptom scale, and (3) each of the 11 content areas listed above. A computer algorithm for generating diagnoses and scale scores is available, as well as a detailed manual to aid in establishing interrater reliability (Hodges, 1983, 1986, 1990).

Reliability. A reliability study with preadolescent inpatients by Hodges, Cools, and McKnew (1989) used a test–retest interrater design (i.e., different interviewers administered the CAS on the two occasions). The median inter-interview time interval was 9 days. Diagnoses were computer-generated, using strict adherence to DSM-III-R. Based on child report on the CAS, the κ values were 1.00 for MDD and 0.71 for DD. In both psychiatric and medically chronically ill samples, the internal consistency for items contributing to the disorders of MDD and DD was found to be high (i.e., α values of 80 or above) (Hodges, Saunders, Kashani, Hamlett, & Thompson, 1990).

Validity

Relationship to Other Measures. A study comparing self-report questionnaires to computer-generated diagnoses on the CAS provided evidence of discriminant and convergent validity (Hodges, 1990b). The self-report measures were administered to preadolescent inpatients by a research assistant who was blind to the results of the interview. Children diagnosed as depressed (either MDD or DD) scored significantly higher on the CDI than did nondepressed children. There was no difference observed for the conduct- vs. non-conduct-disordered and the anxiety- vs. non-anxiety-disordered children on the CDI. Also, the depressed children did not score higher on the State–Trait Anxiety Inventory for Children (Spielberger, 1973) than did the children with an anxiety disorder.

Further analyses were conducted with the preadolescent sample described above (Hodges, 1990b) to examine the relationship between the presence or absence of various diagnoses (i.e., depression, anxiety, conduct disorder) and factor scores on the CDI (Hodges & Craighead, 1990). Previous research with the CDI (Smucker & Craighead, 1990) had identified five factors: dysphoric mood, loss of personal and social interest, self-deprecation, vegetation symptoms, and acting-out behavior. Comparison of children with and without diagnoses revealed that the children with depression scored significantly higher than nondepressed children on dysphoric mood, loss of interest, and self-deprecation. No differences were observed between anxiety- and non-anxiety-disordered or between conduct- and non-conduct-disordered children on these factors.

The relationship between depression, as diagnosed by the CAS, and the Differential Emotions Scale—IV (DES) (Blumberg & Izard, 1985) was examined in a study testing the hypothesis that depressed youngsters are characterized by higher levels of sadness, self-directed hostility, anger, guilt, and shyness (Carey, Finch, & Carey, 1991). The sample was psychiatric inpatients, ranging in ages from 10 to 17, and diagnoses were determined by computer algorithm based on the child version of the CAS. Depressed youths reported higher levels of negative emotions (i.e., sadness, shame, shyness, guilt, self-directed hostility, and anger) as well as lower levels of enjoyment compared to nondepressed youths. A discriminant analysis demonstrated that five DES scales contributed and correctly classified 80% of the depressed subjects, as classified by the CAS.

Comparison to Alternatively Derived Diagnoses. A concordance study compared diagnoses derived with the CAS to the K-SADS in a design using lay interviewers with an inter-interview period of 2 days (Hodges, McKnew, Burbach, & Roebuck, 1987). For each interview, the child and parent were interviewed separately and simultaneously. Diagnoses for both interviews were computed by algorithm, using DSM-III (American Psychiatric Association, 1980) criteria, with no clinical judgment involved. Diagnostic concordance for depression (i.e., MDD or DD) was computed four ways: based on child interview only (κ = 0.52), based on parent interview only (κ = 0.75), based on combining the data (either parent- or child-endorsed) ($\kappa = 0.61$), and based on consensus of parent and child interview (i.e., diagnosis present for both child and parent) ($\kappa = 0.61$). Thus, fair to good concordance was observed, depending on informant.

Course of Illness. Zahn-Waxler, Radke-Yarrow, and their colleagues used the CAS to compare the course of morbidity factors observed in the infants and toddlers of manic–depressive unipolar and control parents (Zahn-Waxler et al., 1988; Radke-Yarrow, Nottelmann, Martinez, Fox, & Belmont, 1992). During the first 2 years of life, the offspring of the affectively ill parents displayed major problems in early relationship formation and in social and emotional development. Four years later, at age 6 years, the children were administered the CAS and the parents completed the CBCL to determine whether the problems identified early in the children's development reflected precursor patterns of later diagnosable disorders. DSM-III diagnoses were determined by a psychiatrist after reviewing the CAS and the CBCL. The psychiatrist and interviewing psychologist were blind to the parental diagnoses. The offspring of the manic–depressive parents were compared to the offspring of nondisturbed control parents, with the results indicating significantly more depression as well as other diagnoses in the manic–depressive group than in the control group (Zahn-Waxler et al., 1988). Furthermore, the offspring of bipolar and unipolar mothers demonstrated different developmental paths from preschool to middle childhood relative to the onset of a clinical level of depression (Radke-Yarrow et al., 1992).

Symptom Scales

Reliability. The test–retest study by Hodges et al. (1989) also evaluated the reliability of the symptom scores. The correlations were significant and satisfactory for MDD ($r = 0.89$) as well as DD ($r = 0.86$). *T*-tests comparing the number of symptoms at time 1 and time 2 revealed no significant differences for MDD or DD.

Interinformant reliability was assessed in a sample of preadolescent inpatients, the children being interviewed by a psychologist and the parents by psychiatric social workers (Hodges, Gordon, & Lennon, 1990). There was an inter-interview interval of 12 days on average. The interviewers were blind to each other's interview results. Correlations between child and parent were significant and moderate for both MDD ($r = 0.46$) and DD ($r = 0.45$). *T*-tests comparing number of symptoms reported by children and parents indicated no significant difference.

Validity
Relationship to Other Measures. In a validity study with mostly preadolescent children, correspondence between the CAS child version and maternal report on the CBCL was examined (Hodges, Kline, Stern, Cytryn, & McKnew, 1982). The CBCL Depression scale correlated significantly with the CAS Depression subscale ($r = 0.51$). In addition, the CAS Depression scale correlated significantly with self-report on the CDI ($r = 0.53$).

The Beck Depression Inventory (BDI) (Beck & Beamesderfer, 1974) was correlated with the CAS Depression symptom scale in two samples of adolescents, psychiatrically hospitalized and a nonreferred school sample (Barrera & Garrison-Jones, 1988). Trained research assistants administered the CAS. In the inpatient sample, the CAS Depression symptom scale was found to correlate significantly with the BDI ($r = 0.49$). Evidence of discriminant validity is offered by the findings that the BDI scores were not significantly related to CAS conduct disorder symptoms ($r = 0.04$) or anxiety symptoms ($r = 0.15$). In the nonreferred school sample of adolescents, the BDI correlated highly and significantly with the CAS Depression syndrome scale ($r = 0.73$). Lower correlations were found between the BDI and other CAS scales, including Conduct Disorder ($r = 0.29$) and Anxiety ($r = 0.29$).

Comparisons among Contrast Groups. A comparison among psychiatric inpatients, outpatients, and normal controls provided evidence of contrast group validity (Hodges et al., 1982). On the Depression symptom scale (consisting of items assessing MDD or DD), inpatients scored significantly higher than psychiatric outpatients, who in turn scored significantly higher than controls. The same analysis was conducted for the CBCL Depression scale, which did not differentiate the inpatient and outpatient groups, as did the CAS.

Psychiatrically disturbed children were compared to pediatric patients as well as nonreferred children in a study of children with cystic fibrosis (Thompson, Hodges, & Hamlett, 1990). The sex, age, and socioeconomic status of the children in the cystic fibrosis group were used as matching variables for the other two groups. The psychiatric patients reported significantly more symptoms on both the MDD and DD symptom scales than the nonreferred group or the cystic fibrosis group.

Developmental Trends. Kashani, Orvaschel, Rosenberg, and Reid (1989) studied developmental trends in a community sample consisting of equal males and females from each of three age groups (i.e., 8-, 12-, and 17-year-olds). Analyses of the symptom scales revealed expected age and gender differences (Rutter, 1986b). According to the children's interviews, symptoms of depression were significantly more frequent in the 17-year-olds. No age effects were observed for the Birleson Depression Self-Rating (Birleson, 1981). Thus, the CAS Depression scale was more sensitive to depression symptoms than a self-report measure (Kashani, Rosenberg, & Reid, 1989).

Intervention Studies. Runyan, Everson, Edelsohn, Hunter, and Coulter (1988) used the CAS to assess the effects of court involvement and testimony for a sample of sexually abused girls. This was a prospective study in which the children were administered the CAS within 2 weeks following disclosure and 5 months after the first interview. Relevant to depression, improvement was defined as a reduction in the CAS Depression symptom scale of 1 standard deviation or more. Children awaiting criminal trial were only 8% as likely to improve, compared to children not involved in the court process. Juvenile court testimony emerged as a positive influence, with a likelihood of improving that was 6–7 times greater for children who testified, in comparison with all other children. Thus, slow movement of criminal proceedings was associated with more depression, while testifying in juvenile court was associated with less depression at follow-up.

Content Scales: Reliability and Validity

Of the 11 content areas, the "Mood" scale has depression-related items that primarily reflect on dysphoria and anhedonia. Reliability data for the content scales are provided in the papers previously cited for the symptom scales. In addition, evidence of contrast group validity for the Mood content scale is provided by two studies conducted by Verhulst and his colleagues (Verhulst, Bieman, Ende, Berden, & Sanders-Woustra, 1990; Verhulst, Althaus, & Berden, 1987). In both of these studies, the Mood content scale contributed significantly to a discriminant analysis between disturbed and nondisturbed children, identified by an independent morbidity criterion. Lee and Gotlib (1991) conducted a 10-month follow-up of symptoms present in offspring of three maternal groups: depressed psychiatric, nondepressed psychiatric, and nondepressed community. At follow-up, the offspring of the psychiatrically disturbed parents continued to evidence more mood problems than the community group.

The CAS has been used in children of all age ranges, including as young as 5 years, with a preponderance of the psychometric data having been established with preadolescent children. Diagnosis can be made via stringent use of computer-scoring algorithm or clinical diagnosis by a professional. The interviewers have ranged from clinicians to highly trained research assistants/graduate students. The CAS can be used in clinical research settings in which it is desirable to use an interview that yields clinically relevant information as well as diagnostic information.

There has been a systematic attempt to study the psychometric properties of the CAS for three sets of variables: presence or absence of diagnosis, symptom score scales, and content scales that reflect on areas of adjustment. The test–retest and internal consistency data for diagnosis as well as for the Depression symptom scale are good. There is evidence of convergent and discriminant validity as well as sensitivity to change in psychological state. The CAS appears to be particularly useful for studying target populations that are younger (pre- and early adolescents) and that vary from healthy to disturbed.

Diagnostic Interview for Children and Adolescents

Early research on the DICA was conducted with the first version, described in Herjanic et al. (1975). The DICA was modeled after the Renard Diagnostic Interview (Helzer, Robins, Croughan, & Welner, 1981), and diagnoses were based on the *International Classification of Psychiatric Disorders* as well as the Feighner criteria (Feighner et al., 1972). A revised version of the DICA was developed in 1981 and included the DSM-III diagnoses. The DICA was again revised in 1988 to provide DSM-III-R diagnoses, and was named the DICA-R.

The DICA-R has separate interviews for children of ages 6–12 and for adolescents of ages 13–17 (DICA-R-A), in addition to the parent interview. For both age groups, the questions are basically the same, with an attempt to make the wording and examples age-appropriate (Reich, 1988). Unfortunately, there are no psychometric data available yet on the DICA-R, and it is hoped that further research will shed light on whether the child and adolescent versions have adequate reliability and validity for the respective age groupings. The organization of the DICA-R remains the same as the earlier version in that the interview is divided according to DSM-III-R diagnostic categories. The psychometric data presented here are for the second version of the DICA.

Diagnosis

Reliability. In a test–retest, interrater reliability study with inpatients, a κ value of 0.90 was reported for "affective disorder" (Welner, Reich, Herjanic, Jung, & Amado, 1987). Apparently, this study included only MDD, since the second version of the DICA did not diagnose DD. Also, the replicability of the study from the information available is questionable because it is not clear to what extent clinical judgment was involved in the diagnostic procedure. Lay interviewers were used; however, two psychiatrists who developed the DICA edited the interviews and made diagnoses using a coding guide prepared for the interview according to DSM-III criteria.

Interinformant reliability was reported in Welner et al. (1987) with a psychiatric outpatient sample. The κ value reflecting on diagnostic concordance between the child and parent interviews was 0.63 for "affective disorder." However, concordance was not based on strict adherence to DSM-III. Only the symptoms were attended to, with duration information ignored. Additionally, the diagnoses were considered concordant even if one symptom was lacking for diagnosis in one of the interviews.

Poor parent–child concordance for the diagnosis of depression was observed in three studies in which the parents were psychiatric patients or controls. Reported κ values were −0.07 (Kashani, Orvaschel, Burk, & Reid, 1985), 0.17 (Earls, Reich, Jung, & Coninger, 1988), and 0.11 (Sylvester, Hyde, & Reichler, 1987). In addition, in Sylvester et al. (1987), diagnostic concordance between parents was determined, yielding a κ value of 0.39. In Brunshaw and Szatmari (1988), the distribution of diagnosis by parent and child interview revealed no cases in common between parent and child. A recent study of psychiatric inpatient children yielded more encouraging results, with a fair level of concordance between parent and child (κ = 0.43) (Vitiello, Malone, Buschle, Delaney, & Behar, 1990).

Validity

Relationship to Other Measures. In Sylvester et al. (1987), the presence or absence of the diagnosis of depression, based on the DICA administered to the child, was compared to the presence or absence of depression based on the Personality Inventory for Children (Lachar & Gdowski, 1979), using a *T* score of 65 or greater as the cutoff point. A κ value of 0.24 was reported, indicating slight concordance.

Comparison to Alternatively Derived Diagnoses. In the Welner et al. (1987) study described above, the presence or absence of diagnosis given by a psychiatrist based on the DICA, as administered to the child, was compared to diagnosis given by a psychiatrist based on all other available information. The κ value for depression was in the moderate range (κ = 0.52). In Vitiello et al. (1990), diagnoses made by a child fellow after administering the DICA to the child were compared to diagnoses made by a child psychiatry fellow who administered an unstructured clinical admission interview. It appears that in both conditions the diagnoses were based on the fellows' judgment. Again, a κ value in the moderate range was reported.

The DICA was compared to the K-SADS in a study that examined correspondence between interview-yielded diagnoses and clinical diagnoses from the chart discharge summary (Carlson, Kashani, Thomas, Vaidya, & Daniel, 1987). Around admission, the DICA child version was administered by a child psychiatrist or graduate student and the DICA parent version by a social worker. Diagnosis made as a result of the interviews was compared to a best-estimate diagnosis made by a psychiatrist on the basis of all available information after the child was discharged. For "all affective disorders," the concordance between the DICA and the discharge best-estimate diagnosis was in the fair range (κ = 0.48 for the child version, κ = 0.43 for the parent version).

Course of Illness. The stability of psychiatric diagnoses 4 years after children were evaluated at a speech and language clinic was investigated by Cantwell and Baker (1989). Clinical diagnoses were made by a psychiatrist on the basis of the parent and child version of the DICA and parent and teacher questionnaires. Relative to the other disorders, low stability was observed for affective disorders; however, one third of the originally diagnosed cases still evidenced depression.

Summary

For the diagnosis of MDD, good test–retest reliability and satisfactory concordance between clinical interview–generated diagnosis and discharge diagnosis have been demonstrated. Few validity data have been generated for the DICA, except for the comparison to alternatively derived diagnoses. In addition, no psychometric data on symptom scores have been reported. Data on dysthymic disorder have not been generated, but should become available when studies on the DICA-R are conducted.

The DICA has been used by numerous researchers, primarily to help document diagnosis for the purposes of subject selection. It has also been used to determine the prevalence of disorders in a community sample, although a tendency to overdiagnose was corrected by identifying cases that both had a disorder and were judged to need treatment by a reviewing psychiatrist (Kashani et al., 1987). However, the need to utilize an impairment measure with any diagnostic interview is increasingly being recognized. While most of the studies have employed clinicians to generate diagnoses or identify cases, diagnoses can be determined by computer algorithm separately for the child and the parent. These methodological procedures can be clearly replicated by others, which in turn facilitates comparisons across studies.

Diagnostic Interview Schedule for Children

The DISC was the result of an effort by the National Institute of Mental Health (NIMH) to generate an interview for epidemiological research that would parallel the Diagnostic Interview Schedule (DIS) (Robins, Helzer, Croughan, & Ratcliff, 1981), which had been developed for epidemiological research with adults. The NIMH report (Costello et al., 1984) on the psychometric properties of the DISC is referred to here as the "original NIMH study" for the sake of clarity, since numerous publications are based on this same subject sample. The results of this first NIMH study were sufficiently disappointing to necessitate continued efforts to improve the DISC before its widespread use was recommended. Another NIMH grant sponsored a study of a revised version of the DISC (DISC-R), which resulted in the generation of another version of the DISC (DISC-2). The psychometric study of the DISC-R is contained in an NIMH report by Shaffer et al. (1988). Since these additional efforts still did not result in an interview that was ready for implementation in a multicenter epidemiological study, similar to the Epidemiologic Catchment Area project conducted on adults, a multicenter project has been sponsored to further develop the instrument.

The DISC is intended to be administered by lay interviewers and to be used in epidemiological research. The response formats are categorical (i.e., "Yes," "No," "Sometimes"). Interrater reliability is considered to be a trivial issue, since the interviewer is supposed to record the child's literal answer (e.g., "Yes") (Costello et al., 1984, p. 22).

Diagnosis

Reliability. Test–retest reliability was assessed in the original NIMH study, with a mean inter-interview interval of 12 days. Diagnoses were computer-generated. Each respondent was interviewed once by a clinician and once by a lay interviewer. The κ values for MDD and DD were 0.44 and 0.47, respectively. The κ values for the parent version were 0.50 for MDD and 0.49 for DD. Because of the large number of diagnoses generated with the DISC in this study, a second scoring algorithm was developed. Because almost all the subsequent work with the DISC uses this second algorithm, it is described here. The modified criteria for presence of diagnosis were as follows: "a) unmodified DSM III criteria were met, and b) the total of scores on symptoms included in the criteria for the disorder exceeded an arbitrary cut-off point, chosen so that the number diagnosed then approximated to the number diagnosed by the clinicians" (Costello et al., 1984, p. 27). The criteria that corresponded to DSM-III criteria were then referred to as "mild," and the criteria artificially set so that clinicians and lay interviewers generated the same number of diagnoses were labeled "severe." Using the "severe" criteria unfortunately did not improve the test–retest reliability, with a κ of 0.36 reported for MDD.

A test–retest study of the DISC was conducted during the pilot work for the Puerto

Rican child psychiatry epidemiological study (Bird et al., 1987). The two interviewers, who were both psychiatrists, administered the DISC to the child and a parent, but were also free to ask any other questions. Diagnoses were their best clinical judgment, based on the interviews (both the DISC and unstructured) and other available information. Fair reliability was observed for MDD ($\kappa = 0.46$) and DD ($\kappa = 0.55$).

The second NIMH study on a revised version of the DISC (DISC-R) used a sample of psychiatric patients, ranging in age from 11 to 17 years (mean 13 years). The design involved each respondent's being interviewed by a lay interviewer and a clinician, with an interval between interviews of 1–3 weeks. At the first assessment, all subjects received both the DISC and a clinical semistructured interview, while at the second assessment, half the sample received the DISC and the other half the clinical interview. No data on DD were generated because of the insufficient number of cases with the diagnosis. The DISC was administered by lay interviewers, while the clinical interview was given by psychiatrists, psychologists, and social workers. Computer algorithm was used to arrive at diagnoses for both the DISC and the clinical interview. The clinician was also asked to give a clinical diagnosis. With this primarily adolescent sample, test–retest reliability for MDD was satisfactory for both the child version ($\kappa = 0.63$) and the parent version ($\kappa = 0.72$).

In the original NIMH study, parent–child concordance was poor for the child version for MDD ($\kappa = 0.14$) and for DD ($\kappa = 0.16$). Use of the "severe" criteria did not improve concordance. In the study of the DISC-R, parent–child concordance for MDD was more encouraging ($\kappa = 0.40$) (Shaffer et al., 1988).

Validity

Relationship with Other Measures. The relationship between diagnosis of depression on the DISC and the Youth Self-Report (YSR) questionnaire (Achenbach & Edelbrock, 1987) was examined in an adolescent inpatient sample (Weinstein, Noam, Grimes, Stone, & Schwab-Stone, 1990). Diagnosis was computer-generated, using the "mild" algorithm in the original NIMH study that followed the DSM-III criteria. The adolescents diagnosed as depressed scored significantly higher than nondepressed adolescents on all the scales on the YSR, including: depressed, somatic complaint, aggressive, delinquent, thought disorder, internalizing, externalizing, and total score. These results lend some support for concurrent validity, but do not reflect well on discriminant validity.

Comparison to Alternatively Derived Diagnoses. In the original NIMH study, concordance between DISC-generated and clinical diagnoses was fair for MDD ($\kappa = 0.44$) and for DD ($\kappa = 0.41$). For the parent version, the findings were similar, with a κ value of 0.50 for MDD and for DD.

In a study conducted at a health maintenance organization with a preadolescent sample, DISC-generated computer diagnoses were compared to diagnoses made by a pediatrician as well as a social worker (Costello, Edelbrock, Costello, Dulcan, & Brent, 1986). The κ values for depression are not given separately; however, summary statistics are given for "emotional diagnoses." Concordance was poor for all comparisons, including the DISC with the social workers' diagnoses ($\kappa = 0.30$) and the DISC with the pediatricians' diagnoses ($\kappa = 0.04$). The values for the parent version of the DISC were similar.

The DISC was compared to clinicians' DSM-III diagnoses in a sample of adolescent inpatients (Weinstein, Stone, Noam, Grimes, & Schwab-Stone, 1989). The clinicians' diagnoses were those made at admission by the staff or training psychiatrists. The DISC interview was conducted within 2 weeks of admission by either a psychiatrist or a psychologist. The κ values were low, indicating poor concordance (i.e., for any affective disorder, $\kappa = 0.09$; for MDD, $\kappa = 0.17$). The authors report that if the modified algorithm, referred to as the "severe level" in the original NIMH study, were used, there was no improvement in correspondence.

In the study of the DISC-R, poor concordance was found for MDD between the DISC-R child version and the clinical interview ($\kappa = 0.39$) as well as between the parent version and the clinical interview ($\kappa = 0.36$) (Shaffer et al., 1988).

The DISC was compared to the K-SADS in a community sample of 9- to 12-year-olds (Cohen et al., 1987). The DISC interviewers were lay, and the K-SADS was administered by clinicians. Both interviews were scored by a computer algorithm. Concordance between the DISC and the K-SADS for MDD was poor ($\kappa = 0.00$–0.10 depending on the criteria used).

Comparisons among Contrast Groups. Contrast group validity was examined in a study by Costello, Edelbrock, and Costello (1985), in which 40 children referred to psychiatry from the original NIMH study (Costello et al., 1984) were matched to 40 children visiting their pediatricians from the HMO study (Costello et al., 1986). Statistical analyses were not generated separately for depression; however, the authors noted that dysthymia was one of the disorders with high endorsements in both groups (40% of the pediatric cases and 47% of the psychiatric cases for the "mild level" and none in either group for the "severe" level).

Data relevant to contrast group validity were generated by the Dunedin multi-disciplinary study, which is a longitudinal study of a representative sample of New Zealand children (McGee & Williams, 1988). At two follow-up times (age 11 and 13), three subject groups (i.e., depressed, pastdepression, and nondepressed) were compared on (1) symptom scales derived from the DISC, (2) scale scores from parent report, and (3) scale scores from teacher report. At age 11, the children were administered the entire DISC, and at age 13, a very abbreviated version of the DISC. At each follow-up, parents completed questionnaires rather than receiving the parent version of the interviews. Since the determination of subject group required self-report on the DISC (for absence or presence of depression), it follows that for the two depressed groups, the children reported more depression. However, the depressed groups differed from the nondepressed comparison group in having significantly higher ratings on the following scales: (1) antisocial/conduct disorder by parent report at ages 9 and 13, teacher report at age 13; (2) worry/anxiety by parent report at ages 9 and 13; (3) psychotic scale by parent report at age 13; and (4) impulsivity/hyperactivity by self-report on the DISC at age 11. These findings raise questions about discriminant validity given the higher levels of nondepressed symptoms in the children identified as depressed, compared to nondepressed children.

Symptom Scores

Reliability. Test–retest reliability of the data in the original NIMH study was analyzed for summed symptom scales by Edelbrock et al. (1985). As mentioned previously, each respondent was interviewed once by a clinician and once by a lay interviewer, both with the DISC. Data for 27 symptom areas were presented for the total sample and by three age groups (6–9, 10–13, 14–18). Intraclass correlation (ICC) for the total score for the depression symptom areas was satisfactory for the total sample (ICC = 0.64); however, it was clearly unsatisfactory for children below age 10 (for ages 6–9, ICC = 0.30; for ages 10–13, ICC = 0.53). The reliabilities for the parent version were in the acceptable range across all age ranges.

Williams, McGee, Anderson, and Silva (1989) reported on the internal consistency of the DISC subscale scores used in Edelbrock, Costello, Dulcan, Conover, and Kalas (1986). For the depression-related scales, moderate α values were reported for the Affective ($\alpha = 0.67$) and Suicidal ($\alpha = 0.66$) scales, whereas poor internal consistency was observed for the Vegetative scale ($\alpha = 0.41$) and the Cognitive scale ($\alpha = 0.45$).

Parent–child agreement for the data collected in the original NIMH study was reported by Edelbrock et al. (1986). The correlation was low for the total sample ($r = 0.28$,

$p < 0.001$), as well as for each of the age groups, including 6–9 ($r = 0.08$), 10–13 ($r = 0.30$, $p < 0.01$), and 14–18 years old ($r = 0.32$, $p < 0.01$).

Validity

Relationship to Other Measures. Parent–child agreement was reported by Williams et al. (1989) for 13 of the subscale scores outlined by Edelbrock et al. (1986). At the follow-up at age 11, the Dunedin children were administered the DISC and the parents completed a questionnaire. The correlations between child-reported and parent-reported depression across the two instruments was significant but in the low range (for boys, $r = 0.25$; for girls, $r = 0.24$).

Comparison among Contrast Groups. Contrast group validity is provided in the study by Costello et al. (1985) cited above. The psychiatric group scored significantly higher than the pediatric group on depression symptoms.

In the HMO study, the health care providers (pediatricians) were asked to provide diagnoses. A comparison of the children with and without a diagnosis, as determined by the pediatricians, was not significant for any of the symptom scales on the child version of the DISC, including the depression-related scales (Costello et al., 1986).

Other Studies. The DISC was administered to both children and parents in three prevalence studies: the Puerto Rico Child Psychiatry Study (Bird, Gould, Yager, Staghezza, & Canino, 1989), the New York Child Longitudinal Study (Velez, Johnson, & Cohen, 1989), and an HMO study (Costello et al., 1988). Since there is so little known about the true prevalence of depression disorders, the results relevant to prevalence cannot be viewed as a criterion for establishing validity. The application of the DISC in these studies and the problem with overinclusiveness will be briefly discussed, since there are implications for users of the DISC. Even though the DISC is intended to be administered by lay interviewers because of the obvious difficulty in using professionals in epidemiological research, the Puerto Rico study used psychiatrists and the HMO study used psychiatric social workers.

Due to the large number of subjects who qualified for a DSM-III diagnosis, additional criteria, besides the presence of a diagnosis, were required in all three studies. These additional criteria, which were needed to reduce the prevalence rates to an expected level, reflected various strategies. In the Puerto Rico study, the additional criterion was impairment, as judged by the psychiatrists who generated a score on the Children's Global Assessment Scale (CGAS) (Shaffer et al., 1983).

In the New York and HMO studies, the additional criteria required that the subject score above a cutoff score that was determined by identifying the extreme scores on the relevant scale (e.g., depression). In the New York study, the value was equal to or greater than 1 standard deviation above the symptom scale mean for the sample. In the HMO study, the value was an arbitrary cutoff point selected in the original NIMH grant report (Costello et al., 1984) so that the number of children diagnosed with this method approximated the number diagnosed by the clinicians.

Certainly a case can be made for applying impairment criteria to children's diagnoses in order to identify cases in need of treatment. However, the solutions used in these studies are problematic. One used the subjective judgment of a highly trained clinician, which is not feasible for epidemiological studies, while the other two studies did not reflect on disorders defined by the DSM-III criteria.

Summary

The DISC has been the subject of considerable study because of the interest in having a version of the DIS that can be used for epidemiological research with youth. Despite this attention, the psychometric data reveal a number of concerns about using the DISC to study depression in children. The reliability for the diagnosis of depression has been unsatisfactory except for the DISC-R, which was tested only with youths aged 11 and older. The results of validity studies in which the DISC has been compared to alternatively derived diagnoses has been disappointing, with mostly poor concordance. The data relevant to contrast group validity were equally disappointing in terms of discriminant validity.

Test–retest reliability for the depression symptom scores was satisfactory only for older youths (>14 years). Parent–child agreement for depression symptoms was clearly unacceptable for younger children (<10 years). The data relevant to validity of the depression symptom scale are very limited, and the few data that do exist are not encouraging.

These data raise questions about the use of the DISC for studying depression in children under 10, or perhaps under 14, years of age. In fact, some researchers have raised the issue that it appeared that younger children (under the age of 10 or 11) had difficulty with the interview (Bird et al., 1987). In addition, there appears to be a consistent problem with overdiagnosis, irrespective of whether the diagnoses are generated by clinicians or a computer algorithm. Furthermore, there is apparently some discomfort in using lay interviewers, since many of the studies used highly trained clinicians. Given the interest in the DISC, it may evolve into a satisfactory instrument for epidemiological research on depression. The DISC clearly performs better for disruptive disorders, as reviewed elsewhere (e.g., Hodges & Zeman, 1993). However, on the basis of the psychometric data currently available, it does not appear to be the interview of choice for diagnosing depression in clinical samples or for monitoring depressive symptoms.

Interview Schedule for Children

The ISC is described as a "semistructured, symptom-oriented" interview that was designed to yield current symptom ratings rather than differential diagnosis (Kovacs, 1985). The ISC was originally developed for research on depression in youths, and thus the "core" of the interview inquires about depression-related symptoms, the duration of these symptoms, and the presence of hallucinations and delusions (Kovacs, 1983). Addenda were developed for other disorders that the ISC did not cover in detail in order to permit differential diagnosis. Most of the coding consists of severity ratings.

The ISC is intended to be administered by a clinician who can make clinical diagnoses. The parent is first interviewed, then the child. The clinician rates each item three times, on the basis of the parent interview, the child interview, and then an overall summary rating for both informants. Information on duration of symptoms is typically gathered only from the parent.

Diagnoses are to be based on all available information. For example, in the longitudinal study conducted by Kovacs, Feinberg, Crouse-Novak, Paulauskas, and Finkelstein (1984), diagnoses were based on the ISC, clinical history, and demographic and environmental data, as well as on academic record and test scores. Other clinicians on the research project reviewed the diagnoses so that diagnoses could be generated by consensus.

For follow-up interviews, an "interim rating" is given for each item to indicate whether clinically significant symptoms (i.e., a rating of 3 or above on a 0- to 8-point scale) have been evident between the time of the last assessment and the 2 weeks preceding the interview. These interim ratings are scored dichotomously, as present or absent.

Diagnosis: Reliability

Last, Strauss, and Francis (1987) conducted a test–retest, interrater reliability study in a sample of children referred to a clinic for child and adolescent anxiety disorders.

Given that the two interviews were administered on the same day (morning and afternoon), the inter-interview interval was a matter of hours at best. The same pair of clinicians administered all the interviews. The κ value for MDD was 0.84 and for DD, 0.66. As pointed out by Last (1987), there were a number of variables that probably enhanced reliability, including the short test–retest interval, the use of the same two interviewers, and the generation of diagnoses based on clinical judgment.

Diagnosis Based on Child and Parent Interviews: Validity

Comparison of Contrast Groups and Course of Illness. Kovacs et al. (1984) conducted a longitudinal study that examined the course of depression in school-age children. This study included a group of depressed children, who were classified into subtypes (MDD, DD, and Adjustment Disorder with Depressed Mood), and a control group (nondepressed psychiatrically disordered children). The mean follow-up interval was 3 years, with a range of 0–8 years. The presence or absence of a depression diagnosis was used to determine group assignment (depressed vs. control group) as well as to assess the major dependent variables. These dependent variables primarily involved determining the timing for the presence or absence of the depression as well as comorbid diagnoses (i.e., pattern of onset and offset or recovery). No diagnostic reliability data were provided for this study. The results of this study have provided a rich source of information about the course of depression in children, which is detailed elsewhere in this volume. With respect to psychometric properties, the differentiation of the three depression subtypes, in terms of onset and pattern of recovery, offers evidence of validity.

Individual Items: Reliability

No report of parent–child concordance, in which the two informants were interviewed by different interviewers, has been made for the ISC for diagnosis or symptom scales. However, in a study in which the same interviewer was used, parent–child agreement on individual depression-related items has been reported. The reliability was poorer for depression items compared to "acting-out" items. Pearson correlations were generated between the severity ratings for parent and child for each item. For example, the mean correlation for mood/affect items was moderate ($r = 0.52$); for cognitively oriented depression items, poor ($r = 0.32$); and for vegetative/psychomotor items, moderate ($r = 0.55$) (Kovacs, 1983). The subject sample in this study was from the longitudinal study of depressed children (Kovacs et al., 1984).

Symptom Scales: Validity

Relationship to Other Measures. Subjects from two longitudinal studies conducted by Kovacs and her colleagues (i.e., depression and diabetes) were used to examine the relationship between the ISC and questionnaires (Paulauskas & Kovacs, 1984). An ISC depression index, which consisted of 11 items and represented the summed and then averaged clinician ratings of the items, was correlated with self-report CDI scores as well as the parent report on the Depression scale on the CBCL. The ISC Depression score correlated significantly but only moderately with the CDI ($r = 0.33$) and with the CBCL Depression scale ($r = 0.38$).

Summary

Few studies have been conducted to assess the psychometric properties of the ISC. There are no test–retest data for diagnosis other than the study with a morning–afternoon design. No parent–child agreement for diagnosis or for symptom scales is available. In fact, there has been no psychometric study of any symptom scales for the ISC. It is ironic that even when the ISC has been administered to assess change over time, self-report on symptom questionnaires (e.g., the CDI) has been used for quantitative analysis, rather than symptom scales from the interview (e.g., Kovacs et al., 1990).

In any case, the results of the longitudinal study on the course of depression suggest that the ISC is sensitive to changes in diagnostic state. However, as pointed out by Rutter (1986a), the fact that the follow-up assessments were not made blind to the original diagnosis argues for replication of this study.

In part, the paucity of psychometric data reflects the perspective that the function of the ISC is to reduce information variance by following a semistructured format and to reduce criterion variance by using diagnostic criteria. The ISC is viewed as a semistructured symptom-oriented interview that is used as an aid to the clinician who makes a clinical diagnosis on the basis of all available information. The disadvantage of this approach is that replicability cannot be assumed because of the degree of subjectivity involved in the diagnostic process. In any case, only highly trained clinicians who are very familiar with differential diagnosis would be acceptable interviewers. In fact, Kovacs points out that the ISC may be most valuable to researchers who need the flexibility offered by the semistructured approach and who desire to use the interview for the purpose of case selection. Also, it can be used successfully to track onset and offset of diagnoses using the procedure set out by Kovacs.

Schedule for Affective Disorders and Schizophrenia in School-Age Children

The K-SADS was modeled after an adult interview, the Schedule for Affective Disorders and Schizophrenia (SADS) (Endicott & Spitzer, 1978). The K-SADS (Puig-Antich & Chambers, 1978), which was developed by Puig-Antich and his colleagues, has been revised twice to make changes in the interview (1984 and 1986) and again to update it for DSM-III-R (1988). There are two versions of the K-SADS: the Epidemiological version (K-SADS-E) and the Present Episode version (K-SADS-P). In the K-SADS-E, each question is basically asked twice to determine whether the symptom is present currently and whether it was present in the past. In the K-SADS-P, each question is also scored twice to determine the symptom severity at its worst during the present episode of the illness (or the previous 12 months, whichever is shorter) and the symptom rating for the last week only. When the K-SADS-P is used to assess change, the rating for the last week is used. The authors suggest that both the Epidemiological and Present Episode versions be administered because the Epidemiological version does not assess levels of symptom severity.

The authors of the K-SADS recommend that the parent and the child each be interviewed by the same interviewer, with the parent seen first. To clarify any discrepancies, the interviewer may choose to see either informant alone or both together. "Summary ratings" are made for both time periods (e.g., at worst time and last week for the Present version), and these ratings are based on all sources of information (e.g., parent, child, school, medical chart) (Ambrosini, 1988). In the case of discrepancies, the interviewer is to use his "best clinical judgment" (Ambrosini, 1988). Thus, for each of the K-SADS versions, the interviewer makes six sets of scorings (Chambers et al., 1985). All diagnoses conform to either research Diagnostic Criteria (RDC) (Spitzer, Endicott, & Robins, 1978) or DSM-III-R. The K-SADS is described as semistructured because the interview questions are meant to be only a guide for questions that can be helpful and informative (Ambrosini, 1988). The rater is to ask as many questions as necessary to arrive at a well-documented rating, yet probing should be as neutral as possible.

Reliability. Test–retest reliability was generated for diagnoses and for symptom scores for a sample of children, ages 6–17, who were referred to a child and adolescent depression clinic (Chambers et al., 1985). The inter-interview interval was within 72 hours for all interviews. The reliability was in the fair range ($\kappa = 0.54$) for MDD and in the good range ($\kappa = 0.70$) for nonmajor depressive disorders, as defined by the RDC.

The same research group reported on the stability of a diagnosis of MDD over a 2-week period in medication studies in a preadolescent sample (Puig-Antich et al., 1987) and in an adolescent sample (Ryan et al., 1986). For the purposes of subject selection, potential subjects were evaluated twice, 2 weeks apart, with only those children who were diagnosed both times as having MDD being retained for the study. In both studies, approximately 20% of the subjects who were diagnosed in the first assessment did not meet diagnostic criteria in the second assessment 2 weeks later.

Parent–child diagnostic concordance was examined for the children of proband parents participating in the Yale family genetic study of depression (Weissman et al., 1987). However, the fact that the same interviewer administered the K-SADS to the parent as well as to the child flaws this study for the purposes of studying child–parent concordance. Also, in this study, approximately one half of the sample were 18–23 years old, and thus would be better described as young adult offspring. In any case, the κ values for MDD ranged from 0.11 to 0.47, depending on the age of the proband. Higher concordance was associated with adolescence and greater impairment, as measured by the CGAS (Weissman, Warner, & Fendrich, 1990). At 2 years after initial interviewing, the battery was readministered, and again the same group of interviewers interviewed the parent and child. The stability of recall of a lifetime diagnosis was moderate ($\kappa = 0.58$) for the cases in which a different interviewer from the group was used in the follow-up from the initial assessment. When strict impairment criteria were included for the diagnosis of depression, the κ value was reduced to 0.36 (Fendrich, Weissman, Warner, & Mufson, 1990).

Validity

Relationship to Other Measures. McCauley, Mitchell, Burke, and Moss (1988) reported a modest and significant correlation ($r = 0.39$) between the CDI and the K-SADS. There was a significant effect for the CDI across three groups of psychiatric patients: currently having MDD, having had an episode of MDD in the past year, and having diagnoses other than depression. Two child psychiatrists and a psychologist interviewed the children and determined diagnoses.

In an interesting study on mood variability in adolescents, Costello, Benjamin, Angold, and Silver (1991) identified three groups in a psychiatric inpatient sample (depressed, nondepressed, and comorbid for depression and disruptive disorders). The K-SADS was used in arriving at a clinical diagnosis. Contrary to expectations, there was no difference among the three groups in self-reported mood, assessed three times a day for 7 consecutive days. All three groups reported high levels of depressive symptoms.

The K-SADS has been used to identify samples of depressed children for studies assessing whether the biological markers that have been examined in depressed adults are observed in children. Potentially, a biological marker could be used as a "gold standard" for determining the presence of MDD. Unfortunately, in general, the findings, especially for sleep EEG and cortisol secretion (i.e., the dexamethasone suppression test), failed to support these biological factors as markers in childhood depression (Rutter, 1988).

Comparison to Alternatively Derived Diagnoses. In Carlson et al. (1987), the K-SADS conducted on admission to an inpatient unit was compared to a best-estimate diagnosis based on chart review at discharge. An experienced child psychiatrist generated diagnoses based on an integration of all available information and after having interviewed both the child and the parent with the K-SADS. Moderate concordance ($\kappa = 0.58$) was observed for "all affective disorders" (defined as MDD, DD, and Adjustment Disorder with Depressed Mood). Both the K-SADS interviewer and the clinician who conducted the chart review may have been highly influenced by the admission and referral records, to which both had access.

Comparison among Contrast Groups. In Garber, Zeman, and Walker (1990), healthy controls were found to have fewer diagnoses than three other groups: psychiatric controls, children with recurrent abdominal pain, and children with organic pain.

Course of Illness. On the basis of the Dunedin longitudinal data, McGee and Williams (1988) identified three groups of 9-year-olds who differed on depressive disorder (current depressive disorder, past depressive disorder, and no depressive disorder). At age 9, the children were administered the K-SADS section for depression by one of three psychiatrists. Diagnoses were consensus diagnoses made by two psychiatrists and were based on all available information. Children from the three groups were compared at ages 11 and 13, using the DISC. Both groups of children identified with depressive disorder, based on the K-SADS at 9 years of age, reported significantly more depressive symptoms than the comparison groups when reassessed at ages 11 and 13. These children also reported more disruptive behaviors. The K-SADS has been used to select subject groups in which follow-up inquiry was made about the children's status. In Asarnow et al. (1988), depressed children were compared to schizophrenia-spectrum disorders for rehospitalization rates. Depressed children had rehospitalization rates of 35% within 1 year and 45% within 2 years.

Hammen, Burge, Burney, and Adrian (1990) used the K-SADS in a study of offspring of depressed women. The K-SADS was administered at initial evaluation and every 6 months, with all follow-up interviews being conducted by telephone. Diagnosis was based on all available information, which included the interview, parent questionnaires, teacher questionnaires, reports from treating therapists, and any other available information. Diagnoses were made by consensus by a research team. While the interviewers, who were graduate students, were blind to parental diagnosis except in cases where it was disclosed by the subjects, it is not clear whether the research team members were. Children of depressed mothers were much more likely to have a diagnosis. The percentages of children receiving at least one lifetime diagnosis in each of the parental comparison groups were as follows: unipolar mothers, 82%; bipolar, 72%; medically ill, 43%; and normal, 32%. Across follow-ups, children of unipolar mothers displayed high rates of chronic and new disorders. When a continuous variable was used to measure outcome, the CDI was used or the presence or absence of diagnosis was converted to a 4-point scale (0 = no depression, 1 = mild nondiagnosable symptoms, 2 = mild dysthymia, and 3 = MDD or marked dysthymic disorder).

Summary and Item Scores Based on Child and Parent Interviews: Reliability

Chambers et al. (1985) reported reliability for depression summary scales, which reflect the final ratings given by the interviewer based on all information, including both child and parent interviews. The derived scales varied from 2 to 17 items, with test–retest reliability correlations ranging from 0.67 to 0.81 and internal consistency from 0.68 to 0.84. Ambrosini, Metz, Prabucki, and Lee (1989) reported on the internal consistency of the 9-, 12-, and 17-item scales for MDD. The α values were satisfactory, ranging from 0.76 to 0.89.

Parent–child agreement on symptom endorsement in the Yale family genetic study of depression is described in Angold et al. (1987). As mentioned earlier, the same interviewer conducted the interviews with the child and the parent. The κ statistics were calculated for the gate question for MDD (i.e., further questions for depression were asked only if the respondent answered positively) and for the remaining symptoms (referred to as Part B in DSM-III). The parent–child concordance for the gate question, which inquires about dysphoria and anhedonia, was fair (κ = 0.40). The agreement for the remaining symptoms was generally poor, with the 21 symptoms having κ values below 0.40 except for diurnal variation (κ = 0.52), thoughts of death (κ = 0.50), suicidal ideas (κ = 0.45), and suicide attempt (κ = 0.46). The authors describe the level of disagreement between parents and children as striking, especially given that they were interviewed by the same interviewer.

In Apter, Orvaschel, Laseg, Moses, and Tyano (1989), different interviewers, who were child psychiatry fellows, interviewed the adolescent and the mother. However, both interviewers reviewed all pertinent referral and emergency room material available, prior to administering the K-SADS. Diagnosis was based on the interviewing clinicians' judgment, based on all available information, as to the primary diagnosis. Parent–child concordance for the diagnosis of depression was not given; however, the agreement for all diagnoses was provided (κ = 0.42). Intraclass correlations for three depression-related scales ranged from 0.55 to 0.62. While the authors made an effort to have independent interviews, the findings may still be inflated by the fact that all interviewers may have been similarly influenced by the prior information that they all reviewed.

Ivens and Rehm (1988) examined child–parent concordance for a list of depression-related items. The κ values comparing mother and child ranged from 0.02 to 0.39, whereas the κ values between child and father ranged from −0.02 to 0.29.

Symptom Scores Based on Parent and Child Interviews: Validity

Intervention Studies. A series of studies on the efficacy of antidepressant medication for childhood and adolescent depression have utilized the K-SADS both to identify subjects (i.e., independent variable) and to measure outcome (e.g., average of the summary ratings for 9 items from the K-SADS). Since the findings of controlled, double-blind studies fail to indicate that antidepressants are clearly effective, these studies do not reflect on the validity of the K-SADS (e.g., Geller, Cooper, Graham, Marsteller, & Bryant, 1990; Geller et al., 1992; Puig-Antich et al., 1987; Ryan et al., 1986). Additionally, the fact that the antidepressant drugs have a documented benefit in the treatment of attention-deficit disorders (Pliszka, 1991; Rutter, 1988) means that any observed response to medication could not be assumed automatically to be validation of depression diagnosis.

The K-SADS was used in a treatment study comparing two types of group therapy for depressed adolescents: social-skills training and therapeutic group (Fine, Forth, Gilbert, & Haley, 1991). The K-SADS and the CDI were administered pretreatment, posttreatment, and at 9-month follow-up. The outcome variable used from the K-SADS was 12 items from the depression section. At posttreatment, there was a significant difference on the K-SADS scale between the groups, in favor of the therapeutic support group, whereas the results for the CDI were nonsignificant. At follow-up, there were no significant differences on either the K-SADS scale or the CDI.

Summary

The K-SADS is probably the most widely used interview for the study of depression. The reliability of the interview is satisfactory for both depression diagnoses and the symptom scales. The strongest validity data are provided by comparison to alternatively derived diagnoses and, to a lesser extent, course of illness. There are some preliminary data indicating the potential usefulness of depression symptom scale scores.

Like the ISC, the K-SADS is meant to be used only by highly trained professionals who are qualified at assigning clinical diagnoses, which are to be based on all available information. These procedures basically use the "LEAD" model described by Spitzer (1983), which is an acronym for using an Expert diagnostician who utilizes All Data collected during more than a single examination (i.e., Longitudinally) to generate diagnoses. Used in this way, the K-SADS appears to be quite acceptable for the purpose of subject selection, which is the typical use.

The disadvantages of this approach include the variability and subjective judgment reflected in the specific techniques for resolving discrepancies (e.g., confronting the child with the mother present), the process of giving differential weights to reports from various informants, and the degree to which the DSM criteria are strictly adhered to (vs. clinical wisdom applied in interpreting the criteria). For purposes of monitoring change in diagnosis or symptoms over time, these subjective elements potentially are much more problematic than when the purpose is solely to distinguish depressed from nondepressed youth.

Children's Depression Rating Scale—Revised

The CDRS (Poznanski et al., 1979) is a clinician-rated scale that yields a summed score indicating severity of depression. It was modeled after the Hamilton Depression Rating Scale (Hamilton, 1960), which was developed to assess depression in adults. In 1984, Poznanski (1984) introduced a revised version of the scale (CDRS-R) that includes a set of questions to ask the child and permits a 7-point, rather than 5-point, rating system for most response items (Poznanski et al., 1984). A subsequent revision added an additional item, resulting in 15 items that are rated on the basis of verbal responses of the interviewees and 3 items that are rated by the clinician on the basis of observation of the child's nonverbal behavior (Poznanski, 1990). The summed total score on the CDRS-R can range between 18 and 118 points, with a score of 40 or more generally indicating clinical depression and a score over 60 indicating severe depression (Poznanski et al., 1984). While Poznanski recommends that the CDRS be based on all available sources of information, she also stresses that emphasis be placed on the child's report.

The psychometric information on the CDRS-R includes data on test–retest reliability, parent–child concordance, and concurrent validity. For a sample of psychiatric outpatients, the CDRS was administered 2 weeks apart by different psychiatrists (Poznanski et al., 1984). Test–retest reliability for the total score was high ($r = 0.86$, $N = 32$).

Data on interinformant reliability have mostly reflected poor child–parent agreement. In a nonclinical sample, children and their parents were independently interviewed, and the CDRS-R was rated by clinicians blind to each other's results (Mokros, Poznanski, Grossman, & Freeman, 1987). For 14 items of the CDRS-R, parent–child agreement was examined in terms of symptom severity (i.e., Pearson correlations between the item ratings) and symptom presence or absence (i.e., a rating of 3 or higher indicating presence of a clinically significant symptom). For the items, the correlations between parent and child ratings ranged from −0.01 to 0.42, with a correlation of 0.38 between child and parent summary scores. The κ values were under 0.40 for all but one item. Similar levels of child–parent agreement were reported for a sample of children referred to a depression clinic (Mokros et al., 1987). In another study (Stark, Reynolds, & Kaslow, 1987), the correlation between the CDRS-R based on the children's report and the Depression scale of the CBCL was poor ($r = 0.09$).

In Shain, Naylor, and Alessi (1990), clinician-rated CDRS-R and self-report on the CDI were compared in an adolescent inpatient sample. A significant correlation ($r = 0.89$) was observed for females, but not for males ($r = 0.41$). The results of a study of depression and anxiety in hospitalized pediatric patients suggest that the CDRS-R may not have good discriminant validity in terms of differentiating depression and anxiety (Eason, Finch, Brasted, & Saylor, 1985).

The CDRS-R has been used in numerous medication treatment studies to assess change in severity of depression. However, as mentioned above, these studies do not provide good evidence of validity (e.g., Geller et al., 1990). The CDRS-R was also used in a treatment study comparing wait-list controls to self-control therapy and behavioral problem-solving therapy (Stark et al., 1987). Group treatment was conducted in the public school with children identified by self-report screening measures. At posttesting, there was no significant difference among the three conditions; however, pre-to-post comparisons revealed significant improvement for the two experimental conditions, but none for the wait-list group.

The CDRS-R was administered on admission and every 2 weeks thereafter in a study of adolescent inpatients, who were classified as either chronically or acutely depressed on the basis of history at admission (Shain, King, Naylor, & Alessi, 1991). Chronically depressed adolescents had a significantly slower initial rate of improvement, as defined by a CDRS-R score of 40 or higher, than did the acutely depressed.

Summary

The CDRS-R is relatively easy to use, either by itself or in conjunction with one of the diagnostic interviews. The test–retest reliability of the total score is satisfactory. Given the usefulness of this scale, there are surprisingly limited data on its psychometric properties, especially validity. It shares some of the same dilemmas as do the interviews that encourage diagnosis by the LEAD model.

Conclusions

Studying the psychometric properties of the diagnostic interviews is an ongoing process. With continued efforts, we will be able to provide better information about the relative strengths and weaknesses of each interview, given the particulars of any given study, including the sample characteristics, the research questions of interest, and the availability of various resources.

For studies in which the interview is used for subject selection (depressed vs. nondepressed), all the interviews could at present be used with some comfort, except perhaps the Diagnostic Interview Schedule for Children (DISC). All of them offer some standardization to the interview content and diagnostic criteria. Additionally, each provides for differential diagnosis, which is critical given the comorbidity observed for depression. For the most part, the Schedule for Affective Disorders and Schizophrenia in School-Age Children (K-SADS) and the Interview Schedule for Children (ISC) have been used when a homogeneous group of depressed youths is to be studied. Very few data exist for validity of the subtypes of depression, except for the ISC. However, replication by other research groups or with a design offering more safeguards against bias would add more weight to these findings with the ISC.

None of the interviews has demonstrated superiority in monitoring change in depression or depression symptoms. In fact, the psychometric properties of depression symptom scales have been studied only for the Child Assessment Schedule (CAS), DISC, and K-SADS. It is surprising that the Children's Depression Inventory (CDI) has been used to assess severity of depression in studies in which these diagnostic interviews have been used.

If information other than diagnosis is of interest, then the CAS is potentially advantageous because of the content scales, reflecting on adjustment across life areas, for which there are psychometric data (see also Hodges & Zeman, 1993). As a result, the CAS has been used in samples that are most likely heterogeneous for diagnosis and that may have subclinical symptoms that would likely be demonstrated via symptom scales (e.g., sexually abused, medically ill, homeless).

If resources are not an issue, then any of the interviews is acceptable. For the K-SADS and the ISC, only highly trained clinicians can be used. However, there need to be enough professionals available so that the diagnoses can be made blind to data relevant to the hypotheses. This is particularly a problem when the interviews are used for purposes other than initial assessment. The CAS and the Diagnostic Interview for Children and Adolescents (DICA) can be administered by trained interviewers who are not necessarily qualified to generate diagnoses, since computer-generated diagnoses as well as clinician-based diagnoses can be made with either. The DISC purportedly can be used with lay interviewers who have no knowledge of diagnostically related issues; however, some users of the DISC (e.g., Breslau, 1987) have demonstrated problems with false-positives when the interview is used in this way.

As the data base about childhood and adolescent depression expands, the task of psychometrically assessing the various interviews will become easier. At present, both the validation of the depression diagnoses and the procedural validation of the interviews are taking place simultaneously. In addition, we are making gains in related issues, including developing guidelines for integrating information from various informants and approaches to assessing impairment. It is to be hoped that these efforts will bring us closer to the goal of understanding the mental health needs of children.

References

Achenbach, T. M., & Edelbrock, C. (1983). *Manual for the Child Behavior Checklist and Revised Child Behavior Profile*. Burlington, CT: Queen City Printers.

Achenbach, T. M., & Edelbrock, C. D. (1987). *Manual for the Youth Self-Report and Profile*. Burlington, Vermont: University Associates in Psychiatry.

Achenbach, T. M., McCounaghy, S., & Howell, C. (1987). Child/adolescent behavioral and emotional problems: Implications of cross informant correlations for situational specificity. *Psychological Bulletin, 101*, 213–232.

Ambrosini, P. J. (1988). Schedule for Affective Disorders and Schizophrenia for School Aged Children— Present version. Unpublished manuscript.

Ambrosini, P. J., Metz, C., Prabucki, K., & Lee, J. (1989). Video tape reliability of the third revised edition of the K-SADS. *Journal of the American Academy of Child and Adolescent Psychiatry, 28*, 723–728.

American Psychiatric Association (1980). *Diagnostic and statistical manual of mental disorders*, 3rd ed. Washington, DC: Author.

American Psychiatric Association (1987). *Diagnostic and statistical manual of mental disorders*, 3rd ed., revised. Washington, DC: Author.

Angold, A., Weissman, M. M., John, K., Merikangas, K. R., Prusoff, B. A., Wickramaratne, P., Gammon, G. D., & Warner, V. (1987). Parent and child reports of depressive symptoms in children at low and high risk of depression. *Journal of Child Psychology and Psychiatry, 28*, 901–915.

Apter, A., Orvaschel, H., Laseg, M., Moses, T., & Tyano, S. (1989). Psychometric properties of the K-SADS-P in an Israeli adolescent inpatient population. *Journal of the American Academy of Child and Adolescent Psychiatry, 28*, 61–65.

Asarnow, J. R., & Carlson, G. A. (1985). Depression self-rating scale: Utility with child psychiatric inpatients. *Journal of Consulting and Clinical Psychology, 53*, 491–499.

Asarnow, J. R., Goldstein, M. J., Carlson, G. A., Perdue, S., Bates, S., & Keller, J. (1988). Childhood-onset depressive disorders: A follow up study of rates of rehospitalization and out-of-home placement among child psychiatric inpatients. *Journal of Affective Disorders, 15*, 245–253.

Barrera, M., Jr., & Garrison-Jones, C. V. (1988). Properties of the Beck Depression Inventory as a screening instrument for adolescent depression. *Journal of Abnormal Child Psychology, 16*, 263–273.

Bartko, J. J., & Carpenter, W. T., Jr. (1976). On the methods and theory of reliability. *Journal of Nervous and Mental Disease, 163*, 307–317.

Beck, A., & Beamesderfer, A. (1974). Assessment of depression: The depression inventory. *Psychological Measurements in Psychopharmacology, 7*, 151–169.

Bird, H. R., Canino, G., Gould, M. S., Ribera, J., Rubio-Stipec, M., Woodbury, M., Huertas-Goldman, S., & Sesman, M. (1987). Use of the Child Behavior Checklist as a screening instrument for epidemiological research in child psychiatry: Results of a pilot study. *Journal of the American Academy of Child and Adolescent Psychiatry, 26*, 207–213.

Bird, H., Gould, M., Yager, T., Staghezza, B., & Canino, G. (1989). Risk factors for maladjustment in Puerto Rican children. *Journal of the American Academy of Child and Adolescent Psychiatry, 28*, 847–850.

Birleson, P. (1981). The validity of depressive disorder in childhood and the development of a self-rating scale: A research report. *Journal of Child Psychology and Psychiatry, 22*, 73–88.

Blumberg, S. H., & Izard, C. E. (1985). Affective and cognitive characteristics of depression in 10- and 11-year-old children. *Journal of Personality and Social Psychology, 49*, 194–202.

Breslau, N. (1987). Inquiring about the bizarre: False positives in Diagnostic Interview Schedule for Children (DISC) ascertainment of obsessions, compulsions, and psychotic symptoms. *Journal of the American Academy of Child and Adolescent Psychiatry, 26*, 639–644.

Brunshaw, J. M., & Szatmari, P. (1988). The agreement between behaviour checklists and structured psychiatric interviews for children. *Canadian Journal of Psychiatry, 33*, 474–480.

Cantwell, D. P., & Baker, L. (1989). Stability and natural history of DSM-III childhood diagnoses. *Journal of the American Academy of Child and Adolescent Psychiatry, 28*, 691–700.

Carey, T. C., Finch, A. J., & Carey, M. P. (1991). Relation between differential emotions and depression in emotionally disturbed children and adolescents. *Journal of Consulting and Clinical Psychology, 59*, 594–597.

Carlson, G., Kashani, J., Thomas, M., Vaidya, A., & Daniel, A. (1987). Comparison of two structured interviews on a psychiatrically hospitalized population of children. *Journal of the American Academy of Child and Adolescent Psychiatry, 26*, 645–648.

Chambers, W. J., Puig-Antich, J., Hirsch, M., Paez, P. Ambrosini, P. J., Tabrizi, M. A., & Davies, M. (1985). The assessment of affective disorders in children and adolescents by semi-structured interview: Test–retest reliability of the Schedule for Affective Disorders and Schizophrenia for School Age Children, Present Episode Version. *Archives of General Psychiatry, 42*, 696–702.

Cohen, P., O'Connor, P., Lewis, S., Velez, C., & Malachowski, B. (1987). Comparison of DISC and K-SADS-P interviews of an epidemiological sample of children. *Journal of the American Academy of Child and Adolescent Psychiatry, 26*, 662–667.

Costello, E. J., Benjamin, R., Angold, A., & Silver, D. (1991). Mood variability in adolescents: A study of depressed, nondepressed & comorbid patients. *Journal of Affective Disorders, 23*, 199–212.

Costello, E. J., Costello, A. J., Edelbrock, C., Burns, B. J., Dulcan, M. K., Brent, D., & Janiszewski, S. (1988). Psychiatric disorders in pediatric primary care. *Archives of General Psychiatry, 45*, 1107–1116.

Costello, E. J., Edelbrock, C. S., & Costello, A. J. (1985). Validity of the NIMH diagnostic interview schedule for children: A comparison between psychiatric and pediatric referrals. *Journal of Abnormal Child Psychology, 13*, 579–595.

Costello, E. J., Edelbrock, C., Costello, A., Dulcan, M., & Brent, D. (1986). *The diagnosis and management of psychopathology in children in an organized primary health care setting.* [Contract No. 278-83-0006 (DB)]. Rockville, MD: Division of Biometry and Applied Sciences, National Institute of Mental Health.

Costello, A. J., Edelbrock, L. S., Dulcan, M. K., Kalas, R., & Klaric, S. H. (1984). *Report on the NIMH Diagnostic Interview Schedule for Children (DISC)*. Washington, DC: National Institute of Mental Health.

Coyne, J., & Downey, G. (1991). Social factors and psychopathology: Stress, social support, and coping processes. *Annual Review of Psychology, 42*, 401–425.

Earls, F., Reich, W., Jung, K. G., & Cloninger, C. (1988). Psychopathology in children of alcoholic and antisocial parents. *Alcoholism: Clinical and Experimental Research, 12*, 481–487.

Eason, L. J., Finch, A. J., Jr., Brasted, W., & Saylor, C. F. (1985). The assessment of depression and anxiety in hospitalized pediatric patients. *Child Psychiatry and Human Development, 16*, 57–64.

Edelbrock, C., & Costello, A. J. (1988). Structured psychiatric interview for children. In M. Rutter, A. H. Tuma, & I. S. Lann (Eds.), *Assessment and diagnosis in child psychopathology* (pp. 87–112). New York: Guilford Press.

Edelbrock, C., Costello, A. J., Dulcan, M., Conover, N. C., & Kalas, R. (1986). Parent–child agreement on child psychiatric symptoms assessed via structured interview. *Journal of Child Psychology and Psychiatry, 27*, 181–190.

Edelbrock, C., Costello, A. J., Dulcan, M., Kalas, R., & Conover, N. C. (1985). Age differences in the reliability of the psychiatric interview of the child. *Child Development, 56*, 265–275.

Endicott, J., & Spitzer, R. L. (1978). A diagnostic interview: The Schedule for Affective Disorders and Schizophrenia. *Archives of General Psychiatry, 35,* 837–844.

Fieghner, J. P., Robins, E., Gerze, S. B., Woodruff, R. A., Winokur, G., & Munoz, R. (1972). Diagnostic criteria for use in psychiatric research. *Archives of General Psychiatry, 26,* 57–63.

Fendrich, M., Weissman, M. M., Warner, V., & Mufson, L. (1990). Two-year recall of lifetime diagnoses in offspring with high and low risk for major depression. *Archives of General Psychiatry, 47,* 1121–1127.

Fine, S., Forth, A., Gilbert, M., & Haley, G. (1991). Group therapy for adolescent depressive disorder: A comparison of social skills and therapeutic support. *Journal of the American Academy of Child and Adolescent Psychiatry, 30,* 79–85.

Fleiss, J. L. (1981). *Statistical methods for rates and proportions,* 2nd ed. New York: John Wiley.

Garber, J., Zeman, J., & Walker, L. S. (1990). Recurrent abdominal pain in children: Psychiatric diagnoses and parental psychopathology. *Journal of the American Academy of Child and Adolescent Psychiatry, 29,* 648–656.

Geller, B., Cooper, T. B., Graham, D. L., Fetner, H. H., Marsteller, F. A., & Wells, J. M. (1992). Pharmaco-kinetically designed double-blind placebo-controlled study of nortriptyline in 6- to 12-year-olds with major depressive disorder. *Journal of the American Academy of Child and Adolescent Psychiatry, 31,* 34–44.

Geller, B., Cooper, T. B., Graham, D. L., Marsteller, F. A., & Bryant, D. M. (1990). Double-blind placebo-controlled study of nortriptyline in depressed adolescents using a "fixed plasma level" design. *Psychopharmacology Bulletin, 26,* 85–90.

Hamilton, M. (1960). A rating scale for depression. *Journal of Neurological and Neurosurgical Psychiatry, 23,* 56–62.

Hammen, C., Burge, D., Burney, E., & Adrian, C. (1990). Longitudinal study of diagnoses in children of women with unipolar and bipolar affective disorder. *Archives of General Psychiatry, 47,* 1112–1117.

Helzer, J. E., Robins, L. N., Croughan, J. L., & Welner, A. (1981). Renard diagnostic interview: Its reliability and procedural validity with physicians and lay interviewers. *Archives of General Psychiatry, 38,* 393–398.

Herjanic, B., Herjanic, M., Brown, F., & Wheatt, T. (1975). Are children reliable reporters? *Journal of Abnormal Child Psychology, 3,* 41–48.

Hodges, K. (1983). Guidelines to aid in establishing inter-rater reliability with the Child Assessment Schedule. Unpublished manuscript.

Hodges, K. (1986). Guidelines to aid in establishing inter-rater reliability with the Child Assessment Schedule, 2nd ed. Unpublished manuscript.

Hodges, K. (1990a). Guidelines to aid in establishing inter-rater reliability with the Child Assessment Schedule, 3rd ed. Unpublished manuscript.

Hodges, K. (1990b). Depression and anxiety in children: A comparison of self-report questionnaires to clinical interview. *Psychological Assessment: A Journal of Consulting and Clinical Psychology, 2,* 376–381.

Hodges, K., Cools, J., & McKnew, D. (1989). Test–retest reliability of a clinical research interview for children: The Child Assessment Schedule (CAS). *Psychological Assessment: A Journal of Consulting and Clinical Psychology, 1,* 317–322.

Hodges, K., & Craighead, W. E. (1990). Relationship of Children's Depression Inventory factors to diagnosed depression. *Psychological Assessment: A Journal of Consulting and Clinical Psychology, 2,* 489–492.

Hodges, K., & Fitch, P. (1979). Development of a mental status examination interview for children. Paper presented at the meeting of the Missouri Psychological Association, Kansas City, MO.

Hodges, K., Gordon, Y., & Lennon, M. (1990). Parent–child agreement on symptoms assessed via a clinical research interview for children: The Child Assessment Schedule (CAS). *Journal of Child Psychology and Psychiatry, 31,* 427–436.

Hodges, K., Kline, J., Stern, L., Cytryn, L., & McKnew, D. (1982). The development of a child assessment interview for research and clinical use. *Journal of Abnormal Child Psychology, 10,* 173–189.

Hodges, K., McKnew, D., Burbach, D. J., & Roebuck, L. (1987). Diagnostic concordance between the Child Assessment Schedule (CAS) and the Schedule for Affective Disorders and Schizophrenia for School-Aged Children (K-SADS) in an outpatient sample using lay interviewers. *Journal of the American Academy of Child and Adolescent Psychiatry, 26,* 654–661.

Hodges, K., & Saunders, W. (1989). Internal consistency of a diagnostic interview for children: The Child Assessment Schedule (CAS) *Journal of Abnormal Child Psychology, 17,* 691–701.

Hodges, K., Saunders, W., Kashani, J., Hamlett, K., & Thompson, R. (1990). Internal consistency of DSM-III diagnoses using the symptom scales of the Child Assessment Schedule (CAS). *Journal of the American Academy of Child and Adolescent Psychiatry, 29,* 635–641.

Hodges, K., & Zeman, J. (1993). Interviewing. In M. Hersen & T. H. Ollendick (Eds.), *Handbook of child and adolescent assessment* (pp. 65–81). Boston, Massachusetts: Allyn & Bacon.

Ivens, C., & Rehm, L. P. (1988). Assessment of childhood depression: Correspondence between reports by child, mother, and father. *Journal of the American Academy of Child and Adolescent Psychiatry, 27,* 738–741.

Kashani, J. H., Beck, N. C., Hoeper, E. W., Fallahi, C., Corcoran, C. M., McAllister, J. A., Rosenberg, T. K., & Reid, J. C. (1987). Psychiatric disorders in a community sample of adolescents. *American Journal of Psychiatry, 144,* 584–589.

Kashani, J. H., Orvaschel, H., Burk, J. P., & Reid, J. C. (1985). Informant variance: The issue of parent–child disagreement. *Journal of the American Academy of Child Psychiatry, 24,* 437–441.

Kashani, J. H., Orvaschel, H., Rosenberg, T. K., & Reid, J. C. (1989). Psychopathology in a community sample of children and adolescents: A developmental perspective. *Journal of the American Academy of Child and Adolescent Psychiatry, 28,* 701–706.

Kashani, J., Rosenberg, T., & Reid, J. (1989). Developmental perspectives in child and adolescent depressive symptoms in a community sample. *American Journal of Psychiatry, 146,* 871–875.

Kovacs, M. (1981). Ratings scales to assess depression in school-aged children. *Acta Paedopsychiatrica (Basel), 46,* 305–315.

Kovacs, M. (1983). The Interview Schedule for Children (ISC): Interrater and parent–child agreement. Unpublished manuscript. University of Pittsburgh.

Kovacs, M. (1985). The Interview Schedule for Children. *Psychopharmacology Bulletin, 21,* 991–994.

Kovacs, M., Feinberg, T. L., Crouse-Novak, M. A., Paulauskas, S. L., & Finkelstein, R. (1984). Depressive disorders in childhood. I. A longitudinal study of characteristics and recovery. *Archives of General Psychiatry, 41,* 229–237.

Kovacs, M., Iyengar, S., Goldston, Obrosky, D. S., Stewart, J., & Marsh, J. (1990). Psychological functioning among mothers of children with insulin-dependent diabetes mellitus: A longitudinal study. *Journal of Consulting and Clinical Psychology, 58,* 189–195.

Kronenberg, Y., Blumensohn, R., & Apter, A. (1988). A comparison of different diagnostic tools for childhood depression. *Acta Psychiatrica Scandinavica, 77,* 194–198.

Lachar, D., & Gdowski, C. L. (1979). *Actuarial assessment of child and adolescent personality: An interpretive guide for the Personality Inventory for Children Profile.* Los Angeles: Western Psychological Services.

Last, C. G. (1987). Developmental considerations. In G. Last & M. Hersen (Eds.), *Issues in diagnostic research* (pp. 201–216). New York: Plenum Press.

Last, C. G., Strauss, C. C., & Francis, G. (1987). Comorbidity among childhood anxiety disorders. *Journal of Nervous and Mental Disease, 175,* 726–730.

Lee, C. M., & Gotlib, I. H. (1991). Adjustment of children of depressed mothers: A 10-month follow-up. *Journal of Abnormal Psychology, 100,* 473–477.

McCauley, E., Mitchell, J. R., Burke, P., & Moss, S. (1988). Cognitive attributes of depression in children and adolescents. *Journal of Consulting and Clinical Psychology, 56,* 903–908.

McGee, R., & Williams, S. (1988). A longitudinal study of depression in nine-year-old children. *Journal of the American Academy of Child and Adolescent Psychiatry, 27,* 342–348.

Mokros, H. B., Poznanski, E., Grossman, J. A., & Freeman, L. N. (1987). A comparison of child and adolescent parent ratings of depression for normal and clinically referred children. *Journal of Child Psychology and Psychiatry, 28,* 613–627.

Paulauskas, S. L., & Kovacs, M. (1984). The Interview Schedule for Children (ISC): A symptom-oriented psychiatric interview. Paper presented at the American Psychology Association Conference, Toronto, Canada, August 1984.

Pliszka, S. R. (1991). Antidepressants in the treatment of child and adolescent psychopathology. *Journal of Clinical Child Psychology, 20,* 313–320.

Poznanski, E. O. (1984). Children's depression rating scale. Unpublished manuscript.

Poznanski, E. O. (1990). Children's depression rating scale, revised ed. Unpublished manuscript.

Poznanski, E., Cook, S. C., & Carroll, B. J. (1979). A depression rating scale for children. *Pediatrics, 64,* 442–450.

Poznanski, E., Grossman, J. A., Buchsbaum, Y., Banegas, M., Freeman, L., & Gibbons, R. (1984). Preliminary studies of the reliability and validity of the children's depression rating scale. *Journal of the American Academy of Child Psychiatry, 23,* 191–197.

Puig-Antich, J., & Chambers, W. (1978). *The Schedule for Affective Disorders and Schizophrenia for School-Age Children (Kiddie-SADS).* New York: New York State Psychiatric Institute.

Puig-Antich, J., Goetz, D., Davies, M., Kaplan, T., Davies, S., Ostrow, L., Asnis, L., Twomey, J., Iyengar, S., & Ryan,

N. D. (1989). A controlled family history study of prepubertal major depressive disorder. *Archives of General Psychiatry, 46,* 406–418.

Puig-Antich, J., Perel, J. M., Lupatkin, W., Chambers, W. J., Tabrizi, M. A., King, J., Goetz, R., Davies, M., & Stiller, R. L. (1987). Imipramine in prepubertal major depressive disorders. *Archives of General Psychiatry, 44,* 81–89.

Radke-Yarrow, M., Nottelmann, E., Martinez, P., Fox, M. B., & Belmont, B. (1992). Young children of affectively ill parents: A longitudinal study of psychosocial development. *Journal of the American Academy of Child and Adolescent Psychiatry, 31,* 68–77.

Reich, W. (1988). *DIS Newsletter, 5(2),* 8–9.

Robins, L. N. (1985). Epidemiology: Reflections on testing the validity of psychiatric interviews. *Archives of General Psychiatry, 42,* 918–924.

Robins, L., Helzer, J., Croughan, J., & Ratcliff, K. (1981). National Institute of Mental Health Diagnostic Interview Schedule: Its history, characteristics, and validity. *Archives of General Psychiatry, 38,* 381–389.

Runyan, D., Everson, M., Edelsohn, G., Hunter, W., & Coulter, M. (1988). Impact of legal intervention on sexually abused children. *Journal of Pediatrics, 113,* 647–653.

Rutter, M. (1986a). Depressive feelings, cognitions, and disorders: A research postscript. In M. Rutter, C. E. Izard, & P. B. Read (Eds.), *Depression in young people* (pp. 491–519). New York: Guilford Press.

Rutter, M. (1986b). The developmental psychopathology of depression: Issues and perspectives. In M. Rutter, C. E. Izard, & P. B. Read (Eds.), *Depression in young people* (pp. 3–30). New York: Guilford Press.

Rutter, M. (1988). Depressive disorders. In M. Rutter, A. H. Tuma, & I. S. Lann (Eds.), *Assessment and diagnosis in child psychopathology* (pp. 347–376). New York: Guilford Press.

Ryan, N. D., Puig-Antich, J., Cooper, T., Rabinovich, H., Ambrosini, P., Davies, M., King, J., Torres, D., & Fried, J. (1986). Imipramine in adolescent major depression: Plasma level and clinical response. *Acta Psychiatrica Scandinavica, 73,* 275–288.

Shaffer, D., Gould, M. S., Brasic, J., Ambrosini, P., Fisher, P., Bird, H., & Aluwahlia, S. (1983). A Children's Global Assessment Scale (CGAS). *Archives of General Psychiatry, 40,* 1228–1231.

Shaffer, D., Schwab-Stone, M., Fisher, P., Davies, M., Piacentini, J., & Gioia, P. (1988). *Results of a field trial and proposals for a new instrument (DISC-R).* Washington, DC: National Institute of Mental Health (Grant Nos. MH 36971 & MH CRC 30906-10).

Shain, B. N., King, C. A., Naylor, M., & Alessi, N. (1991). Chronic depression and hospital course in adolescents. *Journal of the American Academy of Child and Adolescent Psychiatry, 30,* 428–433.

Shain, B. N., Naylor, M., & Alessi, N. (1990). Comparison of self-rated and clinician-rated measures of depression in adolescents. *American Journal of Psychiatry, 147,* 793–795.

Smucker, M. R., & Craighead, W. R. (1990). Factor analysis of the Children's Depression Inventory. Unpublished manuscript.

Spielberger, C. D. (1973). *Preliminary manual for the State–Trait Anxiety Inventory for Children.* Palo Alto, CA: Consulting Psychologists Press.

Spitzer, R. L. (1983). Psychiatric diagnosis: Are clinicians still necessary? *Comprehensive Psychiatry, 24,* 399–411.

Spitzer, R. L., Endicott, J., & Robins, E. (1975). Clinical criteria for psychiatric diagnosis and DSM-III. *American Journal of Psychiatry, 132,* 1187–1192.

Spitzer, R. L., Endicott, J., & Robins, E. (1978). Research diagnostic criteria: Rationale and reliability. *Archives of General Psychiatry, 35,* 773–782.

Stark, K. D., Reynolds, W. M., & Kaslow, N. J. (1987). A comparison of the relative efficacy of self-control therapy and a behavioral problem-solving therapy for depression in children. *Journal of Abnormal Child Psychology, 15,* 91–113.

Sylvester, C., Hyde, T., & Reichler, R. (1987). The Diagnostic Interview for Children and Personality Inventory for Children in studies of children at risk for anxiety disorders or depression. *Journal of the American Academy of Child and Adolescent Psychiatry, 26,* 668–675.

Thompson, R., Hodges, K., & Hamlett, K. (1990). A matched comparison of adjustment in children with cystic fibrosis and psychiatrically referred and nonreferred children. *Journal of Pediatric Psychology, 15,* 745–759.

Velez, C. N., Johnson, J., & Cohen, P. (1989). A longitudinal analysis of selected risk factors for childhood psychopathology. *Journal of the American Academy of Child and Adolescent Psychiatry, 28,* 861–864.

Verhulst, F. C., Althaus, M., & Berden, G. (1987). The Child Assessment Schedule: Parent–child agreement and validity measures. *Journal of Child Psychology and Psychiatry, 28,* 455–466.

Verhulst, F. C., Bieman, H. V., Ende, J. V. D., Berden, G. F. M. G., & Sanders-Woudstra, J. (1990). Problem behavior in international adoptees. III. Diagnosis of child psychiatric disorders. *Journal of the American Academy of Child and Adolescent Psychiatry, 29*, 420–428.

Vitiello, B., Malone, R., Buschle, P. R., Delaney, M. A., & Behar, D. (1990). Reliability of DSM-III diagnoses of hospitalized children. *Hospital and Community Psychiatry, 41*, 63–67.

Weinstein, S. R., Noam, G. G., Grimes, K., Stone, K., & Schwab-Stone, M. (1990). Convergence of DSM-III diagnoses and self-reported symptoms in child and adolescent inpatients. *Journal of the American Academy of Child and Adolescent Psychiatry, 29*, 627–634.

Weinstein, S. R., Stone, K., Noam, G. G., Grimes, K., & Schwab-Stone, M. (1989). Comparison of DISC with clinicians' DSM-III diagnoses in psychiatric inpatients. *Journal of the American Academy of Child and Adolescent Psychiatry, 28*, 153–160.

Weissman, M. M., Warner, V., & Fendrich, M. (1990). Applying impairment criteria to children's psychiatric diagnosis. *Journal of the American Academy of Child and Adolescent Psychiatry, 29*, 789–795.

Weissman, M. M., Wickramaratne, P., Warner, V., John, K., Prusoff, B. A., Merikangas, K. R., & Gammon, G. D. (1987). Assessing psychiatric disorders in children: Discrepancies between mothers' and children's reports. *Archives of General Psychiatry, 44*, 747–753.

Welner, Z., Reich, W., Herjanic, B., Jung, K. G., & Amado, H. (1987). Reliability, validity, and parent–child agreement studies of the Diagnostic Interview for Children and Adolescents (DICA). *Journal of the American Academy of Child and Adolescent Psychiatry, 26*, 649–653.

Williams, S., McGee, R., Anderson, J., & Silva, P. A. (1989). The structure and correlates of self-reported symptoms in 11-year-old children. *Journal of Abnormal Child Psychology, 17*, 55–71.

Zahn-Waxler, C., Mayfield, A., Radke-Yarrow, M., McKnew, D. H., Cytryn, L., & Davenport, Y. B. (1988). A follow up investigation of offspring of parents with bipolar disorder. *American Journal of Psychiatry, 145*, 506–509.

11

Assessment of Depression in Children and Adolescents by Self-Report Questionnaires

William M. Reynolds

Introduction

Virtually all research and clinical work with depressed children and adolescents utilizes assessment procedures. Assessment is a basic process for determining the presence or absence of depression and depressive symptoms in children and adolescents. Assessment as a process encompasses both formal and informal procedures for making decisions about persons. As measures for the assessment of depression are discussed in this chapter, it should be recognized that assessment as a process does not occur in isolation. The assessment of depression in youngsters, as with other clinical domains and populations, is a complex interaction of the individual being evaluated, the assessment methods, the clinician or evaluators, and the setting events, as well as prior experiences and the reason for the assessment.

This chapter describes self-report measures used to evaluate depressive symptoms in children and adolescents. This being the case, the measures reviewed herein do not provide formal diagnosis of depression as a disorder in youngsters. Assessment, whether by self-report, clinical interview, or other methodology, is critical for the clinical evaluation of depression as well as for research designed to enhance our understanding of depression in young people. To help children and youth who are depressed and in a state of significant psychological distress, we must first identify these youngsters. This is an important goal of professionals who are dedicated to the psychological well-being of children and adoles- cents. Because of the importance of assessment, the tools we use to identify distressed youngsters must be psychometrically sound and linguistically appropriate, otherwise we

William M. Reynolds • Psychoeducational Research and Training Centre, University of British Columbia, Vancouver, British Columbia V6T 1Z4, Canada.

Handbook of Depression in Children and Adolescents, edited by William M. Reynolds and Hugh F. Johnston. Plenum Press, New York, 1994.

risk missing those children and adolescents who may be in need of psychological assistance.

Assessment also provides us with a means to evaluate the effectiveness of interventions designed to ameliorate depression in young people. The effectiveness of treatments for psychological disorders such as depression can best be determined by the utilization of valid and reliable assessment procedures (Reynolds & Stark, 1983). This requirement suggests that outcome measures of depression used in treatment research must demonstrate high levels of reliability and validity.

There are a number of characteristics unique to depression that support the use of and need for self-report assessment procedures. Depression as an internalizing disorder encompasses many symptoms that are internal to the youngster and are not easily observable. Cognitive symptoms of guilt, self-deprecation, suicidal ideation, hopelessness, and feelings of worthlessness are among the symptoms of depression that are subjective to the child and hard to notice unless a formal evaluation is conducted. Similarly, some somatic symptoms such as insomnia, appetite loss, and other problems are sometimes difficult for others to observe and may go undetected by parents and significant others. Another aspect of depression in youngsters that points to the need for assessment is the general lack of self-awareness of their psychological condition along with the lack of self-referral for mental health problems by children and adolescents. This circumstance results in many youngsters having a feeling that their life is quite miserable, but unaware that they may have a mental health problem, or that they should let someone know so that some treatment can be provided to remediate this condition. We cannot expect children to know the symptoms of depression and, if these symptoms occur, to tell an adult. Thus, we must have procedures for the formal evaluation of these symptoms, using methods that are reliable and valid for the purpose of our evaluation.

The assessment of depression is a critical component for the identification of affected youngsters, as well as for research designed to enhance our understanding of the nature of this disorder in young people. The manner in which we assess depression in youngsters guides how we operationalize our perspective of depressive phenomena. For the determination of depression according to formal classification criteria that includes both inclusion and exclusion components, the standard practice has been the use of structured clinical interviews. Structured clinical interviews are typically formulated to evaluate all symptoms, their duration, and potential exclusion criteria as specified by a formal set of diagnostic criteria. In this manner, the Schedule for Affective Disorders and Schizophrenia in School-Age Children (Kiddie SADS) (Puig-Antich & Chambers, 1978) was designed to provide diagnostic information on disorders in youngsters according to Research Diagnostic Criteria (RDC) (Spitzer, Endicott, & Robins, 1978). Likewise, the *Diagnostic and Statistical Manual of Mental Disorders* (DSM) (American Psychiatric Association, 1980, 1987) criteria for psychiatric disorders are assessed by other interviews such as the Child Assessment Schedule (Hodges, Kline, Stern, Cytryn, & McKnew, 1982), the Diagnostic Interview for Children and Adolescents (Herjanic & Reich, 1982; Reich, Herjanic, Welner, & Gandhy, 1982), and the Diagnostic Interview Schedule for Children (Costello, Edelbrock, & Costello, 1985) [for a review of these measures see Hodges (Chapter 10)].

The focus of assessment is an important consideration in the evaluation and use of measures of depression with children and adolescents. This relates to the question of "valid for what?" Measures for the assessment of depression may be roughly delineated as either diagnostic or designed to determine severity in their orientation and purpose (Reynolds, 1994b). Diagnostic measures are generally structured clinical interviews that focus on the classification of formal disorders of depression according to specified rules or classification criteria, such as those delineated in DSM (e.g., major depression, dysthymic disorder). Severity measures typically evaluate a range of depressive symptoms with the assessment format specific to the depth of symptom expression (e.g., frequency of occurrence, intensity). Diagnostic measures produce a diagnosis, and severity measures generally provide a total score that may be compared to a derived cutoff score. In this manner, many severity measures of depression allow for the evaluation of a "clinical level" of depressive symptomatology assuming an adequate coverage of the symptom domain (Reynolds, 1994a). Using the formulation of Compas, Ey, and Grant (1993), single-scale self-report depression measures assess *depressed mood* in youngsters, and self-report measures that are components of a comprehensive assessment measure allow for the assessment of *depressive syndromes*.

Self-report measures of depression typically evaluate the depth or severity of depressive symptoms. In this manner, self-report scales may provide useful information as to the level of depressed mood experienced by the youngster. As noted, a youngster's score at or above a cutoff score may be used as an indication that the child demonstrates a clinically significant level of depressive symptomatology. However, the use of a cutoff score based on the severity of symptoms is not equivalent to a diagnosis of depression according to recognized classification systems. The diagnosis of depression requires a more extensive evaluation procedure, incorporating structured diagnostic interviews or other in-depth methods as well as a trained clinician. Likewise, there should be an empirical basis for the delineation of a cutoff score and some evidence for the efficacy of this score.

This chapter focuses on self-report measures of depression for children and adolescents. It is important to recognize that depression in children, and to a somewhat lesser extent in adolescents, is generally best evaluated from a multidimensional perspective, with different measures using diverse sources of information (e.g., parent, child, teacher, peer), as well as different methods (e.g., self-report questionnaires vs. clinical interview) (Reynolds, 1992). As discussed by Kazdin (Chapter 13), there are difficulties inherent in the combination and interpretation of the outcome of depression measures using multiple informants. However, the use of multiple informants, particularly with children, provides a much richer picture of the nature of depressive symptoms.

The use of self-report procedures for the evaluation of children and adolescents has a long history with a great deal of test-development activity during the 1930s and 1940s for a variety of affective and mental health domains (Reynolds, 1993a). The evaluation of depression in children and adolescents is a relatively recent development, at least with regard to the utilization of brief self-report questionnaires. Prior to the 1980s, the Minnesota Multiphasic Personality Inventory (MMPI) (Hathaway & McKinley, 1940), which included a depression scale, had been used with adolescents as well as adults. This chapter will focus on contemporary self-report assessment procedures for the evaluation of depression in children and adolescents. Although clinical interview measures of depression are, for practical purposes, dependent on self-report, this chapter describes those self-report procedures that are self-completed by using either a paper-and-pencil or a card-sort format.

When using self-report measures, it is important to recognize the task demands of the measure, and in particular how these demands fit the metacognitive as well as the reading and language ability of the youngster. Most self-report questionnaires are limited to use with children of age 8 and above. For children below a 4th- or 5th-grade level, it is often necessary to read the items to the child to avoid confounding with reading ability. Reading and comprehension requirements become problematic when measures developed for adults are used with adolescents, particularly young adolescents and youngsters who are reading below grade level. Adult measures include questions or statements that many youngsters do not fully understand (e.g., "I don't feel I look any worse than I used to." "I don't get irritated at all by the things that used to irritate me") or include vocabulary that the youngster may not comprehend (e.g., "constipation").

William M.
Reynolds

Self-Report Measures of Depression for Children and Adolescents

A number of self-report measures have been developed for the assessment of depression in children and adolescents. As noted above, several measures designed for use with adults have also been used with adolescents. The use of self-report questionnaires for the assessment of depressive symptomatology in children and adolescents has seen a rapid growth in research and clinical applications. From a few reports in the early 1980s to the routine use of self-report depression measures in a wide range of child and adolescent mental health disciplines, self-report measures provide a simple and direct method for the evaluation of the clinical severity of depressive symptoms in young people. Table 1 lists those measures described below. These measures are among the most frequently used self-report scales for the assessment of depressive symptomatology in children and adolescents. In addition to these measures, a number of other scales have been developed and are listed at the end of this section.

Children's Depression Inventory

The Children's Depression Inventory (CDI) (Kovacs, 1979, 1992), developed as a downward revision of the Beck Depression Inventory (BDI) (A. T. Beck, Ward, Mendelson, Mock, & Erbaugh, 1961), is one of the most frequently used research measures of depression in children. The early development of the CDI was described by Kovacs and Beck (1977) with a format- and language-modified version of the BDI and a sample of seven children and adolescents aged 9–15 years. The CDI consists of 27 items with each item represented by three statements of varying severity. The youngster responds by selecting the statement that best describes his or her feelings and behavior over the past 2 weeks. Some of the items may be a bit confusing to some children (e.g., "I do not do what I am told most of the time"). A modified 24-item version of the CDI has been used by Edelsohn, Ialongo, Werthamer-Larsson, Crockett, and Kellam (1992) with first-grade children aged 5–9 years.

Table 1. Description of Self-Report Measures of Depression Used with Children and Adolescents

Measure/author(s)	Development target population	Number of items	Response format	Manual available?
Children's Depression Inventory Kovacs (1979)	Children/adolescents	27	3-Alternative	Yes
Children's Depression Scale Lang & Tisher (1978)	Children/adolescents	66	Card sort	Yes
Depression Self-Rating Scale Birleson (1981)	Children	18	Likert 3-point	No
Reynolds Child Depression Scale Reynolds (1989a)	Children	30	Likert 4-point	Yes
Reynolds Adolescent Depression Scale Reynolds (1986a)	Adolescents	30	Likert 4-point	Yes
Center for Epidemiological Studies Depression Scale Radloff (1977)	Adults	20	Likert 4-point	No
Beck Depression Inventory A. T. Beck et al. (1961)	Adults	21	4-Alternative	Yes[a]

[a]The manual for the BDI is specific to the use and characteristics of the BDI with adults.

Over the past decade, the psychometric characteristics of the CDI have been reported in many studies. In general, researchers find internal consistency reliability coefficients in the low to upper 0.80s (Cole & Carpentieri, 1990; Crowley, Worchel, & Ash, 1992; Kazdin, French, & Unis, 1983b; Kovacs, 1983; Nelson, Politano, Finch, Wendel, & Mayhall, 1987; Reynolds, Anderson, & Bartell, 1985; Smucker, Craighead, Craighead, & Green, 1986) and test–retest reliability coefficients ranging from 0.38 to 0.87 (Blumberg & Izard, 1986; Finch, Saylor, Edwards, & McIntosh, 1987; Kazdin, French, Unis, & Esveldt-Dawson, 1983c; Kovacs, 1980/1981, 1983; Nelson & Politano, 1990; Saylor, Finch, Spirito, & Bennett, 1984; Smucker et al., 1986; Weiss et al., 1991; Wierzbicki, 1987). Much of the variability in the test–retest reliability of the CDI is a function of the time interval between assessments and the study sample characteristics. In their sample of first-grade children, Edelsohn et al. (1992) reported an internal consistency of 0.81 and test–retest reliability of 0.60 for a retest interval of 2 weeks and 0.43 over a 4-month interval for the 24-item modified CDI.

Although the CDI is not a diagnostic measure, research has provided information on the use of the CDI in distinguishing between depressed and nondepressed youngsters (e.g., Benfield, Palmer, Pfefferbaum, & Stowe, 1988; Curry & Craighead, 1990; Moretti, Haley, & Marriage, 1985b; Fristad, Weller, Weller, Teare, & Preskorn, 1988; Kazdin, 1987a, 1989; Kazdin, Esveldt-Dawson, Unis, & Rancurello, 1983a; Kazdin et al., 1983c; Lobovits & Handal, 1985; Moretti, Fine, Haley, & Marriage, 1985; Nelson et al., 1987; Saylor et al., 1984; Wendel, Nelson, Politano, Mayhall, & Finch, 1988). The results of these studies are mixed and tend to show a lack of diagnostic efficacy. Results vary as a function of the clinical and comparison population and CDI cutoff score used by the investigators. Because the CDI is a severity measure, this outcome should not be viewed as a failure on the part of the CDI. Furthermore, the diagnostic results reported for the CDI tend to be superior to those found with several other depression measures (Kazdin & Heidish, 1984).

In a study of 70 children with DSM-III-R diagnoses of depression, anxiety, oppositional, attention-deficit, or conduct disorder, Hodges and Craighead (1990) found that depressed children reported greater scores on three of five factors of the CDI. These three factors, dysphoric mood, loss of personal and social interest, and self-deprecation, consisted of 14 of the 27 CDI items. The other two factors, acting-out and vegetative symptoms, were related to diagnoses of oppositional disorder and anxiety disorder, respectively. M. P. Carey, Faulstich, Gresham, Ruggiero, and Enyart (1987) conducted a factor-analytical study of the CDI with a sample of 153 child and adolescent psychiatric inpatients and a control sample of 153 nonreferred youngsters. M. P. Carey et al. (1987) reported on two- and three-factor models, with factors described as depressive affect, oppositional behavior, and personal adjustment. The first two factors were the best fit for describing the CDI with the clinical sample, although both factor models were poor in correctly classifying the inpatient youngsters. Weiss et al. (1991), in a study with a large sample of clinic-referred children and adolescents, examined the factor structure of the CDI, finding difference in factor structure and item loadings between children and adolescents. They also found that the factor models obtained for both age groups accounted for only approximately one third of the variance in CDI scores, thus suggesting that the resultant factors were not representative of the construct assessed by the CDI.

It is important to note that the CDI, like most self-report measures of depression, was not designed as a diagnostic measure. However, the CDI is useful in assessing the severity of depressive symptomatology. As indicated above, the clinical validity of a depression severity measure cutoff score needs to be established. In research and clinical use of the CDI, a question has emerged as to what cutoff score represents a clinically relevant level of depressive symptoms. In research studies, various CDI cutoff scores have been used by investigators to designate clinical groups of youngsters. In an early report, Kovacs (1980/1981) recommended that a score of 19 and above be used to designate a clinical level of depression. A cutoff score of 19 appears to be appropriate given the score distributions for the CDI found with various school-based samples of children. Studies using large samples of youngsters generally report a mean score on the CDI of about 8–10, with a standard deviation of around 7–8 points (e.g., Cole, 1991; Cole & Carpentieri, 1990; Doerfler, Felner, Rowlison, Evans, & Raley, 1988; Finch, Saylor, & Edwards, 1985; Larson, Raffaelli, Richards, Ham, & Jewell, 1990; Ollendick, Yule, & Ollier, 1991; Smucker et al., 1986; Saylor et al., 1984). In general, a score of 19 identifies about 10% of school-based children as demonstrating a clinical level of depressive symptoms.

In research with children who have various psychological disorders, CDI scores in the 12- to 13-point range have been reported (e.g., Joffe, Dobson, Fine, Marriage, & Haley, 1990; Nelson et al., 1987; Weiss et al., 1991). A number of investigators (e.g., Cole, 1991; Cole & Carpentieri, 1990; Doerfler et al., 1988; Hodges, 1990; Kendall, Stark, & Adam, 1990; Larson et al., 1990; Ollendick & Yule, 1990; Smucker et al., 1986; Stark, Reynolds, & Kaslow, 1987; Strauss, Forehand, Frame, & Smith, 1984) have used this cutoff to identify depressed and nondepressed groups of youngsters. In a study of depression in a sample of 752 school children, Worchel et al. (1990) used a cutoff score of 11 on the CDI to select children who were depressed. This cutoff score resulted in the identification of approximately one third of their sample. Kovacs (1983), in an unpublished paper, suggested that a cutoff score of 13 be used to delineate a clinical level of depression, although this score will overidentify a significant number of nondepressed youngsters. A number of investigators (e.g., Handford, Mattison, Humphrey, & McLaughlin, 1986; Kaslow, Rehm, & Siegel, 1984; Larson et al., 1990; Mattison, Handford, Kales, Goodman, & McLaughlin, 1990; Sacco & Graves, 1984) have used scores of 11–13 on the CDI to identify depressed youngsters. This is problematic, since these values are close to the mean CDI score found in the studies of school-based nonreferred youngsters. Thus, these scores should not be considered indicative of a clinically relevant level of depressive symptomatology on the CDI. In other studies, researchers have based CDI cutoff scores on the distribution of scores using relatively small samples. Bodiford, Eisenstadt, Johnson, and Bradlyn (1988) classified their sample as high and low CDI groups on the basis of the sample score distribution, although some youngsters in the high depression group had scores of 10 on the CDI. Other investigators (e.g., Kazdin, 1989) have used scores of 16 and 17 on the CDI to identify depressed youngsters.

A manual for the CDI has recently been published and deserves some note. The availability of a test manual describing the psychometric characteristics, norms, and procedures for administration and interpretation is a critical and necessary component of any psychological test (American Psychological Association, 1985). Thus, it is somewhat reassuring after many years of use to finally see a manual for the CDI. Unfortunately, there are a number of concerns regarding the claims and procedures presented in the manual that are sufficiently problematic to warrant discussion.

The manual presents normative data, a critical issue for the CDI. The CDI normative sample consisted of 1266 children and young adolescents from an unspecified number of schools in Florida. Data were those from a subsample of youngsters from a previously published study by Finch et al. (1985). No data on race or ethnicity of the sample are reported, although it is suggested that the ethnic characteristics of the sample can be estimated from that of the school district. There are no data to support this claim, nor does the manual describe the estimated ethnic makeup of the 23% of the sample of nonwhite ethnicity. Youngsters were from grades 2–8. Thus, the norms do not include high school students. This lack is problematic, and the manual erroneously suggests that the norms are based on a wider age range than is the case. For instance, the age range for boys is listed in the manual as 7–15 years. No mean age is given, and it may be estimated that there were very few 15-year-olds in the sample. Yet, the tables of normative data and score conversions report the norms separately for 7- to 12-year-olds and 13- to 17-year-olds. Given that there were no 16- or 17-year-old boys in the normative sample, the listing of a norm group age range of 13–17 years may be seen as a misrepresentation. Because of the narrow age range of older boys, it may be the case that this norm group is based on a relatively small sample. Contrary to standard and accepted practice, the manual does not report the sample size of the various age-specific normative groups; thus, comparisons are made to an unknown number of youngsters. No norms based on the total sample or separately for boys and girls are presented. The use of age-specific norms based on unknown numbers of youngsters in each group is problematic, especially given that, as the manual notes, the difference in CDI scores between the two age groups used in the norm tables was not statistically significant or even of practical significance (i.e., less than 1 point difference between age groups). An internal consistency reliability of 0.86 is presented for the total normative sample. Reliability coefficients of the CDI for the various norm comparison groups are not provided. The manual also fails to note that the normative sample is based on an oral administration of the CDI as indicated in the original article by Finch et al. (1985).

The manual presents five subscales (factors) for the CDI, with very little evidence for validity and poor reliability. Furthermore, the manual provides a great deal of emphasis on the scoring of these factors on the CDI, to the extent that the CDI protocol provides a scoring template for these factors and tables for conversion of subscale raw scores to standard scores. The five factors, negative mood, interpersonal problems, ineffectiveness, anhedonia, and negative self-esteem, were derived from a factor analysis of the CDI normative sample. The factor loadings of CDI items on factors suggests a less than parsimonious fit that is problematic for the interpretation of factors. For instance, interpersonal problems consists of 4 items, 3 of which are specific to acting-out problems. The item dealing with reduced social interest is included on this scale, although the factor loading of 0.28 is low. Factor loadings on 6 items defining the primary factor of negative mood were generally low, ranging from 0.21 to 0.42, with a median factor loading of 0.33. The anhedonia item that should define the anhedonia factor demonstrated the lowest loading (0.26) of items on this factor, while the items of vegetative–somatic symptoms such as sleep disturbance (0.42) and somatic concerns (0.34) demonstrate more meaning loadings on this factor. Other problems in the interpretability of the factor analysis are evident and suggest that the derived factor structure is inappropriate for the development of clinically useful subscales as presented in the manual. Further, the low internal consistency reliabilities, which range from 0.59 to 0.68, do not support the clinical interpretation of subscale scores on the CDI, at least those subscales presented in the manual.

The manual also presents a 10-item CDI short form based on item–total scale analysis of the normative sample with little evidence for validity. The manual confuses discriminant validity with discriminant efficacy, although with regard to the latter, the manual reports that a discriminant function analysis of CDI scores for the normative sample and a clinical sample of 134 youngsters failed to correctly classify any of the clinical cases. The basis for determining the cutoff scores is also flawed, since it was conducted with the presumption that none of the 1266 children and adolescents in the normative sample were depressed. Given results of epidemiological studies of children and adolescents, this is an erroneous assumption that invalidates the cutoff-score analyses. On the basis of such analyses, the manual recommends a cutoff score of 20 on the CDI that represents a T-score of 60–66 depending on the age and gender of the youngster. Given this reliance on CDI raw scores for determining a cutoff, it is unclear as to the utility of the standard scores or different standard scores by age. The use of different standard scores for males and females and for different ages ignores the absolute distress level indicated by the CDI raw score. Likewise, in the clinical sample, the mean score of the 65 children with major depression was 11.8, which is in the T-score range of 50–54. Thus, most youngsters with major depression would be classified in the normal range on the basis of the norms presented in the manual. It is important to recognize that the foregoing criticism is specific to the CDI manual rather than the CDI as a severity measure of depressive symptomatology in children. Judging from the publisher's preface in the manual, it appears that the manual may have for the most part been written by the publisher rather than by Dr. Kovacs. It is thus somewhat disappointing after years of clinical and research use of the CDI to find a manual that includes analyses, subscale construction, and norms that detract from a clinically useful measure.

Children's Depression Scale

The Children's Depression Scale (CDS) (Lang & Tisher, 1978) is a self-report measure of children's depression that uses a modified card-sort response format. CDS items are individually listed on cards that the child sorts into one of five boxes labeled as follows: "Very Wrong," "Wrong," "Don't Know/Not Sure," "Right," and "Very Right" (Tisher & Lang, 1983). Developed in Australia, the CDS consists of 66 items, 18 of which are considered to encompass a "positive affective experiences" (P score) subscale, and the remaining 48 items constitute a depression subscale (D score). The positive-affect scale includes one subscale of 8 items (Pleasure and Enjoyment), with the remaining items on the P scale described as miscellaneous (Lang & Tisher, 1987). The depression subscale also contains five additional subscales (Affective Response, Social Problems, Self-Esteem, Sickness and Death, Guilt, and Pleasure and Enjoyment) along with 9 additional miscellaneous D items. In addition to the child form, there is also a parent response form. A manual by Lang and Tisher (1987) developed for use in North America was published with norms (decile scores) based on 37 normal children (22 boys and 15 girls of ages 9–16 years) from Australia.

There have been several studies documenting the psychometric characteristics of the CDS. Tisher, Lang-Takac, and Lang (1992) report on a test–retest study by Tonkin and Hudson (1981), who found a 1-week test–retest reliability coefficient of 0.74 for the CDS with a sample of 60 children. Internal consistency reliability has been found to be high, which may be expected, given the large number of items on the scale. Internal consistency reliability coefficients ranging from 0.92 to 0.94 have been reported (e.g., Bath & Middleton, 1985; Kazdin, 1987b; Knight, Hensley, & Waters, 1988; Tonkin & Hudson, 1981), although some of these studies were based on the 66-item total scale and others on the 48-item D scale. Kazdin (1987b) described the psychometric characteristics of the CDS with a clinical sample of 185 children, reporting correlations of 0.48 and 0.51 between child report on the CDS D scale and scores on the CDI and the modified Bellevue Index of Depression, respectively. The correlation between parents' and children's CDS scores was low, $r = 0.04$. Other investigators have found somewhat higher correlations between the CDS and CDI. Knight et al. (1988) and Rotundo and Hensley (1985) reported correlations of 0.76 and 0.84, respectively, with the higher magnitude due to some extent to the heterogeneity of the various sample characteristics (e.g., combined normal and clinical samples).

The CDS has been found to differentiate between diagnosed depressed and non-depressed youngsters. In a study of 35 children seen in a clinical setting, Fine, Moretti, Haley, and Marriage (1984) found that the child-completed CDS differentiated between youngsters with affective disorders and youngsters with other disorders. The authors did not find differences between these groups on the parent-completed form of the CDS. Based on a review of research with the CDS, Tisher et al. (1992) report that the CDS subscales do not appear to be supported by factor analyses conducted by other investigators and suggest that the total D score should be the primary clinical score. Overall, the CDS holds promise with regard to a reliable child self-report measure, although the number of items and format make administration and scoring a bit cumbersome. The lack of sufficient normative data is a limitation for the clinical use of this measure.

Depression Self-Rating Scale

Developed in Scotland, the Depression Self-Rating Scale (DSRS) by Birleson (1981) is an 18-item self-report questionnaire that uses a three-point response format (most of the time, sometimes, never) and is designed for use with children aged 7–13 years. Items are rated on the basis of their occurrence during the past week. The author reports a split-half internal consistency reliability of 0.86 for the 73 children used in the developmental study, with a test–retest reliability of 0.80 for a subsample of 20 youngsters. Birleson, Hudson, Buchanan, and Wolff (1987) provided evidence for the clinical validity of the DSRS, reporting a sensitivity value of 66.7 and a specificity of 76.7 based on a clinical cutoff score of 15 on the DSRS.

In a study of 82 child psychiatric inpatients, Asarnow and Carlson (1985) modified the DSRS by adding 3 additional items and examined both the 21- and the 18-item versions. They found mean differences between depressed and nondepressed youngsters on both forms. However, unlike Birleson (1981), they reported relatively low reliability, with internal consistency of 0.73 for the 18-item and 0.76 for the 21-item versions and split-half reliability coefficients of 0.61 and 0.67 for these two forms, respectively. Asarnow and Carlson (1985) examined the utility of the DSRS cutoff score of 13, finding a sensitivity of 64% and specificity of 88% using the 18-item form of the scale. With a subsample of 24 children, correlations between the CDI and DSRS of 0.81 and 0.82 were found for the 18- and 21-item versions, respectively. However, low correlations were found between the DSRS and the Children's Depression Rating Scale (CDRS), a clinical interview developed by Poznanski, Cook, and Carroll (1979), with both versions of the DSRS demonstrating a correlation of 0.19 (nonsignificant) with the CDRS. In a study of 26 developmentally and educationally delayed youngsters seen in an adolescent psychiatric inpatient setting, D. C. Beck, Carlson, Russell, and Brownfield (1987) reported a correlation of 0.33 between the DSRS and the BDI with a subsample of 15 youngsters who completed both measures. Overall, results examining the psychometric integrity of the DSRS are mixed and suggest that further study is necessary to determine the utility of the DSRS as a self-report measure of depressive symptomatology in children.

Reynolds Child Depression Scale

The Reynolds Child Depression Scale (RCDS) (Reynolds, 1989a,b) is a self-report measure of depressive symptomatology designed for use with children of ages 8–13 years. The RCDS consists of 30 items and includes 29 items specific to symptoms of depression that are rated as to the frequency of their occurrence during the past 2 weeks using a four-point "almost never" to "all the time" response format. Items are worded in the present tense to evaluate current symptom status (e.g., Item 8: I feel like crying; Item 14: I feel like hurting myself). Seven items are reverse-keyed (e.g., Item 25: I feel like having fun) so that a negative response is indicative of depressive status. The last item on the RCDS consists of five "smiley-type" faces ranging from sad to happy, to which the child responds by placing an X over the face that indicates how he or she feels and represents an evaluation of general dysphoric to euphoric mood.

The RCDS has been used in a number of descriptive and intervention studies of depression in children (e.g., Baker & Reynolds, 1994; Bartell & Reynolds, 1986; Crosbie-Burnett & Newcomer, 1990; Rawson, 1992; Rawson & Tabb, 1993; Reynolds et al., 1985; Reynolds & Graves, 1989a,b; Roseby & Deutsch, 1985; Stark et al., 1987). The manual for the RCDS provides normative information on over 1600 children representing heterogeneous ethnic and socioeconomic backgrounds, along with procedures for administration, scoring, and interpretation and data on reliability and validity. As reported in the manual, the internal consistency reliability for the standardization sample was 0.90. The internal consistency reliability of the RCDS with samples of normal and depressed youngsters has ranged from 0.88 to 0.92 (Baker & Reynolds, 1994; Bartell & Reynolds, 1986; Reynolds, 1989b; Reynolds et al., 1985; Reynolds & Graves, 1989a,b; Stark, 1984). Lopez (1985), using a Spanish-language version of the RCDS, reported an internal consistency reliability of 0.83 with a sample of children in Puerto Rico. Reynolds and Graves (1989a) reported a test–retest reliability coefficient of 0.85 for the RCDS using a 4-week interval between testing with an ethnically diverse sample of 220 children from grades 3–6. The mean difference in RCDS scores between the two assessments was less than 2 points. By grade, test–retest reliability coefficients ranged from 0.81 for 3rd grade to 0.92 for 6th grade.

Validity data have been reported in the RCDS manual in the form of high correlations with other self-report and clinical interview measures of childhood depression, as well as content validity, factor analysis, discriminant validity, and clinical utility (Reynolds, 1989b). The RCDS has demonstrated correlations with the CDI ranging from 0.70 to 0.79 across several studies (e.g., Baker & Reynolds, 1994; Bartell & Reynolds, 1986; Benavidez & Matson, 1993; Lopez, 1985; Reynolds, 1989b; Reynolds et al., 1985; Stark, 1984). In addition to correlations with other self-report measures, Reynolds (1989b) reports a correlation between the RCDS and the Children's Depression Rating Scale—Revised (CDRS-R), a semistructured clinical interview by Poznanski et al. (1984), of 0.76 ($p < 0.001$), which can be considered high as a demonstration of criterion-related validity. Using the CDRS-R cutoff score to provide a base rate for a clinical level of depression, Reynolds (1989b) reported a specificity rate of 97%, sensitivity of 73%, a Yule's Y of 0.81 ($p < 0.0001$), and a phi coefficient of 0.73 ($p < 0.0001$) for the RCDS cutoff score with a sample of 82 children. In a study with 25 adolescents with mental retardation and 25 intellectually average youngsters, Benavidez and Matson (1993) reported correlations between the RCDS and CDI of 0.75 and 0.74 for the samples of youngsters with mental retardation and average intellect, respectively. For these two samples, the correlations between the RCDS and the Bellevue Index of Depression, a clinical interview measure developed by Petti (1978), were 0.64 and 0.73, respectively. A number of studies (e.g., Crosbie-Burnett & Newcomer, 1990; Rawson & Tabb, 1993; Stark et al., 1987) have shown the RCDS to be sensitive to treatment outcome as a measure of depression.

Reynolds Adolescent Depression Scale

The Reynolds Adolescent Depression Scale (RADS) (Reynolds, 1986b, 1987a) was developed to evaluate the severity of depressive symptoms in adolescents aged 12–18 years. The RADS consists of 30 items and uses a four-point response format ("almost never" to "most of the time"). Items on the RADS were written to reflect symptomatology specified by the DSM-III for major depression and dysthymic disorder, as well as additional symptoms delineated by the RDC (Spitzer et al., 1978) and by Carlson and Strober (1979) in their study of depression in adolescents. Items evaluate somatic, motivational, cognitive, mood, and vegetative components of depression. Items on the RADS require a 3rd-grade reading level.

The RADS test manual provides documentation of normative information, reliability, validity, and interpretation of test results in studies involving over 11,000 adolescents from various locations in the United States. Norms for the RADS are based on an ethnically diverse sample of 2460 adolescents in grades 7–12. The RADS norms appear to be relatively robust, with similar mean scores reported in a number of other investigations of normal samples of school-based youngsters (e.g., Dalley, Bolocofsky, Alcorn, & Baker, 1992; Reynolds & Miller, 1989; Schonert-Reichl, 1994). Scores on the RADS range from 30 to 120, with a score of 77 used as a cutoff to define a clinically relevant level of depressive symptomatology.

Reliability of the RADS has been high (ranging from 0.91 to 0.96) with samples of normal and depressed adolescents ranging in size from 62 to 2120 (Anderson & Reynolds, 1988; Dalley et al., 1992; Kraemer, 1992; Lapsley, Flannery, Krug, & McGinnis, 1984; Reynolds, 1985a, 1987a, 1989c, 1990; Reynolds & Coats, 1982; Reynolds & Miller, 1989; Schonert-Reichl, 1994). In a study of 26 mildly retarded adolescents (Reynolds & Miller, 1985), the internal consistency reliability of the RADS was 0.87. Nieminen and Matson (1989) reported an internal consistency reliability of 0.88 for the RADS with a sample of 76 youngsters aged 11–18 years with a diagnosis of conduct disorder. Overall, the internal consistency findings support homogeneity of item content on the RADS. Test–retest reliability based on a sample of 104 adolescents who were tested with a 6-week interval between testings was 0.80, which is viewed as acceptable. A 12-week test–retest reliability coefficient of 0.79 was also found for the RADS with a sample of 415 high school students (Reynolds, 1987a). Baron and DeChamplain (1990) reported on a French-language translation of the RADS with a sample of 140 francophone adolescents in Quebec, finding high internal consistency, $r_\alpha = 0.93$, and a 3-week test–retest reliability coefficient of 0.86.

The validity of the RADS has been established in a number of studies that have examined relationships with other depression scales and measures of related constructs. The analyses encompassed by the RADS have demonstrated strong correlations with other self-report measures of depression, including the BDI (A. T. Beck et al., 1961), the Center for Epidemiological Studies—Depression Scale (CES-D) (Radloff, 1977), and the Zung Self-Rating Depression Scale (Zung, 1965) ($r = 0.71$–0.89). Baron and DeChamplain (1990) reported a correlation of 0.80 between French-language versions of the RADS and BDI with a sample of francophone adolescents. Kahn, Kehle, and Jenson (1987), in a study of 349 8th-grade students, found a correlation of 0.75 between the RADS and the CDI. With a sample of 1054 younger adolescents aged 12–14, a correlation of 0.70 was found between the RADS and the CDI (Reynolds, 1987a), while Brown, Overholser, Spirito, and Fritz (1991) reported a correlation of 0.64 between the RADS and the CDI in a sample of adolescent suicide attempters. In samples of 95 conduct-disordered students, Matson and Nieminen (1987) found a correlation of 0.62 between the RADS and the CDI. In a sample of 113 adolescent psychiatric inpatients, T. C. Carey, Finch, and Carey (1991) found a multiple regression coefficient of 0.72 between the RADS and four subscales of the Differential Emotions Scale—IV (DES) (Blumberg & Izard, 1986). In a sample of 45 adolescent inpatients with major depression, Shain, Naylor, and Alessi (1990) reported a correlation coefficient of 0.87 between the RADS and the CDI. M. P. Carey, Lubin, and Brewer (1992) reported correlations between the RADS and the Youth Depression Adjective Checklist (Y-DACL) (Carey et al., 1992) of 0.45 and 0.48 for samples of psychiatric inpatients and nonreferred adolescents, respectively.

Researchers have found higher RADS scores in samples of special education students including those with learning, emotional, and behavioral problems (e.g., Dalley et al., 1992; Hagborg, 1992; Lyon & Bolin, 1988; Nieminen & Matson, 1989; Reynolds & Miller, 1985), although Navarrete (1992) did not find differences in RADS scores between learning-disabled and nondisabled adolescents. M. P. Carey, Finch, Belter, Imm, and Carey (1991), in a sample of 115 adolescents from a psychiatric inpatient sample, found significant relationships between the RADS and the subscales of the Family Assessment Device (FAD) (Epstein, Baldwin, & Bishop, 1983), and Havey and Dodd (1992) reported a difference on the RADS between children of alcoholics and children of nonalcoholic parents. In studies with suicidal youngsters, researchers have found significant differences on the RADS between suicidal and nonsuicidal adolescents and high RADS scores among suicidal adolescents, and significant correlations between the RADS and measures of suicidal behaviors (Brown et al., 1991; King, Raskin, Gdowski, Butkus, & Opipari, 1990; King et al., 1992; Lyon & Bolin, 1988; Mazza & Reynolds, 1991; Reynolds, 1989c, 1990; Sadowski & Kelley, 1993; Spirito, Stark, Fristad, Hart, & Owens-Stively, 1987; Spirito, Stark, Hart, &

Fristad, 1988). In a study of adolescents with major depression and an age- and sex-matched normal control group, Shain et al. (1991) found significant differences in RADS scores between youngsters with major depression (M = 85.5) and normal controls (*M* = 45.5), *t* = 9.02, *p* < 0.0001.

Criterion-related validity of the RADS has been established using semistructured clinical interviews of depression. For the measurement of depression, the structured clinical interview is considered the most sensitive and selective assessment methodology. In a school-based study of 111 adolescents, Reynolds (1987a) found a correlation of 0.83 between the RADS and the Hamilton Depression Rating Scale (HDRS) (Hamilton, 1960, 1967). In their study of adolescents with major depression, Shain et al. (1990) reported a correlation of 0.73 between the RADS and the HDRS and of 0.78 between the RADS and the CDRS-R.

The RADS uses a cutoff score to describe a clinical level of depressive symptom severity. The RADS cutoff score has been validated in several studies, using both HDRS scores and formal diagnosis based on the Schedule for Affective Disorders and Schizophrenia (SADS; Endicott & Spitzer, 1978) as criterion measures (Reynolds, 1987a; Reynolds & Evert, 1991). Using the RADS cutoff score of 77 and an HDRS cutoff score of 15 with a subsample of 32 adolescents from a psychiatric center, T. C. Carey, Kelley, and Carey (1991) found that 78.1% were correctly classified using the cutoff scores on these two measures. Using a more conservative cutoff score of 20 on the HDRS, Reynolds (1987a) reported a correct classification of 89.2% in a sample of 111 school-based adolescents. The RADS has also demonstrated clinical efficacy in its use in a number of adolescent depression treatment studies as an outcome measure of treatment efficacy (Hains, 1992; Kahn, Kehle, Jenson, & Clark, 1990; Reynolds & Coats, 1986).

Beck Depression Inventory

The BDI (A. T. Beck et al., 1961) was developed for adults and is one of the most widely used self-report measures of adult depressive symptomatology (Reynolds & Gould, 1981). The BDI consists of 21 items, each consisting of four statements of varying degrees of symptom severity. A number of investigators have used the BDI with adolescents, although the reading requirements and format of the scale present difficulty for some youngsters. Likewise, users of the BDI often apply cutoff scores used with adults to adolescents without adequate validation.

The internal consistency reliability of the BDI with adolescents has been reported in the 0.70s to 0.80s (Kashani, Sherman, Parker, & Reid, 1990; Reynolds, 1985a; Reynolds & Coats, 1982; Roberts, Lewinsohn, & Seeley, 1991; Strober, Green, & Carlson, 1981; Teri, 1982). Strober et al. (1981) reported a 5-day test–retest reliability of 0.69 in a sample of 78 psychiatric inpatient adolescents. In a study of 37 older adolescents, Kutcher & Marton (1989) reported a 1-week test–retest reliability coefficient of 0.83. Reporting on test–retest data for the BDI in a large sample of adolescents retested between 1 week and 1 month after test, Roberts et al. (1991) found a test–retest reliability of 0.67 which is low to moderate. Overall, the reliability of the BDI with adolescents is lower than that found in other self-report measures of depression developed specifically for youngsters.

Validity evidence for the BDI has been examined in clinical and school-based samples. Barrera and Garrison-Jones (1988) examined the utility of the BDI in samples of hospitalized psychiatric patients (*N* = 65) and school-based adolescents (*N* = 49), finding reasonable sensitivity and specificity in the school sample, but poor results for the psychiatric sample. Kashani et al. (1990) also noted a relatively low sensitivity rate (48%) using the BDI cutoff score of 16 in a sample of 100 clinic-referred adolescents. In a study of 1704 adolescents who were assessed with a number of self-report measures as well as a diagnostic interview, Roberts et al. (1991) reported a correlation of 0.50 between the BDI and a 14-item form of the HDRS, which is relatively low. They also reported low κ coefficients for the BDI in identifying cases of major depression (κ = 0.14) and dysthymia (κ = 0.03). The BDI has been used by a number of investigators for the examination of depression in adolescents (e.g., Baron & Joly, 1988; D. C. Beck et al., 1987; Kaplan, Hong, & Weinhold, 1984), with several studies using the 13-item BDI short form (Friedrich, Reams, & Jacobs, 1982; Rierdan & Koff, 1993; Siegel & Griffin, 1984).

Center for Epidemiological Studies—Depression Scale

The CES-D (Radloff, 1977) consists of 20 items and was designed for use with adults. CES-D items are rated from 0 to 3 on the basis of their frequency of occurrence over the past week. The CES-D includes both positive and negative keyed items. The CES-D has been used by a number of investigators with adolescents (e.g., Doerfler et al., 1988; Garrison, Jackson, Marsteller, McKeown, & Addy, 1990; Garrison, Schluchter, Schoenbach, & Kaplan, 1989; Garrison, Schoenbach, & Kaplan, 1985; Hops, Lewinsohn, Andrews, & Roberts, 1990). In a study of self-report depression in a sample of over 1000 children and adolescents, Doerfler et al. (1988) found a moderate correlation ($r = 0.58$) between the CES-D and the CDI. Roberts et al. (1991) reported a short-term (1- to 4-week) test–retest reliability for the CES-D with adolescents of 0.61, which is low.

The CES-D cutoff score has been found to identify between 40% and 50% of nonclinical youngsters as depressed (e.g., Doerfler et al., 1988; Gjerde, Block, & Block, 1988; Faulstich, Carey, Ruggiero, Enyart, & Gresham, 1986; Manson, Ackerson, Dick, Baron, & Fleming, 1990; Roberts, Andrews, Lewinsohn, & Hops, 1990; Roberts et al., 1991; Schoenbach, Kaplan, Grimson, & Wagner, 1982; Schoenbach, Kaplan, Wagner, Grimson, & Miller, 1983), a distinct problem in the clinical use of this measure. For instance, while the CDI cutoff score of 19 identified approximately 10% of subjects in the Doerfler et al. (1988) study, the CES-D cutoff of 16 identified 46% of their school-based sample as depressed. Setting higher cutoff scores results in significantly more youngsters identified as depressed than are adults (Radloff, 1991). Roberts et al. (1991) found a relatively low correlation of 0.48 between the CES-D and a 14-item form of the HDRS. They also found low κ coefficients for the CES-D in identifying cases of major depression (κ = 0.11) and dysthymia (κ = 0.02). The moderate correlations with other depression measures and the high endorsement proportions found among adolescents, as well as limitations in symptoms assessed by the scale (Rabkin & Klein, 1987) and the 1-week evaluation interval, limit the utility of the CES-D as a measure of depressive symptomatology in youngsters.

Adolescent Psychopathology Scale: Major Depression and Dysthymia Scales

The Adolescent Psychopathology Scale (APS) (Reynolds, in press) is a multidimensional self-report measure of psychopathology designed for use with adolescents aged 13–19. The APS consist of 20 Clinical Disorder scales, 5 Personality Scales, and 11 Content scales, as well as several validity indicators. The development of the APS was based on clinical samples of over 500 adolescents from 31 inpatient and outpatient treatment settings in 21 states and a nonclinical sample of over 2800 adolescents drawn from 11 public junior and senior high schools in 8 states. The APS include scales of major depression and dysthymic disorder. The Major Depression scale consists of 29 items reflecting DSM-IV symptoms, with items rated on the basis of their occurrence over the past 2 weeks. The Dysthymic Disorder scale consists of 16 items rated as to their occurrence over the past 6 months. Reynolds (1993b) reported an internal consistency reliability of 0.95 for both the normal and the clinical samples for the Major Depression scale. The Dysthymia Disorder scale demonstrated internal consistency reliability coefficients of 0.89 and 0.88 for the clinical and school samples, respectively.

Scores on the APS are provided in the form of T-scores, with a mean of 50 and a standard deviation of 10, with clinical levels variable across APS scales to accommodate differences in base rates across disorders. Validity evidence in the form of content validity, contrasted groups validity (normal adolescents vs. those with a diagnosis of major depression), and criterion-related validity as demonstrated by correlations with other self-report (MMPI, RADS) and clinical interview (SADS, HDRS) measures of depression are presented in the APS manual and support the validity of the Major Depression and Dysthymia scales of the APS with adolescents.

Other Self-Report Measures

In addition to the measures described above, there are a number of other self-report measures of depression that will not be discussed. These measures include the Children's Depression Adjective Check Lists (Eddy & Lubin, 1988; Sokoloff & Lubin, 1983); the Face Valid Depression Scale for Adolescents (Mezzich & Mezzich, 1979); the Multiscore Depression Inventory originally designed for use with adults (Berndt, Petzel, & Berndt, 1980); the depressive symptom score of the Hopkins Symptom Checklist (Derogatis, Lipman, Rickels, Uhlenhuth, & Covi, 1974) used by Compas, Slavin, Wagner, and Vannatta (1986); the Self-Rating Depression Scale (Zung, 1965) developed for adults with reports of its use with adolescents (e.g., Lineberger, 1987; Zung, 1974); several short-form modifications of the CDI (Carlson & Cantwell, 1979; Lefkowitz & Tesiny, 1980) and the Zung (1965) Self-Rating Depression Scale (Lefkowitz & Tesiny, 1980); the Childhood Depression Assessment Tool (Brady, Nelms, Albright, & Murphy, 1984), a 26-item yes/no format questionnaire; the General Behavior Inventory (Klein, Depue, & Slater, 1986), a 73-item self-report measure designed to assess symptoms of cyclothymia; the Rating Scale of Dysphoria (Lefkowitz, Tesiny, & Solodow, 1989), a 12-item self-rating adaptation of the Peer Nomination Inventory of Depression (Lefkowitz & Tesiny, 1980); the 66-item Depressive Experiences Questionnaire for Adolescents (Blatt, Schaffer, Bers, & Quinlan, 1992); the Inventory to Diagnose Depression (Zimmerman & Coryell, 1987) used by Ackerson, Dick, Manson, and Baron (1990) with adolescents; the 6-item Depressive Affect self-report scale by Rosenberg (1965); the depression subscale of the Youth Self-Report (Achenbach & Edelbrock, 1987); and the revised self-report version of the depression scale from the Child Behavior Checklist (Achenbach & Edelbrock, 1983) developed by Clarke, Lewinsohn, Hops, and Seeley (1992).

Screening for Depression in Elementary and Secondary Schools

The results of epidemiological investigations of depression in school-based child and adolescent samples provide support for schools in collaboration with mental health professionals to engage in procedures for the identification of distressed youngsters. Without active procedures, the majority of depressed children and adolescents will not be identified or receive treatment [Reynolds & Johnston (Chapter 1)]. In large-sample testings of school-based groups of children and adolescents, between 10% and 18% demonstrate moderate to severe levels of depressive symptomatology (Doerfler et al., 1988; Reynolds, 1985b, 1987a; Reynolds and Coats, 1982).

The outcome of a single administration of self-report depression measures needs to be interpreted with caution. There is a tendency for children and adolescents to score higher on the first administration of self-report depression questionnaires than on a second testing conducted a short time after the initial assessment (Edelsohn et al., 1992; Reynolds, 1987a;

Reynolds & Graves, 1989a). For example, Tharinger and Stark (1990) reported that 40% of children who scored above the cutoff on the CDI on an initial assessment scored below the cutoff when retested a short time after the initial testing. The general inference is that the first testing represents an overendorsement of depressive symptoms. This result is also found in the use of depression measures with adults and is not unexpected, given that depression as a clinical psychopathology is not a stable trait. There is variability in the duration and intensity of depression. A youngster's level of depressive symptomatology may change, sometimes in relationship to a transient stressor, such as a bad grade on a test, or a less defined event or set of circumstances that may temporarily result in the youngster's feeling down for a short period of time. The assessment process itself may result in an overendorsement for some youngsters who on the second testing are more contemplative or view their symptoms as not as severe as they initially thought. The purpose of a multiple-stage assessment is to refine the identification process using self-report severity measures by systematically reducing cases of false positives.

A multiple-stage assessment procedure for the screening and identification of depression in children and adolescents has been developed by Reynolds (1986b) and further validated by Reynolds and Evert (1991) and Kahn, Kehle, and Jenson (1988). This screening procedure consists of three assessment stages or gates. The stages are (1) large-group screening with self-report questionnaires of depression; (2) retesting of youngsters who, on the basis of the initial assessment, meet specified cutoff score criteria for clinical levels of depressive symptomatology; and (3) conducting individual clinical interviews with children and adolescents who demonstrate clinical levels of depression at Stages 1 and 2 assessments. The application of this screening procedure results in one of three identification decisions: not depressed, not clinically depressed but in need of reevaluation at a later date, and clinically depressed.

In the application of this model to screening in high school settings (Reynolds, 1986b), the author has typically identified 18–20% of adolescents as demonstrating a clinically relevant level of depression on the initial assessment. When reassessed at the second stage, between 25% and 30% of these youngsters no longer score in a depressed range on self-report measures. In this manner, the two screenings using self-report, paper-and-pencil measures of depression reduce the proportion of potentially depressed youngsters to approximately 12–15% of the total sample. The last stage of the screening model further reduces the pool of youngsters with clinically relevant levels of self-reported depressive symptoms. At the final stage, the procedure results in the identification of 7–12% of the original sample tested. The application of this procedure and description of each stage are presented below.

Stage 1

The first stage of this screening procedure involves the group assessment of children or adolescents with one or more self-report depression measures. For youngsters aged 8 and above, the assessment can be carried out in the classroom by the teacher. At this stage, all youngsters in a school, grade, or certain classes are tested in their classrooms. Teachers or school personnel who administer the measures need to be trained as to the specifics of administration and have a general understanding of the nature of the screening procedure. Manuals for the RCDS and RADS include appendices of instructions for school psychologists as well as teachers that explain the group administration procedure and caution against such problems as mood induction when administering the questionnaires. In this manner, an entire school can be tested in 15 or 20 minutes. In practice, it has been found that it is advisable to test all classes at the same time, as well as to schedule the assessment around midmorning to ensure the optimal number of students given an observation of tardiness among some depressed youngsters. In addition, a morning assessment allows for the evaluation to take place at a time when some depressed youngsters may be experiencing a diurnal variation with symptoms worsening in the morning.

After the youngsters have been tested, it is important that questionnaires be scored quickly and accurately. This is a critical point because asking a youngster, particularly a distressed one, how he or she is feeling brings an expectation that something will be done to remediate this condition. Thus, the depression measure should be scored and youngsters at or above a clinical level identified for Stage 2 of the screening procedure within 1–2 weeks.

Stage 2

The second stage of this procedure involves the retesting of all youngsters who score at or above a clinical cutoff score on the depression measure. The reassessment should be conducted with the same depression measure and take place 1–2 weeks after the initial assessment [this is a modification of the original time interval suggested by Reynolds (1986b)]. Testing can occur in small groups, with 5–10 youngsters in the elementary school grades and 20–30 youngsters in junior and senior high school settings. In both the initial and second stages of the procedure, it is important not to tell youngsters that they are being tested for signs of depression, in order to avoid the potential induction of depressive mood. We have found it quite sufficient to inform youngsters that the questionnaires they are completing are designed to find out how they are feeling about themselves and things in general. An examination of depression-scale items indicates that this is a reasonable description of the type of questions asked of the youngsters. It is also important not to overdramatize the assessment, especially the second testing, at which awareness of some selection process is often evident to the youngsters.

The second stage is designed to refine the identification process by eliminating youngsters who were experiencing a transient depressed mood, overendorsed depressive symptoms on the initial assessment, or for any other reason manifested a significant level of depressive symptomatology on the first assessment, but will not on the second testing. Youngsters who score depressed on both assessments are then individually interviewed in the third stage of the screening procedure.

Stage 3

The third stage of the screening procedure involves conducting individual clinical interviews with all youngsters who met the criteria for clinically relevant levels of depression at both Stage 1 and Stage 2 evaluations. Clinical interviews should be conducted only by trained professionals, that is, psychologists or others with specific training in the interview measure that is used. Because a formal diagnosis of depression is typically not needed by school personnel, and in some settings may not be desired due to classification implications, it is suggested that an interview measure of severity, such as the CDRS-R or the HDRS, be used in the third stage of this procedure. However, if trained personnel are available, a structured clinical interview such as the Child Assessment Schedule may be administered to obtain diagnostic as well as additional clinical information. It is vital that the clinical interview be administered as soon as possible following the second stage. It is not advisable, and in some cases may be detrimental or exacerbate feelings of hopelessness and abandonment, to allow a youngster who has told of his or her depression to wait weeks before a professional interviewer sees the youngster. Thus, schools must be ready to begin interviews when results of the second screening are available.

The third stage, although time-consuming, is a vital component. The total reliance on self-report measures of depression is less than desirable for identifying clinically depressed children and adolescents who are in need of treatment or referral. Clinical interviews allow for more fine-tuned examination of symptom severity, as well as some definition of the problems that may be causing the depression in the youngster. This latter information is often important in treatment decision-making on the part of the psychologists or school professional.

Limitations and Caveats

The procedure described above for the identification of depressed youngsters has been implemented in numerous school districts with very positive results and responses by parents, teachers, and other school personnel. This three-stage procedure has also been used in the selection of depressed youngsters for inclusion in psychological treatment studies (e.g., Kahn et al., 1990; Marcotte, & Baron, 1993; Reynolds & Coats, 1986; Stark et al., 1987). It should be noted that this model is designed for large-scale screening and not necessarily the testing of individual cases. For individual assessment, a self-report measure, followed several days later by a clinical interview, may be the most efficacious assessment procedure.

It is important to note that this three-stage screening procedure is designed for the identification of depressed youngsters. This procedure is not designed or recommended for the identification of suicidal youngsters. For the identification of suicidal youngsters, a two-stage procedure has been developed (Reynolds, 1988) on the basis of the screening of suicidal ideation using the Suicidal Ideation Questionnaire (Reynolds, 1987b). This procedure is described in more detail by Reynolds [Reynolds, 1991; Reynolds and Mazza (Chapter 24)]. The difference is that once a youngster has admitted to significant thoughts of killing himself or herself at the initial stage, clinical interviews for suicidal behavior (e.g., Reynolds, 1990) are conducted as soon as possible (second stage). It is recommended that school-based screening include both self-report measures of depression and suicidal behavior in order to enhance the fidelity of the selection of depressed as well as suicidal youngsters.

Summary and Conclusions

The assessment of depression in children and adolescents is a complex and often multifaceted procedure. This chapter has presented information on self-report measures of depression designed for or used with children and adolescents. Self-report measures represent one of the primary methods for the evaluation of the severity of depressive symptomatology. As was shown, a number of measures have been developed that demonstrate high levels of reliability and validity. Thus, we can view self-reports of children and adolescents as an important source of clinical information.

A major requirement for determining whether a child or adolescent is depressed is the availability of objective and valid assessment instruments, as well as appropriate procedures for the integration of these measures. The identification of depressed youngsters is a primary concern for psychologists, psychiatrists, counselors, social workers, and school and mental health service providers. It is also important that professionals who utilize depression measures be trained in the application and interpretation of these measures, as well as knowledgeable as to the limitations inherent in each measure.

Self-report measures are a useful means to evaluate depression in children and adolescents. Because of the subjective and internalizing nature of many symptoms of depression, the youngster's direct report provides valuable information. Self-report measures are also relatively brief and do not require the level of training and experience that is necessary for the use of clinical interviews. Although there are numerous positive aspects to self-report depression measures, there are also limitations. Self-report measures evaluate symptoms associated with depression, but typically do not inquire as to whether a symptom is due to depression or an extraneous cause. Thus, the youngster who on a self-report measure endorses weight loss, irritability, difficulty sleeping, aches and pains, self-deprecation, and some evidence of guilt may appear to be somewhat depressive. However, during the course of a clinical interview, inquiry as to the reason for such symptoms may portray a youngster who lost a difficult and important wrestling match at school, was told by the wrestling coach to drop to a lower weight class, and is kept up at night by the cries and feeding schedule of an infant sibling. Clinical interviews also allow for the structuring of questions appropriate to the youngster's developmental level. These are two of a number of characteristics that support the use of clinical interviews.

The author's perspective is that self-report measures are a useful methodology for the initial assessment of youngsters' level of depressive symptomatology. Self-report depression measures can provide reliable and valid information. However, for the comprehensive, detailed investigation of depression in young people, clinical interviews are an important methodology. In clinical practice, it is highly desirable for professionals to follow up with a clinical interview those youngsters who demonstrate clinical levels of depressive symptomatology on a self-report measure.

References

Achenbach, T. M., & Edelbrock, C. (1983). *Manual for the Child Behavior Checklist and Revised Child Behavior Profile*. Burlington: Department of Psychiatry, University of Vermont.

Achenbach, T. M., & Edelbrock, C. (1987). *Manual for the Youth Self-Report and Profile*. Burlington: Department of Psychiatry, University of Vermont.

Ackerson, L. M., Dick, R. W., Manson, S. M., & Baron, A. E. (1990). Properties of the Inventory to Diagnose Depression in American Indian adolescents. *Journal of the American Academy of Child and Adolescent Psychiatry, 29*, 601–607.

American Psychiatric Association (1980). *Diagnostic and statistical manual of mental disorders*, 3rd ed. Washington, DC: Author.

American Psychiatric Association (1987). *Diagnostic and statistical manual of mental disorders*, 3rd ed., revised. Washington, DC: Author.

American Psychological Association (1985). *Standards for educational and psychological testing*. Washington, DC: Author.

Anderson, G, & Reynolds, W. M. (1988). A multivariate investigation of stress, coping, and depression in adolescents. Paper presented at the Annual Meeting of the National Association of School Psychologists, Chicago, April 1988.

Asarnow, J. R., & Carlson, G. A. (1985). Depression Self-Rating Scale: Utility with child psychiatric inpatients. *Journal of Consulting and Clinical Psychology, 53*, 491–499.

Baker, J. A., & Reynolds, W. M. (1994). Enhancing teachers' recognition of depressed children in their classrooms: A teacher training model (submitted).

Baron, P., & DeChamplain, A. (1990, June). Evaluation de la fidélité et de la validité de la version française du RADS auprès d'un groupe d'adolescents francophones. Paper presented at the Annual Convention of the Canadian Psychological Association, Ottawa.

Baron, P., & Joly, E. (1988). Sex differences in the expression of depression in adolescents. *Sex Roles, 18*, 1–7.

Barrera, M., and Garrison-Jones, C. V. (1988). Properties of the Beck Depression Inventory as a screening instrument for adolescent depression. *Journal of Abnormal Child Psychology, 16*, 263–273.

Bartell, N. P., & Reynolds, W. M. (1986). Depression and self-esteem in academically gifted and nongifted children: A comparison study. *Journal of School Psychology, 24*, 55–61.

Bath, H. I., & Middleton, M. R. (1985).The Children's Depression Scale: Psychometric properties and factor structure. *Australian Journal of Psychology, 37*, 81–88.

Beck, A. T., Ward, C., Mendelson, M., Mock, J., & Erbaugh, J. (1961). An inventory for measuring depression. *Archives of General Psychiatry, 4*, 561–571.

Beck, D. C., Carlson, G. A., Russell, A. T., & Brownfield, F. E. (1987). Use of depression rating instruments in developmentally and educationally delayed adolescents. *Journal of the American Academy of Child and Adolescent Psychiatry, 26*, 97–100.

Benavidez, D. A., & Matson, J. L. (1993). Assessment of depression in mentally retarded adolescents. *Research in Developmental Disabilities, 14,* 179–188.

Benfield, C. Y., Palmer, D. J., Pfefferbaum, B., & Stowe, M. L. (1988). A comparison of depressed and nondepressed disturbed children on measures of attributional style, hopelessness, life stress, and temperament. *Journal of Abnormal Child Psychology, 16,* 397–410.

Berndt, D. J., Petzel, T., & Berndt, S. M. (1980). Development and initial evaluation of a multiscore depression inventory. *Journal of Personality Assessment, 44,* 396–404.

Birleson, P. (1981). The validity of depressive disorder in childhood and the development of a self-rating scale: A research report. *Journal of Child Psychology and Psychiatry, 22,* 73–88.

Birleson, P., Hudson, I., Buchanan, D. G., & Wolff, S. (1987). Clinical evaluation of a self-rating scale for depressive disorder in childhood (Depression Self-Rating Scale). *Journal of Child Psychology and Psychiatry, 28,* 43–60.

Blatt, S. J., Schaffer, C. E., Bers, S. A., & Quinlan, D. M. (1992). Psychometric properties of the Depressive Experiences Questionnaire for Adolescents. *Journal of Personality Assessment, 59,* 82–98.

Blumberg, S. H., & Izard, C. E. (1986). Discriminating patterns of emotions in 10- and 11-year-old children's anxiety and depression. *Journal of Personality and Social Psychology, 51,* 852–857.

Bodiford, C. A., Eisenstadt, J. H., Johnson, J. H., & Bradlyn, A. S. (1988). Comparison of learned helpless cognitions and behavior in children with high and low scores on the Children's Depression Inventory. *Journal of Clinical Child Psychology, 17,* 152–158.

Brady, M. A., Nelms, B. C., Albright, A. V., & Murphy, C. M. (1984). Childhood depression: Development of a screening tool. *Pediatric Nursing, 10,* 222–225.

Brown, L. K., Overholser, J., Spirito, A., & Fritz, G. K. (1991). The correlates of planning in adolescent suicide attempts. *Journal of the American Academy of Child and Adolescent Psychiatry, 30,* 95–99.

Carey, M. P., Faulstich, M. E., Gresham, F. M., Ruggiero, L., & Enyart, P. (1987). Children's Depression Inventory: Construct and discriminant validity across clinical and nonreferred (control) populations. *Journal of Consulting and Clinical Psychology, 55,* 755–761.

Carey, M. P., Finch, A. J., Belter, R. W., Imm, P., & Carey, T. (1991). Family Assessment Device: Utility with inpatients and their parents. Paper presented at the Annual Meeting of the American Psychological Association, San Francisco, August 1991.

Carey, M. P., Lubin, B., & Brewer, D. H. (1992). Measuring dysphoric mood in pre-adolescents and adolescents: The Youth Depression Adjective Checklist (Y-DACL). *Journal of Clinical Child Psychology, 21,* 331–338.

Carey, T. C., Finch, A. J., & Carey, M. P. (1991). Relation between differential emotions and depression in emotionally disturbed children and adolescents. *Journal of Consulting and Clinical Psychology, 59,* 594–597.

Carey, T. C., Kelley, M. L., & Carey, M. P. (1991). The relation of cognitions, emotions and behavior to depressive symptomatology. Paper presented at the Annual Meeting of the American Psychological Association, San Francisco, August 1991.

Carlson, G. A., & Cantwell, D. P. (1979). A survey of depressive symptoms in a child and adolescent psychiatric population. *Journal of the American Academy of Child Psychiatry, 18,* 587–599.

Carlson, G. A., & Strober, M. (1979). Affective disorders in adolescents. *Psychiatric Clinics of North America, 2,* 511–526.

Clarke, G. N., Lewinsohn, P. M., Hops, H., & Seeley, J. R. (1992). A self- and parent-report measure of adolescent depression: The Child Behavior Checklist Depression Scale (CBCL-D). *Behavioral Assessment, 14,* 443–463.

Cole, D. A. (1991). Preliminary support for a competency-based model of depression in children. *Journal of Abnormal Psychology, 100,* 181–190.

Cole, D. A., & Carpentieri, S. (1990). Social status and the comorbidity of child depression and conduct disorders. *Journal of Consulting and Clinical Psychology, 58,* 748–757.

Compas, B. E., Ey, S., & Grant, K. E. (1993). Taxonomy, assessment, and diagnosis of depression during adolescence. *Psychological Bulletin, 114,* 323–344.

Compas, B. E., Slavin, L. A., Wagner, B. M., & Vannatta, K. (1986). Relationship of life events and social support with psychological dysfunction among adolescents. *Journal of Youth and Adolescence, 15,* 205–221.

Costello, E. J., Edelbrock, C. S., & Costello, A. J. (1985). Validity of the NIMH Diagnostic Interview Schedule for Children: A comparison between psychiatric and pediatric referrals. *Journal of Abnormal Child Psychology, 13,* 579–595.

Crosbie-Burnett, M., & Newcomer, L. L. (1990). Group counseling children of divorce: The effects of a multimodal intervention. *Journal of Divorce, 13,* 69–78.

Crowley, S. L., Worchel, F. F., & Ash, M. J. (1992). Self-report, peer-report, and teacher-report measures of childhood depression: An analysis by item. *Journal of Personality Assessment, 59,* 189–203.

Curry, J. F., & Craighead, W. E. (1990). Attributional style in clinically depressed and conduct disordered adolescents. *Journal of Consulting and Clinical Psychology, 58,* 109–115.

Dalley, M. B., Bolocofsky, D. N., Alcorn, M. B., & Baker, C. (1992). Depressive symptomatology, attributional style, dysfunctional attitude, and social competency in adolescents with and without learning disabilities. *School Psychology Review, 21,* 444–458.

Derogatis, L. R., Lipman, R. S., Rickels, K., Uhlenhuth, E. H., & Covi, L. (1974). The Hopkins Symptom Checklist (HSCL): A measure of primary symptom dimensions. In P. Pichot (Ed.), *Psychological measurements in psychopharmacology: Modern problems in pharmacopsychiatry,* Vol. 7 (pp. 79–110). Paris: Karger.

Doerfler, L. A., Felner, R. D., Rowlison, R. T., Evans, E., & Raley, P. A. (1988).Depression in children and adolescents: A comparative analysis of the utility and construct validity of two assessment measures. *Journal of Consulting and Clinical Psychology, 56,* 769–772.

Eddy, B. A., & Lubin, B. (1988). The Children's Depression Adjective Check Lists (C-DACL) with emotionally disturbed adolescent boys. *Journal of Abnormal Psychology, 16,* 83–88.

Edelsohn, G., Ialongo, N., Werthamer-Larsson, L., Crockett, L., & Kellam, S. (1992). Self-reported depressive symptoms in first-grade children: Developmentally transient phenomena? *Journal of the American Academy of Child and Adolescent Psychiatry, 31,* 282–290.

Endicott, J., & Spitzer, R. L. (1978). A diagnostic interview: The schedule for affective disorders and schizophrenia. *Archives of General Psychiatry, 35,* 837–844.

Epstein, N. B., Baldwin, L. M., & Bishop, D. S. (1983). The McMaster Family Assessment Device. *Journal of Marital and Family Therapy, 9,* 171–180.

Faulstich, M. E., Carey, M. P., Ruggiero, L., Enyart, P., & Gresham, F. (1986). Assessment of depression in childhood and adolescence: An evaluation of the Center for Epidemiological Studies Depression Scale for Children (CES-DC). *American Journal of Psychiatry, 143,* 1024–1027.

Finch, A. J., Saylor, C. F., & Edwards, G. L. (1985). Children's Depression Inventory: Sex and grade norms for normal children. *Journal of Consulting and Clinical Psychology, 53,* 424–425.

Finch, A. J., Saylor, C. F., Edwards, G. L., & McIntosh, J. A. (1987). Children's Depression Inventory: Reliability over repeated administrations. *Journal of Clinical Child Psychology, 16,* 339–341.

Fine, S., Moretti, M., Haley, G., & Marriage, K. (1984). Depressive disorder in children and adolescents: Dysthymic disorder and the use of self-rating scales in assessment. *Child Psychiatry and Human Development, 14,* 223–229.

Fine, S., Moretti, M., Haley, G., & Marriage, K. (1985). Affective disorders in children and adolescents: The dysthymic disorder dilemma. *Canadian Journal of Psychiatry, 30,* 173–177.

Friedrich, W., Reams, R., & Jacobs, J. (1982). Depression and suicidal ideation in early adolescents. *Journal of Youth and Adolescence, 11,* 403–407.

Fristad, M. A., Weller, E. B., Weller, R. A., Teare, M., & Preskorn, S. H. (1988). Self-report vs. biological markers in assessment of childhood depression. *Journal of Affective Disorders, 15,* 339–345.

Garrison, C. Z., Jackson, K. L., Marsteller, F., McKeown, R., & Addy, C. (1990). A longitudinal study of depressive symptomatology in young adolescents. *Journal of the American Academy of Child and Adolescent Psychiatry, 29,* 581–585.

Garrison, C. Z., Schluchter, M. D., Schoenbach, V. J., & Kaplan, B. H. (1989). Epidemiology of depressive symptoms in young adolescents. *Journal of the American Academy of Child and Adolescent Psychiatry, 28,* 343–351.

Garrison, C. Z., Schoenbach, V. J., & Kaplan, B. H. (1985). Depressive symptoms in early adolescence. In A. Dean (Ed.), *Depression in multidisciplinary perspective* (pp. 60–82). New York: Brunner/Mazel.

Gjerde, P. F., Block, J., & Block, J. H. (1988). Depressive symptoms and personality during late adolescence: Gender differences in the externalization–internalization of symptom expression. *Journal of Abnormal Psychology, 97,* 475–486.

Hagborg, W. J. (1992). Prevalence and correlates of self-reported depressive mood among seriously emotionally disturbed adolescents. *Psychological Reports, 70,* 23–26.

Hains, A. A. (1992). Comparison of cognitive–behavioral stress management techniques with adolescent boys. *Journal of Counseling & Development, 70,* 600–605.

Hamilton, M. (1960). A rating scale for depression. *Journal of Neurology, Neurosurgery, and Psychiatry, 23,* 56–62.

Hamilton, M. (1967). Development of a rating scale for primary depressive illness. *British Journal of Social and Clinical Psychology, 6,* 278–296.

Handford, H. A., Mattison, R. E., Humphrey, R. J., & McLaughlin, R. E. (1986). Depressive syndrome in children entering a residential school subsequent to parent death, divorce, or separation. *Journal of the American Academy of Child and Adolescent Psychiatry, 25,* 409–414.

Hathaway, S. R., & McKinley, J. D. (1940). A multiphasic personality schedule. I. Construction of the schedule. *Journal of Psychology, 10,* 249–254.

Havey, J. M., & Dodd, D. K. (1992). Environmental and personality differences between children of alcoholics and their peers. *Journal of Drug Education, 22,* 215–222.

Herjanic, B., & Reich, W. (1982). Development of a structured psychiatric interview for children: Agreement between child and parent on individual symptoms. *Journal of Abnormal Child Psychology, 10,* 307–324.

Hodges, K. (1990). Depression and anxiety in children: A comparison of self-report questionnaires to clinical interview. *Psychological Assessment: A Journal of Consulting and Clinical Psychology, 2,* 376–381.

Hodges, K., & Craighead, W. E. (1990). Relationship of Children's Depression Inventory factors to diagnosed depression. *Psychological Assessment: A Journal of Consulting and Clinical Psychology, 2,* 489–492.

Hodges, K., Kline, J., Stern, L., Cytryn, L., & McKnew, D. (1982). The development of a child assessment interview for research and clinical use. *Journal of Abnormal Child Psychology, 10,* 173–189.

Hops, H., Lewinsohn, P. M., Andrews, J. A., & Roberts, R. E. (1990). Psychosocial correlates of depressive symptomatology among high school students. *Journal of Clinical Child Psychology, 19,* 211–220.

Joffe, R. D., Dobson, K. S., Fine, S., Marriage, K., & Haley, G. (1990). Social problem-solving in depressed, conduct-disordered, and normal adolescents. *Journal of Abnormal Child Psychology, 18,* 565–575.

Kahn, J. S., Kehle, T. J., & Jenson, W. R. (1987). Depression among middle-school students: Descriptive and correlational analyses. Paper presented at the Annual Convention of the National Association of School Psychologists. New Orleans, March 1987.

Kahn, J. S., Kehle, T. J., & Jenson, W. R. (1988). Assessment and treatment of depression among early adolescents. Paper presented at the Annual Convention of the National Association of School Psychologists, Chicago, April 1988.

Kahn, J. S., Kehle, T. J., Jenson, W. R., & Clark, E. (1990). Comparison of cognitive–behavioral, relaxation, and self-modeling interventions for depression among middle-school students. *School Psychology Review, 19,* 196–211.

Kaplan, S. L., Hong, G. K., & Weinhold, C. (1984). Epidemiology of depressive symptomatology in adolescents. *Journal of the American Academy of Child Psychiatry, 23,* 91–98.

Kashani, J. H., Sherman, D. D., Parker, D. R ., & Reid, J. C. (1990). Utility of the Beck Depression Inventory with clinic-referred adolescents. *Journal of the American Academy of Child and Adolescent Psychiatry, 29,* 278–282.

Kaslow, N. J., Rehm, L. P., & Siegel, A. W. (1984). Social–cognitive and cognitive correlates of depression in children. *Journal of Abnormal Child Psychology, 12,* 605–620.

Kazdin, A. E. (1987a). Assessment of childhood depression: Current issues and strategies. *Behavioral Assessment, 9,* 291–319.

Kazdin, A. E. (1987b). Children's Depression Scale: Validation with child psychiatric inpatients. *Journal of Child Psychology and Psychiatry, 28,* 29–41.

Kazdin, A. E. (1989). Identifying depression in children: A comparison of alternative selection criteria. *Journal of Abnormal Child Psychology, 17,* 437–454.

Kazdin, A. E., Esveldt-Dawson, K., Unis, A. S., & Rancurello, M. D. (1983a). Child and parent evaluations of depression and aggression in psychiatric inpatient children. *Journal of Abnormal Child Psychology, 11,* 401–413.

Kazdin, A. E., French, N. H., & Unis, A. S. (1983b). Child, mother, and father evaluations of depression in psychiatric inpatient children. *Journal of Abnormal Child Psychology, 11,* 167–180.

Kazdin, A. E., French, N. H., Unis, A. S., & Esveldt-Dawson, K. (1983c). Assessment of childhood depression: Correspondence of child and parent ratings. *Journal of the American Academy of Child Psychiatry, 22,* 157–164.

Kazdin, A. E., Heidish, I. E. (1984). Convergence of clinically derived diagnoses and parent checklists among inpatient children. *Journal of Abnormal Child Psychology, 12,* 421–436.

Kendall, P. C., Stark, K. D., & Adam, T. (1990). Cognitive deficit or cognitive distortion in childhood depression. *Journal of Abnormal Child Psychology, 18,* 255–270.

King, C. A., Raskin, A., Gdowski, C. L., Butkus, M., & Opipari, L. (1990). Psychosocial factors associated with urban adolescent female suicide attempts. *Journal of the American Academy of Child and Adolescent Psychiatry, 29,* 289–294.

King, C. A., Segal, H. G., Gargan, S., Ghaziuddin, N., Naylor, M., & Kaminski, K. (1992). Suicidal adolescents' follow-up adjustment. Paper presented at the Annual Convention of the American Association of Suicidology, April 1992.

Klein, D. N., Depue, R. A., & Slater, J. F. (1986). Inventory identification of cyclothymia. IX. Validation in offspring of bipolar patients. *Archives of General Psychiatry, 43*, 441–445.

Knight, D., Hensley, V. R., & Waters, B. (1988). Validation of the Children's Depression Scale and the Children's Depression Inventory in a prepubertal sample. *Journal of Child Psychology and Psychiatry, 29*, 853–863.

Kovacs, M. (1979). *Children's Depression Inventory*. University of Pittsburgh School of Medicine: Author.

Kovacs, M. (1980/1981). Rating scales to assess depression in school-aged children. *Acta Paedopsychiatrica, 46*, 305–315.

Kovacs, M (1983). The Children's Depression Inventory: A self-rating scale for school-aged youngsters. Unpublished manuscript.

Kovacs, M. (1992). *Children's Depression Inventory manual*. North Tonawanda, NY: Multi-Health Systems.

Kovacs, M., & Beck, A. T. (1977). An empirical–clinical approach toward a definition of childhood depression. In J. G. Schulterbrandt & A. Raskin (Eds.), *Depression in childhood: Diagnosis, treatment and conceptual models* (pp. 1–25). New York: Raven Press.

Kraemer, E. S. (1992). Relationship between depressive symptomatology and social functioning in adolescents. Unpublished master's thesis. University of Wisconsin—Madison.

Kutcher, S. P., & Marton, P. (1989). Utility of the Beck Depression Inventory with psychiatrically disturbed adolescent outpatients. *Canadian Journal of Psychiatry, 34*, 107–109.

Lang, M., & Tisher, M. (1978). *Children's Depression Scale*. Victoria: Australian Council for Educational Research.

Lang, M., & Tisher, M. (1987). *Children's Depression Scale Manual, North American Edition*. Palo Alto, CA: Consulting Psychologists Press.

Lapsley, D. K., Flannery, D. J., Krug, J., & McGinnis, C. (1984). Loneliness, depression, and epistemological relativity in early and late adolescence. Paper presented at the Annual Meeting of the Midwestern Psychological Association, Chicago, May 1984.

Larson, R. W., Raffaelli, M., Richards, M. H., Ham, M., & Jewell, L. (1990). Ecology of depression in late childhood and early adolescence: A profile of daily states and activities. *Journal of Abnormal Psychology, 99*, 92–102.

Lefkowitz, M. M., & Tesiny, E. P. (1980). Assessment of childhood depression. *Journal of Consulting and Clinical Psychology, 48*, 43–50.

Lefkowitz, M. M., Tesiny, E. P., & Solodow, W. (1989). A rating scale for assessing dysphoria in youth. *Journal of Abnormal Child Psychology, 17*, 337–347.

Lineberger, M. A. (1987). Pregnant adolescents attending prenatal parent education classes: Self-concepts, anxiety, and depression levels. *Adolescence, 22*, 179–193.

Lobovits, D. A., & Handal, P. J. (1985). Children depression: Prevalence using DSM-III criteria and validity of parent and child depression scales. *Journal of Pediatric Psychology, 10*, 45–54.

Lopez, N. (1985). Assessing depressive symptoms using the Child Depression Scale and the Children's Depression Inventory: A cross cultural comparison of children in Puerto Rico and the United States. Unpublished doctoral dissertation. University of Wisconsin—Madison.

Lyon, M. A., & Bolin, J. A. (1988). Depression in a sample of alternative learning center adolescents. Paper presented at the Annual Meeting of the National Association of School Psychologists, Chicago, April 1988.

Manson, S. M., Ackerson, L. M., Dick, R. W., Baron, A. E., & Fleming, C. M. (1990). Depressive symptoms among American Indian adolescents: Psychometric characteristics of the Center for Epidemiologic Studies Depression Scale (CES-D). *Psychological Assessment: A Journal of Consulting and Clinical Psychology, 2*, 231–237.

Marcotte, D., & Baron, P. (1993). L'efficacité d'une strategie d'intervention emotivo-rationnelle auprès d'adolescents depressifs du milieu scolaire. *Canadian Journal of Counseling, 27*, 77–92.

Matson, J. L., & Nieminen, G. S. (1987). Validity of measures of conduct disorder, depression, and anxiety. *Journal of Clinical Child Psychology, 16*, 151–157.

Mattison, R. E., Handford, H. A., Kales, H. C., Goodman, A. L., & McLaughlin, R. E. (1990). Four-year predictive value of the Children's Depression Inventory. *Psychological Assessment: A Journal of Consulting and Clinical Psychology, 2*, 169–174.

Mazza, J. J., & Reynolds, W. M. (1991). Longitudinal investigation of psychosocial factors and suicidal ideation in adolescents. Paper presented at the Annual Meeting of the American Psychological Association, San Francisco, August 1991.

Mezzich, A. C., & Mezzich, J. E. (1979). Symptomatology of depression in adolescence. *Journal of Personality Assessment, 43*, 267–275.

Moretti, M. M., Fine, S., Haley, G., & Marriage, K. (1985). Childhood and adolescent depression: Child-report versus parent-report information. *Journal of the American Academy of Child Psychiatry, 24,* 298–302.

Navarrete, L. A. (1992). Epidemiology of depressive symptoms in adolescents with learning disabilities and a nonequivalent comparison group. Unpublished doctoral dissertation. University of New Mexico.

Nelson, W. M., & Politano, P. M. (1990). Children's Depression Inventory: Stability over repeated administrations in psychiatric inpatient children. *Journal of Clinical Child Psychology, 19,* 254–256.

Nelson, W. M., Politano, P. M., Finch, A. J., Wendel, N., & Mayhall, C. (1987). Children's Depression Inventory: Normative data and utility with emotionally disturbed children. *Journal of the American Academy of Child and Adolescent Psychiatry, 26,* 43–48.

Nieminen, G. S., & Matson, J. L. (1989). Depressive problems in conduct-disordered adolescents. *Journal of School Psychology, 27,* 175–186.

Ollendick, T. H., & Yule, W. (1990). Depression in British and American children and its relation to anxiety and fear. *Journal of Consulting and Clinical Psychology, 58,* 126–129.

Ollendick, T. H., Yule, W., & Ollier, K. (1991). Fears in British children and their relationship to manifest anxiety and depression. *Journal of Child Psychology and Psychiatry, 32,* 321–331.

Petti, T. A. (1978). Depression in hospitalized child psychiatry patients: Approaches to measuring depression. *Journal of the American Academy of Child Psychiatry, 17,* 49–59.

Poznanski, E. O., Cook, S. C., & Carroll, B. J. (1979). A depression rating scale for children. *Pediatrics, 64,* 442–450.

Poznanski, E. O., Grossman, J. A., Buchsbaum, Y., Banegas, M., Freeman, L., & Gibbons, R. (1984). Preliminary studies of the reliability and validity of the Children's Depression Rating Scale. *Journal of the American Academy of Child Psychiatry, 23,* 191–197.

Puig-Antich, J., & Chambers, W. (1978). *The Schedule for Affective Disorders and Schizophrenia for School-age Children (Kiddie-SADS).* New York: New York State Psychiatric Institute.

Rabkin, J. G., & Klein, D. F. (1987). The clinical measurement of depressive disorders. In A. J. Marsella, R. M. A. Hirschfeld, & M. M. Katz (Eds.), *The measurement of depression* (pp. 30–83). New York: Guilford Press.

Radloff, L. S. (1977). The CES-D Scale: A self-report scale for research in the general population. *Applied Psychological Measurement, 1,* 385–401.

Radloff, L. S. (1991). The use of the Center for Epidemiologic Studies Depression scale in adolescents and young adults. *Journal of Youth and Adolescence, 20,* 149–166.

Rawson, H. E. (1992). The interrelationship of measures of manifest anxiety, self-esteem, locus of control, and depression in children with behavior problems. *Journal of Psychoeducational Assessment, 10,* 319–329.

Rawson, H. E., & Tabb, L. C. (1993). Effects of therapeutic intervention on childhood depression. *Child and Adolescent Social Work Journal, 10,* 39–51.

Reich, W., Herjanic, B., Welner, Z., & Gandhy, P. R. (1982). Development of a structured psychiatric interview for children: Agreement in diagnosis comparing child and parent interviews. *Journal of Abnormal Child Psychology, 10,* 325–336.

Reynolds, W. M. (1985a). Development and validation of a scale to measure depression in adolescents. Paper presented at the Annual Meeting of the Society for Personality Assessment, Berkeley, CA, March 1985.

Reynolds, W. M. (1985b). Depression in childhood and adolescence: Diagnosis, assessment, intervention strategies and research. In T. R. Kratochwill (Ed.), *Advances in school psychology,* Vol. 4 (pp. 133–189). Hillsdale, NJ: Erlbaum Associates.

Reynolds, W. M. (1986a). *Reynolds Adolescent Depression Scale.* Odessa, FL: Psychological Assessment Resources.

Reynolds, W. M. (1986b). A model for the screening and identification of depressed children and adolescents in school settings. *Professional School Psychology, 1,* 117–129.

Reynolds, W. M. (1987a). *Reynolds Adolescent Depression Scale: Professional Manual.* Odessa, FL: Psychological Assessment Resources.

Reynolds, W. M. (1987b). *Suicidal Ideation Questionnaire.* Odessa, FL: Psychological Assessment Resources.

Reynolds, W. M. (1988). *Suicidal Ideation Questionnaire: Professional Manual.* Odessa, FL: Psychological Assessment Resources.

Reynolds, W. M. (1989a). *Reynolds Child Depression Scale.* Odessa, FL: Psychological Assessment Resources.

Reynolds, W. M. (1989b). *Reynolds Child Depression Scale: Professional Manual.* Odessa, FL: Psychological Assessment Resources.

Reynolds, W. M. (1989c). Suicidal ideation and depression in adolescents: Assessment and research. In P. F. Lovibond & P. Wilson (Eds.), *Clinical and abnormal psychology* (pp. 125–135). Amsterdam: Elsevier.

Reynolds, W. M. (1990). Development of a semistructured clinical interview for suicidal behaviors in adolescents. *Psychological Assessment: A Journal of Consulting and Clinical Psychology, 2,* 382–390.

Reynolds, W. M. (1991). A school-based procedure for the identification of adolescents at-risk for suicidal behaviors. *Family and Community Health, 14,* 64–75.

Reynolds, W. M. (1992). Depression in children and adolescents. In W. M. Reynolds (Ed.), *Internalizing disorders in children and adolescents* (pp. 149–254). New York: John Wiley.

Reynolds, W. M. (1993a). Self-report methods. In T. H. Ollendick & M. Hersen (Eds.), *Handbook of child and adolescent assessment* (pp. 98–125). New York: Plenum Press.

Reynolds, W. M. (1993b). *The Adolescent Psychopathology Scales: Initial reliability of clinical disorder* scales. Paper presented at the Annual Meeting of the Society for Personality Assessment, San Francisco, March 1993.

Reynolds, W. M. (1994a). Depression in adolescents: Contemporary issues and perspectives. In T. H. Ollendick & R. J. Prinz (Eds.), *Advances in clinical child psychology*, Vol. 16 (pp. 261–316). New York: Plenum Press.

Reynolds, W. M. (1994b). Depression. In V. B. Van Hasselt & M. Hersen (Eds.), *Handbook of adolescent psychopathology*. New York: Lexington Books.

Reynolds, W. M. (in press). *Adolescent Psychopathology Scale*. Odessa, FL: Psychological Assessment Resources.

Reynolds, W. M., Anderson, G., & Bartell N. (1985). Measuring depression in children: A multimethod assessment investigation. *Journal of Abnormal Child Psychology, 13,* 513–526.

Reynolds, W. M., & Coats, K. I. (1982). Depression in adolescents: Incidence, depth and correlates. Paper presented at the 10th International Congress of the International Association for Child and Adolescent Psychiatry, Dublin, July 1982.

Reynolds, W. M., & Coats, K. I. (1986). A comparison of cognitive–behavioral therapy and relaxation training for the treatment of depression in adolescents. *Journal of Consulting and Clinical Psychology, 54,* 653–660.

Reynolds, W. M., & Evert, T. (1991). Efficacy of a multiple-gate screening strategy for identification of clinical levels of depressive symptomatology in adolescents. Unpublished manuscript.

Reynolds, W. M., & Gould, J. (1981). A psychometric investigation of the standard and short form Beck Depression Inventory. *Journal of Consulting and Clinical Psychology, 49,* 306–307.

Reynolds, W. M., & Graves, A. (1989a). Reliability of children's reports of depressive symptomatology. *Journal of Abnormal Child Psychology, 17,* 647–655.

Reynolds, W. M., & Graves, A. (1989b). Depressive symptomatology in gifted and nongifted children: Teacher and child report comparisons. Paper presented at the Annual Meeting of the American Educational Research Association, San Francisco, March 1989.

Reynolds, W. M., & Miller, K. L. (1985). Depression and learned helplessness in mentally retarded and nonretarded adolescents: An initial investigation. *Applied Research in Mental Retardation, 6,* 295–307.

Reynolds, W. M., & Miller, K. L. (1989). Assessment of adolescents' learned helplessness in achievement situations. *Journal of Personality Assessment, 53,* 211–228.

Reynolds, W. M., & Stark, K. D. (1983). Cognitive behavior modification: The clinical application of cognitive strategies. In M. Pressley & J. R. Levin (Eds.), *Cognitive strategy research: Psychological foundations* (pp. 221–266). New York: Springer-Verlag.

Rierdan, J., & Koff, E. (1993). Developmental variables in relation to depressive symptoms in adolescent girls. *Development and Psychopathology, 5,* 485–496.

Roberts, R. E., Andrews, J. A., Lewinsohn, P. M., & Hops, H. (1990). Assessment of depression in adolescents using the Center for Epidemiologic Studies Depression Scale. *Psychological Assessment: A Journal of Consulting and Clinical Psychology, 2,* 122–128.

Roberts, R. E., Lewinsohn, P. M., & Seeley, J. R. (1991). Screening for adolescent depression: A comparison of depression scales. *Journal of the American Academy of Child and Adolescent Psychiatry, 30,* 58–66.

Roseby, V., & Deutsch, R. (1985). Children of separation and divorce: Effects of a social role-taking group intervention on fourth and fifth graders. *Journal of Clinical Child Psychology, 14,* 55–60.

Rosenberg, M. (1965). *Society and the adolescent self-image*. Princeton, NJ: Princeton University Press.

Rotundo, N., & Hensley, V. R. (1985). The Children's Depression Scale: A study of its validity. *Journal of Child Psychology and Psychiatry, 26,* 917–927.

Sacco, W. P., & Graves, D. J. (1984). Childhood depression, interpersonal problem-solving, and self-ratings of performance. *Journal of Clinical Child Psychology, 13,* 10–15.

Sadowski, C., & Kelley, M. L. (1993). Social problem solving in suicidal adolescents. *Journal of Consulting and Clinical Psychology, 61*, 121–127.

Saylor, C. F., Finch, A. J., Spirito, A., & Bennett, B. (1984). The Children's Depression Inventory: A systematic evaluation of psychometric properties. *Journal of Consulting and Clinical Psychology, 52*, 955–967.

Schoenbach, V. J., Kaplan, B. H., Grimson, R. C., & Wagner, E. H. (1982). Use of a symptom scale to study the prevalence of a depressive syndrome in young adolescents. *American Journal of Epidemiology, 116*, 791–800.

Schoenbach, V. J., Kaplan, B. H., Wagner, E. H., Grimson, R. C., & Miller, F. T. (1983). Prevalence of self-reported depressive symptoms in adolescents. *American Journal of Public Health, 73*, 1281–1287.

Schonert-Reichl, K. A. (1994). Gender differences in depressive symptomatology and egocentrism in adolescence. *Journal of Early Adolescence, 14*, 49–64.

Shain, B. N., Kronfol, Z., Naylor, M., Goel, K., Evans, T., & Schaefer, S. (1991). Natural killer cell activity in adolescents with major depression. *Biological Psychiatry, 29*, 481–484.

Shain, B. N., Naylor, M., & Alessi, N. (1990). Comparison of self-rated and clinician-rated measures of depression in adolescents. *American Journal of Psychiatry, 147*, 793–795.

Siegel, L. J., & Griffin, N. J. (1984). Correlates of depressive symptoms in adolescents. *Journal of Youth and Adolescence, 13*, 475–487.

Smucker, M. R., Craighead, W. E., Craighead, L. W., & Green, B. J. (1986). Normative and reliability data for the Children's Depression Inventory. *Journal of Abnormal Child Psychology, 14*, 25–39.

Sokoloff, R. M., & Lubin, B. (1983). Depressive mood in adolescent, emotionally disturbed females: Reliability and validity of an adjective checklist (C-DACL). *Journal of Abnormal Child Psychology, 11*, 531–536.

Spirito, A., Stark, L. J., Fristad, M., Hart, K., & Owens-Stively, J. (1987). Adolescent suicide attempters hospitalized on a pediatric unit. *Journal of Pediatric Psychology, 12*, 171–189.

Spirito, A., Stark, L. J., Hart, K. J., & Fristad, M. (1988). Overt behavior of adolescent suicide attempters hospitalized on a general pediatrics floor. *Journal of Adolescent Health Care, 9*, 491–494.

Spitzer, R. L., Endicott, J., & Robins, E. (1978). Research diagnostic criteria: Rationale and reliability. *Archives of General Psychiatry, 35*, 773–782.

Stark, K. D. (1984). A comparison of the relative efficacy of self-control therapy and behavior therapy for the reduction of depression in children. Unpublished doctoral dissertation. University of Wisconsin—Madison.

Stark, K. D., Reynolds, W. M., & Kaslow, N. J. (1987). A comparison of the relative efficacy of self-control therapy and behavioral problem-solving therapy for depression in children. *Journal of Abnormal Child Psychology, 15*, 91–113.

Strauss, C. C., Forehand, R., Frame, C., & Smith, K. (1984). Characteristics of children with extreme scores on the Children's Depression Inventory. *Journal of Clinical Child Psychology, 13*, 227–231.

Strober, M., Green, J., & Carlson, G. (1981). Utility of the Beck Depression Inventory with psychiatrically hospitalized adolescents. *Journal of Consulting and Clinical Psychology, 49*, 482–483.

Teri, L. (1982). The use of the Beck Depression Inventory with adolescents. *Journal of Abnormal Child Psychology, 10*, 277–284.

Tharinger, D. J., & Stark, K. (1990). A qualitative versus quantitative approach to evaluating the Draw-A-Person and Kinetic Family Drawing: A study of mood- and anxiety-disorder children. *Psychological Assessment: A Journal of Consulting and Clinical Psychology, 2*, 365–375.

Tisher, M., & Lang, M. (1983). The Children's Depression Scale: Review and further developments. In D. P. Cantwell & G. A. Carlson (Eds.), *Affective disorders in childhood and adolescents—An update* (pp. 181–203). Jamaica, NY: Spectrum Publications.

Tisher, M., Lang-Takac, E., & Lang, M. (1992). The Children's Depression Scale: Review of Australian and overseas experience. *Australian Journal of Psychology, 44*, 27–35.

Tonkin, G., & Hudson, A. (1981). The Children's Depression Scale: Some further psychometric data. *Australian Council for Educational Research Bulletin for Psychologists, 30*, 11–18.

Weiss, B., Weisz, J. R., Politano, M., Carey, M., Nelson, W. M., & Finch, A. J. (1991). Developmental differences in the factor structure of the Children's Depression Inventory. *Psychological Assessment: A Journal of Consulting and Clinical Psychology, 3*, 38–45.

Wendel, N. H., Nelson, W. M., Politano, P. M., Mayhall, C. A., & Finch, A. J. (1988). Differentiating inpatient clinically-diagnosed and normal children using the Children's Depression Inventory. *Child Psychiatry and Human Development, 19*, 98–108.

Wierzbicki, M. (1987). A parent form of the Children's Depression Inventory: Reliability and validity in nonclinical populations. *Journal of Clinical Psychology, 43*, 390–397.

Worchel, F. F., Hughes, J. N., Hall, B. M., Stanton, S. B., Stanton, H., & Little, V. Z. (1990). Evaluation of subclinical depression in children using self-, peer-, and teacher-report measures. *Journal of Abnormal Child Psychology, 18,* 271–282.

Zimmerman, M., & Coryell, W. (1987). The Inventory to Diagnose Depression (IDD): A self-report scale to diagnose major depressive disorder. *Journal of Consulting and Clinical Psychology, 55,* 55–59.

Zung, W. W. K. (1965). A self-rating depression scale. *Archives of General Psychiatry, 12,* 63–70.

Zung, W. W. K. (1974). The measurement of affects: Depression and anxiety. In P. Pichot (Ed.), *Psychological measurements in psychopharmacology: Modern problems in pharmacopsychiatry,* Vol. 7 (pp. 170–188). Paris: Karger.

12

Assessment of Depression in Children and Adolescents by Parents, Teachers, and Peers

Harvey F. Clarizio

The Need for Significant Others as Informants

The limitations of self-report measures and interviews with children dictate the need for data from parents, teachers, and peers. Although children may be the best source of information for rating their inner feelings and self-perceptions, most authorities agree that information should be obtained from other sources. Several limitations of self-report measures are noteworthy, each of which underscores the need for input from significant others in the child's life. Prominent among these limitations are the comprehension of items in self-report scales, the lability of children's moods, and the need for an ecological perspective.

There are two facets of the comprehension problem—readability of the items and sociocognitive immaturity. While reading obstacles associated with self-report scales are readily overcome by presenting the items to the child orally, comprehension may not be easily achieved. The low but inverse relationship between depression and achievement (Stark, 1990) indicates that some depressed youngsters possess below-average reading ability and underscores the need to ensure that they comprehend the items. Fortunately, the readability levels of commonly used self-report scales range from 1st- to 3rd-grade reading level and are below the age levels proposed for the various measures (Kazdin & Petti, 1982). Even if youngsters understand the items, however, it is doubtful that they have sufficient cognitive or experiential maturity to rate accurately the frequency, severity, and duration of such depressive symptoms as self-regard, sleep disturbances, sad looks, and withdrawn posturing.

Harvey F. Clarizio • Department of Counseling and Educational Psychology, Michigan State University, East Lansing, Michigan 48824-1034.

Handbook of Depression in Children and Adolescents, edited by William M. Reynolds and Hugh F. Johnston. Plenum Press, New York, 1994.

There is also the danger that self-report measures may reflect what happened in the child's life that day or week rather than a more general behavioral pattern. The finding that one third of children scored as high on the Children's Depression Inventory (CDI) (Kovacs, 1983) as moderately to severely depressed adults strongly suggests that this scale tends to exaggerate the frequency and severity of depression in children.

Self-report scales provide the perspective of one person, one who, by definition, is developmentally immature. This limitation is particularly problematic because of the low agreement between child reports and adult ratings of childhood depression. Kazdin, French, and Unis (1983), for instance, found that psychiatric inpatient youngsters aged 5–13 years consistently rated themselves as less depressed across various measures of depression than did their parents. This finding indicates the need for different cutoff scores for parent-completed and child-completed inventories (Kazdin, Colbus, & Rodgers, 1986). Unfortunately, there are no well-established cutoff scores that have been used to delineate clinical levels of depression among most self-report scales (Kazdin et al., 1986) or child scales completed by parents.

Direct interviewing of the child has long been known to be feasible, reliable, and valid (Rutter & Graham, 1968). Moreover, it can offer insight into the child's subjective experience, provide opportunities to observe the child's behavioral, emotional, and cognitive functioning, and permit combination of breadth and depth of coverage (Hughes & Baker, 1990). Despite these benefits, the child interview places *general* demands (e.g., recognizing that one has a problem) as well as *specific* demands (e.g., recalling temporal covariation and duration of symptoms) that tax the developmental capabilities of pre-adolescents (Kovacs, 1986). Differences in children's metamemory, communication skills, reliance on contextual cues, and desire to please adults are not insurmountable obstacles, but ameliorating them does demand developmentally sensitive interviewing (Hughes & Baker, 1990) by a highly skilled clinician. Further, children under the age of 10 are not reliable reporters of their own symptoms except for fears (Edelbrock, Costello, Dulcan, Kalas, & Conover, 1985). Finally, interviews are also time-consuming. For example, the Kiddie Schedule for Affective Disorder and Schizophrenia (K-SADS) takes 45–120 minutes to conduct (Orvaschel, 1985). In short, even though the psychiatric interviews with children might well be the method most commonly used to assess childhood depression, many youngsters may not be able to recognize, properly label, accurately monitor, or estimate frequency, severity, and duration of their depressive symptomatology (Kovacs, 1986). Additionally, depressed youngsters are often reluctant or unable to communicate freely, limiting their usefulness as informants. Reports by significant others are needed to fill these voids and to provide a broader perspective.

Perhaps the most important reason for including reports from parents and teachers centers around the reality that parents and teachers are typically the ones who refer children for evaluation and treatment. Children usually do not refer themselves for treatment. Instead, their caregivers are the ones who express concern about children and seek professional assistance on their behalf. Because it is the important adults in a child's life who first call the child to the attention of mental health specialists, it is essential that we have a clear, detailed, reliable, and valid assessment of their concerns about the child.

Advantages and Disadvantages

Parent, teacher, and peer ratings have many disadvantages and advantages. The disadvantages include the (1) inability to rate the unobservable nature of many of the inner aspects of depression (e.g., suicidal ideation, excessive guilt feelings); (2) ambiguity in the meaning of the symptoms to be appraised (e.g., depressed mood); (3) wide individual differences among raters, such as leniency, stringency, or rating everybody average; and

(4) failure to assess antecedent and consequent events surrounding the child's behavior that are often important in determining the why, when, and where factors necessary to effective management.

The advantages of behavior rating scales include (1) drawing on a rater's often substantial previous experience with the child over long periods of time and in different settings; (2) gathering of data on rare and infrequent behaviors; (3) low cost and efficiency in gathering calculable information; (4) normative data to determine the degree of pathology for a given child within the same-age and same-sex group and to show whether treatment has brought the child closer to the average child; (5) the existence of various scales, on which substantial information has been collected regarding their psychometric properties and practical value; (6) ecological validity in that the opinions of various "significant others" are incorporated; and (7) the quantification of qualitative aspects of child behavior not readily available through other means (Barkley, 1990).

Assessment by Parents

General Psychopathology Scales

The scales most commonly used by parents to assess their children's depression are general inventories that cover a multitude of different kinds of symptoms or constellations, among which is depression (Kazdin, 1988). Two of the better-known general childhood psychopathology scales, the Personality Inventory for Children (PIC) and The Child Behavior Checklist (CBCL), are described below.

Personality Inventory for Children. The PIC illustrates how parental reports can be used to obtain accurate information about the child and his or her relationships with others. The PIC (Wirt, Lachar, Klinedinst, & Seat, 1977) contains clinical subscales, one of which is designed to measure depression in children. The PIC can be used with children between 3 and 16 years of age and is to be completed by someone who has had ample opportunity to observe the child, usually the mother. The Depression scale consists of 46 items dealing with such factors as moodiness, social isolation, crying spells, lack of energy, pessimism, serious attitude, indecisiveness, uncommunicativeness, concern with death and separation, and sensitivity to criticism. All the 46 items had to be nominated by at least four of seven judges to be included in the scale. The test–retest reliability of this scale based on 34 psychiatric outpatients was 0.94 over a 15-day average period and 0.93 for 45 normal children over a 2-week interval. No validity data are available for this scale except for data indicating that the scale's scores are high for various clinical samples. Although profile analysis is not yet well developed with the PIC, other scales of the instrument, such as the Anxiety Withdrawal scale and Social Skills scale, should be considered in the interpretation of childhood depression, as the correlation of these three subscales with the Depression subscale is 0.81, 0.62, and 0.62, respectively, due in part to overlap of items on these subscales.

Criticisms questioning the utility of the PIC center around the out-of-date norms, inconsistency between mother, father, and teacher ratings, and whether the scale should be completed at home or at the clinic or school (Leon, Kendall, & Garber, 1980; Reynolds, Anderson, & Bartell, 1985; C. Reynolds & Tuma, 1985; Rothermel & Lovell, 1985). Despite its shortcomings, the PIC remains one of the most sophisticated and best-developed personality scales available for children.

Child Behavior Checklist. The CBCL developed by Achenbach and Edelbrock (1982), also relies on parental report as a means of assessing childhood depression and other clinical conditions. The CBCL is designed to assess in standardized format the social competencies and childhood problems among youngsters aged 4–16 as reported by their parents or teachers. Of the 118 childhood behavior problems, some pertain to depressive phenomena. The items, which are rated on a three-point scale, contain specific observable child behaviors (e.g., talks about killing self) that require more general inferences (e.g., unhappy, sad, or depressed) and behaviors that require considerable judgment on the part of others (e.g., feels too guilty). A 5th-grade reading capability is required to complete the CBCL (Mooney, 1984). It is easy to administer, well normed with respect to age and gender as well as to normal and clinical populations, psychometrically sound, and clearly appropriate for a wide variety of clinic-referred children. It is quite useful in distinguishing clinical from nonclinical groups and in providing a broad overview of the child's problems from the parents' and teachers' perspectives. The usefulness of this checklist in differentiating among clinical samples is reflected in the finding that follow-up scores on social involvement differentiated between suicidal children and depressed children. The depressed tended to withdraw from others, while the suicidal tended to maintain contact with friends and family (Cohen-Sandler, Berman, & King, 1982). While the CBCL is helpful in distinguishing clinically impaired youngsters from the general population, its usefulness with normals may be limited (Mooney, 1984). The reliability of the depression items due to their less observable nature is also lower than the average of other individual scales. And, like most rating scales, the CBCL tends to locate the problems in the individual child's pathology and to neglect the impact on the child's problems of environmental forces such as the family system or classroom. Despite these limitations, the CBCL has deservedly gained a respected role in the psychological assessment of children's problems.

Recent research (Rey & Morris-Yates, 1991) has demonstrated that a measure of depression extracted from the CBCL by Nurcombe et al. (1989) was able to discriminate between adolescents with and without major depression with an accuracy comparable to that reported for the dexamethasone suppression test. The subjects consisted of 667 adolescents aged 12–16 years, referred to the Rivendell Adolescent Unit in Sydney, Australia. Two senior clinicians made independent DSM-III diagnoses. Using analyses of the receiver operating characteristic (ROC) of signal-detection theory, the only technique that yields an overall index of diagnostic accuracy uninfluenced by decision biases and prior probabilities (Swets, 1988), the investigators found that the 22 items of the CBCL-NUR were most accurate when discriminating between patients with and without major depression. The scale discriminates almost as accurately between major depression and separation anxiety. The scale was least accurate when discriminating depression from dysthymia, although even in this instance the scale did better than chance.

Adaptations of Self-Report

Almost all the self-report measures of childhood depression have been reworded so that parents can report on their children's depression. Thus far, no single measure has clearly demonstrated superior reliability and validity (Kazdin, 1990) despite the use of parent-report scales in several investigations. As is the case with self-report scales with children, the primary purpose of these adapted parent-related scales is to rate the *severity* of depression, not to achieve a diagnosis. For instance, both the CDI, the most cited and thoroughly researched questionnaire designed to assess depression in school-aged children and adolescents, and the Children's Depression Scale (CDS) developed by Tisher and Lang (1978) have also been used as parent-rated depression measures. By and large, there seems to be limited consistency across raters. Children's self-report of depression on the CDI and CDS shows a modest relationship with parents' ratings of children's depression (Moretti, Fine, Haley, & Marriage, 1985). In general, there is a reliable but low agreement ($r = 0.25$) for parent and child assessments of problem behavior (Achenbach, Mc-

Conaughy, & Howell, 1987). Children see their impairment as less severe than their parents. Direct observation of overt depressive behavior among child psychiatric inpatients shows that behavioral measures are consistently related to parent-completed ratings of depression and DSM-III diagnoses but not to child-completed ratings (Kazdin, Esveldt-Dawson, Sherick, & Colbus, 1985). This finding does not invalidate parent-rated scales, self-report inventories, and interviews of children. Both parental reports and self-reports might well be valid measures of different external criteria even though they do not correlate highly with each other. There is no need to assume that one source of information is correct and the other inaccurate, given what we know from personality research about the situational specificity of behavior and low relationships between various measures of a construct. Indeed, research indicates that parental reports correlate with decreased social participation on the youngster's part and visible signs of emotion (Kazdin et al., 1985) and that child self-reports of depression correlate with suicide attempt and ideation, low self-esteem, and negative attributional style (Kazdin, French, Unis, & Esveldt-Dawson, 1983). Research in validating rater reports is often plagued by criterion contamination. For instance, clinical ratings are sometimes used as an external criterion to validate parental reports when, in fact, they are based on parental input.

Adaptations of Peer Report

Just as self-report inventories have been revised for use by parents, the peer-nomination technique has been altered for use by parents. For instance, unlike the Peer Nomination Inventory of Depression (PNID), the Rating Scale for Dysphoria (RSD) (Lefkowitz, Tesiny, & Solodow, 1989) was developed to be either a self-rated or an adult-rated scale. The items for the RSD include 12 of the 13 depression-related items on the PNID rewritten using a Likert response format (Table 1). As an example, the PNID item "Who often plays alone?" was rewritten for the self-rating scale to read, "Do you often play alone?" For the adult-rating scale, it would read, "Does [name] often play alone?" Possible answers to each item were one of five choices: never, almost never, sometimes, almost always, always. Scores could range from 12 to 60, with higher scores indicating a greater level of dysphoria. The PNID item "Who sleeps in class?" was not included on the RSD, although no rationale was provided for its deletion.

The psychometric study of the RSD involved two separate studies, each providing data for both contemporaneous and longitudinal analysis. The subjects were 784 children and their 784 mothers. All the children were pupils in the New York City public schools, and the families were predominately of middle socioeconomic status. Ethnic composition was not indicated. Longitudinal data were collected for 124 of these mother–child pairs after an interval of 2 years and for 133 mother–child pairs after 4 years. At the second interval, 82 of the 133 children's fathers also provided RSD data.

Table 1. Items from the Peer Nomination Inventory for Depression Adapted to a Rating Scale of Dysphoria[a]

1. Does [name] play alone?	7. Does [name] worry a lot?
2. Does [name] try again when he/she loses?	8. Does [name] play?
3. Does [name] feel lonely?	9. Does [name] take part in things?
4. Does [name] feel well?	10. Does [name] have much fun?
5. Does [name] feel he/she can't do things?	11. Does [name] think others don't like him/her?
6. Does [name] cry?	12. Does [name] feel sad?

[a]Adapted from Lefkowitz et al. (1989), *Journal of Abnormal Child Psychology, 17,* 337–347. Copyright 1989 by Plenum Publishing Corporation.

Reliability of the RSD was demonstrated by internal consistency, interrater agreement, and temporal (test–retest) stability. The internal consistency for the various groups, as measured by coefficient α, had values ranging from 0.70 to 0.77. Also, the mean scores and variability for the RSD were quite stable across all groups and time periods. Interrater agreement was calculated by correlating the mothers' and fathers' RSD scores, both concurrently and after an interval of 4 years. Scores obtained by the fathers 4 years after the mothers' initial RSD scores yielded an r of 0.45 ($N = 82$, $p < 0.001$). Agreement in both cases was moderately correlated and statistically significant, indicating adequate interrater agreement even over 4 years of child development. Temporal stability was moderately high as reflected by test–retest correlations of 0.73 after 2 years and 0.66 after 4 years.

Content, concurrent, construct, and predictive validity were all determined for the RSD. Because the items for the RSD were obtained from the PNID, the following discussion on content validity for the PNID also applies to the RSD.

Concurrent validity was assessed by correlating the mothers' RSD scores with both the peer nominations of depression and the children's self-rated depression as measured on a mother-completed form of the CDI at modal age of 10 years. These correlations tended to be low, but statistically significant, for peer nomination and self-ratings. Concurrent validity was also assessed by correlating children's RSD scores at modal ages of 12 and 14. In all cases, the resulting coefficients were highly statistically significant. Only the fathers' RSD scores at child age 14 years failed to correlate significantly with the other ratings.

Construct validity was assessed by correlating RSD scores with a set of variables presumed to relate to dysphoria. The variables thought to correspond to higher RSD scores were poor work-study habits, mothers' rejection, parental disharmony, mothers' depression and neuroticism, and children's self-rated neuroticism. Peer-nominated happiness and mothers' and children's extraversion were believed to be inversely related to higher RSD scores. In all cases, the RSD scores showed statistically significant positive correlations with the variables presumed to be associated with dysphoria and statistically significant negative correlations with the measures of happiness and extraversion.

Finally, predictive validity was assessed by examining the relationship between mothers' RSD scores when the children were modal age 10 years and children's RSD scores at ages 12 and 14 years. The correlations were 0.30 ($N = 122$, $p < 0.001$) at age 12 and 0.21 ($N = 133$, $p < 0.001$) at age 14. Overall, the RSD has been shown to possess satisfactory psychometric properties. It would appear that the RSD can reliably and validly assess dysphoria based on a definition implied from the relationship of dysphoria to different variables measured in this study.

Assessment by Teachers

There are several reasons that input from teachers is important for the assessment of childhood depression. First, children and adolescents spend approximately 12,000 hours in school settings during the formative years of their lives. Second, next to parents, teachers know the children better than perhaps any other adult. Third, because young people exhibit different types of behaviors at home and at school (Leon et al., 1980), data from the teacher can aid in developing a broader view of the youngster's adjustment. Teacher-rated scales and direct observation are two methods available to teachers and specialists in the schools for assessing depression in young people.

Teacher-Rated Scales

Behavior Evaluation Scale—2. The Behavioral Evaluation Scale—2 (BES-2) was developed by McCarney and Leigh (1990) in response to the need for an operational definition of emotional impairment as defined under Public Law 101-476, the Individuals with Educational Disabilities Act (IDEA), formerly known as the Education for All Handicapped Act (EHA) or more commonly as Public Law 94-142. This scale, originally developed in 1983 and revised in 1990, devotes 17 of its 76 items to the assessment of depression, which under PL 101-476 is defined as "a general pervasive mood of unhappiness or depression." Items are weighted to reflect the seriousness of the behaviors rated. Each item is rated for frequency from 1 (never or not observed) to 7 (continuously throughout the day). Consistent with the Federal government's definition of emotional impairment, this scale also has a related subscale of 14 items designed to measure "a tendency to develop physical symptoms of fears associated with personal or school problems."

Sample items from the depression subscale of the BES-2 include: lack of interest in activities, facial expressions of sadness or displeasure, crying, low self-image, suicidal thoughts, and feelings of helplessness.

The BES-2 is designed to serve students from kindergarten through grade 12. It has six primary purposes: (1) to screen for behavior problems, (2) to assess the behavior of referred pupils, (3) to aid in the diagnosis of serious emotional disturbance/behavior disorders (e.g., depression), (4) to link assessment with specific behavioral interventions (assessment utility), (5) to evaluate the outcomes of behavioral interventions, and (6) to record data for research (McCarney & Leigh, 1990).

The scale was restandardized on 2772 students in grades K–12 from 31 states selected to provide representation of the demographic characteristics of the United States population reported in the United States Census data. Internal consistency coefficients ranged from 0.87 to 0.89 for four different age groups on the depression subscale. Test–result reliabilities were 0.94 with a group of normal youngsters and 0.90 with a group of behaviorally disordered youth. Standard errors of measurement are reported for the total scale as well as for the subscales. Content validity was established by subjecting the item pool to a sample of 675 professionals from 31 states to judge the appropriateness of each item. All items selected for inclusion on the final scale were deemed appropriate as stated by a minimum of 95% of the respondents. Evidence of criterion-related validity was based on a study that correlated the scores of 26 behaviorally disordered pupils on the BES-2 with scores on the Teacher Rating Scale of the Behavior Rating Profile (BRP) by Brown and Hammill (1978). The resulting correlation coefficient between the depression subscales on these two instruments was 0.44. Although the BES-2 appears to differentiate between behaviorally disordered and normal youngsters, no evidence is available regarding its ability to distinguish among specific groups of psychiatrically disordered youths. Contrary to the authors' assertions (McCarney & Leigh, 1990), the high intercorrelations between the subscales ($r = 0.57–0.90$) suggest that differential diagnosis among various emotionally impaired subgroups would be difficult. Strengths of the scale include an adequate norm group, minimal time to administer (15–20 minutes), and the linkage between assessment and intervention.

Behavior Disorders Identification Scale.   The Behavior Disorders Identification Scale (BDIS) by Wright (1988) is similar to the BES-2 in that it is also modeled after the Federal definition of seriously emotionally disturbed as outlined under Public Law 101-476. As in the BES-2, only one of the five subscales deals with the assessment of depression in young people. This 81-item scale is for use with individuals of ages 4.5–21 years. The BDIS was standardized on 3188 students based on ratings obtained from 867 teachers in 71 school districts across 23 states. Each of the 10 items on the depression subscale rates for frequency but not for severity. Males received higher scores than females on all five subscales. Interrater reliability ranged from 0.88 to 0.94 from all age levels. The test–retest reliability of the depression subscale is 0.92. The intercorrelations among the

BDIS subscales range from 0.67 to 0.75, which indicates that students with problems in one area are likely to also have problems in other areas. Content validity was based on input from the test author and from an unknown number of "diagnosticians and educational personnel." Criterion-related validity was established by correlating the BDIS subscale scores with the BES (original version) subscale scores. The depression subscale on the BDIS showed a 0.65 correlation with the BES depression subscale. This scale is also designed for use with parents. Like the BES-2, teacher-intervention strategies are designed for each elevated item on the depression subscale. The effort to link assessment with intervention is commendable. It remains for future research to establish whether this tie-in between assessment and intervention leads to superior outcomes over traditional approaches to assessment/intervention.

Teacher Report Form. A Teacher Report Form (TRF) of the CBCL is available for classroom use (Achenbach & Edelbrock, 1986). Like the CBCL completed by the parent, the TRF consists of 118 items, the vast majority of which (85) are identical on both forms. Some 9 items were changed only slightly in wording to make them more suitable to the classroom. For example, in TRF Item 25, the word "pupils" was substituted for the word "children" in CBCL Item 25, which reads "Doesn't get along with the other children." For the remaining 24 items, the content was altered so that the items would be appropriate to the classroom setting. For example, an item on allergy in the CBCL might be replaced by "Hums or makes odd noises in class." Each of the 118 items is rated on a 3-point scale (0 = not true; 1 = somewhat or sometimes true; 2 = very true or often true). The TRF can usually be completed in 8–10 minutes. Ratings are based on the previous 2-month period rather than on the previous 6-month period as for the CBCL. When pupils have more than one teacher, as is often the case in secondary schools and departmentalized elementary schools, the opportunity is present to compare students' functioning in different classes and to explore why teacher perceptions vary from one setting to another. It is also possible to average scale scores to form a composite picture. No scales are designed to detect various kinds of informant bias such as denying, exaggeration, and social desirability sets. Because teacher ratings did not prove to provide as a good a basis for typology as do the parent profiles, the TRF does not use "profile types." Socioeconomic and racial differences are regarded as too small to warrant the use of separate norm groups.

Teacher Affect Rating Scale. The three scales discussed above attempt to assess various aspects of student psychopathology, one of which involves depression. There is one scale, however, that is devoted solely to the assessment of depression in children by teachers, namely, the Teacher Affect Rating Scale (TARS) developed by Petti (undated). This scale consists of 26 items, each of which is rated on a scale of 0–3. The ratings are based on the child's behavior during the past week. Sample items, which are rated on a 4-point scale from "not at all" to "very much," include "poor work effort," "irritable, easily annoyed," and "lacks enjoyment." This scale seems to measure three factors: a behavior factor, a learning factor, and a depression factor.

Because this scale is still in the developmental stage, there is little information on its psychometric properties. Like most rating scales, it probably does not differentiate between the *demoralized* child and the child with a depressive *disorder*. For example, many learning-disabled children may be demoralized but do not have depressive disorders. Having the ratings based on the past week, say, vs. the past 4 weeks, will also result in an increased number who are called depressed when, in reality, they are not. Finally, the value of teacher ratings of depression remains to be established. It might well be that teachers are better at identifying disruptive students than they are at identifying depressed students.

Teachers are in a unique position to observe students over an extended period of time, with respect not only to educational performance but also to social interactions with classmates. Thus, a major practical limitation of observational methods—their time-consuming nature—is obviated by the teachers' having to spend so much time with students. Observational techniques are particularly well suited to the assessment of the overt behaviors characteristic of depression, such as diminished social and motor activity, sad facial expression, on-task classroom pursuits, and playground/lunchroom interactions. Despite the obvious and natural suitability of observational methods to assess depression in classrooms, development of observational codes for teachers has been neglected.

Kazdin (1990) reports on an observational system that divides behaviors into three categories: (1) *social*, which in turn consists of talking, playing a (structured) game, and participating in a group activity; (2) *solitary* behavior, which in turn is divided into playing a game alone, working on an academic task, listening and watching, straightening one's room, and grooming (self-care); (3) *affect-related* expression, which subsumes smiling, frowning, arguing, and complaining. Although the behavioral code was developed for use with inpatient children during free-period times, it could easily be adapted for teacher use in a classroom. Such an adaptation would be welcomed, particularly if it were structured so that antecedents and consequences could be systematically studied.

Direct Observation Form. The CBCL has a Direct Observation Form (DOF) that is designed for use by an experienced observer who observes the target child in settings such as classrooms and lunchrooms. The general practice is for the experienced observer to write a narrative description of the student's behavior as it occurs over a 10-minute interval and then to rate the pupil on the 96 behavior problems. The 4-point rating scale capitalizes on the finer-grained discriminations made by experienced observers. Of the 96 items, 49 are similar to those of the TRF, 11 have no direct counterpart on the TRF, and 36 items differ only slightly from items on the TRF. The DOF also permits the scoring of on-task behavior at 1-minute intervals. Interrater agreement based on total problem score is quite acceptable for children both in a residential treatment center ($r = 0.96$) and in public school classes ($r = 0.92$). As no standardized scoring profile yet exists, the authors suggest that a child's deviance be judged by comparing the target student's scores with the scores of two control students of the same sex observed under the same conditions.

DSM-III Criteria. It is also possible for the teacher to use DSM criteria as a basis for observation. Relying on observational data, the teacher might ask the questions presented in Table 2, which relate to diagnostic criteria of major depressive disorder derived from DSM-III.

The questions raised in Table 2 can prove helpful in structuring teacher observations of possible major depressive disorders. Some major limitations should be kept in mind, however. First, teachers might not be able to rate observable behaviors pertinent to depression because they occur outside the school setting (e.g., Does the child have difficulty falling asleep and/or wake up earlier than usual?). Also, teachers might have difficulty in making judgments about certain observable behaviors even though they do occur within the school setting (e.g., the amount of weight gain or loss). Finally, some aspects of major depressive disorder are not observable (e.g., suicidal ideation). An individual's internal states frequently do not lend themselves to observational assessment. Despite these limitations, teachers should be encouraged to be more sensitive observers of depressive states, conditions that teachers might well overlook. No professional group spends more time with young people than teachers, and their observational powers should be honed and tapped in the detection of depressive disorders.

Peer Ratings

Though not widely used, peer nominations offer a fascinating and promising tool for assessing childhood depression. Ratings by peers suffer from the same problems noted earlier in the discussion of ratings by parents, teachers, and clinicians. In addition, raters may tend to overestimate the relationship between popularity and positive mood, as well as the relationship between rejection or neglect and depression. Despite its limitations, this method has numerous advantages that are often overlooked or deemphasized. Many of the symptoms of depression, such as dysphoria, loss of energy, or lack of involvement in activities, can be readily observed by peers in the give-and-take of social interaction. Peers also have the opportunity to observe across a number of settings in the neighborhood and school. There is also the advantage of having several raters rather than just one. Finally, the

Table 2. Symptom Checklist for Major Depressive Disorders (Derived from DSM-111)[a]

Question	Yes	No
1A. Does the student appear sad, unhappy, depressed, low, cranky, or down in the dumps most of the time?	☐	☐
2A. Does the student seem to think that there is nothing to enjoy at all?	☐	☐
3A. Has the student lost interest in homework or the job?	☐	☐
4A. Does the student seem to think that things are not going to work out and are hopeless?	☐	☐
5A. Is the student easily irritated? (Does he/she get mad very easily?)	☐	☐
6B. Has the student lost his/her appetite?	☐	☐
7B. Has his/her appetite increased termendously?	☐	☐
8B. Has the student lost 4 or more pounds during the last year?	☐	☐
9B. Has the student gained 4 or more pounds during the last month or 10 or more pounds during the last year?	☐	☐
10C. Does the student need more sleep than previously?	☐	☐
11D. Does the student feel tired most of the time?	☐	☐
12E. Is the student more restless than before? (Observer should look for inability to sit still, pacing, pulling or rubbing his/her hair, skin, clothing, or pressure of speech.)	☐	☐
13E. Has the student slowed down? (Observer should look for slowed speech, increased pauses before answering, monotonous speech, or slowed body movement.)	☐	☐
14F. Has the student lost interest in activities that were pleasurable in the past? (Hobbies, art, music, TV, sports, social gatherings, sex, etc.)	☐	☐
15G. Does the child often blame himself/herself excessively when things go wrong?	☐	☐
16G. Does the child seem to feel very bad or guilty for minor mistakes?	☐	☐
17G. Does the child feel worthless, useless, or no good at all?	☐	☐
18H. Does the child find it difficult to concentrate and focus on what he/she is doing?	☐	☐
19H. Is it difficult for the student to make decisions quickly?	☐	☐
20I. Has the student been thinking about hurting himself/herself? If yes, please explain.	☐	☐

[a]Adapted from McKnew and Cytryn (1985). To diagnose depression, the person must have at least one symptom from group A and four symptoms from the eight groups lettered B through I.

raters are already knowledgeable about many of the behaviors in question in that they too have experienced them in the process of growing up.

Peer Nomination Inventory of Depression

The best-known technique of this type is the PNID (Lefkowitz & Tesiny, 1980), which consists of 20 items designed to sample four areas of functioning related to depression: affective, cognitive, motivational, and vegetative.

The content validity of these 20 items was determined by the judgment of nine "experts." From a list of 29 potential manifestations of depression gathered from the clinical literature, these experts chose the items they believed most indicative of and relevant to the definition of depression provided. Of the 20 items finally selected, 14 were presumed to measure depression, 4 were presumed to measure happiness, and 2 were presumed to measure popularity. The happiness and popularity items were added to temper the negative tone of the depression items, as well as to assist in the examination of construct validity. Children are asked in a group setting questions such as these: "Who often thinks they are bad?" "Who plays alone?" "Who often looks sad?" "Who often sleeps in class?" "Who doesn't have such fun?" Each child nominates other classmates for each question, with a child's score equaling the total number of nominations received. The scale was originally normed on 452 boys and 492 girls from 61 4th- and 5th-grade classrooms in New York City. Internal consistency reliabilities are good ($r = 0.85$). Test–retest coefficients for the total depression score are adequate ($r = 0.79$). Factor analyses that were cross-validated across samples indicate that the symptoms of childhood depression may be represented by three factors: loneliness, inadequacy, and dejection (Lefkowitz & Tesiny, 1980). The normative data base was later expanded to 3020 youngsters in grades 3–5 in New York City (Lefkowitz & Tesiny, 1985).

PNID performance is predictive of school performance, self-concept, teacher rating of work, skill, and school behavior, peer rating of happiness and popularity, and locus of control (Lefkowitz & Tesiny, 1985; Lefkowitz, Tesiny, & Gordon, 1980; Tesiny & Lefkowitz, 1982), but it is not clear whether the variables predicted by the PNID could be predicted as well or better by other general measures of personality disturbance. Further, the degree of relationship between peer and teacher ratings of depression is moderate at best ($r = 0.41$), and the correlation between peer ratings and self-report on a short form of the CDI is low ($r = 0.23$). Another study by these authors based on 58 3rd- 4th-, and 5th-grade students reported lower correlations between mothers' ratings of depression on the CBCL and PNID ratings for boys ($r = 0.14$) than for girls ($r = 0.26$) (Tesiny & Lefkowitz, 1982).

Later research based on 752 5th-, 6th-, and 9th-grade public school children from a midsize city in central Texas and 142 5th graders from a large metropolitan area in southwest Texas confirmed previous research showing a higher relationship between two other-reports of depression (from peers and teachers) than between self-report and other-reports of depression. For instance, the correlation between teacher reports as measured by the TRF and scores from peer reports as measured by the PNID was 0.35. The correlation between teacher reports and self-report as measured on the CDI was only 0.13, and the correlation between peer and self-report was 0.27 (Worchel et al., 1990). The low correlations might be explained, in part, by the fact that the nature of the items on the three scales used varies appreciably. Whereas the CDI attempts to assess internal states such as not liking oneself, the PNID measures more observable behaviors such as sleeping in class and the TRF includes items of overt and covert nature (Worchel et al., 1990). This same study (Worchel et al., 1990) also raises questions about the generalizability of PNID normative data gathered on pupils in New York City, as scores in both of the Texas samples were significantly lower than those obtained from the New York City samples. Whereas a PNID cutoff score of 4.00 identifies the upper 5% of the New York sample, only 1.2% of the

Texas sample received a PNID score of 4.00 or higher. Whether the differences in normative data can be explained solely on the basis of differences in geographic area and racial difference between the Texas and New York samples awaits further research. One conclusion is clear, however. We will need additional local normative data before a cutoff score can be confidently set for children of different racial/gender groups from a given geographic area.

Use of the PNID in a public school setting can pose other problems. While informed consent is most likely not needed from all classmates and their parents for a preliminary screening of the class, it would be required by Federal guidelines if a given child is suspected of being seriously emotionally handicapped due to depression. Moreover, because this scale has been used with public school populations, we do not know how well the PNID discriminates between children with depressive *symptoms* and children with depressive *disorder*. Finally, the PNID's usefulness within *clinical* settings is severely limited by the absence of a stable peer group whose members know the child well enough to rate accurately. Despite its imitations, the PNID is a well-developed, reliable scale with validity studies showing consistently moderate correlations with such variables as competence (Blechman, McEnroe, Carella, & Audette, 1986), lower social interaction time (even though depressed children initiated a greater number of interactions and were approached more frequently than nondepressed children) (Altmann & Gotlib, 1988), and success on an anagram task (Ward, Friedlander, & Silverman, 1987). It remains a one-of-a-kind scale for assessing depression in children.

Summary

Parents, teachers, and peers play a significant role in the assessment of depression in children and adolescents. Indeed, it is difficult to justify a screening program or diagnostic assessment that does not incorporate the ratings or observations, or both, of significant others with data gathered from the target child. Given that no single measure has been shown to be psychometrically superior, a prudent course of action would dictate use of multiple informants (e.g., parents and teachers) and multiple methods (e.g., checklists and sociometrics) in the assessment and treatment of depression in young people. Areas in need of further research include the sensitivity and specificity rates for various adult-reported scales, the establishment of appropriate cutoff scores for scales rated by significant others, the clinical significance of the disparities among informants, the different external correlates of scales completed by parents, teachers, and classmates, and the treatment utility of measures obtained from significant others.

References

Achenbach, T., & Edelbrock, C. (1982). *Manual for the Child Behavior Checklist and Child Behavior Profile*. Burlington: Department of Psychiatry, University of Vermont.

Achenbach, T., & Edelbrock, C. (1986). *Manual for the Teacher's Report Form and Teacher Version of the Child Behavior Profile*. Burlington: Department of Psychiatry, University of Vermont.

Achenbach, T., McConaughy, S., & Howell, C. (1987). Child/adolescent behavioral and emotional problems: Implications of cross-informant correlations for situational specificity. *Psychological Bulletin, 101*, 213–232.

Altmann, E., & Gotlib, H. (1988). The social behavior of depressed children: An observational study. *Journal of Abnormal Psychology, 16*, 29–44.

Barkley, R. (1990). *Attention deficit hyperactivity disorder: A handbook for diagnosis and treatment*. New York: Guilford Press.

Blechman, E., McEnroe, M., Carella, E., & Audette, D. (1986). Childhood competence and depression. *Journal of Abnormal Psychology, 95*, 223–227.

Brown, L., & Hammill, D. (1978). *Behavior Rating Profile*. Austin, TX: Pro-Ed.

Cohen-Sandler, R., Berman, A., & King, R. (1982). Life stress and symptomatology: Determinants of suicidal behavior in children. *Journal of the American Academy of Child Psychiatry, 21*, 178–186.

Edelbrock, C., Costello, A., Dulcan, M., Kalas, R., & Conover, N. (1985). Age differences in the reliability of the psychiatric interview for the child. *Child Development, 56*, 265–275.

Hughes, J., & Baker, D. (1990). *The clinical child interview*. New York: Guilford Press.

Kazdin, A. (1988). Childhood depression. In E. Mash and L. Terdal (Eds.), *Behavioral assessment of childhood disorders* (pp. 157–195). New York: Guilford Press.

Kazdin, A. (1990). Assessment of childhood depression. In A. LaGreca (Ed.), *Through the eyes of the child: Obtaining self-reports from children and adolescents* (pp. 189–233). Boston: Allyn & Bacon.

Kazdin, A., Colbus, D., & Rodgers, A. (1986). Assessment of depression and diagnosis of depressive disorder among psychiatrically disturbed children. *Journal of Abnormal Child Psychology, 14*, 499–515.

Kazdin, A., Esveldt-Dawson, K., Sherick, R., & Colbus, D. (1985). Assessment of overt behavior and childhood depression among psychiatrically disturbed children. *Journal of Consulting and Clinical Psychology, 53*, 201–210.

Kazdin, A., French, N., & Unis, A. (1983). Child, mother, and father evaluations of depression in psychiatric inpatient children. *Journal of Abnormal Child Psychology, 11*, 167–180.

Kazdin, A., French, N., Unis, A., & Esveldt-Dawson, K. (1983). Assessment of childhood depression: Correspondence of child and parent ratings. *Journal of the American Academy of Child Psychiatry, 22*, 157–164.

Kazdin, A., & Petti, T. (1982). Self-report and interview measures of childhood and adolescent depression. *Journal of Child Psychology and Psychiatry, 23*, 437–457.

Kovacs, M. (1983). The Children's Depression Inventory: A self-rating scale for school-aged youngsters. Unpublished manuscript.

Kovacs, M. (1986). A developmental perspective on methods and measures in the assessment of depressive disorders: The clinical interview. In M. Rutter, C. Izard, & P. Read (Eds.), *Depression in young people* (pp. 435–465). New York: Guilford Press.

Lefkowitz, M., & Tesiny, E. (1980). Assessment of childhood depression. *Journal of Consulting and Clinical Psychology, 48*, 43–50.

Lefkowitz, A., & Tesiny, E. (1985). Depression in children: Prevalence and correlates. *Journal of Consulting and Clinical Psychology, 53*, 647–656.

Lefkowitz, M., Tesiny, M., & Gordon, N. (1980). Childhood depression, family income, and locus of control. *Journal of Nervous and Mental Disease, 168*, 732–735.

Lefkowitz, M., Tesiny, E., & Solodow, W. (1989). A rating scale for assessing dysphoria in youth. *Journal of Abnormal Child Psychology, 17*, 337–347.

Leon, G., Kendall, P., & Garber, J. (1980). Depression in children: Parents, teachers, and child perspectives. *Journal of Abnormal Child Psychology, 8*, 221–235.

McCarney, S., & Leigh, J. (1990). *Behavior Evaluation Scale*. Austin, TX: Pro-Ed.

McKnew, D., & Cytryn, L. (1985). Symptom checklist for major depressive disorders. *Psychopharmacological Bulletin, 21*, 957–958.

Mooney, K., (1984). Child behavior checklist. In D. Keyser & R. Sweetland (Eds.), *Test Critiques*, Vol. 1 (pp. 168–189). Kansas City, MO: Test Corporation of America.

Moretti, M., Fine, S., Haley, C., & Marriage, K. (1985). Childhood and adolescent depression: Child-report versus parent-report information. *Journal of the American Academy of Child Psychiatry, 24*, 298–302.

Nurcombe, B., Seifer, R., Scioli, A., Tramontana, M., Grapentine, W., & Beauchesne, H. (1989). Is major depressive disorder in adolescence a distinct diagnostic entity? *Journal of the American Academy of Child and Adolescent Psychiatry, 28*, 333–342.

Orvaschel, H. (1985). Psychiatric interview suitable for use in research with children and adolescents. *Psychopharmacology Bulletin, 21*, 737–745.

Petti, T. (undated). Teacher Affect Rating Scale (TARS). Indiana University School of Medicine, Indianapolis, Indiana.

Rey, J., & Morris-Yates, A. (1991). Adolescent depression and the child behavior checklist. *Journal of the American Academy of Child and Adolescent Psychiatry, 30*, 423–427.

Reynolds, C., & Tuma, J. (1985). Review of Personality Inventory for Children. In J. Mitchell (Ed.), *The ninth mental measurements yearbook* (pp. 1154–1159). Lincoln, NE: Buros Institute of Mental Measurement.

Reynolds, W. M., Anderson, G., & Bartell, N. (1985). Measuring depression in children: A multimethod assessment investigation. *Journal of Abnormal Child Psychology, 13*, 513–526.

Rothermel, R., & Lovell, M. (1985). Personality Inventory for Children. In D. Keyser & R. Sweetland (Eds.), *Test Critiques*, Vol. 2 (pp. 570–578). Kansas City, MO: Test Corporation of America.

Rutter, M., & Graham, P. (1968). The reliability and validity of the psychiatric assessment of the child. I. Interview with the child. *British Journal of Psychiatry, 114,* 563–579.

Stark, K. (1990). *Childhood depression: School-based intervention.* New York: Guilford Press.

Swets, J. (1988). Measuring the accuracy of diagnostic systems. *Science, 240,* 1285–1293.

Tesiny, E., & Lefkowitz, M. (1982). Assessing childhood depression: Cumulative data. Paper presented at the Annual Meeting of the American Psychological Association, Washington, DC, August 1982.

Tisher, M., & Lang, M. (1978). *Children's Depression Scale,* research ed., Palo Alto, CA: Consulting Psychologists Press.

Ward, L., Friedlander, M., & Silverman, W. (1987). Children's depressive symptoms, negative self-statements and causal attributions for success and failure. *Cognitive Therapy and Research, 11,* 215–227.

Wirt, R., Lachar, D., Klinedinst, J., & Seat, P. (1977). *Multidimensional description of personality.* Los Angeles: Western Psychological Services.

Worchel, F., Hughes, J., Hall, B., Stanton, S., Stanton, H., & Little, V. (1990). Evaluation of subclinical depression in children using self-, peer- and teacher-report measures. *Journal of Abnormal Child Psychology, 18,* 271–282.

Wright, F. (1988). *Behavior Disorders Identification Scale.* Columbia, MO: Hawthorne.

13

Informant Variability in the Assessment of Childhood Depression

Alan E. Kazdin

Introduction

In the assessment of childhood dysfunction, multiple methods of assessment are routinely used. Method of assessment can refer to a variety of characteristics of the measure, including the source of information (e.g., parent, teacher, child), modalities of assessment (e.g., global ratings, projective techniques, "objective" personality tests), assessment format within a given modality (e.g., true/false, multiple choice, forced choice), and the extent to which the subject is aware of the assessment procedures and purposes (e.g., obtrusive vs. unobtrusive assessment), to mention a few. To assess childhood dysfunction, typically information is sought from several sources or informants. Parents, teachers, children, peers, clinicians, and others may be asked to provide information in a standardized way (e.g., psychological tests) regarding child functioning (see Mash & Terdal, 1988; Rutter, Tuma, & Lann, 1988). Understandably, not all informants will provide the same information, which is a primary reason for seeking input from diverse sources. The extent to which alternative sources of information vary in their views of the child is referred to here as *informant variability*.

Informant variability is critically important to evaluation of children.[1] At the same time, it is important to note the broader assessment context. As a rule, assessment is concerned with understanding particular constructs or underlying concepts (e.g., intelligence, depression). A psychological measure is of interest insofar as it operationalizes and

---

[1]For ease of presentation, the term "children" is used generally to refer to children and adolescents, i.e., youths of ages 18 years and under. The common reference is not intended to neglect vast developmental differences. As relevant to separate discussions, the distinctions between childhood and adolescence and specific age groupings will be mentioned.

Alan E. Kazdin • Department of Psychology, Yale University, New Haven, Connecticut 06520-8205.

Handbook of Depression in Children and Adolescents, edited by William M. Reynolds and Hugh F. Johnston. Plenum Press, New York, 1994.

represents the construct. The use of a single measure to represent a construct, sometimes referred to as "single operationism," has a significant liability (see Kazdin, 1992). An individual's score on the measure reflects his or her standing on the characteristic of interest combined with the unique features of the assessment method. Multiple measures are obtained to help separate the influence of a given assessment method from the construct of interest. Ideally, the different measures of the same construct will converge or lead to similar conclusions about a given individual or group of individuals.

Adults play a major role in the assessment of childhood disorders. Young children are not likely to be able to identify many areas of their own dysfunction. The point becomes obvious as the age of the child decreases (e.g., 1 to 3-year-olds) and the severity or pervasiveness of the dysfunction increases (e.g., mental retardation, autism). On common-sense grounds, one does not expect children to be able to report on their "problems" or to report very well. Indeed, many facets of affect, cognition, and behavior would not be regarded as "problems" by children. Hence adults, particularly the parents, usually are relied on to provide assessment information. Second and related, children and adolescents are considered to have limited or less than fully developed cognitive processes to permit the perspective that evaluation of psychological and interpersonal functioning may require. Thus, their capacity to their own functioning in context, in relation to others, and in relation to their own past performance is likely to be limited. For these reasons, adult evaluations of child functioning play a central role. The importance of adult perspectives does not gainsay the significant role that child self-evaluations may play. Indeed, children's views about themselves are critically important (see LaGreca, 1990).

The different perspectives used to evaluate child functioning have led to the issue of informant variability, the extent to which different sources of information vary in their evaluations of the child. The purpose of this chapter is to examine issues related to informant variability in the assessment of depression as well as other emotional and behavioral problems of children. Although diverse informants or sources of information will be mentioned, the primary focus will be on the relation of parent and child agreement in assessment.

There are several reasons for highlighting parent–child agreement as the main focus. To begin, child and parent evaluations are central to the diagnosis of childhood disorders. The standard method of obtaining diagnoses is to seek separate interviews with the parent and child. Diagnosis of disorders is reached by combining the information. Second, research on the nature, characteristics, and course of childhood dysfunction relies heavily on parent evaluations. Parents are sought as the primary informants about child psychopathology because they are considered to be the most knowledgeable about their children's behavior across situations and time. Parents are usually responsible for deciding when child functioning is problematic and hence warrants attention. Finally, parent–child agreement is the main focus here because it serves as a paradigm for conceptualizing informant variability more generally. There may be unique features stemming from the obviously very special relations between parents and children. Even so, substantive and methodological issues that emerge from the study of parent and child agreement can address broader issues about different informants and their use and integration in assessment.

The focus on the parent and child in the context of assessing childhood depression is a matter of emphasis. Other informants (e.g., teachers, peers) and assessment of emotional and behavioral problems more generally will be mentioned as well. The chapter highlights the literature on informant variability; the review is selective to make salient points and to identify areas of ambiguity. The chapter discusses the factors that contribute to such variability and the validity of assessments obtained from alternative sources. Finally, implications of the findings on informant variability for conceptualization of childhood dysfunction, research, and clinical practice with children are also examined.

Agreement among Informants

Informant variability can have different meanings depending on how it is assessed. Variation among informants is examined by obtaining information from different persons (e.g., child, parent, teacher) who evaluate the child. The resulting information can be used to examine agreement or variation among informants in several ways. Typically, Pearson product–moment correlations are computed to examine the covariation (correlation) between two raters. A correlation is used when the scores can vary along some dimensional scale (e.g., for a single item or total score of a questionnaire or inventory). Correlations refer to the pattern of covariation between two raters (e.g., child and parent). It is well known that a correlation can be very high, indeed "perfect" ($r = 1.00$), without the raters ever agreeing in the values they provide. A correlation provides useful information about the relative standing or rank order of the scores between two sets of informants. One would expect, for example, that parents and children would tend to agree in the standing children are accorded in a group of cases. Children who rate themselves as depressed presumably would have parents who also view them as depressed and so on for varying degrees of depression.

When the score is categorical (presence or absence of a particular symptom or disorder), alternative estimates of agreement can be used. The most frequently used measure is kappa (κ), a correlational statistic that measures agreement on a categorical (binary) criterion. Agreement means that the raters agreed exactly on their score (yes or no, present or absent) for whatever is being evaluated. The value of κ varies from 0.00 to 1.00. The statistic is of interest because it considers the agreement over and above "chance." If two raters randomly scored the presence or absence of a symptom on several occasions, they would agree on some occasions as a matter of chance (given the frequencies with which each scored the presence of the symptom). Kappa evaluates agreement over and above the level that would be expected by chance alone.[3]

Another way to assess agreement or informant variability is to consider the absolute scores produced by different raters [e.g., child- and parent-completed Children's Depression Inventory (Kovacs, 1981)] and to examine the differences in their scores. The magnitude and direction of the differences can be examined. The purpose of examining the difference score (amount of difference) is to see the pattern of scores, i.e., whether children tend to report more or fewer symptoms than parents, teachers, and peers and whether this pattern varies systematically. Also, the difference score can itself be correlated with other variables. For example, the difference score can be correlated with such other variables as parent psychopathology, family socioeconomic status, and others. Difference scores as well as the correlational statistics mentioned here are the most commonly used methods to evaluate agreement among informants.

Delineation of a large number of disorders in childhood and adolescence in contemporary diagnosis (American Psychiatric Association, 1994) and developments in diagnostic assessment methods have spawned research on different informants. The reason is that diagnostic assessment routinely relies on child and parent interviews. Hence, disagreement in the nature of the child's symptoms and dysfunction is readily detectable. Also,

---

[3]The formula for κ is

$$\kappa = P_o - P_c/1 - P_c$$

where P_o is the proportion of agreements between observers on the number of times they note the "presence" and absence of the symptoms and P_c is the proportion of expected agreement on the basis of chance. When raters agree at the same level that would be expected by chance, $\kappa = 0$. If agreement surpasses the expected level, κ exceeds zero and approaches a maximum of +1.00. Kappa can also extend from 0 to −1.00. Negative values mean that agreement is less than the level expected by chance.

disorders that are subject to considerable research, such as attention-deficit disorder, often rely more heavily on other informants (teachers) than on parents and children. Consequently, drawing on different informants and weighing their input raises critical research as well as clinical questions.

Agreement among informants in the assessment of children has been a topic of research before the current emphasis on childhood disorders and their assessment. Early findings in the field have previewed many contemporary studies by showing, for example, that there is little or no agreement between child and parent evaluations of child functioning, moderate agreement between parents, and a tendency for parents to underestimate internalizing symptoms of their children (e.g., Guerney, Shapiro, & Stover, 1968; Langford & Alm, 1954; Piers, 1972). Findings from more contemporary research have been culled and evaluated in a meta-analytical review of research that examined the extent to which alternative sources of information agree on the emotional and behavioral problems of children (see Achenbach, McConaughy, & Howell, 1987). Comparisons included studies evaluating the agreement among children, parents, teachers, and mental health workers. Across a variety of studies, Achenbach et al. (1987) found that child and parent evaluations of child behavior showed reliable but relatively low agreement (mean $r = 0.25$). Correspondence between child and teacher and child and mental health worker evaluations was also low ($r = 0.20$ and $r = 0.27$, respectively). The low levels of correspondence are not unique to comparisons in which children are sources of information. Agreement between parent and mental health worker evaluations of children was within the same range (mean $r = 0.24$).

Of interest in this chapter are the findings of variability among informants in the assessment of childhood depression. In one of our own studies, we examined the relations among parent (mothers and fathers) and child ratings of depression in a clinical sample of children ($N = 104$, ages 5–13) hospitalized in a short-term inpatient service (Kazdin, French, Unis, & Esveldt-Dawson, 1983d). As is common in studies of informant variability, all raters completed the "same" measures that focused on the child's dysfunction. In this study, three measures were used to assess depression [Children's Depression Inventory (CDI), Bellevue Index of Depression (BID), and Depression Symptom Checklist (DSCL)]. Children and parents were interviewed separately to complete the measures. The results revealed little correspondence among raters. For example, for the CDI, the correlations between child–mother ratings and child–father ratings were $r = 0.03$ and $r = 0.01$, respectively. Essentially, parent and child views of the child's level of depression on a standard measure bore no relation. For the other measures, the correlations were higher and in the low to moderate range. For the BID, the correlations between child–mother and child–father ratings were higher and statistically significant ($r = 0.21$ and $r = 0.36$, respectively); for the DSCL, the correlations were low ($r = 0.07$ and $r = 0.09$, respectively). Overall, child–parent correlations were extremely low and shared only minute variance. In contrast, mother–father correspondence was reliably higher. For the CDI, BDI, and DSCL, mother–father correlations in rating the child's depression were in the moderate range ($r = 0.56$, $r = 0.66$, and $r = 0.60$, respectively).

Many other studies have been completed on the topic and have extended the breadth of informants to parent, teacher, and peer raters and the scope of dysfunction beyond depression. In a few cases, depression and other constructs (e.g., aggression, social adjustment) have been included in the same study to examine the extent to which the results are unique to depression (e.g., Kazdin, Esveldt-Dawson, Unis, & Rancurello, 1983b; Kazdin, French, & Unis, 1983c; Reynolds, Anderson, & Bartell, 1985; Weissman, Orvaschel, & Padian, 1980). The results show that parent and child ratings of depression show little relation and that other domains are similar in this regard. Extending research to peers, teachers, and psychiatric hospital staff has also yielded low correlations with child self-report of depression (e.g., r's < 0.3) (Jacobson, Lahey, & Strauss, 1983; Lefkowitz & Tesiny,

1984; Sacco & Graves, 1984; Saylor, Finch, Baskin, Furey, & Kelly, 1984a). The generally low agreement between child and other raters who evaluate the child has been fairly consistent. Comparisons with other combinations of informants such as mothers–fathers, parents–teachers, and peers–teachers have shown agreement in the low to moderate range (e.g., 0.2–0.6) (e.g., Jensen, Traylor, Xenakis, & Davis, 1988a; Phares, Compas, & Howell, 1989; Saylor et al., 1984a; Shoemaker, Erickson, & Finch, 1986; Touliatos & Lindholm, 1981). It is worth noting that low correlations are not always found when parents' or teachers' measures are compared with measures obtained from the children. In a few studies with children and adolescents and clinic and nonreferred samples, parent–child and teacher–child correlations have been higher [e.g., r's range from 0.3 to 0.7 (Ines & Sacco, 1992; Romano & Nelson, 1988; Slotkin, Forehand, Fauber, McCombs, & Long, 1988)]. The reasons for discrepancies are not immediately apparent.

The bulk of the literature on informant variability has focused on the correlation between raters for overall scale scores on such measures as the CDI. More fine-grained analyses have examined individual symptoms of depression or individual items rather than total scores for various measures. The focus on individual symptoms or items is potentially instructive if agreement can be shown to vary by type of symptom. Indeed, possibly a few symptoms or types of symptoms account for the relatively low agreement on overall scores.

Agreement does not appear to vary systematically among the various symptoms of depression. For example, Ivens and Rehm (1988) examined outpatient cases (8–12 years old) and their parents. Each child and parent independently completed a diagnostic interview (Schedule for Affective Disorders and Schizophrenia for School-Age Children). Item-by-item agreement was computed (κ) for symptoms of depression. Agreement was low for virtually all symptoms between all rater combinations (median $\kappa \leq 0.2$). For the overall diagnosis of depression, κ's ranged from -0.02 to 0.17 (minimally acceptable agreement beyond chance being usually regarded as ≥ 0.50 or 0.60). Studies have varied on agreement with individual items, individual symptoms, and overall diagnoses with estimates below or above acceptable levels (e.g., Herjanic & Reich, 1982; Kashani, Orvaschel, Burk, & Reid, 1985; Orvaschel, Puig-Antich, Chambers, Tabrizi, & Johnson, 1982; Welner, Reich, Herjanic, Jung, & Amado, 1987). There is no immediate resolution to the differences among studies, although variables that influence agreement are discussed below.

The low to moderate agreement has been scrutinized further by examining the directionality of reporting between parent and child raters. The directionality refers to which source of information yields greater reporting (i.e., higher frequency, greater severity) of the symptom. Parents and teachers tend to report more externalizing symptoms (conduct, attentional, oppositional problems) than children, whereas children often report higher rates of internalizing symptoms (anxiety, fear, obsessions) (Edelbrock, Costello, Dulcan, Conover, & Kalas, 1986; Loeber, Green, Lahey, & Stouthamer-Loeber, 1991). The results regarding depressive symptoms are by no means clear. For example, in one study of children, mothers tended to report more depressive symptoms than children (Ivens & Rehm, 1988). An exception was the reporting of decreased energy, sleep disturbance, and suicidal thought. In another study, children reported more vegetative signs of depression but did not differ from their parents in reporting suicidal or affective symptoms (Edelbrock et al., 1986). The latter authors interpreted this finding to suggest that parents may report fewer symptoms that are not a problem for them.

At present, the most salient conclusion is that agreement between children and their parents on individual symptom areas tends to be low. More factual information and concrete observable behaviors rather than symptom presence or severity are associated with higher agreement (Herjanic & Reich, 1982). Children may report more often on internalizing symptoms, parents more often on externalizing symptoms. Yet these differences are not consistent and are overshadowed by a more pervasive pattern of low to moderate agreement on individual symptoms or scales reflecting symptom constellations.

Variables that Contribute to Informant Agreement

Overview of Major Findings

The low agreement between parents and children in evaluating the emotional and behavioral problems of the children is now fairly well established. It is unlikely that the degree of disagreement is random. The extent to which parents and children and other informants agree is likely to vary as a function of a number of characteristics regarding assessment, including type of symptoms, combinations of informants, type of measures, age of the child, and so on. Indeed, the findings that agreement between parents is usually higher than agreement between parents and children have already been mentioned. Several studies have attempted to identify factors that influence performance of raters and that influence agreement between raters. Studies have differed widely in the characteristics studied and the samples of children (e.g., inpatient, community). Few findings are robust across samples.

Types of Child Symptoms and Dysfunction.   Characteristics of the child's symptoms or domains of dysfunction are likely to influence the patterns of reporting symptoms and agreement among informants. For example, one might expect that children would be better reporters of their internal or emotional states (e.g., sadness). Even though internal states often have overt behavioral referents available to others such as parents and teachers (e.g., fearfulness or crying), it is likely that children would be better able than others to identify the scope, severity, and range of internal states. Evidence suggests that internalizing symptoms such as anxiety, somatic complaints, and suicidal thoughts (symptoms of depression), as well as visual and auditory hallucinations and persecutory delusions, are reported more frequently by children than by parents who rate these symptoms of the children (Ivens & Rehm, 1988; Kashani et al., 1985). Parents are likely to report on externalizing behaviors that are bothersome to them (e.g., hyperactivity, oppositional behaviors). However, it is not possible to formulate a simple rule regarding which rater reports a given symptom more frequently. Children sometimes report more externalizing behaviors than their parents, such as truancy, drinking alcohol, and using drugs (Kashani et al., 1985). Inaccesibility of the information to the parents may contribute to parent underreporting.

The type of symptom or information contributes to the level of agreement. Beginning with the Herjanic and Reich (1982) study on the diagnosis of children, agreement on the majority of symptoms was generally low. Yet agreement on individual items that focused on factual information (school expulsion, repetition of a grade level at school, enuresis) was relatively high; on items that focused on internalizing states (fears, obsessions, hallucinations), relatively low. Some studies suggest that informant agreement is better for externalizing rather than for internalizing behaviors (e.g., Jensen et al., 1988a; Kolko & Kazdin, 1993). For example, parent–child agreement on several conduct-problem scales (each composed of multiple items) was found to be higher ($r = 0.42$) than agreement on scales reflecting affective and neurotic symptoms ($r = 0.19$) (Edelbrock et al., 1986). Higher agreement on externalizing in comparison to internalizing symptoms has been found for child–teacher, child–peer, teacher–peer, and parent–teacher evaluations as well (e.g., Kolko & Kazdin, 1993; Ledingham, Younger, Schwartzman, & Bergeron, 1982). Variations within externalizing behavior have been studied. For example, agreement between children and parents has been found to be greater for oppositional and conduct behaviors in comparison to hyperactive and inattentive behaviors (Loeber, Green, Lahey, & Stouthamer-Loeber, 1990). In general, agreement tends to be higher for externalizing symptoms. The reasons for this finding are not yet clear. The conspicuousness of the behaviors (e.g., the degree to which they are obvious or detectable) was not related to correspondence of parent and child ratings in one study (Kolko & Kazdin, 1993). However, severity of behavior was reliably related to correspondence ($r = 0.35$). Further work is necessary to evaluate agreement for different types of behaviors and to relate agreement to other variables (e.g., rater combinations) with which agreement may interact.

Child Age and Sex. Conceivably, the variability between parents and children could be traced to characteristics of the children. Child age and sex are two prime characteristics that might well influence ratings. It is not merely that age and sex are salient subject variables in general. Rather, age and sex are significant influences in the assessment and manifestations of depression as well as other disorders (e.g., see Kazdin, 1989a; Reynolds, 1992). Given developmental differences in cognitive maturation as well as symptom patterns, age would be a primary candidate among the factors to examine. In light of verbal and cognitive development, young children are less likely to be able to reflect on their behavior, to comprehend the meaning of psychological and diagnostic assessment, and to appreciate the notions underlying assessment of dysfunction (e.g., seeing a change from usual behavior; experiencing facets of their own affect, cognition, and behavior as "problems"). As children become older, they might be expected to recognize problem areas and to agree more, even though not necessarily well, with adult raters. The results for age are inconsistent; all patterns have been shown, with child–parent agreement higher or lower than adolescent–parent agreement and no differences as a function of child age (see Achenbach et al., 1987; Jensen, Xenakis, Davis, & DeGroot, 1988b; Kazdin et al., 1983c; Kolko & Kazdin, 1993). The diverse findings may reflect the interaction of age with other variables. For example, in one study, the effects of child age on agreement varied with the identity of the other informant (parent vs. teacher) and type of behavior (e.g., hyperactivity vs. oppositional and conduct problems) (see Loeber et al., 1990).

Child sex has been studied in relation to agreement. In their review, Achenbach et al. (1987) found that child–parent agreement did not vary as a function of child sex. Agreement between girls and their parents has been found to be greater than between boys and their parents (e.g., Kazdin et al., 1983c; Kolko & Kazdin, 1993). However, the findings have been restricted to selected scales within a given study and do not represent a strong pattern. Because boys and girls may differ on symptoms and the relative frequency of the same symptoms (e.g., aggression), sex differences with these other influences controlled remain unclear.

Parent and Family Characteristics. The influence of parent characteristics on ratings of child dysfunction and parent–child agreement has been examined in several studies. The central finding has been that parent symptoms, stress, and marital discord often influence parent ratings of the child. Several studies have shown that parent stress and psychopathology correlate in the low to moderate range (e.g., $r = 0.20–0.50$) with parent ratings of child depression or overall emotional and behavioral problems of the child (Brody & Forehand, 1986; Fergusson, Lynskey, & Horwood, 1993; Friedlander, Weiss, & Traylor, 1986; Jensen et al., 1988a; Moretti, Fine, Haley, & Marriage, 1985; Phares et al., 1989; Webster-Stratton & Hammond, 1988). Higher parent symptom scores are associated with higher parent ratings of child deviance. Mothers, who are more frequently utilized as raters, have been more well studied than fathers. However, the relation of overall parent symptoms and level of depression has been found to influence father evaluations of child symptoms as well (Ivens & Rehm, 1988; Phares et al., 1989).

Parent dysfunction also relates to agreement of child and parent ratings. For example, mother and father symptom scores (Hopkins Symptom Checklist) correlate significantly ($r \approx 0.20–0.40$) with difference scores of parent–child ratings (Jensen et al., 1988a). The reason for the relation of parent symptoms to ratings of child symptoms and to level of agreement is not clear. Some research has suggested that parent symptoms influence both the perceptions of child maladjustment and parenting behaviors that influence child deviance (Forehand, Lautenschlager, Faust, & Graziano, 1986; Webster-Stratton, 1988).

Limitations of Current Research

A number of other factors have been studied in relation to agreement between raters (see Achenbach et al. 1987; Jensen et al., 1988a,b). Such factors as severity and frequency of behavior, type of behavior (e.g., problem vs. prosocial), socioeconomic status of the family, race, parent contact (familiarity) with the child, number of siblings, child birth order, and child patient status (e.g., patient vs. nonpatient samples) illustrate the range of variables evaluated in relation to agreement between parents and children as well as other informant combinations. Several studies are exemplary in evaluating multiple raters within a given study, alternative methods of assessing agreement, and diverse factors with which agreement is likely to be related (e.g., Jacob, Grounds, & Haley, 1982; Ledingham et al., 1982; Victor, Halverson, & Wampler, 1988). Few differences have been identified that are robust across studies. The paucity of studies on a given variable is one of the reasons that consistencies may be difficult to detect. For a given variable of interest, it is simply difficult to accrue more than a few studies. However, there are more salient problems that conspire against clarify of findings among studies.

First, the selection of variables to investigate in relation to agreement is not guided by conceptualization of the assessment process or characteristics of the informants. Lack of conceptualization refers to the absence of specifying processes or mechanisms that might explain what specifically accounts for disagreement between informants or over- and underreporting. Variables (e.g., socioeconomic status, race) are identified without a view as to why they are important. Pure empiricism without a conceptual framework can wonder needlessly with an unclear yield. Conceptualization of the process may help identify the specific factors that affect agreement. Various subject and demographic variables that are usually studied may be poor approximations of these factors and obscure the relations of individual and multiple influences on agreement.

Second and related, in cases in which variables may have impact on agreement or direction of symptom reporting, the effects might be explained by other uncontrolled variables. For example, familiarity of the rater with the child may influence agreement. Father absence and nonbiological relation to the child were used to operationalize familiarity (exposure to the child) in one study (Jensen et al., 1988b). Agreement between fathers and children was greater for biological fathers than for stepfathers in select comparisons. Analogously, another study found that the correlation between teacher and child ratings was higher for children the teachers rated as more familiar (Ines & Sacco, 1992). One might draw the conclusion that familiarity is indeed relevant to agreement between the child and other adults. Yet interpretation of the variable is difficult without further analysis. What is it about familiarity that would lead to greater agreement? Is familiarity confounded with other variables such as marital status or stress of the parent? Mothers are generally regarded as "familiar" with their children and evince low agreement in general. Would variation in degrees of familiarity within a sample of mothers, or with other factors controlled, show the relation of this variable to agreement?

Similarly, child–parent agreement has been greater for externalizing than for internalizing behavior, as reviewed previously. Severity of the symptom, frequency of occurrence, and conspicuousness would be some of many reasons that could account for this finding. The few studies that have examined possible reasons or different types of externalizing behavior do not yield a clear pattern (Kolko & Kazdin, 1993; Loeber et al., 1991). Interpretation of the finding of greater parent–child agreement on externalizing rather than internalizing symptoms is not obvious. In general, it is not clear that there is interest in the field in this level of conceptualization of the assessment process. Yet investigation of individual variables without this level of conceptual analysis makes the yield very difficult to interpret or to utilize for clinical benefit.

Finally, the literature on agreement focuses heavily on Pearson product–moment correlations. The extent to which a variable is considered to affect agreement may be based on an analysis of correlations, i.e., which correlations are significant and which correlations are more significant than others. As is well known, the statistical significance of a correlation is unusually dependent on sample size. Discrepant findings in the literature of correlations can easily emerge when one study reports a significant correlation and another does not or within a given study when a correlation is significant for one subsample (girls, boys; younger, older; patients, nonpatients) but not for their counterpart. The heavy reliance on statistical significance vs. magnitude of effects (e.g., effect size) is invariably a point of concern in data evaluation (see Kazdin, 1992). In relation to the agreement literature, the matter may be particularly important. Effect size or other such measures of magnitude of effect would be worth reporting as a means of examining consistencies among studies in which statistical significance is more likely to be ephemeral.

Other issues in relation to correlation are noteworthy in passing. The sample within any given study, whether patient or community sample, may show a relatively restricted range of scores on the measure. The restricted range would of course attenuate the correlations and as well could lead to substantial differences across studies. The relatively consistent findings regarding informant variability are noteworthy in this regard. Even so, the restricted range of any individual sample could yield lower bound estimates of agreement in the population. Agreement has been computed primarily in terms of Pearson product–moment correlations. Other correlational statistics (e.g., ρ, κ, intraclass correlation) are less often examined and address different facets of agreement.

Alternative Views and Interpretations of Informant Variability

There are different ways of interpreting low to moderate agreement among raters. The interpretations highlighted below are not necessarily contrasting views or mutually exclusive. Rather, they provide various perspectives on how to consider discrepancies among informants in their evaluations of child functioning.

Accuracy in Reporting

Variability among raters has inevitably led to the notion of accuracy in reporting. On a priori grounds, it is reasonable to assume that the child actually behaves in particular ways that can be assessed "objectively." When reports of two raters differ, it is difficult to avoid the presumption that one of them is correct. For example, if a parent and child are asked to report on the number of tics the child evinces in a 30-minute period or the number of tantrums before bedtime in a given week, it is reasonable to consider there to be a "true" criterion by which to judge accuracy. Definition of the problem and an observable independent criterion (e.g., videotaped record of tics scored by separate observers) could in principle and practice be used to compare child and parent report and to judge the extent to which each hits the mark, i.e., is accurate.

In evaluating informant variability in the assessment of emotional and behavior problems, the notion of accuracy in reporting usually has to be suspended. Usually there is no objective criterion against which to compare child and parent report. Notions such as "under- and overreporting" are also used when one rater's score (e.g., the child's) is lower or higher than the other rater's score. the terms belie an assumption that the individual has misestimated a true score or reality that can be independently checked.

In several studies, child, parent, and teacher reports of dysfunction on various questionnaires have been compared with psychiatric diagnosis (e.g., Kazdin, Colbus, & Rodgers, 1986; Kazdin & Heidish, 1984; Mattison, Bagnato, & Strickler, 1987). Psychiatric diagnosis completed by a clinician is used as the criterion against which to judge accuracy and under- or overreporting of different raters. The results of such studies must be interpreted cautiously. Usually, diagnosis is based on information obtained from the parent and child. Separately completed ratings by child and parent are then examined to see their relation to psychiatric diagnosis. Essentially, child and parent sources of information are in both the predictors (questionnaires) and the criterion (diagnosis). The fact that a clinician may integrate or differentially weight or use information from parents and children to reach a diagnosis does not imbue the result with accuracy. If parent ratings correlate more highly with psychiatric diagnosis of the child, this does not mean that parent ratings are more accurate or valid, only that clinicians and parents agree more or the clinicians weighted parent reports more in the diagnostic process. One can use other criteria against which to evaluate child, parent, teacher, and other rater evaluations. It is likely that scores of child dysfunction obtained from different raters will vary in the extent to which they correlate with or predict other criteria. The correlations of measures obtained from different raters are critically important but raise issues of validity rather than accuracy, as addressed below.

In general in the assessment of child dysfunction, the notion of accuracy has limited value. Accuracy is restricted to those instances in which a criterion can be identified that provides an objective or consensually agreed on standard free from the input of raters whose views are being evaluated. Depending on the question presented to raters and the assessment criterion, accuracy might be identified in relation to depression. For example, a child, parent, and teacher could be asked to estimate how often a child engages in a specific set of activities that the child has identified as enjoyable. If objective measures of performance of these activities were available, then of course accuracy could be assessed. However, in the usual case, we are restricted to comments about whether one rater produces scores that are higher than another and the agreement between these scores.

Validity of Alternative Perspectives

Ratings from different informants can be viewed from a different perspective, namely, one of validity. That is, the concern is not with agreement or differences between informants per se. The question is whether a measure completed by a particular informant meets broader criteria of validity. A given measure completed by a rater (parent or child) can be examined from the standpoint of construct validity (Cronbach & Meehl, 1955). The construct presumed to be assessed by a particular measure leads to tests that in turn validate and elaborate the measure. The measure–informant unit (e.g., the particular scale, such as the CDI, completed by the child) can be evaluated in its own right. In principle, data related to the measure and diverse types of reliability (e.g., internal consistency, test–retest) and validity (e.g., concurrent, predictive) can support or elaborate underlying theory, the construct, and the measure–informant unit.

Agreement or lack of agreement between or among sets of raters is not necessarily troublesome. The issue is one of validity, or the extent to which reports from different informants (child, parent, teacher, peers, clinicians, or others) relate to and predict other criteria. The validity of measures can be assessed in many ways. Typically, validation begins by correlating the measures with other criteria. Predictions are made between the constructs of interest (e.g., depression and various cognitive processes) at a given point in time or over time. The validity of the measure is supported if the correlations are obtained as predicted. For example, the child's self-ratings of depression might well correlate with a host of other measures in a predictable fashion and hence help to validate a given self-report measure of depression. In principle, the validity of reports from all informants could be established in this way.

Research on informant variability has helped to remind us of the cautions required in interpreting correlations between measures. Specifically, research has shown that measures from the same informant (e.g., parent) are often highly correlated independently of whether the constructs that are measured would be expected to go together. Background for this issue pertains to the criteria for establishing construct validity of a given measure.

Trait and Method Variance. To argue that the construct of interest is measured requires a pattern of correlations that is consistent with the construct. Campbell and Fiske (1959) elaborated the notions of convergent and discriminant validity as part of requirements for test validation. Convergent validity refers to evidence that a particular measure correlates with other measures; discriminant validity refers to evidence that the measure does not correlate significantly with other measures with which it would not be expected to correlate.

To examine convergent and discriminant validity, two or more constructs (e.g., personality traits, disorders, symptom areas) each need to be assessed by two or more measures. Ideally, the assessment methods (e.g., self-report or parent or teacher report) would be the same for each construct. As a simple example, a study might assess severity of childhood depression and aggression as two constructs of interest. Mothers and their children each would complete an interview or questionnaire for both depression and aggression. Two constructs (depression, aggression) × two assessment methods (mother, child ratings) would lead to 4 scores for each mother and child pair. For all the subjects, scores are correlated with each other, generating what Campbell and Fiske (1959) referred to as a *multitrait–multimethod matrix*. The intercorrelations permit one to identify the extent to which measures of the same construct (e.g., depression) are correlated with each other. Measures of the same construct should correlate relatively highly. Conversely, measures of quite different constructs should correlate less well and certainly less well than measures designed to assess the same construct. The correlation pattern of convergent and discriminant validity can support the construct validity of a given measure.

The main reason for mentioning the multitrait–multimethod matrix here is that it permits evaluation of common method variance in the correlations between measures. Rater or source of information (e.g., child, parent) can be viewed as method variance and contribute significantly to correlations between two measures. Evaluations of the rater as part of a multitrait–multimethod matrix have yielded interesting information in relation to informant variability.

Consider, as an example, a study that assessed depression and aggression (two constructs) among inpatient children ($N = 120;$) (Kazdin et al., 1983b). Children, mothers, and fathers completed a questionnaire and an interview designed to assess depression and then a parallel questionnaire and interview designed to assess aggression. In all cases, of course, the depression and aggression of the child were being evaluated. Table 1 presents the correlation matrix in the form that permits examination of convergent and discriminant validity and the role of the rater (method variance) in the correlations. First, there are several diagonal rows of numbers (not enclosed in triangles). These numbers are correlations when the rater is different but the construct and measure are the same; they are used to support convergent validity. For example, the correlation for child and mother scores on the CDI was $r = 0.10$. The child–father correlation for this measure was $r = 0.40$. These

TABLE 1. Correlations of Children and Their Parents for the Children's Depression Inventory (CDI), Bellevue Index of Depression (BID), Hostility–Guilt Inventory (HGI), and Interview for Aggression (IA)[a]

		Children (N = 120)				Mothers (N = 120)				Fathers (N = 57)			
		Depression			Aggression	Depression			Aggression	Depression			Aggression
		CDI	BID	HGI	IA	CDI	BID	HGI	IA	CDI	BID	HGI	IA
Children													
Depression	CDI												
	BID	0.62[d]											
	HGI	0.38[d]	0.42[d]										
Aggression	IA	0.41[d]	0.49[d]	0.26[c]									
Mother													
Depression	CDI	0.10	0.24[c]	0.14	0.29[c]								
	BID	0.16[b]	0.27[d]	0.10	0.20[b]	0.71[d]							
	HGI	0.13	0.17	0.24[b]	0.24[b]	0.46[d]	0.56[d]						
Aggression	IA	0.03	-0.04	0.10	0.23[b]	0.26[c]	0.54[d]	0.60[d]					
Fathers													
Depression	CDI	0.40[d]	0.33[c]	0.36[c]	0.27[b]	0.74[d]	0.37[c]	0.36[c]	-0.11				
	BID	0.33[c]	0.41[c]	0.24[b]	0.27[b]	0.65[d]	0.69[d]	0.32[b]	0.25[b]	0.54[d]			
	HGI	0.28[b]	0.28[b]	0.37[c]	0.20	0.55[d]	0.56[c]	0.79[d]	0.46[d]	0.60[d]	0.57[d]		
Aggression	IA	0.14	0.01	0.22	0.37[c]	0.27[b]	0.54[d]	0.54[d]	0.68[d]	0.12	0.55[d]	0.53[d]	

[a]From Kazdin et al. (1983b). The solid-line triangles include correlations of measures completed by the same rater. The dashed-line triangles include correlations of measures completed by different raters. The diagonal rows of numbers between the dashed-line triangles are validity correlations (completion of the same measures by different raters).
[b] p < 0.05; [c] p < 0.01; [d] p < 0.001.

correlations and others in the diagonals indicate what we have discussed already, namely, that child and parent ratings correlate in the low to moderate range. Table 1 merely shows this correlation to be similar for depression and aggression.

Of greater interest are the correlations enclosed in the triangles. The *solid triangles* include measures completed by the same rater. In general, the correlations within a given solid triangle correlate relatively highly. This means that measures completed by the same informant share an important source of variance. Indeed, correlations by the same rater who rates different constructs (depression, aggression) tend to be higher than correlations of the same construct (depression) by different raters. For example, child ratings of depression and aggression on two interviews (BID and IA in Table 1) were correlated at $r = 0.49$ (same rater and measures but different constructs). This is much higher than ratings of depression between mother and child, which were correlated at $r = 0.10$ and $r = 0.27$ (same construct, different raters).

The results of this study and others like it can be used to evaluate the validity of measures of depression. Questions have emerged in selected studies about whether measures of depression assess emotional disturbance, internalizing symptoms, or some other response domain more generally, rather than depression in particular. Such concerns have emerged from efforts to show discriminant validity, namely, that measures of depression and internalizing symptoms correlate more highly with each other than with measures of other constructs (see Cole, 1987; Kazdin et al., 1983b; Saylor, Finch, Spirito, & Bennett, 1984a; Shoemaker et al., 1986; Stanger & Lewis, 1993; Treiber & Mabe, 1987; Wolfe et al., 1987). In relation to informant validity, other facets of these studies are of special relevance here. In studies that permit separation of construct (trait variance) from rater (method variance), the strong contribution of rater variance is consistently demonstrated. That is, measures of different traits within raters are often more likely to correspond that measures of the same traits between different raters. This finding has been consistent across different informants including children, parents, teachers, peers, and hospital staff as sources of information. Stated more succinctly, there is a strong method (rater) component that often pervades the ratings.

The contribution of method variance is critically important when validating measures obtained from the different informants. As we shall see next, several studies have shown that child self-report correlates moderately to highly with other measures. However, if the other measures were also completed by the child, interpretation of the correlations is ambiguous. It is quite likely that the correlations will be high because of the child's being the source of information common to both measures.

Correlates of Informant Ratings. Several studies provide data to suggest that scores from parents, teachers, and children relate in meaningful ways to other criteria. Ratings from children and adolescents have been related to several other measures completed by the youngsters themselves, including anxiety and fear, assertiveness, suicidal attempt and ideation, hopelessness, negative attributional style, and family conflict (e.g., Fauber, Forehand, Long, Burke, & Faust, 1987; Forehand et al., 1988; Haley, Fine, Marriage, Moretti, & Freeman, 1985; Kazdin, French, Unis, Esveldt-Dawson, & Sherick, 1983e; Sacco & Graves, 1984; Strauss, Forehand, Frame, & Smith, 1984; Weissman et al., 1980). For example, in a recent study, children and adolescents (ages 7–17) completed the CDI and several other measures that assessed self-esteem, locus of control, hopelessness, and cognitive attributions (McCauley, Mitchell, Burke, & Moss, 1988). The CDI correlated in the moderate range with these other measures ($r = 0.33–0.76$). These correlations could be used to support the validity of self-report CDI. Yet, these measures were all completed by the youth themselves. The moderate to high correlations might result from the common rater variance rather than or in combination with the constructs embraced by the measures.

Evidence for the validity of child self-report is more persuasive when the criterion does not include a common method component (e.g., child self-report measure). With this more stringent criterion, child self-report of depression has reliable correlates and hence is a valid indicator. For example, child and adolescent ratings of depression correlate with parent or teacher ratings of anxiety and social withdrawal, nonverbal interview behavior, social competence, overt social behavior, cognitive functioning, and poor school performance, including grade point average, and peer ratings of attractiveness, likeability, and social withdrawal (Altmann & Gotlib, 1988; Fauber et al., 1987; Kazdin, 1989b; Kazdin, Sherick, Esveldt-Dawson, & Rancurello, 1985; Slotkin et al., 1988; Strauss et al., 1984). Self-reported depression also relates to past and current experience of physical abuse, as assessed independently of child report (Kazdin, Moser, Colbus, & Bell, 1985). Thus, the correlations of self-report extend to measures that differ in method factors.

Several studies have shown that parent ratings predict other measures in which parental evaluation is not operative to ensure that common method variance does not account for the correlations (e.g., Hinshaw, Han, Erhardt, & Huber, 1992; Offord, Boyle, & Racine, 1989). For example, parent ratings of the children's and adolescents' ratings of depression predicted grade point average; in the same study, only mother CDI ratings predicted teacher evaluations of social adjustment and other anxiety symptoms (Slotkin et al., 1988). Parental reports of their children's depression correlate with diminished social interaction patterns on the part of the child and overt signs of expressive affect (Kazdin, Esveldt-Dawson, Sherick, & Colbus, 1985).

In short, both child and parent ratings can be advanced as valid measures of childhood depression. Each has been shown to relate to other constructs and measures in predictable ways. The same can be said of reports from other informants. For example, teacher and peer reports of childhood depression have been validated with their own correlates, as reflected in overt classroom behavior, academic performance, and popularity (e.g., Kazdin, Esveldt-Dawson, & Loar, 1983a; Lefkowitz & Tesiny, 1980; Tesiny & Lefkowitz, 1982; Tesiny, Lefkowitz, & Gordon, 1980).

In general, research to date has shown that scores obtained from different informants may not correlate highly with each other. Yet evidence indicates that the measures correlate with other criteria in ways consistent with the construct of depression. Thus, data from each informant have demonstrated criterion or concurrent validity. What has not been studied is the extent to which information from one source rather than another is optimal for predicting various criteria longitudinally. For example, child, parent, teacher, and peer ratings might well vary in the extent to which they predict subsequent suicide attempt. The validity and utility of information from alternative informants, alone and in combination, warrant further attention.

Few studies have compared the relative utility of information from alternative sources in predicting an independent criterion. A recent study nicely approximates the type of work that is needed in this regard. In this study, children, parents, and teachers completed measures to assess a variety of disruptive behaviors (Loeber et al., 1991). The extent to which the measures predicted performance 1 year later was examined. Among the findings, child, parent, and teacher ratings of conduct problems at the first assessment varied in their correlation with police contacts ($r = 0.0, 0.20, 0.0$, respectively) and school suspensions ($r = 0.28, 0.19, 0.30$, respectively) 1 year later. The prediction of other outcome criteria was examined as well, including whether children repeated a grade at school and were in a special placement class. In general, parent ratings were more consistent than child and teacher ratings in predicting performance 1 year later. The relations were generally low ($r = 0.03–0.20$) for all parent ratings and the varied outcome criteria. At first glance, the results would suggest the greater predictive utility of parent ratings. However, the criteria here were themselves based on parent report (i.e., parent report of school suspensions, and so on). Thus, the contamination of common method variance in predictors and

criterion could readily explain the results. At the same time, the study illustrates three
needed emphases, namely, the evaluation of multiple raters, the comparison of their
relative utility in relation to other criteria, and a longitudinal perspective in evaluating the
utility of data from different informants.

263

Informant
Variability in
Assessment

Implications

The study of informant variability in assessing childhood dysfunction has become an
area of research in its own right. The routine use of parents and children in diagnostic
assessment and the frequent reliance on others (teachers, peers) in research in developmental psychopathology more generally has made salient the different perspectives on the
child's symptoms. Repeated demonstration of the low to moderate agreement among
raters, with occasional exceptions, has broad implications for the conceptualization of
childhood dysfunction, for research, and for clinical practice.

Conceptual Issues

Symptom constellations such as depression in current diagnostic systems are conceptualized very much like "traits" have been conceptualized in traditional personality
theories. That is, symptoms (or groups of symptoms such as depression) are considered to
reflect patterns of affect, cognition, and behavior that are consistent across situations and
over time. Research on informant variability does not necessarily dispel the view that
individuals show consistent patterns across situations and over time. Yet variation among
raters raises interesting prospects for how disorders are viewed.

Symptom patterns of individuals may be influenced in varying degrees by the context,
situations, and other factors. Perhaps it is not merely different perspectives that different
informants have about the "same" child, but rather some changes in child performance
in the presence of diverse informants. This is not to say that the child changes completely
in the presence of different cues, but rather that there may be some change and that
patterns of performance may vary in salience across situations.

Implicitly, researchers may be surprised or disappointed that two raters (parents,
teachers, children) do not agree on the disorder. Yet the seeming inconsistency that this
disagreement putatively reflects is greatly reduced by conceptualizing disorders somewhat differently. Drawing from personality research, disorders might be viewed from the
standpoint of representing the separate and combined influence of individual characteristics (traits), contexts (situations), and their interaction (Magnusson, 1981). Viewing a
"disorder" as "in" the child may be a narrow conceptualization of dysfunction. The child's
functioning is likely to vary widely across diverse contexts. A depressed child may not
manifest depressive symptoms in all waking moments. Interactions with others, changes in
situations and contexts, and fluctuations within the individual himself or herself can also
contribute to the manifestations and experience of depressive symptoms. The varied
ratings provided by the child and others (parents, teachers) may reflect variation in
manifestations of depression and in the child's experience. The different situations,
contexts, and perceptions are not artifacts or method variance, one might argue, but rather
central features of the interaction of trait × situation variance. A trait view begins with the
notion that there is genuine "trait" variance that can be delineated between individuals so
that in fact the disorder in some sense does "reside" within the individual. At the same
time, the situational influences are not trivial, and patterns of responding that do not
consider contexts and influences are incomplete.

The assumption of stable disorders within individual children has value in the sense
that distinguishing biological and psychological features can be studied and demonstrated.

At the same time, this is not tantamount to gainsaying the role of situational, contextual, and other influences that may greatly influence manifestation and experience of depression. Parent, teacher, and child ratings produce *discrepant* results for evaluations of the child's depression only if it is assumed that child depressive symptoms are driven from within completely and do not vary in how and when they are manifest and in what degree of severity.

Conceptualization of disorders and their manifestations might be developed to incorporate consistent findings about informant variability. Variation across situations and contexts may represent more than mere differences in rater perceptions; they may also reflect differences in presentation and experience of symptoms themselves. The role of situational and contextual influences on disorders is recognized with some disorders. For example, attention-deficit disorders are usually acknowledged as more readily apparent in school settings and by teacher evaluations. This is not to say that dysfunction cannot be assessed by focusing on the children and their performance on a variety of measures outside the classroom; rather, the classroom is a place where hyperactivity and deficits in attention can be readily assessed and perhaps are more likely to be manifest. In principle, the situation and contextual variance is recognized as important. Severity of dysfunction of a disorder and among different disorders also points to the importance of situation variance. For some disorders (severe autism, mental retardation), the dysfunction itself is so pervasive that the effect situational and contextual influences on symptom manifestations may seem minor. The central point is that conceptualization of situations and disorder × situation interactions is made salient by research on informant variability. The focus has been on variability of performance among informants. Further study of influences in variation of symptom manifestation across situations and contexts is important to elaborate possible bases of rater differences. Relatedly, the way in which information in different situations is perceived, weighted, and integrated by different informants may be important to understand as well in relation to informant agreement.

In general, conceptual work is needed to better understand the underpinnings of informant variability. By and large, research has examined the factors that may influence agreement between raters but without conceptual understanding of these factors. For example, in some studies, the child's chronological age has influenced agreement between parents and children, with greater parent–youth correspondence as the child's age increases (Edelbrock et al., 1986). Such a demonstration is a useful initial step. Further work is needed to understand the basis for this difference conceptually. Age itself is not very informative as a construct unless those processes or factors associated with age (e.g., cognitive development) that might explain the differences are assessed and evaluated. In the aforecited study, for example, age of the child could have been highly correlated with age of the parent (i.e., older children tend to have parents who are older), so child age is not necessarily even the variable that accounts for the difference. Similarly, other variables that have been shown to influence degree of agreement between parent and child such as child sex, race, and socioeconomic disadvantage warrant analysis. How and why these variables influence the degree of agreement have yet to receive significant attention in conceptualizations of child dysfunction.

In general, the conceptualization of informant variability has received little attention. Critical questions remain to be addressed. Are there any implications of discrepancies between raters for conceptualizing dysfunction to begin with? Is agreement among alternative raters significant as a substantive finding (e.g., predictor) of clinical course, given the meaning such agreement might have? What is the significance of situations in which child or parent provides higher ratings of a given dysfunction (e.g., suicidal thought)? Research to date has established the lack of agreement and the variation in estimating symptoms within a given area. There is a need for further research that moves beyond empirical demonstration of informant variability to test conceptual models that will advance understanding of that variability.

Informant variability has critically important implications for the conduct of research on childhood depression and of course childhood disorders more generally. Researchers operationalize childhood depression in many ways that must be viewed quite cautiously in light of informant variability. The most common methods of identifying depressed children for research purposes are selection of youth based on one of various criteria: diagnosis of depressive disorder or relatively severe depression based on one informant (usually the child, parent, teacher, or peers). There are critical research implications regarding the criteria that are used to identify depressed and nondepressed children, given the variation due to informants. Essentially, within a given population of children, different samples will be identified as depressed depending on the method of assessment and the informant whose information (child, parent) will be used.

As an illustration, in one investigation, three commonly used selection procedures to identify and characterize depressed children were compared (Kazdin, 1989b). Within a sample of hospitalized children ($N = 231$, ages 7–12), three ways of operationalizing depression were compared: depression defined by psychiatric diagnosis, child-completed measures, and parent-completed measures of depression. The child- and parent-completed measures included questionnaire, interview, and symptom checklist measures. Psychiatric diagnosis was derived separately from a semistructured diagnostic interview. The purpose was to examine the extent to which the different criteria would select a similar group of depressed patients.

Generally, the results indicated that children identified as depressed by one criterion (e.g., diagnosis, or child ratings, or parent ratings) were not identified as depressed by another criterion. For example, of the cases that met DSM-III criteria for a diagnosis of depressive disorder, 31.6% and 67% also met commonly used cutoff scores that define depression on the child- and parent-completed CDI, respectively. This means that who is considered "depressed" depends very much on the criterion. The implications are important for the substantive findings. In this study, other measures were included to evaluate the extent to which different selection criteria would generate different findings. Using *child ratings* to define depressed and nondepressed children, depression was related to negative cognitive processes (e.g., lower aspirations, more internal attributions of negative events), low self-esteem, and hopelessness. Using *parent ratings*, relations between depression and these other domains were not significant. From the standpoint of research, the results indicate that the informant who served as the basis for identifying depressed cases may influence the substantive findings.

A related research implication pertains to the cutoff scores used to identify depressed youth. Research on depression with adults has identified various cutoff scores to delineate groups that are considered low, moderate, or high in severity of depression. The Beck Depression Inventory (Beck, Ward, Mendelson, Mock, & Erbaugh, 1961) is often used in this fashion to identify groups for further comparison. The research supports an implicit view that the *scale* has a cutoff score. There has been a tendency to extend this approach to child depression measures. For example, the Children's Depression Inventory has been evaluated extensively. On the basis of clinical use and normative data, a recommendation has been to use a particular score (≥ 19) to define depressed children (e.g., Smucker, Craighead, Craighead, & Green, 1986). The goal to identify an extreme group based on percentile ranking and standard deviation from mean levels is important for research and clinical purposes. Research on informant variability challenges the tendency to view a particular scale score as a cutoff without considering the informant. Research has shown that for the CDI and other measures, the mean and hence cutoff scores in standard deviation units above the mean differ for children and parents (Kazdin, 1989b; Kazdin et al., 1986). Thus, the identity of the source of information must be taken into account in identifying cutoff scores. (No doubt a number of other factors need to be considered in determining cutoff scores to identify depressed and nondepressed youth such as child age, sex, and ethnicity, although discussion of such factors is beyond the scope of this chapter.)

Clinical Implications

Variability among informants has obvious significance for clinical work. The initial point in clinical work at which discrepancies are likely to arise is in reaching clinical diagnoses. Diagnostic procedures routinely attempt to integrate child and parent, and occasionally teacher, information. Low agreement on individual symptoms and overall diagnoses means that in many cases the clinician will not have the benefit of consistency among raters. Acceptable agreement between parents and children has been demonstrated in some diagnostic studies (e.g., Welner et al., 1987). Even so, diagnostic agreement is not always high and discrepant information can emerge in clinical practice. Precisely how discrepant information ought to be integrated is a matter of clinical judgment.

Researchers have tried to assist the diagnostic process by recommending and exploring ways of integrating information from different raters (e.g., Piacentini, Cohen, & Cohen, 1992; Reich & Earls, 1987; Verhulst & Koot, 1992). For example, Bird, Gould, and Staghezza (1992) compared alternative ways of integrating parent and child information in reaching a diagnosis. Information was used to examine the extent to which child and parent information predicted clinician diagnosis. Parent report was better in predicting diagnoses for more externalizing disorders (attention-deficit and oppositional disorders); child information was better for predicting internalizing disorders (e.g., anxiety disorders, depression). Overall, parent report was slightly more predictive of diagnoses. The results suggest that different informants might be weighted differently on the basis of the domain that is assessed. However, a limitation of this type of work, mentioned earlier, is that diagnosis is derived from a clinician's evaluation of parent and child information. Hence, the predictor and criterion are confounded. As yet, there is no reliable means in use for integrating information in clinical work. One recommendation is to consider the symptom as present if either informant acknowledges the problem (Bird et al., 1992). Such a recommendation ensures that no symptom is overlooked. In clinical work, the decision-making process can be influenced by the nature of the symptom, the consequences of overlooking the symptom, and available treatment.

In one of my own cases, for example, we could not reach agreement regarding an event with a young adolescent girl. Sarah, 13 years old, ran in front of an automobile but was not injured. Whether this was an accident or a suicide attempt was a matter of dispute. A persuasive case was made by the mother that Sarah ran in front of the car purposely. Although the mother was not present, peers with whom Sarah was walking conveyed to the mother the major details of the event (e.g., Sarah's despondency that day, the purposeful exclusion of Sarah from the conversation and interaction). Thus, the mother based her report on the information and discussion with her daughter's peers, who agreed that Sarah intentionally ran in front of the car. In the diagnostic interview, Sarah herself denied suicidal ideation or attempt currently or in relation to the prior event. She explained this specific event as an attempt to cross the street at a point when this was reasonable in light of walking home. No clear rules were available within the diagnostic scheme to resolve the matter. Sarah and her mother disagreed when brought together to discuss the interview.

As is often the case in clinical work, supplementary information was available, including history (e.g., no history of the child in suicidal threats, no family history of suicide attempt) as well as concurrent information from the child (e.g., measures of child depression and hopelessness). The supplementary information suggested that current suicide risk was low, but of course did not help in deciding how to score the diagnostic interview on this point. One item may or may not be critical in scoring a diagnostic interview. The more general question is raised about discrepant information as it emerges in practice and how to reach a resolution. It is possible that better understanding of the utility of reports from different informants in predicting other criteria may reduce the need for and value of reaching an integrated view that combines information from different raters (see Angold, Weissman, John, Wickramaratne, & Prusoff, 1991; Bird et al., 1992).

Research has been helpful in addressing informant variability in clinical work. Generally, child report of internalizing symptoms (e.g., depression, withdrawal) and parent report of externalizing symptoms (e.g., aggression, antisocial behavior) probably warrant greater credence, given findings from studies of informant variability. Measures from different informants are critically important. The different perspectives provide different samples of child functioning. In clinical work, as well as in research, one does not necessarily look for agreement or convergence among alternative sources of information. The sources are valuable precisely because they may reflect discrepancies.

Conclusions

In the study of childhood dysfunction, obtaining measures from multiple informants has become standard. The child's functioning at home and at school and the prospect that the child's perspective is cognitively underdeveloped make information from adults essential. The child's report, too, is important and cannot be viewed as ancillary. Indeed, the literature on informant variability suggests that the child's perspective on functioning may be particularly informative in relation to internalizing symptoms such as depression. Thus, multiple perspectives continue to be critical to the assessment and evaluation process.

The different perspectives provided by informants have yet to be exploited conceptually or clinically. Research to date has focused on reporting discrepancies among different raters who evaluate emotional and behavioral problems of children. Several studies attest to the low to moderate agreement among children and their parents, teachers, and peers. Research has also begun to examine the variables or factors associated with agreement, i.e., that influence the magnitude of agreement or the direction of the discrepancy between two raters. A variety of subject and demographic variables of the child or family (e.g., sex, age, race, socioeconomic status, parent psychopathology, stress) have been studied. This type of research extends beyond demonstrating low to moderate agreement and describes some of the conditions on which agreement depends.

Two other types of research might be identified as logical next steps. To begin, it would be critically important to go beyond description to understand processes leading to agreement and disagreement between alternative informants. We have little understanding of why specific variables may influence disagreement or discrepancies among informants. For example, mothers and fathers sometimes differ in the extent to which their evaluations correlate with their children's self-reports. It is unclear why this discrepancy occurs. Similarly, parent psychopathology and stress have influenced the degree of disagreement among informants. Here again, we have little understanding of the factors that underlie these differences. Understanding the bases of informant differences and variables that contribute to these differences may have important implications regarding perception of functioning that extend beyond the assessment of childhood psychopathology.

To aid research in this area, there might be value in experimental investigations in which standard stimuli (e.g., videotapes of children behaving in home and school settings) are presented. Parents and children can complete assessments to evaluate the children whose behavior has been prerecorded on tape. A laboratory paradigm would permit evaluating parent and child perspectives when stimuli are held constant. Moreover, vignettes presented to parents and children can manipulate variables to determine their influence on perception and on informant agreement. A laboratory approach to research might permit assessment of a broader range of variables to test hypotheses about processes that underlie agreement.

Another line of research that is needed pertains to validation regarding information from different informants. Assessment is completed with regard to some purpose, decision, or criterion. The extent to which information about child dysfunction from different informants is useful in predicting outcomes of interest warrants further attention. Although information may be available from multiple informants, we may wish to weight different informant views differently depending on the criterion in which we are interested. The clinical utility of information from multiple informants does not necessarily come from combining the information. Rather, understanding the relation of information to alternative current and long-term criteria may contribute to better utilization of that information.

ACKNOWLEDGMENT. Completion of this chapter was facilitated greatly by the support of Research Scientist Award MH00353 from the National Institute of Mental Health. The author wishes to express gratitude for the support.

References

Achenbach, T. M., McConaughy, S. H., & Howell, C. T. (1987). Child/adolescent behavioral and emotional problems: Implications of cross-informant correlations for situational specificity. *Psychological Bulletin, 101,* 213–232.

Altmann, E. O., & Gotlib, I. H. (1988). The social behavior of depressed children: An observational study. *Journal of Abnormal Child Psychology, 16,* 29–44.

American Psychiatric Association (1994). *Diagnostic and statistical manual of mental disorders,* 4th ed. Washington, DC: Author.

Angold, A., Weissman, W., John, K., Wickramaratne, P., & Prusoff, B. (1991). The effects of age and sex on depression ratings in children and adolescents. *Journal of the American Academy of Child and Adolescent Psychiatry, 30,* 67–74.

Beck, A. T., Ward, C. H., Mendelson, M., Mock, J., & Erbaugh, J. (1961). An inventory for measuring depression. *Archives of General Psychiatry, 4,* 53–63.

Bird, H. R., Gould, M. S., & Staghezza, B. (1992). Aggregating data from multiple informants in child psychiatry epidemiological research. *Journal of the American Academy of Child and Adolescent Psychiatry, 31,* 78–85.

Brody, G. H., & Forehand, R. (1986). Maternal perceptions of child maladjustment as a function of the combined influence of child behavior and maternal depression. *Journal of Consulting and Clinical Psychology, 54,* 237–240.

Campbell, D. T., & Fiske, D. (1959). Convergent and discriminant validation by the multitrait–multimethod matrix. *Psychological Bulletin, 56,* 81–105.

Cole, D. A. (1987). Utility of confirmatory factor analysis in test validation research. *Journal of Consulting and Clinical Psychology, 55,* 584–594.

Cronbach, L. J., & Meehl, P. E. (1955). Construct validity in psychological tests. *Psychological Bulletin, 52,* 281–302.

Edelbrock, C. S., Costello, A. J., Dulcan, M. K., Conover, N. C., & Kalas, R. (1986). Parent–child agreement on child psychiatric symptoms assessed via structured interview. *Journal of Child Psychology and Psychiatry, 27,* 181–190.

Fauber, R., Forehand, R., Long, N., Burke, M., & Faust, J. (1987). The relationship of young adolescent CDI scores to their social and cognitive functioning. *Journal of Psychopathology and Behavioral Assessment, 9,* 161–172.

Fergusson, D. M., Lynskey, M. T., & Horwood, L. J. (1993). The effect of maternal depression on maternal ratings of child behavior. *Journal of Abnormal Child Psychology, 21,* 245–269.

Forehand, R., Brody, G., Slotkin, J., Fauber, R., McCombs, A., & Long, N. (1988). Young adolescent and maternal depression: Assessment, interrelations, and family predictors. *Journal of Consulting and Clinical Psychology, 56,* 422–426.

Forehand, R., Lautenschlager, G. J., Faust, J., & Graziano, W. G. (1986). Parent perceptions and parent–child interactions in clinic-referred children: A preliminary investigation of the effects of maternal depressive moods. *Behaviour Research and Therapy, 24,* 73–75.

Friedlander, S., Weiss, D., & Traylor, J. (1986). Assessing the influence of maternal depression on the validity of the Child Behavior Checklist. *Journal of Abnormal Child Psychology, 14,* 123–133.

Gurney, B. G., Jr., Shapiro, E. B., & Stover, L. (1968). Parental perceptions of maladjusted children: Agreement between parents and relation to mother–child interaction. *Journal of Genetic Psychology, 113,* 215–225.

Haley, G., Fine, S., Marriage, K., Moretti, M., & Freeman, R. (1985). Cognitive bias and depression in psychiatrically disturbed children and adolescents. *Journal of Consulting and Clinical Psychology, 53,* 535–537.

Herjanic, B., & Reich, W. (1982). Development of a structured psychiatric interview for children: Agreement between child and parent on individual symptoms. *Journal of Abnormal Child Psychology, 10,* 307–324.

Hinshaw, S. P., Han, S. S., Erhardt, D., & Huber, A. (1992). Internalizing and externalizing behavior problems in preschool children: Correspondence among parent and teacher ratings and behavior observations. *Journal of Clinical Child Psychology, 21,* 143–150.

Ines, T. M., & Sacco, W. P. (1992). Factors related to correspondence between teacher ratings of elementary student depression and student self-ratings. *Journal of Consulting and Clinical Psychology, 60,* 140–142.

Ivens, C., & Rehm, L. P. (1988). Assessment of childhood depression: Correspondence between reports by child, mother, and father. *Journal of the American Academy of Child and Adolescent Psychiatry, 27,* 738–741.

Jacob, T., Grounds, L., & Haley, R. (1982). Correspondence between parents' reports on the Behavior Problem Checklist. *Journal of Abnormal Child Psychology, 10,* 593–608.

Jacobson, R. H., Lahey, B. B., & Strauss, C. C. (1983). Correlates of depressed mood in normal children. *Journal of Abnormal Child Psychology, 11,* 29–40.

Jensen, P. S., Traylor, J., Xenakis, S. N., & Davis, H. (1988a). Child psychopathology rating scales and interrater agreement. I. Parents' gender and psychiatric symptoms. *Journal of the American Academy of Child and Adolescent Psychiatry, 27,* 442–450.

Jensen, P. S., Xenakis, S. N., Davis, H., & DeGroot, J. (1988b). Child psychopathology rating scales and interrater agreement. II. Child and family characteristics. *Journal of the American Academy of Child and Adolescent Psychiatry, 27,* 451–461.

Kashani, J. H., Orvaschel, H., Burk, J. A., & Reid, J. C. (1985). Informant variance: The issue of parent–child disagreement. *Journal of the American Academy of Child Psychiatry, 24,* 437–441.

Kazdin, A. E. (1989a). Developmental differences in depression. In B. B. Lahey & A. E. Kazdin (Eds.), *Advances in clinical child psychology,* Vol. 12 (pp. 193–219). New York: Plenum Press.

Kazdin, A. E. (1989b). Identifying depression in children: A comparison of alternative selection criteria. *Journal of Abnormal Child Psychology, 17,* 437–454.

Kazdin, A. E. (1992). *Research design in clinical psychology,* 2nd ed. Needham Heights, MA: Allyn & Bacon.

Kazdin, A. E., Colbus, D., & Rodgers, A. (1986). Assessment of depression and diagnosis of depressive disorder among psychiatrically disturbed children. *Journal of Abnormal Child Psychology, 14,* 499–515.

Kazdin, A. E., Esveldt-Dawson, K., & Loar, L. (1983a). Correspondence of teacher ratings and direct observations of classroom behavior of psychiatric inpatient children. *Journal of Abnormal Child Psychology, 11,* 549–564.

Kazdin, A. E., Esveldt-Dawson, K., Sherick, R. B., & Colbus, D. (1985). Assessment of overt behavior and childhood depression among psychiatrically disturbed children. *Journal of Consulting and Clinical Psychology, 53,* 201–210.

Kazdin, A. E., Esveldt-Dawson, K., Unis, A. S., & Rancurello, M. D. (1983b). Child and parent evaluations of depression and aggression in psychiatric inpatient children. *Journal of Abnormal Child Psychology, 11,* 401–413.

Kazdin, A. E., French, N. H., & Unis, A. S. (1983c). Child, mother, and father evaluations of depression in psychiatric inpatient children. *Journal of Abnormal Child Psychology, 11,* 167–180.

Kazdin, A. E., French, N. H., Unis, A. S., & Esveldt-Dawson, K. (1983d). Assessment of childhood depression: Correspondence of child and parent ratings. *Journal of the American Academy of Child Psychiatry, 22,* 157–164.

Kazdin, A. E., French, N. H., Unis, A. S., Esveldt-Dawson, K., & Sherick, R. B. (1983e). Hopelessness, depression and suicidal intent among psychiatrically disturbed inpatient children. *Journal of Consulting and Clinical Psychology, 51,* 504–510.

Kazdin, A. E., & Heidish, I. E. (1984). Convergence of clinically derived diagnoses and parent checklists among inpatient children. *Journal of Abnormal Child Psychology, 12*, 421–436.

Kazdin, A. E., Moser, J., Colbus, D., & Bell, R. (1985). Depressive symptoms among physically abused and psychiatrically disturbed children. *Journal of Abnormal Psychology, 94*, 298–307.

Kazdin, A. E., Sherick, R. B., Esveldt-Dawson, K., & Rancurello, M. D. (1985). Nonverbal behavior and childhood depression. *Journal of the American Academy of Child Psychiatry, 24*, 303–309.

Kolko, D. J., & Kazdin, A. E. (1993). Emotional/behavioral problems in clinic and nonclinic children: Correspondence among child, parent, and teacher reports. *Journal of Child Psychology and Psychiatry, 34*, 991–1006.

Kovacs, M. (1981). Rating scales to assess depression in school aged children. *Acta Paedopsychiatrica, 46*, 305–315.

LaGreca, A. M. (Ed.) (1990). *Through the eyes of the child: Obtaining self-reports from children and adolescents.* Needham Heights, MA: Allyn & Bacon.

Langford, L. M., & Alm, O. W. (1954). A comparison of parent judgments and child feelings concerning the self adjustment and social adjustment of twelve-year-old children. *Journal of Genetic Psychology, 85*, 39–46.

Ledingham, J. E., Younger, A., Schwartzman, A., & Bergeron, G. (1982). Agreement among teacher, peer, and self-ratings of children's aggression, withdrawal, and likability. *Journal of Abnormal Child Psychology, 10*, 363–372.

Lefkowitz, M. M., & Tesiny, E. P. (1980). Assessment of childhood depression. *Journal of Consulting and Clinical Psychology, 48*, 43–50.

Lefkowitz, M. M., & Tesiny, E. P. (1984). Rejection and depression: Prospective and contemporaneous analyses. *Developmental Psychology, 20*, 776–785.

Loeber, R., Green, S. M., Lahey, B. B., & Stouthamer-Loeber, M. (1990). Optimal informants on childhood disruptive behaviors. *Development and Psychopathology, 1*, 317–337.

Loeber, R., Green, S. M., Lahey, B. B., & Stouthamer-Loeber, M. (1991). Differences and similarities between children, mothers, and teachers as informants on disruptive child behavior. *Journal of Abnormal Child Psychology, 19*, 75–95.

Magnusson, D. (Ed.) (1981). *Toward a psychology of situations: An interactional perspective.* Hillsdale, NJ: Erlbaum Associates.

Mash, E., & Terdal, L. (Eds.) (1988). *Behavioral assessment of childhood disorders*, 2nd ed. New York: Guilford Press.

Mattison, R. E., Bagnato, S. J., & Strickler, E. (1987). Diagnostic importance of combined parent and teacher ratings on the Revised Problem Checklist. *Journal of Abnormal Child Psychology, 15*, 617–628.

McCauley, E., Mitchell, J. R., Burke, P., & Moss, S. (1988). Cognitive attributes of depression in children and adolescents. *Journal of Consulting and Clinical Psychology, 56*, 903–908.

Moretti, M. M., Fine, S., Haley, G., & Marriage, K. (1985). Childhood and adolescent depression: Child-report versus parent-report information. *Journal of the American Academy of Child Psychiatry, 24*, 298–302.

Offord, D. R., Boyle, M. H., & Racine, Y. (1989). Ontario Child Health Study: Correlates of disorder. *Journal of the American Academy of Child and Adolescent Psychiatry, 28*, 856–860.

Orvaschel, H., Puig-Antich, J., Chambers, W., Tabrizi, M. A., & Johnson, R. (1982). Retrospective assessment of prepubertal major depression with the Kiddie-SADS-E. *Journal of the American Academy of Child Psychiatry, 21*, 392–397.

Phares, V., Compas, B. E., & Howell, D. C. (1989). Perspectives on child behavior problems: Comparisons of children's self-reports with parent and teacher reports. *Psychological Assessment, 1*, 68–71.

Piacentini, J. C., Cohen, P., & Cohen, J. (1992). Combining discrepant diagnostic information from multiple sources: Are complex algorithms better than simple ones? *Journal of Abnormal Child Psychology, 20*, 51–63.

Piers, E. V. (1972). Parent prediction of children's self-concepts. *Journal of Consulting and Clinical Psychology, 38*, 428–433.

Reich, W., & Earls, F. (1987). Rules for making psychiatric diagnosis in children on the basis of multiple sources of information: Preliminary strategies. *Journal of Abnormal Child Psychology, 15*, 601–616.

Reynolds, W. M. (Ed.) (1992). *Internalizing disorders in children and adolescents.* New York: John Wiley.

Reynolds, W. M., Anderson, G., & Bartell, N. (1985). Measuring depression in children: A multi-method assessment investigation. *Journal of Abnormal Child Psychology, 13*, 513–526.

Romano, B. A., & Nelson, R. O. (1988). Discriminant and concurrent validity of measures of children's depression. *Journal of Clinical Child Psychology, 17*, 255–259.

Rutter, M., Tuma, A. H., & Lann, I. S. (Eds.) (1988). *Assessment and diagnosis of child psychopathology.* New York: Guilford Press.

Sacco, W. P., & Graves, D. J. (1984). Childhood depression, interpersonal problem-solving, and self-ratings of performance. *Journal of Clinical Child Psychology*, *13*, 10–15.

Saylor, C. F., Finch, A. J., Baskin, C. H., Furey, W., & Kelly, M. M. (1984a). Construct validity for measures of childhood depression: Application of multitrait–multimethod methodology. *Journal of Consulting and Clinical Psychology*, *52*, 977–985.

Saylor, C. F., Finch, A. J., Jr., Spirito, A., & Bennett, B. (1984b). The Children's Depression Inventory: A systematic evaluation of psychometric properties. *Journal of Consulting and Clinical Psychology*, *52*, 955–967.

Shoemaker, O. S., Erickson, M. T., & Finch, A. J., Jr. (1986). Depression and anger in third- and fourth-grade boys: A multimethod assessment approach. *Journal of Clinical Child Psychology*, *15*, 290–296.

Slotkin, J., Forehand, R., Fauber, R., McCombs, A., & Long, N. (1988). Parent-completed and adolescent-completed CDIs: Relationship to adolescent social and cognitive function. *Journal of Abnormal Child Psychology*, *16*, 207–217.

Smucker, M. R., Craighead, W. E., Craighead, L. W., & Green, B. J. (1986). Normative and reliability data for the Children's Depression Inventory. *Journal of Abnormal Child Psychology*, *14*, 25–39.

Stanger, C., & Lewis, M. (1993). Agreement among parents, teachers, and children on internalizing and externalizing behavior problems. *Journal of Clinical Child Psychology*, *22*, 107–115.

Strauss, C. C., Forehand, R. L., Frame, C., & Smith, K. (1984). Characteristics of children with extreme scores on the Children's Depression Inventory. *Journal of Clinical Child Psychology*, *13*, 227–231.

Tesiny, E. P., & Lefkowitz, M. M. (1982). Childhood depression: A 6-month follow-up study. *Journal of Consulting and Clinical Psychology*, *50*, 778–780.

Tesiny, E. P., Lefkowitz, M. M., & Gordon, N. H. (1980). Childhood depression, locus of control, and school achievement. *Journal of Educational Psychology*, *72*, 506–510.

Touliatos, J., & Lindholm, B. W. (1981). Congruence of parents' and teachers' ratings of children's behavior problems. *Journal of Abnormal Child Psychology*, *9*, 347–354.

Treiber, F. A., & Mabe, P. A., III (1987). Child and parent perceptions of children's psychopathology in psychiatric outpatient children. *Journal of Abnormal Child Psychology*, *15*, 115–124.

Verhulst, F. C., & Koot, H. M. (1992). *Child psychiatric epidemiology: Concepts, methods, and findings.* Newbury Park, CA: Sage.

Victor, J. B., Halverson, C. F., Jr., & Wampler, K. S. (1988). Family–school context: Parent and teacher agreement on child temperament. *Journal of Consulting and Clinical psychology*, *56*, 573–577.

Webster-Stratton, C. (1988). Mothers' and fathers' perceptions of child deviance: Roles of parent and child behaviors and parent adjustment. *Journal of Consulting and Clinical Psychology*, *56*, 909–915.

Webster-Stratton, C., & Hammond, M. (1988). Maternal depression and its relationship to life stress, perceptions of child behavior problems, parenting behaviors, and child conduct problems. *Journal of Abnormal Child Psychology*, *16*, 299–315.

Weissman, M. M., Orvaschel, H., & Padian, N. (1980). Children's symptom and social functioning self-report scales: Comparison of mothers' and children's reports. *Journal of Nervous and Mental Disease*, *168*, 736–740.

Welner, Z., Reich, W., Herjanic, B., Jung, K. G., & Amado, H. (1987). Reliability, validity, and parent–child agreement studies of the Diagnostic Interview for Children and Adolescents (DICA). *Journal of the American Academy of Child and Adolescent Psychiatry*, *26*, 649–653.

Wolfe, V. V., Finch, A. J., Jr., Saylor, C. F., Blount, R. L., Pallmeyer, T. P., & Carek, D. J. (1987). Negative affectivity in children: A multitrait–multimethod investigation. *Journal of Consulting and Clinical Psychology*, *55*, 245–250.

IV
TREATMENT APPROACHES

14

Psychological Treatment Approaches for Depression in Children

Kevin D. Stark, Lawrence W. Rouse, and Cynthia Kurowski

Overview

It is acutely apparent from the preceding chapters that depression during childhood is a very serious disturbance that has been formally recognized only since 1980. The research base for understanding this disorder is growing very rapidly, and much exciting research is currently under way. While research on childhood depression has mushroomed, very little research on the treatment of depression during childhood has been completed. In fact, there have been more chapters and books written about how to treat depression than there are studies evaluating the effectiveness of psychological treatments for depressed youths. Furthermore, most of the studies that have been completed could be considered clinical analog studies, since they have involved subclinical populations. In this chapter, we hope to contribute something beyond another review of the existing treatment literature. To this end, we will first evaluate existing treatment programs against their adequacy in addressing the disturbances that may cause or maintain a depressive disorder during childhood and then describe a comprehensive intervention program for depressed youths.

Reflected throughout this chapter is our belief that the treatment programs cited in the literature to date, including our own, are too circumscribed in their focus. They are based on unidimensional models of adult depression that fail to recognize the multitude of possible avenues that lead to the development of a depressive disorder. Furthermore, this unidimensional approach does not adequately recognize the interdependence of the various systems (i.e., cognitive, behavioral, affective, physiological, interpersonal, and environmental) that are hypothesized to be involved in depression. Moreover, existing empirically evaluated interventions represent downward extensions of effective interven-

Kevin D. Stark, Lawrence W. Rouse, and Cynthia Kurowski • Department of Educational Psychology, University of Texas, Austin, Texas 78712.

Handbook of Depression in Children and Adolescents, edited by William M. Reynolds and Hugh F. Johnston. Plenum Press, New York, 1994.

tions for adults. While this approach may have represented a fruitful initial starting point for the development of interventions for depressed youths (Kaslow & Rehm, 1983), at this point it would be wise to take a step back from the adult treatment models and rethink how we are using them. It may be useful to incorporate treatment components that better reflect and address the realities of the depressed youngster's life. For example, children are much more dependent on, and influenced on a daily basis by, their parents and family than are adults who have limited contact with their family of origin. Consequently, adults may no longer live within the milieu that led to and maintained depressogenic schemata; however, children still live within the family that is providing schema-consistent information and other dysfunctional influences. A child with poor social skills receives negative feedback from his or her classmates on a daily basis, while an adult with poor social skills can find solace in a job that requires a minimum of contact with others. In addition, procedures followed for implementing various treatment procedures may have to be altered to make them useful for children. Most children are not engaged in treatment through the traditional verbal interview procedure. They find this procedure to be boring and lose interest in therapy very quickly. Thus, stories, games, and activities have to be used as the vehicle for implementing many of the treatment procedures. Otherwise, the therapeutic process is not engaging enough for many children and the resultant disinterest can lead to premature termination or the failure of the child to benefit maximally from treatment.

This chapter is organized around the various psychosocial disturbances associated with depressive disorders during childhood. The disturbances that are identified and briefly discussed are based on a cognitive–behavioral model of depression that emphasizes both child and environmental variables that interact in a reciprocal fashion to cause and maintain depression during childhood (Stark, Rouse, & Livingston, 1991). More specifically, the child variables hypothesized to be of greatest importance are cognitive, behavioral, emotional, and physiological factors and such environmental variables as parental characteristics, family climate factors, and other environmental variables. Research relevant to each of these specific topics is discussed in other chapters in this book. The discussion in this chapter will reflect our contention that there is no single avenue to the development of depression, but rather that it may result from a variety of disturbances either individually or in combination. Furthermore, it is hypothesized that a disturbance in any one area (e.g., the child's family) will produce and eventually be supported by disturbances in other systems (e.g., the child's information-processing). Likewise, an improvement that is produced by treatment in a given domain may create ripples of change in other areas, but the other disturbances, if left unaddressed, may cause a relapse.

The discussion begins with a description of the empirical evaluations of interventions for depressed children and is followed by a description of an intervention program for children that is designed to improve children's self-esteem but has not been empirically evaluated. Given the very central role of the child's negative sense of self in depressive disorders, we believe that it is of critical importance to specifically target an improvement in self-esteem during treatment. The adequacy of these empirically based treatments and the nonempirical treatment model will be evaluated within the context of what we know from existing research about the disturbances associated with depression during childhood. Finally, a comprehensive treatment program that has grown out of our own treatment-outcome research—research into the disturbances associated with depressive disorders during childhood—and our clinical experiences will be described.

Empirically Based Treatment-Outcome Studies

Several investigators have studied the effects of cognitive–behavioral interventions on depression in children and adolescents (e.g., Kahn, Kehle, Jenson, & Clark, 1990; Reynolds & Coats, 1986; Stark, Reynolds, & Kaslow, 1987). Overall, the results of these studies have indicated that a variety of cognitive–behavioral interventions have been successful in the reduction of depressive symptoms in children from public schools. In this section of the chapter, we will review the existing treatment-outcome research and enumerate the disturbances that are addressed by each intervention. A given treatment was considered to address a certain disturbance if a technique or therapy activity was specifically designed to change that specific variable. For example, if the treatment targeted the increase of social skills, then it was considered to address social-skills deficits. This same treatment was not considered to address a maladaptive schema for social situations. It should be noted that the following analysis is limited by the brevity with which the interventions were described in the articles.

Single-Subject Studies. Petti, Bornstein, Delamater, and Conners (1980) evaluated the effects of a multimodal treatment for a 10-year-old girl who exhibited chronic dysphoria, a high level of anxiety, aggression, poor social skills such as low frequency of eye contact, bossiness, and tense body posture, and somatic complaints including headaches and other physical concerns. Treatment included a successive and additive progression of interventions that included individual therapy, individual help in school, a dramatics group, family therapy, imipramine, and social-skills training. Therapy was conducted during psychiatric hospitalization and was characterized by a milieu approach. Social-skills training consisted of 9 15-minute sessions over a 3-week period and included a male and a female prompter. Assessment took place during a dramatics group meeting. Individual assistance in academics was provided daily. The formats of the individual therapy, group dramatics, and family therapy were not reported. Results indicated minimal change prior to the imipramine regimen. A significant decrease in depressive symptoms was noted after the addition of medication and social-skills training.

The treatment involved some techniques that focused mainly on the aforementioned behavioral social skills associated with depression. More specifically, social- and academic-skills deficits, and the inability to obtain reinforcement, were targeted. Social-skills deficits were addressed through social-skills training, which included modeling, behavioral rehearsal, and corrective feedback. Tutoring and teaching adaptive school behaviors were provided in an attempt to remediate the academic-skills deficits. Inability to obtain reinforcement was addressed by increasing positive social opportunities and a positive family atmosphere through dramatics and family therapy. The family behavioral variable of low rates of positive reinforcement in the family was addressed in family therapy by teaching the mother to attend to positive behaviors.

Frame, Matson, Sonis, Fialkov, and Kazdin (1982) treated a 10-year-old boy with a DSM-III diagnosis of major depression with social-skills training designed to remediate inappropriate body position, poor eye contact, poor speech quality, and bland affect. Treatment consisted of instructions, modeling, role-play, feedback, and verbal praise for each specific behavior. The subject participated in individual training sessions with a single therapist. Each session was 20 minutes long, and treatment was implemented each weekday for 20 days. Session events began with didactic instruction followed by modeling. A sequence of role-play and correction activities was then implemented until skill mastery was achieved. Verbal praise was given for appropriate responses in role-play, and an edible reward was offered for cooperative behavior at the end of the session. Results of a multiple-baseline design across behaviors showed a decrease in each target behavior measured during simulated role-play. Therapeutic gains were maintained at a 12-week follow-up. The child behavioral variable of social-skills deficit was directly addressed and was the main focus of the treatment.

Frame, Johnstone, and Giblin (1988) describe the assessment and treatment of a 9-year-old girl with a diagnosis of dysthymia. Treatment consisted of social-skills training, a reinforcement program, parent training, and pleasant-events scheduling. Therapy was apparently delivered over a 10-week period in an individual format. The specific number of sessions, length of each session, and session format were not reported. Also, the details of the implementation of the school-based reinforcement program were not reported. Treatment was apparently extended into real-life situations through homework assignments for the subject and her mother. Results indicated an improvement in mood ratings, measures of depression, frequency of contact with peers, and academic performance. Maintenance of treatment effects was found at 6-month and 1-year intervals.

The treatment directly addressed child behavioral and family behavioral variables and, to a lesser degree, child affective variables. Social-skills deficits and excess of maladaptive behavior were treated through modeling, rehearsal, and role-play. The youngster's inability to obtain reinforcement was addressed through pleasant-events scheduling, a positive-reinforcement program at school, and increasing social contacts. Academic-skills deficits were addressed through a positive-reinforcement program for increasing grades. The family behavioral variable of obtaining low rates of reinforcement from family interaction was addressed by having the mother increase verbal praise of the child for being in a good mood and for making new friends and participating in group activities. The variable of low rates of family social and recreational behavior was addressed through pleasant-activity scheduling.

Group Studies. Butler, Miezitis, Friedman, and Cole (1980) compared the relative efficacy of cognitive restructuring, a role-play, attention placebo, and a no-treatment control condition for the treatment of 5th and 6th graders who self-reported depressive symptoms. The cognitive-restructuring intervention was related to teaching a rational approach to processing information. The role-play intervention consisted of role-playing adaptive responses to personal or social problems of relevance to the individuals. Treatment for both interventions was delivered in groups over 10 1-hour weekly sessions. The format for the role-play group began with a warm-up exercise followed by review, and a series of role-plays and discussions. Each session ended with a summary discussion and homework assignment. Session events for the cognitive-restructuring group began with an introduction, moved to cognitive-restructuring exercises and discussion, and concluded with a homework assignment. Results indicated that students in the role-playing and cognitive-restructuring conditions improved in their ratings of depression and related constructs as compared to the control or attention placebo conditions. Children receiving the role-playing intervention improved the most and significantly more across measures than those receiving the cognitive-restructuring intervention. No follow-up assessment was completed.

The role-play intervention was designed to address social-skills deficits through role-playing, enactment, and homework assignments. Children were taught how to deal with personal problems such as loneliness and rejection by peers. In addition, children were taught interpersonal problem-solving.

The cognitive-restructuring intervention consisted of teaching subjects the relationship between thoughts and feelings, how to recognize self-depreciating automatic thoughts, and how to generate alternative thoughts. Social-skills deficits were targeted through teaching listening skills and assigning practice of new skills through homework assignments.

Stark et al. (1987) studied the effects of a self-control intervention, a behavioral problem-solving intervention, and a wait-list control condition on 29 4th-, 5th-, and 6th-grade children who were moderately depressed. The self-control intervention consisted of self-evaluation, self-monitoring, self-reinforcement, and attribution retraining. The behavioral problem-solving intervention consisted of training in self-monitoring, pleasant-event scheduling, and problem-solving. Subjects in each experimental condition participated in 12 sessions of 45–50 minutes each over a 5-week period. Treatment sessions were conducted in a group format with a single therapist. The order of session events for a typical meeting was not reported, although a highly structured treatment manual was used for both conditions. The effects of treatment were extended outside the therapy session through homework assignments. At posttesting, subjects in the treatment groups reported significant improvements in depressive and anxious symptoms and related constructs as compared to the control group. The improvements were maintained or extended during a 5-week follow-up period. Subjects in the self-control group also reported higher self-esteem.

The self-control intervention mainly addressed disturbances in information-processing, including disturbances in self-monitoring, negative self-evaluations, an insidious attributional style, and problem-solving deficits. Negative self-evaluations were altered through the development of positive self-evaluative statements. Reattribution training was used to change the youngsters' insidious negative attributional style. The inability to obtain reinforcement was addressed by teaching self-reinforcement techniques, increasing engagement in pleasant activities, and promoting the use of positive self-statements.

The behavioral problem-solving intervention addressed a number of child cognitive, behavioral, and affective variables. The child cognitive variable of problem-solving deficits was addressed. Distorted information-processing was addressed by teaching accurate self-monitoring of engagement in pleasant activities and monitoring of mood. Problem-solving deficits were addressed by teaching interpersonal problem-solving skills via modeling and story exercises that included the generation of alternative pleasant activities. The child behavioral variable of the inability to obtain reinforcement was specifically addressed by promoting involvement in pleasant activities.

Kahn et al. (1990) investigated the effects of a cognitive–behavioral intervention, a relaxation intervention, a self-modeling intervention, and a wait-list control condition on 68 moderately depressed middle school students. The cognitive–behavioral intervention focused on the acquisition of self-control, problem-solving, and social skills. The relaxation treatment was aimed at teaching progressive muscle relaxation. The goal of the self-modeling treatment was to teach behaviors that were incompatible with depression.

Subjects in the cognitive–behavioral and relaxation conditions participated in 12 50-minute therapy sessions over 6–8 weeks. Treatment was implemented in a group format with a single therapist. Subjects in the self-modeling group were seen individually for 12 10- to 12-minute sessions over 6–8 weeks. The presentation formats of the treatment procedures for each group were not reported. Homework was assigned in the cognitive–behavioral and relaxation groups. Results indicated that the treatments were effective at decreasing depression as well as increasing self-esteem at posttest and at a 1-month follow-up assessment. Additionally, the cognitive–behavioral and relaxation groups showed the most improvement across subjects and time.

The cognitive–behavioral intervention addressed distorted information-processing and problem-solving deficits. Distorted information-processing was addressed by teaching the relationship between depression and negative thoughts, self-monitoring of mood and activities, realistic goal-setting, the relationship between mood and thinking, and generating alternative thinking. Problem-solving deficits were addressed by teaching problem-solving skills through examples, role-play, and rehearsal. Social-skills deficits and inability to obtain reinforcement were also targeted in the cognitive–behavioral intervention. Social-skills deficits were addressed by teaching basic social skills, negotiation, and communication skills. Inability to obtain reinforcement was addressed through pleasant-events scheduling and self-reinforcement.

The relaxation intervention addressed child behavioral variables including replacing tension with relaxation via practice of behaviors associated with relaxation. The child affective variable of worry was addressed by teaching relaxation and the relation between stress and depression.

The self-modeling intervention primarily addressed social-skills deficits, which was accomplished by prompting the subjects in the use of adaptive social skills while making a videotape of how to behave in different social situations and then having them observe the videotape. Specific skills taught included eye contact, posture, expression of positive affect, and verbalizations of positive self-attributions.

Analysis. Analysis of the treatment protocols reveals that child cognitive and behavioral variables have been the primary focus of treatment in past investigations. Considering the wide range of variables associated with childhood depression, the current treatments may fail to address the total clinical picture of some youngsters. Future treatment efforts should strive to be more comprehensive and include techniques to address child affective, parent, and family variables.

The studies related to the treatment of childhood depression uncover several issues as to the possible need for a comprehensive treatment protocol. First, the intent of some of the studies was to test the efficacy of short-term interventions only (e.g., Kahan et al., 1990; Stark et al., 1987). The recent emphasis on short-term therapies may exclude important knowledge to be gained from the implementation of comprehensive and thus possibly longer treatments.

Second, many studies included subjects from student populations. Children and adolescents from clinical populations may experience a wider range and more intense impact of the variables involved in the etiology and maintenance of depressive symptoms. Thus, children from clinical populations may benefit from a more comprehensive treatment. It is interesting to note that Frame et al. (1988), whose treatment covered child behavioral and affective variables and family behavioral variables, successfully conducted treatment in a clinical setting with a subject who was formally diagnosed with dysthymia.

Third, most of the investigations reviewed reported follow-up data for only a few weeks after treatment. The long-term impact of short-term treatments addressing mainly child cognitive and child behavioral variables is unknown. Again, it is interesting to note that Frame et al. (1988), whose treatment covered the most variables associated with childhood depression, reported the maintenance of treatment gains at 1 year follow-up.

Another issue related to the development and investigation of a comprehensive treatment plan is brought to the fore by the fact that many of the treatment studies reviewed included subjects from a school population who were treated in a school setting. Also, therapy was aimed at the level of the individual child. Certainly, a child's primary socialization groups in addition to school peers and adults are the parents and family. Impacting these additional variables would provide an ecological approach in therapy, possibly influencing the total clinical picture.

It is interesting to note that the treatments reviewed generally did not directly address child affective variables. Several studies, however, did teach the subjects about the relationship between feelings/mood and thinking and behavior. Additionally, several treatments focusing on increasing pleasant events also impacted anhedonia. The only studies that directly addressed affective variables were those that included a relaxation treatment targeting the child affective variable of worry. Thus, a need exists for future treatment protocols to specifically target affective variables.

Finally, a comprehensive treatment may need to be connected with a more comprehensive assessment procedure. Indeed, some of the studies reviewed did not adequately measure the impact of the treatment on variables the protocol did address. This was especially true for variables that were indirectly targeted. For example, treatments that addressed increasing the understanding of social skills did not measure the subject's change in understanding and knowledge of social skills, let alone the change in the specific schema. Frame et al. (1982), in their social-skills training program, measured the decrease in inappropriate behaviors, but did not include a measure of increases in prosocial behaviors. The measurement of these variables would be important in the development of a prescriptive treatment chosen from a comprehensive treatment protocol.

Non-Empirically Based Treatment-Outcome Studies

A program for children with low self-esteem (Pope, McHale, & Craighead, 1988) will be described and discussed because of the close relationship between self-esteem and depression. We believe that this program includes a number of treatment procedures that may prove useful in the treatment of depressed youths. For example, the authors provide strategies for improving social skills as a means of improving the youngster's social relationships and thus the feedback he or she receives from peers about himself or herself. This positive feedback would help create a more positive sense of self.

The self-esteem program looks at a child's level of self-esteem in five areas: social, academic, family, body image, and global self-esteem. It is assumed by the authors that low self-esteem results from a large discrepancy between the perceived self and the ideal self. Interventions can occur at both ends of this discrepancy. One way to intervene is to help change the child's perceived self. If the child's view is negatively biased, then these cognitive distortions might be targeted. In some cases, the child would be taught skills that would lessen the gap between actual and expected performance. The other way to enhance self-esteem is to examine and modify the child's standards. Perhaps the child's standards are too high or unrealistic. The treatment methods described in the self-esteem program are predominantly associated with the cognitive–behavioral perspective and resemble those often found in the literature on the treatment of depression. For example, the program includes training in social problem-solving, standard-setting, self-control, and attribution and social-skills training in its attempt to enhance a child's self-esteem.

The self-esteem program recognizes the important role that parents play in their children's self-esteem. The authors hypothesize that low rates of positive reinforcement likely contribute to low self-esteem, which is a phenomenon that also has been hypothesized to lead to the development of depression (Lewinsohn, 1974). It would be helpful for the program to include a guideline for parents to use in providing reinforcement to their children for their behavior. In addition, parents who have unrealistic and perfectionistic standards for their children's behavior can cause problems by modeling such maladaptive ways of thinking. The authors explain that children learn to use self-statements from the way their parents talk to themselves. The authors recommend that parents be encouraged to help their children set reasonable standards for themselves. Also, children are taught to reinforce themselves for using positive self-statements. They are also instructed to use negative self-statements and attributions as signals to examine and modify their standards.

The self-esteem program begins by teaching children a systematic approach to identifying and solving difficult social problems. Then, cognitive disturbances such as negative self-evaluations and an insidious attributional style are assessed and treated. Also, at the cognitive level, the program is designed to remediate interpersonal problem-solving deficits. Behavioral disturbances targeted include a social-skills knowledge deficit and an excess of maladaptive social behavior. It seeks to help children increase their ability to obtain reinforcement, which is theorized to be partly dependent on adequate social skills. Noticeably lacking from the program is an acknowledgment of how family factors may impact social skills.

The treatment protocol is divided into separate components, and the authors suggest that treatment be administered in the prescribed order. The apparent reasoning for this suggestion is that each section builds on the information and skills developed in previous sessions. Nevertheless, it seems that the treatment modules are distinct enough so that interventions could be individualized to meet the specific needs of each child. Thus, if a youngster does not need remediation in a certain area, the related modules could be skipped. Perhaps the authors do not recommend taking such an approach because of our limited ability to assess disturbances as specifically as necessary to do so. The program recognizes the problem of generalizability and tries to promote generalization through the use of homework, particularly in the areas of social problem-solving and social-skills training.

One of the strengths of this program is that the child's developmental level is given consideration. The specific implications of developmental characteristics for various treatment procedures, including self-control, standard-setting, and social skills, are explained. For example, children experience changes in standard-setting in terms of who establishes the standard and how the child interprets his or her behavior against the standard. The authors note that early in a child's life, parents and teachers set the standards for children and that praise may be enough to make the child feel good about his or her behavior. As the child develops, peers have greater influence in determining standards and acceptability of performance. A developmental consideration across all interventions is that children tend to be more concrete in their thinking and therefore may need more concrete examples and homework assignments. The authors state the importance of examining the child's developmental level in each of four domains taken from the social learning model: behavior, cognition, emotion, and biology. A goal of the program is to even out the level of development across the domains. Each of the interventions in this program emphasizes one or more of these domains. For example, the authors state that problem-solving includes work in the affective, cognitive, and behavioral domains.

Proposed Procedures for the Treatment of Depressed Children

In the following sections of this chapter, we describe procedures for remediating the disturbances associated with depression during childhood. As noted at the beginning of the chapter, these procedures have developed as we completed treatment-outcome research and more recently through our clinical work. The treatment procedures are described separately as they apply to an area of disturbed functioning. However, the procedures are combined in a systematic and logical fashion so that they build on each other and lead to the remediation of all the disturbances.

The procedures that will be described have been adapted from major adult models for the treatment of depressed adults. The self-control procedures have been adapted from those developed by Rehm (e.g., Rehm, Kaslow, & Rabin, 1987) for the treatment of depressed adults. The behavioral procedures have been adapted from a variety of sources, most notably Beck, Rush, Shaw, and Emery (1979) and Lewinsohn (e.g., Lewinsohn & Graf, 1973), and the cognitive procedures have been adapted from Beck (e.g., Beck et al., 1979). However, they have been specifically altered for children, and the media used to implement these procedures have been changed so that they are engaging for children. Furthermore, in recognition of the need for a multidimensional model of depression, the procedures have been combined into a unique treatment model, and we combine interventions for the child with parent training, family therapy, and teacher consultation.

The intervention program usually begins with affective education. This component provides the child and therapist with a common language and understanding of depression. It also serves as the primary vehicle for helping the youngster tune in to those of his or her emotions, behaviors, and situations that provoke negative thoughts and emotions. Subsequently, the mood-enhancement procedures of activity scheduling and mastery experiences are employed to provide the youngster with some means of controlling his or her emotions and consequently to distance the youngster somewhat from his or her depressogenic thinking. At this point, the therapist employs a number of self-control and behavioral procedures to learn more about the child and to help the child acquire additional skills for controlling his or her depressive symptoms.

The overall goal of treatment is change at the level of core schemata. The cognitive restructuring procedures, and to some extent all the procedures described in this chapter, are used to produce this change. A variety of cognitive procedures are used throughout treatment as opportunities arise, and a number of sessions should be devoted to teaching the youngster how to independently use the procedures. Included among the procedures used with depressed youths are cognitive restructuring, cognitive modeling, behavioral assignments, problem-solving, and self-instructional training.

A number of rules are followed when using the cognitive procedures. The therapist begins by using the techniques in a tentative, probing fashion as he or she tests to see whether the child is ready for cognitive change. In the beginning of treatment, the therapist is primarily responsible for identifying and restructuring the child's thinking. As treatment progresses, the child is taught to identify his or her own maladaptive thoughts and schemas and to restructure them. Third, the therapist and child move from identifying and restructuring automatic thoughts to identifying themes in the child's thoughts that are reflective of depressogenic schemata or core schemata. Finally, the most powerful way to produce cognitive change is through behavioral assignments.

Throughout the work with the child, the therapist is consulting with the youngster's parents and teachers to teach them how they can support the therapeutic efforts. In addition, concurrently, the parents are engaged in parent training. The goals of the training are to teach the parents (1) positive methods for managing their child's behavior, (2) noncoercive methods for disciplining the child, (3) personal anger-management skills, (4) self-esteem enhancement procedures, (5) empathic listening, and (6) recreation. If it is evident that the family is dysfunctional, then family therapy is instituted immediately. After completion of the parent training sessions, the families who need additional assistance are engaged in family therapy. Those who do not need additional help are finished. The following skills are taught to the family members during the meetings: (1) how to communicate more effectively, (2) how to use family problem-solving, (3) how to communicate positive messages and feelings, (4) conflict-resolution skills, and (5) changing interactions that support maladaptive schemata. The description of the treatment program begins with a description of interventions for child disturbances and progresses to interventions for disturbances in parenting skills and dysfunctional families.

Psychological Interventions for the Child

Treatment Process. Our treatment program is conceptually based on a skills-deficit and cognitive-distortion model of depression (Stark et al., 1991). Three important goals of treatment are to teach new skills, influence real-life situations, and achieve practical outcomes. The intervention program is based on two assumptions that provide a foundation for the development of the treatment process for the child, parents, and family: First, it is assumed that a treatment program conceptually based on a skills-deficit and cognitive-distortion model of depression should be couched in principles of learning. Second, it is assumed that children and their parents and families display unique psychotherapy demand characteristics. Therefore, the treatment process reflects an education, skills-acquisition, skills-application framework (Meichenbaum, 1977). The intervention is seen as flexible within the general guidelines of learning principles. The therapeutic relationship between the therapist and child, parents, and family is characterized by collaboration and problem-solving.

We view the group format to be the preferred mode of delivering the treatment. Our past experience suggests that a group setting offers situations that enhance learning, such as decreasing feelings of alienation and isolation, practice with same-age peers with common problems, and ample opportunity for feedback and social reinforcement. The length of each session and of the entire program should be sufficient to cover areas of concern and achieve mastery of skills and short enough to avoid boredom. Concepts, skills, and procedures should be presented in short, simple lessons with small goals to enhance successful memory, understanding, and performance of meaningful materials and activities. Ample feedback and reinforcement should be offered from the therapist or group members, using social praise, descriptions of positive or successful performance, or small rewards. Feedback and reinforcement can also be offered through ongoing monitoring of progress. Treatment should also involve fun activities such as cartoons or video presentations.

The within-session treatment process seems to benefit from being structured in a way that facilitates the achievement of therapy goals. One helpful within-session framework is the instructional model used in the ACCESS social skills training program (Walker, Todis, Holmes, & Horton, 1988). The instructional model is characterized by ordered session activities that reflect guidelines for learning, such as provision of a clear rationale, definition of skills, presentation of examples, gradual presentation of difficult concepts, opportunity for practice until mastery, and correction activities. Sessions begin with a discussion and review of the previous session and the homework assignment. The session ends with a specified homework assignment. Our experience indicates that session events can be modified to accommodate the needs of the children. For example, a review of last session or open discussion may reveal that the children need to acquire a skill that was not planned for that session. In this case, the therapist must quickly identify the new area for instruction, set up examples, and structure role-plays and relevant homework.

The treatment process across sessions should also be flexible and continue with increasing emphasis on homework. At the same time, within-session events such as discussion and role-play should become more related to experiences with homework and other real-life situations. New information and skill-building should continue as needed to deal with the appropriate real-life situations. The treatment process should continue until ongoing therapist, parent, teacher, self-report, and observational evaluations indicate that skill objectives are met and the children report satisfaction with progress. Additionally, assessment should indicate generalization of skills across settings, behaviors, and time and the ability to generate new skills as needed.

We also recognize the need to extend treatment to the natural environment and accomplish this through homework assignments, which, in general, have been shown to be beneficial to therapy outcome (e.g., Fennell & Teasdale, 1987; Persons, Burns, & Perloff, 1988; Zettle & Hayes, 1987). Homework assignments (1) enhance learning by increasing opportunities for practice, (2) provide additional material for within-session discussion, (3) promote generalization, (4) encourage self-regulation, (5) increase the personal meaningfulness of therapy, and (6) bring others into the treatment process (Beck et al., 1979; Kanfer & Phillips, 1969; Shelton, 1979; Shelton & Ackerman, 1974; Shelton & Levy, 1981). Homework should be couched within a collaborative and problem-solving framework, as the exclusive use of therapist-devised homework assignments with children may not be an optimal approach (Rouse, 1994). The process of giving homework assignments may benefit from the approach outlined by the affirmation model (Larrabee, 1988). Therapist behaviors should be characterized by open-ended questions, paraphrasing, reflection of feelings, and summary statements in the generation of homework ideas, planning of homework activities, and discussion of outcome.

Our experience suggests that the homework process should include some structure for reaching goals as outlined by Beck et al. (1979), Martin and Worthington (1982), and Shelton (1979). First, the rationale for the assignment, development of ideas, and specific steps for implementation should be conjointly developed. The format for the actual assignment should include a do statement, a quantity statement, a record statement, a bring statement, and a contingency statement. When developing homework assignments, consideration should be given to the frequency, number of settings, and length of time for practice. Additionally, the time between homework assignments may need to be adjusted so the child can gradually attempt and correct the performance of skills.

Several strategies can be used to counter noncompliance due to cognitive barriers and environmental inducements to noncompliant behaviors (Beck et al., 1979; Larrabee, 1988; Martin & Worthington, 1982; Shelton & Levy, 1981). Homework assignments should at first be small, brief, and nonthreatening and increase in size and difficulty as the client becomes more skillful. Cognitive rehearsal, including a plan to carry out a set of instructions and to cope with barriers or distractions, is useful. To overcome cognitive interferences, one can use a public commitment to comply, which involves having the client enter into a contract or repeat orally what he or she is going to do. The therapist also should reduce the likelihood of embarrassment and danger by scheduling homework carefully and providing support when experiments "backfire." Additionally, Beck et al. (1979) recommend that the therapist help clients distance themselves from the problem by presenting homework as an experiment or as a practice exercise similar to ones used in sports or other activities to acquire new skills.

We have presented some homework assignments as "investigations," having the child assume the role of a detective. To overcome environmental influences, the therapist should incorporate a planned reinforcement in the homework program along with offering verbal and social praise. Other strategies that enhance compliance include cues in the form of providing a notebook to organize and save written material, written instructions, and homework recording sheets. We also believe that significant others should be involved in enhancing compliance. For example, parents can be taught to monitor their child's compliance with homework and to reinforce their child for his or her effort and skill mastery.

Intervening in the Mood Disturbance

General Approach. Depressed youths experience a variety of mood disturbances. The first procedure used in the process of trying to improve a depressed child's mood is affective education. Affective education helps the youngster gain an understanding of the relationship between thoughts, feelings, and behaviors and thereby helps the youngster learn the cognitive–behavioral conceptualization of depression. Furthermore, it is used as a means of helping the youngster develop a sense of trust in the therapist, and if a group format is being used, it facilitates the development of trust in fellow group members and a sense of group cohesion.

We have used a series of games as the medium for teaching children about their emotions. As a result of participating in these games, the youngsters learn: (1) the names of a variety of pleasant and unpleasant emotions, (2) that emotions are experienced along a continuum of intensity, and (3) how to recognize when they are experiencing various emotions as well as signs of what others look like when they are experiencing these emotions. The actual content of the activities is designed to address the child's specific needs. For example, some children may not recognize the spectrum of emotions that they experience or the continuum of severity. These dimensions would then become the primary focus of the activities. In contrast, another child may not be able to recognize how others are feeling. In this case, teaching the child how to recognize the behavioral cues that are associated with various emotions becomes the focus of the activities. A series of activities that are designed to remediate the aforementioned deficits are described below.

A series of games that we refer to as Emotional Vocabulary, Emotional Vocabulary II, Emotion Charades, Emotion Password, Emotion Statues, and Emotion Expression are used as the medium for teaching the children about their emotions. The activities begin by teaching the children the basics about emotions and then progressively build on this knowledge. Progressively more complex skills are taught and finer distinctions between the emotions are made.

During Emotional Vocabulary, a set of cards is constructed with each card bearing the name of an emotion. The number of cards made and the sophistication of the emotions on the cards should vary dependent on the age of the child. With younger and less mature clients, we use fewer cards with more basic emotions on them (e.g., scared, sad, happy). The game is played by placing the deck of cards in the middle of the table. The players take turns drawing cards from the deck. After picking a card, the player states the name of the emotion and then describes how the emotion feels and what was happening the last time he or she felt that emotion. The game can be played a number of times until the child has learned how each of the emotions is experienced.

The therapist starts to teach the child the cognitive–behavioral perspective during Emotional Vocabulary II. More specifically, through this game the child begins to learn about the relationship between thought, behavior, and emotion. The deck of cards is once again used, and the game is played in much the same way as the first one. However, this time, after picking a card and reading it aloud, describing how it feels, and what was going on the last time he or she felt that way, the child also describes what a person who is feeling that emotion might be thinking and how that person might be behaving. The objective is to help the child see that his or her feelings don't arise from nowhere, rather that they are associated with what he or she is thinking.

During Emotional Charades, the link between thoughts, feelings, behaviors, and situations is strengthened, and the child learns how to identify the emotional states of others. Once again, the players take turns drawing cards from the deck, only this time they don't read the name of the emotion out loud; rather, they read it to themselves and think about what a child who is feeling that emotion might look like and how that child might behave. Then, the child acts out the expression of the emotion while the other player or players try to identify it. Once an emotion is correctly identified, the player states what the actor did that clued him or her in to the identity of the emotion, what was happening the last time he himself or she herself felt that way, and what he or she was thinking at that time.

Emotion Password is played following the same rules as the television game show. A second deck of emotion words is constructed. The group of children is divided into two teams. One player on each team reads the card and gives the clues and another player tries to guess the name of the emotion. The teams alternate taking turns, giving clues, and trying to identify the emotion. The point value declines by 1 with each missed guess. If the teams are having a difficult time identifying the word and the point value has declined to zero, then the word is revealed to the players. After a word is correctly identified, the losing team can get 2 bonus points for a member's describing the last time he or she felt that emotion, what it felt like, and what he or she was thinking. Each player gets at least one chance to give the clues and one to guess what the word is. Thus, everyone participates in the game.

Emotion Statues is a game that has to be played with more than two people. During this activity, the players take turns being the statue, the sculptor, and the audience. The child who is the sculptor chooses a card from the deck and informs the statue but doesn't let the audience know what it is. Then, the sculptor works with the statue to arrange his or her facial expression and posture so that the statue looks like a person who is experiencing that emotion. Once the emotion is correctly identified, the player states the cues that he or she used to identify the emotion and what a person experiencing that emotion might be thinking, how that person might be behaving, and what was happening the last time he himself or she herself felt the particular emotion.

Emotion Expression is the final activity. This time, after drawing a card from the deck without divulging the name of the emotion, the actor expresses the emotion vocally but wordlessly. He or she tries to express the emotion through his or her voice. Using no words, the child tries to express the emotion through the sounds that he or she makes. The player who correctly identifies the emotion states what clues he or she used to identify the emotion and describes the last time he or she felt that way, the thoughts he or she had, and what was happening.

It is important to note that the games really serve as a springboard to much useful therapeutic discussion. The therapist has to be alert for opportunities to probe in more depth and for opportunities to connect thoughts and feelings. In addition, it is important to help the youngsters recognize that they experience many emotions over the course of the day and that each emotion is experienced along a continuum of intensity. This continuum can be further elucidated through questions and examples.

Altering Dysphoric Mood through Activity Scheduling. Activity scheduling is the purposeful incorporation of enjoyable and goal-directed activities in the child's day. Engaging in such activities is a powerful coping skill that can be used to moderate depressive affect. It helps the youngster obtain reinforcement and combat the withdrawal, passivity, and sedentary life-style associated with an episode of depression. Pleasant activities seem to lift mood through providing the child with the pleasure (reinforcement) of completing the activity and through distraction from his or her preoccupation with negative thinking. Finally, it may lead to some cognitive restructuring as the child rediscovers that life can be enjoyable and worth living. All these impacts result in an improvement in mood.

Training children to use this coping procedure is relatively easy. The training procedure begins by helping the child recognize the relationship between engagement in pleasant activities and improvement in mood. Most children can readily understand that they feel good when they do fun things. The next step involves identifying mood-enhancing activities. This enhancement can be accomplished through interviewing the chid and parents to determine what activities the child seems to enjoy. In addition, the child can be asked to keep track of activities that he or she enjoyed doing over the next few days or over the week. Once mood-enhancing activities have been identified, the child is instructed to engage in them regularly, especially when he or she is starting to experience a change in mood. For the less compliant or skillful youngster, the therapist may want to add more structure. This can be accomplished by literally scheduling daily pleasant activities on a weekly calendar sheet, taking into account the child's other necessary activities.

We have found that parental support for this schedule is a necessity. First, parental permission needs to be obtained for participation in the activities. Second, parental support through participation, provision of transportation, financial outlay, and supervision may be required. Finally, parents can help by reminding their child to follow the schedule. In addition, they can provide the child with gentle encouragement to get up and follow the schedule. In addition, when a parent notices that the child's mood is becoming worse, he or she can remind the child to cope by doing something pleasant. The final step prior to sending a child off to implement an activity schedule is for the child and therapist to try to identify any impediments to carrying out the plan. As impediments are identified, problem-solving is used to develop plans for overcoming the impediments. It is also important for the child to realize that unforeseen occurrences will sometimes make it difficult for the plan to be carried out as initially conceived. When something comes up, the child is instructed to try to "go with the flow" and alter his or her plans to include as many of the scheduled pleasant events as possible. Finally, the child is instructed to self-monitor completion of the activities.

Another class of activities that is important to work into the scheduling is mastery activities. These are activities that usually have some sort of instrumental value. By completing these tasks, the child gains a sense of accomplishment or mastery. For children, this usually means successfully completing some school assignments, projects, a hobby kit, or household chores. When scheduling mastery activities with depressed children, it is important to recognize that they commonly feel overwhelmed by the thought of trying to complete the task. To combat this, the therapist works with the child to break the task down into manageable components. Subsequently, completion of the components is scheduled on a weekly calendar so that they can be manageably and successfully completed. After scheduling, the therapist and child try to identify any potential impediments to completing the task. Problem-solving is used to develop plans for overcoming the impediments. Once again, parental support is crucial to ensuring that the schedule is followed. Parents can remind the child to stay on schedule, and they can be instructed to help their child complete the component tasks. Following completion of each component task, the parents are asked to reinforce the child's efforts to help the child recognize his or her success by reminding the child of what he or she has accomplished.

In order to increase the likelihood of compliance with the schedule, a number of additional steps can be taken. The child may be asked to sign a contract agreeing to try to carry out the plan. Another procedure that can be used is cognitive rehearsal. When this procedure is used, the child is led through an imagery exercise in which he or she completes the activity plan. While imaging the plan, the child is asked to try to experience the pleasant feelings that are associated with successful accomplishment of the activities.

Interventions for Excessive Anxiety. Deep muscle relaxation is taught to the children as a coping skill that they can use to cope with anxious affect and the related symptoms that commonly co-occur with depression. The state of relaxation that is achieved through a deep muscle relaxation exercise is a positive and peaceful feeling that provides depressed youths with a respite from their anxious and dysphoric moods. Following the suggestions of Ollendick and Cerney (1981), we have modified the relaxation procedure for children. It often takes a number of sessions to teach a child to relax, since each training session is shorter than that for adults to match the children's shorter attention span. In addition, before the actual training begins, children have to be taught the names and locations of various muscles, e.g., "biceps." They also find the procedure somewhat more discomforting than adults, as the procedure seems to be "weird" or "mysterious," "like you're trying to hypnotize me." Consequently, more time is spent preparing the youngster for the actual procedure by explaining what the therapist is going to do and say and how the child is expected to react and behave. In addition, we have found that it is useful to explain the whole procedure to the child's parents beforehand so that they don't end up with a misunderstanding about what the therapist is doing as a result of hearing the child's description of the procedure.

During the training, the child is informed that relaxation is a skill that he or she will learn and that, like any other skill, takes practice to master and be able to use effectively. When reading the relaxation script, we alter the standard protocol to include more visual cues, e.g., "Make your right leg tight like a stretched out rubber band" and then "Now let your leg muscle go completely loose and wiggly like Jello." It is also important to pay very close attention to the child's adherence to the instructions. If the child appears to be having trouble following some of the directives, or is doing the exercise incorrectly, then the therapist has to calmly deviate from the script and help the youngster get on track. In addition, the therapist can watch the child's physical responses and utilize them within the exercise, e.g., "Your arm may begin to twitch as you become more and more relaxed and let go of all your worries and tension." After the child has successfully made it through all the muscle groups, an audiotape of the complete relaxation exercise is made for the child, and the youngster is instructed to listen to it, preferably through headphones, on a daily basis. The child and therapist, sometimes in collaboration with the child's parents, try to set a time when the child can listen to the tape without being disturbed and a place where he or she can get comfortable and won't be disturbed. After each time the child completes the exercise, he or she is instructed to complete a relaxation exercise rating form. This form is used to structure the homework exercise, which seems to enhance compliance, and to help demonstrate to the child that he or she is able to attain a deeper level of relaxation as a result of practicing.

Once the child has clearly mastered the relaxation exercise and can achieve a deep, restful state of relaxation independently by listening to the tape, an abbreviated version of the tape is introduced and the child is taught to use relaxation whenever he or she is just beginning to feel anxious or worried. Typically, this is accomplished by going to a quiet and comfortable spot to listen to the tape. The key to successfully employing relaxation as a coping skill seems to be identifying the first signs of worry or anxiety and using the relaxation before the feeling becomes overwhelming. As a result of the affective education training, the child has learned to identify the early signs of anxiety and the situations in which it usually occurs. These signs and situations serve as cues that it is time to get out the relaxation tape and find a quiet spot to listen to it. The ultimate goal is to teach the child to recognize which of his or her muscles are tense and then to use his or her own internal representation of the section of the tape related to those muscles to relax away the tension. Once again, a parent who is tuned in to the child can be extremely helpful to the coping process by cuing the child that it appears to be a good time to listen to the tape. In addition, the parents can provide the child with activity rewards for demonstrating the effective use of relaxation to cope with stressful situations or anxious feelings.

Some children have difficulty completing homework assignments because of anxiety surrounding the assignment. Relaxation can be combined with positive coping imagery to help the youngsters desensitize themselves to the fear. Once a child can achieve a state of deep relaxation, the therapist combines it with positive coping imagery that is related to the assignment the child is reporting anxiety about trying to complete. For example, the child may be working on being more assertive with his or her parents. First, the child is lead through a relaxation exercise. When the child is relaxed, the therapist guides him or her through an imagery activity in which the child successfully asserts himself or herself. The child is instructed to then focus on the good feeling that accompanies successful completion of the imaginal activity. Parents would be primed for a successful interaction through the therapist explaining to them that their child is learning how to respectfully communicate his or her feelings.

Reducing Excessive Anger. Teaching children to cope with anger begins with helping them recognize the sensations that define anger. Once again, the affective education exercises help the youngsters do so. It is especially important to help the child recognize the initial physical and cognitive cues that he or she is becoming angry. It seems to be critical to identify these early signs, or else the child becomes overwhelmed with anger too quickly to be able to prevent it. In fact, this sudden access of anger seems to be the biggest impediment to successful treatment, as the children seem to become angry in a flash. They also believe that they have no control over their anger. Some children seem to require treatment with an antidepressant in order to be able to slow down the reaction enough to be able to use some of the strategies for coping with it.

Relaxation training is one of the procedures that can be used to help children cope with their anger. A procedure similar to that described above for teaching the youngster to cope with anxiety is used. The child is taught to leave a situation as soon as he or she is beginning to feel angry and to then listen to the relaxation tape and calm down. Once the child is very skilled, he or she is taught to direct his or her attention to the muscle tension and focus on relaxing it away. However, we have found that it is necessary to augment this technique with some self-instructional training and cognitive restructuring, which is described in more detail below in the section entitled "Intervening at the Cognitive Level." The cognitive interventions are used to change the youngster's more inflammatory thinking. In addition, problem-solving is taught to the child as a coping strategy. Anger is considered to be a cue that a problem needs to be solved. The child has to either take action to change the anger-provoking situation or develop and implement plans for coping with anger. Some of the effective coping strategies are to (1) leave the situation; (2) go and do something enjoyable; (3) use words rather than actions to express anger; (4) do something physically demanding, like riding an exercise bike or playing basketball; and (5) express anger through drawing or writing.

It is very difficult for a child to follow through and enact one of these coping strategies. Once again, parental support is crucial. Parents can encourage the child to use a coping strategy by establishing an incentive program for successfully coping with anger. In some instances, it is also possible to make arrangements for a parent to help cue the child that he or she is becoming angry. This is a tricky endeavor, since telling an angry person that he or she is angry can often escalate the problem. Consequently, a great deal of preplanning and rehearsal are usually necessary. A neutral cueing system typically involving some agreed-on noninflammatory phrase can be used to help the youngster without exacerbating the problem.

It is important to note that many of the other procedures, while they do not directly target the child's mood disturbance, are designed to alter and improve mood. For example, the cognitive-restructuring procedures are designed to change the child's thinking that is related to the mood disturbance. The belief is that changing the child's thinking can lead to a change in mood. More specifically, helping the child have a more realistic and less extreme style of thinking will lead to more reasonable emotional reactions.

Intervening in Maladaptive Behavior
Social Skills Disturbances. The source of the social-skills disturbance is often-times unclear and multifaceted. Is the youngster in fact being socially rejected or neglected, or is the child's perception of rejection or neglect the result of distorted thinking? Does the youngster misperceive the behaviors and intentions of others and consequently behave in a way that would naturally lead to rejection or avoidance? Does the child simply not know what is socially desirable behavior? Are parents or other family members modeling and encouraging inappropriate social behaviors? Commonly, the youngster's social problems result from some combination of these variables.

Prior to developing the intervention, it is important to conduct a complete assessment that includes child, teacher, and parent reports as well as an observation. It has been our experience that parents and teachers do not have the training to make the fine observations that contribute to the treatment plan, nor are they aware of the specific beliefs the child has about social situations that are of therapeutic relevance. There seems to be no substitute for observing the child in the actual social situations of interest. Observation allows the therapist to observe the reciprocal relationships between the target child's behavior and that of his or her peers. This observation can be supplemented by interviewing the child's teachers and parents about the child's social behavior. With some children, more of an ongoing assessment is necessary, which requires the assistance of the youngster's teachers. In this case, the teachers are taught to recognize the occurrence or nonoccurrence of specific social behaviors, and the therapist remains in regular phone contact with the teachers as a means of assessment.

The social-skills training usually involves more than simply teaching the child specific skills. In addition to skills training, cognitive-restructuring procedures are used to help the child perceive social situations in a more realistic and less threatening fashion. Anxiety-reduction procedures may be used to help the child feel comfortable entering and staying in social situations as well as to gain the courage to try new interpersonal behaviors.

The content and teaching techniques that we use with depressed children to teach them social skills when a deficit exists are similar to traditional social-skills training procedures. We have taught basic assertiveness, including microskills such as eye contact and facial expression, and advanced assertiveness skills, such as giving compliments, asking others to stop annoying behavior, conversational skills, and conflict resolution. The traditional procedures of education, modeling, role-playing, coaching, feedback, and homework assignments are used to teach the skills. The specific skills taught should be tailored to meet the specific needs of each child.

Assertiveness, one aspect of social skill, can be trained through using several techniques. We begin the training by using a series of cartoons that illustrate the differences between passive, assertive, and aggressive people. During the presentation of the cartoons, the behavioral characteristics of the cartoon characters are noted along with the reactions of others and the results of their behaviors. The therapist and the child then take turns role-playing the different behaviors. The session then turns to having the child provide an example of a fun activity he or she would like to engage in with someone and a role-play of assertively asking the person to engage in the activity. The therapist and the child then take turns in each role. During this time, if the child indicates undue anxiety about making the request, the therapist and child develop coping statements that can be used to decrease any apprehension. Self-instructional training can be used to teach the child to use verbal mediators to successfully accomplish the role-play as well as interactions outside the office. Similar procedures are used to teach other assertive behaviors, such as giving compliments and asking others to stop annoying behaviors.

These behavioral activities naturally lead to the identification of distorted thinking as the child verbalizes his or her perceptions and concerns. These distortions are also evident in the child's descriptions of what took place in other social situations, including homework assignments. When this happens, cognitive restructuring is used. During the role-playing activities, the therapist can query the youngster for his or her automatic thoughts. The youngster's responses can be used to identify the self-statements, schemata, and possible core schemata that are active during social interactions.

An effective medium for assessing and teaching social skills is games. Most of our social rules (e.g., taking turns, following rules) are incorporated into successful game-playing, and most games (excluding video games) represent a structured interpersonal interaction. Thus, a youngster's behavioral deficits and excesses as well as his or her skills are readily apparent during game play. This medium is also engaging. While playing the games, the therapist very systematically points out interpersonal-skills deficits and then educates, models, coaches, and provides the child with feedback about his or her attempt to acquire new skills. In addition, observing the child playing games allows the therapist to access "hot cognitions." When it is evident that the child's mood has changed or that the child has entered a critical situation, the therapist can instruct the child to think out loud. At this point, if maladaptive thoughts are identified, they can be restructured or more adaptive self-instructions can be taught to the child.

Inability to Obtain Reinforcement. A variety of procedures can be used to help a depressed child increase the amount of reinforcement he or she obtains. This goal can be accomplished through the activity-scheduling procedure noted above and through social-skills training. However, in the instances in which the child is being restricted from obtaining reinforcement by parental mandate, it is necessary to work with the child's parents to identify what is causing the restriction. For some parents, it is fear; for others, it is due to practical limitations such as the need for the child to care for siblings. In either case, problem-solving is completed with the family. The problem is defined as the child's or children's being unable to engage in a healthy level of pleasant activities. The factors that are preventing the child from being able to do so are delineated and possible solutions are then brainstormed. Subsequently, the solutions are evaluated for their potential outcome.

We believe that it is important to recognize the parents' legitimate concern for their child's or children's safety and encourage them to give higher ratings to solutions that they can be comfortable with. The parents are not encouraged or coerced into letting their children engage in any activity that they do not believe to be safe. This premise is stated explicitly. In addition, the parents are instructed to tell the therapist when they feel as though they are being ganged up on or coerced into making a decision they don't agree with. Activities that clearly invite a greater probability of danger are noted as being such by the therapist and are discouraged. In the case of the youngster who is restricted because of babysitting duties, the objective of the problem-solving process is to make babysitting less boring and to derive more potent activities for nonbabysitting times.

Teaching children self-reinforcement can help fill a void of external reinforcers. Self-reinforcement is the process of presenting rewards to oneself contingent on successful performance of a desired behavior. It has the same impact on behavior that externally administered rewards have: It increases the probability that the behavior will occur in the future.

Depressed youths not only come from environments that are devoid of external rewards, but also have a very difficult time reinforcing themselves. This difficulty may stem from their generally low level of self-esteem or their tendency to evaluate themselves negatively. When teaching a child self-reinforcement, it is commonly necessary to concurrently use other procedures such as cognitive restructuring and self-evaluation training.

The first step in the training is to identify reinforcers. Doing so can be an especially difficult task to accomplish with anhedonic and severely depressed youngsters. With such children, the therapist tries to identify things that were rewarding prior to the current episode of depression. During this assessment, which can be completed through a self-report questionnaire (Stark, 1990) or through an interview, the therapist tries to identify activities, favorite snacks and beverages, people, objects, and thoughts that are rewarding for the child. While identifying these rewards, it is important for the therapist to determine whether the identified rewards are readily available in the child's environment and whether they can be self-administered, since the emphasis is on self-administration. As rewards are identified, they are compiled into a list that is then used like a menu. Having the rewards written down helps the youngsters remember them and use them.

Since children do not have independent access to, or control over, the delivery and choice of many rewards, it is necessary to involve the parents in the identification and self-administration process. The parents are also interviewed to identify rewards for the child, and any additional rewards are added to the child's menu. Securing parental support is a prerequisite to the success of the procedure. A commitment should be secured from the parents to try to provide their child with access to rewards.

After identifying possible rewards and securing parental support, the training process begins by educating the child about reinforcement and punishment. Concrete examples (e.g., teaching a pet to do tricks) are used to help the youngster gain an understanding of the impact of rewards. The importance of immediacy, contingency, and continuous schedules of reinforcement is discussed and illustrated with examples from the child's everyday life. In addition, the emotional impact of rewards is discussed with the child. The point to be made is that rewarding oneself feels good while punishment feels bad.

The relationship between emotion and self-consequation is an important link for the child to understand. It is especially important for the youngster to recognize that positive self-statements, especially self-evaluative statements, can be rewards and lead to positive affect, while negative self-statements can be self-punitive and lead to unwanted negative affect.

The next characteristic of reinforcement to be taught is that rewards vary along a continuum of potency that is calibrated by how much pleasure is derived from each one. This idea is then applied to the youngster's reward menu by rank-ordering the rewards on the basis of their potency. A hypothetical value between 0 and 100 is assigned to each reward as a way of concretely reflecting its potency. Subsequently, the child is taught to self-administer highly valued rewards for difficult or demanding tasks, medium rewards for moderately demanding tasks, and less valuable rewards for simple tasks.

Once the child understands all the aforementioned characteristics of reinforcement, the therapist models pulling all these concepts together to reinforce himself or herself and encourages the child to do the same during the next few meetings when an appropriate situation arises. The therapist can pose hypothetical situations and ask the child to describe how he or she would use self-reinforcement. The child may also be instructed to choose a behavior that will occur during the session and to demonstrate his or her use of self-reinforcement following enactment of the designated behavior. Finally, the child is given a homework assignment to record his or her use of self-reinforcement.

Acting-Out Behaviors. Treating the acting-out behaviors of depressed children is a very difficult process, since they and the systems of which they are a part are often locked in a negative and coercive cycle. Success seems to hinge on being able to identify the functional value (Alexander & Parsons, 1982) of the acting-out for the child and for one of the major systems in which he or she is involved and creating an integrated treatment plan that involves the child, his or her parents, and school staff. Identifying the functional value means determining the instrumental value of the child's acting-out. Does it achieve some desired goal within the peer group or within the family? Does it serve to support an unhealthy view of the self? Does it relieve anxiety or depression? Once the functional value is determined, the objective becomes to teach the youngster an appropriate means of achieving his or her goals.

Oftentimes, the first step in this process is to discuss with the child what the assessment has revealed about the functional utility of the youngster's behavior. Subsequently, the child and therapist collaboratively develop an understanding of the child's goals. Then a plan is developed for helping the youngster use more adaptive means of achieving the goals.

Intervening at the Cognitive Level. It is apparent that a treatment for depressed children should address the disturbances they are experiencing in their thinking. To successfully accomplish this aim, the intervention must address the disturbances found in the youngster's schemata, their processing errors, negative self-evaluations, and hopelessness. A number of techniques can be used to directly intervene with disturbances in cognition.

Changing Dysfunctional Schemata. One of the ultimate goals of the treatment program is to change the dysfunctional schemata that give rise to the errors in information-processing—i.e., the depressogenic automatic thoughts—and are associated with the dysfunctional emotions and behaviors. The class of procedures that are used to directly change schemata is cognitive-restructuring procedures. Included among these are: (1) What's the evidence? (2) What's another way to look at it? (3) What if? (4) Behavioral experiments.

Cognitive-restructuring procedures are designed to modify the client's thinking and the premises, assumptions, and attitudes that underlie the client's thoughts (Meichenbaum, 1977). We have used a number of the procedures developed by Beck et al. (1979). Children are taught to be "thought detectives" who identify maladaptive thoughts and (1) evaluate the evidence for the thought, (2) consider alternative interpretations, or (3) think about what really would happen if the undesirable event occurred. These procedures are used throughout treatment by the therapist, and the children are taught how to independently use the procedures.

With depressed children, the timing of the use of the cognitive-restructuring procedures is important. Commonly, during the early part of treatment, the child holds negatively distorted thoughts to be true, and he or she cannot achieve the necessary distance from the thoughts to objectively evaluate them. With the development of the therapeutic relationship, and the acquisition of some coping skills, the youngster has the necessary base for beginning to entertain the notion that his or her thoughts and perceptions may not always reflect reality. Another concern stems from the fact that the cognitive-restructuring procedures require the child to pay close attention to his or her thoughts and changes in emotions. This increased attention can lead to an exacerbation of the child's depressive symptoms if the child has not acquired skills for regulating them. Thus, it is important to determine when the child has acquired some coping skills and can use them to moderate the impact of depressive symptoms.

As implied in the previous paragraph, the first step in cognitive restructuring is to identify distorted thoughts. This identification can be accomplished through listening to the youngster's descriptions of what is happening in his or her life and in his or her perceptions of interpersonal situations. It can also be accomplished by having the children tune in to their thoughts in various situations that are associated with negative mood states as well as through having them use a change in mood as a cue to tune in to their thinking. We commonly instruct the children to write down their thoughts in these situations. It is difficult for the children to remember to do this, to recognize that they are in a problematic situation or that their mood is changing, and to remember to keep a diary of their thoughts. Consequently, we have found that it is very helpful to enlist the assistance of parents and teachers in these endeavors. Both parents and teachers are instructed to cue the child that he or she should tune in to his or her thoughts and write them down.

At this point, the overview of the cognitive-restructuring procedure presented in the preceding paragraphs has described the restructuring of automatic thoughts. To restructure schemata, which is the ultimate goal of therapy, since it produces an overall change in the way the child perceives himself or herself and the world, it is necessary for the therapist and the child to identify schemata through watching for themes in the youngster's automatic thoughts and through a number of other procedures outlined in Stark (1990). This identification process relies very heavily on the therapist's skills, as the procedure seems to be too cognitively demanding for children. However, once a schema is identified by the therapist, the therapist checks the validity of the schema with the child by asking the child if it makes sense for him or her. Subsequently, the therapist and child watch for instances in which the schema is actively guiding the processing of information and then direct the cognitive-restructuring procedures against it. With practice, children can learn to recognize the thoughts and behaviors that reflect a particular schema and to try to restructure it. In fact, as children acquire the cognitive-restructuring procedure, they begin to spontaneously ask the same questions of themselves that the therapist asks.

What's the evidence? "What's the evidence?" is a very useful technique that children readily understand. It involves asking the child to work with the therapist to find evidence that supports or refutes the youngster's automatic thoughts and the schemata underlying them. The first step involves defining the premise that encompasses the child's maladaptive thoughts. Once it has been defined, the therapist works with the child to establish the evidence that he or she believes is necessary to support or disconfirm the underlying premise. After agreeing on the necessary and sufficient evidence, the therapist and child evaluate the existing evidence and establish a procedure for collecting additional evidence. Subsequently, the therapist and child review the evidence and process the outcome. Finally, the child is given a homework assignment to collect evidence that supports the revised, more adaptive premise. As the youngster becomes skillful at identifying maladaptive thoughts and schemata, he or she is taught to independently use the procedure as the thoughts arise. It is important to note that it takes a considerable time to teach a child to do this. Once again, the youngster's parents can assist in this process.

What's another way to look at it? Alternative interpretation is a cognitive-restructuring procedure that can be used to broaden the focus of the child's thinking. In this case, the way that the child is interpreting events is altered as the therapist and child work together to identify alternative interpretations. They collaboratively generate a number of plausible, more adaptive, and *realistic* interpretations for what has happened or for a particular belief. Next, they evaluate the evidence for the alternative interpretations, and then the most plausible one is chosen. Once again, the goal is to teach the child to do this on his or her own. This teaching is accomplished through the therapist's modeling the use of the procedure and coaching the child about how to use it. In addition, we ask the children to teach their parents and teachers how to use this procedure and to ask the parents and teachers to help them use it when it is appropriate to do so.

What if? Depressed children often exaggerate the significance of a situation or predict unrealistically dire outcomes. "What if" can be used to help them obtain a more realistic understanding of the meaning of the situation and to see that the probable outcome is not going to be as bad as predicted. When using "What if," the therapist acknowledges the child's distressing situation, but helps the child recognize exaggerated interpretations of the significance of the event. These exaggerations are then countered with evidence for a more realistic outcome.

Behavioral experiments. Perhaps the most efficient way to change a child's thinking is to strategically alter behaviors that serve as the base of evidence for the child's thoughts. The alteration in behavior and the resultant change in outcomes provide the child with immediate, direct, and concrete contradictory evidence for an existing maladaptive schema or supportive evidence for a new, more adaptive schema. This process of assigning personal experiments requires creativity, as the therapist has to be able to first identify a maladaptive thought or schema, bring it to the child's recognition, work with the child to establish the necessary evidence to support or refute it, and then devise a behavioral assignment that directly tests its validity. Furthermore, steps have to be taken to ensure that the experiment is actually carried out as planned. In some instances, role-playing ahead of time, imaginally walking through the assignment, or writing a contract may be used to promote compliance. Once again, parental support and the cooperation of the youngster's teachers are invaluable. After the experiment has been completed, the therapist works with the child to process the results. This is an important step, since the child may distort the results without the therapist's objective input.

Methods for Altering Faulty Information-Processing. Depressed children tend to pay attention to the negative things that are occurring in their lives to the exclusion of positive information. This disturbance in self-monitoring may stem from a variety of errors in information-processing. To counter this tendency, children can be taught to self-monitor positive events. Self-monitoring is the purposeful and conscious act of observing oneself. Depending on the nature of the child's problems, he or she may be taught to observe his or her own behavior, thoughts, feelings, or physical reactions and make a judgment about their occurrence or nonoccurrence. In addition, the youngster may be instructed to monitor what is happening when he or she has a specific thought or emotion. After its occurrence, the youngster is instructed to record the information in some manner.

Teaching a child to self-monitor a behavior or observable event can be relatively easy. The first step is to collaboratively define the phenomenon of interest and to identify examples and nonexamples of it. It is useful to begin the training with a behavior that is likely to occur during the session that gives the therapist an opportunity to help the child tune in to the occurrence of the behavior, check for accuracy of self-monitoring, model the procedure if necessary, and reward the child for successful and accurate self-monitoring. The more opportunities the youngster has to observe the behavior during practice sessions, the better and more rapidly the skill will be acquired.

After identifying and defining the target for self-monitoring, the child and therapist devise a method for recording its occurrence of nonoccurrence. The parameters of self-recording need to be stated in concrete and specific terms that are clearly understood by the child. The child needs to be taught how to record its occurrence (e.g., by narrative or slash mark), as well as when and how often to record. It is important to devise a system that allows the child to immediately record the occurrence of the target. Thus, the system has to be mobile and not so obtrusive that the child will feel as though others will be aware that he or she is doing something unusual. If this happens, the child is often unwilling to complete the task. The importance of immediacy in self-recording for accuracy is emphasized.

When the child seems to be accurately self-monitoring during the session, he or she is then instructed to self-monitor in vivo as a homework assignment. However, before the child is sent out to complete the assignment, the child and therapist collaborate to identify potential impediments to successfully carrying out the homework assignment. After a potential roadblock has been identified, the child and the therapist use problem-solving to develop a plan for overcoming each impediment. The child is encouraged to use this same problem-solving procedure during the actual completion of homework if an impediment arises. Finally, prior to the child's completing the self-monitoring in vivo, the child and the therapist review the homework assignment to be sure that the child understands it. At the beginning of each subsequent session, the child and therapist review the child's efforts and develop plans to overcome any difficulties. The results of the self-monitoring are discussed, and their implications for coping with the depressive symptoms, or for specific beliefs, are highlighted. It is critically important to process the results and help the child understand their implications.

The content of the self-monitoring varies to meet the therapeutic goals. One of the more common targets, as noted earlier in this chapter, is self-monitoring of engagement in pleasant events. Other common targets are thoughts, behaviors, situations, and behaviors of others. It serves as a method for directing the child's attention to more positive things, thus breaking the cycle of negative attention. It helps the child see that there are some positive things going on in his or her life.

Once again, the support of parents and teachers is important for the success of the self-monitoring intervention. Parents and teachers can be informed about the target of the self-monitoring, and they can assist the child in recognizing when it is happening and remind the child to self-record. In the case of the teacher, it is important that he or she cue the child in a very discreet way. Such cueing can be accomplished by establishing a behavioral cue and instructing the teacher to use the cue to quietly and discreetly remind the child.

Children make a number of additional errors in their information-processing that require intervention. Included among these are the errors noted by Beck et al. (1979). These errors are evident in the youngster's daily comments and evaluations. Parents and teachers can be instructed to recognize verbalizations that reflect these errors and to help the youngsters recognize and correct them.

Self-Evaluation. Depressed children evaluate their performances, possessions, and personal qualities more negatively than nondepressed youths, and their self-evaluations tend to be negatively distorted (Kendall, Stark, & Adam, 1990). In other words, they tend to be unrealistically and unreasonably negative in their self-evaluations. Children can be taught to evaluate themselves more reasonably and positively when it is realistic to do so. During this process, they learn to recognize their positive attributes, outcomes, and possessions. The first step of the procedure is to identify the existence and nature of the disturbance. This task can be accomplished through the use of the My Standards Questionnaire—Revised (Stark, 1990). This measure allows the therapist to determine whether the child is setting unrealistically stringent standards for his or her performance.

If the standards are unrealistic and the child is evaluating his or her performance against them, the outcome is inadequacy. When this is the case, cognitive-restructuring procedures are used to help the child accept more reasonable standards. When the child sets realistic standards, but evaluates himself or herself negatively, cognitive restructuring and self-monitoring are used. The cognitive-restructuring procedures of "What's the evidence" and cognitive modeling may be used. Self-monitoring would be used as a means of solidifying the new self-evaluation, as the child is instructed to self-monitor the evidence that supports it. Over the course of treatment, the therapist and child review the evidence that supports the new self-evaluation.

In some instances, the child can benefit from change; the goal of self-evaluation training then becomes helping the child translate personal standards into realistic goals and then develop and carry out a plan for attaining the goals. Typically, this training occurs late in treatment after the child has acquired the other self-control procedures and has gained sufficient distance from his or her negative thinking to allow him or her to make and recognize the changes. Following the translation process, the child prioritizes the areas in which he or she is working toward self-improvement. Initially, a plan is formulated for producing improvement in an area in which success is probable. Problem-solving is used to help develop the plan. The long-term goal is broken down into subgoals, and problem-solving is used to develop a plan that will lead to attainment of the subgoals and eventually the goal. Prior to enacting the plan, the child and therapist try to identify possible impediments to carrying out the plan. Once again, problem-solving is used to develop contingency plans for overcoming the impediments. When the plan, including the contingency plans, has been developed, the child is instructed to self-monitor his or her progress toward change. Alterations in the plan are made along the way.

Altering Automatic Thoughts. The consciousness of depressed children is dominated by negative automatic thoughts. Especially prevalent are negative self-evaluative thoughts. As these thoughts are identified, which is very easily accomplished since they permeate the depressed youngster's conversations, they can be directly altered. Cognitive modeling and self-instructional training are two procedures that can be used to directly alter the automatic thoughts of depressed children.

The first step for using either procedure is to make the child aware of the tendency to think negatively. Doing so is accomplished through education, thinking aloud while playing games that pull for self-verbalizations (e.g., puzzle-building, completing mazes), and helping the child recognize them as they occur during the games and other activities during the sessions. It is especially fruitful to watch for signs that the child's mood has changed within the session and then to ask the child to state what he or she is and was thinking. It typically takes quite a bit of practice before children can independently catch their thoughts. In fact, they often require extended assistance from the therapist, and we solicit help from the child's teachers and parents. We ask them to gently make the child aware of statements that have a negative evaluative component. The adult simply repeats the negative statement using a tone that indicates that it is a question, e.g., "I'll *never* be able to do this?" We also have found it useful to give the children personalized lists of their automatic thoughts and instructions to self-monitor their occurrence by placing a hatch-mark in front of each thought after it occurs. The child is taught to replace a negative thought after catching it. One method of accomplishing this replacement technique is to model more adaptive thoughts.

Cognitive modeling involves the therapist's verbalizing his or her thoughts, or verbalizing more adaptive thoughts, that the child might use to replace existing thoughts or ones that he or she might have the next time a particular situation arises. Typically, the procedure involves modeling more adaptive thoughts and asking the child to put them into his or her own words and then rehearse them. In addition to using cognitive modeling when specific thoughts are being targeted, the therapist thinks aloud whenever he or she confronts a problem or some other situation that enables him or her to model adaptive thoughts for the child. This is done throughout treatment as a means of planting seeds of more adaptive thinking.

When a depressed child is having an especially difficult time replacing thoughts, self-instructional training can be used. Self-instructional training (Meichenbaum, 1977) is used to help a child internalize any set of self-statements that guide the child's thinking and behavior. In our work with depressed children, we have used Kendall's (e.g., Kendall, 1977) adaptation of Meichenbaum's procedure. Any content of the thoughts can be taught. It is especially useful with children who are experiencing a deficit in their verbal mediational skills, such as a child who simply blows up and exerts no control over his or her emotions. It can also be used to help children acquire the problem-solving sequence of self-instructions described below.

Problem-Solving. Depressed children can be taught problem-solving as a direct means of eliminating this deficit. Problem-solving training is designed to counteract the rigidity in depressed children's thinking, as it forces them to consider alternative solutions to situations. It also helps them overcome hopelessness, as they see that there may be some options of which they were previously unaware. The children also gain a sense of self-efficacy as they experience some success and sense of mastery over the environment. It is important for depressed youngsters to learn that problems and disappointing situations are a normal part of life that simply has to be faced and solved on a regular basis. There is no reason to get upset, since it doesn't change the problem. Rather, planned action needs to be undertaken.

The problem-solving procedure that we have used is similar to the one used by Kendall (e.g., Kendall, 1981). Children are taught a series of five problem-solving steps through education, modeling, coaching, rehearsal, and feedback. Games such as checkers, Othello, and Jenga are commonly used. In fact, any game that provides the children with multiple possible moves at the same time can be used. This criterion is necessary to illustrate the concepts and value of looking at *all* of the possibilities, projecting the consequences for each one, and provides the children with immediate consequences for a poor choice that stems from a breakdown in the process. The first step is problem definition. Identifying and placing a label on the problem provides the child with some sense of control, since he or she finally knows what the problem is. Since depressed children often face a multitude of problems, this first step may be repeated a number of times, and the problems are then prioritized and worked on in order of priority.

Generation of alternative solutions is the second step. Children are taught to brainstorm as many possible solutions as they can without evaluating them. When children are first being taught to generate solutions, they are often very limited in the range and number of possibilities that they generate. Consequently, they have to be taught additional possibilities. It is important to teach them not to evaluate the alternatives, since depressed youths have a tendency to believe that nothing will work. Thus, the youngsters will short-circuit the process.

The third step involves predicting the likely outcomes for each possible solution. Early in the training process, this prediction requires the therapist and child to collaboratively evaluate the outcome of each possible solution relative to the desired goals. Oftentimes, the therapist has to help the child recognize potential positive outcomes as well as the limitations and self-defeating consequences of other possibilities. As therapy progresses, the therapist's role is reduced to simply asking probing or reminding questions as the child becomes increasingly responsible for completing the process.

The fourth step involves reviewing the possible solutions, choosing the one that is most consistent with the child's goals, and enacting the plan.

The final step is evaluating the progress the child is making toward goal attainment and the overall outcome of the chosen solution. If the outcome is a desirable one, the child self-reinforces. If the outcome is undesirable, the youngster reconsiders the possible solutions, chooses an alternative one, and enacts it.

Family Intervention

Parent Training
Parental Pathology.   Before describing the parent training component of the intervention program, it is important to note that many depressed children come from families with a parent who is experiencing a psychological disorder. In such cases, after establishing a relationship with the family, the therapist begins working toward getting the disturbed parent to agree to enter treatment with another psychologist and to seek psychiatric treatment when it is necessary. When a parent is uncooperative, and doesn't seek therapy, we minimize the parent's role in assisting the child to implement the treatment procedures. We also believe that the lack of parental cooperation probably decreases the impact of the overall intervention package. In addition to referring parents for their own therapy, at times the parents have to be referred for marital therapy.

Overview
Parents as collaborators in treatment.   Throughout the preceding sections of this chapter, we have alluded to the importance of involving the parents in the treatment process. Prior to describing the parent training component that is designed to enhance overall parenting skills, we will describe how parents are taught during this training to help their children acquire the skills they are being taught in therapy. The parents' level of involvement in their children's treatment is based on how healthy the parents and family are. In the case of healthy parents and family, the parents are brought into a collaborative treatment process to promote their child's acquisition and generalization of new skills. In this way, parent training is viewed as directly impacting the children's treatment. In contrast, we see the parent training modules described later in this chapter as changing parenting practices, parent–child interaction patterns, and the family milieu so that they also support the children's treatment.

When working with the parents to help them support the treatment efforts with their children, the role of the parent is initially one of consultant; however, it gradually turns into one of assistant therapist and then cotherapist, which parallels the role of the children during the course of their therapy. Parents are seen as a central link between the children's acquiring the skills during the sessions and applying them within the natural environment through completion of homework assignments. Parents are taught to be facilitative through setting up opportunities for the child to carry out assignments, reinforcing the child for completion of therapeutic homework and use of coping skills, prompting the child to use the skills, answering questions about something he or she doesn't understand about the treatment program, modeling the use of a coping skill, and assisting in cognitive restructuring and problem-solving. An essential role is to monitor and verify that homework has been completed. Thus, the parent facilitates the child's application of skills whenever possible outside the therapist's office.

Parents begin the parent training at the same time the children enter their treatment groups. In addition to learning the specific parenting skills described later, the parents are apprised by the therapist at the beginning of each meeting what their child is working on and what his or her homework assignments are. At this time, the therapist describes what the parents can do to help their child acquire the skills being taught and to complete the therapeutic homework. Simultaneous learning of the concepts by the parents and child promotes a sense of going through the same experience and the development of a common language and understanding of the goals, rationale, techniques, and process of the child's therapy. Additionally, this situation also helps define child and adult role boundaries, which in turn may lead to adaptive structural changes within the family. We have found that it is essential to provide the parents with a notebook, outlines of training content, and other treatment materials. The notebook serves as a vehicle for the organization of written materials, provides a quick reference guide, and acts as a stimulus for parent involvement.

In order that the parents may assist in promoting the acquisition and generalization of skills by their children, they must understand the nature of depression in children, the skills the children are learning, and the techniques being applied to promote acquisition. The therapist describes the nature of childhood depression, the collaborative, problem-solving nature of the parental group, and the child treatment program. These topics are addressed via didactic instruction, discussion, and group members sharing experiences. Sharing experiences assists with breaking the ice and building group cohesion.

The parents are given an overview of the child treatment program. Basic concepts such as the cognition–emotion–behavior relationship are presented, emphasizing the impact that maladaptive cognitions have on emotion and behavior. The skills that the children are taught including affective, self-control, activity-scheduling, social, relaxation, cognitive-restructuring, self-instruction, and problem-solving are described. The exercises the children complete are described by the trainer and demonstrated in-session for the parents. It is especially important that the parents take the role of their child in order to understand what their child is experiencing.

The therapeutically relevant cognitive constructs are defined for the parents. An explanation is given to the parents concerning typical self-statements depressed children may automatically generate. Examples are solicited and discussed in relation to self-statements that reflect cognitive errors such as overgeneralization and irrational beliefs such as "I should be perfect." Examples of negative self-evaluations are also discussed. Parents are taught how to help their children replace negative self-statements with positive self-statements, and the process of recognizing schemata and using cognitive restructuring is modeled and role-played.

As therapy progresses, more emphasis is placed on the parents' assisting their children to learn and implement the coping skills in the natural environment and on monitoring and verifying the children's completion of homework. Parents are encouraged to discuss their attempts to help their children practice and to complete a diary of their own thoughts, actions, and affect while helping their child. In addition, the success of and barriers to implementation of homework are recorded and discussed.

Parent skills component. At the same time that the child begins individual or group treatment, we initiate a parent training program that is designed to change the child's milieu and to alter dysfunctional parenting practices and interactions. In particular, we are trying to create a more positive environment, in terms of both the affective tone and the means of managing the children. In addition, the program reduces conflict and increases the youngster's role in decision-making within the family. Finally, it is designed to foster positive self-esteem. The parenting skills are taught in 2- to 3-week modules depending on the pace of skills acquisition of the group of parents. Typically, 8–12 parents are included in the groups, and the meetings last between 1½ and 2 hours. All meetings are conducted at the children's schools in the evening.

Positive Behavior-Management Procedures. There is a dearth of research on the parenting practices of parents of depressed children. Our experiences have led us to the conclusion that some parents of these youngsters rely primarily on punitive and coercive methods for managing their children's behavior. Such practices create a negative affective state within the household and lead to the development of a negative sense of self within the children. The message conveyed to the child by such practices is that he or she is "bad" or unworthy of love and affection.

Through a combination of education, modeling, role-plays, coaching, and feedback, parents are taught to use reinforcement for appropriate behavior as the primary means of managing their children's behavior. We also use videotape equipment as frequently as possible. The first step in this process is to help the parents become more effective and active observers of their children's behavior, and in particular of their children's positive behaviors. To accomplish this, we have borrowed from the treatment program devised by Barkley (1987) for defiant children. The therapist asks a volunteer to role-play his or her child while the two of them engage in play. During the demonstration, the therapist verbally mirrors the child's behavior just as a sportscaster would give the play-by-play during a radio broadcast. The point of the exercise is to get parents to attend to what their child is doing. After fielding questions, and there usually are very many, we have the parents form groups of three or four. One member of each group role-plays his or her child, and another member role-plays himself or herself as parent. The parent tries the verbal mirroring procedure as he or she gets help from the observers and the therapist who is going from group to group. In addition, the parents are instructed not to ask any questions or direct the child's play; rather, they are instructed to simply observe and narrate. The exercise continues until all parents have had an opportunity to role-play themselves. This procedure is surprisingly difficult for many parents to acquire, as they have a hard time paying attention and noticing in any detail what their child is doing. In addition, their natural tendency is to be controlling and to ask lots of questions.

At the end of the meeting, the parents are given the homework assignment to spend 15–20 minutes a day playing with their depressed child. They are instructed to let their child choose the activity. The sole purpose of this playtime is to enjoy being with their child and to notice all the positive things that the child does. They are given strict instructions not to ask questions, be directive, or get caught in any coercive interchanges. They are also instructed to pay particular attention to their child's positive qualities during the ensuing week and to write down a list of these qualities and to bring the list with them to the next meeting.

During the next meeting, the parents are taught the principles of reinforcement and the impact it has on their child's self-esteem. Once again, through therapist-planned role-plays and the role-plays of playtime, the parents are given practice at reinforcing their child's appropriate behavior. Parents are given the homework assignment to continue to play with their child and to practice reinforcing the child during this time. In addition, they are instructed to try to manage their child's behavior through reinforcement of appropriate behavior.

Self-Esteem Enhancement. Parents are taught the power of praise. They learn that it helps their child feel good, boosts self-esteem, and can be used to increase the occurrence of desirable behaviors. They are instructed to praise their child a minimum of 3 to 6 times per day. To teach the parents how to praise their children, education, modeling, role-plays, coaching, and feedback are used. Emphasis is placed on praising their child's efforts regardless of the result. Parents often need some help identifying qualities of their child that are worthy of praise. They are instructed to identify multiple aspects of their child to praise, including such things as social skills, appearance, intelligence, coordination, cooperativeness, compliance, affection, and self-expression. They can also scan their child's schoolwork for something to praise. Parents are taught to be concrete and specific when giving praise, especially in the beginning of the process. Being genuine when giving praise is emphasized, and they are taught that it is better to give a small compliment than a big lie. Parents are also instructed to avoid hyperbole. To help support their children's efforts toward improvement, they are taught to watch for opportunities to praise their child's small steps toward this end. For example, "I loved listening to you read to me. It sounds like you really tried hard in school today."

An especially powerful form of praise seems to be written praise. The parents surprise their child with a note in his or her lunchbag, on the bathroom mirror, or on the youngster's door just above the handle at eye level. We have also learned that parents need to be taught to avoid giving their child left-handed compliments, since they really are put downs. In addition to the usual homework, the parents are instructed to (1) praise their child at least 3 to 6 times a day and (2) keep track of how often they criticize their child during the first two days and then reduce the number of criticism by one each day until they hit zero.

Noncoercive Discipline. The first step to teaching parents noncoercive behavior-management skills has been achieved through teaching positive parenting practices. The next step is to teach the parents to avoid the coercive cycle. To do so, they are taught the means by which to give clear and effective directives and the time-out procedure. In addition, use of natural consequences is emphasized. Once again, education, modeling, coaching, role-playing, and feedback are used to help the parents acquire these skills. They are given the homework assignment to continue the positive playtime, to predominantly rely on reinforcement for positive behavior, and to use time-out and natural consequences for inappropriate behavior. Much of the time is spent answering questions about how to handle various situations that the parents have found themselves in during the previous week and incorporating other parents into the discussion through frequent use of role-plays of the situations. The homework following the second training session for this module remains the same as the previous weeks, with the addition of monitoring their effectiveness at using the new disciplinary procedures. They are instructed to write down a description of any especially problematic situations and to bring it along to the next meeting.

Anger Management. One of the more striking and memorable observations of some families with depressed children is that the parents are angry and express it through frequent personal verbal attacks on their children. This behavior is extremely destructive and shatters the child's self-esteem. In such instances, the previous sessions help reduce this tendency toward angry lashing out as the parents acquire better ways to manage their children's behavior. Additional steps are taken to teach the parents to control their own anger. A procedure that is similar to that used with the children is used with the parents. In essence, they are taught to identify the triggers of their anger and the thoughts that underlie it. Subsequently, they are taught to use their anger as a cue to leave the situation and use adaptive coping statements and relaxation to control it. Once it is under control, they can reenter the situation. The homework remains the same as the previous weeks, with the addition of monitoring their use of the coping skills and gauging the impact on their child and family as a result of controlling their anger.

Empathic Listening. To combat depressed children's sense that their parents don't care about them or their feelings, and to help the parents better understand their children's feelings and to open up the channels of communication among family members, the parents are taught empathic listening. Through education, they are taught the meaning of empathy, including the notion that they should care about their children's feelings, even those they disagree with. Empathy both lets the child know that the parents care and that they feel that the child's feelings are important.

Parents are taught a four-step model of empathic listening through education, modeling, role-plays, coaching, and feedback. The first step is active listening, which means teaching the parents to listen to their child without thinking about their own problems or work they have to do. It also means not interrupting the child while he or she is talking by arguing, providing advice, or through one-upmanship. In addition, it means giving the child good eye contact and the other nonverbal signs that they are listening.

The second step involves teaching the parents to repeat what the child just said. Having to repeat forces the parents to listen, and it communicates to the child that he or she has been heard. Some parents have a tendency to editorialize while repeating what the child said, so special attention is paid to watching for this during role-plays, and they are given examples of what not to do that include such editorial remarks.

The third step is teaching the parents to let their child know that they understand how he or she is feeling. They are taught that they don't have to like to or agree with it, they simply have to understand the feeling.

During the final step, the parents are taught how to put all that they learned together to communicate empathy. This component of the parent training tends to be a good deal of fun, as the parents create some humorous situations. The homework assignments for these sessions include continuing to spend time playing with their child and using the previously taught skills. In addition, they are instructed to keep track of their empathic communications.

Recreation. Our own research (Stark et al., 1990) indicates that the families of depressed children are characterized by a failure to engage in recreational activities of any sort. Thus, we try to teach the parents how to have fun. This enlightenment is accomplished primarily through education and the group process. The parents help each other identify low-cost or no-cost enjoyable activities within the community in which families can participate. The importance of engaging in pleasant activities is discussed, as well as excuses for not doing so. Then, through the use of problem-solving, the parents schedule a reasonable number of activities into their week. Their homework assignment, in addition to the usual assignment, is to engage in the pleasant activities and monitor the impact they have on themselves and their family.

Family Therapy

Overview. Consistent with the theme of the rest of the treatment program is an emphasis on teaching the participants skills that will remediate the disturbances in family functioning that research has shown to be associated with depressive disorders during childhood. Open, honest, direct, and congruent communication among family members serves as the base for effective family functioning (Alexander & Parsons, 1982). Such communication is fostered through communication training. It is also presumed to contribute to a sense of the family's being accepting of more expression of feelings and desires as well as input from each family member. To help reduce the amount of conflict evident within the family, the family is taught problem-solving and conflict-resolution skills. It is also hoped that involving the family in problem-solving training will facilitate the child's acquisition of problem-solving skills (Braswell & Bloomquist, 1991). As the family changes and functions more adaptively, and as the family is impacted by improved and more positive parenting practices, the family is directly taught how to communicate positive messages to one another.

While the therapist is working with the family on the aforementioned skills, he or she is actively observing and assessing the family. The therapist is observing the family with the intention of identifying interaction patterns, behaviors, or other forms of communication that would have led to the development of the depressed child's specific maladaptive schemata.

The family therapy sessions are conducted at the children's school in the evening. Sessions are scheduled once a week for ½–1 hour. In some cases when the family seems to be in a great deal of distress, meetings are held twice a week until the situation stabilizes, and then a weekly schedule is arranged. All family members are expected to attend the meetings.

Communication Training. The communication training procedure we employ is based on the procedure outlined in Alexander and Parsons (1982) and consists of teaching nine principles. The first principle taught is to speak in short, clear sentences. The rule that they are to try to follow is to say what they want in ten words or fewer. This brevity seems to promote clarity in communication, as the bottom-line message does not get lost in excess verbiage. It also reduces or eliminates accusatory, blaming, and other provocative statements. The resultant objectivity has the added bonus of reducing conflict and manipulation through guilt. While many family members are not used to such brevity, it is relatively easy to teach them this skill through a combination of education, modeling, coaching, and feedback. Concurrently, family members are taught the second and third principles: how to listen to the speaker and how to communicate that they are actively listening to one another. This training includes teaching the listeners to be attentive to the speaker, which includes providing the speaker with eye contact and appropriate body position and restating or rephrasing the context and feelings expressed by the speaker. Consequently, they are prevented from talking over one another and from thinking about counterarguments rather than listening. At the very least, this procedure sends the other family member the message that he or she cares enough to listen and consider what is being said.

Family members are taught to accept and communicate responsibility for their thoughts, feelings, and requests through making "I" statements, which leads to a reduction in blaming and defensiveness. Hand in hand with teaching family members to use "I" statements is teaching them to be more direct through the use of "you" within their statements, thus directly communicating whom the statement is directed toward.

Once family members are communicating more clearly, concisely, and with direct communication of responsibility, they are ready to add the next component, which is impact statements. They are taught to state what another family member is doing and what it leads the speaker to think and feel. In other words, they are taught to communicate their personal reactions to others' behaviors. The impact and effectiveness of these statements are partially dependent on the acquisition of another communication skill, being concrete and specific in one's statements. Thus, they are taught to state their feelings, thoughts, and requests in very specific terms. If a request is being made, then the desired behavior is described in specific terms, and the context in which it is to occur, including the time parameters, is stated with specificity.

Family members are taught to provide the listener with options whenever possible when making requests, rather than simply making demands. Providing options contributes to a greater sense of a democratic milieu. While listening to another family member talk, other family members are encouraged to interrupt the speaker and obtain clarification when necessary and to provide the speaker with relevant feedback. Finally, the therapist helps the family members attain congruence at the verbal, nonverbal, and contextual levels of their communications.

Family Problem-Solving. Families continually face problems ranging from what television shows to watch to how to cope with a parent's losing a job. To help the family deal most effectively with their day-to-day problems, they are taught the same five-step problem-solving sequence that the children are taught. The therapist helps them learn how to apply the steps to the problems that they bring with them to therapy sessions. Family members are encouraged to apply the process to the problems both as a group and individually outside therapy. The application of problem-solving by family members not only leads to solutions that reduce stress within the family but also provides the depressed child with examples of how to use problem-solving (Braswell & Bloomquist, 1991). Furthermore, it communicates the message that difficulties are simply problems to be solved and that they can be dealt with most effectively through active effort. While family members can learn the steps very quickly, it takes a good deal of practice and monitoring of their use before the process becomes a normal part of their routine.

Conflict Resolution. One of the more consistent results of the research on the families of depressed children is that their households are charaterized by elevated levels of conflict. We have once again borrowed a procedure from Alexander and Parsons (1982) for helping families develop an alternative interaction pattern to reduce conflict within their families. Alexander and Parsons describe a five-step conflict-management strategy. These steps are taught to family members through education, modeling, coaching, rehearsal, and corrective feedback. When first introducing this skill, it is useful to have the family members apply it to less emotionally laden and more easily resolved problems rather than the most controversial ones. Otherwise, the family members may be too passionate in their opinions to allow the skill to be successfully applied. The first step is for the two family members who are in conflict to agree to discuss the point of contention and to designate a time and place for the discussion. The initiator of the discussion states one issue clearly while the other family member uses his or her active listening skills and does not introject any new information. The speaker then gives two recent examples of the situation, this being followed by the listener's repeating what was said. Next, the speaker states the personal impact of the examples, and the listener restates the emotional impact of the examples on the speaker. The final step involves discussion of alternatives that would lead to a solution and choosing and enacting a mutually agreed-on solution.

Positive Communication. Our experiences working with families of depressed youths have led us to incorporate a session or two on communicating positive statements to family members. We do this later in therapy after the conflict and hard feelings have lessened, thus allowing the family members to feel as though they can honestly say something positive about one another. We have often taught this skill through a game. In this game, each family member takes five 3 × 5 cards and writes his or her name on each card. The cards are then collected, shuffled, and placed in a pile in the middle of the seating arrangement. Family members take turns drawing a card from the deck and responding to one of the following directives: (1) Tell the person something that you like about him or her. (2) Tell the person something that he or she did over the past month that you liked. (3) Tell the person something he or she did over the past week that you liked. (4) Tell the person something he or she did tonight that you liked. (5) Tell the person something that you would like him or her to do more often. One of these statements is made during each successive turn around the family. The person drawing a card may draw his or her own name. When this occurs, the person makes a statement about himself or herself. Family members are instructed to keep track of their use of such compliments over the ensuing weeks.

Changing Schema-Consistent Maladaptive Interactions. The final family therapy strategy employed is somewhat more difficult to implement. While interacting with the family, the therapist observes the family members' interaction patterns and communications to try to identify those that are maintaining the depressed youngster's depressogenic schemata. This observation and hypothesis-generation process involves deductive reasoning. Through his or her interactions with the depressed child, the therapist has acquired a knowledge of the depressogenic schemata that the child holds. On the basis of this knowledge, the therapist tries to deduce from the interactions and communications of family members what is happening that would sustain such schemata.

Once the maladaptive interactions are identified, the therapist uses all the therapeutic tools in his or her arsenal to change them.

Summary

Our knowledge of how to treat depressive disorders in children remains at a very early stage. It is the contention of the authors that a multicomponent intervention that involves intervening with the child and family along with parent training is necessary to produce meaningful and lasting change. A cognitive–behavioral treatment model that emphasizes intervening at the affective, behavioral, and cognitive levels with the child was outlined. The ultimate goal of this intervention program is for the child to acquire (1) a set of coping skills for moderating his or her depressive symptoms, (2) a problem-solving set toward daily difficulties, and (3) a new, more adaptive way of processing information, especially information about the self. This intervention has received preliminary support from our research. The parents are taught how to support the therapeutic efforts that are being made with their children, as well as more effective parenting practices. The parenting skills are designed to create a more positive family environment in which behavior is managed through positive procedures. In addition, the parents are taught how to foster positive self-esteem within their children and how to control their own anger and avoid coercive interactions. Finally, the parents are taught how to help their family have fun. The family therapy component is designed to improve communication, reduce conflict, increase the children's role in family decisions, and change the family interactions that lead to and maintain the depressed child's maladaptive schemata.

References

Alexander, J. F., & Parsons, B. (1982). *Functional family therapy*. Monterey, CA: Brooks/Cole.

Barkley, R. A. (1987). *Defiant children: A clinician's manual for parent training*. New York: Guilford Press.

Beck, A. T., Rush, A. J., Shaw, B. F., & Emery, G. (1979). *Cognitive therapy of depression*. New York: Guilford Press.

Braswell, L., & Bloomquist, M. L. (1991). *Cognitive behavior therapy with ADHD children: Child, family and school interventions*. New York: Guilford Press.

Butler, L., Miezitis, S., Friedman, R., & Cole, E. (1980). The effect of two school-based intervention programs on depressive symptoms in preadolescents. *American Educational Research Journal, 17*, 111–119.

Fennell, M. J. V., & Teasdale, J. D. (1987). Cognitive therapy for depression: Individual differences and the processes of change. *Cognitive Therapy and Research, 11*, 253–271.

Frame, C. L., Johnstone, B., & Giblin, M. S. (1988). Dysthymia. In M. Hersen & C. G. Last (Eds.), *Child behavior therapy casebook* (pp. 63–81). New York: Plenum Press.

Frame, C., Matson, J. L., Sonis, W. A., Fialkov, M. J., & Kazdin, A. E. (1982). Behavioral treatment of depression in a prepubertal child. *Journal of Behavior Therapy and Experimental Psychiatry, 3*, 239–243.

Kahn, J. S., Kehle, T. J., Jenson, W. R., & Clark, E. (1990). Comparison of cognitive–behavioral, relaxation, and self-modeling interventions for depression among middle-school students. *School Psychology Review, 19*, 196–211.

Kanfer, F. H., & Phillips, J. S. (1969). A survey of current behavior therapies and a proposal for classification. In C. Franks (Ed.), *Behavior therapy: Appraisal and status* (pp. 445–475). New York: McGraw-Hill.

Kaslow, N. J., & Rehm, L. P. (1983). Childhood depression. In R. J. Morris & T. R. Kratochwill (Eds.), *The practice of child therapy* (pp. 27–51). New York: Pergamon Press.

Kendall, P. C. (1977). On the efficacious use of verbal self-instructional procedures with children. *Cognitive Therapy and Research, 1*, 331–341.

Kendall, P. C. (1981). Cognitive–behavioral interventions with children. In B. B. Lahey & A. E. Kazdin (Eds.), *Advances in clinical child psychology*, Vol. 4 (pp. 53–90). New York: Plenum Press.

Kendall, P. C., Stark, K. D., & Adam, T. (1990). Cognitive deficit or cognitive distortion in childhood depression? *Journal of Abnormal Child Psychology, 18*, 267–283.

Larrabee, M. J. (1988). How to encourage students to take responsibility: Affirmation to promote counseling homework. *School Counselor, 35,* 220–228.

Lewinsohn, P. M. (1974) A behavioral approach to depression. In R. J. Friedman & M. M. Katz (Eds.), *The psychology of depression: Contemporary theory and research* (pp. 50–87). New York: Guilford Press.

Lewinsohn, P. M., & Graf, M. (1973). Pleasant activities and depression. *Journal of Consulting and Clinical Psychology, 41,* 261–268.

Martin, G. A., & Worthington, E. L. (1982). Behavioral homework. *Progress in Behavior Modification, 13,* 197–226.

Meichenbaum, D. (1977). *Cognitive–behavior modification.* New York: Plenum Press.

Ollendick, T. H., & Cerney, J. A. (1981). *Clinical behavior therapy with children.* New York: Plenum Press.

Persons, J. B., Burns, D. D., & Perloff, J. M. (1988). Predictors of dropout and outcome in cognitive therapy for depression in a private practice setting. *Cognitive Therapy and Research, 12,* 557–575.

Petti, T. A., Bornstein, M., Delamater, A., & Conner, C. K. (1980). Evaluation and multimodality treatment of a depressed prepubertal girl. *Journal of the American Academy of Child Psychiatry, 19,* 690–702.

Pope, A. W., McHale, S. M., & Craighead, W. E. (1988). *Self-esteem enhancement with children and adolescents.* New York: Pergamon Press.

Rehm, L. P., Kaslow, N. J., & Rabin, A. (1987). Cognitive and behavioral targets in a self-control therapy program for depression. *Journal of Consulting and Clinical Psychology, 55,* 60–67.

Reynolds, W. M., & Coats, R. I. (1986). A comparison of cognitive–behavioral therapy and relaxation training for the treatment of depression in adolescents. *Journal of Consulting and Clinical Psychology, 54,* 653–660.

Rouse, L. W. (1994). Psychotherapeutic homework and treatment outcome: A study of social skills training with early adolescent males (in prep.).

Shelton, J. L. (1979). Instigation therapy: Using therapeutic homework to promote treatment gains. In A. P. Goldstein & F. H. Kanfer (Eds.), *Maximizing treatment gains: Transfer enhancement in psychotherapy* (pp. 225–245). New York: Academic Press.

Shelton, J. L., & Ackerman, J. M. (1974). *Homework in counseling and psychotherapy.* Springfield, IL: Charles C. Thomas.

Shelton, J., & Levy, R. (1981). *Behavioral assignments and treatment compliance: A handbook of clinical strategies.* Champaign, IL: Research Press.

Stark, K. D. (1990). *Childhood depression: School-based intervention.* New York: Guilford Press.

Stark, K. D., Reynolds, W. M., & Kaslow, N. J. (1987). A comparison of the relative efficacy of self-control therapy and a behavioral problem-solving therapy for depression in children. *Journal of Abnormal Child Psychology, 15,* 91–113.

Stark, K. D., Rouse, L. W., & Livingston, R. (1991). Treatment of depression during childhood and adolescence: Cognitive–behavioral procedures for the individual and family. In P. C. Kendall (Ed.), *Child and adolescent therapy: Cognitive–behavioral procedures* (pp. 165–208). New York: Plenum Press.

Walker, H. M., Todis, B., Holmes, D., & Horton, G. (1988). *The ACCESS program: Adolescent curriculum for communication and effective social skills.* Austin, TX: ProEd.

Zettle, R. D., & Hayes, S. C. (1987). Component and process analysis of cognitive therapy. *Psychological Reports, 61,* 939–953.

15

Psychological Approaches to the Treatment of Depression in Adolescents

Peter M. Lewinsohn, Gregory N. Clarke, and Paul Rohde

Introduction

This chapter focuses on the psychological treatment of adolescents with nonbipolar, nonpsychotic depression, e.g., major depressive disorder (MDD) or dysthymia (DY), as specified in the *Diagnostic and Statistical Manual of Mental Disorders*, third edition—revised (DSM-III-R) (American Psychiatric Association, 1987). Although bipolar disorder is known to occur in adolescence, albeit at a very low prevalence (Bashir, Russell, & Johnson, 1987; Carlson, 1982; Lewinsohn, Hops, Roberts, Seeley, & Andrews, 1993a), the available evidence suggests that its etiology is primarily biological or genetic or both (Medlewicz, 1985).

The study and treatment of depression in adolescents have moved from being relatively neglected areas to being very active areas of professional and scientific attention, and many textbooks (e.g., Cantwell & Carlson, 1983; Clarizio, 1989; Klerman, 1986; Lewis, 1991; Lewis & Miller, 1990; Matson, 1989; Oster & Caro, 1990; Patros & Shamoo, 1989; Rutter, Izard, & Read, 1986; Stark, 1990) have been partially or entirely devoted to these topics. In addition, a number of treatment manuals (Clarke, Lewinsohn, & Hops, 1990; Moreau, Mufson, Weissman, & Klerman, 1991) have been developed. Another important development is that depression in children and adolescents has been identified as a high-priority area by the National Institute of Mental Health (1990).

The increased interest in adolescent depression has been fueled by an increase in relevant research investigations. Epidemiological studies (e.g., Lewinsohn et al., 1993a)

Peter M. Lewinsohn and Paul Rohde • Oregon Research Institute, Eugene, Oregon 97403-1983. **Gregory N. Clarke** • Division of Child Psychology, Oregon Health Sciences University, Portland, Oregon 97201.

Handbook of Depression in Children and Adolescents, edited by William M. Reynolds and Hugh F. Johnston. Plenum Press, New York, 1994.

indicate that the point and lifetime prevalence of affective disorders in this population is surprisingly high and comparable to adult levels as reported in the Epidemiologic Catchment Area Study (Robins & Regier, 1991). Other reasons for interest in the topic include the fact that depressed adolescents are at very high risk for relapse (Kovacs et al., 1984; Lewinsohn et al., 1993a), that early-onset depression may have a protracted course (Kovacs, Paulauskas, Gatsonis, & Richards, 1988), and that adolescent depression may be a more serious form of the disorder (Weissman et al., 1984c). Adolescent depressives also have been found to have such future adjustment problems as marital problems, school attrition, hospitalization, unemployment, drug involvement, delinquent behavior, arrest and criminal conviction, and being in a car accident (Carlson & Strober, 1979; Chiles, Miller, & Cox, 1980; Kandel & Davies, 1986; Newcomb & Bentler, 1988; Paton, Kessler, & Kandel, 1977).

Our efforts in this area in the past decade have consisted of a large prospective epidemiological study (the Oregon Adolescent Depression Project) in which a large number of high school students were followed over a period of 1 year (Lewinsohn et al., 1993a); a randomized, controlled clinical trial to evaluate the efficacy of a cognitive–behavioral group intervention for adolescent depression (Lewinsohn, Clarke, Hops, & Andrews, 1990); and a controlled pilot investigation of the school-based prevention of depression in adolescents with an elevated risk of future depression (Clarke, Hawkins, Sheeber, Lewinsohn, & Seeley, 1994). In this chapter, we will make use of the results of these studies.

It is sobering to note that up to 70–80% of depressed teenagers do not receive treatment (Keller, Lavori, Beardslee, Wunder, & Ryan, 1991; Rohde, Lewinsohn, & Seeley, 1991). This low treatment rate may be attributed to a lack of adolescent, parent, and teacher information regarding the basic facts about adolescent depression. Few adults and even fewer adolescents are aware of the wide range of physical, cognitive, and behavioral manifestations that constitute the depression syndrome. Also, given the high degree of comorbidity of depression with disruptive behavior disorders and substance abuse (Rohde et al., 1991), the other syndrome may become the focus of attention and the coexisting depression may be overlooked (Clark & Mokros, 1991). Our experience has been that many clinically depressed teenagers typically do not label themselves as depressed or as requiring help. They often do not know that help relevant to their problems is available.

In the balance of this chapter, we first review the most frequently observed psychosocial, personal, and psychopathological problems associated with unipolar depression. The depression-related problematic behaviors are often the focus of treatment and as such merit examination to determine the extent to which existing treatments address the particular pattern of deficits and strengths associated with adolescent depression. While the psychosocial problems associated with adult depression have become relatively well known (e.g., Barnett & Gotlib, 1988), those associated with depression in adolescents have received much less attention.

We then review most of the major psychological approaches currently used in the treatment of adolescent depression, providing for each a brief summary of the major theoretical premises and their relationship to the specific strategy and tactics of the treatment. We also provide case illustrations of several of these approaches and, when available, summaries of empirical outcome data.

Finally, we discuss special issues pertinent to the treatment of unipolar affective disorders in adolescents. These include treatment-relevant issues such as assessment, prevention, group vs. individual therapy, relapse prevention, the treatment of special populations (e.g., depression secondary to medical illness, racial minorities), parental involvement in treatment, the impact of gender, and issues relevant to research, including future directions.

Importance of Functional Assessment

As the diagnostic assessment of depressive disorders has become more rigorous [exemplified by the DSM-III-R and semistructured diagnostic interviews such as the Schedule for Affective Disorders and Schizophrenia in School-Age Children (K-SADS) and the Diagnostic Interview Schedule for Children], the role of functional assessment in treatment planning has diminished. The diminution of interest in functional assessment is unfortunate, since pinpointing specific problematic areas of functioning as an integral part of treatment has been a hallmark of cognitive–behavior therapy (Kanfer & Phillips, 1970; Kazdin, 1975; Lewinsohn & Rohde, 1987). Functional assessment directs the design of treatment interventions and provides the basis for an evaluation of the efficacy of treatment. Functional assessment is especially important in the treatment of depression, because outside the core symptom of sad affect, depressed individuals are quite heterogeneous in their symptom presentation.

Availability of Two Data Sets

The availability of two large data sets provides us an opportunity to shed light on the functional problems associated with adolescent depression, as well as on differences in the functional problems between community-residing depressed teens and those seeking treatment. The Epidemiological Data Set consists of a representative sample of 1710 high school adolescents who completed a diagnostic interview and an extensive questionnaire on entry into the study. Additional detail is provided in Lewinsohn et al. (1993a). On the basis of DSM-III-R diagnostic information, three groups were created: 44 adolescents in an episode of MDD, 272 adolescents who had previously met criteria for MDD (formerly MDD), and 1076 adolescents who had never met criteria for any of the assessed DSM-III-R diagnoses [Never Mentally Ill (NMI)].

The Treatment Data Set consists of data for 91 depressed adolescents who participated in a controlled randomized clinical trial designed to evaluate the efficacy of a cognitive–behavioral group treatment intervention. The study is described in greater detail in Lewinsohn, et al. (1990).

Adolescents in both data sets completed questionnaire batteries that measured the following constructs: stress (daily hassles and major life events), current depression, other psychopathology (internalizing and externalizing behavior problems, suicidal behavior), depressotypic cognitions (pessimism and attributions), self-consciousness, self-esteem, social self-confidence, emotional reliance, aspirations (academic, family, and occupational), coping skills, social support (family and friends), conflict with parents, interpersonal attractiveness, physical health, and maturational level (for more details, see Lewinsohn, Rohde, & Seeley, 1993b). These constructs were chosen because they are known to be problematic for depressed adults.

The Currently Depressed, Formerly Depressed, and NMI diagnostic groups from the Epidemiological Data Set were compared on all the psychosocial constructs. Results are shown in Fig. 1. With only three exceptions (family aspirations, occupational aspirations, and maturational level), differences between the three groups were highly significant (all $p < 0.01$). The negative findings indicate that adolescent depression is *not* associated with the importance placed on marrying the right person and having a family, the importance attached to finding steady work and being successful in one's employment field, or stage of pubertal development. The positive findings indicate that a consistent pattern of differences was found for the other constructs. In general, the NMI group exhibited the most

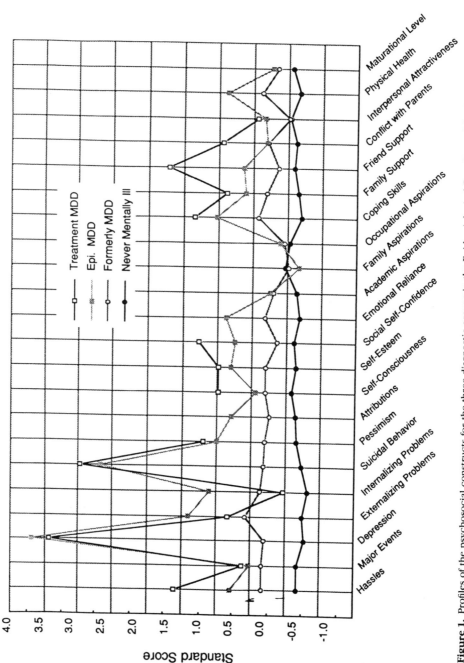

Figure 1. Profiles of the psychosocial constructs for the three diagnostic groups in the Epidemiological Data Set and for the MDD group in the Treatment Data Set.

adaptive functioning and significantly differed in comparison to the Currently Depressed group, which was the most pathological or dysfunctional. The Formerly Depressed group was intermediate. With only one exception (interpersonal attractiveness), the Formerly Depressed also differed significantly from the NMI on each of the constructs, indicating that the psychosocial problems of depressed adolescents linger even after the adolescent has clinically recovered.

Difficulties also extended to the academic area. The three groups differed significantly on grade point average (GPA), with the NMI subjects reporting a significantly higher mean GPA (3.05) compared to both the Formerly (2.88) and the Currently Depressed (2.81) groups, which did not significantly differ from each other. Other school-related problems that were more frequently reported by the two depressed groups included repeating a grade, being late for school, missing school, failing to complete homework, and dissatisfaction with grades.

Information from the parents was consistent with the teens' report. The three groups differed on the parent-report Child Behavior Checklist (Achenbach & Edelbrock, 1978). As expected, the Currently Depressed group had the highest scores on measures of internalizing and externalizing problems.

Differences between Treated and Nontreated Depressed Adolescents

The MDD group in the Treatment Data Set was compared to the 44 nontreated depressed adolescents from the Epidemiological Data Set on the assessed constructs, and the results for this group are also shown in Fig. 1. Although both groups met criteria for MDD and did not differ on a self-report construct of current depression, the treated adolescents did report greater levels of major stressful events, heightened self-consciousness, less social self-confidence and less perceived social support from their friends, and more conflicts with parents. These findings suggest that treatment-seeking in depressed teens may be triggered by stressful life events in the context of low social support. In other words, it appears that the circumstances surrounding a depressive episode, rather than the severity of the depression, set the stage for treatment-seeking.

Target Complaints for Treated Adolescents

As part of the intake interview, the teenagers and the parents in the treatment study indicated which difficulties they wanted addressed in treatment. The most common complaint categories reported by teens were dysphoric mood, generalized interpersonal difficulties, poor self-esteem, and decreased effectiveness and coping. These same four problem categories were also the most frequently reported target complaints of the parents.

Conflicts with Parents

The degree and types of conflicts between parents and adolescents in both data sets were assessed with the Issues Checklist (Robin & Weiss, 1980), in which separate parent and teen ratings are made regarding the occurrence and intensity of discussions regarding 45 issues (e.g., cleaning up bedroom, coming home on time). A factor analysis with varimax rotation computed on the teen's cross-product score identified eight factors: noise level around the house, drug and alcohol use, choice of friends/free time, school-related problems, household chores, clothes, eating habits, and money. The diagnostic groups from both data sets were compared on these factors. Differences between the four groups on the eight factors were all highly significant ($p < 0.001$). For each factor, the NMI teenagers reported the lowest level of conflict, followed by the Formerly and Currently Depressed groups, who reported comparable levels of conflict. The depressed adolescents from the Treatment Study were significantly higher than the depressed adolescents from the Epidemiological Study on three factors: noise level (e.g., playing stereo or radio too loud), school-related activities (e.g., doing homework), and issues around eating (e.g., what teenager eats). These findings suggest that certain kinds of adolescent–parent conflict may act as triggers for treatment-seeking.

Gender Differences

We were especially interested in determining whether depressed boys and girls had similar psychosocial problems. Comparisons on the psychosocial constructs revealed several differences. The elevations for externalizing problem behaviors and for pessimism, and the lowered level for academic aspirations, were greater for depressed boys than for depressed girls. When boys and girls were examined separately on academic problems, school problems were most severe for the currently depressed boys and for the formerly depressed girls. Formerly depressed girls also reported more health problems.

Although the treated boys and girls did not differ on the average number of reported target complaints, a few gender differences were noted in the frequency of various types of complaints. Girls reported relatively more problems with dysphoric mood, poor self-esteem, irritability/anger, and concentration, while boys reported relatively greater decreased effectiveness and coping, generalized interpersonal difficulties, concern about the future, and problems with anxiety.

Implications for Treatment

To summarize, consistent with other research findings (e.g., Asarnow & Bates, 1988; Hirschfeld & Blumenthal, 1986), our results indicate that depressed adolescents manifest the same pattern of problems associated with adult depression. To wit, depressed adolescents report themselves as having experienced stressful life events, being pessimistic and making depressotypic attributions for failure experiences, being more self-consciousness and emotionally dependent on others, having lower self-esteem and social self-confidence and poorer coping and social skills, receiving less perceived social support from family and friends, experiencing more conflict with parents, and having other mental and physical problems. The fact that depressed and even formerly depressed had academic problems has implications for assessment. In contrast to research with adults (Blackburn & Smyth, 1985; Rohde, Lewinsohn, & Seeley, 1990), formerly depressed adolescents appear to continue to show many of the depression-related psychosocial deficits after recovery.

Major Approaches to the Treatment of Adolescent Depression

As indicated earlier, systematic study of the etiology and treatment of adolescent depression is of relatively recent vintage. In addition, only a small proportion of depressed teenagers receive treatment. Ideally, the design of treatment-intervention strategies for use with adolescents should be sensitive to the developmental issues critical for this transitional period between childhood and adulthood. For example, according to a popular theory (Erikson, 1968), the major task that needs to be accomplished during adolescence is for the young person to establish a unique identity. While certain types of problems may be especially, and perhaps even uniquely, important for adolescents, the symptom pattern shown by depressed adolescents is very similar to that shown by depressed adults (e.g., Carlson & Kashani, 1988; Friedman et al., 1983; Puig-Antich & Weston, 1983; Ryan et al., 1987). Furthermore, as we reported earlier in this chapter, the psychosocial problems associated with depression in adolescents appear to be very similar to those found with adults. Therefore, it seems reasonable to take the position that etiological models developed for use with adult depressives can be usefully applied to depression in adolescents, even though this position risks disregarding potentially important developmental considerations (Malmquist, 1977).

Acknowledging the aforementioned caveats, there currently exist a variety of psychological treatment approaches that have been shown to be effective with adult depression (Beckham & Leber, 1985; American Psychiatric Association, 1989; McLean & Carr, 1989). Several of these interventions have been recently modified for use with adolescents.

The major treatment approaches in current use are psychoanalytical–psychodynamic, cognitive–behavioral, problem-solving, interpersonal, self-control, and family therapies. We will review each of these interventions, as well as several less commonly used approaches. Because each of these psychological interventions was developed from specific etiological hypotheses, we will briefly present their theoretical underpinnings.

Psychodynamic Therapy

The psychodynamic approach to depression may be traced back to the influential paper by Freud (1917) "Mourning and Melancholia," in which he pointed to some of the important differences and similarities between bereavement and depression. A subsequent paper by Abraham (1927) pointing to the importance of dependency needs in the etiology of depression was also very influential. Beginning with these early papers, psychoanalytical models of depression have emphasized the importance of early mother–infant interaction, the loss (real or imagined) of a love object toward whom the person has ambivalent feelings (Fenichel, 1945; Spitz, 1946), and the conversion of aggressive or hostile feelings into self-hatred (Abraham, 1927; Freud, 1917/1964). Later authors, such as Bibring (1953), extended the psychoanalytical model by postulating that the importance of being unable to achieve one's ego ideals is a cause of depression. Blatt (1974) attempted to integrate earlier work by proposing two forms of depression: *anaclitic depression*, in which the person feels helpless, fears abandonment, and wants to be cared for and loved, and *introjective depression*, a developmentally more advanced disorder in which the person feels intensely inferior, guilty, and worthless.

Recently, Bemporad (1988) has conceptualized depression as a reaction to the deprivation of anything that is important to the maintenance of the depression-prone individual's self-esteem or self-worth (e.g., failure on an exam, personal rejection). Due to a lack of internal psychological resources, depression-prone individuals rely excessively on external support and help to deal with stressful life events. External support is inherently less dependable than internal resources and leaves the person more vulnerable to blows to his or her sense of self-worth.

An important aspect of psychodynamic as well as other older approaches to depression has been the hypothesis that adolescence is a time of increased conflict and turmoil. For one, the internal stabilizers of childhood are no longer available or appropriate. As relationships outside the family become increasingly important, some teenagers become overly reliant on peers and other extrafamilial sources of support. In addition, mental and sexual maturation are occurring. Sexual maturation opens up a new area for exploration, as well as the potential for peer rejection. Mental maturation allows the teenager to more objectively and realistically perceive his or her abilities and liabilities. Thus, Blos (1983) believes that de-idealization of the self and of other objects in the teen's environment represents the most difficult task of adolescence. All the aforementioned pressures and sources of conflict are postulated to create an elevated potential for depression during this period of life. The depression, in turn, may be accompanied by a host of acting-out behaviors, such as truancy, antisocial behavior, drug abuse, and promiscuity.

Perhaps more than others, psychodynamic therapists recognize the importance of attending to developmental issues. Because treatment is undertaken in a person who is still developing, the goal of therapy is to unblock developmental movement and redirect it toward achieving adult status and maturity (Blos, 1983). One of the goals of the psychodynamic treatment of adolescent depressives is to prevent them from making mistaken choices in crucial and far-reaching decisions, such as getting married or dropping out of school, that may reduce anxiety but may also diminish the chances for future individuation.

Psychodynamic treatment is generally individual and long-term, often beginning with an initial phase during which the therapist provides support and reassurance to develop the therapeutic alliance. Sessions typically occur twice a week to develop the therapist–patient relationship and to maintain the momentum of treatment. In addition to understanding of the present condition, exploration of the patient's developmental history is an important component. As in psychoanalytical therapy with adults, interpretation of the transference (in which previous conflicts are reexperienced in relation to the therapist) becomes important in the middle phase of treatment (Lewis, 1991). For transient depressions, i.e., those that occur in teenagers who have the resources to deal with the dysphoria, the creation of a supportive and nonjudgmental "holding environment" by the therapist may be sufficient for the adolescent to find new meaning in his or her life and to restore the sense of self-worth. For others, a longer course of treatment may be necessary to help them develop new mechanisms of maintaining self-worth.

The following case example, adapted from Bemporad (1988), illustrates the psychodynamic approach: The patient, Jane, a 16-year-old young woman, presented symptoms of confusion, anxiety, and panic. When she entered therapy, her initial anxiety subsided and a picture emerged of more long-standing depression, with feelings of alienation and loneliness. Jane had grown up in a wealthy family and had experienced only limited affection and emotional support from a succession of nannies and from her sister.

As Jane and her boarding school peers approached adolescence, the other young women began wearing makeup, dating boys, and occasionally drinking alcohol. Jane experienced all these behaviors as threatening, and she withdrew into her studies. Eventually, even her two closest friends became interested in participating in these activities, which left Jane feeling abandoned. This turn of events was the beginning of intense feelings of dysphoria.

One of the first goals of therapy was to make Jane feel safe and comfortable in her relationship with the therapist. During this initial phase, the therapist attempted to focus on areas of strength and common interests in order to increase the therapeutic alliance. Assuming the role of surrogate parent, the therapist not only showed interest but also encouraged autonomy, supported creative ventures, and accepted setbacks without criticism.

One area of strength for Jane was her fine writing skills. With the encouragement of her therapist, she joined the staff of the school newspaper and a writing club. Her contributions in both groups were valued by her peers. These activities also provided Jane with friendly interactions with boys and girls in a task-oriented, nonthreatening group setting. As a function of these achievements, there was a reduction of her symptoms.

Having made progress, Jane was able to tolerate more introspective explorations of her past. She shared old fears and feelings of inferiority with her therapist, who primarily listened rather than providing interpretations. Gradually, Jane experienced a greater sense of freedom and confidence, which in turn increased her ability to take risks. She sought out new friends and, after initial hesitation, even began dating.

Jane continued therapy in which the therapist assumed a variety of roles. He conceptualized his role, first as a surrogate parent, then as a mentor, and finally as a friend. With this kind of foundation, the therapist began to offer interpretations and to advance the "working through" of unresolved conflicts (Lewis, 1991).

While psychodynamic therapy is one of the most venerable and long-standing treatment approaches, there is unfortunately no controlled research on its effectiveness with depressed adolescents. Nonetheless, given its long history in clinical practice, it is safe to assume that the psychodynamic approach or variations thereof will continue to be employed in the treatment of adolescents. This approach therefore merits closer empirical examination, preferably in controlled treatment-outcome investigations.

Cognitive–Behavioral Therapy

Although the term cognitive–behavioral therapy is often used as though it referred to a single approach, historically it has two distinct and initially separate roots, one in the cognitive theories of Beck (1967), Ellis (1962), and Seligman (1975), the other in the behavioral theories of Skinner (1953), Ferster (1966), Lewinsohn (1974), and Coyne (1976). While more recent interventions often combine aspects of both cognitive and behavioral treatments (e.g., Clarke et al., 1990; Reynolds & Coats, 1986), it is worthwhile to review their underlying assumptions.

Cognitive therapies for depression were originally derived from the theories of Aaron Beck, Albert Ellis, Martin Seligman, and their respective colleagues. Albert Ellis (Ellis & Harper, 1961; Ellis, 1962), the first major cognitive therapist, postulated that irrational beliefs (e.g., one must always be successful) caused people to overreact emotionally (with affects such as depression) to certain antecedent events (e.g., the termination of a relationship). The model of Beck (1967) focuses on a negative cognitive triad that consists of negative views of oneself, one's environment, and the future. These pessimistic cognitions, which arise from a maladaptive developmental history, lead to hopelessness and depression. This theory was followed by the learned-helplessness model of Seligman (1975), which theorized that depression results from experiencing uncontrollable negative events. After encountering an uncontrollable event, the individual develops "learned helplessness," i.e., the belief that his or her behavior has no influence on outcomes. In 1978, in an attempt to address shortcomings of the original learned-helplessness model, Abramson, Seligman, and Teasdale (1978) reformulated it to include assumptions about the way people explain causation, i.e., attribution theory. According to the reformulated model, one's attributional style determines whether aversive experiences actually lead to depression. The "depressogenic" attributional style includes internal, global, and stable attributions for negative events (e.g., "Steve didn't call me tonight because I'm a very unattractive person") and external, specific, and unstable attributions for positive events (e.g., "Steve invited me to his party because the people he really cares about were out of town"). The goals of cognitive therapy are to help the person to become aware of his or her negative cognitions and their destructive impact and to learn to replace these negative thoughts with positive and constructive ways of thinking about experiences.

Modifications of cognitive therapy have been suggested to facilitate its use with adolescents (Emery, Bedrosian, & Garber, 1983; Wilkes & Rush, 1988). The modifications include: (1) emphasis on developing a therapeutic alliance because the adolescent has usually not sought treatment voluntarily; (2) awareness of the developmental facts about adolescence (e.g., the fact that strong emotions are often expressed nonverbally); (3) involvement of the family, given that beliefs and rules about life are developed in that context; and (4) suitable task assignments and the use of reinforcement for homework completion. Rush and colleagues have developed a treatment protocol for cognitive treatment of depressed adolescents (Wilkes, Belsher, Rush, & Frank, 1994).

The central feature of the behavioral theory of depression is the focus on the reduced frequency of behavior of depressives and the conceptualization of depression as an extinction phenomenon. The behavioral model of depression was first introduced by Skinner (1953) and elaborated by Ferster (1966), who suggested that sudden environmental changes, punishment and aversive control, and shifts in reinforcement contingencies can all contribute to the reduced rate of behavior seen in depressives. Lewinsohn and colleagues (Lewinsohn & Shaw, 1969; Lewinsohn, 1974) emphasized the causal impact of a lack of positive reinforcement from pleasurable activities, especially the lack of reinforcement that is contingent on responses of the individual. Deficient social skills were hypothesized to act as important antecedents to the low rate of reinforcement. In addition to a low rate of positive reinforcement, a high rate of aversive experiences was also hypothesized as an antecedent (Lewinsohn & Talkington, 1979). Coyne (1976) complemented this formulation by suggesting that the depressive episode is maintained by the negative responses of significant others to the depressed person's behavior. Although people in the social environment may at first respond to the depressed person with genuine concern and support, over time and with an increase in symptoms, others find the depressed person's behavior increasingly aversive. In other words, the behavioral theory suggests that the depressed adolescent may be subject to any or any combination of the following influences: living in an environment that lacks positive reinforcers or has an excess of aversive contingencies, lacking the skills to elicit positive reinforcement from important others or to terminate aversive contingencies from others, or emitting behaviors that are aversive to others. The goal of behavior therapy is to teach the depressed adolescent skills to change the quality of his or her interaction with the environment.

The following case studies are illustrative of behavioral interventions that have been successfully used with depressed adolescents. McCabe, Mallon-Wenzel, Reid, and Pinkston (1982) report on the use of social-skills training in the treatment of a 19-year-old "neurotically depressed" young woman. On the basis of the patient's presenting complaints of a lack of intimate personal relationships and an inability to initiate and maintain conversations, three behaviors were identified as intervention targets: eye contact, audible speech, and upper body relaxation. The intervention consisted of exercises designed to increase target behavior rates, role-plays in which the targeted behaviors were further reinforced, and homework assignments to generalize the target behaviors to extratherapy settings. All three behaviors showed significant improvement at posttreatment and at a 2-week follow-up. More important, the young woman's depression had significantly abated and her self-esteem had increased.

In a novel use of the Premack principle, Johnson (1971) contracted with a 17-year-old depressed boy to read from a list of positive self-statements as a prerequisite to urination. This intervention was intended to increase a low-frequency behavior (positive self-statements) by making it a precondition for the occurrence of a high-frequency behavior (urination). After 2 weeks, the patient reported that his depressed mood had lifted and that he was experiencing spontaneous positive self-cognitions at times other than before urination. Note that although the behavior targeted for change was increasing positive thoughts, the mechanism through which therapeutic change was effected was based on behavioral theory. This case illustrates the sometimes blurry boundaries between cognitive and behavioral interventions.

McDonald and Campbell (1981) employed a self-administered differential-reinforcement program with a 19-year-old girl with a long-standing history of depression. Over a 7-week period, the patient was taught to self-administer aversive consequences (e.g., cleaning the oven) in response to the onset of depressive mood and to self-reward (e.g., eating chocolate pudding) contingent on the termination of her depressed feelings. At the end of treatment, the young woman had almost completely eliminated her depressed mood, and this improvement was maintained at 6-month follow-up. Specifically, her mean daily rate of depressive ruminations was reduced from 5.5 hours to 15 minutes at follow-up.

Adolescent Coping with Depression Course. Our own earlier research regarding the treatment of depression in adults (Zeiss, Lewinsohn, & Muñoz, 1979) indicated that a variety of cognitive–behavioral interventions were equally effective in decreasing depression level. On the basis of these results, Zeiss et al. (1979) hypothesized that any short-term cognitive–behavioral therapy for depression would be successful if it included an elaborated, well-planned rationale, the provision of skills to handle daily life, the independent use of these skills outside the therapeutic context, and the patient's internal attribution for improvement. These findings and the resulting hypotheses were incorporated into the adult Coping with Depression (CWD) Course (Lewinsohn, Antonuccio, Steinmetz, & Teri, 1984). More recently, we have revised this intervention for use with adolescents. The balance of this section describes, in some detail, the Adolescent Coping with Depression (CWD-A) Course (Clarke et al., 1990).

The CWD-A Course is a short-term, cognitive–behavioral, group intervention for depressed adolescents. An earlier version of the CWD-A Course (Clarke & Lewinsohn, 1986) consisted of 14 2-hour sessions, conducted on a schedule of twice each week for 7 weeks. The revised version (Clarke et al., 1990) consists of 16 2-hour sessions conducted over an 8-week period. Although the CWD-A Course was developed as a group intervention, it can be used in individual therapy.

Treatment sessions are conducted in a classlike fashion, with group leaders teaching adolescents methods of controlling their depressed mood through a variety of skills. Each adolescent is provided with a participant workbook (Clarke et al., 1990), which contains brief readings, structured learning tasks, short quizzes, and forms for homework assignments.

The first CWD-A session reviews guidelines for the group, the rationale of the treatment, and the social-learning view of depression. Participants are taught that being depressed generally results from difficulty in dealing with the stresses of life and that the goal of the course is to learn new skills to better deal with these stresses and thereby gain control over their mood. Figure 2 identifies the specific skills that are taught during each session.

Given that tension and anxiety are frequently reported as problematic by many depressed adolescents, especially in social situations, relaxation training is the first skill taught. Relaxation skills, consisting of the Jacobson (1929) progressive muscle relaxation method, are taught early in the course because they are relatively easy to learn. Providing adolescent participants with an initial success experience may enhance their sense of perceived self-efficacy (Bandura, 1977), which is hypothesized to be a critical component of successful psychotherapeutic interventions (e.g., J. D. Frank, 1957; Zeiss et al., 1979).

Relaxation training is followed by sessions focused on pleasant activities. The goal is to increase the quantity and quality of positive activities. In addition to teaching adolescents basic self-change skills (e.g., monitoring specific behaviors, establishing a baseline, setting realistic goals), these sessions make use of the Pleasant Events Schedule (PES) (Mac-Phillamy & Lewinsohn, 1982), which has been revised for use with adolescents. The PES assesses the frequency and actual or potential enjoyment of 320 potentially pleasant activities (e.g., taking a walk, reading a book) and provides each adolescent with an individualized list of pleasant activities to increase.

The next sessions focus on increasing positive and decreasing negative thoughts. The cognitive sessions focus on identifying, challenging, and changing negative and irrational thoughts. The specific techniques incorporate tactics developed by Rush, Shaw, and Emery (1979) and Ellis and Harper (1961), which were simplified for use with adolescents. Cartoon strips with popular characters (e.g., Garfield the Cat, Bloom County) are employed to illustrate how negative thoughts and beliefs contribute to depression and how positive counterthoughts can be used to challenge or offset the negative beliefs. Through a series of progressively more advanced exercises, adolescents are taught how to apply cognitive techniques to their thoughts.

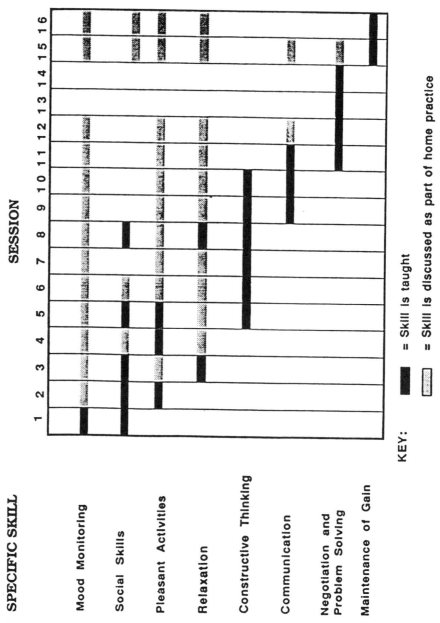

Figure 2. Overview of the Adolescent Coping with Depression Course.

The social-skills sessions focus on conversation techniques, planning more social activities, and strategies for making more friends. In contrast to the other skill areas, social-skills training occurs throughout the CWD-A Course (see Fig. 2), in order to better integrate these skills with the other techniques taught in the class.

The final two sessions focus on integrating the skills learned, anticipating future problems, maintaining therapy gains, developing a life plan and goals, and how to avoid becoming depressed again. Participants identify the skills that they found to be most effective for overcoming their depressed mood. Aided by the therapist, each adolescent develops a written, personalized "emergency plan," detailing the steps he or she will take to counteract feelings of depression should they ever be experienced again.

In addition to the skills described above, which were all modified from the adult CWD Course (Lewinsohn et al., 1984), the CWD-A Course incorporates the teaching of basic communication, negotiation, and conflict-resolution skills, primarily for use with parents. The rationale for teaching communication skills is that familial conflicts normally escalate as teenagers progressively assert their independence and that unsuccessful resolution of these conflicts often leads to reciprocally punishing interactions that in turn may contribute to or maintain the adolescent's depression. The specific negotiation and communication techniques used in the CWD-A Course were adapted from materials developed by Arthur Robin (Robin, 1979; Robin, Kent, O'Leary, Foster, & Prinz, 1977) and John Gottman (Gottman, Notarius, Gonso, & Markman, 1976). The communication training includes feedback, modeling, and behavior rehearsal to correct negative habits (e.g., accusations, interruptions, put-downs). The negotiation and problem-solving skills training uses a four-step model: (1) concisely define the problem, (2) brainstorm alternative solutions, (3) decide on one or more mutually satisfactory solutions, and (4) specify the details for implementing the agreement.

The following case example illustrates the implementation of the CWD-A: Alan was a 14-year-old boy of above-average intelligence whose parents divorced with he was 3 years old. At the time of treatment referral, Alan was living with his mother, stepfather, and a 9-year-old half-brother. His mother sought treatment for Alan to address complaints of dysphoria, socially inappropriate behavior with peers, and extreme daydreaming. Alan often sought out younger children to play with and had underdeveloped self-care skills; e.g., in contrast to most of his same-age peers, he was unable to ride the bus by himself.

Alan participated in a CWD-A group during his summer vacation. Although initially reluctant, Alan offered little resistance to his mother's insistence that he attend the group. During the initial sessions, Alan showed some of his inappropriate behavior (e.g., grimacing, throwing pens or pencils, ignoring comments), which precipitated teasing by the other group members. This teasing was addressed and limited by the group leader, but did not completely cease until Alan's behavior improved later in the course.

Alan learned the social skills quickly, responding positively to role-plays and constructive feedback. His interpersonal behavior, however, reverted to previous age-inappropriate levels during social breaks, suggesting a failure to generalize beyond the role-plays. In the pleasant-activities sessions, Alan complied with all homework assignments, although he was not interested in increasing his level of pleasant activities and did not make any substantial increase in either the number or the type of pleasant events.

In the cognitive-therapy sessions, Alan quickly identified several highly self-denigrating thoughts (e.g., "I'm always going to be a failure"). He understood the concepts of identifying and challenging irrational thoughts and did very well on his homework, spontaneously generating several positive rebuttals to negative beliefs. Alan's overall mood had improved about 50% by this time and continued to improve throughout the remainder of the course. While he still exhibited occasional inappropriate interrupting in the group, prompting from the leader led him to start asking other teens about their interests and hobbies. Over several sessions, he became better at alternating between listening and talking and became increasingly accepted by other group members.

In the final sessions of the group, Alan responded positively to the negotiation-skills training and became quite accomplished in problem-solving and negotiation. He used these skills to achieve limited but tangible objectives with his parents, particularly with his mother, who was more willing to negotiate with him than was his stepfather. The problem-solving paradigm helped Alan to establish a more constructive pattern of interaction with his mother. By the end of treatment, Alan's depression had improved substantially and he was exhibiting much higher rates of prosocial and developmentally appropriate behaviors. At a 4-year posttreatment brief telephone follow-up contact, Alan was attending college, was actively involved in the campus radio station, and had established a small but stable social support network of same-age peers. He had not experienced any further depressive episodes.

In addition to the adolescent CWD-A group, we have developed a separate treatment protocol for the parents of depressed teenagers (Lewinsohn, Rohde, Hops, & Clarke, 1991a,b) that consists of 9 2-hour sessions over an 8-week period. Our rationale for developing the parent protocol was twofold: (1) to provide the parents with an overview of the skills and techniques taught to the adolescents and thereby promote parental acceptance and support for the changes expected of the teenagers and (2) to provide parents with training in the same communication, negotiation, and problem-solving techniques taught to their teenagers.

Problem-Solving Therapy

Nezu, Nezu, and Perri (1989) have formulated a transactional, social problem-solving model of depression and a corresponding treatment approach. The model posits that depressed individuals have poor problem-solving skills, which leave them especially vulnerable to the disruptive effects of major life stressors. Failure to successfully ameliorate the effects of these stressors leads to increased depression, an increased perceived aversiveness of the stressors, and even an increased likelihood that other stressors will occur. These unsuccessful problem-solving experiences are hypothesized, in turn, to lead to an inhibited motivation to engage in future social problem-solving and an even greater vulnerability to future depression. The approach of Nezu and colleagues is consistent with the views of Cicchetti and Schneider-Rosen (1984), who have argued that psychopathology in children and adolescents should be conceptualized in terms of failure to negotiate the important tasks of social–cognitive competency in development. Stage-relevant task mastery is seen as the mechanism by which children and adolescents progress to new levels of cognitive organization.

Nezu et al. (1989) outline a social problem-solving intervention that specifically targets depressive symptomatology. This treatment shares many features with the problem-solving sessions in the CWD-A Course, including problem definition, solution generation (brainstorming), and solution selection and implementation. Nezu et al. (1989) review empirical support for the efficacy of problem-solving treatment (PST) with depression in adults. Unfortunately, PST has not yet been examined as a treatment for depression in adolescents. However, given our clinical experience that problem-solving techniques represent a powerful component of the CWD-A Course, we anticipate that PST will eventually prove to be an effective intervention for adolescent depressive disorders.

Interpersonal Psychotherapy

An intervention that may also prove to be effective for depressed adolescents is interpersonal psychotherapy (IPT) (Klerman, Weissman, Rounsaville, & Chevron, 1984). IPT is a brief psychological treatment originally developed and evaluated for the treatment of depression in adults (Klerman et al., 1984). IPT posits that depression occurs in the context of maladaptive interpersonal relationships, and thus therapy sessions focus on identifying and modifying problematic social circumstances (e.g., prolonged grief, familial conflict, role transitions, interpersonal skill deficits). Therapy focuses on current rather than past interpersonal relationships and is administered in an individual rather than a group format. In the NIMH Collaborative Treatment Study for Depression in adults (Elkin et al., 1989), IPT demonstrated effectiveness equal to antidepressant medication and equal to and perhaps even slightly superior to cognitive therapy.

Moreau et al. (1991) recently modified IPT for use with depressed adolescents (IPT-A). IPT-A is a brief intervention in which weekly therapy sessions are interspersed with telephone contacts between therapist and patient. While treatment focuses primarily on the teenager, parents play an integral role in the initial phase, during which the therapist discusses with them the adolescent's symptoms and need for treatment. The parents may also be seen during the course of therapy regarding changes needed at home and at school. As with IPT, therapy sessions concentrate on interpersonal relationships, but social circumstances particularly salient in adolescence are addressed in more detail, including parent–adolescent conflicts (particularly regarding authority and autonomy), peer pressures (e.g., pressure to engage in drug use), and the problems of single-parent families. In addition to an uncontrolled pilot study of an "IPT-like" psychotherapy conducted by Robbins, Alessi, and Colfer (1989), Moreau et al. (1991) reported that an uncontrolled trial of IPT with depressed adolescents is currently in progress and will direct further modifications and the development of a treatment manual and associated materials such as videotapes.

Moreau et al. (1991) provide case examples of IPT-A, including the following case: Diane, a 16-year-old high school student, sought treatment for recurrent depression. She had been hospitalized at the age of 15, receiving a diagnosis of MDD with psychotic features. During the hospitalization, Diane acknowledged that she had been sexually molested several years earlier by her mother's boyfriend. Diane's mother blamed her for the sexual abuse, and since that time, their relationship had been tense and estranged. After hospitalization, Diane began to have repeated brief sexual encounters with various young men. She thought of herself as a "slut" and a "failure." During this time, she experienced dysphoria, guilt, fatigue, irritability, decreased appetite, hypersomnia, poor concentration, and a lack of interest in usual activities except sex, which she had without pleasure. These problems contributed to her failure to complete the 10th grade.

Therapy focused on Diane's interpersonal deficits, identified by the therapist as confusion between affection and sex; intense dependency needs more appropriate for a child than for an adolescent; and an inability to effectively articulate her needs. In therapy, Diane identified the maladaptive communication patterns in her interpersonal relationships and became more aware of her effect on others. The therapist then helped her develop alternative, more effective, methods of communication. The therapist also helped Diane to recognize the intensity of her dependency needs and to create attainable relationship goals. Diane decreased her number of sex partners and attempted to establish a single, monogamous relationship. As Diane became more aware of her problems, she initially became more dysphoric. However, she felt increasingly less depressed as she began to feel more in control of her problems. Her functioning in other areas improved midway through therapy, and she began to make serious plans for returning to school. As Diane better understood her mother's own problems and became more effective in finding her own sources of love and support, she was less disappointed with her mother, although some tension remained in their relationship.

Self-Control Therapy

Another treatment approach that merits closer examination as an intervention for depressed adolescents is based on the self-control model of depression developed by Rehm (1977). In the self-control model, depression is hypothesized to result from deficits in self-monitoring (e.g., selective attention to negative events), self-evaluation (e.g., unrealistic or perfectionistic standards), or self-reinforcement (e.g., excessive self-punishment). As a treatment approach, patients are taught in a structured, time-limited, group format to identify the specific antecedents and consequences of their behaviors, and then to self-administer reinforcement or punishment or both to increase positive behaviors and decrease depressive behaviors. The efficacy of self-control therapy for adult depression has been demonstrated in a number of studies (e.g., Fuchs & Rehm, 1977; Rehm, Fuchs, Roth, Kornblith, & Romano, 1979). Because aspects of self-control therapy are similar to, and consistent with, other cognitive–behavioral therapies for depression, components of self-control therapy such as self-monitoring and self-reinforcement have been integrated into several treatment programs (e.g., Clarke et al., 1990; Reynolds & Coats, 1986).

Family Therapy

Given the findings that maladaptive parent–child interactions are associated with child and adolescent depression (e.g., Biglan et al., 1985), family therapy is a potentially appealing treatment modality and will be discussed briefly here [the reader is referred to Kaslow and Racusin (Chapter 16) for a more detailed discussion of family therapy].

A variety of theoretical orientations for family therapy exist, including structural or systems therapy (Minuchin, 1974), behavioral family therapy (Alexander, Barton, Schiavo, & Parsons, 1976; Robin, 1979, 1981), and strategic family therapy (Madanes, 1981). A cogent review of these different models as adapted for use with adolescents is provided by Oster and Caro (1990). Although these models clearly differ in specific aspects, the underlying assumption of each is that the adolescent's depression is an expression of more general dysfunction in the family system. In the systems model, the depressed adolescent acts as the identified "symptom bearer" in the family. By expressing overt depressive symptoms, the adolescent distracts the attention of both family members and others away from other disturbed functioning (e.g., the parents' marital problems). According to systems theory, it is inadvisable to address the adolescent's problem behaviors outside the social context in which the behaviors occur (e.g., the family).

The aim of family therapy varies depending on the specific model, but in many cases treatment focuses on the following goals: improving communication among family members, altering dysfunctional patterns of behavior (e.g., a mother keeping the adolescent out of school whenever the teen feels blue, subtly reinforcing expression of depressive symptomatology), and changing maladaptive alliances in the family structure (e.g., a father and daughter allied against the mother, thus splitting and vitiating the normative parental alliance).

Given its greater structure and reasonably explicit treatment manuals, the behavioral family therapy of Robin (1979, 1981) is probably the most likely candidate for research evaluation as a treatment for adolescent depression. While behavioral family therapy has not yet been examined as an independent treatment for adolescent depression, it has been used in the treatment of parent–adolescent conflict (Robin, 1981) and delinquent behavior (Alexander et al., 1976).

Miscellaneous Therapies

Our review of current treatment interventions for adolescent depression is intended to cover the major theoretical orientations rather than to be an exhaustive review. Treatments we did not review include the existential therapies, as represented, for example, by Becker (1964) and Yalom (1980). In existential therapies, "loss of meaning," "authenticity," and "death anxiety" are central constructs. We are not aware of any reports of the use of existential therapy with depressed adolescents.

Another therapeutic approach, kinetic psychotherapy (KPT), has been described by Schacter (1984). KPT is a group approach designed for young adolescents and children that emphasizes nonverbal, gamelike exercises, particularly oriented toward youths who have difficulty identifying and verbalizing their feelings. As depressive reactions come out during the game play, the therapist "stops the action" to facilitate verbalization of the feeling, as well as relevant extragroup experiences. Self-esteem is targeted through repeated emotion-sharing success experiences in the group, as well as success in the game exercises.

A relatively inexpensive and easy intervention that may be effective in treating depression is a program of physical exercise. Aerobic exercise has been shown to be effective in reducing mild to moderate depression in middle-aged as well as older adults (Doyne et al., 1987; Klein et al., 1985). Given its low cost and potential efficacy, physical exercise treatments for adolescent depression should be evaluated.

Treatment-Outcome Research

In the last decade, several investigators have begun examining psychological treatments (primarily cognitive–behavioral interventions) for depressed adolescents in a randomized controlled design. Relatively few studies have been completed, but several are in progress.

In an uncontrolled pilot study of 38 hospitalized adolescents 13–17 years old, Robbins et al. (1989) examined the efficacy of an intensive, multimodal intervention program that included psychodynamically and IPT-oriented individual therapy sessions three times weekly, group therapy sessions twice weekly, and family therapy sessions weekly, combined with cognitive–behavioral-oriented inpatient ward therapeutic milieu. After 6 weeks of psychotherapy intervention, 18 (47%) of these patients exhibited a positive response. The remaining psychotherapy-nonresponsive patients were entered in a subsequent trial of antidepressant medication with continued psychotherapy, with a 92% positive-response rate. The multicomponent intervention makes it difficult to attribute the results to any specific component. Nevertheless, this study is probably representative of what is actually done in many inpatient settings.

Fine, Forth, Gilbert, and Haley (1991) compared two short-term group treatments for depressed adolescents. In their study, 66 teenagers aged 13–17 were assigned to either a social skills training group or a more unstructured therapeutic support group. At the conclusion of the 12-week treatment, adolescents in the therapeutic support groups evidenced greater improvements in depressive symptoms and self-concept. However, the two groups were comparable at 9 months posttreatment.

To our knowledge, only three published studies have addressed the treatment of adolescent depression in randomized controlled trials with a nontreated control condition. In the first study, Reynolds and Coats (1986) identified depressed adolescents on the basis of elevated scores on two schoolwide administrations of the Beck Depression Inventory (BDI) (Beck, Ward, Mendelson, Mock, & Erbaugh, 1961), the Reynolds Adolescent Depression Scale (RADS) (Reynolds, 1987), and a single administration of the Bellevue Index of Depression (BID) (Petti, 1978). The 30 subjects (mean age 15.6 years) culled from this case-finding process were randomly assigned to one of three conditions: (1) a cognitive–behavioral, self-control therapy group; (2) a relaxation therapy group; and (3) a wait-list control. The active treatments were highly structured and were administered in 10 50-minute sessions conducted over a 5-week period. Substantial attrition (30%) occurred over the course of the study, with dropout being disproportionately high in the treatment conditions. Retained subjects in both active treatments showed substantial and equal improvement, which was maintained at a 5-week follow-up. Subjects in the wait-list control group exhibited little improvement at any of the assessments, suggesting that spontaneous recovery is uncommon among untreated adolescent depressives.

Kahn, Kehle, Jenson, and Clark (1990) examined the effectiveness of three active interventions and a wait-list control in the treatment of depressive symptomatology in middle school adolescents aged 10–14 years. Potential subjects were identified using a two-stage, school-based screening procedure similar to that employed by Reynolds and Coats (1986). Two initial screening administrations of the Children's Depression Inventory (CDI) (Kovacs, 1980/1981) and the RADS (Reynolds, 1987) identified an initial pool of subjects, who were then administered the BID (Petti, 1978). Subjects were not diagnostically interviewed. The identified 68 subjects were randomly assigned to one of four conditions: (1) a progressive muscle relaxation group therapy; (2) a cognitive–behavioral group therapy, modeled after the CWD-A (Clarke, Lewinsohn, & Hops, 1990); (3) a self-modeling intervention (Prince & Dowrick, 1984) in which subjects watched videotaped samples of their own behavior, selectively edited to show only desired, nondepressive behaviors; and (4) a wait-list control condition. Significant treatment effects were obtained for all three active treatments relative to the control condition. While the difference was not statistically significant, the cognitive–behavioral intervention exhibited greater positive effects across all outcome measures. Intervention gains were maintained at a 1-month posttreatment follow-up.

In Lewinsohn, et al. (1990), a total of 59 adolescents who met Research Diagnostic Criteria (RDC) (Spitzer, Endicott, & Robins, 1978) for MDD or Intermittent Depression were randomly assigned to one of three conditions: (1) a group for adolescents only ($N = 21$); (2) an identical group for adolescents, but with their parents enrolled in a separate parent group ($N = 19$); and (3) a wait-list condition ($N = 19$). Adolescents and their parents participated in extensive follow-up interviews at intake, posttreatment, and 1, 6, 12, and 24 months posttreatment.

Overall multivariate analyses demonstrated significant pre- to posttreatment change on all dependent variables across treatment conditions. Subsequent planned comparison indicated that all significant subject improvement was accounted for by the two active treatment conditions. Contrary to expectation, there were no significant differences between the adolescent only and the adolescent and parent conditions on diagnostic and self-report outcome variables. The 6- and 24-month follow-up interview data collected for the adolescents in the two active interventions showed that treatment gains were maintained.

Currently, a second clinical trial of CWD-A is in progress. Over a 2-year period, approximately 125 adolescent participants meeting DSM-III-R criteria for MDD or DY will have been entered into the study. Results to date replicate the findings of the earlier study.

Suicide-Treatment-Outcome Research

Several treatment interventions have been specifically developed to address suicidal behavior in adolescents. It is well known that there is a substantial correlation between depression and suicidal behavior (e.g., Crumley, 1979; Andrews & Lewinsohn, 1993), and suicidal behaviors of various kinds are often problematic for depressed adolescents.

A pilot study of cognitive–behavioral family therapy for suicidal adolescents and children has been reported by Sanchez-Lacay, Trautman, and Lewin (1991). The treatment is based on a model described by Trautman and Rotheram-Borus (1988) that incorporates elements of cognitive therapy, social problem-solving, relaxation, self-monitoring, and family communications-skills training designed to reduce conflict (Magana, Goldstein, Karno, Miklowitz, & Jenkins, 1986). All pertinent family members are asked to take part in treatment. In their study, Sanchez-Lacay et al. (1991) randomly assigned female adolescent suicide attempters to either the treatment described above or an "unstructured treatment." Adolescents in both conditions showed equal improvement at posttreatment and at a 5-week follow-up assessment.

Another promising treatment intervention for suicidal behavior is a social problem-solving therapy developed by Lerner and Clum (1990). The treatment is based on the assumption that the key deficit of suicidal individuals is poor interpersonal problem-solving ability in the face of high stress. In this study, 18 subjects, ages 18–24, were assigned to either problem-solving therapy or supportive therapy. Both treatments consisted of 10 sessions conducted over a 5- to 7-week period. Subjects in problem-solving therapy showed greater improvement in regard to depression and problem-solving self-efficacy than those in supportive therapy. Improvements in problem-solving ability and in suicidal ideation were greater for the problem-solving condition, but the differences were not statistically significant. Future research is needed to determine whether comparable findings can be obtained with younger adolescents.

Future Directions

Spectrum of Care

As various interventions are shown to be effective in treating depressed adolescents, it will become possible to incorporate them into a vertically organized "spectrum of care" paradigm in which interventions are ranked or ordered in terms of frequency of required contacts and cost. Specific interventions could then be matched to severity level and to other diagnostic considerations (e.g., suicide risk, existence of comorbid disorder, and the family context in which the depression occurs). In this model, more costly and demanding interventions would be applied only after less costly ones have been ineffective. An example of this approach is the program currently being tested in several schools in Portland, Oregon, by Clarke et al. (1994). Information about depression and suicide (two sessions) is offered to all students in 5 45-minute health class sessions. Then, a modified prevention-oriented CWD-A Course (15 45-minute sessions) is offered to those who have elevated Center for Epidemiological Studies—Depression Scale (CES-D) scores but whose depression is not severe enough to meet diagnostic criteria. Finally, the entire CWD-A Course is offered to those in a current episode of MDD. In a spectrum of care paradigm such as this, adolescents are triaged to the appropriate intervention level on the basis of empirically determined risk or severity factors. Overall, the intent is to minimize inappropriate care, maximize effectiveness, and keep costs low.

Prevention of Adolescent Depression in At-Risk Populations

The intervention efforts reviewed in this chapter have focused on the treatment of adolescents who are already depressed (i.e., tertiary prevention). While the clinically depressed should be provided with treatment, it is clinically and economically preferable to *prevent* depression and to prevent those who are mildly depressed from developing a more severe and prolonged episode (Lewinsohn et al., 1984). Prevention programs should especially be aimed at teenagers who are at increased risk for future depression (i.e., secondary prevention). Examples of populations at risk for clinical depression include "demoralized" adolescents, i.e., those with low levels of persistent but subdiagnostic depressed affect (Lewinsohn, Hoberman, & Rosenbaum, 1988), and adolescents who have depressed parents (Beardslee, Bemporad, Keller, & Klerman, 1983; Downey & Coyne, 1990; Weissman et al., 1984a,b).

Two depression-prevention interventions have been developed for adolescents. Klein, Greist, Bass, and Lohr (1987) developed a school-based "wellness" prevention intervention that was tested in a Midwestern high school. The program emphasized aerobic exercise and made use of an interactive computer program to provide information about depression and other health problems (e.g., venereal disease, drug use/abuse). The aerobic exercise program included before- and after-school jogging, indoor roller-skating, and soccer. Other group activities offered as part of the program included classroom demonstrations, canoeing, and nature trips. Near the end of the school year, 89% of the students had heard of the program and 34% had participated in at least one aspect of the program. Participation was greater for females and for the younger students. Although the program attracted some of the more depressed adolescents, there was no evidence that participation in the program reduced depression. Depression was measured with the depression cluster of the Symptom Checklist-90—Revised (Derogatis, Lipman, & Covi, 1973). For an investigation that was recently completed Clarke et al. (1994) developed a school-based program aimed at reducing the incidence of depression among "demoralized" high-school adolescents. At-risk 9th and 10th grade adolescents are identified by a two-stage screening procedure. A self-report depression scale, the CES-D (Radloff, 1977), is administered schoolwide (stage 1), followed by a diagnostic interview (the K-SADS) with adolescents reporting elevated CES-D scores (stage 2). Those adolescents with a current DSM-III-R depressive disorder are diverted to a CWD-A tertiary treatment group. The remaining subdiagnostic but demoralized adolescents are randomly assigned to either (1) a 15-session cognitive–behavioral preventive intervention, modified from the CWD-A Course; or (2) a "usual care" control condition. All subjects are followed at 6 and 12 months postintervention to evaluate the impact of the secondary preventive intervention on depression symptoms, appropriate treatment-seeking, suicide attempts, school attendance, and other individual and community indices of health and prosocial behaviors. Survival analyses indicated a significant 12-month advantage for the prevention program, with affective disorder total incidence rates of 14.5% for the active intervention vs. 25.7% for the central control. More detail is provided in Clarke et al. (1994).

Relapse Prevention

Although several treatment interventions have already been shown to be effective for adolescent depression and others are currently being evaluated, little systematic information is available regarding the rate of depression relapse in the recovered. Among adult patients, depression is often a recurrent disorder (Belsher & Costello, 1988), with depressed patients having an average of five to six episodes during their lifetime (Angst et al., 1973). Furthermore, it appears that successful treatment is no guarantee against subsequent relapse; approximately 50% of adult patients who are recovered at the end of cognitive–behavioral treatment relapse within 1 year (Gonzales, Lewinsohn, & Clarke, 1985; Keller, Shapiro, Lavori, & Wolfe, 1982). Preliminary results from our adolescent data sets indicate that formerly depressed adolescents also tend to relapse, although the rate may be less elevated. On the basis of incomplete data, approximately 23% of the adolescents in our Treatment Data Set and approximately 15% of those who had recovered from an episode of depression in our community adolescent sample (Epidemiology Data Set) relapsed within the first year.

The importance of developing strategies to prevent depression relapse has been stressed by Peter Wilson and his colleagues (Wilson, 1992). In an early study (Baker & Wilson, 1985), individuals who participated in cognitive–behavioral group treatment for depression received "booster" sessions at 2 weeks, and 1, 2, and 3 months posttreatment. There was no evidence that the additional interventions reduced relapse rates. E. Frank (1986) has suggested the ongoing use of IPT as a maintenance treatment for recurrent depression in adults. Relapse prevention has received considerable attention in other areas, such as substance abuse (e.g., Donovan & Ito, 1988; Emmons, Emont, Collins, & Weidner, 1988; Marlatt & Gordon, 1985; O'Connell & Shiffman, 1988) and schizophrenia

329

Psychological
Approaches in
Adolescents

(e.g., Mintz, Mintz, & Goldstein, 1976; Parker, Johnston, & Hayward, 1988). The methodological and conceptual advances that have been reported in these studies may guide the development of effective relapse-prevention programs for depressed patients.

Unique Needs of Dysthymics

Research and clinical work has not attended to the potentially different treatment needs of those with MDD, those with dysthymia (DY), and those who have "double depression" [an episode of MDD superimposed on a long-standing dysthymic disorder (see Keller & Lavori, 1984)]. While the distinction between MDD and DY has been recognized since DSM-III (American Psychiatric Association, 1980), treatment studies generally have either ignored this distinction or focused exclusively on MDD. McCullough (1991) is one of a growing number of investigators to suggest that treatments specifically aimed at DY need to be developed. He has developed a three-stage cognitive–behavioral intervention in which adult dysthymics are encouraged to accept responsibility for their depression (i.e., it is something that they can control) and to develop strategies to achieve and maintain control over their mood level. The three stages of this program consist of (1) baselining cognitive and behavioral patterns of functioning, (2) learning a six-step situational-analysis task to evaluate the efficacy of their behavior, and (3) generalizing this learning to everyday situations.

Delivery of Treatment Services

Depressed adolescents seek and receive treatment in a wide variety of settings, including inpatient psychiatric hospitals, day hospitals, community clinics, private practice offices, school counselor offices, and general medical clinics. Given the low rate at which depressed adolescents are treated, the relative attractiveness of these varied settings should be studied. Characteristics of the patient (e.g., gender, developmental level) and of the depression (e.g., severity, presence of suicidal behavior) would appear to be potentially relevant factors for future investigation.

An underutilized service delivery setting that warrants exploration is the school. Adolescents are a "captive audience" during the school day (with the important exception of dropouts). Thus, efforts to detect and treat depression in the school setting may be more successful than those using standard mental health service delivery settings. Reynolds and Coats (1986) have successfully used this paradigm, administering a self-report depression screener to all students as a case-finding method, a procedure described in more detail by Reynolds (1986).

One way of introducing depression interventions into the school may be through the auspices of school-based health clinics, which are being developed in many locations (Dryfoos, 1988). Originally developed to address issues of teen sexuality and physical health, surveys indicate that the teen health clinic may be a very good setting for addressing other disorders, such as depression. In a study conducted during the implementation of a comprehensive school-based adolescent clinic, Riggs and Cheng (1988) asked students about their willingness to use a school-based clinic for various health and emotional problems. Interestingly, students who reported depressed mood or past suicide attempt or both were significantly more willing to use the clinic than those who did not report depression. In another survey regarding the kinds of services adolescents would be most likely to seek at a school-based health clinic, Hawkins, Spigner, and Murphy (1990) found that 20% of the sample indicated a desire for a "clinic to treat the blues."

Individual vs. Group Intervention

Most therapists, either by choice or by necessity, work with adolescents in individual or family therapy (Cohen-Sandler & Berman, 1980). The reason for this preference may be theoretical considerations or the difficulty of recruiting the minimum number (three or four) depressed adolescents to begin a group. On the other hand, most treatment-outcome studies have evaluated the efficacy of group interventions, probably because groups are more cost-effective. We have previously compared individual and group cognitive–behavioral therapy for adults with depression and found them to be equally efficacious (Brown & Lewinsohn, 1984; Teri & Lewinsohn, 1986).

The issue of individual vs. group therapy has been difficult to resolve in the treatment literature. The advantages and disadvantages of group and individual therapy have been discussed (e.g., Yalom, 1985). In individual therapy, clients receive more personal attention, enjoy a higher degree of confidentiality, and do not have to "share" the therapist with others. Individual therapy may be necessary for some depressed adolescents because their degree of social withdrawal makes it difficult for them to function in a group context. On the other hand, group therapy may be more effective for interpersonal difficulties, in that groups provide many opportunities to interact with others and to acquire greater skill in interpersonal interaction. Another advantage of group therapy is that the participants often discover that their problems are not unique to them, as they had previously believed. They can also exchange suggestions and support with other group members. Our experience with teen groups has been that feedback from other adolescents regarding irrational cognitions, social skills, and other problems is almost always perceived by the target adolescent as more "believable," and thus often has greater impact, than the same feedback provided by an adult therapist. Group treatments are almost always more cost-effective and probably produce less therapist burnout, which is a problem in any therapy with depressed individuals.

While our experience with groups has been limited to the CWD-A Course, group therapy appears more acceptable to most teenagers than individual therapy. Some report having felt very uncomfortable in prior individual therapy and finding it difficult to form a therapeutic alliance with the adult therapist. Not surprisingly, the degree of perceived group cohesiveness (Yalom, 1985) is a good predictor of outcome among depressed adults (Hoberman, Lewinsohn, & Tilson, 1988). Similarly, preliminary analyses with adolescents in the CWD-A Course reveal that greater group cohesiveness by the third session was significantly associated with recovery by the end of treatment, even after controlling for initial depression level ($r = 0.28$, $p < 0.05$). In conclusion, more treatment-outcome research is needed to evaluate the relative efficacy (and cost) of individual vs. group therapy.

Assessment

Several issues regarding assessment deserve comment. The first involves the sources from which assessment data should be obtained. That is, to what extent do therapists need to gather diagnostically important information from sources other than the adolescent, such as the parents and the school? While information from adult patients is generally considered sufficient, children are considered less reliable sources of information, especially regarding externalizing problems (Loeber, Green, & Lahey, 1990). However, adolescents (ages 14–18) have been shown to be as reliable as adults, showing good test–retest reliability of diagnostic information (Edelbrock, Costello, Dulcan, Kalas, & Conover, 1985) about depression. At the same time, agreement between parent and adolescent is lower than for parent–child dyads (Achenbach, McConaughy, & Howell, 1987). It appears that the adolescent is probably most qualified to report on her or his depression. Nevertheless, it is important to interview parents to understand their perception of the problem.

Another assessment issue is not unique to adolescence. For the most part, diagnoses of depression and other psychopathology have focused exclusively on labeling or categorizing the depressed individual. This practice does not incorporate information about the context in which the depression occurs, i.e., the depressed adolescent's family or living situation. Information about family interaction and the adolescent's role in the family should be assessed. However, because there is no generally accepted methodology for assessing family interactions, this task is not easy. Given the important role of families in adolescent depression, development of an interpersonal diagnostic system might be especially useful for therapeutic work with children and adolescents.

Depression in Medically Ill Adolescents

Although it is often unrecognized and untreated (Perez-Stable, Miranda, Muñoz, & Ying, 1990), a diagnosable depressive disorder is present in approximately 15–20% of seriously medically ill adults (Katon & Roy-Byrne, 1988; Petty, 1989; Thompson, Stoudemire, Mitchell, & Grant, 1983). Consistent with these findings, adolescents with cancer (Kashani & Hakami, 1982; Rait et al., 1988) and chronic diseases such as sickle cell disease, asthma, and diabetes also report significantly more depressive symptomatology than a matched comparison group of healthy teens (Seigel, Golden, Gough, Lashley, & Sacker, 1990). The diagnosis of depression in medically ill adolescents is complicated by the fact that many diseases and medications produce depression-like symptoms, such as fatigue, pain, weight change, and insomnia (Corkery, 1987; Dilsaver, Votolato, & Coffman, 1988; Duer, Schwenk, & Coyne, 1988; Hayes, 1991). Kathol (1985) provides an excellent overview of the difficulties in differentially diagnosing depression in medically ill populations. However, even when medical professionals recognize that a medically ill patient is depressed, they may not see the depression as needing to be treated because the affective disorder is considered to be an "understandable" reaction to the medical illness. Treating the depression in medically ill patients may be especially important because recent and still somewhat controversial findings in the field of psychoimmunology suggest that negative emotional states such as depression may diminish the body's immunological defenses against disease (e.g., Hall, 1987; Syvalahti, 1987). To the extent that such findings are replicated, treating the depression may help maximize immune system functioning, thus improving the chances of survival.

A few studies have reported the results of treatment in adults in whom depression is secondary to a medical condition. Behavioral interventions have been adapted for treating depression in patients with severe rheumatoid arthritis (Appelbaum, Blanchard, Hickling, & Alfonso, 1989) and myocardial infarction (Brown, Munford, & Munford, in press). The CWD Course has been modified for use with patients who have Alzheimer's disease and their caretakers (Reifler, Larson, Teri, & Poulsen, 1986).

We know of no investigations examining the efficacy of psychological treatments for depression in medically ill children or adolescents. Given the substantial comorbidity of depression and physical symptoms and diseases in adolescents (Seeley, 1991), clearly this is a high-priority area deserving more research.

Delinquent Youth

A potentially important target population for depression treatment are adolescents who enter the juvenile court system, because they are at high risk for depression (Alessi, McManus, Grapentine, & Brickman, 1984) and suicidal behavior (Hendren & Blementahl,

1989). The high rate of depression is probably related to the fact that these adolescents have experienced and are experiencing a great deal of stress and frustration, such as constraints on their behavior, legal problems, frequent changes in residence (including being detained), school problems, family conflict, peer conflict, and criminal victimization, and to their inadequate ability to cope with the stressful life events they experience. When treatment is provided to delinquent teenagers, it often focuses on the externalizing problem behaviors, which are typically responsible for their coming to the attention of the court and are perceived as needing remediation.

Bereavement and Depression

The symptoms of mourning occasioned by the loss of a loved one are similar to the symptoms of depression (Clayton, 1979). The acute phase of uncomplicated bereavement generally remits without professional intervention after 6 months to a year (Worden, 1982). If symptoms persist beyond that time, however, health-care utilization tends to increase (McHorney & Mor, 1988) and some form of intervention may be recommended.

Weller, Weller, Fristad, and Bowes (1991) report that 37% of a sample of 38 recently bereaved children met criteria for MDD. Osterweis, Solomon, and Green (1984) reviewed the literature regarding risk factors for increased psychopathology during bereavement in children and adolescents and concluded that early adolescents are especially vulnerable. Other factors that were associated with increased risk for psychiatric disorder following bereavement included the loss of a father for adolescent boys, a conflict-ridden relationship with the deceased, a vulnerable and excessively dependent surviving parent, an unstable living environment, and an unanticipated death (e.g., suicide or homicide).

There are many publications on the use of support groups and other therapeutic interventions with mourners (e.g., Worden, 1982; Melges & DeMaso, 1980; Rogers, Vachon, Lyall, Sheldon, & Freeman, 1980). Although not deemed essential, supportive psychotherapy may be useful even for uncomplicated bereavement to help the person normalize the experience, accept the loss, and redirect interpersonal activities toward the living. It is worth noting that IPT-A includes grief as an area of interpersonal functioning that can be the focus of intervention.

Early behavioral treatments for bereavement typically consisted of habituation exposure to the bereavement cues (Kavanagh, 1990), which often led to reductions in avoidance and distress but no change in the associated depression. Thus, Sireling, Cohen, and Marks (1988) concluded that depressed mood associated with grief was more affected by "nonspecific" efforts to get individuals to engage in and enjoy more pleasant activities. We are unaware of any controlled investigations specifically addressing the efficacy of cognitive–behavioral treatments for depression associated with bereavement in adolescents.

Racial Minorities

The cultural makeup of our nation is becoming increasingly diverse. Tharp (1991) discusses the impact of this cultural diversity on the general theory and practice of psychotherapy with children and adolescents. It is an important issue, given that in the adult literature, nonwhite clients have been found to have much higher rates of therapy dropout, even when the services appear to be similar (Sue, Allen, & Conaway, 1978). Tharp suggests that therapy is most effective when it is compatible with the client's culture and that therapists should modify their approach depending on whether the client is African-American, Asian-American, Hispanic, or Anglo.

Almost all the reported research and case studies in the area of adolescent depression have focused on middle or upper class white adolescents. Given that depression may be accentuated by those negative life stressors that are associated with poverty and nonwhite racial status (Davis, 1990; Lorion & Felner, 1986), one can question the generalizability of the results of current research to adolescents who are nonwhite and of low socio-economic status.

Several investigators have modified interventions for use with minority groups, and we are most aware of modifications of the CWD and CWD-A. The CWD Course has been modified for use as a preventive intervention with Native Americans aged 45 and older who have chronic physical illnesses (Manson, Moseley, & Brenneman, 1988; Manson, 1988). The course was modified to be culturally relevant for reservation tribes and was simplified to accommodate the limitations imposed by the physical illnesses of the participants.

The CWD-A Course is currently being modified for use for the treatment of depression in poor African-American adolescents (Jeanne Robinson, personal communication). Dr. Robinson believes that both the underlying theory and the format of the CWD-A Course make it potentially appropriate, with necessary modifications, for use with this population. Among the proposed changes are modifying the format to include a wider range of language competency, use of more in-session work and less home practice due to a lack of privacy at home, recognition of the increased responsibilities for care of family members that these teenagers may bear, anticipating difficulty with getting to the treatment site, and possible use of financial incentives to reward participation. Dr. Robinson's examination of the CWD-A Course should provide valuable insights into the kinds of modifications that may be indicated.

Comorbidity

The results of numerous studies show that depressed adolescents (as well as adults) have high rates of other psychiatric disorders (Maser & Cloninger, 1990; Biederman et al., 1987; Bernstein, Borkovec, & Coles, 1986). Our own research (Rohde et al., 1991) found that depressed adolescents, compared to nondepressed controls, were at elevated risk for most psychiatric disorders but especially anxiety disorders (18% in the depressed vs. 3% in the nondepressed), disruptive-behavior disorders (8% vs. 2%), and substance-abuse/dependence disorders (14% vs. 2%). Given the high degree of comorbidity, therapists working with depressed adolescents need to carefully assess the possible presence of other psychiatric disorders.

To create homogeneous research samples, most investigations have employed stringent exclusion criteria, which typically exclude from the study depressed adolescents who have psychiatric diagnoses other than depression. Consequently, little is known about the efficacy of treatment with comorbid depressives. Future studies need to examine outcome when depressives are categorized as having or not having another disorder. At this point we do not have answers to many questions, among them these: Given comorbidity, to what extent are standard intervention packages more or less effective? What modifications, if any, are needed to effectively address the complications added by comorbidity?

Parents

An important question in the treatment of adolescent depression is the degree to which parents, siblings, and teachers should be included in the intervention planning and implementation. Many of the treatments reviewed in this chapter recommend the involvement of parents. Given that parental involvement is encouraged, the degree and nature of this involvement vary (Kendall & Morris, 1991). Even though several therapies emphasize the involvement of the parent, only one controlled treatment-outcome investigation (Lewinsohn et al., 1990) has included offering treatment to the parents as part of the experimental design.

On the basis of their review of the outcome literature for family-based and individual psychotherapy with children and adolescents, Fauber and Long (1991) conclude that current research findings do not provide support for the importance of including the parents. Nevertheless, they suggest that if the initial assessment indicates that family processes and issues (e.g., parenting practices, parent–adolescent conflict, inadequate supervision at home) are thought to contribute to the adolescent's problems, family involvement is recommended. Individual therapy may be preferred in those cases in which skill deficits in the adolescent are seen as having a primary etiological role.

It may be hypothesized that parents can positively or negatively impact the maintenance of treatment gains and influence relapse. In the adult treatment literature, there has been a good deal of research regarding the influence of family members (either parents or spouse) in predicting relapse of schizophrenia and depression. Emotional expressiveness (EE) appears to be the most relevant measure of this family influence. EE is a measure of the degree of criticism, hostility, and overinvolvement expressed by relatives toward the patient. Several studies have shown that adult psychiatric patients living with high EE relatives were significantly more likely to relapse than patients living with low EE relatives (Vaughn & Leff, 1976; Hooley, Orley, & Teasdale, 1986). In a sample of 7- to 14-year-old patients hospitalized for depression, Asarnow, Tompson, Hamilton, Goldstein, and Guthrie (1994) found a strong association between EE and outcome 1 year posthospitalization. Children returning to high EE homes were less likely to recover and more likely to relapse.

Confidentiality

An important concern in therapy with adolescents is the extent to which they have a right to and can expect confidentiality. Can the therapist share information obtained from the adolescent with the patient's parents? This issue is complicated by the fact that it is usually the parent who brings the adolescent in for treatment and who pays for it. There are no simple answers to these questions. People *in loco parentis* have a right to some information, such as whether in the therapist's opinion the adolescent is making progress in therapy. Parents also have a right to be informed if their son or daughter is talking about engaging in dangerous behavior. Because of these and other constraints on confidentiality, it is essential to have explicit ground rules that are understood by both the teenager and the parent(s) regarding the boundaries of confidentiality. In cases in which the adolescent's confidentiality is to be broken, the necessity for doing so should be discussed with the patient beforehand. In our clinics, we specify the extent of and the exceptions to confidentiality in an intake letter of informed consent. While consent letters have traditionally been associated with research rather than clinical settings, the complicated nature of the confidentiality issue makes providing such a document useful for all patient-care settings.

Gender Differences

Several issues arise regarding the interaction of adolescent gender and the treatment of depression. First, what, if any, is the impact of same-sex vs. mixed-sex treatment groups? Are there special circumstances in which same-sex or mixed-sex groups would be more appropriate? One way of looking at this issue is within the broader context of homogeneity of groups, in that same-sex groups are, at least in one important respect, more homogeneous than mixed-sex groups. Yalom (1985) suggests that participants in homogeneous groups become cohesive and mutually supportive more quickly, have better attendance, and show more immediate symptom relief. On the negative side, homogeneous groups are thought to remain more superficial. Yalom notes that individuals in heterogeneous groups have a greater potential for growth in long-term therapy. All this, of course, is based on experiences with adults.

Another gender issue is whether the sex of the therapist impacts rate of recovery. Same-sex therapist–client dyads may be perceived by the client as more helpful (Jones & Zoppel, 1982), and a possible solution for group therapy is to use female and male cotherapists. Regarding treatment outcome, Beutler, Crago, and Arizmendi (1986) reviewed the literature pertaining to the effect of therapist variables and concluded that no consistent relation has been found between the gender or sex role identity of the therapist and treatment outcome.

Yet another gender-related issue is that the assessment and treatment of depression be sensitive to gender differences. Carter and Kaslow (1992) review the available research findings in the presentation of depression in adult women. On the basis of these findings, they discuss potential modifications of existing treatments to specifically address sociocultural aspects that may be especially important in the treatment of depressed women (e.g., the central importance of relationships in women's sense of self, the balance between autonomy and intimacy needs). The extent to which these differences and concerns are applicable to adolescent females has not been examined.

Finally, one may ask whether gender-specific treatments or at least treatment components are indicated. This would be the case if etiological agents were found to operate differently in males and females. For example, self-esteem and self-image were closely associated with depression in girls (Allgood-Merten, Lewinsohn, & Hops, 1990). In addition, Friedrich, Reams, and Jacobs (1988) found that in adolescents ages 13–16, depression scores on the BDI were more closely associated with stressful life events in males and with lower social support from peers and family in females. On the other hand, depression in both genders was correlated equally with lower grade point averages. Thus, gender-specific treatment components may yield better results than an intervention that ignores gender differences.

Methodological and Conceptual Issues in Outcome Research

The available results regarding treatments of adolescent depression are encouraging, often achieving an effect size (i.e., mean difference between treatment and control subjects divided by standard deviation for the control group) of 1 or more. However, methodological improvements can strengthen our confidence in the findings of future studies. The relevant issues in conducting treatment-outcome research with depressed adolescents are in many ways similar to those important in conducting clinical trials with adults (e.g., Elkin, Pilkonis, Docherty, & Sotsky, 1988a,b). For instance, the clear specification of what constitutes remission or recovery, relapse, and recurrence will make it easier to compare the results from different studies. The relevance of the recent recommendations (E. Frank et al., 1991) for a consistent terminology regarding the course of depression for adult depressives should be evaluated vis-à-vis their appropriateness for use with adolescents.

Future research should include both diagnostic (dichotomous) and continuous measures of depression for evaluating outcome. In several previous studies (e.g., Reynolds & Coats, 1986; Kahn et al., 1990), self-report measures were the sole criterion to define depression caseness. Although self-report depression scales have been shown to possess good psychometric properties with children and adolescents (e.g., Roberts, Andrews, Lewinsohn, & Hops, 1990; Roberts, Lewinsohn, & Seeley, 1991), they yield many false-positives when contrasted with formal diagnoses.

A related methodological issue is the use of self-report measures as the only measure of change. Conclusions regarding outcome drawn only from patient self-report may be subject to various response biases. Assessment of outcome should employ measures that include reports from the teens, clinical experts who have not been part of the treatment, parents, and perhaps even peers and teachers (Kendall & Morris, 1991) to represent many different perspectives, each of which is important.

A conceptual issue needing attention is the delineation of specific treatment components necessary for improvement and the process(es) that mediate therapeutic change. A general model of therapeutic improvement should include pretreatment variables (e.g., level of depressotypic cognitions, coping skills, adolescent–parent relationship), specific aspects of the treatment, and treatment process variables (e.g., group cohesiveness or therapeutic alliance, therapist skill, participation, and skill acquisition). Relevant to these issues are adult studies examining the mechanisms and processes of change in cognitive therapy (e.g., Jarrett & Nelson, 1987; Persons & Burns, 1985) and dismantling studies of self-control therapy (Rehm et al., 1979) and problem-solving therapy (Nezu & Perri, 1989). Progress in this area has been slow, but similar types of questions need to be raised about the necessary and sufficient conditions for therapeutic change on the part of depressed adolescents. Questions include whether change corresponds to the specific areas targeted by the intervention or is improvement-nonspecific.

Prediction of Outcome in the Treatment of Adolescent Depression

A number of writers have discussed the possibility of matching patients to specific therapies (Paul, 1966; Nelson, 1988). Once it has been shown that a given treatment is more effective than no treatment, research can move toward identifying those patients who are most (and least) likely to benefit from the treatment.

Clarke et al. (1992) investigated the characteristics of depressed adolescents who improved most at the end of treatment with the CWD-A Course. Analyses were conducted examining treatment response via diagnostic and continuous outcome measures. In a discriminant function analysis predicting posttreatment recovery as per diagnosis, the overall canonical correlation was $R = 0.63$ ($p < 0.005$). Better outcome (e.g., no diagnosis of affective disorder) was associated with (1) lower initial levels of self-reported depression, (2) lower initial state anxiety, (3) higher initial enjoyment and frequency of pleasant activities, and (4) more rational thoughts at intake. The second outcome measure consisted of change on the BDI from pre to post. In a simultaneous multiple regression analysis predicting change on the BDI, the multiple R was 0.84 ($p < 0.0001$). Improvement was significantly associated with (1) a greater number of past psychiatric diagnoses, (2) parent involvement in treatment, and (3) younger age at onset of first depressive episode.

Concluding Comment

Considering the relatively short period of time for which the psychological treatments of adolescent depression have been studied, much progress has been made. But even more research needs to be done. We hope this chapter will serve as an impetus to such research.

References

Abraham, K. (1927). *A short study of the development of the libido: Selected papers on psycho-analysis* (D. Bryan and A. Strachey, translators). London: Hogarth Press.

Abramsom, L. Y., Seligman, M. E. P., & Teasdale, J. (1978). Learned helplessness in humans: Critique and reformulation. *Journal of Abnormal Psychology, 87,* 49–74.

Achenbrock, T. M., & Edelbrock, C. S. (1978). The classifications of child psychopathology: A review and analysis of empirical efforts. *Psychological Bulletin, 85,* 1275–1301.

Alessi, N. E., McManus, M., Grapentine, W. L., & Brickman, A. (1984). The characterization of depressive disorders in serious juvenile offenders. *Journal of Affective Disorders, 6,* 9–17.

Alexander, J. F., Barton, C., Schiavo, R. S., & Parsons, B. V. (1976). Systems–behavioral intervention with families of delinquents: Therapist characteristics, family behavior, and outcome. *Journal of Consulting and Clinical Psychology, 44,* 656–664.

Allgood-Merten, B., Lewinsohn, P. M., & Hops, H. (1990). Sex differences and adolescent depression. *Journal of Abnormal Psychology, 99,* 55–63.

American Psychiatric Association (1980). *Diagnostic and statistical manual of mental disorders,* 3rd ed. Washington, DC: Author.

American Psychiatric Association (1987). *Diagnostic and statistical manual of mental disorders,* 3rd ed., revised. Washington, DC: Author.

American Psychiatric Association (1989). *Treatment of psychiatric disorders: A task force report of the American Psychiatric Association,* Vols. 1–3. Washington, DC: Author.

Andrews, J. A., & Lewinsohn, P. M. (1992). Suicidal attempts among older adolescents: Prevalence and co-occurrence with psychiatric disorders. *Journal of the American Academy of Child and Adolescent Psychiatry, 31,* 655–662.

Angst, J., Baastrup, P., Grof, P., Hippius, H., Poldinger, W., & Weis, P. (1973). The course of monopolar depression and bipolar psychoses. *Psychiatricia, Neurologica, et Neurochirurgia, 76,* 489–500.

Appelbaum, K. A., Blanchard, E. B., Hickling, E. J., & Alfonso, M. (1988). Cognitive behavioral treatment of a veteran population with moderate to severe rheumatoid arthritis. *Behavior Therapy, 19,* 489–502.

Asarnow, J. R., & Bates, S. (1988). Depression in child psychiatric inpatients: Cognitive and attributional patterns. *Journal of Abnormal Child Psychology, 16,* 601–615.

Asarnow, J. R., Tompson, M., Hamilton, E. B., Goldstein, M. J., & Guthrie, D. (1994). Family-expressed emotion, childhood-onset depression, and childhood-onset schizophrenia spectrum disorders: Is expressed emotion a nonspecific correlate of child psychopathology or a specific risk factor for depression? *Journal of Abnormal Psychology* (in press).

Baker, A. L., & Wilson, P. H. (1985). Cognitive–behavior therapy for depression: The effects of booster sessions on relapse. *Behavior Therapy, 16,* 335–344.

Bandura, A. (1977). Self-efficacy: Toward a unifying theory of behavioral change. *Psychological Review, 84,* 191–215.

Barnett, P. A., & Gotlieb, I. H. (1988). Psychosocial functioning and depression: Distinguishing among antecedents, concomitants, and consequences. *Psychological Bulletin, 104,* 97–126.

Bashir, M., Russell, J., & Johnson, G. (1987). Bipolar affective disorder in adolescence: A 10-year study. *Australian and New Zealand Journal of Psychiatry, 21,* 36–43.

Beardslee, W. R., Bemporad, J., Keller, M. B., & Klerman, G. L. (1983). Children of parents with affective disorders: A review. *American Journal of Psychiatry, 140,* 825–831.

Beck, A. T. (1967). *Depression: Clinical, experimental, and theoretical aspects.* New York: Harper & Row.

Beck, A. T., Rush, A. J., Shaw, B. F., & Emery, G. (1979). *Cognitive therapy of depression.* New York: Guilford Press.

Beck, A. T., Ward, C. H., Mendelson, M., Mock, J. E., & Erbaugh, J. K. (1961). An inventory for measuring depression. *Archives of General Psychiatry, 4,* 561–571.

Becker, H. S. (1964). *The other side.* New York: Free Press.

Beckham, E. E., & Leber, W. R. (1985). *Handbook of depression: Treatment, assessment, and research.* Homewood, IL: Dorsey Press.

Belsher, G., & Costello, C. G. (1988). Relapse after recovery from unipolar depression: A critical review. *Psychological Bulletin, 104,* 84–96.

Bemporad, J. R. (1988). Psychodynamic treatment of depressed adolescents. *Journal of Clinical Psychology, 49(a)*(Supplement), 26–31.

Bernstein, D. A., Borkovec, T. D., & Coles, M. G. H. (1986). Assessment of anxiety. In A. R. Ciminero, K. S. Calhoun, & H. E. Adams (Eds.), *Handbook of behavioral assessment* (pp. 353–403). New York: John Wiley.

Beutler, L. E., Crago, M., & Arizmendi, T. G. (1986). Research on therapist variables in psychotherapy. In S. L. Garfield & A. E. Bergin (Eds.), *Handbook of psychotherapy and behavior change,* 3rd ed. (pp. 257–310). New York: John Wiley.

Bibring, E. (1953). The mechanism of depression. In P. Greenacre (Ed.), *Affective disorders* (pp. 13–48). New York: International Universities Press.

Biederman, J., Munir, K., Knee, D., Armentrano, M., Autor, S., Waternaux, C., & Tsaung, M. (1987). High rate of affective disorders in probands with attention deficit disorder in their relatives: A controlled family study. *American Journal of Psychiatry, 144,* 330–333.

Biglan, A., Hops, H., Sherman, L., Friedman, L., Arthur, J., & Osteen, V. (1985). Problem solving interactions of depressed women and their spouses. *Behavior Therapy, 16,* 431–451.

Blackburn, I. M., & Smyth, P. (1985). A test of cognitive vulnerability in individuals prone to depression. *British Journal of Clinical Psychology, 24,* 61–62.

Blatt, S. (1974). Levels of object representation in anaclitic and introjective depression. *Psychoanalytic Study of the Child, 29,* 107–157.

Blos, P. (1983). The contribution of psychoanalysis to the psychotherapy of adolescents. *Psychoanalytic Study of the Child, 38,* 577–600.

Brown, M. A., Munford, A. M., & Munford, P. R. (in press). Comparison of behavior and supportive therapy of psychological distress in myocardial infarction/bypass patients. (in press).

Brown, R. A., & Lewinsohn, P. M. (1984). A psychoeducational approach to the treatment of depression: Comparison of group, individual, and minimal contact procedures. *Journal of Consulting and Clinical Psychology, 52,* 774–783.

Cantwell, D. P., & Carlson, G. A. (1983). *Affective disorders in childhood and adolescence: An update.* New York: Spectrum Publications.

Carlson, G. A. (1982). Bipolar illness in adolescents. *Archives of General Psychiatry, 39,* 549–555.

Carlson, G. A., & Kashani, J. H. (1988). Phenomenology of major depression from childhood through adulthood: Analysis of three studies. *American Journal of Psychiatry, 145,* 1222–1225.

Carlson, G., & Strober, M. (1979). Affective disorders in adolescence. *Psychiatric Clinics of North America, 2,* 511–526.

Carter, A. S., & Kaslow, N. J. (1992). Phenomenology and treatment of depressed women. *Psychotherapy, 29,* 603–609.

Chiles, C. A., Miller, M. L., & Cox, G. B. (1980). Depression in an adolescent affective disorder. *Journal of Operational Psychiatry, 37,* 1179–1184.

Cicchetti, D., & Schneider-Rosen, K. (1984). Toward a transactional model of childhood depression. In D. Cicchetti & K. Schneider-Rosen (Eds.), *Childhood depression* (pp. 5–28). San Francisco: Jossey-Bass.

Clarizio, H. F. (1989). *Assessment and treatment of depression in children and adolescents.* Brandon, VT: Clinical Psychology Publishing.

Clark, D., & Mokros, H. (1991). Depression and suicidal behavior. In P. H. Tolan and B. J. Cohler (Eds.), *Handbook of clinical research and practice with adolescents* (pp. 333–358). New York: John Wiley.

Clarke, G. N., Hawkins, W., Murphy, M., Sheeber, L. B., Lewinsohn, P. M., & Seeley, J. R. (1994). Targeted prevention of unipolar depressive disorder in an at-risk sample of high school adolescents: A randomized trial of a group cognitive intervention. *Journal of the American Academy of Child and Adolescent Psychiatry,* in press.

Clarke, G. N., & Lewinsohn, P. M. (1986). *Instructor's manual for the Adolescent Coping with Depression Course.* Unpublished manuscript. Oregon Health Sciences University, Portland, Oregon.

Clarke, G. N., Lewinsohn, P. M., & Hops, H. (1990). *Instructor's manual for the Adolescent Coping with Depression Course.* Eugene, OR: Castalia Press.

Clarke, G. N., Hops, H., Lewinsohn, P. M., Andrews, J. A., Seeley, J. R., & Williams, J. (1992). Cognitive behavioral group treatment of adolescent depression: Prediction of outcome. *Behavior Therapy, 23,* 341–354.

Clayton, P. J. (1979). The sequelae and nonsequelae of conjugal bereavement. *Psychiatry, 136,* 1530–1534.

Cohen-Sandler, R., & Berman, A. L. (1980). Diagnosis and treatment of childhood depression and self-destructive behavior. *Journal of Family Practice, 11,* 51–58.

Corkery, J. C. (1987). Recognition and treatment of depression. *American Family Physician, 35,* 197–200.

Coyne, J. C. (1976). Toward an interactional description of depression. *Psychiatry, 39,* 28–40.

Crumley, F. E. (1979). Adolescent suicide attempts. *Journal of the American Medical Association, 241,* 2404–2407.

Davis, L. (1990). Trends in themes of African-American family research 1939–1989. *Western Journal of Black Studies, 14,* 191–195.

Derogatis, L. R., Lipman, R. S., & Covi, L. (1973). SCL-90: An outpatient rating scale—Preliminary report. *Psychopharmacology Bulletin, 9,* 13–26.

Dilsaver, S. C., Votolato, N., & Coffman, J. (1988). Depression in medical practice. *American Family Physician, 38,* 117–124.

Donovan, D. M., & Ito, J. R. (1988). Cognitive behavioral relapse prevention strategies and aftercare in alcoholism rehabilitation. *Psychology of Addictive Behavior, 2,* 74–81.

Downey, G., & Coyne, J. C. (1990). Children of depressed parents: An integrative review. *Psychological Bulletin, 108,* 50–76.

Doyne, E. J., Ossip-Klein, D. J., Bowman, E. D., Osborn, K. M., McDougall-Wilson, I. B., & Neimeyer, R. A.

(1987). Running versus weight lifting in the treatment of depression. *Journal of Consulting and Clinical Psychology, 55*, 748–754.

Dryfoos, J. G. (1988). School based clinics and their role in helping students meet the 1990 objectives. *Health Education Quarterly, 15*, 71–80.

Duer, S., Schwenk, T. L., & Coyne, J. C. (1988). Medical and psychosocial correlates of self-reported depressive symptoms in family practice. *Journal of Family Practice, 27*, 609–614.

Edelbrock, C., Costello, A. J., Dulcan, M. K., Kalas, R., & Conover, N. C. (1985). Age differences in the reliability of the psychiatric interview of the child. *Child Development, 56*, 265–275.

Elkin, I., Pilkonis, P. A., Docherty, J. P., & Sotsky, S. M. (1988a). Conceptual and methodological issues in comparative studies of psychotherapy and pharmacotherapy. I. Active ingredients and mechanisms of change. *American Journal of Psychiatry, 145*, 909–917.

Elkin, I., Pilkonis, P. A., Docherty, J. P., & Sotsky, S. M. (1988b). Conceptual and methodological issues in comparative studies of psychotherapy and pharmacotherapy. II. Nature and timing of treatment effects. *American Journal of Psychiatry, 145*, 1070–1076.

Elkin, I., Shea, M. T., Watkins, J. T., Imber, S. D., Sotsky, S. M., Collins, J. F., Glass, D. R., Pilkonis, P. A., Leber, W. R., Docherty, J. P., Fiester, S. J., & Parloff, M. B. (1989). National Institute of Mental Health Treatment of Depression Collaborative Research Program: General effectiveness of treatments. *Archives of General Psychiatry, 46*, 971–982.

Ellis, A. (1962). *Reason and emotion in psychotherapy*. New York: Lyle Stuart.

Ellis, A., & Harper, R. A. (1961). *A guide to rational living*. Hollywood: Wilshire Book.

Emery, G., Bedrosian, R., & Garber, J. (1983). Cognitive therapy with depressed children and adolescents. In D. P. Cantwell & G. A. Carlson (Eds.), *Affective disorders in childhood and adolescence* (pp. 445–471). New York: Spectrum Publications.

Emmons, K. M., Emont, S. L., Collins, R. L., & Weidner, G. (1988). Relapse prevention versus broad spectrum treatment for smoking cessation: A comparison of efficacy. *Journal of Substance Abuse, 1*, 79–89.

Erikson, E. H. (1968). *Identity: Youth and crisis*. New York: W. W. Norton.

Fauber, R. L., & Long, N. (1991). Children in context: The role of the family in child psychotherapy. *Journal of Consulting and Clinical Psychology, 59*, 813–820.

Fenichel, O. (1945). *The psychoanalytic theory of neurosis*. New York: W. W. Norton.

Ferster, C. B. (1966). Animal behavior and mental illness. *Psychological Record, 16*, 345–356.

Fine, S., Forth, A., Gilbert, M., & Haley, G. (1991). Group therapy for adolescent depressive disorder: A comparison of social skills and therapeutic support. *Journal of the American Academy of Child and Adolescent Psychiatry, 30*, 79–85.

Frank, E. (1986). Interpersonal psychotherapy as a maintenance treatment for patients with recurrent depression. Unpublished manuscript.

Frank, E., Prien, R. F., Jarrett, R. B., Keller, M. B., Kupker, D. J., Lavori, P. W., Rush, A. J., & Weissman, M. M. (1991). Conceptualization and rationale for consensus definitions of terms in major depressive disorder. *Archives of General Psychiatry, 48*, 851–855.

Frank, J. D. (1957). Some determinants, manifestations, and effects of cohesiveness in therapy groups. *International Journal of Group Psychotherapy, 7*, 53–63.

Freud, S. (1917/1964). Mourning and melancholia. In *Collected Works* (Vol. 14, pp. 243–258). London: Hogarth Press.

Friedman, R. C., Hurt, S. W., Clarkin, J. F., Corn, R., & Aronoff, M. S. (1983). Symptoms of depression among adolescents and young adults. *Journal of Affective Disorders, 5*, 37–43.

Friedrich, W., Reams, R., & Jacobs, J. (1988). Sex differences in depression in early adolescents. *Psychological Reports, 62*, 475–481.

Fuchs, C. Z., & Rehm, L. P. (1977). A self-control behavior therapy program for depression. *Journal of Consulting and Clinical Psychology, 45*, 206–215.

Gonzales, L. R., Lewinsohn, P. M., & Clarke, G. N. (1985). Longitudinal follow-up of unipolar depressives: An investigation of predictors of relapse. *Journal of Consulting and Clinical Psychology, 33*, 461–469.

Gottman, J., Notarius, C., Gonso, J., & Markman, M. (1976). *A couple's guide to communication*. Champaign, IL: Research Press.

Hall, J. G. (1987). Depression, stress, and immunity (letter). *Lancet, 334*, 1467–1468.

Hawkins, W. E., Spigner, C., & Murphy, M. (1990). Perceived use of health education services in a school-based clinic. *Perceptual and Motor Skills, 70*, 1075–1078.

Hayes, J. R. (1991). Depression and chronic fatigue in cancer patients. *Primary Care Clinics, 18*, 327–339.

Hendren, R. L., & Blumenthal, S. J. (1989). Adolescent suicide: Recognition and management in the forensic setting. *Forensic Reports, 2*, 47–63.

Hirschfeld, R. M. A., & Blumenthal, S. J. (1986). Personality, life events, and other psychosocial factors in adolescent depression and suicide. In G. L. Klerman (Ed.), *Suicide and depression among adolescents and young adults* (pp. 213–254). Washington, DC: American Psychiatric Press.

Hoberman, H. M., Lewinsohn, P. M., & Tilson, M. (1988). Group treatment of depression: Individual predictors of outcome. *Journal of Consulting and Clinical Psychology, 56*, 393–398.

Hooley, J. M., Orley, J., & Teasdale, J. D. (1986). Levels of expressed emotion and relapse in depressed patients. *British Journal of Psychiatry, 148*, 642–647.

Jacobson, E. (1929). *Progressive relaxation,* Chicago: University of Chicago Press.

Jarrett, R. B., & Nelson, R. O. (1987). Mechanisms of change in the cognitive therapy of depression. *Behavior Therapy, 18*, 227–241.

Johnson, W. G. (1971). Some applications of Homme's covenant control therapy: Two case reports. *Behavior Therapy, 2*, 240–248.

Jones, E. E., & Zoppel, C. L. (1982). Impact of client and therapist gender on psychotherapy process and outcome. *Journal of Consulting and Clinical Psychology, 50*, 259–272.

Kahn, J. S., Kehle, T. J., Jenson, W. R., & Clark, E. (1990). Comparison of cognitive–behavioral, relaxation, and self-modeling interventions for depression among middle-school students. *School Psychology Review, 19*, 196–211.

Kandel, D. B., & Davies, M. (1986). Adult sequelae of adolescent depressive symptomatology. *Archives of General Psychiatry, 43*, 255–262.

Kanfer, F. H., & Phillips, J. S. (1970). Learning foundations of behavior therapy. New York: John Wiley.

Kashani, J., & Hakami, N. (1982). Depression in children and adolescents with malignancy. *Canadian Journal of Psychiatry, 27*, 474–477.

Kathol, R. G. (1985). Depression associated with physical disease. In E. E. Beckham & W. R. Leber (Eds.), *Handbook of depression: Treatment, assessment, and research* (pp. 745–762). Homewood, IL: Dorsey Press.

Katon, W., & Roy-Byrne, P. P. (1988). Antidepressants in the medically ill: Diagnosis and treatment in primary care. *Clinical Chemistry, 34*, 829–836.

Kavanagh, D. J. (1990). Towards a cognitive–behavioural intervention for adult grief reactions. *British Journal of Psychiatry, 157*, 373–383.

Kazdin, A. E. (1975). *Behavior modification in applied settings.* Homewood, IL: Dorsey Press.

Keller, M. B., & Lavori, P. W. (1984). Double depression, major depression, and dysthymia: Distinct entities or different phases of a single disorder? *Psychopharmacology Bulletin, 20*, 399–402.

Keller, M. B., Lavori, P. W., Beardslee, W. R., Wunder, J., & Ryan, N. (1991). Depression in children and adolescents: New data on "undertreatment" and a literature review on the efficacy of available treatments. *Journal of Affective Disorders, 21*, 163–171.

Keller, M. B., Shapiro, R. W., Lavori, P. W., & Wolfe, N. (1982). Relapse in major depressive disorder: Analysis with the life table method. *Archives of General Psychiatry, 39*, 911–915.

Kendall, P. C., & Morris, R. J. (1991). Child therapy: Issues and recommendations. *Journal of Consulting and Clinical Psychology, 59*, 777–784.

Klein, M. H., Greist, L. H., Bass, S. M., & Lohr, M. (1987). Autonomy and self-control: Key concepts for the prevention of depression in adolescents. In R. F. Muñoz (Ed.), *Depression prevention: Research directions* (pp. 103–124). Washington, DC: Hemisphere.

Klein, M. H., Griest, J. H., Gurman, A. S., Neimeyer, R. A., Lesser, D. P., Bushnell, N. J., & Smith, R. E. (1985). A comparative outcome study of group psychotherapy vs. exercise treatments for depression. *International Journal of Mental Health, 13*, 148–175.

Klerman, G. L. (Ed.) (1986). *Suicide and depression among adolescents and young adults.* Washington, DC: American Psychiatric Press.

Klerman, G. L., Weissman, M. M., Rounsaville, B. J., & Chevron, E. S. (1984). *Interpersonal psychotherapy of depression.* New York: Basic Books.

Kovacs, M. (1980/1981). Rating scales to assess depression in school-aged children. *Acta Paedopsychiatrica, 46*, 305–315.

Kovacs, M., Feinberg, T. L., Crouse-Novack, M. A., Paulauskas, S. L., Pollock, M., & Finkelstein, R. (1984). Depressive disorders in childhood. II. A longitudinal study of the risk for a subsequent major depression. *Archives of General Psychiatry, 41*, 643–649.

Lerner, M. S., & Clum, G. A. (1990). Treatment of suicide ideators: A problem-solving approach. *Behavior Therapy, 21*, 403–411.

Lewinsohn, P. M. (1974). Manual of instructions for the behavior ratings used for the observation of interpersonal behavior. In E. J. Mash & L. G. Terdal (Eds.), *Behavior therapy assessment* (pp. 335–345). New York: Springer.

Lewinsohn, P. M., Antonuccio, D. O., Steinmetz, J., & Teri, L. (1984). *The coping with depression course: A psychoeducational intervention for unipolar depression.* Eugene, OR: Castalia Press.

Lewinsohn, P. M., Clarke, G. N., Hops, H., & Andrews, J. (1990). Cognitive–behavioral group treatment of depression in adolescents. *Behavior Therapy, 21*, 385–401.

Lewinsohn, P. M., Hoberman, H. M., & Rosenbaum, M. (1988). A prospective study of risk factors for unipolar depression. *Journal of Abnormal Psychology, 97*, 251–264.

Lewinsohn, P. M., Hops, H., Roberts, R. E., Seeley, J. R., & Andrews, J. (1993). Adolescent psychopathology: I. Prevalence and incidence of depression and other DSM-III-R disorders in high school students. *Journal of Abnormal Psychology, 102*, 133–144.

Lewinsohn, P. M., & Rohde, P. (1987). Psychological measurement of depression: Overview and conclusions. In A. J. Marsella, R. M. A. Hirschfeld, & M. Katz (Eds.), *The measurement of depression* (pp. 240–266). New York: Guilford Press.

Lewinsohn, P. M., Rohde, P., Hops, H., & Clarke, G. N. (1991a). *Instructor's manual for course for parents of adolescents enrolled in the Adolescent Coping with Depression Course.* Eugene, OR: Castalia Press.

Lewinsohn, P. M., Rohde, P., Hops, H., & Clarke, G. (1991b). *Leader's manual for parent groups: Adolescent Coping with Depression Course.* Eugene, OR: Castalia Press.

Lewinsohn, P. M., Rohde, P., & Seeley, J. R. (1993). Psychosocial characteristics of adolescents with a history of suicide attempt. *Journal of the American Academy of Child and Adolescent Psychiatry, 32*, 60–68.

Lewinsohn, P. M., & Shaw, D. (1969). Feedback about interpersonal behavior as an aspect of behavior change: A case study in the treatment of depression. *Psychotherapy and Psychosomatics, 17*, 82–88.

Lewinsohn, P. M., & Talkington, J. (1979). Studies on the measurement of unpleasant events and relations with depression. *Applied Psychological Measurement, 3*, 83–101.

Lewis, M. (1991). Intensive individual psychodynamic psychotherapy: The therapeutic relationship and the technique of interpretation. In M. Lewis (Ed.), *Child and adolescent psychiatry: A comprehensive textbook* (pp. 796–812). Baltimore: Williams & Wilkins.

Lewis, M., & Miller, S. M. (Eds.) (1990). *Handbook of developmental psychopathology.* New York: Plenum Press.

Loeber, R., Green, S. M., & Lahey, B. B. (1990). Mental health professional's perceptions of the utility of children, parents and teachers as informants on childhood psychopathology. *Journal of Clinical Child Psychology, 19*, 136–143.

Lorion, R., & Felner, R. (1986). Research on mental health interventions with the disadvantaged. In S. Garfield and A. Bergin (Eds.), *Handbook of psychotherapy and behavior change*, 3rd ed. (pp. 739–776). New York: John Wiley.

MacPhillamy, D. J., & Lewinsohn, P. M. (1982). The pleasant events schedule: Studies on reliability, validity, and scale intercorrelation. *Journal of Consulting and Clinical Psychology, 50*, 363–380.

Madanes, C. (1981). *Strategic family therapy.* San Francisco: Jossey-Bass.

Magana, A. B., Goldstein, M. J., Karno, M., Miklowitz, D. J., Jenkins, J., & Falloon, I. R. H. (1986). A brief method for assessing expressed emotion in the relatives of psychiatric patients. *Psychiatry Research, 17*, 203–212.

Malmquist, C. P. (1977). Childhood depression: A clinical and behavioral perspective. In J. G. Schulterbrandt and A. Raskin (Eds.), *Depression in childhood: Diagnosis, treatment, and conceptual models* (pp. 33–59). New York: Raven Press.

Manson, S. M. (1988). *Overview: A preventive intervention trial for older American Indians.* Unpublished manuscript. University of Denver.

Manson, S. M., Moseley, R. M., & Brenneman, D. L. (1988). *Physical illness, depression, and older American Indians: A preventive intervention trial.* Unpublished manuscript. Oregon Health Sciences University, Portland, Oregon.

Marlatt, G. A., & Gordon, J. R. (Eds.) (1985). *Relapse prevention: Maintenance strategies in the treatment of addictive behaviors.* New York: Guilford Press.

Maser, J. D., & Cloninger, C. R. (1990). *Comorbidity of mood and anxiety disorders.* Washington, DC: American Psychiatric Press.

Matson, J. L. (1989). *Treating depression in children and adolescents.* New York: Pergamon Press.

McCabe, M. M., Mallon-Wenzel, C., Reid, W. J., & Pinkston, E. M. (1982). Social Skills training for a depressed woman. In E. M. Pinkston, J. L. Levitt, G. R. Green, N. L. Linsk, and T. L. Rzepnicki (Eds.), *Effective social work practice* (pp. 139–157). San Francisco: Jossey-Bass.

McCullough, J. P. (1991). Psychotherapy for dysthymia: A naturalistic study of ten patients. *Journal of Nervous and Mental Disease, 179*, 734–740.

McDonald, L., & Campbell, D. R. (1981). Operant treatment of depression: A case study. *Psychological Reports, 49*, 327–333.

McHorney, C. A., & Mor, V. (1988). Predictors of bereavement depression and its health services consequences. *Medical Care, 26*, 882–893.

McLean, P. D., & Carr, S. (1989). The psychological treatment of unipolar depression: Progress and limitations. *Canadian Journal of Behavioural Science, 21*, 452–469.

Medlewicz, J. (1985). Genetic research in depressive disorders. In E. E. Beckham & W. R. Leber (Eds.), *Handbook of depression: Treatment, assessment, and research* (pp. 795–815). Homewood, IL: Dorsey.

Melges, F. T., & DeMaso, D. R. (1980). Grief resolution and therapy: Reliving, revising, and revisiting. *American Journal of Psychiatry, 34,* 51–61.

Mintz, J., Mintz, L., & Goldstein, M. J. (1976). Expressed emotion and relapse in first episodes of schizophrenia: A rejoinder to MacMillan et al. *British Journal of Psychiatry, 151,* 314–320.

Minuchin, S. (1974). *Families and family therapy.* Cambridge, MA: Harvard University Press.

Moreau, D., Mufson, L., Weissman, M. M., & Klerman, G. L. (1991). Interpersonal psychotherapy for adolescent depression: Description of modification and preliminary application. *Journal of the American Academy of Child and Adolescent Psychiatry, 30,* 642–651.

National Institute of Mental Health (1990). *National Plan for Research on Child and Adolescent Mental Disorder: A report requested by the U.S. Congress submitted by the National Advisory Mental Health Council.* DHHS Publication No. (ADM) 90-1683.

Nelson, R. O. (1988). Relationships between assessment and treatment within a behavioral perspective. *Journal of Psychopathology and Behavioral Assessment, 10,* 155–170.

Newcomb, M. D., & Bentler, P. M. (1988). Impact of adolescent drug use and social support on problems of young adults: A longitudinal study. *Journal of Abnormal Psychology, 97,* 64–75.

Nezu, A. M., Nezu, C. M., & Perri, M. G. (1989). *Problem solving therapy for depression: Theory, research, and clinical guidelines.* New York: John Wiley.

Nezu, A. M., & Perri, M. G. (1989). Social problem-solving therapy for unipolar depression: An initial dismantling investigation. *Journal of Consulting and Clinical Psychology, 57,* 408–413.

O'Connell, K. A., & Shiffman, S. (1988). Negative affect smoking and smoking relapse. *Journal of Substance Abuse, 1,* 25–33.

Oster, G. D., & Caro, J. E. (1990). *Understanding and treating depressed adolescents and their families.* New York: John Wiley.

Osterweis, M., Solomon, F., & Green, M. (Eds.) (1984). *Bereavement: Reactions, consequences, and care.* Washington, DC: National Academy Press.

Parker, G., Johnston, P., & Hayward, L. (1988). Parental "Expressed Emotion" as a predictor of schizophrenic relapse. *Archives of General Psychiatry, 45,* 806–813.

Paton, S., Kessler, R., & Kandel, D. (1977). Depressive mood and adolescent drug use: A longitudinal analysis. *Journal of Genetic Psychology, 131,* 267–289.

Patros, P. G., & Shamoo, T. K. (1989). *Depression and suicide in children and adolescents.* Needham Heights, MD: Allyn & Bacon.

Paul, G. (1966). *Insight versus desensitization in psychotherapy: An experiment in anxiety reduction.* Stanford, California: Stanford University Press.

Perez-Stable, E. J., Miranda, J., Muñoz, R. F., & Ying, Y. (1990). Depression in medical outpatients: Underrecognition and misdiagnosis. *Archives of Internal Medicine, 150,* 1083–1088.

Persons, J. B., & Burns, D. D. (1985). Mechanisms of action of cognitive therapy: The relative contributions of technical and interpersonal interventions. *Cognitive Therapy and Research, 9,* 539–551.

Petti, T. A. (1978). Depression in hospitalized child psychiatry patients: Approaches to measuring depression. *Journal of the American Academy of Child Psychiatry, 17,* 49–59.

Petty, F. (1989). Depression and medical illness. *American Journal of The Medical Sciences, 298,* 59–68.

Prince, D., & Dowrick, P. W. (1984). Self modeling in the treatment of depression: Implications for video in behavior therapy. Paper presented at the annual conference of the Association for the Advancement of Behavior Therapy, Philadelphia, November 1984.

Puig-Antich, J., & Weston, B. (1983). The diagnosis and treatment of major depressive disorder in childhood. *Annual Review of Medicine, 34,* 231–245.

Radloff, L. S. (1977). The CES-D Scale: A self-report depression scale for research in the general population. *Applied Psychological Measurement, 1,* 385–401.

Rait, D. S., Jacobsen, P. B., Lederberg, M. S., & Holland, J. C. (1988). Characteristics of psychiatric consultations in a pediatric cancer center. *American Journal of Psychiatry, 145,* 363.

Rehm, L. P., Fuchs, C. Z., Roth, D. M., Kornblith, S. J., & Romano, J. M. (1979). A comparison of self-control and assertion skills treatments of depression. *Behavior Therapy, 10,* 429–442.

Reifler, B. V., Larson, E., Teri, L., & Poulsen, M. (1986). Alzheimer's disease and depression. *Journal of the American Geriatrics Society, 34,* 855–859.

Reynolds, W. M. (1986). A model for the screening and identification of depressed children and adolescents in school settings. *Professional School Psychology, 1,* 117–129.

Reynolds, W. M. (1987). *Reynolds Adolescent Depression Scale: Professional Manual.* Odessa, FL: Psychological Assessment Resources.

Reynolds, W. M., & Coats, K. I. (1986). A comparison of cognitive–behavioral therapy and relaxation training for the treatment of depression in adolescents. *Journal of Consulting and Clinical Psychology, 54*, 653–660.

Riggs, S., & Cheng, T. (1988). Adolescents' willingness to use a school-based clinic in view of expressed health concerns. *Journal of Adolescent Health Care, 9*, 208–213.

Robbins, D. R., Alessi, N. E., & Colfer, M. V. (1989). Treatment of adolescents with major disorder: Implications of the DST and the melancholic subtype. *Journal of Affective Disorders, 17*, 99–104.

Roberts, R. E., Andrews, J. A., Lewinsohn, P. M., & Hops, H. (1990). Assessment of depression in adolescents using the Center for Epidemiologic Studies Depression Scale. *Journal of Consulting and Clinical Psychology, 2*, 122–128.

Roberts, R. E., Lewinsohn, P. M., & Seeley, J. R. (1991). Screening for adolescent depression: A comparison of depression scales. *Journal of the American Academy of Child and Adolescent Psychiatry, 30*, 58–66.

Robin, A. L. (1979). Problem-solving communication training: A behavioral approach to the treatment of parent–adolescent conflict. *American Journal of Family Therapy, 7*, 69–82.

Robin, A. L. (1981). A controlled evaluation of problem-solving communication training with parent adolescent conflict. *Behavior Therapy, 12*, 593–609.

Robin, A. L., Kent, R. N., O'Leary, K. D., Foster, S., & Prinz, R. J. (1977). An approach to teaching parents and adolescents problem-solving communication skills: A preliminary report. *Behavior Therapy, 8*, 639–643.

Robin, A. L., & Weiss, J. G. (1980). Criterion-related validity of behavioral and self-report measures of problem-solving communication skills in distressed and nondistressed parent–adolescent dyads. *Behavioral Assessment, 3*, 339–352.

Robins, L., & Regier, D. (1991). *Psychiatric disorders in America*. New York: Free Press.

Rogers, J., Vachon, M. L. S., Lyall, W. A., Sheldon, A., & Freeman, S. J. J. (1980). A self-help program for widows as an independent community service. *Hospital and Community Psychiatry, 31*, 844–847.

Rohde, P., Lewinsohn, P. M., & Seeley, J. R. (1990). Are people changed by the experience of having an episode of depression? A further test of the scar hypothesis. *Journal of Abnormal Psychology, 99*, 264–271.

Rohde, P., Lewinsohn, P. M., & Seeley, J. R. (1991). Comorbidity with unipolar depression. II. Comorbidity with other mental disorders in adolescents and adults. *Journal of Abnormal Psychology, 100*, 214–222.

Rutter, M., Izard, C. E., & Read, P. B. (Eds.) (1986). *Depression in young people: Developmental and clinical perspectives*. New York: Guilford Press.

Ryan, N. D., Puig-Antich, J., Ambrosini, P., Rabinovich, H., Robinson, D., Nelson, B., Iyengar, S., & Twomey, J. (1987). The clinical picture of major depression in children and adolescents. *Archives of General Psychiatry, 44*, 854–861.

Sanchez-Lacay, A., Trautman, P. D., & Lewin, N. (1991). Expressed emotion and cognitive family therapy of suicide attempters. Paper presented at the annual meeting of the American Academy of Child and Adolescent Psychiatry, San Francisco, October 1991.

Schachter, R. (1984). Kinetic psychotherapy in the treatment of depression in latency age children. *International Journal of Group Psychotherapy, 34*, 83–91.

Seeley, J. R. (1991). Adolescent depression and physical illness: Causal predominance and the mediational role of coping. Unpublished master's thesis. Eugene: University of Oregon.

Seigel, W. M., Golden, N. H., Gough, J. W., Lashley, M. S., & Sacker, I. M. (1990). Depression, self-esteem, and life events in adolescents with chronic diseases. *Journal of Adolescent Health Care, 11*, 501–504.

Seligman, M. E. P. (1975). *Helplessness: On depression, development, and death*. San Francisco: Freeman.

Sireling, S. B., Cohen, D., & Marks, I. (1988). Guided mourning for morbid grief: A replication. *Behavior Therapy, 19*, 121–132.

Skinner, B. F. (1953). *Science and human behavior*. New York: Free Press.

Spitz, R. A., (1946). Anaclitic depression. *Psychoanalytic Study of the Child, 5*, 113–117.

Spitzer, R. L., Endicott, J., & Robins, E. (1978). Research Diagnostic Criteria: Rationale and reliability. *Archives of General Psychiatry, 35*, 773–782.

Stark, K. D. (1990). *Childhood depression: School-based intervention*. New York: Guilford Press.

Sue, S., Allen, D. B., & Conaway, L. (1978). The responsiveness and equality of mental health care to Chicanos and Native Americans. *American Journal of Community Psychology, 6*, 137–146.

Syvalahti, E. (1987). Endocrine and immune adaptation in stress. *Annals of Clinical Research, 19*, 70–77.

Teri, L., & Lewinsohn, P. M. (1986). Individual and group treatment of unipolar depression: Comparison of treatment outcome and identification of predictors of successful treatment outcome. *Behavior Therapy, 17*, 215–228.

Tharp, R. G. (1991). Cultural diversity and treatment of children. *Journal of Consulting and Clinical Psychology, 59*, 799–812.

Thompson, T. L. L., Stoudemire, A., Mitchell, W. D., & Grant, R. L. (1983). Underrecognition of patients' psychosocial distress in a university hospital medical clinic. *American Journal of Psychiatry, 140,* 158–161.

Trautman, P. D., & Rotheram-Borus, M. J. (1988). Cognitive behavior therapy with children and adolescents. In A. Frances and R. Hales (Eds.), *Review of psychiatry,* Vol. 7 (pp. 584–607). Washington, DC: American Psychiatric Press.

Vaughn, C. E., & Leff, J. P. (1976). The influence of family and social factors on the course of psychiatric illness: A comparison of schizophrenic and depressed neurotic patients. *British Journal of Psychiatry, 129,* 125–137.

Weissman, M. M., Gershon, E. S., Kidd, K. K., Prusoff, J. F., Leckman, J., Dibble, E., Hamovit, J., Thompson, W. D., Pauls, D. L., & Guroff, J. J. (1984a). Psychiatric disorders in the relatives of probands with affective disorder. *Archives of General Psychiatry, 41,* 13–21.

Weissman, M. M., Prusoff, B. A., Gammon, P. D., Merikangas, K. R., Leckman, J. F., & Kidd, K. K. (1984b). Psychopathology of children (ages 6–18) of depressed and normal parents. *Journal of the American Academy of Child Psychiatry, 23,* 78–84.

Weissman, M. M., Wickramaratne, P., Merikangas, K. R., Leckman, J. F., Prusoff, B. A., Caruso, K. A., Kidd, K. K., & Gammon, G. D. (1984c). Onset of major depression in early adulthood: Increased familial loading and specificity. *Archives of General Psychiatry, 41,* 1136–1143.

Weller, R. A., Weller, E. B., Fristad, M. A., & Bowes, J. M. (1991). Depression in recently bereaved prepubertal children. *American Journal of Psychiatry, 148,* 1536–1540.

Wilkes, T. C. R., Belsher, G., Rush, A. J., & Frank, E. (Eds.) (1994). *Cognitive therapy for depressed adolescents.* New York: Guilford Press.

Wilkes, T. C. R., & Rush, J. A. (1988). Adaptations of cognitive therapy for depressed adolescents. *Journal of the American Academy of Child and Adolescent Psychiatry, 27,* 381–386.

Wilson, P. (Ed.) (1992). *Principles and practice of relapse prevention.* New York: Guilford Press.

Worden, J. W. (1982). *Grief counseling and grief therapy: A handbook for the mental health practitioner.* New York: Springer.

Yalom, I. D. (1980). *Existential psychotherapy.* New York: Basic Books.

Yalom, I. D. (1985). *The theory and practice of group psychotherapy,* 3rd ed. New York: Basic Books.

Zeiss, A., Lewinsohn, P. M., & Muñoz, R. F. (1979). Nonspecific improvement effects in depression using interpersonal skills training, pleasant activity schedules, or cognitive training. *Journal of Consulting and Clinical Psychology, 47,* 427–439.

16

Family Therapy for Depression in Young People

Nadine J. Kaslow and Gary R. Racusin

Despite increasing evidence that "depression runs in families" (Hammen, 1991) and assertions that family therapy is the treatment of choice for a variety of childhood disorders (e.g., Johnson, Rasbury, & Siegel, 1986), little attention has been paid to utilizing family therapy with depressed children and adolescents. To address this deficiency, we begin this chapter with a brief review of the literature regarding the families of depressed children and the linkage between parental depression and the emergence of depressive symptoms in children (for detailed review see Kaslow, Deering, & Racusin, 1994). These streams of literature are reviewed because any discussion of family therapy techniques with this population must be rooted in current knowledge about these families. Due to space considerations, the related body of research focusing on parent–child relations and the etiology of adult depression will not be reviewed here (for a review, see Burbach & Borduin, 1986). Our attention will then turn to a delineation of an interpersonal family therapy (IFT) model that we have developed specifically for work with depressed youths and their families (Kaslow & Racusin, 1988; Racusin & Kaslow, 1991). This model, predicated on family systems theory, cognitive–behavioral psychology, the tenets of object relations theory, and developmental psychopathology, integrates other authors' approaches to family interventions with depressives.

Literature Review

Families of Depressed Children

Depressed children are members of families in which there are high levels of depression, anxiety, substance abuse, and antisocial pathology in mothers and fathers (e.g.,

Nadine J. Kaslow • Department of Psychiatry and Behavioral Sciences, Emory University School of Medicine, Atlanta, Georgia 30322.   **Gary R. Racusin** • Connecticut Mental Health Center, Yale University, New Haven, Connecticut 06516.

Handbook of Depression in Children and Adolescents, edited by William M. Reynolds and Hugh F. Johnston. Plenum Press, New York, 1994.

Mitchell, McCauley, Burke, Calderon, & Schloredt, 1989; Orvaschel, Weissman, & Kidd, 1980; Strober, 1984; Puig-Antich et al., 1989). More specifically, some empirical data suggest that a maternal history of anxiety disorders, substance abuse, and suicidality better differentiates depressed from nondepressed children than does a simple maternal history of depression (Mitchell et al., 1989). Depressed child probands are more likely than their nondepressed psychiatric counterparts to have two parents with a history of a mood disorder (Mitchell et al., 1989). Additionally, these children have members of their extended families who evidence high rates of psychopathology, particularly mood and substance abuse disorders (Puig-Antich et al., 1989). In addition to familial risk factors of parental psychopathology that increase the child's risk for affective disorder, there are child factors (e.g., increased age, prior history of anxiety disorder) that contribute significantly to the family prediction (Lavori, Keller, Beardslee, & Dorer, 1988).

In some families with a depressed child or adolescent, serious family dysfunction and negative life events have been reported, including family conflict; parent–child conflict; marital conflict, particularly regarding child-rearing; parental death, divorce, or separation; and child maltreatment or physical abuse (e.g., Beck & Rosenberg, 1986; Burbach & Borduin, 1986; Forehand et al., 1988; Handford, Mattison, Humphrey, & McLaughlin, 1986; Hoyt, Cowen, Pedro-Carroll, & Alpert-Gillis, 1990; Kaslow, Rehm, Pollack, & Siegel, 1988; Kazdin, Moser, Colbus, & Bell, 1985; Puig-Antich et al., 1985a,b; Trad, 1987; Wallerstein & Corbin, 1991). A modest relationship has been found between childhood depression and maternal rejection (Lefkowitz & Tesiny, 1984), and depressed adolescents report receiving low levels of parental support (Simons & Miller, 1987). Depressed adolescents report less secure attachment to their parents than do nondepressed psychiatric patients and non-psychiatric controls, and there is a significant negative correlation between severity of depression and security of attachment to parents (Armsden, McCauley, Greenberg, Burke, & Mitchell, 1990). However, on remission from a depressive episode, adolescents report levels of security in attachment to their parents approximating that of normal controls. In adolescents who become depressed, difficulties in resolving past familial traumas (e.g., death of a parent, divorce, deprivation) may be salient (Oster & Caro, 1990). This emergence of depression may reflect increased biological vulnerability secondary to experiencing early loss. The increased likelihood of reexperiencing prior traumas during adolescence may complicate the successful negotiation of separation and individuation issues (Oster & Caro, 1990).

Depressed children perceive their families more negatively than do normal children (Kaslow et al., 1988; Stark, Humphrey, Crook, & Lewis, 1990). Specifically, depressed children report their families as less cohesive, more conflictual, and less expressive. They indicate that their parents are more autocratic and thus feel they have little input in decision-making. These families engage in less social, recreational, or intellectual cultural activities (Stark et al., 1990). Additionally, children who are both depressed and anxious report more family dysfunction than noted in families in which the child is only anxious (Stark et al., 1990). Kashani, Burbach, and Rosenberg (1988) compared depressed and nondepressed adolescents' perceptions of family conflict resolution. Results from this study indicated that although both adolescents with depressive symptomatology and psychiatric control subjects reported more verbal aggressiveness and violence during intrafamilial conflict than did normal adolescents, difficulties with conflict resolution were associated with more severe levels of depressive symptoms, irrespective of diagnostic status. Contrary to the aforementioned findings, Asarnow, Carlson, and Guthrie (1987) found no differences in perceived family environments of depressed children and children with a variety of nonpsychotic disorders. However, the suicidal children in this sample did indicate that their families were less cohesive, more conflictual, and less controlled. These conflicting findings indicate that to date, it remains unclear whether or not depressed children report more family dysfunction than nondepressed psychiatric controls, if the nature of this dysfunction is different, or whether or not both circumstances exist.

Mothers of depressed children report less communication with their children than do mothers of normal or neurotic nondepressed children, and the affective tone of the communication appears more negative (e.g., hostile, tense, punitive) (Puig-Antich et al., 1985a,b). This impaired communication, however, improves on remission of the child's depressive episode. Similar communication patterns were reported by mothers in describing the father–depressed child dyad. However, these results were not specific to the child's diagnostic status, but rather were associated with the presence or absence of pathology in the child.

D. A. Cole and Rehm (1986) compared parental standards for depressed and nondepressed children's performance, as well as parent reward strategies for achievement. Few differences emerged in the standards for performance set by the parents of depressed/clinic children, nondepressed/clinic children, and normal controls, and high standards were set for all children. However, the parents of the depressed/clinic children provided lower rates of positive reinforcement and less positive affect for their children's performance.

Amanat and Butler (1984) compared the interaction patterns of families with a depressed child with those of families with an overanxious child. Results revealed that parents of depressed children tended to be dominant and controlling and did not involve the child in the decision-making process. This finding is consistent with the previously noted report by Stark et al. (1990) in which depressed youth described having minimal input in decision-making. The parents of depressed children engaged in such oppressive behaviors as control of the child's life goals, suppression of self-expression in the child, control of the child's choice of friends, and automatic preferences of adult convenience. The depressed children's attempts at self-expression were negated, resulting in submission and feelings of helplessness. In a related vein, a depressed child's pattern of symptom onset is related significantly to the mother's level of emotional involvement (Asarnow, Ben-Meir, & Goldstein, 1987). Children with an acute onset of their depressive episode typically have mothers who exhibit low levels of emotional involvement, whereas children with a more gradual onset of their depressive symptoms typically have mothers who express high levels of emotional overinvolvement.

In addition to the aforementioned empirical studies focusing on family interactions with depressed children, some notions from clinical theory regarding these family interactions deserve note. Clinical theory suggests that characteristic forms of conflict and maladaptive conflict resolution occur in these families (e.g., Racusin & Kaslow, 1991). The most clearly articulated conflictual interactions are parental ambivalence regarding the child's achievements (Slipp, 1984), an alternating pattern of overprotection and rejection (Parker, 1979), and a highly critical and controlling parental stance that results in feelings of helplessness and incompetence in the child (Benjamin, 1974; Racusin & Kaslow, 1991). Further, it is reasonable to hypothesize that similar to families with a depressed adult, families with a depressed child engage in interactions reinforcing depression that can be illustrated in the following way: depression → hostility → rejection → depression (Coyne, 1976, 1984). In other words, a child's depression elicits hostile and rejecting responses from parents who feel unable to provide the support and satisfaction of demands desired by the child. This parental hostility, in turn, contributes to the child's sense of rejection, further exacerbating the depression.

More recent research, however, reveals that the relationship between depressed individuals and others in their lives may present a more complex picture than a pervasive negative reaction characterized by hostility and rejection. Specifically, in addition to feeling angry toward a depressed person, others in that person's life will retain feelings of concern and a willingness to provide concrete support comparable to that offered to nondepressives. This mixture of positive and negative responses to a depressed individual has been observed in the relationships between depressed pregnant adolescents and their primary caregivers (Sacco & Macleod, 1990). Depressed adolescents are likely to feel confused by these mixed messages of anger and rejection on one hand and care and concern on the other. This interpersonal confusion may increase depressed adolescents' feelings of helplessness and decrease their capacity to accept the care that is offered, thus prolonging their depressive state.

Extrapolating from related models (e.g., Feldman, 1976; Teichman & Teichman, 1990) that integrate the cognitive model and family systems theory of Beck (1967), behaviors and cognitive schemata in children and parents are understood to interact in complex ways that perpetuate the depressive cycle. Specifically, the depressed child acts helpless to gain reassurance from the parents. This helplessness triggers the nondepressed parents' cognitive schema of omnipotence, and they reassure the child, thereby further enhancing their own self-esteem. However, this parental behavior subtly reaffirms the child's inadequate sense of self, thus exacerbating the child's depressive cognitions, which further serve to reinforce the child's depression. As a result, the depressed child becomes more hostile and withdrawn in interactions with parents, engendering feelings of rejection and a cognitive schema of depreciation in the parents. To manage these feelings, the parents are likely to engage in depression-inducing behaviors toward their child (e.g., criticism), which exacerbate the child's sense of weakness, thus sustaining the depressive cycle.

Children of Depressed Parents

Results from family and epidemiological research reveal a genetic predisposition in a significant percentage of individuals who develop mood disorders (for a review, see Cytryn, McKnew, Zahn-Waxler, & Gershon, 1986). If one parent has a major depression or if there is a family history of a major depression, there is approximately a 15% risk that any single child will develop depression (Goodwin, 1982). If both parents have a history significant for major depression, the risk rises to 40% for any given child (Goodwin, 1982). To date, however, data from studies attempting to delineate inherited biological factors in these disorders remain inconclusive. Thus, the increased risk for depression in children of depressed parents appears to be a function of environmental variables in addition to genetic factors.

During the past decade, a plethora of literature has examined the influence of maternal depression on children's development (e.g., Beardslee, Bemporad, Keller, & Klerman, 1983; Downey & Coyne, 1990; Gelfand & Teti, 1990; Hammen, 1991; Minde, 1991). At the same time, there has been a dearth of studies examining the impact of paternal depression on children's psychological functioning. The data that do exist suggest that maternal depression is more strongly associated with the overt manifestation of children's psychological symptomatology, particularly affective disorder, than is paternal depression (Keller et al., 1986). However, paternal alcoholism is associated with increased risk for depression in the child (Welner & Rice, 1988). Further, parental concordance for diagnoses, particularly for mood or anxiety disorders, significantly increases the risk for a mood or anxiety disorder in the child (Merikangas, Prusoff, & Weissman, 1988).

Children of depressed mothers evidence a range of behavior-management problems, emotional difficulties, academic deficits, and impaired social competence throughout the course of their lives, even on remission of their mothers' depressive episodes (e.g., Weintraub, Winters, & Neale, 1986). While some of these children appear depressed, others display symptom pictures consistent with diagnoses of conduct disorder, attention-deficit hyperactivity disorder, or anxiety disorder and are at increased risk for suicidal behavior. Other empirical data indicate that young children of depressed mothers exhibit insecure attachments (Radke-Yarrow, Cummings, Kuszynski, & Chapman, 1985). This finding, however, is tempered by similar findings of insecure attachments in children whose mothers evidence a range of psychiatric disorders (e.g., Benoit, Zeanah, & Barton, 1989). Children of depressed mothers have also been reported to exhibit more negative self-concepts (Jaenicke et al., 1987), and researchers have speculated that this low self-esteem may be attributable to children's internalization of the criticism that they receive from their mothers. Further, these negative beliefs about oneself may contribute to a predisposition for later depressive experiences (Hammen, Gordon, Burge, Adrian, & Jaenicke, 1987). The psychological adjustment of these children is mediated by the severity and course of the mother's affective disorder and comorbid psychiatric conditions, level of maternal expressed emotion, severity of marital discord, level of marital strain and stressful life events, problematic parenting behaviors associated with maternal depression, and adequacy of familial social supports (Hammen, 1991; Schwartz, Dorer, Beardslee, Lavori, & Keller, 1990).

Not all children whose parents have serious affective and other psychiatric disorders become symptomatic themselves (e.g., Weintraub et al., 1986). Indeed, a recently emerging body of literature attempts to articulate the individual mediating factors that account for why these children are apparently more resilient and do not develop emotional and behavioral difficulties themselves. Beardslee and Podorefsky (1988) found that youth who were self-aware, invested in interpersonal relationships, and able to function relatively autonomously vis-à-vis their parents were less likely to develop affective symptomatology.

Depressed women experience difficulties in effectively parenting their children. These women tend to be self-absorbed and consequently less attentive to their children's emotional needs (e.g., Anthony, 1983; Billings & Moos, 1983; Cox, Puckering, Pound, & Mills, 1987; Zekowski, O'Hara, & Wills, 1986). They evidence a less consistent style of discipline, are more controlling in their interaction patterns, and are more critical and negative yet conflict-avoidant when they encounter resistance in their children (e.g., Gordon et al., 1989; Kochanska, Kuczynski, Radke-Yarrow, & Welsh, 1987). Additionally, these women perceive their children as more problematic to parent (Whiffen & Gotlib, 1989). The increased incidence of emotional and behavioral difficulties in children of depressed mothers often complicates parenting demands (e.g., Weintraub et al., 1986). These problematic childhood behaviors may be experienced by depressed mothers as stressful and difficult to manage, as their depression interferes with the flexibility and creativity of their parenting strategies (Kaslow & Carter, 1991).

Despite the aforementioned findings, it is important to underscore the considerable variability in interactional patterns between depressed mothers and their children. While some of these dyads manifest impairments, a significant percentage of depressed women appear very warm and appropriately involved with their children (Cox et al., 1987).

Hops et al. (1987) have discussed findings from a methodologically sophisticated investigation examining the interactions between depressed women, their spouses, and their children. Their results revealed a reciprocally suppressing interaction between depressed mothers' dysphoric affect and family members' aggressive affect. Children of these depressed mothers displayed more irritable affect than did children of normal mothers, but only in the presence of concomitant marital distress (Hops et al., 1987). These findings suggest that families with a depressed mother are engaged repetitively in an interactional pattern characterized by alternating negative interactions and avoidance. This pattern perpetuates the individual's depression by preventing expressions of positive affects and adaptive problem-solving that would lead out of this depressogenic interaction. It is interesting to note that in those families with depressed mothers, the children's fathers appeared more caring toward the children than did the husbands of the nondepressed mothers (Hops et al., 1987). A similar pattern of increased caring has been noted in mothers of infants whose fathers are depressed (Zaslow, Pedersen, Cain, Suwalsky, & Kramer, 1985). While this dynamic may sustain beneficial nurturant caretaking to the child, it may also perpetuate the depressed parent's feelings of inadequacy and incompetence (Teichman & Teichman, 1990).

Family Therapy for Depressives

Research over the past decade has revealed that depression is intrinsically bound to a social context (Klerman, Weissman, Rounsaville, & Chevron, 1984), namely, the family (e.g., Keitner & Miller, 1990). Thus, it is not surprising that a number of writers have developed models for marital and family therapy interventions designed to ameliorate major depression in adults (e.g., Beach, Sandeen, & O'Leary, 1990; Clarkin, Haas, & Glick, 1988; Coyne, 1984, 1988; Falloon, Hole, Mulroy, Norris, & Pembleton, 1988; Gotlib & Colby, 1987; Holder & Anderson, 1990; Kaslow & Carter, 1991; Klerman et al., 1984; Teichman, 1986) or to intervene preventatively with families with parental affective disorders (Beardslee, 1990). However, only two empirical studies could be located that examine the efficacy of marital or family therapy or both when the index person is a depressed adult (Friedman, 1975; Glick et al., 1985). These studies provide only partial support for the superior efficacy of marital/family therapy relative to pharmacotherapy and multimodal treatment. Despite this paucity of empirical findings, family interventions with a depressed adult family member are indicated strongly because ongoing family problems and an unsupportive family environment are associated with a more chronic and relapsing course of the family member's depression and an increased risk for suicidal behavior (Keitner & Miller, 1990).

While some writers have underscored the importance of developing a family model for working with depressed youths (Oster & Caro, 1990; Stark, 1990), the only comprehensive model developed to date is that described in our prior writings on interpersonal family therapy (IFT) (Kaslow & Racusin, 1988; Racusin & Kaslow, 1991). There are some data that support the superior efficacy of treatment for depressed youngsters with parental involvement as compared to treatment for the depressed adolescents only. Specifically, Lewinsohn, Clarke, Hops, and Andrews (1990) compared a cognitive–behavioral group intervention for depressed adolescents with an intervention that incorporated this same intervention for the depressed adolescents with a separate treatment module for the parents of these adolescents. A strong trend was found favoring the concurrent adolescent–parent intervention vs. the adolescent-only condition; however, the statistical significance of this difference was minimal.

Family therapy approaches for treating childhood psychopathology have become increasingly popular with accumulating data revealing the association between maladaptive parent–child interactions and child maladjustment. In the specific case of mood disorders, it has been argued that the affective problems of the child are determined and maintained within the context of dysfunctional interactional processes within the family system (Oster & Caro, 1990). Those children who manifest depressive symptoms may be biologically and genetically predisposed to depression as well as responding to family turmoil (Oster & Caro, 1990). Further, the depressed child's difficulties may serve to exacerbate the family problems. Although it is generally agreed that one's family environment influences one's affective development, the specificity of the "depressogenic environment" remains largely uninvestigated (Clarizio, 1989). Despite theoretical writings advocating the implementation of family therapy for depressed individuals and reports describing positive response to such interventions, there remains a paucity of empirical data regarding the efficacy of family interventions for children and adolescents with internalizing disorders (Fauber & Long, 1991).

Model for Assessment and Family Intervention: Interpersonal Family Therapy

IFT, a psychosocial model for clinical assessment and family intervention for depressed school-age children and adolescents, is predicated on family systems theory, cognitive–behavioral psychology, object relations theory, and developmental psycho-pathology. Consistent with the underlying principles of interpersonal therapy (IPT) for depression enumerated by Klerman et al. (1984), IFT assumes that alleviation of children's depressive symptoms is best accomplished by a focus on current problems as they reflect dysfunctional family interactional processes. The intervention focuses on ameliorating psychological symptomatology, enhancing the quality of family interactions, and improving functioning in cognitive, affective, interpersonal, and adaptive behavior domains. In this section, we articulate the assessment process and intervention techniques associated with the model. This presentation also incorporates the work of other clinical researchers regarding the treatment of depression in a family context.

Beginning Phase. The initial phase of IFT has several tasks. These include joining with the family in a way that permits subsequent assessment and therapeutic intervention, conducting the assessment, providing the family with the results of the assessment, and educating the family about the depressive syndrome as it pertains specifically to that individual family. We understand joining with the family as being related to the attachment process that may be particularly salient in working with depressed families. Much of this work entails generic family therapy skills that we will not reiterate here. Rather, we will focus on those skills that are specific to work with depression.

The clinician must demonstrate an empathic understanding of the family's and the child's depression and feelings of helplessness, while also maintaining sufficient emotional distance so as not to be rendered impotent. To achieve this therapeutic stance, the clinician may adjust the pacing of the interview to match family members' own rates of verbal expressiveness, modulate his or her tone of voice, and attend to expressions of distress while simultaneously communicating understanding that implies a sense of hope. Additionally, the therapist must be cognizant of depressed families' propensities to feel helpless, incompetent, and self-blaming and to fear negative evaluation by the therapist. Accordingly, the clinician must communicate respect both for the family members' distress and for their potential to effect positive change. From the beginning, a context should be offered in which engaging in a negative act does not imply that the individual is a failure and in which problematic acts on the part of one family member are not considered a negative reflection of other family members' inadequacies.

Assessment. Those who are present for the assessment and treatment phases are the identified patient child, the parent(s) or principal caretakers, and any siblings. The assessment focuses on understanding the individual child, other family members, and their reciprocal interactions. Thus, for each family member, we recommend assessing psychological symptomatology, life events, and functioning across cognitive, affective, interpersonal, adaptive behavior, and family domains. These domains were selected on the basis of the research demonstrating their relevance to the assessment of childhood depression (Kaslow & Racusin, 1990a). The rationale for assessing parallel behaviors in all family members stems from several variables that potentially contribute to childhood depression. These variables include modeling of depressive behaviors, the influence of parental depression on parenting behaviors, and the operation of a depressive family style exhibited in difficulties modulating sadness and family member's propensity to reinforce and perpetuate the child's depression.

To paint a comprehensive picture of a child's depression, it is essential to utilize a multitrait, multimethod, multiinformant approach to assessment. Assessment data regarding symptoms and functioning across domains can be collected either through a clinical interview format, through more empirically based methods (i.e., semistructured clinical interviews or questionnaires), or through both. Information should be gleaned from a variety of sources (e.g., child, parents, siblings, teachers, peers, clinicians).

Disposition Decision and Guidelines for Therapeutic Modality Choice. Once the assessment data have been organized into a clinical formulation, it is necessary to decide whether or not clinical intervention with the depressed child is required. If such intervention is indicated, we have found several guidelines useful for determining whether or not family therapy is the treatment of choice (Kaslow & Racusin, 1990b). When there are adequate parental resources *and* the identified patient (IP) child has a reasonable degree of ego strength, family treatment is the treatment of choice. When *neither* of these conditions is met, individual treatment is the treatment of choice, as family sessions may prove toxic and exacerbate the child's symptoms. When adequate parental resources are available *or* the child has a reasonable degree of ego strength, then the therapist's predilections are more justifiably utilized for modality selection. To clarify this position, we consider parents to have adequate resources when they love and care for their child, have some capacity to view child behavior from a developmental perspective, evidence the ability to learn from experience, are able to assume a relatively individuated position permitting reflection on their child's thoughts and feelings, and display reasonable frustration tolerance. Children who have adequate ego strength do not evidence serious behavioral or cognitive disorganization. Specifically, with increased internal and external stimulation, their mental status is not significantly compromised and they retain some age-appropriate capacity to modulate verbal and behavioral impulsivity. Additionally, children with adequate ego strength either possess or evidence the potential to acquire age-appropriate adaptive behavior skills.

Additional guidelines pertain to those conditions under which individual and family therapies may best be provided either concurrently or sequentially (Racusin & Kaslow, in press). For example, concurrent treatments should be considered when parents are able to assist their children with some aspects of their development, but not all (e.g., parental discomfort with the child's sadness). In such cases, individual therapy with the child focuses primarily on areas of functioning in which the child cannot obtain adequate parental assistance. Concurrent family work entails providing conditions of safety for expressing strong and painful affects, assisting parents in empathizing with and communicating their understanding of their child's pain, and promoting the family's acquisition of more adaptive interpersonal, cognitive, and behavioral strategies for affect regulation. Another condition under which both modalities may be provided is when the depressed child evidences severe symptoms (e.g., suicidal actions) interfering with age-appropriate functioning, including basic activities of daily living (e.g., personal hygiene, nutrition, school attendance). In some of these cases, hospitalization may be required for the safety of the child, and in such instances, concurrent individual and family work is essential.

In a supportive relationship, individual therapy addresses both intrapsychic and interpersonal issues associated with the child's depression. More adaptive strategies for coping with distressing feelings, thoughts, and situations are explored, practiced, and evaluated. Family work focuses on identifying and modifying dysfunctional interactional patterns exacerbating the youth's depression and associated feelings of hopelessness and suicidality, as well as addressing the reciprocal effects of the youth's depression on family members.

Feedback. Once the assessment phase has been completed, the clinician provides the family with results and recommendations. When family therapy has been deemed the treatment of choice, emphasis during the feedback process is placed on understanding presenting symptomatology and deficits in functional domains as they express the individual child's development, other individual family members' development, and the functioning of the family as a whole. The presenting problem is reframed in terms of an interactional process between the child's symptomatology and the family's functioning. To emphasize that decreased depression in the child or adolescent may require change in each family member, problems and goals are defined in behavioral and interpersonal terms

(Shaffi & Shaffi, 1992). At this point, the clinician utilizes the presentation of assessment results to provide a more general understanding of the phenomenon of depression. This work entails helping family members understand the interpersonal family therapy perspective and how it applies to their unique family and encouraging them to be active observers of their own thoughts, feelings, behaviors, and family interactions. The therapist is active during this phase, noting examples of dysfunctional interactions as they occur and modeling how to recognize messages communicated and the thoughts and feelings of the recipient of the message. In reviewing the treatment plan with the family, the clinician explains that the treatment is a collaborative venture between family and clinician. This clarity is particularly important in families of depressed individuals, in whom a sense of helplessness and hopelessness may be pervasive. Such a collaborative stance empowers the family to assume greater control and hopefulness in alleviating family members' symptomatology and general family distress.

Middle Phase.   Because the domain of family functioning is critical to children's functioning in this age group, we feel that effecting change within the family is essential to the child's overall improvement. To effect improvements in psychological symptomatology, quality of family interactions, and functioning across domains, structural changes may need to occur in the family. These structural changes may include strengthening the executive subsystem, restructuring the familial hierarchy, and facilitating changes in family rules and interaction sequences that support undesirable behaviors (Minuchin, 1974). The family is supported in developing more adaptive interaction patterns, effective coping skills, and approaches to family problem-solving, and these new patterns and skills are practiced within the sessions. This in-session practice provides a context in which the therapist can provide feedback and the effects of these new patterns can be discussed and understood (Holder & Anderson, 1990). Additionally, the family is encouraged to implement these new patterns and strategies outside the therapy session so as to ready family members for ultimate departure from the therapeutic interaction.

Psychological Symptomatology.   In planning interventions for psychological symptoms associated with depression, it is important to evaluate whether or not specialized procedures and reliance on other resources is necessary. For example, suicidal ideation may necessitate involvement of community resources, or hospitalization may be indicated. Similarly, neurovegetative symptomatology may require referring the child to a child psychiatrist for evaluation of the potential efficacy of adjunct pharmacotherapy.

Our underlying assumption is that psychological symptomatology and deficits across other domains reflect systemic dysfunction, with priority placed on family systems dysfunction. In initiating interventions designed to reduce symptomatology, we inquire about potentially precipitating family events. This inquiry includes examining parents' experiences in their families of origin that may have rendered them vulnerable to depressive experiences. The purposes of these inquiries and this work in the middle intervention stage are to establish the correlation between depressive symptoms and family dysfunction, to assist family members in articulating affects associated with systemic dysfunction, and to permit opportunity to work through these affects. Further, this work assists the family in learning more adaptive ways of expressing these affects and of creatively solving problems as a group.

Family therapy that addresses psychological symptomatology focuses on helping the depressed child and the family to develop an understanding of the child's current depressive episode, identifying precipitating stressors, ascertaining potential future stressors both within and outside the family, elucidating family interactional sequences that are producing stress for the depressed child, and planning strategies to cope with future stresses and their impact (Clarkin et al., 1988; Holder & Anderson, 1990). Family members are helped to see that the nature of their responses to their depressed child may either mitigate or exacerbate the child's depressive symptoms and the course of the disorder (Holder & Anderson, 1990). The therapist works to block scapegoating of the depressed child. This scapegoating may reflect parents' frustration that their efforts to reassure their child have not resulted in rapid amelioration of the child's depressive symptoms and that the child cannot make these symptoms disappear simply by an act of will (Bedrosian, 1988).

In educating the family about the child's depression and associated interactional patterns, the therapist assumes the role of expert and teaches the family about depressive processes through a socratic dialogue (Bedrosian, 1988), rather than lecture in an autocratic manner that fosters feelings of helplessness and incompetence. This educational process typically empowers families by reducing their bewilderment regarding their child's difficulties and increasing their sense of hope for change (Holder & Anderson, 1990). Similar processes also set the stage for facilitating changes in the cognitive, affective, interpersonal, adaptive behavior, and family domains.

When the family history is positive for mood disorders and the child's depression is therefore partially an expression of an underlying biological vulnerability, family therapy also includes education regarding the genetics and biological vulnerability of mood disorders (Holder & Anderson, 1990; Klerman et al., 1984). While this education may be sobering for the family, if conducted in an emotionally empathic manner it may reduce the extent to which the child is blamed or feels guilty for depressive symptoms. This appreciation of the child's ongoing risk for depression can sensitize the family to the potential impact of life stressors on the family as a whole and the child in particular. Additionally, when the depressed child's parents experience significant affective disorders, the preventive intervention strategies of Beardslee (1990) for such families may be instituted. Beardslee's approach entails meeting alone with the parents to provide information regarding the etiology of depression, its psychosocial manifestations, the risks to the children, and the adaptive capacities of the child that may enhance resilience. Parents also are helped to discuss their illness with their children and develop future plans for coping with parental depression and its manifestations in family functioning. These children are offered information explaining their parents' difficulties, supported in asking questions, and helped to relieve themselves of any blame for their parents' illness.

Cognitive Functioning. Depressed children have deficits in instrumental responding, feel negatively about themselves and their future, make maladaptive attributions for explaining events, and cognitively distort information [Kaslow, Brown and Mee (Chapter 6)]. It has been hypothesized that these maladaptive thought patterns emerge from family and extrafamilial interpersonal contexts over the course of the individual's development (Stark, 1990; Teichman, 1986). Indeed, a number of researchers have found that the negative explanatory style of depressed children is also observed in their mothers, although not in their fathers (e.g., Seligman et al., 1984). Given that parents' responses to their child affect the way their child thinks, it is important to enlist parents as part of the cognitive-therapy component of the work (DiGiuseppe, 1986).

Depressed children and adolescents may receive repeated messages from family members that contribute to and maintain their depressogenic thinking. Parents may communicate verbally or nonverbally that they are critical or rejecting of their child, which may result in the child's developing a negative self-schema (Stark, 1990). Further, parents may be critical and controlling in communicating their perceptions of the social environment and the unlikelihood that their child will improve, perceptions that when assimilated by the child contribute to negative schemata about the world and the future (Stark, 1990).

Cognitive–behavioral techniques can be integrated effectively with standard family therapy interventions (Schrodt, 1992). Thus, in the cognitive domain, interventions proceed from developmentally informed family systems and cognitive–behavioral perspectives. At one level, this work involves educating all family members concerning the irrational beliefs, cognitive distortions, and depressogenic attributions associated with the child's depression (Stark, 1990). At a second level, it is necessary to challenge and change those cognitive distortions that maintain or exacerbate the child's depression and are evidenced in maladaptive parent–child interactions, verbal communications, and covert or overt rules (Stark, 1990). These cognitive distortions must be addressed wherever they occur in the family so as to ameliorate individual depressive experiences and to alter parent's child-rearing practices that may be reinforcing and perpetuating their child's depression (DiGiuseppe, 1986). Cognitive-restructuring techniques are often useful in modifying these maladaptive family beliefs and rules (Stark, 1990). At a third level, if cognitive distortions reside principally within the child, the therapist may teach the parents to assist their child in identifying and modifying faulty cognitions (DiGiuseppe, 1986). As parents are present more often than is the therapist when the child is acutely depressed, the parents and the child himself or herself can be helped to challenge collaboratively the child's depressive cognitions when evidenced. This process enlists the support of parents in addressing the child's distorted cognitions and educates parents about cognitive strategies for helping their child cope with affectively distressing situations (DiGiuseppe, 1986).

Cognitive-therapy interventions, conducted individually or within a family context, must provide genuine, realistic, and developmentally appropriate interpretations. To do so, the therapist must assess the goodness of fit between the child's perception and the reality of family and environmental circumstances. It is not helpful to a child to reframe his or her negative perceptions in an inaccurate fashion. Rather, when a child is confronted with a negative situation, the therapist and the family must help the child come to terms with the reality of the problem and place the problem in perspective.

Affective Functioning. Sad or dysphoric affect has been considered the sine qua non of the clinical diagnosis of depression in children and adolescents (Poznanski, 1982). The experience and expression of sad affect change over the course of development (Garber & Kashani, 1991). Garber and Kashani (1991) organized the myriad potential elicitors of sad affect in youth into five broad categories: interpersonal losses, material deprivation, victimization, achievement/competence concerns, and physical illness or injury. The first three categories are associated with the family environment and thus deserve specific attention in family therapy interventions. Although the linkage between the latter two categories and the family environment is less immediately apparent, ambivalent family responses to achievement and failure (Slipp, 1984) and family difficulties coping with physical illness or impairment (Seligman & Darling, 1989) may induce or exacerbate a child's sadness. In addition to manifesting negative affects, depressed children also have difficulties regulating these affects in an adaptive and developmentally appropriate manner (P. M. Cole & Kaslow, 1988). Whether they evidence overly enmeshed or disengaged family systems, depressed children's families have difficulties expressing and modulating emotions and conflict (Oster & Caro, 1990). These dysfunctional family processes contribute to dysphoric affect, anhedonia, and affect-regulation difficulties in depressed children and adolescents.

Family interventions in the realm of affective functioning are framed according to the assessment of the developmental capacities of the child and family members (P. M. Cole & Kaslow, 1988; Cicchetti & Schneider-Rosen, 1984, 1986), the nature of the event, and the degree of associated affective intensity. When a depressed youngster presents with deficits in the affective domain, parents are assisted in helping the child ascertain circumstances under which feelings may be expressed appropriately, toward whom, and the correct labels for these subjective experiences. Therapeutic interventions should help the child acquire developmentally appropriate capacities for affect regulation. This process entails assisting the family and other support systems in appreciating the emotional impact of life events on the child and helping the child comprehend and cope with these events. These aims can be accomplished via aiding the child's acquisition of cognitive, behavioral, and interpersonal strategies for affect regulation (Garber & Kashani, 1991).

Children learn about emotions within the context of interpersonal interactions through observation of and direct instruction from their parents. These processes continue over the course of development. Accordingly, if children exhibit deficits in affective regulatory capacities through underexpression of feelings (e.g., anhedonia) or unmodulated expression of sadness (e.g., frequent crying spells), change must be affected in parent–child interactions. Specifically, parents must provide their child response-contingent positive reinforcement, offer a realistic understanding of those events that the child may control, and ensure that the child assumes control where appropriate. Emphasis is placed on helping parents provide direct instruction in developmentally appropriate affect rules. Specifically, they may encourage their child to discuss feelings when upset, rather than act out in behaviorally maladaptive ways or withdraw and emotionally "shut down." Children are also socialized in affect expression via observation of others. Thus, parents may need to demonstrate to children, by their own behavior, appropriate conditions under which to express particular emotions, methods for expressing and regulating these emotions, and consequences that follow on such emotional expression (Garber & Kashani, 1991).

The therapist must attend to the presence of parental depression and its effects on the child. In some cases, children of depressed parents imitate their parents' depressed mood state and exhibit sadness themselves. In other instances, these children may be reluctant to express distressing affects in an effort to protect their depressed parent. In either case, family intervention entails helping the depressed parent modulate affective distress more adaptively in order to provide a context that will support healthy emotional development in the child. Concurrent with the aforementioned efforts with the parents and the family unit, the therapist works directly with the child to develop self-regulating cognitive and personal strategies for coping with emotions and for accepting nurturant caretaking in a developmentally appropriate manner.

Interpersonal Functioning. Depressed children often exhibit deficits in interpersonal functioning with siblings and peers and engage in few pleasurable activities with their age-mates. IFT emphasizes the importance of parents' providing the child opportunities to engage in age-appropriate peer activities and practice peer-relationship skills. Engaging in pleasurable family activities, some involving all family members and others only the sibship, is also stressed. Activity scheduling can be used to increase the activity level of the family in which depression prevails (Stark, 1990). Activity scheduling must incorporate input from all family members and appreciate the family's financial resources and the practical constraints imposed by work and school (Stark, 1990). As models for peer-interaction skills, the importance of parents' participating in adult activities as a couple and with peers is underlined. Family members are also encouraged to help one another with interpersonal problem-solving. Should parents manifest marital or individual deficits that impede their capacity to undertake the aforementioned behaviors, it may be necessary to address these deficits prior to focusing on enhancing their parenting skills. When parents are unable to facilitate improved interpersonal functioning for their child or when children exhibit more profound peer-relationship deficits, the potential efficacy of child group treatment should be considered.

Adaptive Behavior. IFT in the adaptive behavior domain educates parents and children about age-appropriate adaptive behaviors and how their acquisition has been compromised secondary to the child's depression and the depressive process of the family as a whole. Specifically, the child's deficits in communication skills are addressed by pointing out ways family members speak for the depressed child, ignore the child's efforts to communicate, or refute or devalue the child's assertions. The child's impaired utilization of age-appropriate daily living skills is addressed in two principal ways. First, for those children who have not acquired these skills because of inadequate parenting, the parents are helped to teach their child these skills systematically. The parenting deficit associated with the depressed child's lack of appropriate daily living skills is understood to reflect the parents' own depression (e.g., lack of available energy) or a dysfunctional family system (e.g., the parents' need to sustain the child's dependence). Second, for those children who fail to utilize acquired age-appropriate daily living skills, parents are supported in developing creative strategies for encouraging and reinforcing their child's use of these skills. Treatment regarding impaired socialization skills was discussed earlier in the interpersonal domain.

Family Functioning.   IFT for the family domain addresses the needs of all family members by identifying problematic family patterns and their origins and facilitating alternative interactional patterns that will lead out of the depressive cycle. Dysfunctional verbal and nonverbal patterns and discrepancies between the two are delineated, and family members are encouraged to communicate in a more congruent fashion. Whenever possible, more affectively positive communications are encouraged, with particular attention paid to decreasing critical tone and rejecting comments and to increasing positive reinforcement and adaptive conflict resolution. Further, parents are assisted in bolstering their own self-esteem in ways that do not inhibit the child's development and in supporting the child's self-expression and involvement in decision-making, which decrease the child's sense of helplessness. Interventions in the family domain view cognitions, emotions, behaviors, and interactions as interrelated and focus on helping the family discover the intrapsychic and interpersonal mechanisms that are maintaining depressogenic interrelations between these variables (Teichman & Teichman, 1990). This information is then used to aid the family in developing alternative and more adaptive modes of reciprocal interaction. The therapist's task is to promote this change process.

The first step in addressing family systems difficulties is to "map" the family structure, focusing on subsystems, boundaries, and family members' roles (Minuchin, 1974). When a family map reveals that a child's depression is a function of the role played in the family (e.g., mediator of parental marital conflict), the therapist helps the family redefine the child's role to reduce associated stresses that are contributing to the child's depression (Freeman, Epstein, & Simon, 1986). If the depressed youth is triangulated either by having to buffer two conflicting family members or by detouring his or her conflict with another family member through a third party, the therapist helps the child disengage from the triangle and encourages the conflicting parties to engage each other directly (Bedrosian, 1988). In addition to implementing these structural changes, the therapist assists family members in changing their cognitions so as to prevent the depressed child from resuming a triangulated position.

As noted earlier, there are a variety of problematic interactional patterns that characterize families of depressed children, each of which requires unique intervention planning. In families in which conflict entails parents' ambivalence regarding the child's achievement, parents are assisted in exploring sources of this ambivalence, which typically lie in their families of origin. As this work progresses, the depressed child is less likely to be employed as an object of the parents' projection residual to their family of origin experiences, thus freeing the parents to be more genuinely reinforcing of their child's developmental strivings for achievement and actual accomplishments. Work with the children focuses initially on feelings of helplessness and hopelessness in the achievement domain, and the therapist helps them feel empowered to pursue higher levels of achievement. As the parents become more able to fulfill the role of empowering and rewarding their children for social, academic, athletic, and artistic achievements, the children are assisted in perceiving more accurately these changes in their parents' ways of interacting with and reinforcing them.

Other families are characterized by oscillation between parental overinvolvement with and distancing from the child, parental belittling and controlling of their children, or familial neglect and indulgence of the depressed child's needs. In these families, therapeutic intervention focuses on illuminating these patterns and assisting parents in maintaining a more evenly present and positive attachment to their child. This change results in the child's feeling more lovable, less depressed, and more supported. In order to accomplish this change, parents are assisted in providing more consistent and nurturing caretaking and in positively reinforcing the child's accomplishments and acquisition of developmentally appropriate adaptive behaviors. Work with the child often challenges the distorted inferences that the child frequently draws from his or her own behavior and performance and fosters the child's ability to respond to the differences in the parents' behavior and to reward the parents for their increased support and encouragement. In addition, this work attempts to engender more integrated, developmentally appropriate internal representations of the parent in the child. In doing so, the child's capacity to sustain attachment to the parents, despite the parents' periodic expressions of negative affect, is enhanced. This attachment in turn increases the likelihood that the child will recognize and accept nurturance and positive reinforcement when they are forthcoming from the parents.

Through this work, family members develop a more positive sense of themselves and their self-efficacy, increased comfort with intimacy and attachment, and a more differentiated and cohesive sense of self. It is to be hoped that the frequency and intensity of unresolved conflictual interactions will decrease and the family's ability to effectively problem-solve, cope with crises, and negotiate differences will increase. Additionally, if the effort is successful, each family member feels an enhanced sense of personal and family identity and esteem, experiences age-appropriate involvement in personal and family decision-making, and derives a greater sense of hope and a more positive outlook on the future.

Concluding Phase.   The several tasks of the concluding phase of IFT derive from the description by Klerman et al. (1984) of the termination phase of interpersonal therapy for depression. The first task entails explicitly acknowledging the impending conclusion of treatment. It is essential to clarify this reality and the conclusion of the therapeutic relationship so that the additional work of the concluding phase may proceed. The second task is focusing on the grief evoked at the conclusion of treatment. This grief reaction may reflect a generic response to loss of relationships with others and a more immediate loss of the connection between the therapist and the family. The third task emphasizes the family's acquired competence to deal more adaptively with distressing life events, capitalizing on the family unit as a resource for coping with such events.

Typically, the concluding phase of family intervention with depressed youngsters entails the reemergence of psychological symptomatology and dysfunction across domains of functioning. In general, it is hypothesized that this regression manifests the family's question as to the appropriateness of concluding the work. It is helpful to note the particular domain(s) in which the greatest regression occurs, as particular areas of dysfunction can point to possible additional required interventions meriting discussion with the family. For example, group treatment may be recommended to address peer-relationship deficits residual to depressive episodes. Regression in one or more family members is interpreted as reflecting a reemerging family-wide depressive experience, in this instance associated with loss and anxiety about facing the future without the therapist's support. Additionally, then, the family's previously demonstrated capacity to problem-solve is reiterated, and the concluding phase becomes a laboratory for practicing acquired skills prior to the family's final termination of therapy. Bringing these issues to the family's awareness typically suffices to return the family to a more competent and less depressed stance. Therapists must entertain the possibility, however, that additional interventions may be required to assist the family in dealing with the complexities that contribute to depression in children and families.

Concluding Comments

Our review of the literature indicates an emerging understanding of the complexities of the families of depressed children. However, further research is needed to shed light on the unique and differentiating characteristics and interaction patterns of these families. A particularly glaring absence of knowledge pertains to the siblings of depressed children and to the sibling subsystem. One potentially fruitful approach to carrying out research on these families is to ascertain the applicability of conceptual and empirical models of the interpersonal functioning of depressed adults to depressed children and adolescents. In doing so, it is essential that a developmental appreciation of both the child and the family life cycle be brought to bear.

With this emerging picture of the dynamics of families with a depressed child, interventions specific to this population can be articulated better. As an example, in this chapter we presented a model of interpersonal family therapy (IFT) based on the extant literature on the symptomatology and functional deficits observed in depressed youths and their families and other authors' writings regarding family therapy for depressed individuals. Our clinical experience and pilot research suggest that this model of family therapy for depressed children is efficacious in ameliorating the children's depression and maladaptive family interaction patterns. However, it remains for larger-scale treatment-outcome studies to ascertain which family interventions, either alone or in combination with other modalities (e.g., individual or group therapy, pharmacotherapy), are most efficacious for which depressed youths and their families. It is our conviction that given the primacy of the family in the lives of children and adolescents, the association between dysfunctional family interactional patterns and depression in a youth, and the demonstrated efficacy of family therapy for a variety of childhood disorders, family therapy may be the treatment of choice for many depressed children and adolescents.

References

Amanat, E., & Butler, C. (1984). Oppressive behaviors in the families of depressed children. *Family Therapy*, *11*, 65–75.

Anthony, E. J. (1983). An overview of the effects of maternal depression in the infant and mother. In H. L. Morrison (Ed.), *Children of depressed parents: Risk, identification, and intervention* (pp. 1–16). New York: Grune & Stratton.

Armsden, G. C., McCauley, E., Greenberg, M. T., Burke, P. M., & Mitchell, J. R. (1990). Parent and peer attachment in early adolescent depression. *Journal of Abnormal Child Psychology*, *18*, 683–697.

Asarnow, J. R., Ben-Meir, S. L., & Goldstein, M. J. (1987). Family factors in childhood depressive and schizophrenia-spectrum disorders: A preliminary report. In K. Hahlweg and M. J. Goldstein (Eds.), *Understanding major mental disorder: The contribution of family interaction research* (pp. 123–138). New York: Family Process Press.

Asarnow, J. R., Carlson, G. A., & Guthrie, D. (1987). Coping strategies, self-perceptions, hopelessness, and perceived family environments in depressed and suicidal children. *Journal of Consulting and Clinical Psychology*, *55*, 361–366.

Beach, S. R. H., Sandeen, E.E., & O'Leary, K. D. (1990). *Depression in marriage: A model for etiology and treatment.* New York: Guilford Press.

Beardslee, W. R. (1990). Development of a preventive intervention for families in which parents have serious affective disorder. In G. I. Keither (Ed.), *Depression and families: Impact and treatment* (pp. 101–120). Washington, DC: American Psychiatric Press.

Beardslee, W. R., Bemporad, J., Keller, M. B., & Klerman, G. L. (1983). Children of parents with major affective disorder: A review. *American Journal of Psychiatry, 140*, 825–832.

Beardslee, W. R., & Podorefsky, D. (1988). Resilient adolescents whose parents have serious affective and other psychiatric disorders: Importance of self-understanding and relationships. *American Journal of Psychiatry, 145*, 63–69.

Beck, A. T. (1967). *Depression: Clinical, experimental and theoretical aspects.* New York: Hoeber.

Beck, S., & Rosenberg, R. (1986). Frequency, quality and impact of life events in self-rated depressed, behavioral-problem and normal children. *Journal of Consulting and Clinical Psychology, 54*, 863–864.

Bedrosian, R. C. (1988). Treating depression and suicidal wishes within the family context. In N. Epstein, S. E. Schlesinger, & W. Dryden (Eds.), *Cognitive–behavioral therapy with families* (pp. 292–324). New York: Brunner/Mazel.

Benjamin, L. S. (1974). Structural analysis of social behavior. *Psychological Review, 81*, 392–425.

Benoit, D., Zeanah, C. H., & Barton, M. L. (1989). Maternal attachment disturbances in failure to thrive. *Infant Mental Health Journal, 10*, 185.

Billings, A. G., & Moss, R. H. (1983). Comparisons of children of depressed and nondepressed parents: A social–environmental perspective. *Journal of Abnormal Child Psychology, 11*, 463–485.

Burbach, D. J., & Borduin, C. M. (1986). Parent–child relations and the etiology of depression: A review of methods and findings. *Clinical Psychology Review, 6*, 133–153.

Cicchetti, D., & Schneider-Rosen, K. (1984). Toward a transactional model of childhood depression. In D. Cicchetti and K. Schneider-Rosen (Eds.), *Childhood depression* (pp. 5–27). San Francisco: Jossey-Bass.

Cicchetti, D., & Schneider-Rosen, K. (1986). An organizational approach to childhood depression. In M. Rutter, C. E. Izard, & P. B. Read (Eds.), *Depression in young people: Developmental and clinical perspectives* (pp. 71–135). New York: Guilford Press.

Clarizio, H. F. (1989). *Assessment and treatment of depression in children and adolescents.* Brandon, VT: Clinical Psychology Publishers.

Clarkin, J. F., Haas, G. L., & Glick, I. D. (Eds.) (1988). *Affective disorders and the family: Assessment and treatment.* New York: Guilford Press.

Cole, D. A., & Rehm, L. P. (1986). Family interaction patterns and childhood depression. *Journal of Abnormal Child Psychology, 14*, 297–314.

Cole, P. M., & Kaslow, N. J. (1988). Interactional and cognitive strategies for affect regulation: A developmental perspective on childhood depression. In L. B. Alloy (Ed.), *Cognitive processes in depression* (pp. 310–343). New York: Guilford Press.

Cox, A. D., Puckering, C., Pound, A., & Mills, M. (1987). The impact of maternal depression in young children. *Journal of Child Psychology and Psychiatry, 28*, 917–928.

Coyne, J. C. (1976). Toward an interactional description of depression. *Psychiatry, 39*, 28–40.

Coyne, J. C. (1984). Strategic therapy with married depressed persons: Initial agenda, themes, and interventions. *Journal of Marital and Family Therapy, 10*, 53–62.

Coyne, J. C. (1988), Strategic therapy. In J. F. Clarkin, G. L. Haas, and I. D. Glick (Eds.), *Affective disorders and the family: Assessment and treatment* (pp. 89–114). New York: Guilford Press.

Cytryn, L., McKnew, D. H., Zahn-Waxler, C., & Gershon, E. S. (1986). Developmental issues in risk research: The offspring of affectively ill parents. In M. Rutter, C. E. Izard, and P. B. Read (Eds.), *Depression in young people: Developmental and clinical perspectives* (pp. 163–188). New York: Guilford Press.

DiGiuseppe, R. (1986). Cognitive therapy for childhood depression. In A. Freeman, N. Epstein, & K. M. Simon (Eds.), *Depression in the family* (pp. 153–172). New York: Haworth Press.

Downey, G., & Coyne, J. C. (1990). Children of depressed parents: An integrative review. *Psychological Bulletin, 108*, 50–76.

Falloon, I. R. H., Hole, V., Mulroy, L., Norris, L. J., & Pembleton, T. (1988). Behavioral family therapy. In J. F. Clarkin, G. L. Haas, & I. D. Glick (Eds.), *Affective disorders and the family: Assessment and treatment* (pp. 117–133). New York: Guilford Press.

Fauber, R. L., & Long, N. (1991). Children in context: The role of the family in child psychotherapy. *Journal of Consulting and Clinical Psychology, 59*, 813–820.

Feldman, L. B. (1976). Depression and marital interaction. *Family Process, 15*, 389–395.

Forehand, R., Brody, G., Slotkin, J., Fauber, R., McCombs, A., & Long, N. (1988). Young adolescent and maternal depression: Assessment, interrelations, and family predictors. *Journal of Consulting and Clinical Psychology, 56,* 422–426.

Freeman, A., Epstein, N., & Simon, K. M. (Eds.) (1986). Depression in the family. *Journal of Psychotherapy and the Family, 2,* 1–196.

Friedman, A. S. (1975). Interaction of drug therapy with marital therapy in depressive patients. *Archives of General Psychiatry, 32,* 619–637.

Garber, J., & Kashani, J. H. (1991). Development of the symptom of depression. In M. Lewis (Ed.), *Child and adolescent psychiatry: A comprehensive textbook* (pp. 293–310). Baltimore: Williams & Wilkins.

Gelfand, D. M., & Teti, D. M. (1990). The effects of maternal depression on children. *Clinical Psychology Review, 10,* 329–353.

Glick, I. D., Clarkin, J. F., Spencer, J. H., Haas, G. L., Lewis, A. B., Peyser, J., DeMane, N., Good-Ellis, M., Harris, E., & Lestello, V. (1985). A controlled evaluation of inpatient family interventions. I. Preliminary results of the six-month follow-up. *Archives of General Psychiatry, 42,* 882–886.

Goodwin, F. (1982). *Depression and manic–depressive illness.* Bethesda, MD: National Institutes of Health.

Gordon, D., Burge, D., Hammen, C., Adrian, C., Jaenicke, C., & Hiroto, D. (1989). Observations of interactions of depressed women with their children. *American Journal of Psychiatry, 146,* 50–55.

Gotlib, I. H., & Colby, C. A. (1987). *Treatment of depression: An interpersonal systems approach.* New York: Pergamon Press.

Hammen, C. (1991). *Depression runs in families: The social context of risk and resilience in children of depressed mothers.* New York: Springer-Verlag.

Hammen, C., Gordon, D., Burge, D., Adrian, C., & Jaenicke, C. (1987). Children of depressed mothers: maternal strain and symptom predictors of dysfunction. *Journal of Abnormal Psychology, 96,* 190–198.

Handford, H. A., Mattison, R., Humphrey, F. J., & McLaughlin, R. E. (1986). Depressive syndrome in children entering a residential school subsequent to parent death, divorce, or separation. *Journal of the American Academy of Child Psychiatry, 25,* 409–414.

Holder, D., & Anderson, C. M. (1990). Psychoeducational family intervention for depressed patients and their families. In G. I. Keitner (Ed.), *Depression and families: Impact and treatment* (pp. 157–184). Washington, DC: American Psychiatric Press.

Hops, H., Biglan, A., Sherman, L., Arthur, J., Friedman, L., & Osteen, V. (1987). Home observations of family interactions of depressed women. *Journal of Consulting and Clinical Psychology, 55,* 341–346.

Hoyt, L. A., Cowen, E. L., Pedro-Carroll, J. L., & Alpert-Gillis, L. J. (1990). Anxiety and depression in young children of divorce. *Journal of Clinical Child Psychology, 19,* 26–32.

Jaenicke, C., Hammen, C., Zupan, B., Hiroto, D., Gordon, D., Adrian, C., & Burge, D. (1987). Cognitive vulnerability in children at risk for depression. *Journal of Abnormal Child Psychology, 15,* 559–572.

Johnson, J. H., Rasbury, W. C., & Siegel, L. J. (1986). *Approaches to child treatment: Introduction to theory, research and practice.* New York: Pergamon Press.

Kashani, J. H., Burbach, D. J., & Rosenberg, T. K. (1988). Perception of family conflict resolution and depressive symptomatology in adolescents. *Journal of the American Academy of Child and Adolescent Psychiatry, 27,* 42–48.

Kaslow, N. J., & Carter, A. S. (1991). Depressed women in families: The search for power and intimacy. In T. J. Goodrich (Ed.), *Women and power* (pp. 166–182). New York: W. W. Norton.

Kaslow, N. J., Deering, C. G., & Racusin, G. R. (1994). Depressed children and their families. *Clinical Psychology Review, 14,* 39–59.

Kaslow, N. J., & Racusin, G. R. (1988). Assessment and treatment of depressed children and their families. *Families Therapy Today, 3,* 1–5.

Kaslow, N. J., & Racusin, G. R. (1990a). Childhood depression: Current status and future directions. In A. S. Bellack, M. Hersen, & A. E. Kazdin (Eds.), *International handbook of behavior: Modification and therapy* 2nd ed. (pp. 649–667). New York: Plenum Press.

Kaslow, N. J., & Racusin, G. R. (1990b). Family therapy or child therapy: An open or shut case. Journal of Family Psychology, 3, 273–289.

Kaslow, N. J., Rehm, L. P., Pollack, S. L., & Siegel, A. W. (1988). Attributional style and self-control behavior in depressed and nondepressed children and their parents. *Journal of Abnormal Child Psychology, 16,* 163–175.

Kazdin, A. E., Moser, J., Colbus, D., & Bell, R. (1985). Depressive symptoms among physically abused and psychiatrically disturbed children. *Journal of Abnormal Psychology, 94,* 298–307.

Keitner, G. I., & Miller, I. W. (1990). Family functioning and major depression: An overview. *American Journal of Psychiatry, 147,* 1128–1137.

Keller, M. B., Beardslee, W. R., Dorer, D. J., Lavori, P. W., Samuelson, H., & Klerman, G. R. (1986). Impact of severity and chronicity of parental affective illness and adaptive functioning and psychopathology in children. *Archives of General Psychiatry, 43*, 930–937.

Klerman, G. L., Weissman, M. M., Rounsaville, B. J., & Chevron, E. S. (1984). *Interpersonal psychotherapy of depression*. New York: Basic Books.

Kochanska, G., Kuczynski, L., Radke-Yarrow, M., & Welsh, J. D. (1987). Resolutions of control episodes between well and affectively ill mothers and their young children. *Journal of Abnormal Child Psychology, 15*, 441–456.

Lavori, P. W., Keller, M. B., Beardslee, W. R., & Dorer, D. J. (1988). Affective disorder in childhood: Separating the familial component of risk from individual characteristics of children. *Journal of Affective Disorders, 15*, 303–311.

Lefkowitz, M. M., & Tesiny, E. P. (1984). Rejection and depression: Prospective and contemporaneous analyses. *Developmental Psychology, 20*, 776–785.

Lewinsohn, P. M., Clarke, G. N., Hops, H., & Andrews, J. (1990). Cognitive–behavioral treatment for depressed adolescents. *Behavior Therapy, 21*, 385–401.

Merikangas, K. R., Prusoff, B. A., & Weissman, M. M. (1988). Parental concordance for affective disorders: Psychopathology in offspring. *Journal of Affective Disorders, 15*, 279–290.

Minde, K. (1991). The effect of disordered parenting on the development of children. In M. Lewis (Ed.), *Child and adolescent psychiatric: A comprehensive textbook* (pp. 394–407). Baltimore: Williams & Williams.

Minuchin, S. (1974). *Families and family therapy*. Cambridge, MA: Harvard University Press.

Mitchell, J., McCauley, E., Burke, P., Calderon, R., & Schloredt, K. (1989). Psychopathology in parents of depressed children and adolescents. *Journal of the American Academy of Child and Adolescent Psychiatry, 28*, 352–357.

Orvaschel, H., Weissman, M. M., & Kidd, K. K. (1980). Children and depression: The children of depressed parents; the childhood of depressed patients; depression in children. *Journal of Affective Disorders, 2*, 1–6.

Oster, G. D., & Caro, J. E. (1990). *Understanding and treating depressed adolescents and their families*. New York: John Wiley.

Parker, G. (1979). Parental characteristics in relation to depressive disorders. *British Journal of Psychiatry, 134*, 138–147.

Poznanski, E. O. (1982). The clinical phenomenology of childhood depression. *American Journal of Orthopsychiatry, 52*, 308–313.

Puig-Antich, J., Goetz, D., Davies, M., Kaplan, T., Davies, S., Ostrow, L., Asnis, L., Twomey, J., Iyengar, S., & Ryan, N. D. (1989). A controlled family history study for prepubertal major depressive disorder. *Archives of General Psychiatry, 46*, 406–418.

Puig-Antich, J., Lukens, E., Davies, M., Goetz, D., Brennan-Quattrock, J., & Todak, G. (1985a). Psychosocial functioning in prepubertal major depressive disorder. I. Interpersonal relationships during the depressive episode. *Archives of General Psychiatry, 42*, 500–507.

Puig-Antich, J., Lukens, E., Davies, M., Goetz, D., Brennan-Quattrock, J., & Todak, G. (1985b). Psychosocial functioning in prepubertal major depressive disorder. II. Interpersonal relationships after sustained recovery from affective episode. *Archives of General Psychiatry, 42*, 511–517.

Racusin, G. R., & Kaslow, N. J. (1991). Assessment and treatment of childhood depression. In P. A. Keller & S. R. Heyman (Eds.), *Innovations in clinical practice: A sourcebook*, Vol. 10 (pp. 223–243). Sarasota, FL: Professional Resource Exchange.

Racusin, G. R., & Kaslow, N. J. (in press). Child and family therapy combined: Indications and implications. *American Journal of Family Therapy*.

Radke-Yarrow, M., Cummings, E. M., Kuczynski, L., & Chapman, M. (1985). Patterns of attachment in two- and three-year olds in normal families and families with parental depression. *Child Development, 36*, 884–893.

Sacco, W. P., & Macleod, V. A. (1990). Interpersonal responses of primary caregivers to pregnant adolescents differing on depression level. *Journal of Clinical Child Psychology, 19*, 265–270.

Schrodt, G. R. (1992). Cognitive therapy of depression. In M. Shaffi & S. L. Shaffi (Eds.), *Clinical guide to depression in children and adolescents* (pp. 197–217). Washington, DC: American Psychiatric Press.

Schwartz, C. E., Dorer, D. J., Beardslee, W. R., Lavori, P. W., & Keller, M. B. (1990). Maternal expressed emotion and parental affective disorder: Risk for childhood depressive disorder, substance abuse, or conduct disorder. *Journal of Psychiatric Research, 24*, 231–250.

Seligman, M., & Darling, R. B. (1989). *Ordinary families, special children: A system approach to childhood disability*. New York: Guilford Press.

Seligman, M. E. P., Peterson, C., Kaslow, N. J., Tanenbaum, R. L., Alloy, L. B., & Abramson, L. Y. (1984).

Attributional styles and depressive symptoms among children. *Journal of Abnormal Psychology, 93,* 235–238.

Shaffi, M., & Shaffi, S. L. (Eds.) (1992). *Clinical guide to depression in children and adolescents.* Washington, DC: American Psychiatric Press.

Simons, R. L., & Miller, M. G. (1987). Adolescent depression: Assessing the impact of negative cognitions and socioenvironmental problems. *Social Work, July-August,* 326–330.

Slipp, S. (1984). *Object relations: A dynamic bridge between individual and family treatment.* New York: Jason Aronson.

Stark, K. (1990). *Childhood depression: School-based intervention.* New York: Guilford Press.

Stark, K. D., Humphrey, L. L., Crook, K., & Lewis, K. (1990). Perceived family environments of depressed and anxious children: Child's and maternal figure's perspective. *Journal of Abnormal Child Psychology, 18,* 527–547.

Teichman, Y. (1986). Family therapy of depression. In A. Freeman, N. Epstein, & K. M. Simon (Eds.), *Depression in the family* (pp. 9–39). New York: Haworth Press.

Teichman, Y., & Teichman, M. (1990). Interpersonal view of depression. *Journal of Family Psychology, 3,* 349–367.

Trad, P. V. (1987). *Infant and childhood depression.* New York: John Wiley.

Wallerstein, J. S., & Corbin, S. B. (1991). The child and the vicissitudes of divorce. In M. Lewis (Ed.), *Child and adolescent psychiatry: A comprehensive textbook* (pp. 1108–1117). Baltimore: Williams & Wilkins.

Weintraub, S., Winters, K. C., & Neale, J. M. (1986). Competence and vulnerability in children with affectively disordered parents. In M. Rutter, C. E. Izard, and P. B. Read (Eds.), *Depression in young people* (pp. 205–220). New York: Guilford Press.

Welner, Z., & Rice, J. (1988). School-aged children of depressed parents: A blind and controlled study. *Journal of Affective Disorders, 15,* 291–302.

Whiffen, V. E., & Gotlib, I. H. (1989). Infants of postpartum depressed mothers: Temperament and cognitive status. *Journal of Abnormal Psychology, 98,* 274–279.

Zaslow, M. J., Pederson, F. A., Cain, R. L., Suwalsky, J. T. D., & Kramer, E. L. (1985). Depressed mood in new fathers: Associations with parent–infant interactions. *Genetic, Social and General Psychology Monographs, 111,* 133–150.

Zekowski, E., O'Hara, M., & Wills, K. E. (1986). The effects of maternal mood on mother–infant interaction. *Journal of Abnormal Child Psychology, 15,* 361–378.

17

Pharmacotherapy for Depression in Children and Adolescents

Hugh F. Johnston and J. Jay Fruehling

Introduction

Knowledge in child psychiatry is generated primarily from two sources, systematic research and clinical practice. These two activities create different kinds of knowledge that are collected and communicated in distinct ways. Research-generated knowledge tends to be gathered at academic institutions and is disseminated largely through articles in scientific journals, meeting presentations, and textbooks. Clinical knowledge is amassed through practice and experience and tends to be imparted through "hands-on" training activities. Much of psychiatry in general, and child psychiatry in particular, is taught via an apprenticeship model, largely to facilitate the transfer of clinical knowledge across generations of physicians.

In this chapter, we present an overview of the available knowledge about the medication treatment of childhood depression. Out of necessity, this knowledge includes a mixture of information gleaned from systematic research and information generated from our own experience and imparted to us by our teachers. The reader will find both authoritative "facts," with appropriate citations, and clinical "lore" we have garnered from our colleagues, our own clinical experience, and our patients and their families. All are important ingredients in the successful treatment of depressed children.

In 1958, Kuhn (1958) ushered in a new era with his report on the effectiveness of imipramine in depressed adults. It wasn't long before bold clinicians tried using this medication in children and adolescents. These early pioneers have been followed by a host of energetic researchers and clinicians, yet the practice of prescribing antidepressant

Hugh F. Johnston • Division of Child and Adolescent Psychiatry, Department of Psychiatry, University of Wisconsin Medical School, Madison, Wisconsin 53792.   **J. Jay Fruehling** • Child Psychopharmacology Information Center, Department of Psychiatry, University of Wisconsin, Madison, Wisconsin 53792.

Handbook of Depression in Children and Adolescents, edited by William M. Reynolds and Hugh F. Johnston. Plenum Press, New York, 1994.

medication in the treatment of child and adolescent depression is *still* controversial. The controversy stems from inadequate knowledge in three specific areas: (1) the validity and reliability of the diagnosis of depression, (2) the efficacy of antidepressants in the pediatric population, and (3) the safety of antidepressant medications for children in both the short and long term. The validity and reliability of the diagnosis of childhood depression are reviewed elsewhere in this book. This chapter will focus primarily on the issues of medication efficacy, safety, and use in clinical practice.

In addition, this chapter provides a forum for discussion of several topics related to medication treatment of child and adolescent depression. These include ethical considerations, identification of social and economic forces affecting practice patterns, and the regulation and approval process for antidepressant compounds. Finally, it offers some practical clinical guidelines.

It is important to note that in this chapter, unless stated otherwise, the term "child" refers to both children and adolescents.

Depression

It is impossible to discuss the role of antidepressant medication for depressed children without first briefly discussing the disorder itself. Debate continues about whether childhood depression exists as a distinct disorder or whether it is a constellation of signs and symptoms that might be a nonspecific response to stress [Nurcombe (Chapter 4); Nurcombe et al., 1989]. Clinicians are no more confident than researchers about these general issues. however, clinicians are exquisitely aware of the suffering and disability that are sustained by children with a pervasively bad mood, significant sleep disruption, irritability, and an inability to experience pleasure.

These childhood depressive symptoms can be the direct result of parental divorce, family illness, child abuse, or other stressors. They also may occur in the absence of, or out of proportion to, significant stressors. The *Diagnostic and Statistical Manual of Mental Disorders*, fourth edition (DSM-IV) (American Psychiatric Association, 1994), has termed this constellation of signs and symptoms Major Depression *Episode* (MDE) allowing the syndrome to be applied as a clinical entity regardless of its relationship to most medical conditions, psychosocial stresses, or other psychiatric diagnoses. While discussion continues as to whether Major Depressive *Disorder* (MDD) is a valid clinical entity in children, there has been little controversy regarding MDE, simply because it has enormous face validity. Nearly everyone who works with emotionally disturbed children has seen individuals who appear to be suffering from a depressive syndrome, whether or not this syndrome can be elevated to the status of a distinct disorder.

At first it may seem to be hairsplitting to argue the existence of MDD vs. MDE, but if neither clinicians nor researchers can agree on the boundaries and dimensions of MDD, it makes little sense to discuss pharmacological remedies for the disorder. Furthermore, as long as the validity of MDD remains in question, efficacy studies of antidepressant medications in populations of children who are deemed to have this putative disorder will be methodologically suspect.

However, clinicians regularly encounter individual children with MDE of such severity that it is sensible to entertain the idea of medication treatment. Even if the existence of MDD as a discrete disorder is not a valid construct, using a medication to ameliorate some of the child's more troubling symptoms (such as sleep disturbance, irritability, and anhedonia) is often clinically sensible and humane. Furthermore, MDE may be a significant complicating factor in disorders such as separation anxiety (Kendall, Kortlander, Chansky, & Brady, 1992), overanxious disorder (Strauss, 1988), and conduct disorder (Puig-Antich, 1982), as well as medically ill children [Kashani and Breedlove (Chapter 19)] and those with special needs [Schloss, Sher, and Wisniewski (Chapter 20)]. In these situations, treatment of coexisting MDE should be considered in order to (1) reduce the child's suffering and (2) help make interventions for the underlying disorder(s) or disability more successful.

DSM-IV criteria for MDE in children are very similar to those for MDE in adults except that an irritable mood may be substituted for a sad/depressed mood (American Psychiatric Association, 1994). There follows a condensation of the criteria defining MDE taken from the DSM-IV:

At least five of the following, with at least one being either (1) depressed mood or (2) loss of interest or pleasure:

1. Depressed or irritable mood most of the day, nearly every day (as indicated by either subjective account or observation by others).
2. Markedly diminished interest or pleasure in almost all activities most of the day, nearly every day (as indicated by either subjective account or observation by others of apathy most of the time).
3. Significant failure to make expected weight gains.
4. Insomnia or hypersomnia nearly every day.
5. Psychomotor agitation or retardation nearly every day (observable by others, not merely subjective feelings of restlessness or being slowed down).
6. Fatigue or loss of energy nearly every day.
7. Feelings of worthlessness or excessive or inappropriate guilt (which may be delusional) nearly every day.
8. Diminished ability to think or concentrate, or indecisiveness, nearly every day.
9. Recurrent thoughts of death, recurrent suicidal ideation, a suicide attempt, or a specific plan for committing suicide.

For the convenience of the reader, we will use conventional terminology in the remainder of this chapter. Children and adolescents with MDE will be referred to as "depressed children" or "children suffering from depression." However, we ask the reader to appreciate that this convention tends to lend *unwarranted* credibility to the notion that depression is a firmly established diagnostic entity in children.

Developmental Factors and Antidepressant Medication

Before we discuss developmental factors that affect medication response, it is worthwhile mentioning several issues regarding childhood development and depression [these are explored further by Cicchetti, Rogosch, and Toth (Chapter 7)]. At various levels of physical, emotional, and social development, it is reasonable to expect that the symptoms of affective illness in children will vary as compared to those in adults. These development-related variations are *in addition to* the variations expected to occur from individual to individual. It is also reasonable to expect that the underlying causal mechanisms of affective illness (both biological and psychosocial) will operate somewhat differently according to stage of development. Given that affective illness affects children somewhat differently than it affects adults, it is reasonable to expect that antidepressant medication might also affect children differently as compared to adults. Conversely, some aspects of affective illness seem to transcend developmental age. These aspects include sleep disturbance, anhedonia, and dysphoria. This overlap suggests that there is some measure of commonality in affective illness regardless of the individual's developmental stage. Clearly, more research is needed to elucidate the developmentally dependent variations of depression that impact on response to medication.

The discipline of pharmacology can be divided into two broad categories: pharmacokinetics and pharmacodynamics. *Pharmacokinetics* is concerned with how drugs are absorbed, distributed, metabolized, and eliminated. *Pharmacodynamics* is concerned with the effects that drugs have on physiology. For example, the effects that drugs produce on various organ systems (including therapeutic effects, toxic effects, and side effects) are examples of pharmacodynamic factors, while the rate of absorption and the serum half-life are pharmacokinetic factors.

Age has important effects on pharmacokinetic factors. Almost all the antidepressant compounds are metabolized via oxidative or hydroxylating pathways, or both, in the liver. Relative to body weight, younger children tend to metabolize drugs in the liver faster than older children and adults (Perel, 1978). This circumstance suggests that children should need higher doses (relative to body weight) and perhaps more frequent dosing to achieve the same medication blood and tissue concentrations as adults. Such has indeed been the finding for those drugs that have been systematically studied in children, such as imipramine (Preskorn, Bupp, Weller, & Weller, 1982) and nortriptyline (Geller, Perel, Knitter, Lycaki, & Farooki, 1983). This research has also demonstrated that there is *enormous* variability in rates of metabolism from child to child. This finding suggests that the optimum medication dose will also vary substantially from one child to another.

Only limited information is available regarding the influence of child development on pharmacodynamics, particularly in regard to the central nervous system. It seems likely that a child's immature nervous system might respond differently to antidepressant medications than a mature adult nervous system. Clinical experience suggests that young children are more likely to become paradoxically excited by sedating medications such as phenobarbital and the benzodiazepines. Also, a recent report by Riddle et al. (1990) suggests that children may be more likely than adults to experience behavioral side effects from fluoxetine. These two examples help confirm that neurological development can affect drug response in some cases and that these differential effects may be *clinically significant*. Unfortunately, systematic research in this area is an extremely difficult undertaking, yet at the same time critically important to progress in the field.

There is some suggestion that the cardiovascular pharmacodynamics of the tricyclic antidepressants (TCAs) in children are different that in adults (Wagner & Fershtman, 1993), and it has been hypothesized that children may be more vulnerable than adults to TCA-induced cardiac arrhythmias. This issue is discussed in greater detail in the following section on safety. Since many antidepressant medications have wide-ranging effects on hormone levels, sleep architecture, and metabolism, it is reasonable to expect that these effects might translate into side effects that are different in children as compared to adults. Our clinical experience suggests that these differences (if they exist) are not medically significant in acute treatment. (Whether they impact on long-term development remains unknown.)

In general, children seem to complain less about anticholinergic side effects. Whether this is because they experience fewer side effects or because they do not attribute their experiences to medication is unknown.

Safety and Side-Effect Issues

Because antidepressant medications are neither developed nor marketed for use in children, there are few systematic data on their safety. Consequently, an analysis of the safety of these drugs in children must be inferred from a generalization of adult safety data, from the presence (or absence) of reports in the professional literature regarding adverse events, and from the small number of published research studies that have used child subjects.

A complete discussion of safety and side-effect issues relative to antidepressant medication is beyond the scope of this chapter. This being the case, we will focus on those issues that are particularly relevant to children, presuming that the reader has some general familiarity with these compounds. Broadly speaking, the TCAs appear reasonably safe. The safety of the monoamine oxidase inhibitors appears to be compromised due to dietary compliance issues, and the experience with the newer antidepressant compounds such as sertraline or paroxetine is simply too limited to make generalizations regarding safety. Lithium alone is not commonly used to treat childhood depression; however, in reports of its use in treating children with bipolar disorder, or in augmenting an antidepressant, it appears to be fairly well tolerated.

Side-effect data are typically generated in two contexts: (1) in the course of premarketing safety and efficacy studies and (2) in postmarketing drug surveillance, in which the focus of the report is an unusually severe or idiosyncratic side effect. Because premarketing efficacy studies do not include children, side-effect data that may be unique to this population are not gathered. On the other hand, side effects reported in postmarketing surveillance are often difficult to interpret because of the uncontrolled nature of these reports. The common side effects associated with each class of antidepressant medications are described below. In addition, the medication tables list the common side effects from the 1993 *Physician's Desk Reference* (PDR). While these data are gathered primarily from studies of adults, they are clearly relevant to the treatment of children.

Perhaps the most troubling issue regarding safety is the question of whether antidepressant drugs impact development in children, especially young children. There are historical precedents for concerns of this nature. Tetracycline antibiotics are relatively innocuous in adults, but will permanently stain the developing teeth of young children (Chiappinelli & Walton, 1992; Haring, 1992). Another example is environmental lead exposure. Limits that were initially found to be safe for adults have been shown to result in significant neurotoxicity for children (Lovejoy, Shannon, & Woolf, 1992; Needleman, 1993). As with all treatments, the issue of safety cannot be considered in isolation, but must be weighted against the risks of the disorder(s) left untreated or inadequately treated.

Classes of Medication

Antidepressant medications can be broadly grouped into four categories: the tricyclic antidepressants (TCAs), the monoamine oxidase inhibitors (MAOIs), the selective serotonin reuptake inhibitors (SSRIs), and a fourth group of novel compounds that do not fit well into any of the preceding categories. Each of these classes is discussed in more detail below. We will begin our discussion with several general comments that are applicable to all antidepressant medications.

In studies of depressed adults, antidepressants usually take at least 2 weeks to manifest therapeutic effects distinct from placebo. Clinical experience indicates that a delay in response also occurs in children. This delay strongly suggests that the antidepressant benefit does not result *directly* from the drug's effects on neurotransmitter systems. Instead, it can be hypothesized that the antidepressant effect is a result of some adaptation (taking up to several weeks) to a neurophysiological perturbation caused by the drug. This hypothesis also helps explain how drugs that act on different neurotransmitter systems can have comparable antidepressant effects. Thus far, the search for this putative biological adaptation common to all antidepressants has been disappointing. Although we know a great deal about how various medications affect the nervous system at the level of the synapse, our understanding of how this effect translates into improved mood is woefully incomplete.

None of the antidepressant medications appears to be a "cure" for depression in the common meaning of the word. While these medications are often very potent in reducing or eliminating the symptoms of depression during active treatment, the symptoms often return quickly if the drug is discontinued prematurely. Thus, it can also be hypothesized that the pathophysiological underpinnings of depression are attenuated by medication, but not eliminated.

The clinical response to medications is quite idiosyncratic from individual to individual and difficult to predict. One child will have a robust response to a particular medication, while another child of the same age with similar symptoms will have no response. This idiosyncratic pattern also pertains to side effects. Some children will experience severe side effects from a particular medication, while others may experience no side effects whatsoever. This wide and unpredictable individual variation in medication response again underscores our lack of knowledge regarding the mechanisms by which antidepressant medications produce their therapeutic and nontherapeutic effects.

Tricyclic Antidepressants

The TCA class of medications includes eight chemically related compounds available in the United States and additional drugs available in other countries. Those available in the United States include:

- amitriptyline (Elavil)
- amoxapine (Asendin)
- clomipramine (Anafranil)
- desipramine (Norpramin, Pertofrane)
- imipramine (Tofranil)
- nortriptyline (Pamelor, Aventyl)
- protriptyline (Vivactil)
- trimipramine (Surmontil)

These drugs are believed to exert their therapeutic effects as a result of blocking the reuptake of monoamine neurotransmitters, most particularly norepinephrine and serotonin. They also have, depending on the specific compound, significant effects on other neurotransmitter systems, including histamine, dopamine, acetylcholine, and others. Due to these wide-ranging effects, the TCAs frequently cause unwanted side effects such as sedation, dry mouth, constipation, and electrocardiographic (EKG) changes. As a group, the TCAs are all closely related chemically and share very similar therapeutic effects and side effects. The TCAs are all extremely dangerous in overdose, causing arrhythmias, hypotension, seizures, and cardiovascular collapse. This danger has limited their usefulness, since depressed individuals are often at increased risk for taking medication overdoses. The individual TCAs in common usage for children are each briefly discussed below.

Imipramine is the TCA that has been most widely used in children. The reasons are that it was one of the first compounds available and that it has been approved by the Food and Drug Administration (FDA) for treatment of nocturnal enuresis in children. Imipramine is demethylated in the liver, forming another active compound, desipramine. Thus, its therapeutic effects are likely the result of both the imipramine and the desipramine.

Amitriptyline has also been used extensively in children because it too has been available in the United States for many years. Like imipramine, it has an active demethylated metabolite, nortriptyline, which also has therapeutic effects. Amitriptyline has potent anticholinergic properties, and the associated side effects such as sedation, dry mouth, blurred vision, and constipation make it a less than ideal medication for most children.

Nortriptyline, the demethylated metabolite of amitriptyline, has several advantages over the other TCAs. It has been systematically studied in children (Geller, Cooper, Graham, Getner, & Marsteller, 1992), it is probably less likely to cause cardiovascular side effects than other TCAs (Wilens, Biederman, Spencer, & Geist, 1993), and it is not as sedating as amitriptyline or imipramine.

Desipramine has been shown in controlled studies to be efficacious for the treatment of attention-deficit hyperactivity disorder (ADHD) (Biederman, Baldessarini, Wright, Keenan, & Faraone, 1993; Biederman, Baldessarini, Wright, Knee, & Harmatz, 1989; Gualtieri, Keenan, & Chandler, 1991), making it an attractive alternative for children with both depressive and ADHD symptoms. Unfortunately (see below), desipramine has been recently implicated as rarely causing sudden death in children, making it a very questionable choice in the treatment of depressed children.

Clomipramine is a TCA that has been available outside the United States for many years. It was originally developed and marketed for depression, but was found to have efficacy for the treatment of obsessive–compulsive disorder (OCD). This led to its introduction into the United States market as a treatment for OCD. It has been studied in children (down to age 10) for treatment of OCD (DeVeaugh-Geiss et al., 1992). Although it is not marketed for treatment of depression, clomipramine is mentioned here because it is reasonable to assume that it also has efficacy for depression in children, although its use for this purpose has not been well studied.

The remaining TCAs (amoxapine, protriptyline, and trimipramine) have received little attention in the child psychopharmacology literature and probably do not offer any special advantages over the other TCAs. For this reason, they will not be discussed further.

TCA-Related Safety and Side-Effect Issues. As alluded to above, the TCAs have cardiac-related effects, particularly at higher dosage or in overdose. To date, there have been four cases of sudden death associated with desipramine (Riddle, Geller, & Ryan, 1993; Riddle et al., 1991) and one with imipramine (Saraf, Klein, Gittelman-Klein, & Groff, 1974). Each of these deaths occurred (with the exception of the imipramine case) at approximately *therapeutic* doses. These occurrences suggest that there is a risk, but leaves great uncertainty about the magnitude of this risk and what factors affect it, either positively or negatively. In such a rarely occurring serious phenomenon, it is difficult to be certain whether the drug caused these deaths and, if it did, how. It has been speculated to be cardiac-related (Wagner & Fershtman, 1993). Of all the TCAs, nortriptyline may have some advantages in this area because it appears to affect cardiac conduction less than the others (Geller et al., 1992; Wilens et al., 1993).

Another serious concern has been the risk of a mania being precipitated by TCAs (Geller, Fox, & Fletcher, 1993; Kashani, Hodges, & Shekim, 1980). This occurrence has also been reported with fluoxetine (Venkataraman, Naylor, & King, 1992). Clinical experience suggests that this risk may be greater for teens than for prepubertal children, but clearly more research is needed.

A number of rarely occurring side effects have been reported when TCAs are used in children, including: tics with imipramine (Parraga & Cochran, 1992), exacerbation of asthma by imipramine (Kanner, Klein, Rubinstein, & Mascia, 1989; Miller, 1987), hyperpyrexia related to desipramine (Squires, Neumeyer, Bloomberg, & Krishnamoorthy, 1992), cutaneous reactions from desipramine (Biederman, Gonzalez, Bronstein, DeMonaco, & Wright, 1988), paranoid and aggressive behavior from clomipramine (Alarcon, Johnson, & Lucas, 1991), and alopecia also from clomipramine (Warnock, Sieg, Willsie, Stevenson, & Kestenbaum, 1991).

Although not precisely a side effect, drug-withdrawal effects can be of concern when antidepressant medication is stopped abruptly in children (Geller, Cooper, Carr, Warham, & Rodriguez, 1987; Law, Petti, & Kazdin, 1981). These effects are manifest as malaise, vomiting, and flu-like symptoms. Children may be more susceptible than adults to withdrawal effects because of their relatively more rapid clearance of these compounds once the medication has been discontinued.

The commonly prescribed TCAs are described in Table 1 and a few of the less commonly prescribed ones are described in Table 2.

Table 1. Commonly Prescribed Tricyclic Antidepressants in Children[a]

Generic name (Brand name)	Adverse effects (most common)	FDA age recommendation	Initial dosage	Maintenance dosage	Contraindications	Dose limits
Amitriptyline (Elavil)	Note text at end of Table 1[b]	Not recommended for children under 12 years of age.	Adults: 75–150 mg/day in divided doses Adolescents: 10 mg 3 times a day and 20 mg at bedtime	50–100 mg/day in single dose given at bedtime	Not to be given with MAOI antidepressants.	Up to 300 mg/day for hospitalized patients
Clomipramine (Anafranil)	From child/adolescent studies: dry mouth (63%), somnolence (46%), fatigue (35%), tremor (33%), headache (28%), weight loss (23.2%), anorexia (22%), constipation (22%), abdominal pain (13%), dyspepsia (13%), insomnia (11%), dysmenorrhea (10%).	Approved for use in children and adolescents over age 10	25 mg/day	25–200 mg/day; initially in divided doses. Once titrated to steady state, may be given in one daily dose, in evening, to avoid daytime drowsiness.	History of seizures or brain damage of various etiology; alcoholism; concomitant use with other drugs that lower the seizure threshold; hypersensitivity to Anafranil or other TcAs; in combination or within 14 days before or after an MAOI; during the acute recovery period after a myocardial infarction.	3 mg/kg or 200 mg/day, whichever is smaller
Desipramine (Norpramin, Pertofrane)	Note text at end of Table 1[b]	Safety and effectiveness in children have not been evaluated. Adolescents: Doses lower than those given to adults may be prescribed (no age range listed).	No information on initial dosing listed.	25–100 mg/day based on clinical response	Not to be given in conjunction with, or within 2 weeks of, treatment with an MAOI, or during the acute recovery period after a myocardial infarction. Cautionary use: patients with cardiovascular disease, urinary retention, thyroid disease, those with a preexisting seizure disorder, or patients who abuse alcohol.	More severely ill patients may be dosed up to 150 mg/day. Initially divided dosing, but thereafter once-daily dosing is okay.

Drug		Clinical use	Dosing	Dosing (detailed)	Contraindications/cautions	Maximum dose
Imipramine (Tofranil)	Note text at end of Table 1[b]	May be used as a temporary adjunctive therapy for nocturnal enuresis for children age 6 and above. The effectiveness of the drug in children for conditions other than nocturnal enuresis has not been established. May be used in adolescents for depression.	30–40 mg/day for adolescent depression; 25 mg/day for enuresis	30–100 mg/day for adolescent depression, in a divided dose; 25–50 mg for childhood enuresis for children 6–12. Studies indicate that a 50 mg divided dose (given in midafternoon, repeated at bedtime) may be more effective for early-night bedwetters. Children 12 and over may be given 75 mg nightly.	Not to be given in conjunction with, or within 2 weeks of, treatment with an MAOI, or during the acute recovery period after myocardial infarction. Cautionary use: patients with cardiovascular disease, urinary retention, thyroid disease, those with a preexisting seizure disorder, or patients who abuse alcohol.	Generally not necessary to exceed 100 mg/day.
Nortriptyline (Aventyl, Pamelor)	Note text at end of Table 1[b]	Not recommended for children. May be used in adolescent depression.	No dosing recommendations for children; Adolescents: 30–50 mg/day, in divided doses, or the total daily dose may be given once a day	25–150 mg/day in divided dose or single daily dose; Plasma levels falling in the 50–150 ng/m range are recommended.	Not to be given in conjunction with, or within 2 weeks of, treatment with an MAOI, or during the acute recovery period after a myocardial infarction. Cross-sensitivity between nortriptyline and other dibenzazepines is a possibility.	Not listed for children or adolescents; adult doses above 150 mg/day are not recommended.

[a]This table was prepared using the 1993 *Physicians Desk Reference* (PDR). Every effort was exerted to make it as accurate as possible. It is not meant to be used as a replacement for the PDR when making medication-prescribing decisions.

This is a combination table prepared by taking the first two adverse effects, by category, from the PDR. No percentages were available for the following adverse effects: skin rash, urticaria, petechiae; anticholinergic: paralytic ileus, hyperpyrexia, dry mouth, blurred vision; cardiovascular: myocardial infarction, stroke, orthostatic hypertension; CNS/neuromuscular: coma, seizures; endocrine: testicular swelling and gynecomastia in the male, breast enlargement and galactorrhea in the female; gastrointestinal: nausea and vomiting, anorexia; hematological: bone marrow depression including agranulocytosis, leukopenia, eosinophilia; neurological: numbness, tingling; other: alopecia, edema, jaundice (simulating obstructive), altered liver function, rarely hepatitis; psychiatric: confusional states with hallucinations, disorientation; withdrawal syndrome of malaise, nausea, malaise, and headache on abrupt withdrawal.

[b]As a class of medications, the tricyclics have been linked to the following list of adverse effects, roughly categorized by body system: **Cardiovascular:** Hypotension, hypertension, tachycardia, palpitation, myocardial infarction, arrhythmias, heart block, stroke; **Mental status:** Confusional states with hallucinations (especially in elderly), disorientation, delusions, anxiety, panic, restlessness, agitation, hypomania, exacerbation of psychoses; **CNS:** Ataxia, tremors, peripheral neuropathy, extrapyramidal symptoms, seizures, alterations in EEG patterns; **Visual:** Blurred vision, mydriasis; **Digestive:** Constipation, nausea, vomiting, epigastric distress or cramps, diarrhea, xerostomia, sublingual adenitis, paralytic ileus; **Dermatologic:** Itching, skin rash, urticaria, alopecia, photosensitization, edema, petechiae, perspiration, flushing; **Hemopoietic system:** Bone marrow depression, agranulocytosis, eosinophilia, purpura, thrombocytopenia; **Nervous system:** Numbness, tingling or other paresthesias of extremities, incoordination, drowsiness, dizziness, weakness, fatigue; **Sexual/Hormonal:** Gynecomastia in the male, breast enlargement and galactorrhea in the female, increased or decreased libido, impotence, testicular swelling, parotid swelling, syndrome of inappropriate ADH secretion; **Sleep:** Insomnia, nightmares. **Urologic:** Delayed micturition, urinary retention, urinary frequency, dilation of the urinary tract, nocturia; **Miscellaneous:** Peculiar taste, tinnitus, stomatitis, black-tongue, elevation or depression of blood sugar levels, disturbances of accommodation, drug-withdrawal malaise, headache and nausea, drug fever, cross-sensitivity with other tricyclic drugs.

Table 2. Less Commonly Prescribed Tricyclic Antidepressants in Children[a]

Generic name (Brand name)	Adverse effects (most common)	FDA age recommendation	Initial dosage	Maintenance dosage	Contraindications	Dose limits
Amoxapine (Asendin)	From adult studies: sedation (14%), dry mouth (14%), constipation (12%)	Safety and effectiveness in those under 17 have not been evaluated.	50 mg t.i.d., up to 100 mg t.i.d. by end of first week	Adults: Single dose of up to 300 mg, given at bedtime	Not to be used in patients with prior hypersensitivity to dibenzoxazepine compounds. Should not be given concurrently with MAOIs or within 14 days of the discontinuation of an MAOI. Not recommended during the acute recovery phase of a myocardial infarction.	400–600 mg/day for hospitalized patients (divided dose)
Protriptyline (Vivactil)	In adults (first two for each body system category): Cardiovascular: myocardial infarction, stroke Psychiatric: Confusional states (especially in the elderly) with hallucinations, disorientation Neurological: seizures, incoordination Anticholinergic: paralytic ileus, hyperpyrexia Allergic: drug fever, petechiae Gastrointestinal: nausea and vomiting, anorexia Hematological: agranulocytosis, bone marrow depression Endocrine: impotence, increased or decreased libido Other: jaundice, altered liver function, parotid swelling, alopecia, flushing, weight gain or loss, urinary frequency, nocturia, perspiration	Children: Not recommended for use due to lack of safety and effectiveness studies. Adolescents: Use in depression.	Adolescents: 5 mg t.i.d.	Usual adult dosage 15–40 mg a day in 3 or 4 doses daily	Should not be given concurrently with MAOI. Not to be used within 14 days of the discontinuation of an MAOI medication. Not to be used in the acute recovery phase of a myocardial infarction.	Up to 60 mg a day in divided doses 3 or 4 times a day Doses above this are not recommended.

Generic (Trade)	Children		Adolescents/Adults	Adverse Reactions	Contraindications/Precautions
Protriptyline (Vivactil) (*cont.*)				Withdrawal syndrome of nausea, headache, and malaise with abrupt drug discontinuation. More likely than other tricyclics to aggravate cardiovascular agitation and anxiety and produce cardiovascular reactions such as tachycardia and hypotension.	
Trimipramine (Surmontil)	Not recommended for use in children. May be used in adolescents.	50 mg/day	Adolescents: 50–100 mg/day based on patient response and tolerance. Usually dosed at bedtime. Lowest dose that will maintain remission	In adults (first two for each body system category): Cardiovascular: hypotension, hypertension. Psychiatric: confusional states (especially in the elderly) with hallucinations, disorientation. Neurological: numbness, tingling. Anticholinergic: dry mouth and associated sublingual adenitis (rarely), blurred vision. Allergic: skin rash, petechiae. Hematological: bone marrow depression including agranulocytosis, eosinophilia. Endocrine: gynecomastia in the male, breast enlargement and galactorrhea in the female. Gastrointestinal: nausea and vomiting, anorexia. Other: jaundice, altered liver function, parotid swelling, alopecia, flushing, weight gain or loss, urinary frequency, nocturia, perspiration. Withdrawal syndrome of nausea, headache, and malaise with abrupt drug discontinuation. More likely than other tricyclics to aggravate cardiovascular agitation and anxiety and produce cardiovascular reactions such as tachycardia and hypotension.	Doses above 200 mg/day in adults are not recommended; 250–300 mg/day in hospitalized adults. Should not be given concurrently with MAOI. Allow 2 weeks to elapse after discontinuation of these drugs before Surmontil is initiated. Not to be given in the acute recovery period after a myocardial infarction.

*a*This table was prepared using the 1993 *Physicians Desk Reference* (PDR). Every effort was exerted to make it as accurate as possible. It is not meant to be used as a replacement for the PDR when making medication-prescribing decisions.

Selective Serotonin Reuptake Inhibitors

Hugh F. Johnston
and J. Jay Fruehling

The drugs in this class include:

- fluoxetine (Prozac)
- fluvoxamine (Luvox)
- paroxetine (Paxil)
- sertraline (Zoloft)

The SSRIs have revolutionized the treatment of affective disorders in adults. Whether this will hold true for children remains to be seen. In adults, these drugs have efficacy comparable to that of the TCAs, but have fewer physical side effects and are much safer in overdose. Currently, there are three chemically unrelated compounds available in the United States: fluoxetine, sertraline, and paroxetine. Fluvoxamine, which is currently available only outside the United States, is expected to receive FDA approval by the time this book is printed. Evaluations of pediatric efficacy of sertraline in childhood OCD are in progress, and preliminary results are promising (Johnston, unpublished data).

The SSRIs are a unique class of antidepressant compounds because their direct neurophysiological effects are limited almost exclusively to inhibiting the reuptake of serotonin at the synapse. Because of this limited effect, these compounds do not produce the myriad of side effects commonly seen with other antidepressant medications. In addition, as noted, the SSRIs have demonstrated efficacy in the treatment of depression in adults that is comparable to the efficacy of the TCAs. Clinical experience and preliminary research data suggest that they may have similar efficacy for the treatment of childhood depression.

An open-label trial of fluvoxamine in adolescents with either OCD or depression by Apter et al. (1994) included 6 adolescents diagnosed with MDD. The authors noted that during this 8-week trial, the majority of subjects showed a substantial improvement in their depressive symptoms; however, the drug's impact on impulsive, suicidal, or anorectic symptoms was less clear. They further noted that study participants were in an inpatient psychiatric facility and were provided psychosocial interventions that may have served to improve their clinical condition.

SSRI-Related Safety and Side-Effect Issues.   Fluoxetine (FLX) was the first SSRI introduced in the United States. Although only one controlled trial has been completed (summarized below in the section entitled "Antidepressant Medication Efficacy"), this medication is in widespread use in children. Physician interest in the use of FLX, sertraline (SRT), and paroxetine (PRX) in children is high. Unfortunately, there is essentially no literature on the use of PRX and SRT for the treatment of childhood depression. This being the case, our overview of the SSRIs is limited to FLX only.

The popular media have enthusiastically reported the controversy regarding potential behavioral side effects of FLX, especially suicidality and hypersexuality. Although increased suicidality has not been seen in comparisons of FLX with placebo and with TCAs (Beasley et al., 1991), it does appear that behavioral side effects such as nervousness, hypomania, suicidal ideation, and disinhibition are relatively common in children treated with FLX (Riddle et al., 1990). Data also suggest that severe behavioral side effects may be more common than generally assumed in adults as well (Fava & Rosenbaum, 1990). Our clinical experience suggests that children have a greater risk of experiencing behavioral side effects from FLX than do adults.

The three SSRIs currently available in the United States are described in Table 3.

Monoamine Oxidase Inhibitors

In the United States, the three antidepressant MAOIs commercially available are:

- isocarboxazid (Marplan)

Table 3. Selective Serotonin Reuptake Inhibitors[a]

Generic name (Brand name)	Adverse effects (most common)	FDA age recommendation	Initial dosage	Maintenance dosage	Contraindications	Dose limits
Fluoxetine (Prozac)	In adults: nausea (21.1%), headache (20.3%), nervousness (14.9%), insomnia (13.8%), diarrhea (12.3%), drowsiness (11.6%)	No recommendations are made regarding use in children or adolescents 17 or under.	Adults: 20 mg/day for	Adults: 20–80 mg/day	Contraindications: Not to be used with MAOIs or within 14 days of stopping an MAOI. An MAOI should not be started within 5 weeks of stopping fluoxetine.	Has been dosed up to 80 mg/day in controlled trials of adults. Doses above 20 mg should be given on a morning/noon b.i.d. schedule.
Paroxetine (Paxil)	In adult, placebo-controlled studies: nausea (25.7%), dry mouth (18.1%), headache (17.6%), asthenia (15.0%), constipation (13.8%), dizziness (13.3%), insomnia (13.3%), ejaculatory disturbances (12.9%), diarrhea (11.6%), sweating (11.2%), other male genital disorders (10.0%)	Safety and effectiveness in children have not been established. (This apparently includes adolescents as well, since no mention is made to the contrary)	In adults: 20 mg/day in single daily dose	Potential for interaction with MAOIs Not to be administered within 14 days of discontinuing treatment with a MAOI Wait 2 weeks after stopping an MAOI before administering Paxil	Nonresponders can have dose increased by 10 mg/day; (at one week intervals) to a maximum of 50 mg/day	
Sertraline (Zoloft)	From adult controlled studies: nausea (26.1%), headache (20.3%), diarrhea/loose stools (17.7%), insomnia (16.4%), xerostomia (16.3%), male sexual dysfunction (15.5%), somnolence (13.4%), dizziness (11.7%), tremor (10.7%), fatigue (10.6%)	Safety and effectiveness in children or adolescents have not been established.	Adults: 50 mg once daily	50–200 mg/day in single dose, either in morning or in evening	Not to be used with MAOI's or within 14 days of stopping an MAOI.	20 mg/day

[a]This table was prepared using the 1993 *Physicians Desk Reference* (PDR). Every effort was exerted to make it as accurate as possible. It is not meant to be used as a replacement for the PDR when making medication-prescribing decisions.

- phenelzine (Nardil)
- tranylcypromine (Parnate)

As their category name implies, the MAOIs all inhibit the oxidative degradation of monoamine neurotransmitters, increasing the availability of these neurotransmitters at the synapse. These drugs are infamous for their capacity to produce hypertensive emergencies when foods containing significant amounts of tyramine are ingested. Normally, tyramine is oxidized in the gut; however, when the oxidating enzyme is inhibited by an MAOI, tyramine is absorbed and acts as a vasopressor. This effect has led to cerebral vascular accidents and death in adult patients. If the patient is able to adhere to a special tyramine-free diet, the MAOIs appear to be quite safe.

Children are less likely to follow a strict diet, making MAOI treatment a risky enterprise in this population (O'Regan, 1971; Ray, 1971; Shamsie & Barriga, 1971). This danger is unfortunate, since MAOIs may have unique efficacy for some individuals, especially those with "atypical" depressions, those found unresponsive to standard TCA therapies (Ravaris, Robinson, Ives, Nies, & Bartlett, 1980; Ryan, 1992; Ryan et al., 1988b), or those with depression compounded by significant social phobia (Kelly, Guirguis, Frommer, Mitchell-Heggs, & Sargant, 1970; Liebowitz, Schneier, Hollander, Welkowitz, & Saoud, 1991; Sargant, 1969). Because of these safety issues, MAOIs have fallen from common usage in adults, are very rarely used in children, and will not be discussed further.

The MAOIs are described in Table 4.

Other Compounds

Trazodone, maprotiline, and bupropion are three additional antidepressant medications marketed in the United States. Bupropion has generated considerable interest, since it has shown promise as an antidepressant medication (Arredondo, Streeter, & Docherty, 1992) and has demonstrated efficacy for ADHD (Clay, Gualtieri, Evans, & Gullion, 1988). Perhaps because it is highly sedating, trazodone is rarely used to treat depression in children. However, in an open trial of trazodone for aggressive adolescents (some of whom had depressive symptoms), benefit was seen (N. Ghaziuddin & Alessi, 1992). Although the use of maprotiline in children has shown some promise (Forrest, 1977; Minuti & Gallo, 1991; Okasha & Sadek, 1976; Watanabe, Yokoyama, Kubo, Iwai, & Kuyama, 1978), maprotiline is also rarely used for treatment of childhood depression. The reason may be that maprotiline seems to offer few advantages over other compounds and has been associated with at least one occurrence of sudden death in a child (Popper & Elliott, 1990).

Last, lithium is occasionally considered when treating depressed children. It is usually added to augment the efficacy of a currently prescribed antidepressant. In a recent update on the psychiatric uses of lithium in children by Alessi, Naylor, Ghaziuddin, and Zubieta (1994), no mention is made regarding its use as a sole therapeutic agent in childhood depression. To our knowledge, no controlled studies of lithium have been conducted in childhood depression. Complicating such a study would be the speculation that certain depressed children may be suffering from a variant of bipolar disorder with depressive symptomatology and not a true depression (Delong, 1978, 1990; Delong & Nieman, 1983). Thus, an accurate diagnosis would be critical to the evaluation of the therapeutic role of lithium in depressed children. To date, two open studies have been conducted in which lithium has been used as an augmentation agent (Ryan, Meyer, Dachille, Mazzie, & Puig-Antich, 1988a; Strober, Freeman, & Rigali, 1990). The results of these preliminary studies are encouraging; however, double-blind, placebo-controlled trials (as have been conducted in adult refractory depressives) would help confirm the efficacy of this approach.

Abe and Ohta (1992) have reported on three adolescent girls in whom lithium seemed to be helpful for preventing *cyclical* depressive symptoms. Lithium has also been widely used to treat symptoms of aggressivity and irritability in children with a variety of

Table 4. The Monoamine Oxidase Inhibitors[a]

Generic name (brand name)	Adverse effects (most common)	FDA age recommendation	Initial dosage	Maintenance dosage	Contraindications	Dose limits
Isocarboxazid (Marplan)	In adults: No percentages available: orthostatic hypotension, cardiac rate and rhythm changes, dizziness, vertigo, constipation, headache, overactivity, hyperreflexia, tremor, muscle twitching, mania, hypomania, peripheral edema, weakness, fatigue, dry mouth, blurred vision, hyperhidrosis, anorexia, body weight changes, gastrointestinal disturbances, skin rashes	No recommendations are made regarding use in children or adolescents 17 or younger.	30 mg/day for adults in single or divided doses	Generally unnecessary to exceed 30 mg/day. Since this medication has a cumulative effect, once steady state is achieved, dosing should be at as low a level as possible to control symptoms.	Those with impaired liver or renal functioning or those taking sympathomimetic drugs. Not to be coadministered with or immediately following other MAOI drugs. Not to be used with buspirone until at least 10 days have elapsed since discontinuation. Not to be used in conjunction with clomipramine, tryptophan, dextromethorphan, or fluoxetine. Allow 5 weeks to elapse after discontinuation of fluoxetine before isocarboxazid is initiated.	30 mg/day

(Continued)

Table 4. (*Continued*)

Generic name (brand name)	Adverse effects (most common)	FDA age recommendation	Initial dosage	Maintenance dosage	Contraindications	Dose limits
Phenelzine (Nardil)	Common side effects: nervous system: dizziness, headache, drowsiness gastrointestinal: constipation, xerostomia metabolic: weight gain cardiovascular: postural hypotension, edema genitourinary: anorgasmia, ejaculatory disturbances Less common, not including the categories above: dermatological: skin rash, sweating special senses: blurred vision, glaucoma Severe Side effects, not including the categories above: respiratory: edema of the glottis general: fever associated with increased muscle tone withdrawal syndrome following abrupt withdrawal consisting of vivid nightmares with agitation, possibly frank psychosis, and convulsions	Not recommended for children under age 16 due to lack of controlled studies.	Adolescents: 15 mg t.i.d.	Rapid escalation to 60 mg/day as tolerated by patient. Clinical response may not become apparent until treatment at 60 mg has been continued for at least 4 weeks	Those with known sensitivity to phenelzine, pheochromocytoma, congestive heart failure, a history of liver disease, or abnormal liver function tests. Not to be used with other MAOIs, any sympathomimetic drugs, or related compounds. Avoid foods containing tyramine or dopamine, or excessive caffeine or chocolate intake. Should not be used with meperidine or dextromethorphan or with CNS depressants such as alcohol and certain narcotics. Should not be used in combination with buspirone. Allow 10 days to elapse between the discontinuation of this drug and the institution of another antidepressant, or the discontinuation of another MAOI and beginning treatment with Nardil.	May be necessary to increase early treatment dosage to 90 mg/day to obtain sufficient MAO inhibition.

| Tranylcypromine (Parnate) | Adults: overstimulantion, which may include anxiety, agitation and manic symptoms restlessness or insomnia, weakness, drowsiness, dizziness, xerostomia, nausea, diarrhea, abdominal pain, or constipation, tachycardia, anorexia, edema, palpitation, blurred vision, chills, impotence, headaches, hepatitis, skin rash, impaired water excretion, tinnitus, muscle spasm, tremors, myoclonic jerks, numbness, paresthesia, urinary retention and retarded ejaculation, anemia, leukopenia, agranulocytosis, and thrombocytopenia

postintroduction reports that have not been clearly linked to Parnate therapy:

localized scleroderma, flare-up of cystic acne, ataxia, confusion, disorientation, memory loss, urinary frequency, urinary incontinence, urticaria, fissuring in corner of mouth, akinesia

The most serious reaction associated with Parnate is the occurrence of hypertensive crises, which have sometimes been fatal. | Safety and effectiveness in those below 18 years of age have not been established.

This drug is not recommended as a first-line medication for MDD.

Appears more successful as a second-line medication for drug nonresponders, especially those with major depression without melancholia. | 30 mg/day, usually in divided doses | 30 mg/day, usually in divided doses | Parnate should not be administered in combination with any of the following: MAOI's, dibenzazepine derivatives, sympathomimetics (including amphetamines), some CNS depressants (including narcotics and alcohol), antihypertensive, diuretic, antihistaminic, sedative, or anesthetic drugs, buspirone, dextromethorphan, cheese or other foods with a high tyramine content, or excessive quantities of caffeine.

This drug should not be administered to any patient with a confirmed or suspected cerebrovascular defect or to any patient with cardiovascular disease, hypertension, or history of headache. | Gradual 10 mg/day increments at intervals of 1–3 weeks, the dosage may be increased to a maximum of 60 mg/day. |

*a*This table was prepared using the 1993 *Physicians Desk Reference* (PDR). Every effort was exerted to make it as accurate as possible. It is not meant to be used as a replacement for the PDR when making medication-prescribing decisions.

psychiatric diagnoses (Campbell, Perry, & Green, 1984; Carroll, Jefferson, & Greist, 1987). Whether this represents treatment of symptoms that are a "depressive equivalent" or a "bipolar variant" remains highly speculative.

Several miscellaneous antidepressant medications are described in Table 5.

Antidepressant Medication Efficacy

In this section, we present summaries of the major *placebo-controlled, double-blind* studies of depressed children or adolescents, or both, including pilot studies. These studies are highlighted because, by design, their purpose is to determine medication efficacy. Due to the variations in study designs, inclusion criteria, and efficacy assessment, each is examined according to a standardized outline to facilitate comparison.

Kramer and Feiguine (1981)

Medication studied: Amitriptyline (AMI). Inpatient study.

Study design: Double-blind.

Dose and/or plasma level range: 25 mg q.i.d., increased by 25 mg to a maximum dose of 200 mg/day in divided doses.

Total patients enrolled/study completers: 20 total; 10 on AMI (1 M, 9 F) and 10 on placebo (6 M, 4 F).

Age range/sex: 3.0–16.1 years old/see above.

Entrance criteria: A social worker first identified patients with symptoms of depression (i.e., suicidal ideation or attempts, sadness, insomnia, withdrawal, and dysphoria). Participants had to have a score above 7 on the Psychiatric Rating Scale (PRS) administered by a psychiatrist (patient score range: 7–14). Global impression of dysphoric symptoms was also necessary. Minnesota Multiphasic Personality Inventory (MMPI) (form R) and the Psychiatric Rating Scale (PRS) (form A) were administered. Last, the participant had to have been depressed for 6 months prior to admission and nonfunctional in relation to school.

Comorbid conditions of study participants: None mentioned.

Criteria used to determine satisfactory response: Repeat psychiatric examination during 3rd and 6th weeks. The Depression Adjective Check List was administered at the 3rd, 5th, and 6th weeks. The MMPI was administered during the 6th week. Each test was administered randomly during the weeks stated.

Statistical significance/trends: Marked improvement in both treatment groups at week 6 when compared to week 1.

Conclusions: No significant statistical difference between AMI and placebo.

Comments: Individual therapy was provided to all study participants while the study was in progress. The authors stated that ". . . hospitalization, with its attendant therapeutic modalities, [could have been] the main factor in improvement."

Petti and Law (1982)

Medication studied: Imipramine (IMI). Inpatient study.

Study design: Double-blind, placebo-controlled 7-week pilot study (2-week drug washout, 1 week titration, 3 weeks on maximum dose, 1 week drug taper and withdrawal).

Dose and/or plasma level range: B.i.d. dosing to achieve 5 mg/kg per day.

Total patients enrolled/study completers: 7 enrolled/6 completed [3 IMI (3 M); 3 placebo (2 M, 1 F)].

Age range/sex: 6–12 years old/see above.

Entrance criteria: Entrants were designated as depressed by the Bellevue Index of

Table 5. Miscellaneous Antidepressant Medications[a]

Generic name (Brand name)	Adverse effects (most common)	FDA age recommendation	Initial dosage	Maintenance dosage	Contraindications	Dose limits
Bupropion (Wellbutrin)	From adult studies: agitation (31.9%), dry mouth (27.6%), weight loss (26%), nausea/vomiting (22.9%), dizziness (22.3%), excessive sweating (22.3%), insomnia (18.6%), anorexia (18.3%), blurred vision (14.6%), weight gain (13.2%), tachycardia (10.8%)	The safety and effectiveness in those under age 18 have not been established.	100 mg b.i.d.	200–300 mg/day in divided doses of 100 mg each	Patients with seizure disorder, anorexia nervosa bulimia (due to these patients having an increase in seizure problems). Not to be used concurrently with an MAOI.	Maximum of 450 mg/day given in divided doses of no more than 150 mg each
Maprotiline (Ludiomil)	Apparently from adult studies: dry mouth (22%), dizziness (16%)	No information regarding use in children or adolescents.	Adults: 75 mg/day Elderly: 25 mg/day Single daily doses may be an alternative to divided dosing.	Adults: 75–150 mg/day Elderly: 50–100 mg/day	Not to be used in patients hypersensitive to maprotiline or in patients with known or suspected seizure disorders. Should not be given concomitantly with an MAOI or within 14 days of the discontinuation of an MAOI. Not recommended during the acute recovery phase of a myocardial infarction.	Gradual increase to maximum of 225 mg/day
Trazodone (Desyrel)	Adult inpatient studies: drowsiness (23.9%), dizziness/lightheadedness (19.7%), nervousness (14.8%), xerostomia (14.8%), fatigue (11.3%), nausea/vomiting (9.9%) Has been associated with the occurrence of priapism, which may require surgical intervention. This could result in permanent impairment of erectile function.	Safety and effectiveness in those below 18 years of age have not been established.	Adults: 150 mg/day in divided doses	After an adequate response is achieved, maintenance dosing should be the lowest possible dose that still maintains therapeutic response.	Hypersensitivity to dyserel	Outpatient adults: 400 mg/day in divided doses Inpatient adults: 600 mg/day in divided doses

[a]This table was prepared using the 1993 *Physicians Desk Reference* (PDR). Every effort was exerted to make it as accurate as possible. It is not meant to be used as a replacement for the PDR when making medication-prescribing decisions.

Depression (BID) and the Weinberg Index of Depression. In the 3rd week of the study (1st week on drug/placebo), the Children's Depression Inventory (CDI) was administered and a structured interview, the School Age Depression Listed Inventory (SADLI), was completed, in which the children had to be rated as moderately or more severely depressed.

Comorbid conditions of study participants: None mentioned.

Criteria used to determine satisfactory response: The SADLI and CDI were administered on the last week of maximum dose (end of week 6). The BID was administered during the final week, which was medication taper and withdrawal.

Statistical significance/trends: Of the 3 patients on active drug, 2 showed dramatic improvement on the three measures employed and 1 showed some improvement. However, because the study sample was so small, statistical analysis was not used for hypothesis testing.

Conclusions: IMI is not statistically superior to placebo.

Comments: As part of their clinical care, study participants were provided active milieu therapy, individual dynamic psychotherapy, and initial family work in addition to medication. All 3 patients on IMI experienced withdrawal symptoms, 2 mild and 1 marked consisting of agitation, gastrointestinal distress, increased depression, and hostility.

Kashani, Shekim, and Reid (1984)

Medication studied: Amitriptyline (AMI).

Study design: Double-blind, placebo-controlled crossover study. Inpatient study.

Dose and/or plasma level range: Fixed dosage strategy. Began with 1 mg/kg per day t.i.d. dosing, increased after 3 days to 1.5 mg/kg per day. This dosage was then maintained throughout the remaining 8 weeks of the study (4 on AMI, 4 on placebo).

Total patients enrolled/study completers: 9/9.

Age range/sex: 9–12 years old/8 M, 1 F.

Entrance criteria: Independent diagnostic evaluation by two child psychiatrists and a total score of 20 or higher on the Bellevue Index of Depression (BID). Items associated with aggression were not included in scoring.

Comorbid conditions of study participants: None mentioned.

Criteria used to determine satisfactory response: BID scores dropped below 20 in 6 of the 9 children. These 6 were also noted to have a subjective increase in overall interest level.

Statistical significance/trends: Failed to achieve statistical significance when comparing difference of BID scores between placebo and active drug.

Conclusions: The authors stated that results "looked encouraging" and that a larger trial of AMI was justified.

Comments: The authors mentioned that carryover effects could have affected results at the cross-over phase of this study or milieu therapy could have affected results overall. The dose of AMI could have been too low due to the fixed dosage regimen employed. One patient with a maternal family history of bipolar disorder became hypomanic on AMI.

Puig-Antich et al. (1987)

Medication studied: Imipramine (IMI).

Study design: Double-blind, placebo-controlled study. Accepted cases were randomly assigned to drug or placebo.

Dose and/or plasma level range: After completing the baseline protocol, the patient was given IMI, 1.5 mg/kg per day divided into three daily, roughly equal doses. On the 3rd day, if EKG, blood pressure, and IMI side effects scale were passed, the dose was raised to 3 mg/kg per day. On the 6th day, the same laboratory tests were run before increasing the dose to 4 mg/kg per day. On the 9th day, tests were completed and the dose was increased up to 4 mg/kg per day. On the 12th day, the tests were completed again. If the results were satisfactory, the dose was maintained at 5 mg/kg per day, and the tests were run weekly for the following 35 days.

Total patients enrolled/study completers: In all, 53 children with MDD completed the baseline protocol, of whom 38 completed the double-blind study. All 22 children in the placebo group completed the protocol. Of the 20 children assigned to the drug group, 16 completed the protocol (1 failed to comply with the protocol, 2 refused to come in to the clinic at midprotocol, and 1 child moved). In the follow-up plasma level protocol, 15 of the 16 children who completed the drug protocol completed the plasma protocol. A group of 15 children who were not in the double-blind study were recruited for the plasma study, and all completed the protocol.

Age range/sex: All children were preadolescents. Age and gender ratios were not specified for the double-blind study. There were 18 boys and 12 girls in the plasma protocol. The mean age of these children was 9.56 ± 1.46 years.

Entrance criteria: Children were considered who were reported by at least one source, even self-report, to have at least one of the following four criteria: persistently looks sad, frequently says he or she feels sad, suicidal statement or behavior, school refusal. These children were then assessed by two physicians using the Schedule for Affective Disorders and Schizophrenia for School-Age Children (K-SADS). The child was finally included if both psychiatrists agreed that the child fit the Research Diagnostic Criteria for MDD (summary ratings), the pediatrician found no medical criteria for exclusion, and the parent signed informed consent for the study.

Comorbid conditions of study participants: The authors did not identify any comorbid diagnoses for any of the subjects.

Criteria used to determine satisfactory response: The researchers used the K-SADS—Present Episode version (K-SADS-P) and Kiddie Global Assessment Scale (K-GAS) scores from the 5th week for outcome measurements in the double-blind study. Statistics were used to compare the K-SADS-P scores from the week before IMI administration to those taken in the 5th week. In the plasma protocol, plasma levels were compared to K-SADS scores.

Statistical significance/trends: There were no significant differences between the placebo and drug groups at the midprotocol point. Before/after differences, response/nonresponse differences, and differences between psychotic depressives and endogenous depressives were all insignificant. As a result, the double-blind study was terminated and a plasma protocol was developed and instituted in its place.

Conclusions: On the basis of the results from their plasma study, the authors concluded that during the proper course of IMI treatment, prepubertal major depressive children are the more likely to respond, the higher their plasma concentrations of imipramine and desipramine and the lower the severity of their depressive symptomatology. The negative prediction of response could have been related to the depressive hallucinations/delusions experienced during the protocol or to the overall severity of the depressive symptomatology.

Comments: The authors concluded that the IMI doses may have been too low and that the placebo washout period may not have been long enough.

Geller, Cooper, McCombs, Graham, and Wells (1989)

Medication studied: Nortriptyline (NT). Outpatient study.

Study design: Double-blind, placebo-controlled with a "fixed plasma level." Two-week single-blind washout phase, 8-week "core."

Dose and/or plasma level range: Individualized dosing to achieve steady-state plasma levels between 60 and 100 ng/ml.

Total patients enrolled/study completers: 72 studied, 12 dropouts during the washout phase, 10 dropouts after beginning the 8-week double-blind, placebo-controlled portion/50 completers [26 NT (73.1% M, 26.9% F)], 24 placebo (66.7% M, 33.3% F).

Age range/sex: 5–12 years old/see above.

Entrance criteria: A rating of 4 or more on the MDD criteria items of the K-SADS-P. Participants were dropped if Children's Depression Rating Scale (CDRS) scores were 25 or less at the week 1 or week 2 evaluation (washout phase). Delusional subjects and substance abusers were excluded.

Comorbid conditions of study participants: Those with other major medical, psychiatric, or neurological illnesses were excluded.

Criteria used to determine satisfactory response: A CDRS score of 20 or less or a score of 1 or 2 on MDD criteria items on the K-SADS-P.

Conclusions: No significant difference in response rate between active and placebo groups.

Comments: These patients were chronically ill (96% for more than 2 years, 50% for more than 5 years), and this circumstance may have negatively affected response. The authors speculate that the fixed plasma level range used may have been too low for optimal effect in children.

Simeon, Dinicola, Ferguson, and Copping (1990)

Medication studied: Fluoxetine (FLX). An 8-week study.

Study design: Placebo-controlled, double-blind study. Both outpatients and inpatients.

Dose and/or plasma level range: Initial 20 mg/day dose increased to 40 mg/day after 4–7 days and to 60 mg/day during the 2nd week. Further dose changes were individually titrated in a flexible dose design.

Total patients enrolled/study completers: 40 patients/15 active and 15 placebo completers.

Age range/sex: 13–18 years old/not identified.

Entrance criteria: Baseline Hamilton Depression Score (HAM-D) of 20 or more.

Comorbid conditions of study participants: None mentioned. Patients with schizophrenia, substance abuse, or other psychotic illnesses were excluded.

Criteria used to determine satisfactory response: Not clearly delineated. In addition to the HAM-D, Clinical Global Impressions (CGI), the Raskin Depression Scale, the COVI Anxiety Scale, and the Hopkins Symptom Checklist were employed at screening, baseline, and during weekly visits. The authors stated that "improvements in the fluoxetine group exceeded those in the placebo group on 9 of the 10 clinical variables; all of the HAM-D (5), CGI (3), Raskin (1), and COVI (1), except for the sleep disturbance factor of the HAM-D."

Conclusions: FLX was superior on all clinical measures except for sleep disorder, but the differences were not statistically significant. The authors suggested that long-term treatment trials be initiated.

Comments: A follow-up study was conducted of these study participants after, on average, 24 months.

Geller, Cooper, Graham, Marsteller, and Bryant (1990)

Medication studied: Nortriptyline (NT).

Study design: Double-blind, placebo-controlled using a "fixed plasma level."

Dose and/or plasma level range: Dosed to achieve 80 ng/ml (± 20 ng/ml).

Total patients enrolled/study completers: 52/31; 12 NT (75% M, 25% F), 19 placebo (42.1% M, 57.9% F).

Age range/sex: 12–17 years old/see above.

Entrance criteria: Duration of depressive illness of at least 2 months. Autism, child-onset pervasive developmental disorder, and other major medical psychiatric or neurological illnesses or substance-use disorders were excluded. A total of 17 placebo washout responders were dropped from the study, as were delusional depressives.

Comorbid conditions of study participants: Of those on active drug, 58% had comorbid separation anxiety and 50% antisocial behavior.

Criteria used to determine satisfactory response: Study entrants needed a score of 31 or above on the Children's Depression Rating Scale (CDRS) to continue into the 8-week placebo-controlled, double-blind phase. Drug responders were those whose CDRS score was at or below 25 and who scored less than or equal to 2 on DSM-III criteria items on the K-SADS-P at week 8 of the double-blind phase. An exception could be the DSM-III Concentration item of the K-SADS-P, which could be 3 or less.

Conclusions: The two treatment groups had similar protocol severity ratings. In addition, higher plasma levels of NT resulted in a worsening of their pathology.

Comments: Of the study subjects, 83% had a duration of illness of at least 2 years and 50% had a 5-year duration of illness prior to the start of the protocol. One active responder to NT went on to have a bipolar course.

Geller, Cooper, Graham, Getner, and Marsteller (1992)

Medication studied: Nortriptyline (NT).

Study design: Pharmacokinetically designed double-blind, placebo-controlled, outpatient study. A 10-week protocol that included a 2-week single-blind placebo washout phase.

Dose and/or plasma level range: Participants had to reach a steady-state plasma level of 60–100 ng/ml.

Total patients enrolled/study completers: 72/50; 26 NT (73.1% M, 26.9% F), 24 placebo (66.7% M, 33.3% F).

Age range/sex: 6–12 years old/see above.

Entrance criteria: Needed a score of 40 or greater on the Children's Depression Rating Scale (CDRS) and a duration of depressive illness of 2 months or more. Subjects were dropped if they scored 25 or less on the CDRS at week 1 or 2 of the washout phase. Participants were not enrolled if they were delusional, autistic, or had childhood-onset pervasive developmental disorder (PDD) or other major medical, psychiatric, or neurological illness or a substance-use disorder.

Comorbid conditions of study participants: Of those on active drug, 80.8% had comorbid separation anxiety and 15.4% antisocial behavior.

Criteria used to determine satisfactory response: Responders had a CDRS score of 20 or less and scores of 1 or 2 on all the DSM-II criteria items for MDD on the Depression scale of the K-SADS-P at the end of the double-blind, placebo-controlled phase of the study.

Conclusions: There was a poor rate of response in both treatment groups (30% active, 16.7% placebo).

Comments: None of the 50 patients enrolled had ever received TCA medication before. Of those on active drug, 42% had a duration of depressive illness of 2–5 years and 57% had a duration of more than 5 years.

Summary and Conclusions Regarding Double-Blind, Placebo-Controlled Trials

As indicated by these summaries, the major controlled trials of antidepressant medication to date have failed to demonstrate a significant advantage of active medication over placebo. This result may be attributable to inappropriate patient selection criteria, high placebo response rates, small study power, or other methodological problems. Much of the controversy surrounding medication treatment of depressed children would evaporate if the question of efficacy could be more clearly answered. Since none of these studies has provided compelling evidence that antidepressants are more efficacious than placebo, some workers have been led to erroneously state that "studies show antidepressants don't work in kids." Because of widespread misunderstanding regarding the meaning of these studies, we present a brief digression on interpreting medication efficacy studies.

To conclude that "antidepressants don't work in kids" on the basis of the research presented above is analogous to saying, "A brief search of my bedroom shows that my sunglasses don't exist." The existence of my sunglasses in analogous to the existence of medication efficacy, and the brief search for my sunglasses is analogous to the research studies searching for efficacy. Once I have completed a brief search of my bedroom and failed to find my sunglasses, I really do not know whether they exist or not. All I know is that I have failed to find them. Of course, it is possible that my sunglasses do not exist, but it is more likely that I simply failed to search for them carefully enough or in the right places.

Examined with this in mind, these studies suggest two possibilities: (1) Antidepressant medications are not effective for childhood depression. (2) An antidepressant effect exists, but these studies have failed to detect it. We believe that possibility number 2 will ultimately be borne out, for several reasons. Perhaps the most persuasive reason is the widespread clinical use of these medications in depressed children. It seems unlikely (but possible) that clinicians would continue to prescribe these medications if no clinical benefit were being realized. Second, the studies completed thus far are all methodologically compromised, yet many of them show trends toward efficacy that are not statistically significant. Third, clomipramine and sertraline have been shown to be efficacious in childhood OCD (DeVeaugh-Geiss et al., 1992; Johnston, unpublished data), and it is counterintuitive that anti-OCD effect would exist in the absence of antidepressant effects. Last, antidepressant response in children correlates to blood levels (Preskorn, Weller, & Weller, 1982), and measurable cognitive improvements have been determined with antidepressant treatment (Rapport, Carlson, Kelly, & Pataki, 1993; Stanton, Wilson, & Brumback, 1981).

The issue of efficacy will remain controversial until further data are generated. However, we believe that when future studies are conducted, with methodological refinements in patient selection, dosage optimization, and rating instruments, an antidepressant effect will be detected. Whether this effect will be seen as clinically significant remains to be seen.

Medication Combinations

If the use of antidepressant medication in children is relatively uncharted territory, then drug combinations in the juvenile population truly represent a foray into the unknown. When medications are mixed, a potential for unexpected adverse effects is created. Such effects could come about as a result of either pharmacokinetic or pharmacodynamic interactions. Some theoretical examples of interactive pharmacokinetic effects are competition for metabolic enzymes, induction of higher rates of metabolism, and competition for protein binding. For example, March, Moon, and Johnston (1990) report a case in which fluoxetine appears to have elevated amitriptyline plasma levels in a child. Pharmacodynamic interactions occur when two compounds affect one or more neurotransmitter systems in a similar manner. One such example is when an SSRI and an MAOI are used together (a potentially dangerous combination). Through differing pharmacodynamic mechanisms, each of these drugs tends to increase the amount of serotonin at the synaptic cleft. MAOIs inhibit enzymes that degrade serotonin and SSRIs inhibit serotonin reuptake. When these drugs are used together, patients may develop a constellation of side effects—including a decreased level of consciousness, muscular rigidity, and even death—has been termed the "serotonin syndrome" (Sternbach, 1991).

On the other hand, medication combinations may also produce therapeutic effects superior to either medication used alone. This synergistic phenomenon was suggested in a study reported by Rapport et al. (1993) in which desipramine and methylphenidate were used alone and in conjunction for 16 hospitalized children with both ADHD and mood symptoms. Neuropsychological testing suggested that each medication affected distinct cognitive domains, and when the two were used together, they appeared to have the potential to produce greater clinical improvement than either drug alone. The side effects of this combination are identified in a companion article (Pataki, Carlson, Kelly, Rapport, & Biancaniello, 1993). This theory is often invoked when medication combinations are considered for treatment-resistant depression. The term "augmentation" is frequently used to describe these medication combinations.

Treatment with medication combinations is most often considered under the following circumstances: treating comorbid conditions, augmenting a partial drug response, and possibly managing the troubling side effects of another medication that is working well.

Children who have both psychotic and depressive symptoms may benefit from a combination of a neuroleptic and an antidepressant (Geller, Cooper, Farooki, & Chestnut, 1985).

Augmentation strategies are considered when usual treatments are not adequate, as in the case of partial responders to a single pharmacological agent. Attempting to boost a partial TCA response by adding lithium has been utilized with conflicting efficacy (Ryan et al., 1988a; Strober et al., 1990; Strober, Freeman, Rigali, Schmidt, & Diamond, 1992). Further research is needed to clarify the usefulness of this medication approach.

Ryan et al. (1988a) have added MAOIs to TCA partial responders with some success and have outlined the proper administration of these medication combinations. However, they report dietary compliance difficulties, both deliberate and accidental, as important limiting factors to this treatment approach.

Psychological Issues

In our review, we encountered little regarding the possible psychological implications for children and their families when antidepressant medications are used. While this is a relatively neglected area of research, we believe it has important clinical significance. For example, most children have difficulty understanding that their mood disturbances are the result of an illness. Instead, they tend to see their problems as a result of (1) their own "badness" or (2) the "mean" things done to them by others. The potential psychiatric underpinnings of medication noncompliance in this population should also be explored. We suspect these issues have important implications for antidepressant medication treatment. Research in this area might identify how children and their families are affected when antidepressant medications are prescribed and how these effects should be addressed clinically.

Ethical, Regulatory, and Forensic Considerations

It has been said that good ethics begin with good information. Well-intended concerns, if based on inaccurate or incomplete information, can masquerade as ethical dilemmas.

For example, treating depressed children with medication frequently results in raised eyebrows on the part of well-meaning relatives, teachers, and friends. A commonly voiced opinion is: "Children should learn to solve their problems without resorting to pills." Such concerns are more often knee-jerk vocalizations of popular belief than carefully considered and informed decisions. At their root are mistaken assumptions that mental illness is no different than common unhappiness and that using antidepressant medications is akin to escaping with a bottle of whiskey. Few would suggest that children solve their problems of pneumonia or diabetes without resorting to medication. However, the public's perception of mental illness remains colored by stigma, and ignorance about depression and its treatment is widespread.

Several legitimate ethical concerns do arise commonly. The decision to proceed with antidepressant treatment should result from a considered analysis of the risks and benefits of drug treatment vs. the risks and benefits of treatment without drugs. In truth, this analysis is somewhat ambiguous, since many of the factors under consideration are vague or represent value judgments. For example, the long-term effects of antidepressants on the nervous system are unknown, but probably benign. Can this risk be balanced against a benefit such as improved sleep? Does informing the parents and child of the myriad of uncertainties improve the decision-making process or simply cause alarm? Many parents want to trust their child's doctor because they feel inadequate in their understanding of the technology to make a good decision. On the other hand, doctors feel increasingly compelled to involve parents in the decision process because of their own uncertainties or perhaps because of legal liability concerns.

As though these difficulties were not enough, there are a whole host of subtle pressures influencing the psychiatric treatment. These pressures include pharmaceutical company advertisements directed at physicians, managed care influences to treat as cheaply as possible, and parents demanding a fast and safe remedy, to name just a few.

Clinical Guidelines

Even though there is a relative paucity of systematic study of psychiatric medication use in children, antidepressants are widely prescribed by many child psychiatrists (Child Psychopharmacology Information Center, unpublished data). This curious situation is fostered by several political and regulatory factors. Once a medication is approved by the Food and Drug Administration for the United States market, physicians may prescribe it for any age group and for any clinical purpose they deem appropriate. Pharmaceutical companies are forbidden by law to promote their products for uses beyond the approved indication; however, adherence to this standard appears variable.

The training of child psychiatrists is also a factor. Child psychiatrists are first trained as general psychiatrists and develop a familiarity with the wide range of antidepressant medications. At that time, the patient's age is not commonly a factor to consider, excepting for elderly patients. The clinical experience and prescribing patterns of psychiatrists thus have the potential to be generalized to their practice in children. For these and possibly other reasons, there appears to be little financial advantage for the pharmaceutical industry to study these medications in children, since they are already in widespread use.

Many child psychiatrists are routinely prescribing antidepressants to children and believe (we hope!) that they are doing well by their patients. We suspect that this practice is due to a belief that depression in children is enough like depression in adults to respond similarly to medication therapy.

The practicing clinician is the individual called on to make the decision whether to begin antidepressant medication treatment or not. While a comprehensive treatment algorithm is nearly impossible to articulate, several recurring clinical questions warrant consideration and may provide guidance. The recommendations given below are derived primarily from our clinical practice and experience guided by the research literature. As such, they are a synthesis of experience, research, and common sense. The reader is referred to Ryan (1990) or Rancurello (1986), who have also offered guidelines in this area.

At What Point in an Overall Treatment Plan Should Medication Be Considered?

In the vast majority of child cases of depression, antidepressant medication should not be the "first-line" treatment. Given the uncertainty of efficacy and the paucity of safety data, we reserve medication treatment for a select minority of depressed children. We are less inclined to prescribe if the child's mood difficulties can be ascribed to a recent and (one hopes) temporary stressful situation such as a move or family discord. An initial plan of treatment usually includes some blend of individual and family psychotherapy along with psychosocial intervention. For most children with mild to moderate depressive symptoms, these interventions provide adequate relief.

Children who have extreme symptoms of sleep disturbance, irritability, or anhedonia or those who have not responded to the interventions described above are candidates for a trial of antidepressant medication.

Which Medication Is Best?

In makes *intuitive* sense that one antidepressant medication should be at least slightly more efficacious than the others. If this is true, we do not yet have enough data to determine which drug is best. However, it probably does not matter. We know that the available medications are approximately equivalent regarding efficacy in adults, and there is little reason to expect the situation to be different in children. Given equivalence in efficacy, the best medication is the one that is the safest and produces the mildest side effects *in the particular patient*. These factors vary considerably from situation to situation. For example, the SSRIs clearly have an advantage if there is significant risk of an accidental or intentional overdose. On the other hand, the best choice for a 7-year-old child with depressive symptoms and enuresis is typically a TCA (usually imipramine).

In summary, although there isn't a single "best" medication overall, there is almost always a "best" medication (or at least class of medications) for any given clinical situation. We consider the age of the child, comorbid symptoms, concurrent physical illness, family history, past treatment history, and concomitant medications when choosing an antidepressant.

How Is the Proper Dose Determined?

On the basis of pharmacokinetics alone, it is expected that the proper dose of medication will vary considerably from child to child. Furthermore, some children will experience dose-limiting side effects, while others will experience a therapeutic response at lower than expected doses. Still others will not improve no matter what dose (or type) of medication is used. In every case, the dose regimen must be tailored to the individual child. We ascribe to the principle that the lowest dose of medication that produces satisfactory symptom resolution is best.

In the case of TCAs, we typically escalate the dose gradually until one of three outcomes occurs: (1) The child begins to experience benefit. (2) Side effects become dose-limiting. (3) The blood level of medication approaches the upper range considered therapeutic for adults. (*Note*: There are no systematic studies that have established therapeutic blood levels for antidepressants in children.) When one of these outcomes occurs, the dose is not increased and we simply wait at least 2 weeks for further signs of improvement. The utility of therapeutic blood monitoring of TCAs in children is somewhat controversial. For example, Popper (1992) advocates ignoring TCA blood levels. However, we feel they have utility in assessing compliance and making dose adjustments (Johnston & Swift, 1992). Blood levels can also provide useful information when children are experiencing puzzling side effects or inadequate treatment response. There does appear to be a relationship between TCA blood levels and the presence of CNS toxicity (Preskorn & Jerkovich, 1990), although an occasional child appears to require high blood levels for an adequate response (Johnston, Swift, & March, 1993).

Children who metabolize TCAs rapidly often require divided dosing to prevent the transient uncomfortable side effects resulting from ingesting too much medication at once. As a matter of course, we do not exceed 100 mg TCA per dose.

The proper dose of SSRIs is even more ambiguous due to several factors. Because these drugs are newer, there is simply much less experience with them in children. In addition, there are no systematic pharmacokinetic studies in children that would help clarify whether the dosing used in adults results in comparable blood levels when used in kids. Even given this ambiguity, however, dosing is somewhat less critical with the SSRIs than with the TCAs because the SSRIs are generally better tolerated due to their wider margin of safety in overdose and limited anticholinergic and cardiac effects. Similar to the situation with the TCAs, we start with a modest dose and gradually escalate (over weeks to months) until a treatment response is seen, side effects emerge, or the dose exceeds the current recommendations for adults.

How Should Children Be Monitored during Treatment?

When children begin antidepressant treatment, they should be seen weekly to monitor for the emergence of side effects or adverse reactions. This is especially important during the early phase of medication treatment when the dose is being increased. Inquiries should be made of both the child and the parent regarding possible side effects such as constipation, upset stomach, difficulty urinating, blurred vision, headaches, and so forth. One area that clinicians often fail to ask children about is sexual side effects. This inquiry is often best accomplished with the parent(s) out of earshot, as many children may be embarrassed to discuss their sexuality in front of them.

Children on TCAs should have follow-up EKGs each time the dose is substantially increased. How frequently EKGs are done thereafter is controversial and is best individualized to the patient. For example, young children, children with longer than usual cardiac conduction at baseline, children who complain of cardiovascular symptoms, or children who have had EKG changes emerge while on the antidepressant should have more frequent follow-up EKGs. At the other extreme are children with no complaints and no EKG changes. It is unclear whether these children *ever* require routine periodic EKG monitoring and, if they do, how frequently.

How Long Should Children Be Treated with an Antidepressant?

This is a particularly thorny question that demands further study. Recent research has shown that for many adults, depression is a chronically relapsing disorder that may be best treated by long-term maintenance antidepressant medication. The data of Kovacs, Feinberg, Crouse-Novak, Paulauskas, and Finkelstein (1984) on the natural history of depression in children suggest that episodes tend to be approximately 7 months in duration. In our practice, if a child has a good medication response, we generally treat for 6 months and then begin a gradual medication taper. If depressive symptoms return, the dose is restored to the pretaper level and another taper is attempted 4–6 months later.

Given the paucity of research data, the use of antidepressant medications in children is likely to be viewed as either "cutting edge technology" or "dangerous quackery," depending on the legal circumstances of the moment or a particular lawyer's agenda. This ambiguity should give every clinician involved in treating depressed children pause to consider the legal implications of their actions. Several concepts worth considering are these: informed consent, standard of care, and medical malpractice.

It is important that parents be fully informed of the risks, benefits, and alternatives available when their child's physician is considering prescribing an antidepressant. Although we do not typically require written consent, we carefully document that complete information was provided. Our trainees are often surprised to find that we inform parents that serious side effects (such as seizures and death) are possible. While some may see this practice as unnecessarily alarming, we feel that it is important, especially given the current malpractice situation in the United States. We try to place this information in the proper context by pointing out to parents that they easily accept the risks associated with having their children ride in automobiles and that the risk of medication treatment is probably less. We also routinely inform parents that these drugs are not FDA-approved for treating depression in children. Many parents read medication package inserts. Since antidepressant package inserts typically say "not approved for use in children," parents may wonder about the competence of their doctor. While this frightening information is sobering for most parents, they are usually grateful they were informed.

As a rule, physicians are expected to practice a standard of medicine that is consistent within their local community and specialty. This has been termed the "standard of care." What this means is that a given type of medical practice could be viewed as acceptable in one community, yet be seen as deficient in another. The local standard of care is a particularly important consideration when treating children with antidepressant medication, since most of these compounds are not FDA-approved for treating depression in childhood. This fact makes the local standard all the more important, since there is little else on which to base prescribing practices.

The best strategy for avoiding medical malpractice problems is simply to practice good medicine. While it is true that in some specialties physicians are at high risk to be sued for medical misfortunes that they cannot control, this is generally not the case for psychiatry and especially not for child psychiatry. In the vast majority of instances, a child psychiatrist can avoid malpractice difficulties by (1) practicing in a medically sound, sensible fashion; (2) communicating frequently and honestly with parents; and (3) consulting with colleagues for a second opinion in cases that are particularly troublesome.

Conclusions

Antidepressant treatment for children has emerged as a common clinical practice despite the lack of systematic research demonstrating efficacy. In the authors' opinion, this alone should be considered a clarion call for increased funding for research in child psychopharmacology. In addition, we believe there is a need for revision of FDA policy. The current policy has not protected children by failing to ensure these drugs are systematically evaluated for safety and effectiveness in the pediatric population. Although the current conditions of inadequate research and regulation are troubling, antidepressant medication use remains a clinically practical, often crucial, part of treatment for depressed children.

References

Abe, K., & Ohta, M. (1992). Intermittent lithium administration for prophylaxis of periodic depression of puberty. *Lithium*, *3*, 263–268.

Alarcon, R. D., Johnson, B. R., & Lucas, J. P. (1991). Paranoid and aggressive behavior in two obsessive–compulsive adolescents treated with clomipramine. *Journal of the American Academy of Child and Adolescent Psychiatry*, *30*, 999–1002.

Alessi, N., Naylor, M. W., Ghaziuddin, M., & Zubieta, J. K. (1994). Update on lithium carbonate therapy in children and adolescents. *Journal of the American Academy of Child and Adolescent Psychiatry*, *33*, 291–304.

American Psychiatric Association (1994). *Diagnostic and statistical manual of mental disorders*, 4th ed. Washington, DC: Author.

Apter, A., Ratzoni, G., King, R. A., Weizman, A., Iancu, I., Binder, M., & Riddle, M. A. (1994). Fluvoxamine open-label treatment of adolescents with obsessive–compulsive disorder or depression. *Journal of the American Academy of Child and Adolescent Psychiatry*, *33*, 342–348.

Arredondo, D. E., Streeter, M., & Docherty, J. P. (1992). Bupropion treatment of adolescent depression (NR-315). *APA Annual Meeting, Scientific Proceedings*, p. 125.

Beasley, C. M., Jr., Dornseif, B. E., Bosomworth, J. C., Sayler, M. E., Rampey, A. H., Jr., Heiligenstein, J. H., Thompson, V. L., Murphy, D. J., & Masica, D. N. (1991). Fluoxetine and suicide: A meta-analysis of controlled trials of treatment for depression. *British Medical Journal*, *303*, 685–692.

Biederman, J., Baldessarini, R. J., Wright, V., Keenan, K., & Faraone, S. (1993). A double-blind placebo controlled study of desipramine in the treatment of ADD. III. Lack of impact of comorbidity and family history factors on clinical response. *Journal of the American Academy of Child and Adolescent Psychiatry*, *32*, 199–204.

Biederman, J., Baldessarini, R. J., Wright, V., Knee, D., & Harmatz, J. S. (1989). A double-blind placebo controlled study of desipramine in the treatment of ADD. I. Efficacy. *Journal of the American Academy of Child and Adolescent Psychiatry*, *28*, 777–784.

Biederman, J., Gonzalez, E., Bronstein, B., DeMonaco, H., & Wright, V. (1988). Desipramine and cutaneous reactions in pediatric outpatients. *Journal of Clinical Psychiatry*, *49*, 178–183.

Campbell, M., Perry, R., & Green, W. H. (1984). Use of lithium in children and adolescents. *Psychosomatics*, *25*, 95–101.

Carroll, J. A., Jefferson, J. W., & Greist, J. H. (1987). Psychiatric uses of lithium for children and adolescents. *Hospital and Community Psychiatry*, *38*, 927–928.

Chiappinelli, J. A., & Walton, R. E. (1992). Tooth discoloration resulting from long-term tetracycline therapy: A case report. *Quintessence International*, *23*, 539–541.

Clay, T. H., Gualtieri, C. T., Evans, R. W., & Gullion, C. M. (1988). Clinical and neuropsychological effects of the novel antidepressant bupropion. *Psychopharmacology Bulletin*, *24*, 143–148.

DeLong, G. R. (1978). Lithium carbonate treatment of select behavior disorders in children suggesting manic–depressive illness. *Journal of Pediatrics*, *93*, 689–694.

DeLong, R. (1990). Lithium treatment and bipolar disorders in childhood. *North Carolina Medical Journal*, *51*, 152–154.

DeLong, G. R., & Nieman, G. W. (1983). Lithium-induced behavior changes in children with symptoms suggesting manic–depressive illness. *Psychopharmacology Bulletin*, *19*, 258–265.

DeVeaugh-Geiss, J., Moroz, G., Biederman, J., Cantwell, D., Fontaine, R. Greist, J. H., Reichler, R., Katz, R., & Landau, P. (1992). Clomipramine hydrochloride in childhood and adolescent obsessive–compulsive disorder—a multicenter trial. *Journal of the American Academy of Child and Adolescent Psychiatry*, *31*, 45–49.

Fava, M., Rosenbaum, J. F. (1990). Suicidality and fluoxetine: Is there a relationship? New Research Abstract No. 475. Presented at the Annual Meeting of the American Psychiatric Association, New York, New York.

Forrest, W. A. (1977). Maprotiline (Ludiomil) in depression: A report of a monitored release study of 10,000 patients in general practice. *Journal of International Medical Research*, *5*, 42–47.

Geller, B., Cooper, T. B., Carr, L. G., Warham, J. E., & Rodriguez, A. (1987). Prospective study of scheduled withdrawal from nortriptyline in children and adolescents. *Journal of Clinical Psychopharmacology*, *7*, 252–254.

Geller, B., Cooper, T. B., Farooki, Z. Q., & Chestnut, E. C. (1985). Dose and plasma levels of nortriptyline and chlorpromazine in delusionally depressed adolescents and of nortriptyline in nondelusionally depressed adolescents. *American Journal of Psychiatry*, *142*, 336–338.

Geller, B., Cooper, T. B., Graham, D. L., Fetner, H. H., & Marsteller, F. A. (1992). Pharmacokinetically designed double-blind placebo-controlled study of nortriptyline in 6- to 12-year olds with major depressive disorder. *Journal of the American Academy of Child and Adolescent Psychiatry*, *31*, 34–44.

Geller, B., Cooper, T. B., Graham, D. L., Marsteller, F. A., & Bryant, D. M. (1990). Double-blind, placebo-controlled study of nortriptyline in depressed adolescents using a "fixed plasma level" design. *Psychopharmacology Bulletin*, *26*, 85–90.

Geller, B., Cooper, T. B., McCombs, H. G., Graham, D., & Wells, J. (1989). Double-blind, placebo-controlled study of nortriptyline in depressed children using a "fixed plasma level" design. *Psychopharmacology Bulletin*, *25*, 101–108.

Geller, B., Fox, L. W., & Fletcher, M. (1993). Effect of tricyclic antidepressants on switching to mania and on the onset of bipolarity in depressed 6- to 12-year olds. *Journal of the American Academy of Child and Adolescent Psychiatry*, *32*, 43–50.

Geller, B., Perel, J. M., Knitter, E. F., Lycaki, H., & Farooki, Z. Q. (1983). Nortriptyline in major depressive disorder in children: Response, steady-state plasma levels, predictive kinetics, and pharmacokinetics. *Psychopharmacology Bulletin*, *19*, 62–64.

Ghaziuddin, N., & Alessi, N. E. (1992). An open trial of trazodone in aggressive children. *Journal of Child and Adolescent Psychopharmacology*, *2*, 291–297.

Gualtieri, C. T., Keenan, P. A., & Chandler, M. (1991). Clinical and neuropsychological effects of desipramine in children with attention deficit hyperactivity disorder. *Journal of Clinical Psychopharmacology*, *11*, 155–159.

Haring, J. I. (1992). Case 6: Tetracycline staining. *RDH*, *12*, 12, 16.

Johnston, H. F., & Swift, W. J. (1992). A response to Dr. Popper's article on disregarding antidepressant blood levels. *American Academy of Child and Adolescent Psychiatry Newsletter*, *Spring*, 25–26.

Johnston, H. F., Swift, W. J., & March, J. S. (1993). High plasma level tricyclic therapy in children: A case report and commentary. *Journal of Child and Adolescent Psychopharmacology*, *3*, 115–125.

Kanner, A. M., Klein, R. G., Rubinstein, B., & Mascia, A. (1989). Use of imipramine in children with intractable asthma and psychiatric disorders: A warning. *Psychotherapy and Psychosomatics*, *51*, 203–209.

Kashani, J. H., Hodges, K. K., & Shekim, W. O. (1980). Hypomanic reaction to amitriptyline in a depressed child. *Psychosomatics*, *21*, 867, 876.

Kashani, J. H., Shekim, W. O., & Reid, J. C. (1984). Amitriptyline in children with major depressive disorder: A double-blind crossover pilot study. *Journal of the American Academy of Child and Adolescent Psychiatry*, *23*, 348–351.

Kelly, D., Guirgiis, W., Fromer, E., Mitchell-Heggs, N., & Sargent, W. (1970). Treatment of phobic states with antidepressants: A retrospective study of 246 patients. *British Journal of Psychiatry*, *116*, 387–398.

Kendall, P. C., Kortlander, E., Chansky, T. E., & Brady, E. U. (1992). Comorbidity of anxiety and depression in youth: Treatment implications. *Journal of Consulting and Clinical Psychology*, *60*, 869–880.

Kovacs, M., Feinberg, T. L., Crouse-Novak, M. A., Paulauskas, S. L., & Finkelstein, R. (1984). Depressive disorders in childhood. I. A longitudinal prospective study of characteristics and recovery. *Archives of General Psychiatry*, *41*, 229–237.

Kramer, A. D., & Feiguine, R. J. (1981). Clinical effects of amitriptyline in adolescent depression: A pilot study. *Journal of the American Academy of Child and Adolescent Psychiatry*, *20*, 636–644.

Kuhn, R. (1958). Treatment of depressive states with G22355 (imipramine hydrochloride). *American Journal of Psychiatry*, *115*, 459–464.

Law, W., III, Petti, T. A., & Kazdin, A. E. (1981). Withdrawal symptoms after graduated cessation of imipramine in children. *American Journal of Psychiatry*, *138*, 647–650.

Liebowitz, M. R., Schneier, F. R., Hollander, E., Welkowitz, L. A., Saoud, J. B., Feerick, J., Campeas, R., Fallon, B. A., Street, L., & Gitow, A. (1991). Treatment of social phobia with drugs other than benzodiazepines. *Journal of Clinical Psychiatry*, *52*(Suppl.), 10–15.

Lovejoy, F. H., Jr., Shannon, M., & Woolf, A. D. (1992). Recent advances in clinical toxicology. *Current Problems in Pediatrics*, *22*, 119–129.

March, J. S., Moon, R. L., & Johnston, H. (1990). Fluoxetine–TCA interaction. *Journal of the American Academy of Child and Adolescent Psychiatry*, *29*, 985–986.

Miller, B. D. (1987). Depression and asthma: A potentially lethal mixture. *Journal of Allergy and Clinical Immunology*, *80*, 481–486.

Minuti, E., & Gallo, V. (1982). Use of antidepressants in childhood: Results of maprotiline (Ludiomil) treatment in 20 cases. *Advances in Biochemical Psychopharmacology*, *32*, 223–227.

Needleman, H. L. (1993). The current status of childhood low-level lead toxicity. *Neurotoxicology*, *14*, 161–166.

Nurcombe, B., Seifer, R., Scioli, A., Tramantana, M. G., Grapentine, W. L., & Beauchesne, H. C. (1989). Is major depressive disorder in adolescence a distinct diagnostic entity? *Journal of the American Academy of Child and Adolescent Psychiatry, 28,* 333–342.

Okasha, A., & Sadek, A. (1976). A controlled double-blind clinical trial between maprotiline and amitriptyline in depressive illness. *Journal of the Egyptian Medical Association, 59,* 557–562.

O'Regan, J. B. (1971). The hazards of use of monoamine oxidase inhibitors in disturbed adolescents. *Canadian Medical Association Journal, 105,* 133.

Parraga, H. C., & Cochran, M. K. (1992). Emergence of motor and vocal tics during imipramine administration in two children. *Journal of Child and Adolescent Psychopharmacology, 2,* 227–233.

Pataki, C. S., Carlson, G. A., Kelly, K. L., Rapport, M. D., & Biancaniello, T. M. (1993). Side effects of methylphenidate and desipramine alone and in combination in children. *Journal of the American Academy of Child and Adolescent Psychiatry, 32,* 1065–1072.

Perel, J. M. (1978). Review of pediatric and adult pharmacology of imipramine and other drugs: Report of chairman, ad hoc committee on tricyclic antidepressant cardiotoxicity. In D. S. Robinson (Ed.), *FDA Report* (pp. 1–4).

Petti, T. A, & Law, W., III (1982). Imipramine treatment of depressed children: A double-blind pilot study. *Journal of Clinical Psychopharmacology, 2,* 107–110.

Popper, C. W. (1992). Disregarding antidepressant blood levels. *American Academy of Child and Adolescent Psychiatry Newsletter, Winter,* 19–20.

Popper, C. W., & Elliott, G. R. (1990). Sudden death and tricyclic antidepressants: Clinical considerations for children. *Journal of Child and Adolescent Psychopharmacology, 1,* 125–132.

Preskorn, S. H., Bupp, S. J., Weller, E. B., & Weller, R. A. (1989). Plasma levels of imipramine and metabolites in 68 hospitalized children. *Journal of the American Academy of Child and Adolescent Psychiatry, 28,* 373–375.

Preskorn, S. H., & Jerkovich, G. S. (1990). Central nervous system toxicity of tricyclic antidepressants: Phenomenology, course, risk factors, and role of therapeutic drug monitoring. *Journal of Clinical Psychopharmacology, 10,* 88–95.

Preskorn, S. H., Weller, E. B., & Weller, R. A. (1982). Depression in children: Relationship between plasma imipramine levels and response. *Journal of Clinical Psychiatry, 43,* 450–453.

Puig-Antich, J. (1982). Major depression and conduct disorder in prepuberty. *Journal of the American Academy of Child Psychiatry, 21,* 118–128.

Puig-Antich, J., Perel, J. M., Lupatkin, W., Chambers, W. J., Tabrizi, M. A., King, J., Goetz, R., Davies, M., & Stiller, R. L. (1987). Imipramine in prepubertal major depressive disorders. *Archives of General Psychiatry, 44,* 81–89.

Rancurello, M. (1986). Antidepressants in children: Indications, benefits, and limitations. *American Journal of Psychotherapy, 40,* 377–392.

Rapport, M. D., Carlson, G. A., Kelly, K. L., & Pataki, C. (1993). Methylphenidate and desipramine in hospitalized children. I. Separate and combined effects on cognitive function. *Journal of the American Academy of Child and Adolescent Psychiatry, 32,* 333–342.

Ravaris, C. L., Robinson, D. S., Ives, J. O., Nies, A., & Bartlett, D. (1980). Phenelzine and amitriptyline in the treatment of depression: A comparison of present and past studies. *Archives of General Psychiatry, 37,* 1075–1080.

Ray, I. (1971). The hazards of use of monoamine oxidase inhibitors in disturbed adolescents. *Canadian Medical Association Journal, 105,* 21.

Riddle, M. A., Geller, B., & Ryan, N. (1993). Another sudden death in a child treated with desipramine. *Journal of the American Academy of Child and Adolescent Psychiatry, 32,* 792–797.

Riddle, M. A., King, R. A., Hardin, M. T., Scahill, L., Ort, S. I., Chappell, P., Rasmusson, A., & Leckman, J. F. (1990). Behavioral side effects of fluoxetine in children and adolescents. *Journal of the American Academy of Child and Adolescent Psychopharmacology, 1,* 193–198.

Riddle, M. A., Nelson, J. C., Kleinman, C. S., Rasmusson, A., Leckman, J. F., King, R. A., & Cohen, D. J. (1991). Sudden death in children receiving Norpramin: A review of three reported cases and commentary. *Journal of the American Academy of Child and Adolescent Psychiatry, 30,* 104–108.

Ryan, N. D. (1990). Heterocyclic antidepressants in children and adolescents. *Journal of Child and Adolescent Psychopharmacology, 1,* 21–31.

Ryan, N. D. (1992). The pharmacologic treatment of child and adolescent depression. *Psychiatric Clinics of North America, 15,* 29–40.

Ryan, N. D., Meyer, V., Dachille, S., Mazzie, D., & Puig-Antich, J. (1988a). Lithium antidepressant augmentation in TCA-refractory depression in adolescents. *Journal of the American Academy of Child and Adolescent Psychiatry, 27,* 371–376.

Ryan, N. D., Puig-Antich, J., Rabinovich, H., Fried, J., Ambrosini, P., Meyer, V., Torres, D., Dachille, S., & Mazzie,

D. (1988b). MAOI's in adolescent major depression unresponsive to tricyclic antidepressants. *Journal of the American Academy of Child and Adolescent Psychiatry, 27*, 755–758.

Saraf, K. R., Klein, D. F., Gittelman-Klein, R., & Groff, S. (1974). Imipramine side effects in children. *Psychopharmacologia, 37*, 265–274.

Sargant, W., (1969). Treatment of the phobic anxiety state. *British Medical Journal, 2*, 49.

Shamsie, S. J., & Barriga, C. (1971). The hazards of use of monoamine oxidase inhibitors in disturbed adolescents. *Canadian Medical Association Journal, 104*, 715.

Simeon, J. G., Dinicola, V. F., Ferguson, H. B., & Copping, W. (1990). Adolescent depression: A placebo-controlled fluoxetine treatment study and follow-up. *Progress in Neuropsychopharmacology and Biological Psychiatry, 14*, 791–795.

Squires, L. A., Neumeyer, A. M., Bloomberg, J., & Krishnamoorthy, K. S. (1992). Hyperpyrexia in an adolescent on desipramine treatment. *Clinical Pediatrics, 31*, 635–636.

Stanton, R. D., Wilson, H., & Brumback, R. A. (1981). Cognitive improvement associated with tricyclic antidepressant treatment of childhood major depressive illness. *Perceptual and Motor Skills, 53*, 219–234.

Sternbach, H. (1991). The serotonin syndrome. *American Journal of Psychiatry, 148*, 705–713.

Strauss, C. C. (1988). Behavioral assessment and treatment of overanxious disorder in children and adolescents. *Behaviour Modification, 12*, 234–251.

Strober, M., Freeman, R., & Rigali, J. (1990). The pharmacotherapy of depressive illness in adolescence: I. An open label trial of imipramine. *Psychopharmacology Bulletin, 26*, 80–84.

Strober, M., Freeman, R., Rigali, J., Schmidt, S., & Diamond, R. (1992). The pharmacotherapy of depressive illness in adolescence. II. Effects of lithium augmentation in nonresponders to imipramine. *Journal of the American Academy of Child and Adolescent Psychiatry, 31*, 16–20.

Venkataraman, S., Naylor, M., & King, C. (1992). Mania associated with fluoxetine treatment in adolescents. *Journal of the American Academy of Child and Adolescent Psychiatry, 31*, 276–281.

Wagner, K. D., & Fershtman, M. (1993). Potential mechanism of desipramine-related sudden death in children. *Psychosomatics, 34*, 80–83.

Warnock, J. K., Sieg, K., Willsie, D., Stevenson, E. K., & Kestenbaum, T. (1991). Drug-related alopecia in patients treated with tricyclic antidepressants. *Journal of Nervous and Mental Disease, 179*, 441–442.

Watanabe, S., Yokoyama, S., Kubo, S., Iwai, H., & Kuyama, C. (1978). A double-blind controlled study of clinical efficacy of maprotiline and amitriptyline in depression. *Folia Psychiatrica Neurologica de Japan, 32*(1), 1–31.

Wilens, T. E., Biederman, J., Spencer, T., & Geist, D. E. (1993). A retrospective study of serum levels and electrocardiographic effects of nortriptyline in children and adolescents. *Journal of the American Academy of Child and Adolescent Psychiatry, 32*, 270–277.

V

DEPRESSION IN SPECIAL POPULATIONS

18

Depression in Infants

Paul V. Trad

Introduction

Since 1980, the *Diagnostic and Statistical Manual of Mental Disorders* (DSM) (American Psychiatric Association, 1980) has included criteria for diagnosing *depression* in infants. These criteria are substantially the same as the criteria used to describe depression in adults. If the editions of the DSM reflect an accurate evolution in the nosology of psychopathology, the merging of diagnostic criteria in infants and adults may be construed to mean that depression in these two widely disparate age groups is now viewed as being fundamentally the same disorder.

The concept of depression in infancy has undergone significant revision over the years. Initially, theorists denied that depression was possible during infancy; more recently, however, the use of adult-like criteria for diagnosing the presence of depression in early life has become accepted. The theoretical stance has therefore evolved from the early psychoanalytic position that infant depression could not exist due to the lack of "superego" (Rie, 1966; Rochlin, 1959) to notions of "masked depression" and "depressive equivalents" (Cytryn & McKnew, 1974), in which children were thought to manifest depression through behaviors and disorders different from those seen in adults (Glaser, 1968), to the current nosology, which posits that infants are capable of experiencing an affective disorder that may mirror depression in adults.

This nosological progression strongly suggests continuity in the conceptualization of mood disorders throughout the life span (Trad, 1986, 1987). Each hypothesis that depression either cannot exist in infancy or is somehow fundamentally different from the adult disorder has met with strong theoretical and experimental evidence to the contrary (Fish, Stifter, & Belsky, 1991; Kazdin, 1990). Thus, the formation of a "unified theory of depression" lends support to the assumption of developmental researchers that individuals may

Paul V. Trad • Department of Psychiatry, New York Hospital–Cornell University Medical Center—Westchester Division, White Plains, NY 10605.

Handbook of Depression in Children and Adolescents, edited by William M. Reynolds and Hugh F. Johnston. Plenum Press, New York, 1994.

experience continuity in the function of emotional mood throughout the life span (Rutter, 1986).

This continuity of mood implies that severe depressive feelings may exist on the same continuum as "normal feelings" of sadness; furthermore, both may be part of the continuum containing feelings of contentment and happiness (Izard, Huebner, McGinnis, & Dougherty, 1980). Evidence of such continuity has motivated the search for markers of psychopathology in early life, so that the researchers can confirm that depression and other mood disorders exist from the earliest days of life (Rutter, 1991).

Unfortunately, simple deductive reasoning does not provide proof that depression occurs during the infancy years. Neither does it resolve the question of whether such depression mimics the adult version of the disorder. Because of the numerous theoretical and experimental concerns that prevent verification of these hypotheses, theorists now maintain that the similarity in depressive nomenclature in DSM-III-R simply reflects the most convenient way for clinicians to view mood disorders during infancy (Trad, 1986). Nevertheless, some theoretical barriers still preclude us from definitively identifying depression in infancy. For example, some researchers may argue that depression can be experienced only after the process of self-formation or self-recognition has been completed at the end of infancy (Burland, 1986). Proponents of this view maintain that the infant's inability to conceptualize experience prior to the achievement of a sense of self precludes the development of full-fledged depression. A second problem—or set of problems—in identifying a definitive state of depression in infancy concerns other developmental parameters. Carlson and Garber (1986), for instance, point to three complications associated with identifying depressive symptoms in prepubertal children. First, the clinician encounters difficulty in assessing the subjective status of young children whose language and intellectual abilities are not yet fully developed. Second, it is not clear that symptoms that signify pathology at one developmental stage do so at another developmental stage. Finally, there may be signs of depression unique to very young children that may go unnoticed and undetected if only adult depressive criteria are applied.

If these barriers to identifying depression in infancy are considered as a group—cognitive immaturity relating to self-identity, lack of access to the child's subjective perceptions, lack of symptom specificity over time, and the presence of symptoms unique to childhood—it becomes apparent that a different diagnostic approach may be warranted: Diagnostic criteria for depression, like most other major nosologies, were originally developed to interpret and classify adult psychopathology. Since criteria for depression were initially formulated to apply to developmentally advanced individuals, it is not surprising that these criteria may be inadequate for addressing the diagnostic complexities of the developmental events that infants and young children confront.

Indeed, even among a developmentally mature population, defining depression is no simple task. In one thorough developmental analysis of adult depression, Carlson and Garber (1986) were able to construct only three relatively indistinct categories: (1) severe, episodic depression with vegetative symptoms, psychomotor retardation, diurnal mood variation, anhedonia, and difficulty concentrating; (2) less severe, but the depressive condition is either chronic or part of a personality disorder; (3) short-lived depression related to stress. The lack of specificity of these three categories did not escape Carlson and Garber, who noted that "[A]s with impressionist paintings . . . it is obvious that closer inspection reveals less rather than greater clarity between these distinctions" (Carlson & Garber, 1986, p. 412). Thus, the goal of defining depression in infancy becomes an ambitious one.

Nevertheless, given the acceptance of the developmental continuity reflected in DSM-III-R nomenclature (American Psychiatric Association, 1987), it seems plausible to suggest that a depressive-like state might be found in a more descriptive or fundamental state during infancy. Identifying the presence of such a condition might be of benefit not only for detecting and treating depression during infancy, but also for classifying depressive conditions at later stages of development. Tracing a fundamental depressive state in infancy along the developmental pathway to other states in adulthood might also be more revealing than relying solely on symptomatology that has been validated in adults.

If depressive states during infancy are related to the fundamental differences between adults and infants—the minimal cognitive and emotional status of infants as opposed to the enhanced cognitive and emotional status of adults—one may posit that because infants are at the low end of the developmental continuum, they would experience raw mood states (e.g., rage), while adults might use more sophisticated skills to regulate their emotional states. Thus, adults might be expected to experience more variations on the theme of depression.

We may suspect that infancy is a good place to begin searching for the etiology of depression, but the problem of detecting or describing this condition in its entirety remains. A theory encompassing the origins of depression should be sufficiently flexible to allow for movement up or down the affective scale. We are searching for a basic set of prerequisite conditions that may set the stage for a negative depressogenic response.

While a specific description of all these conditions is probably beyond reach at this early stage, we can attempt to identify some criteria that are known to be associated with a depressive response. For example, one such criterion is neuroendocrine change, a biological response that has been correlated with behavior resembling depression. Specific changes in neuroendocrine function have been identified in young infants subjected to stress or distressing conditions. These neuroendocrine changes have been associated with physical alterations that resemble depressogenic responses, such as prolonged crying and eventual apathy. Another criterion that has been associated with depression is withdrawal. Withdrawal has been widely recognized as a component in infant depressive states (Bowlby, 1960; Spitz, 1945) and has an analog in its adult counterpart, lack of interest or apathy. In addition to its frequency as a symptom of early depression, withdrawal has other characteristics that enhance its candidacy as an apt starting point in the search for the developmental origins of depression.

Withdrawal may be defined as a disengagement from the environment that allows the organism to generate fundamental self-protective strategies. An organism that withdraws from the external world and turns inward cannot be harmed. Neither can it advance its own cause, however, and it is thus in a kind of neutral state. In the absence of positive outside intervention, the state of withdrawal can eventually proliferate to movement further down the continuum of depression, since all chances for coping with the environment have been nullified by inward retreat and nonparticipation with the outside world. Extended disengagement may be interpreted as a primary indicator of chronic depression. On the other hand, the state of withdrawal may be less severe, as the organism selectively responds to a decrease in stressors and other positive environmental feedback.

Because both neuroendocrine changes and behavioral withdrawal have been reasonably well documented in infants, these criteria may offer a means of detecting depression anywhere along the depressive continuum, particularly among young populations, such as infants.

The discussion below will focus on the use of neuroendocrine changes and behavioral withdrawal as markers or indicators of depression, as well as on the dynamics surrounding the onset and dissipation of the disorder in infancy. In order to demonstrate that the neonate is biologically prepared to respond to episodes of stress in a coherent fashion, it is important to identify the occurrence of neuroendocrine changes under certain conditions, with or without accompanying withdrawal.

The Infant's Neuroendocrine Capacity

Biogenic Amine Theories

Insight into the biological underpinnings of depression was initially achieved through a circuitous route. A flurry of investigations into the biological basis of depression was triggered when researchers became aware that reserpine, an antihypertensive agent, occasionally caused a severe depressive reaction in a small but persistent fraction of patients receiving this drug (Achor, Hanson, & Gifford, 1955). Subsequently, researchers demonstrated a marked correlation between the reserpine and depression when they established that the depressive effect of reserpine was dose-dependent and that the depression remitted if the patient stopped using the reserpine (Bunney & Davis, 1965). Related studies conducted at approximately the same time suggested that when derivatives of iproniazid, an antituberculosis agent, were metabolized by the body, mood elevation was likely to result (Pare & Sandler, 1959). Hydrazine compounds, such as isoniazid, were known to inhibit the enzyme monoamine oxidase (MAO) (Zeller, Barsky, Berman, & Fouts, 1952). In turn, MAO's main function had been reported to be the inactivation of biogenic amines (Coppen, 1967). This observation received more support from a related finding that established that imipramine, an effective antidepressant, blocked the reuptake of catecholamines (norepinephrine and dopamine) into the synaptic cleft (Charney, Menkes, & Heniger, 1981; Rosenblatt & Chanley, 1965). Thus, mounting evidence in this area indicated that drugs such as reserpine and iproniazid were responsible for dramatic changes in the brain's endocrine regulation of such hormones as catecholamines, indoleamines, and endorphins. These findings strongly indicated a link between the activity of monoamines in the brain and the individual's psychological status (Bunney & Davis, 1965; Carlsson, Lindvist, & Magnusson, 1957; van Praag, 1977).

Armed with these insights, researchers began to focus on a neuroendocrine theory of depression. Among the first neuroendocrine theories proposed was that depression was associated with a deficiency of catecholamines, while mania was tied to an excess of catecholamines (Brodie, Murphy, Goodwin, & Bunney, 1971). Another theory posited that serotonin deficits were the etiological cause of depression (Åsberg, Thoren, Traskman, Berllsson, & Ringberger, 1976). This latter theory gained credence from a study establishing a relationship between inhibitory maturation and the existence of serotonin in the brain (Lidov & Molliver, 1982). Studies implicating serotonin in the onset of depression hypothesize that low levels of this hormone, along with defects in the neural transport mechanisms, may spark a depressive episode.

A broader bioamine theory has been proposed by Siever and Davis (1985). These researchers focused on the dysregulation of bioamine neurotransmitters as the etiological trigger of depression. According to Siever and Davis, impairment of one or more regulatory mechanisms causes dysregulation of the neurotransmitters. This dysregulation is reflected in erratic patterns of basal output, disruption of normal periodicities including circadian rhythmicities, diminished selective response, and a sluggish return of the system to basal activity after disturbance. Specifically, noradrenergic neuronal firing is elevated and erratic, while the norepinephrine reuptake is decreased.

One major drawback of these neuroendocrine amine hypotheses is that they attempt to correlate blood and urinary concentrations of amine metabolites with depression. Since these concentrations may not reflect brain metabolism accurately, their validity remains unclear (Blombery, Koplin, Gordon, Markey, & Ebert, 1980). As one example, the blood–brain barrier inhibits the escape of serotonin, calling into question the accuracy of the correlation between brain and blood concentrations of this hormone. Moreover, serotonin metabolism is sensitive to dietary tryptophan (van Praag & de Haan, 1980).

One challenging finding concerning affective disorders has been that the secretion rate of cortisol over a 24-hour period remains elevated in most depressed patients (Gibbons, 1964; Sachar, 1975). The hypersecretion of cortisol is believed to reflect malfunction of the limbic system, in addition to the patient's subjective sense of distress (Carroll, 1972). Moreover, a complex relationship between stress and cortisol release has been identified (Carroll, 1976). This relationship may be summarized as follows: The ascending reticular activating system receives input from the diverse areas of the body. Stress triggers the limbic system and perhaps the amygdala. In turn, the limbic system activates the hypothalamus, which then releases a corticotropin-releasing factor (CRF). CRF causes the secretion of corticotropin (ACTH) from the anterior pituitary. When ACTH enters the blood, it promotes the secretion of cortisol from the adrenal cortex. Finally, as the amount of cortisol in the blood becomes elevated, it inhibits hypothalamic neuroendocrine receptors from releasing further CRF (Depue & Evans, 1981; Ganong, 1979).

Cortisol release appears to be dependent on serotonergic function in the hypothalamic–pituitary–adrenal (HPA) axis (Heninger, Charney, & Sternberg, 1984). The strong connection between serotonin and cortisol release was confirmed by two studies in which the metabolic precursor of serotonin, 5-hydroxytryptophan (5-HTP) was administered to patients with aggressive disorders. It was determined that the serum cortisol levels were significantly higher in depressed patients than in controls (Meltzer, Lowy, Robertson, Goodnick, & Perline, 1984a). In another study, the efficacy of antidepressant drugs was tested in groups of depressed patients (Meltzer, Perline, & Tricov, 1984b). After several weeks of treatment with lithium carbonate or an MAO inhibitor, cortisol levels rose when 5-HTP was administered. Moreover, tricyclic antidepressants appeared to normalize the cortisol responses to serotonin. These findings point to a permissive role of serotonin in which abnormally low levels of serotonin may make an individual more vulnerable to depression.

Several researchers have determined that failure of the feedback-inhibitory influence on ACTH–cortisol regulation may be a neuroendocrine marker of depression (Carroll, Curtis, & Mendels, 1976; Depue & Evans, 1981). However, the question pertinent to this discussion remains whether cortisol plays the same role in infants and children as in adults. The following studies focus on this issue.

Knight et al. (1979) examined changes in the cortisol levels of children subjected to stress. In this study, the stress was posed by the anticipation of elective surgery. Cortisol levels were measured at three times. At Time One, 2 weeks before surgery, the children were interviewed and instructed to collect urine samples over the weekend. These samples were later used to estimate the amount of cortisol secretion. Time Two occurred after the child's admission to the hospital and 1 day prior to surgery. Time Three occurred on the day following surgery. Cortisol levels during Time Two were determined to be markedly elevated. The researchers interpreted the lack of cortisol elevation at Time One and Three as suggesting that unconscious defenses such as denial and displacement had been triggered to buffer the stress of hospitalization. The fact that about 50% of adult depressives hypersecrete cortisol has been cross-validated with prepubertal children meeting diagnostic criteria for major depressive disorder (Puig-Antich, Chambers, Halpern, Hallon, & Sachar, 1979). Although all the steps in the infant's neuroendocrine regulation have not yet been documented, it is now believed that a developmental analysis of these factors may allow researchers to identify similarities as well as differences that have been tied to specific emotional states and their regulation.

Integrally related to the question of cortisol production is the level of function in the HPA axis. Dysfunction in the HPA axis has repeatedly been demonstrated to be a key correlate of depression. Among the signs of this dysfunction are cortisol hypersecretion, flattened cortisol circadian periodicity, and the inability to suppress plasma cortisol levels following the administration of the dexamethasone suppression test (DST). These disturbances are common in endogenously depressed patients and are viewed as highly specific markers for a wide range of primary affective disorders. In addition, the DST has been found to be a reliable marker in children with diagnostically confirmed depression (Geller, Rogol, & Knitter, 1983).

Recent studies have shown that the HPA axis also operates in neonates and that, as with adults and older children, changes in cortisol level during infancy are correlated with stress (Gunnar, 1989). It remains to be demonstrated, however, whether cortisol response in connection with depression-evoking stimuli in infants is similar to cortisol secretion in adults. In the following section, the criteria for identifying early markers of depression will be outlined in order to depict depression in infants.

Substantial evidence suggests that the HPA axis responds to the environment at or shortly after the time of birth. For example, Anders, Sachar, Kream, Rolfwang, and Hellman (1970) studied four infants in the first 4 months of life. These researchers found significant elevations in plasma cortisol occurring after 20 minutes of crying, while levels remained low during quiescent periods. Tennes and Carter (1973) studied 40 full-term infants on the 3rd day of life and found low cortisol levels to be associated with sleep, while high cortisol levels were associated with periods of fussing and crying. Gunnar, Fisch, and Malone (1984) investigated 18 healthy newborn boys aged 2–5 days who were about to undergo circumcision. Half these infants were given pacifiers during the procedure, while the other half received no pacifiers. Blood samples for cortisol were taken just before the operation and 30 minutes later. Pretrial cortisol levels did not differ between the two groups. The researchers observed the infants 30 minutes before, during, and after the procedure. Although the group with pacifiers displayed 40% less crying, serum levels of cortisol after circumcision did not differ between the two groups. Moreover, marked cortisol elevations were noted in both groups 30 minutes after the procedure. A longitudinal study of the adrenocortical response to stress was conducted by Hughes et al. (1987). Measurements of cortisol were taken in 10 ill preterm infants. Cortisol levels far exceeded those found in children and adults subjected to surgical stress.

According to Mantagos, Koulouris, and Vagenakis (1991), even simple stress tests have proven effective in evaluating the functioning of the HPA axis during the first months of life. Plasma cortisol was measured in a group of 33 infants aged 1–6 months. After the infants received the painful stimulus of a venipuncture, it was noted that plasma cortisol increased significantly 30 and 60 minutes after the procedure. The researchers concluded that the HPA axis was functionally intact in infants of this age and that the infants responded to the painful stimulus of the venipuncture by a significant increase in plasma cortisol. Another method of measuring the severity of surgical stress was devised by Anand and Aynsley-Green (1988). This method was applied to 94 neonates undergoing surgery. Hormonal levels were measured in blood samples drawn preoperatively, at the end of the operation, and at 6, 12, and 24 hours after the operation. Stress scores were correlated significantly with plasma levels of epinephrine, norepinephrine, insulin, and cortisol. This method predicted the severity of surgical stress in 89.4% of cases.

In an effort to relate behavioral manifestations to distress and adrenocortical activity in newborns, Gunnar, Isensee, and Fust (1987) administered a Brazelton Neonatal Assessment Scale (Brazelton, 1973) midway between feedings to 60 newborns ranging in age from 32 to 122 hours old. Fully 35 of the newborns were normal, while 25 had perinatal problems. This latter group displayed more behaviors indicative of distress and arousal on the Brazelton test and had higher levels of plasma cortisol. Gunnar, Malone, Vance, and Fisch (1985) obtained behavioral and plasma cortisol levels in 80 healthy, full-term, 2 to 3-day old male newborns scheduled for circumcision. Behavioral distress during circumcision was correlated with elevated levels of plasma cortisol. Bacigalupo, Langner, Schmidt, and Saling (1987) found that neonates who had endured a longer delivery period prior to birth had higher concentrations of ACTH, cortisol, and β-endorphins than infants who had undergone a short period of labor. Moreover, all infants had higher plasma levels of these metabolites than their mothers, suggesting that the birth process is experienced by the infant as being stressful. More recently, Lewis and Thomas (1990) tested salivary cortisol in infants aged 2, 4, and 6 months prior to and 15 minutes after the infants received an inoculation. The tests revealed that cortisol rose significantly following inoculation.

A summary of the research findings on the adrenocortical response in normal infants has yielded certain specific findings (Gunnar, 1989). First, this system seems active and response to stimulation from the time of birth. Second, under certain stressful conditions, the infant responds with elevated cortisol. Finally, the infant's adrenocortical system appears to rapidly habituate to repeated exposure to the same event.

Neuroendocrine Challenge of the Hypothalamic–Pituitary–Adrenal Axis

Another method of identifying neuroendocrine changes that may signify dysregulation is through the use of the DST. The DST is used to determine whether dexamethasone can inhibit cortisol output (Carroll, 1984). The test involves administering dexamethasone late in the day before sleep. The following day, two blood samples are drawn to analyze plasma cortisol levels. A positive response is indicated by a persistence of elevated plasma cortisol concentration in both samples. This positive response means that despite an agent known to inhibit cortisol production (i.e., dexamethasone), the patient is unable to regulate endocrine production effectively on his or her own.

The sensitivity of the DST varies. In this context, sensitivity refers to the rate of positive tests among those suspected of being depressed, while specificity refers to the rate of negative tests in a control population. In recent investigations, DST sensitivity has ranged from 22% to 75% (Asnis et al., 1981; Poznanski, Carroll, Banegas, Cook, & Gross, 1982), while specificity has ranged from 85% to 100% (Baldessarini, 1983).

The DST has been investigated less extensively with children than with adults (Geller et al., 1983). In one study, Petty, Asarnow, Carson, and Lesser (1985) administered the DST to 30 children. Of the group, 7 had major depression, 6 had dysthymia, and 17 had other, nonaffective disorders. The study found that similar rates of nonsuppression were displayed by the major depressives (86%) and the dysthymic group (83%). The test demonstrated a sensitivity for major depression (87%) but a low specificity (53%). These trials have nonetheless found the DST helpful for diagnosing depression in children.

In this regard, it is important to realize that serotonin regulates neuroendocrine changes, particularly cortisol secretion (Heniger et al., 1984). To verify this observation, Meltzer et al. (1984b) administered an oral precursor of serotonin to 25 patients with major depression, 6 schizoaffective depressed patients, and 6 bipolar manic patients. They found that serum cortisol levels were significantly higher after administration of the precursor in depressed patients than in normal controls. The researchers noted that their data may confirm the correlation between the increased activity of serotonin metabolites and the violent suicide attempts observed in depressed patients. Moreover, when Meltzer et al. (1984a) tested the effects of tricyclic medication in 8 unipolar and 7 bipolar depressed patients, as well as in 7 manic patients, they found that tricyclics, the major psychopharmacological effect of which is to increase the reuptake of serotonin, reduced the cortisol response in patients with major depression. These investigations substantiate the growing body of data indicating that downward changes in serotonin levels can predispose an individual to depression.

Another means of exploring the relationship between the HPA axis and affective regulation is by analyzing response to growth hormone (GH). Normal patients typically display heightened levels of GH after insulin-induced hypoglycemia. In contrast, unipolar depressives have been shown to have an inadequate GH response to hypoglycemia (Depue & Evans, 1981; J. B. Jensen & Garfinkel, 1990).

Researchers have also demonstrated that the neonatal HPA axis is responsive to stress and negative-feedback systems (Okuno, Nishimura, & Kawarzaki, 1972). Using ACTH and an insulin as stimulation tests, Okuno and colleagues measured plasma 11-hydrocortico-steroid (11-OCHS) (corticosterone and cortisol) response levels. Subjects included infants aged 1–5 days. For comparison, the researchers used a control group that consisted of children between the ages of 4 and 15. Prior to the experiment, the two groups were found to be comparable in terms of resting plasma 11-OCHS levels. Infant subjects were initially given ACTH and insulin. Following this administration, plasma levels of 11-OCHS were found to be elevated.

When the DST was administered next, plasma 11-OCHS levels were reduced. Okuno and colleagues noted that the insulin tolerance test revealed that infants as young as 1–5 days old were able to respond to the insulin challenge and that the decrease in 11-OCHS following the DST demonstrated the viability of a feedback mechanism responsible for the inhibition of cortisol release. Thus, it appears that both the stress response and the negative-feedback inhibitory mechanism in infants are essentially analogous to the regulatory responses demonstrated by children (McKnew & Cytryn, 1973; Puig-Antich, 1986) and adults (Carroll et al., 1976; Matthews, Akil, Greden, & Watson, 1982; Schildkraut, 1965). This non-age-specific cortisol response to stress provides strong evidence of the infant's innate readiness for interacting with environmental stress in ways that may result in homeostasis and self-regulation (Trad, 1987).

Researchers such as Money (1977) have reported a correlation between emotional abuse and psychological disorder manifested in the form of failure to thrive. Patton and Gardner (1975) noted that the growth retardation of infants and young children from disturbed homes has frequently been traced to specific hormonal or metabolic disorders, while an abnormal response to insulin-induced hypoglycemia has been demonstrated in children who have been neglected by primary caregivers (Powell, Brasel, & Blizzard, 1967a,b). The connection between the hormonal dysregulation of unipolar depressives and maternally deprived children may help explain the high incidence of depression among children who sustain a dysfunctional (stressful) relationship with their parents.

Greenberg and Gardener (1960) administered insulin to 7 male infants during the first week of life and found, along with the reduction in blood glucose, a rise in urinary epinephrine excretion. Not only are these results consistent with catecholamine responses to hypoglycemia in adults (Christenson, Alberti, & Brandsborg, 1975; Phillippe, 1983), but also they are in accord with the responses to crying in the neonate (Anders et al., 1970; Tennes & Carter, 1973). Moreover, a relationship between adrenocortical activity and crying has demonstrated that factors that reduce crying may also lessen the hormonal response to stress in infants. To test this hypothesis, Gunnar et al. (1984) studied 18 healthy male newborns between 2 and 5 days old who underwent circumcision. Half this group were given pacifiers, the other half were not. Blood samples for cortisol were taken immediately before circumcision and 30 minutes after. The pacifier appeared to reduce crying by 40%. Both groups, however, showed marked elevations in serum cortisol 30 minutes after circumcision. Gunnar, Connors, Isensee, and Wall (1988) demonstrated that nonnutritive sucking could be used to effectively reduce behavioral distress, but was not associated with a reduction in the adrenocortical response to stimulation.

Opioid System

Another aspect of neuroendocrine function in adults that responds to stress and appears to be related to manifestations of depression is the endogenous opioid system. The primary hormone involved in this system is [β]-endorphin, secreted by the adeno-hypophysis in response to stress. Both [β]-endorphin and ACTH derive from a common precursor, pro-opiomelanocortin (Facchinetti, Petraglia, & Nappi, 1983). Moreover, Guillemin et al. (1977) found that [β]-endorphin and ACTH are secreted concomitantly in elevated amounts in response to acute stress. These hormones are secreted in response to CRF (Vale, Spiess, Rivier, & Rivier, 1981). It has been posited that [β]-endorphin regulates ACTH secretion and that it contributes to the inhibition of hypothalamic secretion (Rose, 1985).

Cohen, Pickar, and Dubois (1981) determined that plasma [β]-endorphin secretion rose in adults who were undergoing stressful conditions, such as surgery. One research team, Risch, Janowsky, Judd, Gillin, and McClure (1983), found that morning plasma levels of [β]-endorphin immunoreactivity were significantly higher in depressed patients and patients with affective disorders than in age- and sex-matched normals and psychiatric patients without affective disorder. Using a radioimmunoassay technique to measure [β]-endorphin response, Matthews et al. (1982) found that dexamethasone may be ineffective in suppressing [β]-endorphinlike material in depressed patients. Reporting on endorphin evaluation in 92 patients with major depression, Agren and Terenius (1983) encountered elevated endorphin levels in this population as compared to normal controls. Moreover, depressed adults have been shown to have a lower ratio of plasma endorphins to cortisol than normal adult patients, while patients with nonmajor depression have lower [β]-endorphin levels than patients with a diagnosis of major depression (Cohen, Pickar, Extein, Gold, & Sweeney, 1984). It appears, then, that adults with depression may be hypersecreting [β]-endorphin or disinhibiting its release.

Many theorists believe that the production of endogenous opioids, including [β]-endorphin, is merely one example of a complex system of neuroendocrine regulation. In this regard, the endogenous opioids may be considered modulators of other hormonal responses. For example, Risch (1982) has noted that the endogenous opioids modulate response to such physiological stimuli as stress, sucking, and lactation. Preliminary reports have determined that the endogenous opioids may also lower production of dopamine. Since dopamine is known to be a prolactin inhibitor, the endogenous opioids, through the suppression of dopamine, may indirectly stimulate prolactin production and ACTH release. Significantly, in adults, [β]-endorphin and ACTH are secreted contemporaneously during stressful situations. In addition, the endogenous opioids have been associated with an increase in serotonin turnover, which stimulates a release of prolactin, GH, and ACTH, as well as a reduction of norepinephrine turnover, which inhibits ACTH release. Elevations in the production of ACTH have also been tied to endogenous opioid production and increases in plasma concentrations of [β]-endorphin, while other endogenous opioids have been found to elevate plasma concentrations of cortisol. Since the hypersecretion of cortisol has been correlated with major depression, this correlation may be significant.

In order to prove the participation of endogenous opioids during reactions to stress, the issue of when endogenous opioid regulation is first functional becomes significant. Facchinetti, Bagnoli, Bracci, and Genazzani (1982) examined plasma opioid production during the first hours of life and determined that neonates produce neuroendocrine opioids. For example, ACTH levels are elevated during the first 6 hours of life, but decline to normal adult levels approximately 18 hours later. Elevated plasma cortisol levels have also been reported during the first 3 hours of life. Gradually, cortisol drops to normal adult levels by the 2nd day of life. Facchinetti et al. (1982) drew umbilical blood samples. Further samples were obtained from the jugular vein of the infants at ½, 6, 12, and 24 hours after birth. [β]-Endorphin blood levels were found to be consistently higher than normal adult levels. Moreover, they parallel the high levels of ACTH. These findings support the evidence that [β]-endorphin is released during stressful events (Levy, McIntoxh, & Black, 1986; Lloyd, Teich, & Rowe, 1991) such as apnea or other apparent life-threatening situations (Myer, Morris, Adams, Brase, & Dewey, 1987).

More recently, it has been found that within the first few days of postnatal life, infants exhibit the ability to regulate diurnally both cortisol and endorphin levels in the same manner as their adult counterparts (Hindmarsh, Tan, Sankaran, & Laxdal, 1989). Researchers have also detected signs of an elaborate neuroendocrinological feedback mechanism during the neonatal period. This feedback mechanism consists of interaction among CRF, mediated cortisol, and ACTH. Theorists have inferred this mechanism from the neonate's ability to secrete cortisol in response to ACTH stimulation or during insulin-induced hypoglycemia coupled with ACTH suppression after dexamethasone administration.

Neuroendocrine Changes and Helplessness

The theory of learned helplessness may further illustrate how stress may predispose an individual to depression. The learned-helplessness model posits that after a series of uncontrollable events are experienced, major emotional, cognitive, and motivational deficits undermine the individual's perception of future responses (Abramson, Seligman, & Teasdale, 1978). For example, animals repeatedly subjected to inescapable shock who are later given the opportunity to escape seem unwilling to do so. This inability to avoid adverse situations appears to stem from the lack of control the individual experienced during the shock of initial exposure. The symptoms exhibited during learned-helplessness reactions resemble the symptoms of depression. These symptoms include a low rate of behavior initiation, negative cognitions, low levels of aggression, and loss of appetite, as well as physiological changes in norepinephrine regulation (Seligman, 1975).

To measure the effects of learned-helplessness-induced depression on brain norepinephrine levels, Weiss and co-workers tested the hypothesis in a series of studies (Weiss, Glazer, & Pohorecky, 1974; Weiss, Glazer, Pohorecky, Bailey, & Schneider, 1979; Weiss, Stone, & Harrell, 1970). In one experiment, some animals were able to avoid receiving a shock to their tails. A second group of animals were yoked and shocked no matter how they reacted. Finally, a third group received no shocks. Weiss and colleagues found that the avoidance-escape animals showed higher levels of norepinephrine in the brain than the nonshocked controls, a result consistent with studies associating brain norepinephrine with the application of a severe stressor. It is probable that inescapable shock depletes brain norepinephrine by causing a precipitously high norepinephrine release rate that prevents the animal from being able to regulate this hormone.

To some degree, these findings may also apply to humans. Van der Kolk, Greenberg, Boyd, and Krystal (1985) posit that the response of animals subjected to unavoidable shock may parallel the behavior of patients diagnosed with posttraumatic stress disorder (PTSD). The apathy and lack of motivation shown by PTSD patients is associated with norepinephrine depletion secondary to unavoidable trauma. Whether an infant's response to behavioral disorganization would be sufficiently traumatizing to allow us to draw a parallel between this phenomenon and inescapable shock is unknown. Nonetheless, studying examples of infant withdrawal in relation to neurotransmitters seems warranted.

Attachment behaviors or their converse, such as withdrawal, may offer a further means of identifying depression at an early age. The experience of a secure attachment to the caregiver has been related to self-esteem, the ability to explore the environment, independence, the capacity to cope with fear and failure, and ability to cooperate with press (Arend, Gove, & Sroufe, 1979; Lewis, Feiring, McGuffog, & Jaskir, 1984). Matas, Arend, and Sroufe (1978) studied play and problem-solving in 48 2-year-old infants. The infants in this group who manifested a secure attachment were found to be more cooperative, persistent, and enthusiastic than the insecurely attached infants, indicating that security of attachment may facilitate the infant's ability to cope more adaptively with the environment. In contrast, separation from the caregiver has been found to result in a dramatic grief response, along with negative physiological functioning, including negative changes in sleep patterns, heart rate, temperature, endocrine function, and immune function (Kalin & Carnes, 1984). Bowlby (1960) has described a syndrome manifested by the infant following separation from the caregiver. First, the infant protests and is distressed. Despair follows, and finally, after several days, the infant lapses into a state of withdrawal and inactivity from which it is difficult to arouse him or her.

The infant's reaction to separation from the caregiver may provide an excellent developmental paradigm for studying depression in this young population. Measures of neuroendocrine function in 1-year-old infants separated from their mothers for 1 hour correlated with similar results seen in adults separated from loved ones. Such infants secrete increased levels of cortisol, as do adults undergoing psychological stress (Bliss, Migeon, Branch, & Samuels, 1956; Tennes & Mason, 1982). Moreover, infants who displayed the most distress excreted the highest cortisol levels. A further correlation between maternal separation and increased cortisol levels in infants has been reported by Larson, Gunnar, and Hertsgaard (1991). These researchers exposed healthy 9-month-old infants to three conditions: morning naps, car rides of 40 minutes, and episodes of maternal separation lasting for 30 minutes. The first two situations resulted in a lowering of salivary cortisol, while maternal separation resulted in significantly higher salivary concentrations of cortisol.

Considered together, these studies seem to suggest that the reaction to separation leading to the infant's withdrawal may provide insight into the origins of depression in infancy. Interestingly enough, this outward behavior has also been tied to neuroendocrine change. For example, challenges to the attachment bond trigger a behavioral syndrome associated with several neuroendocrine correlates, including, most significantly, elevated cortisol. Further investigations of the interplay of ACTH, cortisol, serotonin, and endorphins will most likely provide further insight into the role of neuroendocrine function in the regulation of disordered affect early in life.

Other Affective Influences within the Interpersonal Arena

Discrepancy Awareness

While the infant appears to possess the biological capacity to experience and regulate response to environmental stress during the early days of life, we may ask whether there are also other interpersonal mechanisms that govern the interaction between infant and environment. That is, how does the neonate engage the environment and does the neonate derive satisfaction or dissatisfaction from efforts at interaction?

The capacity of the infant to engage, motivate, and thus control the environment in quest of meeting needs has been demonstrated by cognitive developmentalists investigating infant awareness of discrepancies and contingencies. McCall and McGhee (1977) define discrepancy as the degree of disparity between two stimuli. When charted, infant responses to gradations of discrepancy fall along an inverted U curve.

The infant's perception of a moderate degree of discrepancy from a familiar, standard stimulus triggers an optimal level of both attention and positive affect (Parry, 1982). Extreme discrepancy, in contrast, results in low levels of attention, accompanied by negative affect. Thus, moderate discrepancy registers on the highest portion of the inverted U distribution curve. This hypothesis has been verified by several independent investigators. For example, Hopkins, Zelazo, Jacobson, and Kagan (1976) investigated discrepancy awareness in 7.5-month-old infants and found that reactivity—defined as instrumental responding, fixation, vocalization, and smiling—was maximal to a moderately discrepant stimulus.

While most of the data confirming discrepancy awareness during the early months of life have involved infants between 2 and 6 months of age, Friedman, Bruno, and Vietze (1974) found that neonates as young as 28 hours of age are capable of responding to variations in stimuli according to the predictions of the inverted U curve observed by McCall and McGhee (1977). Conners (1964), who tested undergraduate adult volunteers, demonstrated that this cognitive skill is uniform across age groups. Using eye-movement fixation and verbal report, these subjects displayed the greatest preference for slightly discrepant figures and the least preference for the most extremely discrepant figures. Thus, it appears that the individual's ability to perceive and react emotionally to discrepancies becomes evident during infancy and remains a fundamental component of cognitive functioning throughout life.

Contingency Awareness

Another capability that reveals the infant's proclivity to engage the environment in pursuit of security through relatively sophisticated cognitive processing (i.e., comparative analysis, immediate and remote memory) is contingency awareness. Contingency awareness emerges at around 2–3 months of age and has been defined as a behavioral strategy designed to achieve control over one stimulus by connecting two or more stimuli and perceiving a cause-and-effect relationship between them (Watson, 1966, 1971, 1972).

Prior to being able to demonstrate contingency awareness, infants must possess sufficient memory to enable them to associate a particular stimulus with a particular response. Recent evidence demonstrates that even very young infants possess enough memory to allow for the storage and retrieval of contingency relationships. For example, neonates can learn contingencies and retain learning for 24 hours (DeCasper & Carstens, 1981; Fagen, Morrongiello, Rovee-Collier, & Gekowski, 1984).

Davis and Rovee-Collier (1983) taught a contingency relationship to 2-month-old infants in training sessions and found that memory of the contingency could be retrieved by the infants nearly 3 weeks after the initial trials. Finkelstein and Ramey (1977) conducted a series of experiments to demonstrate that infants can indeed transfer the learning of contingency relationships across tasks. Two groups of infants, one exposed to contingent stimuli and one exposed to noncontingent stimuli, were compared. Infants who received prior contingent stimulation became more competent and efficient learners in new situations, while prior exposure to a noncontingent stimulus was correlated with the disruption of a learned relationship.

Affective Correlates of Discrepancy and Contingency Awareness

The infant's active engagement of the environment through early perceptions of discrepancy and contingency suggests a fundamental drive for survival and an urge to exert control over the environment in order to achieve an adaptive response. If such a drive exists, infants might be expected to react by manifesting positive emotions in response to known contingencies and mild (interesting, but not threatening) discrepancies, while negative reactivity would be exhibited when the infants were confronted with dramatically threatening discrepancies or a disruption in learned contingencies (Fox, 1989; Lewis, Worobey, & Thomas, 1989).

In fact, these responses are common. Blass, Ganchrow, and Steiner (1984) demonstrated how contingency learning and affect are interrelated in infants. In experimental groups, infants as young as 2 hours old were gently stroked on their foreheads during 18 2-minute conditioning trials. Following the stroking sessions, each infant received intra-oral sucrose. Members of a control group received sucrose in each trial, but were not stroked beforehand. After the trials, infants in both groups were exposed to 9 1-minute extinction trials during which they were just stroked. Infants in the control group showed no evidence of conditioning, but 7 of the 9 infants in the experimental group cried during the extinction trials, as compared to only 1 of the 16 in the control group. Thus, the disruption of a contingency relationship—and of the infant's expectation of future contingency—produces negative affect.

As is the case with the perception of contingencies, discrepancy awareness also generates an important affective reaction. Awareness of a discrepancy triggers feelings of uncertainty as the infant struggles to formulate a response to the new situation (Kagan, 1974, 1984). If a discrepant event can be successfully processed by the infant internally (which is most likely to occur with moderately discrepant stimuli), a positive affect is experienced.

On the other hand, encountering an extreme discrepancy is likely to evoke stressful processing, which generates negative affect. McCall and McGhee (1977) note that while negative affect occurs during the processing of extremely discrepant stimuli, positive affect results after processing has been successfully completed. In this manner, the same stimuli may evoke both a negative and a positive emotional response. The interaction between negative and positive emotions during the period of subjective uncertainty the infant undergoes represents the infant's first emotional challenge to regulate the internal state in response to an external stimulus. Success in this regulatory attempt is a marker indicating an ability to cope, i.e., to gain control of the environment.

If the stimulus event is particularly threatening or extremely discrepant, the infant's fragile regulatory capacity may be disrupted. Negative affect will not be successfully regulated and may well engulf the infant, engendering the diffused experience of loss of control and triggering an urge for self-protection through the basic mechanism of withdrawal.

The Infant's Interpersonal Ability to Cope with Stress: Loss of Control and the Urge to Withdraw

To suggest that disturbances in contingency and discrepancy awareness can lead to a depressive state characterized by behavioral withdrawal and neuroendocrine abnormality may appear somewhat simplistic and overdramatic at first. It should be realized, however, that the biological and psychological condition of the unborn and neonate infant is inherently a dramatic one (T. Field, 1989). Opportunities for learning and mastery are limited at this early state of differentiation, bestowing great significance on the few opportunities that do exist and causing a global interpretation of events.

As Stern (1985) points out, many experiences in young children are generalized and do not involve specific memories. Rather, multiple specific memories are incorporated into an abstract formulation of the likely course of events based on typical experiences. Since infants have fewer life experiences to rely on and less expertise in consolidating these experiences—although they are nevertheless able to develop internal working models (Main, Kaplan, & Cassidy, 1985)—they may be prone to interpreting negative events as a global loss of control. As a result, such infants may become vulnerable to a global, or primary, depressive state.

This hypothesis gains support from Rothbaum (1980), who indicates that the motivation for control during infancy may be a phenomenon even more basic than the drives, since control is a chronic condition, whereas the drives emerge in brief energetic bursts. While research on the desire for control remains in its early stages, the universality and diversity of control behaviors are already well documented (Trad, 1986). Rothbaum and Weisz (1989) point out that control, which they define as "causal influence in an intended direction" (p. 18), is so much a part of life that it is difficult to dissociate from it so that it can be observed. Kopp (1982) provides an example of the profound urge for the control by recounting the anecdote in Holmes (1976) about a 5-year-old girl who had to undergo a series of painful injections. At one point, in frustration and fear, the child said, "Let me get control!" (Kopp, 1982, p. 210). If behavioral withdrawal represents a fundamental marker and mediator of depression, it seems likely that the experience that triggers this withdrawal is equally fundamental and global, e.g., lack of control. Thus, consistent thwarting of an infant's attempts at experiencing control may well result in a withdrawal that is indicative of a depressive state.

In their reformulation of the learned-helplessness model of depression, Peterson and Seligman (1984) provide a useful paradigm for examining the elements of withdrawal and depression discussed thus far. Noting that the original learned-helplessness model centered primarily on loss of control and failed to distinguish among types of depression, these investigators offered a reformulation in which behavior is viewed as being dependent on the person's interpretation of why he or she encountered an uncontrollable event.

If the cause of the uncontrollable event is perceived as being global (such as loss of control as experienced by the infant), deficits associated with helplessness (i.e., affective, cognitive, and motivational deficits) will tend to be transferred across a variety of different domains. If a specific factor is singled out as being a causal agent, however, deficits will tend to be more limited. As in the previous learned-helplessness model, the reformulated model proposes that the expectation of future uncontrollability (e.g., for infants this would include expectancies of discrepancy and noncontingency) is sufficient for the production of the majority of depressive symptoms. In addition, internal, stable, and global explanations for bad events are viewed as risk factors for depression. Chronic depression results from explanations that remain stable. Finally, the learned-helplessness reformulation posits that the underlying mechanism for depression remains the same across the life span, but that specific manifestations of depression indicate developmental differences in the use of such explanations.

While the evidence indicates that infants are capable of perceiving contingencies and discrepancies, we know little about infants' internal explanatory system. Nevertheless, it seems reasonable to hypothesize that this system would be global in nature, magnifying the importance and consequences of adverse events, as compared to those experienced by adults. Of course, the infant is highly susceptible to outside interventions, which can quickly eradicate a developing state of withdrawal/depression. Nonetheless, in light of the reformulated learned-helplessness theory, the absence of these positive events may lead to a depressive state deriving from the accumulated expectations of failure and, hence, lack of trying—or withdrawal.

Such a situation may be exhibited during anaclitic depression (e.g., Spitz, 1954; Spitz & Wolf, 1946). The infants in these cases display sadness and weepiness with eventual withdrawal and stupor. Not surprisingly, this syndrome is attributed to disruptions in the infant–caregiver bond, since the relationship with the parent is the primary source of learning and the main source for the infant to experience control.

The effect of a disrupted infant–caregiver bond has been reported in a case discussed by Adler and Buie (1979). The patient, an adult diagnosed with borderline psychopathology, remembered that as a very young child she would lie in her crib feeling desperately alone. She did not attempt to capture her mother's attention by calling out, however, since she had learned through repeated noncontingency experiences that her mother generally did not respond. This case presents a clear example of withdrawal as a symptom of depression in infancy and one that would have perhaps predicted a psychopathological outcome in adulthood.

It is important to note that the manifestations of depression (e.g., helplessness and withdrawal) discussed thus far appear to evolve slowly in the very young. Rholes, Blackwell, Jordan, and Walters (1980) studied 20 children of different ages from kindergarten, 1st, 3rd, and 5th grades. Their susceptibility to learned helplessness was examined by exposing them to either repeated failure or repeated success on hidden figures problems. The study revealed that the experience of failure had significantly less influence on the level of helplessness manifested in these younger children's behavior. Older children were more deeply affected by failure. Like Seligman (1975), Rholes and co-workers hypothesize that the difference in the age groups depends on attributional capabilities.

In another study, Seligman et al. (1984) correlated attributional style and depressive symptoms among children and concluded (p. 238) that

> . . . children with depressive symptoms share some characteristics of adults with depressive symptoms. Both have an attributional style in which bad events are seen as caused by internal, stable, and global factors. Both may be put at risk for future depression by processing information about bad events through this insidious attributional style.

Thus, it appears that a rewarding area of investigation concerning the etiology of depression in infants might be the intersection between younger children's "immunity" to helplessness and the gradual erosion of that immunity. It seems likely that the transition from a lesser to a greater susceptibility to depression might occur as a by-product of cognitive changes in attributional style.

Table 1 summarizes the findings of a series of clinical studies of infant depression.

Tracing the Course of Depressive Manifestations

This section addresses the course of depressive disorders during infancy. DSM-III-R asserts that a major depressive episode may begin at any age, including infancy. The onset and course of the disorder are believed to be variable in their duration. Data gathered from diverse sources regarding risk factors that can trigger depression in infants are contrasted in order to begin addressing the course of depressive disorders during infancy. Although there is a controversy regarding the long-term effects of some of these risk factors (Biringen & Robinson, 1991; Ernst, 1988), a review of the subjects of hospitalization, parental depression, and child abuse demonstrates that evidence regarding the course of depression during infancy already exists. Each of these factors implicates some of the environmental phenomena described above. For example, parental depression may cause the parent to withdraw from interaction with the infant, leading to the experience of disrupted contingency and extreme discrepancy. Abuse can also cause the child to experience extreme discrepancy and a state of helplessness because of inability to escape from the situation. Finally, during hospitalization, children are separated from their caregivers and made to feel as though they no longer can control bodily functions. Each of these factors may result in the perception of learned helplessness along with its concomitant deficits.

Hospitalization

Hospitalization has long been suspected of being a risk factor for infant depression. Researchers have documented numerous affective and cognitive deficits associated with hospitalization during the childhood years (Prugh, 1983; Prugh, Staub, Sands, Kirschbaum, & Lenihan, 1953). Depressive symptoms are evident in virtually every description of hospitalization in infants and children. Susceptibility to depression appears to be a function of many factors, including age at the time of hospitalization, length of stay, and the purpose of hospitalization. Phrased simply, infants and children hospitalized early, repeat-

Table 1. Clinical Studies of Infant Depression

Findings	Spitz (1945)	Spitz & Wolf (1946)	Engel & Reischman (1956)	Emde, et al. (1965)	Meyendorf (1971)	Ossofsky (1974)	Gaensbauer (1980, 1982)	Harmon et al. (1982)
Affective deficits	Depression Feeble smile	Depression Apprehension Sad face Weepiness	Depression Sad face	Depression Sad face Irritable/angry Demanding Fussiness	— Sad face Irritable Monotonous cry	Depression — — Temper tantrums	Depression Sad face Irritable	— — — Temper tantrums
Interpersonal deficits	Withdrawal Apathy Avoidancy	Withdrawal	Withdrawal Avoidancy	Withdrawal Avoidancy	Withdrawal	Withdrawal Apathy	Withdrawal Apathy Avoidancy	—
Attentional deficits	Unresponsive	Unresponsive Stupor	—	—	Unresponsive	Short attention span	Hypervigilance	—
Psychomotor deficits	—	—	Loss of tone Immobility D. posture	D. posture	Restlessness Retardation Fidgeting Ataxia	Hyperactivity Clumsiness	Retardation Lethargy	—
Neurovegetative deficits	—	Weight loss Insomnia	—	—	Eating disturbances	—	Eating disturbances, food refusal Sleep disturbances	—
Developmental deficits	Dev. retardation	Dev. retardation	—	Dev. retardation	Dev. retardation	Dev. retardation	—	—
Abnormal stranger reactions	Abnormal stranger reactions	Abnormal stranger reactions	Abnormal stranger reactions	—	—	—	Abnormal stranger reactions	—
Deficits in immune function	Deficits in immune function	—	—	—	Allergies	—	—	Multiple viral infections
Miscellaneous	— — —	— — —	— — —	Ptosis Change in voice	Enuresis/encopresis Colic	— — —	— — —	Atopic dermatitis Occult GI bleeding

edly, and for long periods face one of the most serious risks for depression. Developmental research categorizes the 0 to 5-year age group as being at high risk. Infants less than 1 year old appear to spend more time in the hospital than any other group of children. Earlier admissions and longer stays combine to expose this group to a higher incidence of depression. As noted, age at time of admission, length of stay, and the purpose of hospitalization represent three other significant variables in determining the likelihood of triggering a depressive episode. Moreover, surgery may be characterized as another risk factor, particularly among children under 5 years old.

Studies have concluded that hospitalization during the first 5 years of a child's life predisposes the child to the development of depressive illness or may actually cause a depressive episode (Blumberg, 1977; Pilowsky, Bassett, Begg, & Thomas, 1982). Most of the DSM-III-R (American Psychiatric Association, 1987) symptoms for major depressive episode have been identified among sick and hospitalized children, substantiating the view that hospitalization can trigger an episode of childhood depression (Burke, Kocoshis, Chandra, Whiteway, & Sauer, 1990). For example, such children show signs of eating and sleeping disturbances (Douglas, 1975; Ferguson, 1979; Mrazek, 1984), psychomotor retardation, apathy (Mrazek, 1984), lethargy (Kashani, Barbareo, & Bolander, 1981), self-reproach/guilt, and even suicidal ideation (Kashani et al., 1981).

Hospitalization can even engender its own set of depressive symptoms, as has been documented since Spitz (1945) described the hospitalism syndrome in British institutions during World War II. The impact of hospitalization may be seen both as isolated symptoms and as a full-fledged depressive syndrome. In the study by Kashani et al. (1981), researchers found that 7% of children admitted to a pediatric ward were depressed and 38% displayed dysphoric mood. Among the most vivid DSM-III-R depressive symptoms in hospitalized infants are changes in emotional tone. Chronic crying and fretfulness begin around the 6th or 7th month, as reported by Spitz and Wolf (1946) and Schaffer and Callender (1959). According to Bowlby, Robertson, and Rosenbluth (1952), this is the infant's "protest" at the hospitalization experience, characterized by high agitation and an attempt to return to the caregiver. "Despair," which follows, is characterized by weeping and other despondent behaviors. Finally, the "detachment" stage brings a general withdrawal from activity and a rejection of attempts by the caregiver to reestablish a relationship. Studies of younger infants do not report these behaviors but comment on the behavioral withdrawal and the conspicuous lack of expression in these children (Schaffer, 1958). Some hospitalized children respond with dulled affect, rather than with emotional extremes. Research indicates that dulled affect may appear as early as 3 weeks of age among hospitalized infants. Hollenbeck et al. (1980) found that cancer patients ages 1.5–4 years placed in a germ-free isolation room acquired an affectless expression over a period of weeks. Schaffer (1958) labeled this phenomenon "global syndrome" and identified it in infants less than 7 months old. Apathetic behavior of this type has also been associated with the child's separation from the parents. A review of the literature indicates that a young child traumatized by repeated or lengthy hospitalization may develop symptoms of depression, be at risk for a major depressive disorder, and generally withdraw from interaction, even with the parents. Overall, the symptoms encountered among hospitalized children include feeding and sleep disturbances, depressed affect, excessive crying, apathy, social avoidance, and withdrawal.

Parental Depression

Parental psychopathology, particularly of the primary caregiver, can have an equally detrimental effect on the child's development (Goodyer, 1990; P. S. Jensen, Bloedau, Degroot, Ussery, & Davis, 1990; Orvaschel, 1990; van Baar, 1990). Weissman et al. (1984a–d), for example, compared the offspring of depressed parents with children whose parents had no psychiatric illness. They discovered that depression in parents resulted in a 3-fold greater risk of having some DSM-III (American Psychiatric Association, 1980) diagnosis— although not necessarily depression—for the child. Major depression was the most common diagnosis found among the children of adults with depression. Fully 13% of such children received this diagnosis. In contrast, none of the controls exhibited the symptoms of major depression.

The children of depressed parents display a number of different types of behavior that distinguish them from more adaptive counterparts. Attachment behaviors are, for example, distinctively different among the children of depressed parents. Gaensbauer, Harmon, Cytryn, and McKnew (1984) encountered disturbed attachment patterns among the offspring of depressed parents. In a sample of 2- to 3-year olds, Radke-Yarrow, Cummings, Kuczynski, and Chapman (1985) found that twice as many children of parents with major depression had insecure attachments as did children with clinically normal parents. R. Field et al. (1985) analyzed the interactions of 3- to 5-month-old infants of postpartum depressed and nondepressed mothers. The infants of depressed mothers had a less optimal mode of interaction that was characterized by frequent drowsiness and the tendency to withdraw. Moreover, depressed mothers also described their children's mood as being more labile. Elevated levels of anxiety, manifested in the form of either a separation anxiety or a phobia, have also been documented among the offspring of parents with affective disorders (Weissman et al., 1984a–d).

While the rate of depression is higher among the children of depressed parents, it is by no means certain that such children will become depressed. Numerous other factors in the environment are likely to contribute to a depressogenic outcome. The sharing of affective states between parent and child is a significant dynamic through which young children, even infants, may experience depression (Hoffman & Drotar, 1991). Researchers such as T. M. Field (1984a,b) have suggested that the manifestation of depressed affect among some infants may reflect a mirroring of their depressed mothers' behaviors. Thus, changes in a mother's affective behavior have been connected to specific interpersonal changes in the infant, while continuity in maternal behavior tends to predict continuity in the infant. But the transmission of depression may be so potent that it does not actually require faithful duplication of the parents' depressed interactional style. Rather, transmission of the parents' perceptions may occur as a result of an empathic exchange by which parent and child are privy to subjective states. Concepts such as "intersubjectivity" (Trevarthan & Hubley, 1978) and "affect attunement" (Stern, 1984) describe a general process by which the parent's emotional state informs the infant how the parent is feeling. These phenomena may also be used to understand how depression may be transmitted between parent and child. In sum, parental psychopathology, particularly depression, signifies an important risk factor for child and infant depression. Evidence indicates that depressed caregivers can induce psychopathology in their offspring more frequently than can their normal counterparts.

Child Abuse. Child abuse and neglect are becoming increasingly more frequent in our society. C. H. Kempe, Silverman, and Steele (1962) pioneers in the field, coined the phrase "battered child syndrome" to describe the situation of young children who have suffered serious physical abuse, generally from a parent or foster parent. Nevertheless, only recently have government and social service agencies begun to compile reliable statistics on the magnitude and severity of child abuse. Moreover, abuse commonly victimizes the very young, with infants and toddlers being disproportionately represented, perhaps because of their more vulnerable status. Some early studies found abusive behavior to be most common among children between 3 months and 3.5 years old (Galdston, 1965).

Researchers have asserted that abuse and neglect are among the most significant causes of infant and childhood depression (Barnett, Manly, & Cicchetti, 1991; Bible & French, 1979; Blumberg, 1981). Abusive behaviors are intimate, personal, familial, and infused with highly ambivalent emotions (Galdston, 1981). The outcome of abuse can be overwhelming for the young child and might include nonorganic failure to thrive—a significant growth retardation that cannot be attributed to organic causes. A child may be suffering from this condition if height and weight fall below the 3rd percentile for the child's expected weight according to chronological age (Pollitt & Eichler, 1976). While the causal relationship between the condition and abuse is not entirely clear, Pollitt, Eichler, and Chon (1975) found that the mothers of such infants are less affectionate and more likely to employ physical punishment. Researchers have also detected developmental deficits in virtually every area of the functioning of abused children (Newberger & Cook, 1983; Sandgrund, Gaines, & Green, 1974; Steele, 1976). The development of motor skills may be particularly susceptible to the effects of abuse. Abused children will often regress developmentally and stop practicing such skills as walking and reaching for objects. Speech and language disorders have also been reported in these children (R. S. Kempe & Kempe, 1978; McGee & Wolfe, 1991). Abused infants between 12 and 19 months of age displayed less pleasure, less interaction, less exploration, and a lower affective repertoire than normals (Gaensbauer, 1982). Moreover, abused infants approached their caregivers only about half as frequently as did nonabused infants, and these infants actually avoided their caregivers 3 times more often than did control infants. Withdrawal was also more notable in these infants than in controls (George & Main, 1979). Abuse retards development of a child's capacity for self-representation (Schneider-Rosen & Cicchetti, 1984). The researchers found a significant relationship between the quality of attachment and the capacity for visual self-recognition.

All these investigations indicate that abuse and neglect are prominent risk factors for depression in young populations. This behavior can leave an indelible imprint on the child, invariably perpetuating a cycle of depression that will linger into childhood and beyond, disrupting developmental progress.

Conclusion

Needless to say, the development of a nosology of depression would be greatly facilitated by the discovery of a fundamental state of depression in infancy, since such a state, once identified, could be charted with relative ease through various developmental periods all the way to the differentiated depressive states observed in adults. Neuroendocrine studies that provide evidence of the preparedness of the infant to respond to stress and to provide self-regulation, in combination with cognitive abilities such as discrepancy and contingency awareness, strongly suggest the possibility that the infant can experience depression. This notion wins further support from the global way in which infants view failure, as well as from the similarity in the characteristics of learned helplessness and anaclitic depression, both of which carry strong components of withdrawal.

With regard to arriving at a definition of a fundamental state of depression postulated to exist during early development, the characteristic or symptom of withdrawal appears to be a good starting point. Withdrawal appears emblematic of depression across the developmental continuum and serves as a marker and mediator for the condition. The search for more refined definitions of depression might prove profitable if the phenomenon of withdrawal is studied in tandem with the internal explanatory systems of infants encountering uncontrollable events.

References

Abramson, L. Y., Seligman, M. E. P., & Teasdale, J. D. (1978). Learned helplessness in humans: Critique and reformulation. *Journal of Abnormal Psychology, 87*, 49–74.

Achor, R. W. P., Hanson, N. O., & Gifford, R. W., Jr. (1955). Hypertension treated with *Rauwolfia serpentina* (whole root) and with reserpine: Controlled study disclosing occasional severe depression. *Journal of the American Medical Association, 159,* 841–845.

Adler, G., & Buie, D. H., Jr. (1979). Aloneness and borderline psychopathology: The possible relevance of child development issues. *International Journal of Psycho-Analysis, 60,* 83–96.

Agren, J., & Terenius, L. (1983). Depression and CSF endorphin fraction I: Seasonal variation and higher levels of unipolar than bipolar patients. *Psychiatry Research, 10,* 303–311.

American Psychiatric Association (1980). *Diagnostic and statistical manual of mental disorders,* 3rd ed. Washington, DC: Author.

American Psychiatric Association (1987). *Diagnostic and statistical manual of mental disorders,* 3rd ed., revised. Washington, DC: Author.

Anand, K. J., & Aynsley-Green, A. (1988). Measuring the severity of surgical stress in newborns. *Journal of Pediatric Surgery, 23(4),* 297–305.

Anders, T. F., Sachar, E. J., Kream, J., Rolfwang, H. P., & Hellman, L. (1970). Behavioral state and plasma cortisol response in the human newborn. *Pediatrics, 46,* 532–537.

Arend, R., Gove, F., & Sroufe, L. A. (1979). Continuity of individual adaptation from infancy to kindergarten: A reductive study of ego resilience and curiosity in pre-schoolers. *Child Development, 50,* 950–959.

Asberg, M., Thoren, P., Traskman, L., Berllsson, L., & Ringberger, V. (1976). 5-HIAA in the cerebrospinal fluids: A biological suicide predictor? *Archives of General Psychiatry, 33,* 1193–1197.

Asnis, G. M., Sachar, E. J., Halbreich, U., Nathan, R. S., Ostrow, L., & Halpern, F. S. (1981). Cortisol secretion and dexamethasone response in depression. *American Journal of Psychiatry, 138,* 1218–1221.

Bacigalupo, G., Langner, K., Schmidt, S., & Saling, E. (1987). Plasma immunoreactive beta-endorphin, ACTH and cortisol concentrations in mothers and their neonates immediately after delivery—their relationship to the duration of labor. *Journal of Perinatal Medicine, 15(1),* 45–52.

Baldessarini, R. J. (1983). *Biomedical aspects of depression and its treatment* (pp. 22–160). Washington, DC: American Psychiatric Press.

Barnett, D., Manly, J. T., & Cicchetti, D. (1991). Continuing toward an operational definition of psychological maltreatment. *Development of Psychopathology, 3,* 19–29.

Bible, C., & French, A. P. (1979). Depression in the child abuse syndrome. In A. P. French & I. N. Berlin (Eds.), *Depression in children and adolescents* (pp. 184–209). New York: Human Sciences Press.

Biringen, Z., & Robinson, J. (1991). Emotional availability in mother–child interactions: A reconceptualization for research. *American Journal of Orthopsychiatry, 61(2),* 258–271.

Blass, E. M., Ganchrow, J. R., & Steiner, J. E. (1984). Classical conditioning in new born humans 2–48 hours of age. *Infant Behavior and Development, 7,* 223–235.

Bliss, E. L., Migeon, C. H., Branch, C. H., & Samuels, L. T. (1956). Reaction of the adrenal cortex to emotional stress. *Psychosomatic Medicine, 18,* 56–76.

Blombery, P. A., Koplin, I. J., Gordon, E. K., Markey, S. P., & Ebert, M. H. (1980). Conversion of MHPG to vanillylmandelic acid. *Archives of General Psychiatry, 37,* 1095–1098.

Blumberg, M. L. (1977). Depression in children on a general pediatric service. *American Journal of Psychotherapy, 32,* 20.

Blumberg, M. L. (1981). Depression in abused and neglected children. *American Journal of Psychotherapy, 35,* 342–355.

Bowlby, J. (1960). Grief and mourning in infancy and early childhood. *Psychoanalytic Study of the Child, 15,* 9–52.

Bowlby, J., Robertson, J., & Rosenbluth, D. (1952). A two-year-old goes to the hospital. *Psychoanalytic Study of the Child, 7,* 82–94.

Brazelton, T. B. (1973). Neonatal behavioral assessment scale. *Clinics in Developmental Medicine, 50,* 1–66.

Brodie, H. K. H., Murphy, D. L., Goodwin, F. K., & Bunney, W. E. (1971). Catecholamines and mania: The effect of alpha-methyl-para-tyrosine on manic behavior and catecholamine metabolism. *Clinical Pharmacology and Therapeutics, 12,* 218–224.

Bunney, W. E., & Davis, J. M. (1965). Norepinephrine in depressive reactions. *Archives of General Psychiatry, 13,* 483–494.

Burke, P., Kocoshis, S. A., Chandra, R., Whiteway, M., & Sauer, J. (1990). Determinants of depression in recent onset pediatric inflammatory bowel disease. *Journal of the American Academy of Child and Adolescent Psychiatry, 29,* 608–610.

Burland, J. A. (1986). The vicissitudes of maternal deprivation. In R. F. Lax, S. Bach, & J. A. Burland (Eds.), *Self and object constancy: Clinical and theoretical perspectives* (pp. 324–347). New York: Guilford Press.

Carlson, G. A., & Garber, J. (1986). Developmental issues in the classification of depression in children. In M. Rutter, C. E. Izard, & P. B. Read (Eds.), *Depression in young people* (pp. 399–434). New York: Guilford Press.

Carlsson, A., Lindvist, M., & Magnusson, T. (1957). 3,4-Dihydroxyphenylalanine and 5-hydroxytryptophan as reserpine antagonists. *Nature, 180*, 1200.

Carroll, B. J. (1972). The hypothalamic pituitary adrenal axis in depression. In B. Davies, B. J. Carroll, & R. M. Mowbray (Eds.), *Depressive illness: Some research studies* (pp. 143–159). Springfield, IL: Charles C. Thomas.

Carroll, B. J. (1976). Limbic system pituitary adrenal cortex regulation in depression and schizophrenia. *Psychosomatic Medicine, 38*, 106–121.

Carroll, B. J. (1984). Dexamethasone suppression test for depression. In E. Usdin et al. (Eds.), *Frontiers in biochemical and pharmacological research in depression* (pp. 179–188). New York: Raven Press.

Carroll, B. J., Curtis, G. C., & Mendels, J. (1976). Neuroendocrine regulation in depression: I. Limbic system adrenocortical dysfunction. *Archives of General Psychiatry, 33*, 1039–1044.

Charney, D. S., Menkes, D. B., & Heniger, G. R. (1981). Receptor sensitivity and the mechanism of action of antidepressant treatment. *Archives of General Psychiatry, 38*, 1160–1180.

Christenson, N. J., Alberti, K. G., & Brandsborg, O. (1975). Plasma catecholamines and blood substrate concentrations: Studies in insulin induced hypoglycemia after adrenaline infusions. *European Journal of Clinical Investigation, 5*, 415.

Cohen, M. R., Pickar, D., & Dubois, M. (1981). Surgical stress and endorphins. *Lancet, 1*, 213–214.

Cohen, M. R., Pickar, D., Extein, I., Gold, M. S., & Sweeney, D. R. (1984). Plasma cortisol and beta-endorphin immunoreactivity in nonmajor and major depression. *American Journal of Psychiatry, 141*, 628–632.

Conners, C. K. (1964). Visual and verbal approach motives as a function of discrepancy from expectancy level. *Perceptual and Motor Skills, 18*, 457–464.

Coppen, A. (1967). The biochemistry of affective disorders. *British Journal of Psychiatry, 113*, 1237–1264.

Cytryn, L., & McKnew, T. (1974). Factors influencing the changing clinical expression of the depressive process in children. *American Journal of Psychiatry, 131*, 879–881.

Davis, J. M., & Rovee-Collier, C. K. (1983). Alleviated forgetting of a learned contingency in an 8-week-old infant. *Developmental Psychology, 19*, 353–365.

DeCasper, A. J., & Carstens, A. A. (1981). Contingencies of stimulation: Effects of learning and emotion in neonates. *Infant Behavior and Development, 4*, 19–35.

Depue, R. A., & Evans, R. (1981). The psychobiology of depressive disorders: From pathophysiology to predisposition. In B. A. Maher & W. B. Maher (Eds.), *Progress in experimental personality research* (pp. 1–114). New York: Academic Press.

Douglas, J. W. B. (1975). Early hospital admissions and later disturbances of behaviour and learning. *Developmental Medicine and Child Neurology, 17*, 456–480.

Emde, R. N., Polak, P. R., & Spitz, R. A. (1965). Anaclitic depression in an infant raised in an institution. *Journal of the American Academy of Child Psychiatry, 4*, 545–553.

Engel, G. L., & Reischman, F. (1956). Spontaneous and experimentally induced depressions in an infant with gastric fistula: A contribution to the problem of depression. *Journal of the American Psychiatric Association, 4*, 428–452.

Ernst, C. (1988). Are early childhood experiences overrated? A reassessment of maternal deprivation. *European Archives of Psychiatry and Neurological Sciences, 237*, 80–90.

Facchinetti, F., Bagnoli, F., Bracci, R., & Genazzani, R. (1982). Plasma opioids in the first hours of life. *Pediatric Research, 16*, 95–98.

Facchinetti, F., Petraglia, F., & Nappi, G. (1983). Different patterns of central and peripheral [β]-ED, [β]-LPH and ACTH throughout life. *Peptides, 4*, 469–474.

Fagen, J. W., Morrongiello, B. A., Rovee-Collier, C., & Gekowski, M. J. (1984). Expectancies and memory retrieval in three-month-old infants. *Child Development, 55*, 936–943.

Ferguson, B. F. (1979). Preparing young children for hospitalization: A comparison of two methods. *Pediatrics, 64*, 656–664.

Field, R., Sandberg, D., Garcia, R., Vega-Lahr, N., Goldstein, S., & Guy, L. (1985). Pregnancy problems, postpartum depression and early mother–infant interactions. *Developmental Psychology, 21*, 1152–1156.

Field, T. (1989). Stressors during pregnancy and the postnatal period. *New Directions for Child Development, 45*, 19–32.

Field, T. M. (1984a). Early interactions between infants and their postpartum depressed mothers. *Infant Behavior and Development, 7*, 517–522.

Field, T. M. (1984b). Perinatal risk factors for infant depression. In J. D. Call, E. Galenson, & R. L. Tyson (Eds.), *Frontiers in psychiatry*, Vol. 2 (pp. 152–159). New York: Basic Books.

Finkelstein, N. W., & Ramey, C. T. (1977). Learning to control the environment in infancy. *Child Development, 48*, 806–819.

Fish, M., Stifter, C. A., & Belsky, J. (1991). Conditions of continuity and discontinuity in infant negative emotionality: Newborn to five months. *Child Development, 62,* 1525–1537.

Fox, N. A. (1989). Infant response to frustrating and mildly stressful events: A positive look at anger in the first year. *New Directions for Child Development, 45,* 47–64.

Friedman, S., Bruno, L. A., & Vietze, P. (1974). Newborn habituation to visual stimuli: A sex difference in novelty detection. *Journal of Experimental Child Psychology, 18,* 242–251.

Gaensbauer, T. J. (1980). Anaclitic depression in a three- and one-half month-old child. *American Journal of Psychiatry, 137,* 841–842.

Gaensbauer, T. J. (1982). Regulation of emotional expression in infants from two contrasting caretaker environments. *Journal of the American Academy of Child Psychiatry, 21,* 163–171.

Gaensbauer, T. J., Harmon, R. J., Cytryn, L., & McKnew, D. (1984). Social and affective development in infants with a manic–depressive parent. *American Journal of Psychiatry, 141,* 223–229.

Galdston, R. (1965). Observations of children who have been physically abused and their parents. *American Journal of Psychiatry, 122,* 440–443.

Galdston, R. (1981). The domestic dimensions of violence: Child abuse. *Psychoanalytic Study of the Child, 36,* 391–414.

Ganong, W. F. (1979). *Review of medical physiology,* 9th ed. Los Altos, CA: Lange Medical Publications.

Geller, B., Rogol, A. D., & Knitter, E. F. (1983). Preliminary data on the dexamethasone suppression test in children with major depressive order. *American Journal of Psychiatry, 140,* 620–622.

George, C., & Main, M. (1979). Social interactions of young abused children: Approach, avoidance and aggression. *Child Development, 50,* 306–318.

Gibbons, J. L. (1964). Cortisol secretion rate in depressive illness. *Archives of General Psychiatry, 10,* 572–575.

Glaser, K. (1968). Masked depression in children and adolescents. *Annual Progress in Child Psychiatry and Child Development, 1,* 345–355.

Goodyer, I. M. (1990). Family relationships, life events and childhood psychopathology. *Journal of Child Psychology and Psychiatry, 31,* 161–192.

Greenberg, R. E., & Gardener, E. I. (1960). The excretion of free catecholamines by newborn infants. *Journal of Clinical Endocrinology, 20,* 1207.

Guillemin, R., Vargo, T., Rossier, J., Minick, S., Ling, N., Rivier, C., Vale, W., & Bloom, F. (1977). [β]-Endorphin and adrenocorticotropin are secreted concomitantly by the pituitary gland. *Science, 197,* 1367–1369.

Gunnar, M. R. (1989). Studies of the human infant's adrenocortical response to potentially stressful events. *New Directions for Child Development, 45,* 3–18.

Gunnar, M. R., Connors, J., Isensee, J., & Wall, L. (1988). Adrenocortical activity and behavioral distress in human newborns. *Developmental Psychobiology, 21(4),* 297–310.

Gunnar, M. R., Fisch, R. O., & Malone, S. (1984). The effects of pacifying stimulus on behavioral and adrenocortical responses to circumcision in the newborn. *Journal of the American Academy of Child Psychiatry, 23,* 34–38.

Gunnar, M. R., Isensee, J., & Fust, L. S. (1987). Adrenocortical activity and the Brazelton Neonatal Assessment Scale: Moderating effects of the newborn's biomedical status. *Child Development, 58(6),* 1448–1458.

Gunnar, M. R., Malone, S., Vance, G., & Fisch, R. O. (1985). Coping with aversive stimulation in the neonatal period: Quiet sleep and plasma cortisol levels during recovery from circumcision. *Child Development, 56,* 824–834.

Harmon, R. J., Wagonfeld, S., & Emde, R. N. (1982). Anaclitic depression: A follow-up from infancy to puberty. *Psychoanalytic Study of the Child, 37,* 67–94.

Heniger, G. R., Charney, D. S., & Sternberg, D. E. (1984). Serotonergic function in depression. *Archives of General Psychiatry, 41,* 398–402.

Hindmarsh, K. W., Tan, L., Sankaran, K., & Laxdal, (1989). Diurnal rhythms of cortisol, ACTH, and [β]-endorphin levels in neonates and adults. *Western Journal of Medicine, 151,* 153–156.

Hoffman, Y., & Drotar, D. (1991). The impact of postpartum depressed mood on mother–infant interaction: Like mother like baby? *Infant Mental Health Journal, 12,* 65–80.

Hollenbeck, A. R., Susman, E. J., Nannis, E. D., Strope, B. E., Herson, S. P., Levine, A. S., & Pizzo, P. A. (1980). Children with serious illness: Behavioral correlates of separation and isolation. *Child Psychiatry and Human Development, 11,* 3–11.

Holmes, S. (1976). The use of control by a hospitalized five-year-old girl. *Maternal–Child Nursing Journal, 5,* 189–197.

Hopkins, J. R., Zelazo, P. R., Jacobson, S. W., & Kagan, J. (1976). Infant reactivity to stimulus–schema discrepancy. *Genetic Psychology Monographs, 93,* 27–62.

Hughes, D., Murphy, J. F., Dyas, J., Robinson, J. A., Riad-Fahmy, D., & Hughes, I. A. (1987). Blood spot glucocorticoid concentrations in ill preterm infants. *Archives of Disease in Childhood, 62(10)*, 1014–1018.

Izard, C. E., Huebner, R. R., McGinnis, G., & Dougherty, L. (1980). The young infant's ability to produce discrete emotion expressions. *Developmental Psychology, 16*, 132–140.

Jensen, J. B., & Garfinkel, B. D. (1990). Growth hormone dysregulation in children with major depressive disorder. *Journal of the American Academy of Child and Adolescent Psychiatry, 29*, 295–301.

Jensen, P. S., Bloedau, M. S., Degroot, J., Ussery, T., & Davis, H. (1990). Children at risk: I. Risk factors and child symptomatology. *Journal of the American Academy of Child and Adolescent Psychiatry, 29*, 51–59.

Kagan, J. (1974). Discrepancy, temperament, and infant distress. In M. Lewis & L. A. Rosenblum (Eds.), *The origins of fear* (pp. 229–248). New York: John Wiley.

Kagan, J. (1984). Continuity and changes in the opening years of life. In R. N. Emde & R. J. Harmon (Eds.), *Continuities and discontinuities in development* (pp. 15–39). New York: Plenum Press.

Kalin, N. H., & Carnes, M. (1984). Biological correlates of attachment bond disruption in human and nonhuman primates. *Progress in Neuropsychopharmacology and Biological Psychiatry, 8*, 459–469.

Kashani, J., Barbareo, G. J., & Bolander, F. (1981). Depression in hospitalized pediatric patients. *Journal of the American Academy of Child Psychiatry, 20*, 123–134.

Kazdin, A. E. (1990). Childhood depression. *Journal of Child Psychology and Psychiatry, 31*, 121–160.

Kempe, C. H., Silverman, F. N., & Steele, B. F. (1962). The battered child syndrome. *Journal of the American Medical Association, 181*, 217–240.

Kempe, R. S., & Kempe, C. H. (1978). *Child abuse.* Cambridge, MA: Harvard University Press.

Knight, R. B., Atkins, A., Eagle, C. J., Evans, N., Finkelstein, J. W., Fukushima, D., Katz, J., & Weiner, H. (1979). Psychological stress, ego defenses, and cortisol production in children hospitalized for elective surgery. *Psychosomatic Medicine, 41*, 40–49.

Kopp, C. B. (1982). Antecedents of self-regulation: A developmental perspective. *Developmental Psychology, 18*, 199–214.

Larson, M. C., Gunnar, M. R., & Hertsgaard, L. (1991). The effects of morning naps, car trips, and maternal separation on adrenocortical activity in human infants. *Child Development, 62(2)*, 362–372.

Levy, E. M., McIntoxh, T., & Black, P. H. (1986). Elevation of circulating β-endorphin levels with concomitant depression of immune parameters after traumatic injury. *Journal of Trauma, 26*, 246–249.

Lewis, M., Fiering, C., McGuffog, C., & Jaskir, J. (1984). Predicting psychopathology in six-year-olds from early social relations. *Child Development, 55*, 123–136.

Lewis, M., & Thomas D. (1990). Cortisol release in infants in response to inoculation. *Child Development, 61(1)*, 50–59.

Lewis, M., Worobey, J., & Thomas, D. (1989). Behavioral features of early reactivity: Antecedents and consequences. *New Directions for Child Development, 45*, 33–46.

Lidov, H. G. W., & Molliver, M. E. (1982). An immunohistochemical study of serotonin neuron development in the rat: Ascending pathways and terminal fields. *Brain Research Bulletin, 8*, 389–430.

Lloyd, D. A., Teich, S., & Rowe, M. I. (1991). Serum endorphin levels in injured children. *Surgery, Gynecology, and Obstetrics, 172*, 449–452.

Main, M., Kaplan, N., & Cassidy, J. (1985). Security in infancy, childhood and adulthood: A move to the level of representation. *Monographs of the Society for Research in Child Development, 50*, 66–104.

Mantagos, S., Koulouris, A., & Vagenakis, A. (1991). A simple stress test for the evaluation of the hypothalamic–pituitary–adrenal axis during the first 6 months of life. *Journal of Clinical Endocrinology and Metabolism, 72*, 214–216.

Matas, L., Arend, R. A., & Sroufe, L. A. (1978). Continuity of adaptation in the second year: The relationship between quality of attachment and later competence. *Child Development, 49*, 547–556.

Matthews, J., Akil, H., Greden, J., & Watson, S. (1982). Plasma measures of beta-endorphin-like immunoreactivity in depressives and other psychiatric subjects. *Life Sciences, 31*, 1867–1870.

McCall, R. B., & McGhee, P. E. (1977). The discrepancy hypothesis of attention affect in infants. In I. C. Uzgiris & F. Weizmann (Eds.), *The structuring of experience* (pp. 179–210). New York: Plenum Press.

McGee, R. A., & Wolfe, D. A. (1991). Psychological maltreatment: Toward an operational definition. *Development and Psychopathology, 3*, 3–18.

McKnew, D. H., & Cytryn, L. (1973). Historical background in children with affective disorders. *American Journal of Psychiatry, 130*, 178–180.

Meltzer, H. Y., Lowy, M., Robertson, A., Goodnik, P., & Perline, R. (1984a). Effect of 5-Hydroxytryptophan on serum cortisol levels in major affective disorders. III. Effects of antidepressants and lithium carbonate. *Archives of General Psychiatry, 41*, 391–397.

Meltzer, H. Y., Perline, R., & Tricov, B. J. (1984b). Effect of 5-hydroxytryptophan on serum cortisol levels in major affective disorders. II. Relation to suicide, psychosis, and depressive symptoms. *Archives of General Psychiatry, 41,* 379–387.

Meyendorf, R. (1971). Infant depression due to separation from siblings syndrome or depression retardation starvation and neurological symptoms: A reevaluation of the concept of maternal deprivation. *Psychiatric Clinics, 4,* 321–335.

Money, J. (1977). The syndrome of abuse dwarfism (psychosocial dwarfism or reversible hyposomatotropism). *American Journal of Diseases of Children, 131,* 508–513.

Mrazek, D. A. (1984). Effects of hospitalization on early child development. In R. N. Emde and R. J. Harmon (Eds.), *Continuities and discontinuities in development* (pp. 211–228). New York: Plenum Press.

Myer, E. C., Morris, D. L., Adams, M. L., Brase, D. A., & Dewey, W. L. (1987). Increased cerebrospinal fluid [β]-endorphin immunoreactivity in infants with apnea and in siblings of victims of sudden infant death syndrome. *Journal of Pediatrics, 111(5),* 660–666.

Newberger, C. M., & Cook, S. J. (1983). Parental awareness and child abuse: A cognitive developmental analysis of urban and rural samples. *American Journal of Orthopsychiatry, 53,* 512–524.

Okuno, A., Nishimura, Y., & Kawarzaki, T. (1972). Changes in plasma 11-hydroxycorticosteroids after ATCH, insulin and dexamethasone in neonatal infants. *Journal of Clinical Endocrinology, 34,* 516–520.

Orvaschel, J. (1990). Early onset psychiatric disorder in high risk children and increased familial morbidity. *Journal of the American Academy of Child and Adolescent Psychiatry, 29,* 184–188.

Ossofsky, H. J. (1974). Endogenous depression in infancy and childhood. *Comprehensive Psychiatry, 15,* 19–25.

Pare, C. M. B., & Sandler, M. (1959). A clinical and biochemical study of a trial of iproniazid in the treatment of depression. *Journal of Neurology, Neurosurgery and Psychiatry, 22,* 247–251.

Parry, G. (1982). Paid employment to enhance the mental health of working class mothers. Paper read at the British Psychological Society, University of York, April 1982.

Patton, R. G., & Gardner, L. I. (1975). Deprivation dwarfism (psychosocial deprivation): Disordered family environment as a cause of so-called idiopathic hypopituitarism. In L. I. Gardner (Ed.), *Endocrine and genetic diseases of childhood and adolescence,* 2nd ed. (pp. 85–98). Philadelphia: W. B. Saunders.

Peterson, C., & Seligman, M. E. (1984). Causal explanations as a risk factor for depression: Theory and evidence. *Psychological Review, 91,* 347–374.

Petty, L. K., Asarnow, J. R., Carson, G. A., & Lesser, L. (1985). The dexamethasone suppression test in depressed dysthymic and nondepressed children. *American Journal of Psychiatry, 142,* 631–633.

Phillippe, M. (1983). Fetal catecholamines. *American Journal of Obstetrics and Gynecology, 146,* 840–855.

Pilowsky, I., Bassett, D. L., Begg, M. W., & Thomas, P. G. (1982). Childhood hospitalization and chronic intractable pain in adults: A controlled retrospective study. *International Journal of Psychiatry and Medicine, 12,* 75–84.

Pollitt, E., & Eichler, A. (1976). Behavioral disturbances among failure to thrive children. *American Journal of Diseases of Children, 130,* 24–29.

Pollitt, E., Eichler, A. W., & Chon, C. (1975). Psychosocial development and behavior of mothers of failure to thrive children. *American Journal of Orthopsychiatry, 45,* 525–537.

Powell, G. F., Brasel, J. A., & Blizzard, R. M. (1967a). Emotional deprivation and growth retardation stimulating idiopathic hypopituitarism: I. Clinical evaluation of the syndrome. *New England Journal of Medicine, 276,* 1271–1278.

Powell, G. F., Brasel, J. A., & Blizzard, R. M. (1967b). Emotional deprivation and growth retardation stimulating idiopathic hypopituitarism. II. Endocrinologic evaluation of the syndrome. *New England Journal of Medicine, 276,* 1279–1283.

Poznanski, E. O., Carroll, B. J., Banegas, M. C., Cook, S. C., & Gross, J. A. (1982). The dexamethasone suppression test in prepubertal children. *American Journal of Psychiatry, 139,* 321–324.

Prugh, D. G. (1983). *The psychosocial aspects of pediatrics.* Philadelphia: Lea & Febiger.

Prugh, D. G., Staub, E. M., Sands, H. H., Kirschbaum, R. M., & Lenihan, E. A. (1953). A study of the emotional reactions of children and families to hospitalization and illness. *American Journal of Orthopsychiatry, 23,* 70–106.

Puig-Antich, J. (1986). Psychological markers: Effects of age and puberty. In M. Rutter, C. E. Izard, & P. B. Read (Eds.), *Depression in young people* (pp. 341–382). New York: Guilford Press.

Puig-Antich, J., Chambers, W., Halpern, F., Hallon, C., & Sachar, E. J. (1979). Cortisol hypersecretion in prepubertal depressive illness: A preliminary report. *Psychoneuroendocrinology, 4,* 191–197.

Radke-Yarrow, J., Cummings, E. M., Kuczynski, L., & Chapman, M. (1985). Patterns of attachment in two- and three-year-olds in normal families and families with parental depression. *Child Development, 56,* 884–893.

Rholes, W. S., Blackwell, J., Jordan, C., & Walters, C. (1980). A developmental study of learned helplessness. *Developmental Psychology, 16*, 616–624.

Rie, H. E. (1966). Depression in childhood: A survey of some pertinent contributions. *Journal of the American Academy of Child Psychiatry, 5*, 653–685.

Risch, S. C. (1982). Beta-endorphin hypersecretion in depression: Possible cholinergic mechanisms. *Biological Psychiatry, 17*, 1071–1079.

Risch, S. C., Janowsky, D. S., Judd, L. L., Gillin, J. C., & McClure, S. F. (1983). The role of endogenous opioid systems in neuroendocrine regulation. *Psychiatric Clinics of North America, 6*, 429–441.

Rochlin, G. (1959). The loss complex. *Journal of the American Psychoanalytic Association, 7*, 299–316.

Rose, R. M. (1985). Psychoendocrinology. In J. D. Wilson & D. W. Foster (Eds.), *Williams textbook of endocrinology*, 7th ed. (pp. 653–681). Philadelphia: W. B. Saunders.

Rosenblatt, S., & Chanley, J. D. (1965). Differences in the metabolism of norepinephrine in depression. *Archives of General Psychiatry, 13*, 495–502.

Rothbaum, F. (1980). Children's clinical syndromes and generalized expectations of control. In H. W. Reese & L. P. Lipsett (Eds.), *Advances in child development and behavior*, Vol. 15 (pp. 207–246). New York: Academic Press.

Rothbaum, F., & Weisz, J. R. (1989). *Child psychology and the quest for control*. New York: Sage Publications.

Rutter, M. (1986). The developmental psychopathology of depression: Issues and perspectives. In M. Rutter, C. E. Izard, & P. B. Read (Eds.), *Depression in young people* (pp. 3–30). New York: Guilford Press.

Rutter, M. (1991). Nature, nurture, and psychopathology: A new look at an old topic. *Development and Psychopathology, 3*, 125–136.

Sachar, E. G. (1975). Twenty-four-hour cortisol secretory patterns in depressed and manic patients. *Progress in Brain Research, 42*, 81–91.

Sandgrund, A., Gaines, R., & Green, A. (1974). Child abuse and mental retardation: A problem of cause and effect. *American Journal of Mental Deficiency, 79*, 327–330.

Schaffer, H. R. (1958). Objective observations on personality development in early infancy. *British Journal of Medical Psychology, 31*, 174–183.

Schaffer, H. R., & Callender, W. M. (1959). Psychologic effects of hospitalization in infancy. *Pediatrics, 25*, 528–539.

Schildkraut, J. J. (1965). The catecholamine hypothesis of affective disorders: A review of supporting evidence. *American Journal of Psychiatry, 122*, 509–522.

Schneider-Rosen, K., & Cicchetti, D. (1984). The relationship between affect and cognition in maltreated infants: Quality of attachment and the development of visual self-recognition. *Child Development, 55*, 648–658.

Seligman, M. E. P. (1975). *Helplessness: On depression, development and death*. San Francisco: Freeman.

Seligman, M. E., Peterson, C., Kaslow, N. J., Tanenbaum, R. L., Alloy, L. B., & Abramson, L. Y. (1984). Attributional style and depressive symptoms among children. *Journal of Abnormal Psychology, 93*, 235–238.

Siever, L. J., & Davis, K. L. (1985). Overview: Toward a dysregulation hypothesis of depression. *American Journal of Psychiatry, 142*, 1017–1031.

Spitz, R. A. (1945). Hospitalism: An inquiry into the genesis of psychiatric conditions in early childhood. *Psychoanalytic Study of the Child, 1*, 53–74.

Spitz, R. A. (1954). Infantile depression and the general adaptation syndrome—On the relation between physiologic model and psychoanalytic conceptualization. In P. H. Hoch & J. A. Zubin (Eds.), *Depression* (pp. 93–108). New York: Grune & Stratton.

Spitz, R. A., & Wolf, K. M. (1946). Anaclitic depression. *Psychoanalytical Study of the Child, 314*, 85–119.

Steele, B. F. (1976). Violence within the family. In R. E. Helfer & C. H. Kempe (Eds.), *Child abuse and neglect: The family and the community* (pp. 3–23). Cambridge, MA: Ballinger.

Stern, D. N. (1984). Affect attunement. In J. D. Call, E. Galenxon, & R. L. Tyson (Eds.), *Frontiers of infant psychiatry* Vol. 2 (pp. 3–14). New York: Basic Books.

Stern, D. N. (1985). *The interpersonal world of the infant*. New York: Basic Books.

Tannes, K., & Carter, D. (1973). Plasma cortisol levels and behavioral states in early infancy. *Psychosomatic Medicine, 35*, 121–128.

Tennes, K. H., & Mason, J. W. (1982). Developmental psychoendocrinology: An approach to the study of emotions. In C. E. Izard (Ed.), *Measuring emotions in infants and children* (pp. 21–37). Cambridge, MA: Cambridge University Press.

Trad, P. V. (1986). *Infant depression: Paradigms and paradoxes*. New York: Springer-Verlag.

Trad, P. V. (1987). *Infant and childhood depression: Developmental factors*. New York: John Wiley.

Trevarthen, C., & Hubley, P. (1978). Secondary intersubjectivity: Confidence, confiding and acts of meaning in the first year. In A. Lock (Ed.), *Action, gesture and symbol: The emergence of language* (pp. 183–229). London/New York: Academic Press.

Vale, W., Spiess, J., Rivier, C., & Rivier, J. (1981). Characterization of a 41-residue ovine hypothalamic peptide that stimulates secretion of corticotropin and [β]-endorphin. *Science, 213,* 1394–1397.

van Baar, A. (1990). Development of infants of drug dependent mothers. *Journal of Child Psychology and Psychiatry, 31,* 911–920.

Van der Kolk, B., Greenberg, M., Boyd, H., & Krystal, J. (1985). Inescapable shock, neurotransmitters, and addition to trauma: Toward a psychology of post traumatic stress. *Biological Psychiatry, 20,* 314–325.

van Praag, H. M. (1977). Significance of biochemical parameters in the diagnosis, treatment, and prevention of depressive disorders. *Biological Psychiatry, 12,* 101–131.

van Praag, H. M., & de Haan, S. (1980). Depression vulnerability and 5-hydroxotryptophan prophylaxis. *Psychiatry Research, 3,* 75–83.

Watson, J. S. (1966). The development of and generalization of "contingency awareness" in early infancy. *Merrill Palmer Quarterly, 12,* 123–125.

Watson, J. S. (1971). Cognitive–perceptual development in infancy: Setting for the seventies. *Merrill Palmer Quarterly, 12,* 123–125.

Watson, J. S. (1972). Smiling, cooing and "the game." *Merrill Palmer Quarterly, 18,* 323–339.

Weiss, J. M., Glazer, H. I., & Pohorecky, L. A. (1974). Neurotransmitters and helplessness: A chemical bridge to depression? *Psychology Today, 8,* 58–62.

Weiss, J. M., Glazer, H. I., Pohorecky, L. A., Bailey, W. H., & Schneider, L. H. (1979). Coping behavior and stress-induced behavioral depression: Studies of the role of brain catecholamines. In R. A. Depue (Ed.), *The psychobiology of the depressive disorders: Implications for the effects of stress* (pp. 125–160). New York: Academic Press.

Weiss, J. M., Stone, E. A., & Harrell, N. (1970). Coping behavior and brain norepinephrine level in rats. *Journal of Comparative Physiological Psychology, 72,* 153–160.

Weissman, M. M., Gershon, E. S., Kidd, K. K., Prusoff, B. A., Leckman, J. F., Dibble, E., Hamovit, J., Thompson, W. D., Pauls, D. L., & Guroff, J. J. (1984a). Psychiatric disorders in the relatives of probands with affective disorders: The Yale University–National Institute of Mental Health collaborate study. *Archives of General Psychiatry, 41,* 13–21.

Weissman, M. M., Leckman, J. F., Merikangas, K. R., Gammon, G. D., & Prusoff, B. A. (1984b). Depression and anxiety disorders in parents and children: Results from the Yale family study. *Archives of General Psychiatry, 41,* 845–852.

Weissman, M. M., Prusoff, B. A., Gammon, G. D., Merikangas, K. R., Leckman, J. F., & Kidd, K. K. (1984c). Psychopathology in the children (ages 6–18) of depressed and normal parents. *Journal of the American Academy of Child Psychiatry, 23,* 78–84.

Weissman, M. M., Wickramaratne, P., Merikangas, K. R., Leckman, J. F., Prusoff, B. A., Caruso, K. A., Kidd, K. K., & Gammon, G. D. (1984d). Onset of major depression in early adulthood: Increased familial loading and specificity. *Archives of General Psychiatry, 41,* 1136–1143.

Zeller, E. A., Barsky, J., Berman, E. R., & Fouts, J. R. (1952). Action of isonicotinic acid hydrazine and related compounds on enzymes involved in the autonomic nervous system. *Journal of Pharmacology and Experimental Therapeutics, 106,* 427–428.

19

Depression in Medically Ill Youngsters

Javad H. Kashani and Lori Breedlove

Review of Psychiatric Disorders in the Medically Ill

Before beginning a discussion about depression in medically ill children, it is important first to briefly examine depression and other psychiatric disorders in medically ill adults, as there tends to be more research in this area than in children, and some of this information may also be applicable to children, or at least worth investigating in this age group.

It is well known that there is a close link between physical and emotional symptoms, each with the potential to exacerbate the other (Thompson, 1988). In light of this link, it is interesting to note that psychiatric patients have an increased incidence of physical morbidity and mortality compared to the general population and that these physical ailments may contribute to their psychiatric symptoms. These medical problems often go unrecognized, as these patients are likely to provoke frustration and anxiety in the clinician (Bunce, Jones, Badger, & Jones, 1982). Although it is important to keep this possibility in mind, this discussion will focus primarily on psychiatric disorders found in those patients with a known medical disorder.

Although secondary major depression is the most common psychiatric complication of severe medical illness (Petty, 1989), many other conditions occur as well, including other mood disorders, grief reactions, adjustment disorders, anxiety disorders, delirium, somatoform disorders, sleep disorders, sexual disorders, alcohol and drug abuse or dependence, and other organic mental disorders. Homicidal and especially suicidal ideations are also not uncommon in these individuals (Davidson, 1987). Due to space limitations, these disorders will not be specifically addressed, except for those with the primary symptom of depression, which will be discussed in the following section.

When evaluating medically ill patients for a possible psychiatric disorder, it is imperative that a biopsychosocial approach be taken because of the potential interplay

Javad H. Kashani • Department of Psychiatry, University of Missouri, Columbia, Missouri 65207. **Lori Breedlove** • Burrell Center, Springfield, Missouri 65804.

Handbook of Depression in Children and Adolescents, edited by William M. Reynolds and Hugh F. Johnston. Plenum Press, New York, 1994.

between the biological and the psychosocial aspects of the illness (Green, 1987). The clinician needs to be familiar with the medical disorder itself and with the medications the patient is taking and to feel comfortable working as part of a multidisciplinary team. A thorough history including family history, which may indicate a genetic predisposition to a particular mental disorder, and past psychiatric history must be completed. As with any evaluation, illicit drug or alcohol abuse or withdrawal from such abuse must also be ruled out.

Frequently, these patients feel a loss of control, and the hospital environment may worsen this feeling, causing additional stress and possibly exacerbating a preexisting psychiatric disorder. An extreme example of how hospitalization can have such a strong effect on the patient's emotional state is that of the "intensive care unit syndrome," in which a person, usually with a life-threatening illness, encounters helplessness, little privacy, poor sleep, and an often noisy, fast-paced technical setting. These patients experience a wide variety of psychiatric symptoms and syndromes, including severe anxiety, mood disorders, delirium, and psychosis. Although many such cases are environmentally induced, they need to be diagnosed and treated aggressively with biological and psychosocial modalities (Goldstein, 1987).

In addition to depressive disorders, it is not uncommon to see personality disorders in the medical setting. These patients are often referred for evaluation because they may (1) display hostile, manipulative, or destructive behavior; (2) evoke frustration in the health care staff; (3) develop other psychiatric disorders and have numerous physical complaints; (4) exhibit poor compliance with medical recommendations; and (5) abuse drugs or alcohol (Fogel & Martin, 1987). Since this is such a difficult and challenging population, care must be taken to educate their primary care physicians and other health care providers through close consultation/liaison so that they get quality medical care. This task is not easy, especially for those patients who evoke anger and other strong emotional reactions in the caregiver, such as those with borderline and antisocial personality disorder. In such cases, the consultant must address the reactions of the staff by allowing them to ventilate their feelings and then attempt to make them aware that these reactions provide diagnostic clues that can be useful in treatment (Fogel & Martin, 1987). These patients must also be followed closely by the psychiatrist in order to facilitate proper treatment and to rule out concurrent mental disorders.

Depression in Medically Ill Adults

Unless otherwise specified, the term "depression" will refer to the DSM-III-R classification of major depression, and more specifically to secondary depression, which has been defined as a depression that occurs after the establishment of the diagnosis of a preexisting, nonaffective psychiatric disorder or medical condition (Winokur, Black, & Nasrallah, 1988).

In this particular population, a dysphoric mood may result from organic mood syndrome, adjustment disorder with depressed mood, dysthymia, dementia, or a major depression (Cohen-Cole & Harpe, 1987). It is important to differentiate between reactive depression that is relatively transient, usually requiring no intervention, and other treatable depressive syndromes. One must also carefully rule out organic causes including medications. The clinician must also be aware of the certain medical conditions that pose a greater risk for depression, some of which are shown in Table 1 (Klerman, 1981).

Various studies have shown depressive symptoms present in 12–36% of outpatients and approximately 33% of inpatients in the medical setting. Depressive syndromes occurred in 11–26% of hospitalized medically ill (Rodin & Voshart, 1986). Some findings suggest that depression is more likely to occur if the medical illness is severe and has a poor prognosis (Moffic & Paykel, 1975).

The diagnosis of depression in this population is often difficult because the stress of an illness or hospitalization may precipitate symptoms resembling major depression, and the somatic and vegetative symptoms needed for a diagnosis of major depression may result from the physical illness. Because of this possible causal link, Cavanaugh (1986) has suggested that the affective and cognitive symptoms of depression are the best indicators for the severity of depression, rather than the vegetative and somatic symptoms.

It is easy for a clinician to justify and possibly minimize depressive symptoms in light of the patient's medical illness, but care must be taken to distinguish between transient symptoms and those of longer duration and greater severity, for several reasons. First and most important is that the depression frequently will not be resolved after the medical illness improves and, surprisingly, these patients usually respond well to standard psychiatric treatments. Second, depressed medically ill patients are at greater risk to have poor compliance and less participation in their medical care. Third, these patients are prone to increased medical morbidity and mortality (Cavanaugh, 1986). Fourth, these patients may have more frequent and costly hospitalizations (Cavanaugh, Clark, & Gibbons, 1983).

Specific treatments in adults will not be addressed, but it is important to stress that if a diagnosis of major depression is made, treatment considerations should include both biological and psychosocial therapies.

Clinical Manifestations of Depression in Children

When discussing depression in medically ill children, we will be referring primarily to those children with medical conditions that are chronic, and sometimes life-threatening.

Table 1. Medical Conditions Associated with Greater Risk for Depression

Cardiovascular diseases	Malignancies
Cardiomyopathy	Central nervous system
Cerebral ischemia	Pulmonary
Congestive heart failure	Mineral/vitamin deficiency or excess
Myocardial infarction	Beri-beri
Connective tissue diseases	Hypervitaminosis A
Polyarteritis nodosa	Pellegra
Systemic lupus erythematosus	Pernicious anemia
Chronic renal disease or dialysis	Wernicke's encephalopathy
Endocrine disorders	Neurological diseases
Adrenal disease	Cerebral vascular accident
Parathyroid abnormalities	Dementia
Pituitary disorders	Huntington's chorea
Thyroid dysfunction	Multiple sclerosis
Infections	Myasthenia gravis
Encephalitis	Parkinson's disease
Hepatitis	Postconcussive syndrome
Human immunodeficiency virus	Temporal lobe epilepsy
Malaria	Wilson's disease
Mononucleosis	
Pneumonia	
Postinfluenza	
Syphilis	
Tuberculosis	

The diagnosis of depression in children can be difficult to make under the best of circumstances, but when added to the complications that go along with a medical disorder, the diagnosis may become even more difficult to make. The clinical manifestations in various age groups are important to consider, as it is known that there are different presentations of depression for particular age groups or developmental levels. Although there are exceptions to these presentations, the groups examined in general will include infants and preschoolers, preadolescents, and adolescents. Much of the literature in this area involves hospitalized medically ill children with depression; therefore, much of the information presented will be about hospitalized children.

As most medically ill children will have at least one hospital admission and many will have frequent hospitalizations, it is important to look at the hospital environment itself. There are numerous stressors at the hospital for anyone, but these stressors may have a profound effect on the child and may go relatively unnoticed by hospital personnel or other adults involved in the child's care, as they may be seen as routine. The degree to which a child is affected by these stressors varies with age, development, and personality traits. Separation from the parent is the first stressful event a child undergoes when hospitalized. Separation may be especially difficult for the younger child and will be discussed more later. The sights, sounds, and smells of the hospital may also be very frightening for the child. The actual illness itself, with possible pain, surgery, and other procedures, is difficult for children to understand and may cause intense anxiety. Various restraints and restrictions that are often necessary may be seen as punishment, causing a number of emotional reactions. Caregivers' attitudes can cause a great deal of stress if they are rude, cold, or uncaring. If staff or family do not speak at the child's level, what they say may be misunderstood or misinterpreted. And finally, if parents fail to visit or are not allowed frequent contact, the child may misperceive their absence as rejection (Blumberg, 1978).

The first group to be discussed in some detail are infants and preschoolers. Over the years, there has been some controversy as to whether the diagnosis of depression can even be made in this age group due to their lack of ego and the lack of verbal abilities to express themselves. Most experts now agree that depression can affect all age groups, but that the diagnosis is much more difficult to make in the very young. In a large study of depressed preschoolers, Kashani and Carlson (1987) concluded that younger children are more likely to present their depression through somatic complaints. According to Blumberg (1978), somatic symptoms, such as crying, enuresis, encopresis, sleep disturbance, and anorexia, which have been referred to as "masked depression" by some authors, seem to be common in these youngsters. Such a collection of symptoms poses a special problem when looking at medically ill children, as it can be a laborious task to determine which symptoms are related to the medical illness itself and which represent depressive symptomatology.

The infant is egocentric and aware of only his own needs; therefore, separation from the mother or maternal figure, as with hospitalization, prior to the age of 2 can result in extreme depression and anxiety (Blumberg, 1978) that may be manifested as helplessness and passivity, possibly similar to Seligman's animal model of learned helplessness (Milavic, 1985). This passive stance may predispose an infant to depression. A 3- to 5-year-old can normally separate from his or her mother and accept a maternal substitute, but may be unable to do so under stressful situations such as being ill or hospitalized. This regression to a previous developmental level may also present itself in other ways if a child fails to adapt to hospitalization or to his or her illness (Nagera, 1978). These children are often restricted by hospital rules, by the medical condition itself, or by parents who have extreme concern for the child's health, all of which may limit normal exploratory behavior. As a result, the child may act out with anger and oppositional behavior or may become withdrawn, apathetic, and passive. In either scenario, the child may be mistakenly perceived by hospital personnel as a bad child or brat if acting out or a model child and perfect patient if passive (Blumberg, 1978). It is therefore important to recognize the various presentations so that depressive symptoms will not go unnoticed and possibly cause adverse developmental consequences. The 3- to 5-year-old is especially sensitive to hospitalizations, and three factors contribute to this increased vulnerability, as reported by Mrazek (1991):

1. The parent is the primary attachment object and is unable to control much of what happens to the child in the hospital.
2. The child wishes to establish independence and autonomy, which is not accepted, as a more passive role is needed in the hospital.
3. Preoperational cognitive abilities exist, making the entire ordeal difficult, if not impossible, for the child to comprehend.

Although preadolescents can better understand explanations and have less difficulty adjusting to hospitalizations (Blumberg, 1978), they can also become depressed. In a study by Kashani, Venzke, and Miller (1981b) of 100 physically handicapped children, ages 7–12 years, admitted for orthopedic procedures, 23% showed evidence of depression. They all experienced a chronic loss of health. The researchers found that the most frequent symptom of depression in this group was loss of interest, followed by guilt and self-reproach. Symptoms were increased if severely traumatic events had caused their condition. With increased peer relations and concern for peer approval, children become increasingly concerned with body image and potential disfigurement or loss of function. Such concerns may lead to hopelessness, a loss of sense of purpose, isolatedness, and school refusal (Milavic, 1985).

Medically ill adolescents are at high risk for developing depression, as they are very aware of their body image and may be extremely fearful and frustrated by the thought of disability, loss of function, or death. They often experience a great deal of guilt feelings and worry about being a burden to others (Blumberg, 1978). These feelings contribute to low self-esteem, which is one of the primary features of depression in adolescence (Milavic, 1985). If the onset of the illness was prior to adolescence and even if the child adapted well to the illness initially, there may be more coping problems during adolescence due to increased concern about sexual identity and the need for more independence from the family (Mrazek, 1991). Those struggling for independence may have great difficulty in doing so due to physical limitations imposed by the illness; thus, they can become angry, resentful, and rebellious, which may lead to depression. Those with deformity and disfigurement are at particular risk for depression, and the clinician must also remember that adolescents are at increased risk for suicide (Mrazek, 1991). A number of coping mechanisms are used by medically ill adolescents, including regression, denial, projection, intellectualization, compensation, and displacement (Hofmann, 1975).

As with adults, but especially with children, it is important to remember that the emotional trauma that may be encountered in medically ill children may have long-term effects and can be as much of a handicap as the medical condition itself (Hofmann, 1975).

Epidemiology of Depression in Medically Ill Children and Adolescents

Various studies have provided an estimated prevalence of children with moderate to severe chronic, handicapping illness or disability to be 5–10% (Perrin & Gerrity, 1984). At any given time, 1 of every 6 children will have a chronic handicapping condition that may range from relatively minor to life-threatening (Graham, 1991).

Studies looking at the prevalence of depression in these chronically ill children have revealed some conflicting results, with some suggesting an increased frequency of depression and others indicating no higher rates of depression. This discrepancy may be due in part to the use of different measures for depression or variation of the actual incidence of depression within specific medical disorders. The setting in which the studies have been conducted (i.e., inpatient vs. outpatient) and the onset and chronicity of the illness can also possibly account for these varying results.

An earlier study conducted by Kashani, Barbero, and Bolander (1981a) looked at 100 children between the ages of 7 and 12 who were admitted to a pediatric ward for suspected or known medical conditions, and not necessarily with a chronic illness. These children and their parents were interviewed by a child psychiatrist using a semistructured interview, DSM-III criteria, and the Bellevue Index of Depression. Investigators found that 7% met criteria for major depression and 38% had a dysphoric mood. It was also of interest that 85.7% of those with major depression had experienced the loss of a significant adult figure.

In a separate study of 80 chronically ill adolescent outpatients with controls, Seigel, Golden, Gough, Lashley, and Sacker (1990) examined depression using the Beck Depression Inventory (BDI), self-esteem using the Rosenberg Scale of Self-Esteem, and life events using the McCutcheon Life Events Checklist. They found moderate to severe depression in 65% of the chronically ill compared to 13% of the control group. This difference was due to the psychological BDI scores and not somatic scores. The medically ill group also had lower self-esteem, at 79% compared to 19% of the control group. There were no significant differences in life events between the two groups. This study included three disease groups, sickle cell anemia, asthma, and diabetes, and no significant difference was found in depression, self-esteem, or life events between the three groups.

In a study examining life events and depressive symptoms in hospitalized ill adolescents, Kaplan, Grossman, Landa, Shenker, and Weinhold (1986) administered the Coddington Life Events Survey and the BDI to 43 acutely ill adolescents, 42 chronically ill adolescents, and 140 adolescents from the general population. They found no differences in the total BDI scores, psychological BDI scores, or life events survey between the three groups; however, the somatic BDI scores were greater in the acutely and chronically ill, and it was felt that these increased somatic symptoms were due to the physical illness itself, not necessarily to increased depression.

A number of studies have looked at depression in specific illnesses in children and adolescents. Several studies have been done involving youngsters with cancer. Kashani and Hakami (1982) conducted a small study in which 35 children and adolescents with cancer, between the ages of 6 and 17, and their parents were interviewed during outpatient visits. Major depression was found in 17% of children and adolescents with cancer, compared to 1.9% of child controls and 4% of adolescent controls. By doing retrospective chart reviews, Rait, Jacobsen, Lederberg, and Holland (1988) found major depression in 12% of 58 child and adolescent inpatients with cancer who were referred for psychiatric consultation.

These findings of an increased prevalence of depression in youngsters with cancer are contradicted by other studies. Kaplan, Busner, Weinhold, and Lenon (1987) administered the Children's Depression Inventory (CDI) to 21 children and the BDI to 17 adolescents with cancer. They found self-reported depression to be equal in adolescent oncology patients and the control population. Childhood cancer patients had lower CDI scores than those of the general population. Kaplan and colleagues (1987) felt that depressive symptoms in cancer patients and the general population were more related to psychosocial life events than to chronic illness. In another study, Tebbi, Bromberg, and Mallon (1988) administered self-reported depression inventories, the BDI, and the Schedule for Affective Disorders and Schizophrenia to 30 adolescents with cancer. They concluded that there were no greater rates of depression in these cancer patients compared to norms. This finding also raises the possibility of masked depression, which was addressed in a study of 76 children by Worchel et al. (1988), which revealed similar findings with no increased depression and, interestingly, lower depression rates in children and adolescents with cancer using the CDI when compared to normal schoolchildren and children who were psychiatric inpatients. Worchel and colleagues (1988) hypothesized that these children with cancer were using denial, thus probably underreporting depressive symptoms. This hypothesis was supported by the observation that the cancer patients' reports of ratings of severity of the disease were unrealistic considering their actual medical condition and by the discrepancy between the nurses' and parents' reports when compared to the patients' reports. These studies of cancer patients do raise interesting questions, which have yet to be answered, regarding the possibility of the increased use of denial or the presence of masked depression.

In looking at depression in those with chronic, handicapping musculoskeletal disorders, Kashani et al. (1981b) found that of 100 children, ages 7–12, who were hospitalized for orthopedic procedures, 23% showed evidence of depression using DSM-III criteria, which is considerably higher than reports of depression in children in the general population.

In a study of 41 youngsters with Crohn's disease, 12 with ulcerative colitis, and 52 with cystic fibrosis, Burke et al. (1989) found a lifetime prevalence of depression, using the Kiddie Schedule for Affective Disorders and Schizophrenia, to be 29% in Crohn's disease, 21% in ulcerative colitis, and 11.5% in cystic fibrosis.

As can be seen from these few studies, a number of different measures and subjects were used. It would at least seem reasonable that these ill children and adolescents would be at higher risk for depressive illness, but further studies need to be done. Very few studies have been done regarding race and sex ratios in the occurrence of depression in medically ill children.

Various factors can negatively influence psychosocial adjustment, all of which can predispose a youngster to an increased risk for depression. The time of onset of the disease may be important, as there can be more problems if the onset occurs during difficult developmental periods, such as early childhood (6 months to 5 years) or early adolescence (Mrazek, 1991). Those in early childhood face special difficulties previously mentioned with separation from their mothers or maternal figures and lack of verbal skills (Nagera, 1978). Immobilization and sensory deprivation can also make adjustment difficult and can easily lead to helplessness (Milavic, 1985). Some children may have a psychiatric history prior to the onset of their illness or a history of responding poorly to new situations and thus may have a greater likelihood of emotional problems with the illness (Nagera, 1978).

The visibility of the illness or the presence of deformity can negatively affect adjustment, as these children are labeled as "disabled" (Pless, 1984) and may have more difficulty obtaining much-needed support (Mrazek, 1991). The nature of the illness itself can have an impact, as some believe that those illnesses that are chronic, but unpredictably episodic rather than persistent, such as rheumatoid arthritis, asthma, and hemophilia, may place increased stress on the child (Steinhauer, Mushin, & Rae-Grant, 1974). Burn patients and those with gastrointestinal symptoms may also be predisposed to depression (Milavic, 1985). Those illnesses in which the diagnosis was delayed or missed initially can certainly create greater amounts of stress and can cause problems establishing a good therapeutic alliance with the patient and family, thus possibly interfering with appropriate treatment (Mrazek, 1991).

Family issues play a role in adaptation, including a family history of psychiatric disorders, especially depression, or poor family adjustment, which may particularly be a problem if the child's prognosis is grim or if the etiology of the child's illness is hereditary or environmental, for which the parents may blame themselves (Mrazek, 1991). An overall lack of strengths and assets can also contribute to maladjustment (Pless, 1984).

The long-term risk of depression and maladjustment in those medically ill children and adolescents who survive to adulthood has also been examined. Teta et al. (1986) interviewed 450 cases from the Connecticut Tumor Registry who had childhood or adolescent cancer and 587 of their siblings, all of whom were adults over the age of 21. They concluded that the cancer survivors did not show an increased risk for lifetime major depression over their siblings. The frequency of major depression in male cancer survivors was 15% and in females was 23%, compared to their siblings at 12% for males and 24% for females. The cancer survivors did, however, have more difficulty reaching some major socioeconomic goals.

Problems Clinicians Encounter in Diagnosing Depression in Medically Ill Children

As mentioned previously, diagnosing depression in medically ill children and adolescents is often an arduous task, and there are a number of potential problems a clinician may encounter when attempting to do so. These problems will be reviewed in this section.

The first major problem encountered is to distinguish which somatic complaints are symptoms of depression and which are a result of the medical condition itself. Due to the illness, these youngsters will often have more physical symptoms, and it must also be remembered that preverbal children with depression will display more somatic symptoms as well. Thus, the clinician is placed in the position of sorting out this dilemma. This being the case, it is very important that the clinician work closely with the pediatrician, and other involved specialists, who have expertise in the area of the physical condition, to help determine whether the physical symptoms are out of proportion to the medical condition, suggesting a stronger probability that the symptoms are psychiatric manifestations. The parents, nursing staff, or others who spend a great deal of time interacting with and observing the child can also give possible clues to the etiology of somatic symptoms.

The use of standardized rating instruments may not be of much use in clarifying this matter, as most of these instruments include somatic symptoms. This problem has been addressed in the adult literature and less so in studies involving children and adolescents. In studying depression in 24 children and adolescents with cancer, Heiligenstein and Jacobsen (1988) suggested that rating scales that contain somatic complaints can potentially overestimate the severity of depression in this population. Using the Children's Depression Rating Scale—Revised (CDRS-R) to assess the presence and severity of depression, the Global Rating of Depression, the Pediatric Performance Scale to monitor pediatric oncology patients' functional status, and clinical interviews with parents and children, these investigators concluded that there was significant overlap between the severity of depression and the amount of functional impairment. This overlap was attributed to the Somatic subscale of the CDRS-R, which included questions regarding appetite, sleep, fatigue, physical complaints, and psychomotor retardation, all of which can be affected by illness. Thus, a modified CDRS-R that eliminated the somatic items was evaluated and found not to correlate with the functional impairments, but maintained diagnostic sensitivity for depression. Therefore, the CDRS-R minus the somatic items may be useful when dealing with childhood oncology patients, and possibly those with other medical illnesses.

Worchel et al. (1988) drew similar conclusions using the CDI in measuring depression in children and adolescents with cancer. In addition to probable underreported depressive symptoms in this group, these investigators found that somatic items and those items addressing self-esteem were not good discriminators between depressed and non-depressed children with cancer. Most other rating scales used to diagnose depression, including the BDI and the Bellevue Index of Depression, also include somatic symptoms, so the clinician must be aware when using these measures that these somatic items may be addressed due either to depression or to the illness itself.

Another potential problem that can arise when evaluating these children is that of countertransference reactions, which can interfere with making an appropriate diagnosis. These medically ill children and their families are often emotionally draining to deal with; thus, the clinician may want to normalize or justify the child's symptoms in order to avoid getting involved, especially if the child is terminally ill or severely disfigured. The primary care physician and others involved in providing care to the youngster may feel helpless, hopeless, and guilty, particularly if there is no cure for the illness. These feelings can lead to withdrawal from the patient and family at a time when increased support is needed. On the contrary, the clinician may overidentify with the patient or family, resulting in overinvolvement (Steinhauer et al., 1974). If not identified and dealt with, all these factors can lead to inaccurate diagnoses and inadequate treatment.

Determining whether psychiatric symptoms are manifestations of a normal grief or adjustment reaction, or the result of major depression, is another potential problem encountered. In this situation, the duration of symptoms and the degree to which they cause dysfunction or interfere with interpersonal relations, play activities, and school activities need to be taken into account. The differential diagnosis will be discussed further in the following section.

The final problem to be discussed is that of determining the onset of depression. Although it may or may not change the intervention, it is an important and interesting question whether the onset of depression occurred after the diagnosis of the medical condition was made, as common sense would suggest, or before the onset of the illness. Failure to recognize that a child was depressed prior to the illness may impede treatment by eliminating potential useful therapeutic interventions, such as addressing previous family problems, prior psychosocial stressors, and possible dysfunctional personality traits of the child. Since depression often goes unrecognized by children and their parents, it is easy for them to blame the medical condition for causing the depression in order to avoid further exploration of the matter.

These are only a few of the numerous potential problems that can arise within individual cases afflicted with medical illness.

Differential Diagnosis

When evaluating a medically ill child or adolescent with depressive symptoms, the differential diagnosis can be extensive. The clinician not only needs to evaluate for psychiatric disorders seen in healthy children, but must also consider an even wider array of potential organic etiologies, which is usually of significantly greater extent than with healthy children. There are certain symptoms and conditions that may be more prevalent in specific medical disorders, which will not be discussed. When evaluating these children and adolescents, it is important to distinguish between primary affective disorders, organic affective disorders, and those depressive symptoms that are situational (Waller & Rush, 1983).

The primary affective disorders that need to be considered include major depression, dysthymia, and bipolar disorder, all of which can present with a dysphoric mood and some of the vegetative symptoms of depression. Particular attention needs to be given to the time of onset, the patient's prior psychosocial history, and the family history of any of these disorders, all of which can help clarify the diagnosis. As with any patient, prior to making any of the aforementioned diagnoses, one must rule out organic factors, which may be especially prevalent in this patient population.

Organic mood disorders with depressive symptoms can be caused by many factors. The first to be considered is drug-induced. The physician must carefully investigate current and past pharmacological agents that have been used in treating the medically ill child or adolescent. A few of the medications that are particularly known to cause depression include antihypertensives, corticosteroids, benzodiazepines, antiinflammatory drugs, anticonvulsants, barbiturates, some antibiotics, cimetidine, and some chemotherapeutic agents. In addition to those medications prescribed in the treatment of the child's condition, abusable drugs must also be taken into account, although it may be easy to forget to inquire about substance abuse in this population. These ill children and especially adolescents may resort to drug or alcohol abuse as a form of self-medication to treat underlying psychiatric or physical symptoms. Metabolic abnormalities, to which these youngsters may be prone to due to their illness or the treatment they are undergoing, can also precipitate depressive symptoms and need to be taken into consideration. These abnormalities might include thyroid and parathyroid dysfunction, adrenal abnormalities, and electrolyte or calcium abnormalities. Another organic etiology for depression is neoplasms, especially if the central nervous system is involved. Besides cancer, other chronic illnesses with which the patient is suffering can also cause depressive features. In some cases, seizure disorders can have symptoms of depression.

Infections, to which these patients are often more prone due to their illness or immunosuppressant medication, can mimic depression, especially if the central nervous system is involved, such as with meningitis or encephalitis. In recent years, studies have suggested that viruses can cause depressive features, such as the studies by Meijer, Zakay-Rones, and Morag (1988), which found higher rates of psychiatric disorders in post-influenza adolescent patients, and the study by Wilson, Kusumakar, McCartney, and Bell (1989), which found increased rates of dysphoria among children who were seropositive for Coxsackie B virus. It is also well known that those who test positive for human immunodeficiency virus and have AIDS can also manifest a number of neuropsychiatric conditions including depression, and dementia, which may resemble depression. Other conditions that affect the immune system also need to be considered.

Besides the more serious psychiatric and organic conditions that cause depression, situational depression can also result. In ill children and adolescents, grief reactions and adjustment disorders need to be distinguished from more serious disorders. According to DSM-III-R, adjustment disorders are reactions to an identifiable psychosocial stressor. With these patients, it may be difficult to establish a specific stressor, as they often have numerous stressors with the onset and course of their illness. The diagnosis itself may precipitate an adjustment disorder, but symptoms should not persist for more than 6 months. Grief reactions or bereavement may be normal occurrences in these children as well but, as with adjustment disorders, must be distinguished from more serious psychiatric conditions. These children must also be given increased support and frequent monitoring for potential progression of their symptoms.

In addition, there are a number of other psychiatric disorders that may display depressive features, including anxiety disorders, such as separation anxiety disorder and posttraumatic stress disorder. It is often difficult to differentiate between anxiety and depression, as anxiety is often a prominent feature of depressive illness, and it is difficult to determine whether the anxiety is a secondary feature or a symptom of the primary disorder. To complicate matters more, those with anxiety disorders also often have depressive symptoms (Roth & Mountjoy, 1982). It is important, though, to make the distinction between anxiety disorders and depressive disorders and, if necessary, to make both diagnoses, in order to treat these patients adequately.

In conclusion, it is impossible to include all the conditions that can cause symptoms of depression. Overall, it is most important to take a very thorough medical and psychiatric history and to order the appropriate diagnostic studies. Biological markers, such as the dexamethasone suppression test, are of limited value due to the increased difficulty of interpreting the test in the face of medical conditions, but future research in this area is needed (Waller & Rush, 1983).

Psychology of Illness

Psychological aspects of medical illnesses have been mentioned in general throughout this chapter as to how they may relate to depression. A few more specific aspects will be looked at in this section, including grieving, parent–child interaction, and emotional trauma that may result from procedures and hospitalizations.

It is first important to acknowledge the potentially devastating impact chronic illnesses pose as compared to acute illnesses in children. These serious and long-term illnesses stress and often physically and emotionally drain the child and family members for an indefinite amount of time. This stressful environment can eventually lead to an altered self-image and low self-esteem in the child (Battle, 1975).

Grieving in children and adolescents over loss of function or possibly in the face of death depends somewhat on the particular developmental level that the child has attained. A child under the age of 5–7 may not understand the ramifications of death, as this is the usual age at which the child acquires understanding of three important concepts related to death: irreversibility, nonfunctionality or finality, and universality or inevitability (Speece & Brent, 1984). The younger child's understanding of the disease or death may be very concrete, although this understanding may not be obvious initially to the clinician; thus, spending extra time with the child talking or in play activities can help determine the child's perception, which in turn can better enable those around the child to help with the grieving process.

In order to grieve, a child must first be aware of his or her diagnosis, although for younger children, the decision as to whether or not to inform them may need to be left up to the parents and physician. After being informed of the diagnosis, the youngster should be allowed time to ask questions and to assess his or her understanding, in order to help alleviate any misperceptions. The child should also be given some hope and reassurance that the treatment team will make every effort to fight the disease and keep the child from suffering unnecessary pain (Lewis, Lewis, & Schonfeld, 1991).

As with adults, there are no specific stages or sequences that children experience when grieving; however, the five-stage sequence described years ago by Kübler-Ross (1969) may help the clinician gain some insight into some of what the patient might be experiencing. These stages include denial and isolation, anger, bargaining, depression, and acceptance. Grieving children and adolescent patients and their families may experience some or all of these stages. In addition to these more common feelings related to grieving, the ill adolescent may have unspoken concerns that he or she is hesitant to voice related to normal developmental needs, such as planning the future, sexuality, life-style, and physical limitations (Blum, 1984). It may put the youngster at ease somewhat if the clinician addresses these issues openly and directly, so the adolescent will feel more comfortable discussing them.

Reactions to death or chronic illness in children are at least partially determined by the reactions of those around them, including family members, friends, and health care workers (Lewis et al., 1991). Parents or siblings may unconsciously withdraw from the chronically ill or dying child to prevent extreme anguish, which can leave the child feeling isolated with no one to talk to about the illness. Parents may experience unacceptable thoughts, such as wishing the child would die in order to relieve the suffering of the child and family. Thoughts such as this can be very upsetting to the parents and lead them to feel extremely guilty, thus possibly causing them to mobilize defense mechanisms, such as reaction formation, in which they may become overly protective of the dying child (Lewis et al., 1991). These factors need to be addressed and normalized to a certain degree, as they can place significant strain on the parent–child relationship.

Regardless of whether or not a child has a terminal illness, the stress surrounding procedures and hospitalization can be enormous for any child with acute or chronic illnesses. Medical procedures may be very frightening and painful, such as wound care of the burn patient. It is possible for these stresses to be so severe as to precipitate a posttraumatic stress reaction similar to that experienced by any child who has undergone a violent traumatic event. A pilot study (Stuber, Nader, Yasuda, Pynoos, & Cohen, 1991) examined a small number of children, ages 3–6 who had undergone a bone marrow transplant. They found that posttraumatic stress disorder (PTSD) symptoms, especially reexperiencing the event, denial, and avoidance of reminders, persisted after 1 year. This is probably also the case with other procedures; therefore, the clinician must be ready to diagnose and treat these children for PTSD and use preventative measures when possible.

Although it is impossible to eliminate pain and frightening experiences in these ill youngsters, certain steps can be taken to better prepare the child for hospitalization and procedures, which may in turn improve coping and tolerance in the child (Nagera, 1978). These preparatory measures include the following: (1) Explain to the child what to expect of an upcoming hospitalization or procedure, being as descriptive as is appropriate for the child's age and developmental level. (If possible, this information should be given so that enough time is allowed for the child to ask questions, which should then be answered accurately.) (2) Enable the child to visit the hospital prior to a scheduled admission. (3) Allow liberal visiting hours and frequent phone calls from family and friends to help support the child's morale. (4) Modify strict preoperative and postoperative rules so that a parent can be present just prior to anesthesia and at the child's awakening in the recovery room. (5) Allow and encourage the child to partake in play activities, preferably with other children. In some cases, it may not be possible to follow these steps, or they may need to be modified in order to accommodate those injuries or illnesses that require more acute or emergent intervention.

The issues mentioned in this section only begin to address the potentially numerous psychological aspects of chronic illness.

Treatment

Treating depression in medically ill children can be very complicated; however, it is important that appropriate treatments not be overlooked or avoided due to the potentially complex task at hand. A number of different approaches can be utilized depending on the individual patient's needs. Those methods might include individual therapy, group therapy, family therapy, and pharmacotherapy. The simultaneous use of several approaches should also be considered, as it is important to treat these children, as with any depressed children, in a timely manner because the course may become relatively chronic. An older study by Poznanski, Zrull, and Krahenbuhl (1976) revealed that on reevaluation of depressed children after an average of 6½ years, clinical depression persisted in 50%.

Before the specific treatment modalities are considered, prevention and strategies to improve coping in these ill children will be mentioned in brief. In looking at ill adolescent inpatients, Hofmann (1975) emphasized the importance of helping these children to cope by recognizing their increasing need for independence, reassuring them about their body integrity, and helping them maintain a sense of self-worth. In order to achieve these goals, the author offered a number of suggestions, which include allowing the adolescents to have as much input into their care as possible, maintaining as much autonomy in their care as possible, establishing peer groups on the wards, and continuing their participation in activities with friends outside the hospital if physically able to do so. With children and adolescents, it is important for them to be given at least minor responsibilities as soon as possible, which may help avoid excessive helplessness (Waller & Rush, 1983). In addition, it is important for professionals involved with the youth to work as a team in a cooperative way and to avoid undermining the efforts of others.

The first specific therapy to be discussed is individual psychotherapy, which will be discussed in general terms. Various methods can be utilized, including play therapy for the younger age group, cognitive therapy, behavioral approaches, and supportive psychotherapy. Initially, it may be necessary to inquire about the children's understanding of their illness and allow them to ventilate their concerns. Due to the families' anxieties, they may not yet have been allowed to do this at home. They, too, need to deal with their own concerns, and this can be facilitated in psychotherapy (Steinhauer et al., 1974). This individual one-to-one time with the therapist is very important, as these children may feel left out of their medical care, since caretakers may have spent little time talking directly to them. Instead, many conversations about their illness may have been directed at the parents. This time can also be spent helping the children to understand their illness in order to promote compliance and better coping, but explanations must be kept at a developmentally appropriate level (Schonfeld, 1991). For younger children, play therapy may be an appropriate way to enable them to express and deal with these fears and anxieties, but it must be kept in mind that the use of play therapy may need to be modified to activities that involve little physical effort, as these children may be limited in terms of physical activity due to their medical condition. In children and adolescents, the physical condition may also limit the length of time they can tolerate a session; thus, more flexibility on the therapist's part may be needed. Otherwise, the usual techniques may be applied in psychotherapy as with other children. For example, the strategies of Bedrosian (1981) when working with depressed adolescents are just as applicable, and possibly more important, when used with medically ill adolescents. The strategies include shortening the traditional 50-minute session, focusing on the development of rapport while minimizing threatening situations, tolerating some noncompliance, maintaining ongoing contact with the family, respecting the patient's privacy, creating an atmosphere that is collaborative, and avoiding difficult "homework" assignments.

Family therapy is another important therapeutic tool that can be utilized to help the ill child. Families of medically ill children and adolescents can face many potentially overwhelming stressors, which can disrupt the family balance and cause even more complex difficulties. Jacobs (1991) outlines common problems faced by families of medically ill children, which include intrafamilial and family interface problems. Intrafamilial problems would include organizational difficulties, such as increased rigidity with problem-solving, difficulty expressing grief or conflict, and reorganization of the family to focus on the illness. Developmental problems also occur within the family, such as limiting the development of the ill child due to constraints, and possibly delaying other family members' development, as they may feel it necessary to spend excessive amounts of time with the ill child. Family interface problems include those dealing with the medical team caring for the child, those dealing with the child's peer group, and financial difficulty imposed by the illness.

If the degree of family dysfunction is not severe, a supportive intervention provided by the child's medical team with psychiatric consultation is probably the best approach; however, this intervention should be time-limited, and if problems persist or progress, formal family therapy with a psychiatrist or other mental health professional may be needed. Formal family therapy needs to include a definition of the problem as it relates to the illness, treatment objectives so that there can be a realistic balance between taking care of the requirements of the illness and maintaining those family priorities that are not related to the illness, and progressive interventions as needed by the particular family (Jacobs, 1991).

Peer support groups or group psychotherapy may also be useful. Since children and especially adolescents are so peer-oriented, criticism or rejection from their peers can have profound effects and can possibly cause as much distress as the illness itself. Thus, it is important to get these ill youngsters involved with their peers as quickly as possible in order to normalize their situation to some extent and to prevent social isolation. Hospitalized children can benefit from support groups with peers who are also ill. In addition, invariably some of those belonging to the group will have adapted well, thus providing positive role models to others. For those children who have longer-term difficulty adapting, more formal individual psychotherapy along with group therapy may be of benefit.

Pharmacological management of depressed medically ill children and adolescents is another important treatment, although it must be modified and used with caution, depending on the specific illness and other treatments the child is receiving. Although clinicians often use psychoactive drugs in this patient population successfully, few studies have documented the actual effectiveness of these drugs in ill children and adolescents; therefore, the clinician must base treatment decisions on those studies involving physically health children and adults (Pfefferbaum, 1991). Prior to starting medications in these children, the usual thorough premedication workup needs to be completed, including a detailed history and mental status exam, a thorough review of the medical record, lab work, and an EKG and EEG as needed. Other special tests or consultation with various specialists may also be necessary prior to instituting medication, depending on the child's illness and complications. It is imperative to work closely with the pediatrician or primary caregiver and the family so that they are well aware of the potential side effects and goals of medication intervention. It is also necessary to identify target symptoms and monitor these symptoms carefully throughout the course of treatment (Pfefferbaum, 1991).

When starting any of the psychotropic medications in this population, very low doses and small dosage increments should be used. The lowest effective dose should then be maintained and adjusted if necessary to prevent or minimize possible adverse side effects, as the illness itself or other medications being used can alter the psychiatric drug's absorption, distribution, metabolism, and excretion (Pfefferbaum, 1991).

Tricyclic antidepressants (TCAs) are the most commonly used medication for depressed children. Monoamine oxidase inhibitors and newer drugs should probably be used with extreme caution, as there are fewer studies and less clinical experience with these agents.

Since TCAs are the most widely used, they will be the area of focus. Even in healthy children, there have been few studies and some conflicting results as to their efficacy vs. placebo; however, some studies (Kashani, Shekim, & Reid, 1984; Petti & Law, 1982; Pfefferbaum-Levine, Kumor, Cangir, Choroszy, & Roseberry, 1983; Preskorn, Weller, & Weller, 1982; Puig-Antich et al. 1987) support the use of tricyclics in depressed children. In addition to their antidepressant effect, Fields (1987) has also shown them to possess analgesic properties, which might be especially helpful in these children. The necessary dosage of tricyclics in ill children may be significantly lower than those in healthy children, as one small study by Pfefferbaum-Levine et al. (1983) of children with cancer showed positive responses at doses less than 2 mg/kg per day. Side effects of TCAs, such as anticholinergic effects, cardiovascular effects, orthostatic hypotension, and rare agranulocytosis, all need to be monitored very closely in ill children. In children with illnesses such as cardiac disease and seizure disorders, special caution with close monitoring must be used when initiating and maintaining tricyclic therapy. Monitoring of blood levels can also be helpful and has been recommended by Orsulak (1986) in a number of situations, some of which include when dealing with potential toxicity, treatment failure, and concurrent hepatic, renal, or cardiovascular disorders.

In addition to antidepressants, there has been recent evidence that stimulants may be effective in treating the depressed medically ill, especially the elderly. Although not well studied and the results are yet to be seen in children, this may be a short-term alternative for the treatment of depression in seriously ill patients who are unable to tolerate the adverse side effects of antidepressants or in whom a rapid response is crucial (Pfefferbaum, 1991).

When using any of the modalities discussed, once again it is important that the clinician maintain contact not only with the child, the parents, and nursing staff, but also with the pediatrician and other treatment team members so that changes in the child's condition can be dealt with immediately.

Future Directions

Acknowledging that it has been only over a decade that there has been convincing evidence of the presence of depression in children and adolescents, there is a great deal to learn about depression in youngsters who are medically ill. An interesting area is the use of various treatment modalities such as family therapy, individual therapy, or a combination of both, as well as the inclusion of pharmacotherapy. The use of each combination requires an appropriate number of subjects to carry out a double-blind study. To further complicate this situation, the use of various medications (e.g., imipramine, amitriptyline, trazodone, fluoxetine, and newer drugs) would indicate the major task that is at hand. Of special consideration is the use of any of the aforestated models for a specific illness (e.g., systemic illness, genetics, infectious diseases). Another area for future consideration would be the development of more standardized measurements of depression that take into account the somatic symptoms that are often present in these ill youngsters. In addition, most of the studies of depressed, medically ill children have dealt with inpatients, and it remains to be seen whether these findings will hold true for outpatients. The information presented in this chapter illustrates the complexity of the task and an exciting future pathway to explore.

References

Battle, C. U. (1975). Chronic physical disease—behavioral aspects. *Pediatric Clinics of North America, 22,* 525–531.

Bedrosian, R. C. (1981). The application of cognitive therapy techniques with adolescents. In G. Emery, S. D. Holton, & R. C. Bedrosian (Eds.), *New directions in cognitive therapy: A casebook* (pp. 168–182). New York: Guilford Press.

Blum, R. W. (1984). The dying adolescent. In R. W. Blum (Ed.), *Chronic illness and disabilities in childhood and adolescence* (pp. 159–176). Orlando, FL: Grune & Stratton.

Blumberg, M. L. (1978). Depression in children on a general pediatric service. *American Journal of Psychotherapy, 32,* 20–32.

Bunce, D. F. M., II, Jones, L. R., Badger, L. W., & Jones, S. E. (1982). Medical illness in psychiatric patients: Barriers to diagnosis and treatment. *Southern Medical Journal, 75,* 941–944.

Burke, P., Meyer, V., Kocoshis, S., Orenstein, D. M., Chandra, R., Nord, D. J., Sauer, J., & Cohen, E. (1989). Depression and anxiety in pediatric inflammatory bowel disease and cystic fibrosis. *Journal of the American Academy of Child and Adolescent Psychiatry, 28,* 948–951.

Cavanaugh, S. V. A. (1986). Depression in the hospitalized inpatient with various medical illnesses. *Psychotherapy and Psychosomatics, 45,* 97–104.

Cavanaugh, S., Clark, D. C., & Gibbons, R. D. (1983). Diagnosing depression in the hospitalized medically ill. *Psychosomatics, 24,* 809–815.

Cohen-Cole, S. A., & Harpe, C. (1987). Diagnostic assessment of depression in the medically ill. In A. Stoudemire & B. S. Fogel (Eds.), *Principles of medical psychiatry* (pp. 23–36). Orlando, FL: Grune & Stratton.

Davidson, L. (1987). Suicide and violence in the medical setting. In A. Stoudemire & B. S. Fogel (eds.), *Principles of medical psychiatry* (pp. 219–235). Orlando, FL: Grune & Stratton.

Fields, H. L. (1987). *Pain*. New York: McGraw-Hill.

Fogel, B. S., & Martin, C. (1987). Personality disorders in the medical setting. In A. Stoudemire & B. S. Fogel (Eds.), *Principles of medical psychiatry* (pp. 253–270). Orlando, FL: Grune & Stratton.

Goldstein, M. G. (1987). Intensive care unit syndromes. In A. Stoudemire & B. S. Fogel (Eds.), *Principles of medical psychiatry* (pp. 403–421). Orlando, FL: Grune & Stratton.

Graham, P. J. (1991). Psychiatric aspects of pediatric disorders. In M. Lewis (Ed.), *Child and adolescent psychiatry: A comprehensive textbook* (pp. 977–994). Baltimore: Williams & Wilkins.

Green, S. A. (1987). Principles of medical psychotherapy. In A. Stoudemire & B. S. Fogel (Eds.), *Principles of medical psychiatry* (pp. 3–21). Orlando, FL: Grune & Stratton.

Heiligenstein, E., Jacobsen, D. B. (1988). Differentiating depression in medically ill children and adolescents. *Journal of the American Academy of Child and Adolescent Psychiatry, 27*, 716–719.

Hofmann, A. D. (1975). The impact of illness in adolescence and coping behavior. *Acta Paediatrica Scandinavica, 256(Supplementum)*, 29–33.

Jacobs, J. (1991). Family therapy in the context of childhood medical illness. In A. Stoudemire & B. S. Fogel (Eds.), *Medical psychiatric practice*, Vol. 1 (pp. 483–506). Washington, DC: American Psychiatric Press.

Kaplan, S. L., Busner, J., Weinhold, C., & Lenon, P. (1987). Depressive symptoms in children and adolescents with cancer: A longitudinal study. *Journal of the American Academy of Child and Adolescent Psychiatry, 26*, 782–787.

Kaplan, S. L., Grossman, P., Landa, B., Shenker, I. R., & Weinhold, C. (1986). Depressive symptoms and life events in physically ill hospitalized adolescents. *Journal of Adolescent Health Care, 7*, 107–111.

Kashani, J. H., Barbero, G. J., & Bolander, F. D. (1981a). Depression in hospitalized pediatric patients. *Journal of the American Academy of Child Psychiatry, 20*, 123–134.

Kashani, J. H., & Carlson, G. A. (1987). Seriously depressed preschoolers. *American Journal of Psychiatry, 144*, 348–350.

Kashani, J., & Hakami, N. (1982). Depression in children and adolescents with malignancy. *Canadian Journal of Psychiatry, 27*, 474–477.

Kashani, J., Shekim, W. O., & Reid, J. C. (1984). Amitriptyline in children with major depressive disorder: A double-blind crossover pilot study. *Journal of the American Academy of Child Psychiatry, 23*, 348–351.

Kashani, J. H., Venzke, R., & Millar, E. A. (1981b). Depression in children admitted to hospital for orthopaedic procedures. *British Journal of Psychiatry, 138*, 21–25.

Klerman, G. L. (1981). Depression in the medically ill. *Psychiatric Clinics of North America, 4*, 301–317.

Kübler-Ross, E. (1969). *On death and dying*. New York: Macmillan.

Lewis, M., Lewis, D. O., & Schonfeld, D. J. (1991). Dying and death in childhood and adolescence. In M. Lewis (Ed.), *Child and adolescent psychiatry: A comprehensive textbook* (pp. 1051–1059). Baltimore: Williams & Wilkins.

Meijer, A., Zakay-Rones, Z., & Morag, A. (1988). Post-influenzal psychiatric disorder in adolescents. *Acta Psychiatrica Scandinavica, 78*, 176–181.

Milavic, G. (1985). Do chronically ill and handicapped children become depressed? *Developmental Medicine and Child Neurology, 27*, 677–682.

Moffic, H. S., & Paykel, E. S. (1975). Depression in medical inpatients. *British Journal of Psychiatry, 126*, 346–353.

Mrazek, D. A. (1991). Chronic pediatric illness and multiple hospitalizations. In M. Lewis (Ed.), *Child and adolescent psychiatry: A comprehensive textbook* (pp. 1041–1050). Baltimore: Williams & Wilkins.

Nagera, H. (1978). Children's reactions to hospitalization and illness. *Child Psychiatry and Human Development, 9*, 3–19.

Orsulak, P. J. (1986). Therapeutic monitoring of antidepressant drugs: Current methodology and applications. *Journal of Clinical Psychiatry, 47*, 39–50.

Perrin, E. C., & Gerrity, P. S. (1984). Development of children with a chronic illness. *Pediatric Clinics of North America, 31*, 19–31.

Petti, T. A., & Law, W. (1982). Imipramine treatment of depressed children: A double-blind pilot study. *Journal of Clinical Psychopharmacology, 2*, 107–110.

Petty, F. (1989). Southwestern internal medicine conference: Depression and medical illness. *American Journal of the Medical Sciences, 298*, 59–68.

Pfefferbaum, B. (1991). Psychopharmacology in medically ill children and adolescents. In A. Stoudemire & B. S. Fogel (Eds.), *Medical psychiatric practice*, Vol. 1 (pp. 455–482). Washington, DC: American Psychiatric Press.

Pfefferbaum-Levine, B., Kumor, K., Cangir, A., Choroszy, M., & Roseberry, E. A. (1983). Tricyclic antidepressants for children with cancer. *American Journal of Psychiatry, 140*, 1074–1076.

Pless, I. B. (1984). Clinical assessment: Physical and psychological functioning. *Pediatric Clinics of North America, 31*, 33–45.

Poznanski, E., Zrull, J. P., & Krahenbuhl, V. (1976). Childhood depression. *Journal of the American Academy of Child Psychiatry, 15*, 491–501.

Preskorn, S. H., Weller, E. B., & Weller, R. A. (1982). Depression in children: Relationship between plasma imipramine levels and response. *Journal of Clinical Psychiatry, 43*, 450–453.

Puig-Antich, J., Perel, J. M., Lupatkin, W., Chambers, W. J., Tabrizi, M. A., King, J., Goetz, R., Davies, M., & Stiller, R. L. (1987). Imipramine in prepubertal major depressive disorders. *Archives of General Psychiatry, 44*, 81–89.

Rait, D. S., Jacobsen, P. B., Lederberg, M. S., & Holland, J. C. (1988). Characteristics of psychiatric consultations in a pediatric cancer center. *American Journal of Psychiatry, 145*, 363–364.

Rodin, G., & Voshart, K. (1986). Depression in the medically ill: An overview. *American Journal of Psychiatry, 143*, 696–705.

Roth, M., & Mountjoy, C. Q. (1982). The distinction between anxiety states and depressive disorders. In E. S. Paykel (Ed.), *Handbook of affective disorders* (pp. 70–92). New York: Guilford Press.

Schonfeld, D. J. (1991). The child's cognitive understanding of illness. In M. Lewis (Ed.), *Child and adolescent psychiatry: A comprehensive textbook* (pp. 949–953). Baltimore: Williams & Wilkins.

Seigel, W. M., Golden, N. H., Gough, J. W. Lashley, M. S., & Sacker, I. M. (1990). Depression, self-esteem, and life events in adolescents with chronic disease. *Journal of Adolescent Health Care, 11*, 501–504.

Speece, M., & Brent, S. (1984). Children's understanding of death: A review of three components of a death concept. *Child Development, 55*, 1671–1686.

Steinhauer, P. D., Mushin, D. N., & Rae-Grant, Q. (1974). Psychological aspects of chronic illness. *Pediatric Clinics of North America, 21*, 825–840.

Stuber, M. L., Nader, K., Yasuda, P., Pynoos, R. S., & Cohen, S. (1991). Stress responses after pediatric bone marrow transplantation: Preliminary results of a prospective longitudinal study. *Journal of the American Academy of Child and Adolescent Psychiatry, 30*, 952–957.

Tebbi, C. K., Bromberg, C., & Mallon, J. C. (1988). Self-reported depression in adolescent cancer patients. *American Journal of Pediatric Hematology/Oncology, 10*, 185–190.

Teta, M. J., Del Po, M. C., Kasl, S. V., Meigs, J. W., Meyers, M. H., & Mulvihill, J. J. (1986). Psychosocial consequences of childhood and adolescent cancer survival. *Journal of Chronic Disease, 39*, 751–759.

Thompson, T. L., II, (1988). Psychosomatic disorders. In J. A. Talbott, R. E. Hales, & S. C. Yudofsky (Eds.), *Textbook of psychiatry* (pp. 493–532). Washington, DC: American Psychiatric Press.

Waller, D. A., & Rush, A. J. (1983). Differentiating primary affective disease, organic affective syndromes, and situational depression on a pediatric service. *Journal of the American Academy of Child Psychiatry, 22*, 52–58.

Wilson, P. M. J., Kusumakar, V., McCartney, R. A., & Bell, E. J. (1989). Features of Coxsackie B virus (CBV) infection in children with prolonged physical and psychological morbidity. *Journal of Psychosomatic Research, 33*, 29–36.

Winokur, G., Black, D. W., & Nasrallah, M. A. (1988). Depressions secondary to other psychiatric disorders and medical illnesses. *American Journal of Psychiatry, 145*, 233–237.

Worchel, F. F., Nolan, B. F., Willson, V. L., Purser, J. S., Copeland, D. R., & Pfefferbaum, B. (1988). Assessment of depression in children with cancer. *Journal of Pediatric Psychology, 13*, 101–112.

20

Depression in Special Education Populations

Patrick Schloss, Holly Sher, and Lech Wisniewski

Depression in children and youth is analogous in many ways to depression in adulthood (Reynolds, 1984). Defining features include a dysphoric mood occurring in combination with cognitive, motivational, and psychomotor changes or disturbances. These changes in mood and behavior may range from a mild degree of reactive sadness to intensely experienced feelings of dysphoria that may include suicidal ideation or lead to suicide attempts. Among the general population of children and youth, unique age-specific features have emerged due to the influence of schools, family, and peer groups occurring during this developmental period.

Depression is also becoming recognized as an important feature of students with special needs. Unique factors in the development and maintenance of depression complicate the diagnostic and treatment process for these students. Depressive features have been observed among several categories of disabilities and at rates significantly higher than in the general student population. This chapter will focus on depression among students receiving special education services. Special attention is given to issues related to defining depression in special education populations, the incidence of depression in these populations, and biological, social, and cognitive theories associated with the etiology and treatment of depression in students with disabilities.

Defining Depression in Special Populations

Contemporary definitions of depression generally address cognitive, motivational, and psychomotor aspects of the disorder (see Table 1). These symptoms include feelings of

Patrick Schloss • Assistant Vice President, Graduate Studies and Research, Bloomsburg University, Bloomsburg, Pennsylvania 17815.   **Holly Sher** • Department of Special Education, University of Missouri, Columbia, Missouri 65211.   **Lech Wisniewski** • Department of Special Education, Eastern Michigan University, Ypsilanti, Michigan 48197.

Handbook of Depression in Children and Adolescents, edited by William M. Reynolds and Hugh F. Johnston. Plenum Press, New York, 1994.

worthlessness and restlessness, changes in appetite, loss of interest in activities, diminished concentration, and repeated thoughts of death or dying.

Authors have provided a framework for categorizing distinct depressive characteristics (Milavic, 1985). Depressive syndromes with unique etiologies, courses of development, maintaining features, and treatment prognoses include psychoanalytical depression (Rie, 1966), manic–depression (Jones & Berney, 1987), anaclitic depression (Spitz, 1946), transitory depression (Lefkowitz & Burton, 1978), dysthymia (depressive neurosis), and major depressive episode (cf., American Psychiatric Association, 1987; Weinberg, Rutman, Sullivan, Penick, & Dietz, 1973).

Identification of depression among children and youth with special needs may be complicated by the diagnostic criteria developed for the general population. Overlapping features that define depression and specific disabilities limit diagnostic accuracy. For example, many depressive features outlined in Table 1 are also associated with learning disabilities, mental retardation, sensory impairments, and physical handicaps.

A second issue is the stability of symptoms being observed. *Stability* is an essential in the diagnostic criteria for children and youth in the general population. Among students with special needs, *changes* in these response patterns, rather than stability, may define a depressive episode. For example, it is not sufficient to simply note high rates of psychomotor agitation in a child with Attention Deficit Disorder with hyperactivity (ADD/HA).

Table 1. Depressive Symptomatology

Sleep disturbances	Negative feelings toward self
Insomnia	Self-deprecation
Nightmares	Frequent verbalizations of worthlessness
Fitful sleep	Frequent verbalizations of inadequacy
Frequent waking	Negative statements about self and world
Early morning awakening	Statements of guilt
Appetitive disturbances	Anhedonia
Changes in appetite	Talk of death or dying
Changes in weight	Somatic complaints
Agitation	Headaches
Hand-wringing	Abdominal pains
Pacing	Nonverbal communication
Restlessness	Slouched posture
Pulling, rubbing, or twisting skin, clothes, and objects	Frowning
Aggression toward others	Infrequent smiling
Aggression toward teachers	Grooming and self-care deficits
Psychomotor disturbances	Failure to respond to previous reinforcing events, people, or interests
Slowed speech	Distorted mood state
Disturbing speech pattern	Limited range or intensity of expression of emotions
Low or monotonous speech	Verbalizations of death or suicide
Decreased speech	Withdrawal from family and friends
Muteness	Avoidance of usual sources of pleasure
Slowed or increased body movements	Outbursts of complaining or shouting
Cognitive disturbances	Talking incessantly
Reported inability to concentrate	Sulking
Indecisiveness	Loss of interest in school or usual activities
Decrease in energy level	
Sustained tiredness	
Lying down	
Indecisiveness	

Since psychomotor agitation is an essential feature of children with ADD/HA, changes in the level of agitation may be a more important aspect in the identification process.

Incidence and Prevalence in Special Populations

Depression appears to be common in students with serious emotional/behavioral difficulties (Colbert, Newman, Ney, & Young, 1982; Cullinan, Schloss & Epstein, 1987; Simonds, 1975; A. A. Silver, 1984), specific learning disability (Hall & Haws, 1989), and physical or health impairments [such as cerebral palsy and general physical handicaps (Breslau, 1990), cystic fibrosis (Drotar, 1978), multiple sclerosis (McIvor, Riklan, & Reznikoff, 1984), orthopedic impairments (Harper, 1983), and congenital/acquired limb deficiencies (Varni, Rubenfeld, Talbot, & Setoguchi, 1989a,b)].

The incidence and prevalence rates reported in these studies varied considerably. Incidence estimates among special needs students range from 2% to 60%. Mean estimates among the general category of special needs students average 14–18%. Several reasons exist for this variability. First, the criteria for identifying depression vary across studies. Procedures have included self-reports, reports from others, formal inventories, and projective methods. The reliability and validity of these procedures produce uncertain results.

Methodological problems also account for the wide variance in incidence/prevalence reports. Studies often fail to control for threats to internal validity. Failure to employ random sampling, comparison groups, reliable measurement, and other design conventions suggests that history, maturation, regression instrumentation, and subject attrition may account for inaccurate conclusions.

Finally, overlap in features that define depression and the specific disabilities obscure research conclusions. For example, some students with a specific learning disability also experience motivational or cognitive difficulties as symptoms of impairment. Students with speech disorder have language or communication difficulties. These difficulties may lead clinicians to determine the existence of depression. The student's critical value (cutoff score) on the assessment measure may be inflated due to the symptoms that are shared with the disability. This procedure may lead to false-positives that may inflate the overall incidences of depression among students with disabilities.

Despite these limitations, the research literature offers several important conclusions. First, children and youth who receive special education services are at greater risk for developing depressive features than their nondisabled peers. Second, depression exists in higher rates among individuals in some specific special needs categories than in others. Students with learning disabilities and emotional disturbance may be especially prone to developing depressive characteristics. The incidence of depression in these groups may be from 10 to 15 times higher than the incidence found in the general student population.

Epistemological Factors in Special Populations

Several studies provide unique epidemiological variables among students with disabilities. Schloss, Epstein, and Cullinan (1988) reported, on the basis of teacher ratings, that severely emotionally disturbed (SED) and educable mentally retarded (EMR) students were observed to have significantly more depressive responses than either learning disabled (LD) or nonhandicapped students. Other variables were also reported. Regardless of age groupings (6–11 or 12–18 years old), SED males were reported to have more depressive symptoms than nonhandicapped males, whereas SED females aged 6–11 were rated as having more symptoms than nonhandicapped females of the same age. Among EMR students, only females, ages 6–11, were rated as having more symptoms than nonhandicapped females. Finally, the authors reported that SED males across both age groupings were more likely to receive higher scores, while females showed a marked decline by age.

Maag and Behrens (1989) reported conflicting findings, based on student self-reports. Maag and Behrens (1989) indicated that while a substantial number of SED students and students with a specific learning disability were experiencing depressive features, no significant differences were found between the student's label (SED or LD) or age grouping (ages 12–14, 15–16, or 17–18).

The findings from these studies (Maag & Behrens, 1989; Schloss et al., 1988) suggest that complex variables are influencing depressive features. In Schloss et al. (1988), SED and EMR students were more likely to be isolated from their nondisabled peers, to have social-skills deficits, and to lack social support. These behavioral cues may be more readily identifiable by the teacher. In contrast, self-reports (Maag & Behrens, 1989) may not be a reliable indicator of depression (cf. Crandall, Crandall, & Katkovsky, 1965), or differences in setting, environmental support, or other factors may influence the occurrence of depression.

Theoretical Approaches Relating to depression in Persons with Disabilities

A number of factors may contribute to the onset, development, and maintenance of depression. Those most directly related to depression in students with disabilities generally fall into three categories: biological factors (Gershon & Nurnberger, 1982; Puig-Antich & Rabinovich, 1985), social/behavioral factors (Altmann & Gotlib, 1988; Cantwell & Baker, 1987; Coyne, 1976; Horne, 1985; Lamen & Reiss, 1987; Lewinsohn, 1974), and cognitive factors (Asarnow & Bates, 1988; Beck, 1972; Benfield, Palmer, Pfefferbaum, & Stowe, 1988; Weiner, 1985).

Empirical support for these theoretical models has been derived from analogue research with animals, laboratory research involving human subjects, and research involving human subjects in applied settings (Asarnow & Bates, 1988; Benfield et al., 1988). We will briefly describe each model, review supporting research, and discuss prevention and treatment implications for students with special needs.

Biological Theories

Biological theories emphasize the role of biophysiological factors as a basis of depressive features. Several biological parameters have been identified, including dysfuncitonal central nervous system (Breslau, 1990; Silver, Hales, & Yudofsky, 1990; Brumback & Stanton, 1983; Colbert et al., 1982), biochemical abnormalities (Puig-Antich et al. 1984), genetic endowment (Cadoret, 1978; Winokur & Coryell, 1991; Mendlewicz & Rainer, 1977), nutritional deficiencies (Whybrow, Akiskal, & McKinney, 1984).

The relationship between biological factors and depressive responses can be direct or indirect. Hormone deficiencies, for example, may have a direct impact on sleep and appetite (Talbott, Hales, & Yudofsky, 1988). Additional interaction with a stressful environment may intensify the depressive response. The social environment may further reinforce the development and maintenance of depressive features—all contributing to the development of childhood depression.

Empirical Support. The presence of a biological component of depression has been well established (Puig-Antich, & Rabinovich, 1985). Researchers have noted concomitant changes in affect, as well as biophysiological disorders (Shelton, Hollon, Purdon, & Loosen, 1991). Further support has been drawn from genetic studies (Blehar, Weissman, Gershon, & Hirschfeld, 1988).

Akiskal (1989) suggests that a dysfunctional limbic system is associated with unique depressive symptoms (disturbances of mood, appetite, sleep, and libido; seasonal, cyclic, and diurnal variation; and changes in the autonomic nervous system). In addition, physical illnesses as well as medications that affect the limibic system have been found to produce depressive symptoms in a significant proportion of patients, while total or rapid eye movement (REM) sleep deprivation has been shown to reduce symptoms of depression (Shelton et al., 1991). Increased risk of depression at puberty has also been found in the children of subjects having early-onset depression (Blehar et al., 1988).

Familial studies of depression report a genetic link (Winokur & Coryell, 1991). Studies that have employed identical and fraternal twins support the genetic link (Talbott et al. 1988). Baron (1991) reports that the risk for the development of depression is 7 times greater among family members where depression has been diagnosed. Shelton et al. (1991) report that the environment and precipitating biological factors also contribute to the development of depression (Whybrow et al., 1984).

Relationship to Children and Youths with Disabilities. There has been an absence of research directly focused at biological parameters of depression among students with disabilities. However, several conclusions can be drawn from a broad review of related literature. Unique biophysical features may predispose a child or youth to develop depressive responses. Environmental stress associated with disability may result in the eventual manifestation of depressive responses. For example, illness and other chronic health impairments may produce feelings of helplessness and hopelessness. Further, persons with developmental disabilities may be relegated to lower social status, lacking the prosocial skills or the ability to obtain satisfaction from others. These environmental events may interact with concomitant biological factors to produce depressive responses.

Prevention and Treatment. Pharmacological therapies have been demonstrated to be effective with adults who exhibit depressive responses. These approaches are receiving increasing attention in the treatment of depression among children and youth. Medications used effectively with children and youths include trycyclic antidepressants, monoamine oxidase inhibitors, selective serotonin reuptake inhibitors, and lithium (Rancurello, 1985).

It is important to note that Werry (1982) reports a tendency by professionals to rely on pharmacological therapies in the face of increasing risks. Serious side effects (e.g., tremor, cardiac conduction, dizziness, and lethargy) and withdrawal symptoms (e.g., gastrointestinal complaints, decreased appetite, withdrawn behaviors, and irritability) require careful monitoring. The long-term effects on growth and cognition are unknown. Consequently, while potentially effective, pharmacological therapies may be used as a treatment of last resort and always in conjunction with social learning approaches.

Social-Learning Theories

Social-learning theorists such as Lewinsohn (1974), Coyne (1976), and Rehm (1977) examined the loss of positive reinforcements as the antecedent to the development of depressive responses. This loss can occur as a result either of one's inability to maximize reinforcing events or of a skill deficit in obtaining available reinforcers.

Lewinsohn (1974) proposes that insufficient reinforcement is the result of social-skills deficits. In the absence of prosocial skills, an individual may not have the social competence to manage the social demands of others. He or she may be oversensitive to negative responses from others or unable to communicate negatives to others. These deficits either reduce the availability of positive interpersonal interactions or increase the rate of noxious interpersonal interactions.

Rehm (1977) hypothesizes that individuals with depressive features tend to have unrealistic expectations for themselves. They tend to evaluate themselves very strictly, reward themselves infrequently, and punish themselves frequently. They also attend selectively to negative events and to immediate rather than long-term consequences of their behavior.

Finally, Coyne (1976) suggests that interpersonal characteristics of people with depressive characteristics may cause increased feelings of unhappiness or hostility in others. The initial reactions of others to the depressed person may appear to be supportive, but are detrimental in the long term.

Empirical Support. Social-learning theorists emphasize the student's reinforcement history as the basis for the development and maintenance of depressive features. Considerable support for the social-learning paradigm of depression can be found in the literature. Peterson, Wonderlich, Raeven, and Mullin (1987) reported that depressive features in youngsters influence adult perceptions of these youngsters. Teachers rated students with depressive responses more negatively than the nondepressed students. Altmann and Gotlib (1988), observing depressed and nondepressed children in free play, reported that children with depressive behaviors solicited social contact more often than nondepressed children and were in turn approached more often by others. However, they also spent more time alone or engaging in negative interactions with others.

Wierzbicki and McCabe (1988) investigated the relationship between social skills and depression. They report the predictive validity of a social-skills measures for the development of depressive responses 1 month later.

Cole and Rehm (1986) proposed a more comprehensive theory, integrating self-control and social-learning theory. The authors reported that the parents of depressed children had substantially higher expectations and provided less reinforcement than did parents of children who were not depressed.

In these studies, the occurrence of stress, the lack of coping skills, and the difficulty in managing social cues can precipitate the development of depressive responses. The effect of these circumstances is singular—a reduction in positive reinforcement. With this reduction, the student is placed on an extinction schedule. Prosocial skills are reinforced less often, and over time desired behaviors occur infrequently. Depressive responses are reinforced and become an integral aspect of the behavioral repertoire.

Relationship to Children and Youths with Disabilities. Once identified as handicapped, students may be relegated to a lower social status by school personnel, family members, and peers (Horne, 1985). A student's social status will influence the quality of his or her interpersonal interactions with peers, school, community, and family (Johnson, 1981). Lower-status students experience fewer positive social interactions. They are more likely to be neglected, ignored, or actively rejected. These interactions influence the student's social, emotional, and cognitive development and reduce other important sources of social support at a critical time (Cole & Milstead, 1989).

Beyond the loss of social status, the literature consistently acknowledges that children with disabilities are more likely to have social deficits that may lead to increased risk for the development of depressive features (Schloss & Schloss, 1987; Schloss, Schloss, Wood, & Kiehl, 1986). Cole and Rehm (1986) reported that students receiving special education services experienced higher failure rates and were less likely to be reinforced that their nondisabled peers. As a consequence of this reinforcement history, these students were more likely to become self-critical. The development of depressive features may be a direct consequence of this failure.

Prevention and Treatment. A variety of environmental events may account for the loss of positive reinforcement. Students with disabilities may lack appropriate social skills, have difficulty identifying and managing social cures, or have difficulty modifying previous response patterns. Several social-learning training programs are available to mediate the antecedent events that lead to a major depressive episode. In addition, the consequences of disruptive and prosocial behaviors may be managed to modify student behavior.

Students may be taught to use specific social skills when the social environment presents specific cues that the student finds challenging. The student may be taught to modify his or her voice or use more complicated interpersonal negotiation strategies in stressful social interactions. The purpose of these skills is to obtain reinforcement from the social environment.

Schloss, Schloss, and Harris (1984) used modeling, behavior rehearsal, feedback, and contingent reinforcement to increase the social-interaction skills or depressed adolescents. The researchers noted an increase in positive social interactions in training conditions as well as during generalization settings. Plienis et al. (1987) employed a conversational-skill and a social problem-solving training program. The program improved the youths' interpersonal communication and social problem-solving skills. Teachers rated the youth as more socially adjusted and reported improvements in their ability to interact socially during unstructured class times. These improvements in social skills also produced concomitant improvements on measures of depression, self-esteem, and loneliness.

Cognitive Theories

Cognitive theorists attribute the formation of depressive reactions to thoughts about oneself regarding past or impending events in which the outcome was or is feared to be negative. They argue that negative attributions increase the likelihood for developing depressive features (Beck, 1976; Weiner, 1985). For example, the student may develop a self-defeating attitude, unrealistic and distorted images of physical attributes, and expectations that the future will be fraught with failure, hardship, frustration, and uncertainty. Unfortunately, this view may be circular with definitions of depression that includes these features.

Cognitive distortions developed during an earlier developmental period are reactivated by later events. Feelings of helplessness or hopelessness (Abramson, Seligman, & Teasdale, 1978; Abramson, Metalsky, & Alloy, 1989) are developed in response to these beliefs. Weiner (1985) examined the role of one's attributional style in the development of depression. Experiences are selectively recorded as being essentially positive or negative, based on a person's attributional style. The symptoms associated with depression are the result of an attributional style that selectively filters environmental events—recording these events as being negative. As a student develops a negative attributional style, he or she may misperceive the relative frequency of adverse and favorable environmental outcomes. The student is more likely to exaggerate the occurrence of negative events while minimizing positive outcomes.

Empirical Support. A number of studies have examined attributional styles, feelings of helplessness and hopelessness, and cognitive self-statements. Beck (1976) reported that depressed individuals perceived and interpreted their environment more negatively. Zarantonello, Johnson, and Petzel (1979) reported that students with depressive features rated their performance on difficult tasks more negatively than nondepressed students. Benfield et al. (1988) assessed attributional style, hopelessness, life stress, and temperament of clinically depressed and nondepressed children. Finally, they reported that children with depressive features tended to make a greater number of specific and unstable attributions regarding positive events when compared to nondepressed children. Finally, Asarnow and Bates (1988) reported that students with depressive features made a number of negative self-reports across a broad spectrum of abilities. They reported more statements of hopelessness, more negative self-perceptions of athletic and scholastic ability and physical appearance, and internal attributions for negative events and external attributions for positive events.

In summary, these students demonstrate that students with depressive features make more negative statements about their performance. They are more negative in their recall of feedback. They develop failure attributions. Finally, they indicate that the future holds frustration and uncertainty.

Relationship to Children and Youths with Disabilities. Children and youths who develop negative attributions about themselves distort their perceptions of their environment. Children and youths who receive special education services do so primarily due to school failure. Schools define handicaps on the basis of failure. Failure at home, when expectations for adequate cognitive and social development are not met, leads parents to subtly communicate their disappointment (see Horne, 1985). One consequence of this failure is the loss of social status (see Horne, 1985). Inability to succeed in meeting adult and peer expectations and a reduction of reinforcement will become a continual source of frustration and failure. These expectations of parents, teachers, and peers may become a continual source of anxiety and frustration. The student's cognitions, reinforcement history, and loss of social status lead to the development of negative attributions and subsequent depressive reactions.

Prevention and Treatment. Cognitively based therapies focus on negative self-evaluation, low rates of self-reinforcement, and increased rates of self-punishment. These antecedents lead to the development of depression and are the focus of intervention strategies. In this strategies, children and youths may learn how unrealistic beliefs and irrational consequences influence their affect. Cognitive therapies have included cognitive problem-solving (Spivack & Shure, 1974), rational–emotive therapy (Waters, 1982), self-instructional training (Meichenbaum & Burland, 1979), and attributional retraining (Dweck, 1975).

Cognitive therapies are short-term interventions that deal primarily with reeducating the student on the issues associated with depression. Students are taught specific skills to identify and change dysfunctional cognitions. Kaslow and Rehm (1983) employed several techniques to identify the relationship between cognition, affect, and behavior; to monitor negative cognitions; to examine the evidence for and against these cognitions; and to establish realistic interpretations for and against unrealistic cognitions. The cognitive therapist helps the student restructure current cognitions while he or she learns several interpersonal problem-solving skills to be applied in stressful situations.

There is little research on the efficacy of this approach among students and even less involving students with disabilities (see Butler, Miezitis, Friedman, & Cole, 1989). However, it is hypothesized that cognitive therapies will present certain challenges for students with disabilities. Students must have several skills if cognitive therapy is to be successful in the prevention and treatment of depression. First, a certain degree of abstract reasoning and cognitive development is necessary. Students typically do not achieve the capacity for abstract reasoning and thought until the formal operation stage of cognitive development during early adolescence. This stage may be delayed in some students with disabilities.

A second potential problem for persons with disabilities is linguistic development. Deficits in speech and language are common among students with disabilities. Beliefs and perceptions that are based on past, present, and future events require a certain degree of language skills. Students will need to possess these skills if they are to articulate their thoughts about their environment.

It is important to note that the student's learning and behavioral characteristics should be considered prior to selecting this approach. Personality and learning styles are variables that will influence the efficacy of cognitive approaches. In the next section, factors that influence the development and maintenance of depressive symptomatology in special populations are discussed.

453

Depression in Special Education Populations

Integrating Theoretical Models

The currently most promising clinical practices for the identification and treatment of depression view depression as a multifaceted problem (Carlson & Cantwell, 1980). Complex intraindividual variables operate in a social environment to develop depressive features. Additional environmental variables lead to the maintenance of these responses. Criterion lists (Table 1) are only observable behaviors of an aggregate syndrome. While several depressive nosologies have been developed by recombining symptoms into unique syndromes, common principles are believed to be operating in the development and maintenance of depression in special populations. These principles have added implications to the overall theory on depression in children and adults. An ecobehavioral model that employs systems analysis may unify current biological, social, and cognitive perspectives of depression, influencing current service delivery systems, particularly school systems, that serve children and youth.

Recent research has identified various biophysiological factors and environmental events that have been associated with depressive features. The development of these features is an iterative process—predisposing factors, antecedents, and consequences alternate to increase the frequency, duration, and intensity of depressive symptoms. These predisposing factors and environmental events serve as antecedents. Once the symptoms have developed, other events occur in the student's environment that reinforce and maintain the depressive symptomology. A schematic of the process is presented in Table 2.

Predisposing Factors

Development and maintenance of the depressive syndrome may depend on several intraindividual variables (see Table 2). In addition to the current official recognition of sex and age differences associated with depressive symptomatology (cf., American Psychiatric Association, 1987; Weinberg et al., 1973), additional language and cognitive differences have been noted (Brumback, 1985; Brumback, Jackoway, & Weinberg, 1980; Colbert et al., 1982; Cullinan et al., 1987; Osborn & Meador, 1990; Plienis et al., 1987). Students with disabilities may be at greater risk of developing depressive features, since language and cognitive deficiencies provide the basis for special education services.

In schools, children and adolescents are required to develop competencies in a variety of language and cognitive tasks, achieve social competence, and attain healthy personal adjustment. Students who fail to demonstrate these competencies are typically referred for diagnostic evaluation and, if appropriate, to receive special education services. Once students with disabilities are identified as handicapped, several variables may predispose them to develop depressive symptoms (Rourke, 1989). In addition, these students are relegated to a lower social status by their peers, school personnel, and family members (see Horne, 1985).

A student's social status will influence the quality of his or her interpersonal interactions with peers, school, community, and family (Johnson, 1981). Lower-status students experience fewer positive social interactions. They are more likely to be ignored, neglected, or actively rejected. These negative interactions interfere with the student's social, emotional, and cognitive development and reduce other important sources of social support during a time of need (Cole & Milstead, 1989), leading to development of lower

Table 2. Development and Maintenance of Depressive Symptomatology

Predisposing factors	Antecedent events	Depressive symptomatology	Maintenance factors
Disability	Antecedent control	Sleep disturbances	Positive reinforcement
Deficient familial patterns	Unable to maximize reinforcement.	Appetitive disturbances	Sympathy
Psychological variables	Unable to rearrange environment.	Agitation	Support
Physiological variables	Reinforcement history	Psychomotor retardation	Assurance
	Unable to avoid/escape unpleasant conditions.	Cognitive disturbances	Attention (suicidal attempt)
	Depressive symptoms may generalize across behaviors, setting, or time.	Decreased energy level	Negative reinforcement
		Negative feelings toward self	Avoidance of school, home, or social responsibilities
	Social-skills deficits	Nonverbal communication	Compliance demands
	Interpersonal deficiencies	Distorted mood state	
	Reduced positive reinforcement gained from interpersonal and other social interactions		
	Personal attributions		
	External control		

self-esteem. Pearce (1977) has argued that these interactions are the probable basis for the development of depressive symptomatology.

Other factors are also believed to influence the development of depressive symptomatology. A number of biophysiological factors, dysfunctional central nervous system (Breslau, 1990; Brumback & Stanton, 1983; Colbert et al., 1982) or abnormal biochemistry (Puig-Antich et al., 1984), and psychosocial factors (such as dysfunctional families, marital discord, or intrafamily conflicts) (Milavic, 1985; Robins, 1978; Rutter, 1966) have been reported in the study of depression. However, given the marked variability of the depressive symptomatology across individuals in these studies, these predisposing factors alone cannot account for the development of depression. These factors interact with the social environment and lead to the development of depressive features. A complex interplay of predisposing factors and unfavorable social environments increases the risk of developing various disorders, including depression.

Antecedent Events

Several antecedent events are associated with the development of depressive symptoms. These events further the iterative process that leads to the major depressive episode. The student's repertoire of coping skills and environmental support determines how depressive symptoms develop. As depressive behaviors emerge, they interfere with daily functioning and attenuate the level of personal competence (Reynolds & Baker, 1988).

Social skills and related-task deficits of students with disabilities are important factors that contribute to depressive features. Social competence enables an individual to establish friendships, form social support networks, and gain acceptance from peers. These support networks are an important buffer against stress, allowing students to cope more effectively with those aspects of human development and the social difficulties that they may face.

Numerous studies have examined social-skills deficits in children and youths experiencing depressive features (Altmann & Gotlib, 1988; Benson, Reiss, Smith, & Laman, 1985; Blechman, McEnroe, Cardella, & Audette, 1986; Helsel & Matson, 1984; Lamen & Reiss, 1987; Sacco & Graves, 1984; Schloss, 1982; Varni et al., 1989a,b). These studies reported that children and adolescents with disabilities often lacked peer-valued social skills. They were reported to have difficulty in establishing gratifying relationships, receiving reinforcement from others, or participating fully in social activities. They performed less skillfully on some tasks involving interpersonal problem-solving. They were preferred less often as playmates or workmates. They were also reported to have difficulties in self-monitoring and in recognizing the interpersonal consequences of their social deficits.

In addition to students' interpersonal difficulties with their nondisabled peers, these studies also reported interpersonal deficiencies manifested by their classroom teachers. Teachers who failed to engineer the learning or social environment were reported to contribute to the social-skills deficits and the negative attitudes that their peers displayed toward students with disabilities. These teachers tended not to focus on developing positive classroom relationships. They were noted to ignore the use of group strategies designed to facilitate prosocial skill development. Finally, these teachers also failed to provide adequate modeling of desired prosocial behaviors (cf., Horne, 1985). In the absence of prosocial responses, students with disabilities may be unable to elicit positive reinforcement from the learning and social environment and may resort to depressive reactions to elicit sympathy and assurance.

Personal attributions—feelings of helplessness and hopelessness—also influence the development of depressive symptoms (Bodiford, Eisenstadt, Johnson, & Bradlyn, 1988; Seligman et al., 1984). A student's affective and cognitive reactions for his or her successes or failures are a function of the causal attributions that the student develops as to why an event occurred (Weiner et al., 1971). These causes include ability, effort, task difficulty, and luck. Ability and task difficulty are considered to be stable, whereas effort and luck are unstable events. When considering the nature of self-attributes about successes and failures, students with a mild handicap tend to be more selective, filtering out and minimizing positive events. They tend to blame themselves for their failures (MacMillan, Keogh, & Jones, 1986). They view the cause of their failures as a lack of ability rather than a lack of effort, while teachers attribute student failure to lack of effort (Tollefson, Melvin, & Thippavajjala, 1990; Seligman & Peterson, 1986).

Maintenance of Depressive Symptomatology

The attitudes of students with disabilities toward interpersonal interactions may reinforce and maintain depressive reaction. Students with disabilities are again at a particular disadvantage. They often stand out as different by demonstrating fewer social or cognitive skills that are valued by teachers or peers (Horne, 1985). In the absence of these valued skills, depressive responses may be reinforced by compliance or escape behaviors that reinforce the student's maladaptive interpersonal interactions.

Schools provide important sources for cognitive and social development. The skills that students acquire become important determinants for success in school, and for later in adult life. By definition, students with disabilities have experienced considerable failure in their cognitive development, and this failure is associated with depressive features (Osborn & Meador, 1990).

Brumback and Weinberg (1977) reported that children with disabilities who exhibit depressive symptoms lose interest in activities and fail to perform assigned tasks. Finally, Reynolds and Miller (1985) reported that students labeled educable mentally retarded attribute their failure to their inability to master the school curriculum. The authors also reported that this sense of failure may generalize to other aspects of their development and vocational training. This failure is directly linked to the difficulty that teachers have in engineering the learning environment.

Students who experience school and social failure that is consistent and sustained are regulated to lower status by their peers and teachers. Depressive features diminish social support in ways not mediated by social-skills deficits. This diminution results in an overall reduction of coping skills and increased social rejection. Students who are experiencing failure hold negative attitudes toward themselves and interact with the environment differently. In the interest of preserving their sense of personal worth, students establish patterns of interactions that become self-defeating. Schloss (1982) reported that students with disabilities were more likely to gain compliance or resist requests from others by exhibiting negative affect and that others were more likely in their interactions to exhibit negative affect toward the student with the disability. Consequently, interpersonal relations and social support are negatively affected. Parents and family may also react in ways that the student finds frustrating and may also manifest depressed responses themselves (Gowen, Johnson, & Goldman, 1989; Pueschel, 1986).

In summary, teachers, students, and family may reinforce the depressive symptoms by failing to provide reassurance, to comply with the students' requests for help, or to counter the students' tendency to withdraw. The failure of these students to gain control over their environment and to receive reinforcement for adequate cognitive and social development is an aspect of their reinforcement history (Wolpe, 1971). These students learn that they cannot determine their own future. Self-determination becomes impossible, given their social and reinforcement history. Over time, the depressive symptoms are strengthened, given the students' limited repertoire of interpersonal, cognitive, and social skills. Consequently, social relationships and social support are negatively affected.

Conclusions

Depression among children and adolescents is essentially analogous to that in adults. For children with special needs, depression is a common complicating factor. Depression appears to occur at a higher rate among children with emotional and behavioral disorders and those with mental retardation. These conclusions must be viewed cautiously, as diagnostic criteria for depression may overlap with criteria for other disorders.

Biological factors, social and behavioral factors, and cognitive factors all appear to contribute to the onset and maintenance of depression. Thus, an integrated approach to the diagnosis and treatment of depression is necessary.

Biological factors and factors related to a disabling condition may predispose students to the development of depression. Stressful events such as school failure, identification of disability, and initiation of special education services may interact with these factors to precipitate a depressive episode. Lack of social skills, faulty attributions, and lack of a support network may contribute to the maintenance of depression. Behaviors resulting from depression may also be reinforced by an excess of sympathy and reduction of demands made on the student.

Effective treatment involves a careful study of the learner. Of particular importance is the extent to which changes in biological, social, and cognitive factors may influence future reactions. In many cases, a number of factors may interact. Therefore, an integrated treatment approach is advocated.

References

Abramson, L., Metalsky, G., & Alloy, L. (1989). Hopelessness depression: A theory-based subtype of depression. *Psychological Review, 96*, 358–372.

Abramson, L., Seligman, M., & Teasdale, J. (1978). Learned helplessness in humans: Critique and reformulation. *Journal of Abnormal Psychology, 87*, 49–74.

Akiskal, H. S. (1989). New insights into the nature and heterogeneity of mood disorders. *Journal of Clinical Psychiatry, 50(5)(Supplement)*: 6–9.

Altmann, E. D., & Gotlib, I. H. (1988). The social behavior of depressed children: An observational study. *Journal of Abnormal Child Psychology, 16*, 29–44.

American Psychiatric Association (1987). *Diagnostic and statistical manual of mental disorders*, 3rd ed., revised. Washington DC: Author.

Asarnow, J., & Bates, S. (1988). Depression in child psychiatric inpatients: Cognitive and attribution patterns. *Journal of Abnormal Child Psychology, 16*, 601–615.

Baron, M. (1991). Genetics of manic depressive illness: Current status and evolving concepts. In P. R. McHugh & V. A. McKusick (Eds.), *Genes, brain and behavior*. New York: Raven Press.

Beck, A. T. (1972). *Depression: Causes and treatment*. University of Philadelphia Press.

Beck, A. T. (1976). *Cognitive therapy and the emotional disorders*. New York: International Universities Press.

Benfield, C., Palmer, D., Pfefferbaum, B., & Stowe, M. (1988). A comparison of depressed and nondepressed disturbed children on measures of attribution style, hopelessness, life stress and temperament. *Journal of Abnormal Child Psychology, 16*, 397–410.

Benson, B., Reiss, S., Smith, D., & Laman, D. S. (1985). Psychosocial correlates of depression in mentally retarded adults. II. Poor social skills. *American Journal of Mental Deficiency, 89(6)*, 657–659.

Blechman, E. A., McEnroe, M. J., Cardella, E. T., & Audette, D. P. (1986). Childhood competence and depression. *Journal of Abnormal Psychology, 95(3)*, 223–227.

Blehar, M. C., Weissman, M. M., Gershon, E. S., & Hirschfeld, R. M. (1988). Family and genetic studies of effective disorders. *Archives of General Psychiatry, 45*, 289–292.

Bodiford, C. A., Eisenstadt, T. H., Johnson, J. H., & Bradlyn, A. A. (1988). Comparison of learned helpless cognitions and behavior in children with high and low scores on the Children's Depression Inventory. *Journal of Clinical Child Psychology, 17(2)*, 152–158.

Breslau, N. (1990). Does brain dysfunction increase children's vulnerability to environmental stress? *Archives of General Psychiatry, 47(1)*, 15–20.

Brumback, R. A. (1985). Wechsler performance IQ deficits in depressed children. *Perceptual and Motor Skills, 61* 331–335.

Brumback, R. A., & Weinberg, N. A. (1977). Childhood depression: An explanation of a behavior disorder of children. *Perceptual and Motor Skills, 44*, 911–916.

Brumback, R. A., Jackoway, M. K., & Weinberg, W. A. (1980). Relation of intelligence to childhood depression in children in an educational diagnostic center. *Perceptual and Motor Skills, 50(1)*, 11–17.

Brumback, R. A., & Stanton, D. R. (1983). Learning disability and childhood depression. *American Journal of Orthopsychiatry, 53*, 264–281.

Butler, L. F., Miezitis, S., Friedman, R. J., & Cole, E. (1989). The effect of two school-based intervention programs on depressive symptoms in pre-adolescent children. *American Educational Research Journal, 17*, 111–119.

Cadoret, R. J. (1978). Evidence for genetic inheritance of primary affective disorder in adoptees. *American Journal of Psychiatry, 135*, 463–466.

Cantwell, D. P., & Baker, L. (1987). Prevalence and type of psychiatric disorder and developmental disorders in speech and language groups. *Journal of Communication Disorders, 20*, 151–160.

Carlson, G. A., & Cantwell, D. P. (1980). Unmasking masked depression in children and adolescents. *American Journal of Psychiatry, 137*, 445–499.

Colbert, P., Newman, B., Ney, P., & Young, J. (1982). Learning disabilities as a symptom of depression in children. *Journal of Learning Disabilities, 15(6)*, 333–336.

Cole, D. A., & Milstead, M. (1989). Behavioral correlates of depression: Antecedents or consequences? *Journal of Counseling Psychology, 36(4)*, 408–416.

Cole, D. A., & Rehm, L. P. (1986). Family interaction patterns and childhood depression. *Journal of Abnormal Child Psychology, 14(2)*, 297–314.

Coyne, J. C. (1976). Depression and the response of others. *Journal of Abnormal Psychology, 85*, 186–193.

Crandall, V. C., Crandall, V. J., & Katkovsky, W. (1965). A children's social desirability questionnaire. *Journal of Counseling Psychology, 29*, 27–36.

Cullinan, D., Schloss, P. J., & Epstein, M. H. (1987). Relative prevalence and correlates of defensive characteristics among seriously emotionally disturbed and nonhandicapped students. *Behavior Disorders, 12*, 90–98.

Drotar, D. (1978). Adaptational problem of children and adolescents with cystic fibrosis. *Journal of Pediatric Psychology, 3(1)*, 45–50.

Dweck, C. S. (1975). The role of expectations and attributions in the alleviation of learned helplessness. *Journal of Personality and Social Psychology, 31*, 674–685.

Gershon, E. S., & Nurnberger, J. I. (1982). Inheritance of major psychiatric disorders. *Trends in Neurosciences, 5*, 241–242.

Gowen, J. W., Johnson, M. N., & Goldman, B. D. (1989). Feelings of depression and parenting competence of mothers of handicapped and nonhandicapped mothers of infants: A longitudinal study. Special Issue: Research on families. *American Journal on Mental Retardation, 94(3)*, 259–271.

Hall, C. W., & Haws, D. (1989). Depressive symptomatology in learning-disabled and nonlearning-disabled students. *Psychology in the Schools, 26(4)*, 359–364.

Harper, D. C. (1983). Personality correlates and degree of impairment in male adolescents with progressive and nonprogressive physical disorders. *Journal of Clinical Psychology, 39(6)*, 859–867.

Helsel, W. J., & Matson, J. L. (1984). The assessment of depression in children: The internal structure of the Child Depression Inventory (CDI). *Behavior Research and Therapy, 22(3)*, 289–298.

Horne, M. D. (1985). *Attitudes toward handicapped students: Professional, peer, and parent reactions.* Hillsdale, NJ: Erlbaum Associates.

Johnson, D. W. (1981). Student–student interactions: The neglected variable in education. *Education Researcher, 10*, 5–10.

Jones, P. M., & Berney, T. P. (1987). Early onset rapid cycling bipolar affective disorder. *Journal of Child Psychology and Psychiatry and Allied Disciplines, 28(5)*, 731–738.

Lamen, D. S., & Reiss, S. (1987). Social skill deficiencies associated with depressed mood of mentally retarded adults. *American Journal of Mental Deficiency, 92(2)*, 224–229.

Lefkowitz, M. M., & Burton, N. (1978). Childhood depression: A critique of the concept. *Psychological Bulletin, 85*, 716–726.

Lewinsohn, P. M. (1974). A psychoeducational approach to the treatment of unipolar depression. *Psychotherapy in Private Practice, 1*, 5–8.

Maag, J. W., & Behrens, J. T. (1989). Epidemiologic data on seriously emotionally disturbed and learning disabled adolescents. Reporting extreme depressive symptomatology. *Behavioral Disorders, 15(1)*, 21–27.

McIvor, G. P., Riklan, M., & Reznikoff, M. (1984). Depression in multiple schlerosis as a function of length and severity of illness, age, remission, and perceived social support. *Journal of Clinical Psychology, 40(4)*, 1028–1033.

Meichenbaum, D., & Burland, S. (1979). Cognitive behavior modification with children. *School Psychology Digest, 8*, 426–433.

Mendlewicz, J., & Rainer, J. D. (1977). Adoption study supporting genetic transmission in manic–depressive illness. *Nature, 268*, 327–329.

Milavic, G. (1985). Do chronically ill and handicapped children become depressed? *Developmental Medicine and Child Neurology, 27(5)*, 677–682.

Osborn, R. G., & Meador, D. M. (1990). The memory performance of selected depressed and nondepressed nine to eleven-year-old-male children. *Behavioral Disorders, 16(1)*, 32–38.

Pearce, J. (1977). Depressive disorder in childhood. *Journal of Child Psychology and Psychiatry and Allied Disciplines, 18(1)*, 79–82.

Peterson, L., Wonderlich, S., Reaven, N., & Mullin, L. (1987). Adult educators' response to depression and stress in children. *Journal of Social and Clinical Psychology, 5*, 51–58.

Plienis, A. J., Hamsen, D. J., Ford, F., Smith, S., Stark, L. J., & Kelly, J. A. (1987). Behavioral small group training to improve the social skills of emotionally disordered adolescents. *Behavior Therapy, 18*, 17–32.

Pueschel, S. M. (1986). The impact on the family: Living with the handicapped child. *Issues in Law and Medicine, 2(3)*, 171–187.

Puig-Antich, J., Goetz, R., Davies, M., Fein, M., Hanlon, C., Chambers, W. J., Tabrizi, M. A., Sachar, E. J., & Weitzman, E. D. (1984). Growth hormone secretion in prepubertal children with major depression. II. Sleep-related plasma concentrations during depressive episode. *Archives of General Psychiatry, 41*, 463–466.

Puig-Antich, J., & Rabinovich, H. (1985). Biological factors in prepubertal major depression. *Psychiatric Annals, 15*, 390–397.

Rancurello, M. (1985). Clinical application of antidepressant drugs in childhood behavioral and emotional disorders. *Psychiatric Annals, 15*, 88–100.

Rehm, L. P. (1977). A self-control model of depression. *Behavior Therapy, 8*, 787–804.

Reynolds, W. M. (1984). Depression in children and adolescents: Phenomenology, evaluation, and treatment. *School Psychology Review, 13*, 171–182.

Reynolds, W. M., & Baker, J. A. (1988). Assessment of depression in persons with mental retardation. *American Journal of Mental Retardation, 93*, 93–103.

Reynolds, W. M., & Miller, K. L. (1985). Depression and learned helplessness in mentally retarded and nonretarded adolescents: An initial investigation. *Applied Research in Mental Retardation, 6*, 295–307.

Rie, H. E. (1966). Depression in childhood: A survey of some pertinent contributions. *Journal of the American Academy of Child Psychiatry, 5*, 653–685.

Robins, L. N. (1978). Sturdy childhood predictors of adult outcomes. Replications from longitudinal studies. *Psychological Medicine, 8*, 611–622.

Rourke, B. P. (1989). A childhood learning disability that predisposes those afflicted to adolescent and adult depression and suicide risk. *Journal of Learning Disabilities, 22(3)*, 169–174.

Rutter, M. (1966). *Children of sick parents: An environment and psychiatric study*. New York: Oxford University Press.

Sacco, W. P., & Graves, D. J. (1984). Childhood depression, interpersonal problem-solving, and self-ratings of performance. *Journal of Clinical Child Psychology, 13(1)*, 10–15.

Schloss, P. J. (1982). Verbal interactions patterns of depressed and nondepressed institutionalized mentally retarded adults. *Applied Research in Mental Retardation, 3*, 12–18.

Schloss, P. J., Epstein, M. H., & Cullinan, D. (1988). Depression characteristics among mildly handicapped students. *Journal of the Multihandicapped Person, 1(4)*, 293–302.

Schloss, P. J., & Schloss, C. N. (1987). A critical review of social skills research in mental retardation. In S. E. Breuning, J. L. Matson & R. P. Barrett (Eds.), *Advances in mental retardation and developmental disabilities: A research annual* (pp. 107–151). Greenwich, CT: JAI Press.

Schloss, P. J., Schloss, C. N., Wood, C. E., & Kiehl, W. S. (1986). A critical review of social skills research with behavior disordered students. *Behavioral Disorders, 11(1)*, 1–14.

Schloss, P. J., Schloss, C. N., & Harris, L. (1984). A multiple baseline analysis of an interpersonal skills training program for depressed youth. *Behavioral Disorders, 9(3)*, 182–188.

Seligman, M., & Peterson, C. (1986). A learned helplessness perspective on childhood depression: Theory and research. In M. Rutter, C. Izard, & P. Read (Eds.), *Depression in young people: Developmental and clinical perspective* (pp. 223–249). New York: Guilford Press.

Seligman, M. E., Peterson, C., Kaslow, N. J., Tanenbaum, R. L., Alloy, L. B., & Abramson, L. Y. (1984). Explanatory style and depressive symptoms among school children. *Journal of Abnormal Psychology, 93*, 235–238.

Shelton, R. C., Hollon, S. D., Purdon, S. E., & Loosen, P. T. (1991). Biological and psychological aspects of depression. *Behavior Therapy, 22*, 201–228.

Silver, A. A. (1984). Children in classes for the severely emotionally handicapped. *Developmental and Behavioral Pediatrics, 5(2)*, 49–54.

Silver, J. M., Hales, R. F., & Yudofsky, S. C. (1990). Psychopharmacology of depression in neurologic disorders. *Journal of Clinical Psychiatry, 51(Supplement)*, 33–39.

Simonds, J. F. (1975). Hallucinations in nonpsychotic children and adolescents. *Journal of Youth and Adolescence, 4(2)*, 171–182.

Spitz, R. A. (1946). Anaclitic depression: An inquiry into the genesis of psychiatric conditions in early childhood. *Psychoanalytic Study of the Child, 2*, 313–342.

Spivack, G., & Shure, M. (1974). *Social adjustment of young children: A cognitive approach to solving real-life problems.* San Francisco: Jossey-Bass.

Talbott, J. A., Hales, R. E., & Yudofsky, S. C. (Eds.), (1988). *The American Psychiatric Press textbook of psychiatry.* Washington, DC: American Psychiatric Press.

Tollefson, N., Melvin, J., & Thippavajjala, C. (1990). Teachers' attributions for students' low achievement: A validation of Cooper and Good's attributional categories. *Psychology in the Schools, 27*, 75–83.

Varni, J. W., Rubenfeld, L. A., Talbot, D., & Setoguchi, Y. (1989a). Stress, social support, and depressive symptomatology in children with congenital/acquired limb deficiencies. *Journal of Pediatric Psychology, 14(4)*, 515–530.

Varni, J. W., Rubenfeld, L. A., Talbot, D., & Setoguchi, Y. (1989b). Determinants of self-esteem in children with congenital/acquired limb deficiencies. *Journal of Developmental and Behavioral Pediatrics, 10(1)*, 13–16.

Waters, V. (1982). Other therapies for children: Rational–emotive therapy. In C. Reynolds & T. Gutkin (Eds.), *Handbook of school psychology* (pp. 510–519). New York: Wiley.

Weinberg, W. A., Rutman, J. R., Sullivan, L., Penick, E. C., & Dietz, S. G. (1973). Depression in children referred to an educational diagnostic center: Diagnosis and treatment. *Journal of Pediatrics, 83*, 1065–1072.

Weiner, B. (1985). An attributional theory of achievement motivation and emotion. *Psychological Review, 92*, 548–573.

Weiner, B., Frieze, I., Kukla, A., Reed, L., Rest, S., & Rosenbaum, R. M. (1971). *Perceiving the cause of success and failure.* New York: General Learning Press.

Werry, J. S. (1982). Pharmacotherapy. In B. B. Lahey & A. E. Kazdin (Eds), *Advances in clinical child psychology*, Vol. 5 (pp. 189–203). New York: Plenum Press.

Whybrow, P. C., Akiskal, H. S., & McKinney, W. T. (1984). *Mood disorders: Toward a new psychobiology.* New York: Plenum Press.

Wierzbicki, M., & McCabe, M. (1988). Social skills and subsequent depressive symptomatology in children. *Journal of Clinical Child Psychology, 17*, 203–208.

Winokur, G., & Coryell, W. (1991). Familial alcoholism in primary unipolar major depressive disorder. *American Journal of Psychiatry, 148*, 184–188.

Wolpe, J. (1971). Neurotic depression. *American Journal of Psychology, 25*, 362–368.

Zarantonello, M. W., Johnson, J. E., & Petzel, T. P. (1979). The effects of age, involvement and task difficulty on actual and perceived performance of depressed college students. *Journal of Clinical Psychology, 5*, 273–281.

VI

SELECTED TOPICS IN
THE STUDY OF DEPRESSION
IN YOUNG PEOPLE

21

Children of Parents with Affective Disorders

Empirical Findings and Clinical Implications

William R. Beardslee and Ingrid Wheelock

For decades, it has been well-established by empirical studies that severe mental illness in parents is associated with an increased rate of psychiatric disorder in their offspring (Buck and Laughton, 1959; Ekdahl, Rice, & Schmidt, 1962; Rutter, 1966; Landau, Hauth, & Othnay, 1972). Recently, a series of rigorous empirical studies have been conducted with the children of parents with serious affective disorder. These studies are a result of both the recognition of the entity of childhood depression and the awareness that children of parents with affective disorders are themselves at particularly heightened risk for depression. Even though the studies employ different conceptual frameworks and methods, there is a clear consensus in the empirical research literature that children of parents with affective disorders fare much more poorly than comparison samples. A variety of reviews have appeared over the last decade or so documenting these findings (Beardslee, Bemporad, Keller, & Klerman, 1983; Waters, 1987; Zuckerman & Beardslee, 1987; Orvaschel, Walsh-Allis, & Ye, 1988; Lee & Gotlib, 1989), and, most recently and extensively, there have been reviews by Downey and Coyne (1990), Rutter (1990), and Keitner and Miller (1990). While studies up until the middle of the last decade used very different approaches and measures and hence are difficult to compare (Beardslee et al., 1983), recent studies have concentrated on the use of structured diagnostic interviews of the parents scored according to standard criteria and standardized systematic assessments of the children's functioning (Downey and Coyne, 1990).

The purpose of this chapter is to review the substantive findings in the major domains relevant to children of parents with affective disorders. Only studies that have employed rigorous empirical designs and clear theoretical conceptualizations are described. This review has not concentrated on methodological issues in the study of such children,

William R. Beardslee and Ingrid Wheelock • Judge Baker Children's Center, Department of Psychiatry, Harvard University Medical School, Boston, Massachusetts 02115.

Handbook of Depression in Children and Adolescents, edited by William M. Reynolds and Hugh F. Johnston. Plenum Press, New York, 1994.

although they are important. Methodological issues are more fully discussed elsewhere (Beardslee et al., 1983; Lee & Gotlieb, 1989; Downey & Coyne, 1990; Keitner & Miller, 1990; Rutter, 1990; Keitner & Miller, 1990). Clearly, much more research is needed, particularly long-term follow-up studies. Many investigators have included both unipolar and bipolar parental affective disorder when studying offspring. Both categories of parental affective disorder are included in this review. In reporting diagnostic assessments of children, the focus has been mostly on lifetime rates of disorder.

A large number of studies using cross-sectional and retrospective designs have reported considerably higher rates of diagnosable psychopathology in the children of parents with affective disorders than in the children of comparison samples (Welner, Welner, McCrary, & Leonard, 1977; McKnew, Cytryn, Efron, Gershon, & Bunney, 1979; Decina et al., 1983; Weissman et al., 1984, 1987a; Weissman, Leaf, & Bruce, 1987b; Beardslee, Keller, & Klerman, 1985; Beardslee et al., 1988; Gershon et al., 1985; Klein, Clark, Dansky, & Margolis, 1988; Orvaschel et al., 1988; Welner & Rice, 1988). These studies also indicate that children of parents with affective disorders are specifically at risk for developing affective illness; in particular, there are higher rates of childhood depression than in comparison samples. In terms of rates of disorder, McKnew et al. (1979) reported that 14 of 30 children whose parents had serious affective disorder met criteria for depression in at least one interview. In a study of manic–depressive parents, Decina et al. (1983) reported on 31 children of bipolar parents ages 7–14 and 18 children of normal parents. Approximately half the children of bipolar parents received DSM-III or RDC diagnoses, while only 6% of the control children did. Orvaschel et al. (1988) found that 41% of children of depressed parents met criteria for at least one psychiatric disorder compared to 15.2% of children in a control group, and 21.3% of the children of depressed parents had affective illness compared to 4.3% of the children of controls. In 1984, Weissman et al. (1984) studied 194 children of parents with major depression, parents with minor depression, and nondepressed parents, and found that 3 times as many children of depressed parents as children of nondepressed parents received diagnoses (24.2% vs. 8.1%). A later study, including both parent and child reports (Weissman et al., 1987a), showed significantly higher lifetime incidence rates for major depression, although high rates for controls were also found. Klein et al. (1988) reported a DSM-III diagnosis rate of 32% for children of depressed parents compared to 0% for children of nondepressed parents in children of ages 14–22. Beardslee and colleagues (Beardslee et al., 1985, 1988; Beardslee, Schultz, & Selman, 1987; Keller et al., 1986; Schwartz, Dorer, Beardslee, Lavori, & Keller, 1990) have indicated substantially higher rates of diagnoses in various subgroups of a large sample (275 individuals in 143 families) and in the large sample as a whole. In their review, Downey and Coyne (1990) note that children of unipolar depressed parents were at particularly high risk for major depressive disorder, as their rate was several times that of control children across a wide range of studies. Determination of the precise rate of disorder in children at risk due to parental affective disorder must await large-scale epidemiological studies.

Furthermore, examination of 9 cases of depression (Beardslee et al., 1985) in children of parents with affective disorder in a risk study has demonstrated that many of the disorders identified through risk studies are serious and impairing and similar to those identified in clinical practice. Studies of the course and outcome of depressions in children identified through risk samples indicate that the course and outcome are similar to those in clinical samples (Keller et al., 1988).

Of particular interest is the lack of attention to treatment for children with serious affective disorder when it has been identified (Beardslee et al., 1985; Keller, Lavori, Beardslee, & Wunder, 1991). In a large study, fewer than one third of the children received any treatment for their depression (Keller et al., 1991). This finding parallels findings of the underrecognition and undertreatment of disorder in epidemiological studies (Offord et al., 1987) and in pediatric practices (Costello et al., 1988).

Almost all studies have employed parent subjects who present for clinical treatment. Beardslee et al. (1988) assessed parents without reference to whether they had sought treatment or not, but rather selected through random sampling from subjects enrolled in a prepaid health plan. This study was undertaken in part to see whether the effects of parental disorder on child outcome held true for affective disorders that have not been referred or treated. The parents and children were assessed with a standard battery used in risk research. A random sample from a prepaid health plan was obtained, and 80% of those eligible consented to be assessed. In 153 children, ages 6–9, in 81 families, psychopathology (lifetime) was found in 64% of the children of parents with a history of affective disorder, in 53% of children whose parents had nonaffective disorder, and in only 35% of parents with no history of psychiatric disorder. With an average sample age of 14.5, the rate of affective disorder in the children of parents with affective disorder was 30% compared with 2% in children of parents with no affective disorder. The children whose parents had affective disorder were more impaired in adaptive functioning and also had a higher rate of most other diagnoses (Beardslee et al., 1988). Follow-up of this sample 4 years later indicated even more impairment (Beardslee, Keller, Lavori, Stanley, & Sacks, 1993a). Of those originally assessed, 91% were followed up; there was an even higher number of families with parental affective disorder because a number of parents had developed affective disorder in the interval between first and second assessment. At follow-up, overall, children of parents with affective disorders were more impaired than children whose parents had experienced no disorders. Children of parents with nonaffective disorders were in between the two groups. This follow-up study also heightened awareness of the need to look within the category of parents who had experienced affective disorders. Parents who had experienced major depressive disorder had youngsters who had more episodes of major depressive disorder than did parents who had experienced affective disorders that were not as serious as major depressive disorder or parents who had no disorder.

The few existing prospective studies support the high rates of risk found in cross-sectional and retrospective designs (Hammen, Burge, Burney, & Adrian, 1990). Hammen et al. (1990) examined children, ages 8–16, of unipolar mothers, bipolar mothers, medically ill mothers, and normal controls with measurements every 6 months for 3 years. Using life table estimates, they show that the cumulative estimated probability of an episode of a major psychiatric diagnosis for the children of unipolar depressed mothers in their sample is 80% by late adolescence and between 70% and 80% for the children of bipolar mothers.

Overall Functional Impairment

Pioneering work by Weissman and colleagues introduced the concept that children of depressed parents experienced different kinds of conflicts and functional impairments at different developmental epochs (Weissman, Paykel, & Klerman, 1972). In addition to studies that focus on diagnosable disorder in offspring of affectively ill parents, studies examining general difficulties in functioning have been conducted (Beardslee et al., 1987; Forehand & McCombs, 1988). While data across the life span of children indicate difficulties at each developmental stage, early childhood (0–5 years) and early to mid-adolescence appear to be times of particularly heightened risk to children.

Infancy

During infancy, children of depressed parents appear to have more cognitive, emotional, and interpersonal problems than children of nondepressed parents (Field et al., 1985; Sameroff, Seifer, Zax, & Barocas, 1987; Whiffen & Gotlib, 1989), as well as more disturbed affiliative and attachment behavior (Gaensbauer, Harmon, Cytryn, & McKnew, 1984). Other studies indicate that the preschool years are also a time of considerable difficulty for children of parents with affective disorders, including both emotional and cognitive developmental problems (Richman, Stevenson, & Graham, 1982), delayed expressive language development, and higher rates of problem behaviors (Zahn-Waxler, McKnew, Cummings, Davenport, & Radke-Yarrow, 1984; Cox, Puckering, Pound, & Mills, 1987). A higher rate of accidents and medical complaints has also been reported (Brown & Davidson, 1978). In pediatric practice, children presenting with stomachaches are more likely to have mothers who are depressed (Zuckerman, Stevenson, & Bailey, 1987). A number of studies (Gaensbauer et al., 1984; Zahn-Waxler et al., 1984, 1988; Sameroff et al., 1987) have conducted extensive follow-ups that indicate that these difficulties persist into the preschool years.

School-Age Functioning

Researchers have emphasized that school-age children of depressed parents have greater cognitive and emotional vulnerability than children of well mothers. Adolescence is a time of particularly heightened risk. Studies that have examined diagnoses and adaptive functioning have reported difficulties in both areas in school-age children. In addition, Jaenicke et al. (1987) report that children (ages 8–16) of depressed and manic–depressed women express more negative views about themselves and display a more negative attributional style than do children of well mothers. Zahn-Waxler, Kochanska, Krupnick, and McKnew (1990) found that when presented with hypothetical scenarios of interpersonal conflict and distress, young children of depressed mothers displayed patterns of overarousal in addition to high levels of responsibility and involvement. The narratives of these children often contained extreme contents or distortions that appeared to reflect guilt feelings or defenses against guilt feelings. The authors suggest that such guilt may place them at increased risk for depression.

A sample of adolescent children of depressed parents studied by Hirsch, Moos, and Reischl (1985) had lower self-esteem and more symptomatology than did children of normal or arthritic parents. Forehand and McCombs (1988) found similar deficits in adolescent functioning. They report a relationship between maternal depression and difficulties in four areas of adolescent functioning: internalizing problems, externalizing problems, prosocial behavior, and cognitive functioning. Beardslee et al. (1987) have reported that a large group of adolescents whose parents have experienced affective disorders show impairments in overall adaptive functioning in addition to diagnosable difficulties. Some show limitations in their ability to conceptualize interpersonal relationships. The same study showed that there were significant effects for IQ, age, sex, and severity of parental illness in addition to parental diagnostic category, emphasizing the need for understanding the complex interplay of variables in the children of parents with affective disorder.

Weissman et al. (1986) have documented a wide array of serious medical conditions that are more likely to occur in the children of parents with depression, including more head injuries, birth complications, and higher rates of hospitalization and utilization of medical services compared to children of non-ill parents.

A longitudinal study by Billings and Moos (1983, 1985) assessed the health and adjustment of children (ages 18 and under) of depressed parents at two points in time, 1 year apart. Impairment in the children continued to be significant at follow-up. These researchers report that while the family environments of remitted parents improved, the children of remitted parents continued to function more poorly than children of controls, displaying more psychological symptoms and behavioral problems. In a follow-up study of children of manic–depressive parents assessed early in life, Zahn-Waxler et al. (1988)

found that the children of bipolar parents who had experienced adjustment problems as infants and toddlers continued to show evidence of substantial behavioral problems when assessed 4 years later. In a longitudinal study of maternal depression and adolescent functioning, Forehand and McCombs (1988) found that maternal depression at initial assessment served as an antecedent for poor adolescent functioning measured 1 year later. Hammen (1988) found that poor self-image and lowered self-esteem in children whose parents have experienced depression or other serious psychopathology predicted subsequent poorer functioning and poorer outcome.

In summary, the children of parents with affective disorders have much higher rates of diagnosis, in particular of affective disorders, than do children of parents without affective disorders. They are also at risk for a variety of other impairments, including problems with self-esteem, guilt, poorer overall functioning, and behavioral difficulties. The cumulative rate of lifetime diagnosis is high. It is important to note that most assessments are lifetime-based in retrospective recall and that the number of children acutely ill at the time of assessment is much smaller than the overall rate of diagnosis.

Resiliency and Understanding in the Children of Parents with Affective Disorder—One Model for the Design of Preventive Intervention

Not only are many children not ill at any one time, but also a significant number manifest resiliency in the face of the stress of having a parent with an affective illness. These children provide examples of how children do survive such stress. It is as important to understand that non-ill, resilient children exist in samples of high-risk children, and to be able to characterize and understand their resiliency, as it is to recognize impairment (Richmond & Beardslee, 1988). Interest in the resiliency in children of parents with affective disorders comes from an awareness of the importance of protective factors that have been identified in a large number of studies of high-risk children (Rutter, 1986; Garmezy, 1987). Rutter (1987) has emphasized a range of factors, including good physical and high intellectual ability, an easygoing temperament in early life, the presence of positive relationships, particularly with parents, and opportunities for involvement outside the home. Inner psychological qualities such as a sense of control over one's surroundings and high self-esteem are also important. Unfortunately, few studies have examined resiliency in children of parents with affective disorders.

In terms of psychological characteristics, factors studied include individuals' modes of thought, action, and response, self-esteem, and coping styles. Pellegrini et al. (1986) have emphasized the importance of social problem-solving ability, sense of control, high self-esteem, and the presence of social networks. Having a best friend particularly protected against episodes of depression. In a cautionary essay, Radke-Yarrow and Sherman (1994) have described children who survive difficult family environments. They indicate that these children were able to engage with others, were intelligent, and to some extent matched parental expectations; these children functioned better than children in the high-risk situation who did not have these attributes. They point out that these children may develop disorders later.

Within the domain of inner psychological attributes falls self-understanding. In a series of studies, Beardslee and colleagues have demonstrated a strong association between resiliency and self-understanding in civil rights workers, survivors of cancer, and children of parents with affective disorders (Beardslee, 1981, 1983, 1989; Beardslee & Podorefsky, 1988). The study by Beardslee & Podorefsky (1988) of the role of self-understanding in resilient children was undertaken in an effort to learn about what children understood and remembered from experiences with affectively ill parents. In this study, 18 children were selected because of their good functioning from a group of over 120 children at risk, all of whose parents had experienced serious affective disorder. Of these 18 youngsters (average age 18), 15 were functioning well at interview. These 15 youngsters had close, confiding relationships with a wide variety of individuals. They performed well in work and school and participated in a variety of activities. They were activists and doers, not overwhelmed by the helplessness of their parents' situations. They credited their relationships as being very helpful in dealing with the parents' disorder, and they also reported that understanding of the parents' illness system was an essential component of their resiliency. Their understanding was extensive—they were well aware that their parents were not functioning normally. They were aware of the vicissitudes and impairments of their parents' disorder. They tended to focus on the changes in their lives— e.g., moves, divorces, difficult economic circumstances that the illnesses had caused— rather than on the details of their parents' diagnoses. They were saddened by the parents' illnesses, but not overwhelmed. Their caretaking of their parents was extensive and often extended into other relationships, i.e., helping out friends. In fact, remarkable, two thirds were engaged in either the helping professions or in caretaking. Fundamentally, they were clear that they had not caused their parents' disorder and were not to blame for it. They believed that this understanding was crucial in coping with the parental illness. More generally, they saw themselves as separate both from the parents' illness system and from their parents. They also saw themselves as able to take independent action. Self-understanding, separateness, and the ability to take action are psychological qualities associated with resiliency in the adolescent children of parents with affective disorder. Exploration of the concept of self-understanding has suggested three elements that are fundamental to understanding: adequate appraisal of the stress to be dealt with, realistic appraisal of the capacity to act and of the consequences of the action, and action congruent with the understanding (Beardslee, 1989).

As noted above and to be reemphasized, it is as essential to be able to understand and recognize risk and resiliency in these youngsters as it is to recognize pathology. In fact, all too often, resilient capacities are obscured, and children at risk are equated with children who are ill. The recognition of resilient qualities may serve as one model for the development of preventive-intervention programs.

Mechanisms of Transmission

The strong association between parental affective disorder and depression in off-spring, at least in adolescence, suggests an influence at least in part specific to affective disorder. Most studies have found that the exposure of the child to both genetic and psychosocial influences within the family makes it impossible to definitively separate the influence of these two predictors or to determine their relative weight in the causation of disorder in childhood.

The classic epidemiological studies of Rutter (1990) have established parental risk factors across broad domains. These risk factors include maternal psychiatric disorder (including depression), paternal criminality, large family size, overcrowding, marital discord, and placement of a child in foster care. These risk factors have been shown to potentiate one another; i.e., they are not simply additive. The presence of a single risk factor does not necessarily lead to poor outcome, but the existence of several heightens the likelihood of poor outcome to a greater degree than simply a sum of the risk factors would suggest. Sameroff and colleagues (Sameroff & Chandler, 1975; Sameroff, Seifer, & Zax, 1982), in a pioneering study of mentally ill mothers followed from pregnancy for 4 years, have shown that severity and chronicity of parental illness in combination with social disadvantage, rather than type of diagnosis, led to the poorest outcome in the children. In fact, children of depressed parents fared somewhat more poorly than children of schizophrenic parents. In a recent essay, Sameroff et al. (1987) emphasized again that risk factors potentiate one another and that multiple risk factors are far worse for children than only one or two.

Nature of Affective Disorder in Adults

Given that the child's experience is so heavily influenced by the presence of parental affective disorder, a review of the relevant characteristics of affective disorders in adults is in order. Affective disorders afflict women at higher rates than men. There are greater rates of affective disorder in the community, assessed by epidemiological studies, than present for treatment. This finding suggests that a large number of people with affective disorder are untreated. While estimates of the rate of affective disorder vary depending on the methodologies and sampling frames used, it is clear that a substantial number of individuals will experience affective disorder. Data from the NIMH Epidemiologic Catchment Area (ECA) Study using lay interviewers suggest an overall lifetime disorder rate of approximately 10% (Robins & Regier, 1991). Data collected from community samples with the Schedule for Affective Disorders and Schizophrenia—Lifetime Version (SADS-L) (Endicott & Spitzer, 1978) using highly trained raters, suggest substantially higher rates, 8–12% for men and 20–26% for women (Beardslee, 1990). Weissman et al. (1987b) have estimated that approximately 8% of mothers are clinically depressed. Others have estimated that this rate increases to 12% in mothers who have recently given birth (O'Hara, 1986; Weissman et al., 1987b; Downey & Coyne, 1990).

Both genetic and life-stress factors are important in the etiology of affective disorders. Genetic evidence gathered from studies of monozygotic twins reared apart shows high concordance rates. This finding indicates a strong genetic influence in some affective disorders (Nurnberger & Gershon, 1982). These rates are generally higher for bipolar disorder than for unipolar disorder. Family history studies have demonstrated that relatives of adults with affective disorders are themselves at higher risk for affective disorders (Gershon et al., 1982). This higher risk also holds true for childhood affective disorder (Strober et al., 1988). It is clear from adopted-away studies of monozygotic twins that there is a significant genetic component for both manic–depressive and depressive disorder. There is a higher rate of concordance for manic–depressive than for depressive disorder (Allen, 1976). In adopted-away offspring studies, there is strong evidence that family environment plays a substantial role in the expression of affective disorders (Von Knorring, Cloninger, Bohman, & Siguardsson, 1983; Cadoret, O'Gorman, Heywood, & Troughton, 1985). At present, there is no way to know whether a child who develops affective disorder does so from genetic or psychosocial effect because so many children who develop depression are exposed to both significant psychosocial stressors and genetic influence from depressed parents (Beardslee, 1990; Downey & Coyne, 1990). There is great promise for more definitive genetic evidence through future linkage and marker studies, but at present, definitive evidence about the relative weight of etiological factors does not exist.

Affective disorders are strongly associated with loss, and indeed the criteria for bereavement reaction are the same as those for depression in DSM-III-R. Job loss, extended bereavement reactions, and marital breakup are all strongly associated with depression (Kessler, Turner, & House, 1987). Brown, Bifulco, Harris, and Bridge (1986) have demonstrated one useful model for understanding the onset of depression in adult woman, a risk–vulnerability model. The loss of a parent in childhood increases the likelihood that depression will be expressed in the face of stressors in adulthood (Brown et al., 1986). There is an extensive literature to suggest that social networks are protective against the emergence of disorder (Eisenberg, 1979). The absence of such networks or their loss, particularly of a close, confiding relationship, may precipitate a depression, exacerbate the course of affective disorder, and limit recovery.

There are biological changes in individuals with depression that are present whether the etiology appears to be primarily genetic, primarily environmental, or a combination of the two influences. There is frequently comorbidity with other psychiatric disorders, particularly alcoholism, the anxiety disorders, and substance abuse. Of particular interest is a recent report form the ECA study, which emphasizes that it is essential to treat underlying psychiatric disorder, such as affective illness, when treating substance abuse. If such underlying disorders are not addressed, treatment for substance abuse is likely to be unsuccessful (Regier et al., 1990).

Affective disorders, whether unipolar or bipolar, are most often chronic, with periods of good functioning interspersed with periods of poor functioning (Keller et al., 1986; Strober et al., 1988). Unfortunately, it appears that the treatment received by affectively ill parents is often less than optimal (Keller et al., 1982). There is reason to believe that early treatment is essential (Kupfer, Frank, & Perel, 1989). Furthermore, there is now evidence that high-quality maintenance therapy substantially increases the likelihood of good outcome for depression (Frank et al., 1990). The need for continued ongoing treatment of adult disorder must be recognized and be part of any intervention for children of parents with affective disorders.

Course of Disorder and Dual Parent Disorder

Factors such as chronicity of illness have a large impact on child functioning and, indeed, have been shown to differentiate children who will do more poorly from those who will do well within samples of affectively ill parents and their children. Keller et al. (1986) examined factors predictive of poorer outcome within a group of parents all of whom had experienced unipolar depression. Greater chronicity and severity of illness were highly associated with poorest child outcome. In particular, duration of episodes of depression in either parent, including dysthymia, number of episodes of major depression, number of times treated for major depression, number of times hospitalized, and suicide attempts, all correlated strongly with poorest outcome and poorest adaptive functioning. This corresponds with the finds of Sameroff et al. (1987), Rutter (1966), and others about the importance of describing parental disorders fully, particularly chronicity of disorder.

Weissman, Warner, Wickramaratne, and Prusoff (1988) have emphasized that an early age of onset (under 20) of major depression in parents increases their children's risk of major depression and increases the likelihood that their children will also experience an early-onset major depression. In their study, they found that children whose parents had an onset of depression before age 20 experienced a 14-fold increased risk of depression before the age of 13.

Given the high rate of comorbidity in adults with affective disorder, it is important to note that children whose parents had not only affective disorder but also another disorder are more at risk and experience more disorder than those whose parents had only a single disorder (Weissman et al., 1987a).

Further, a number of studies have reported that there is a higher than expected concordance rate for affective disorders and psychopathology in the spouse when one parent has an affective illness (Merikangas, Prusoff, & Weissman, 1988). In one study, 69% of the depressed individuals studied had spouses who met criteria for major depression, anxiety disorder, or alcoholism, while 37% of controls had spouses with such diagnoses. Coyne et al. (1987) have found that in examining depressed individuals, nearly 40% of spouses manifest signs of depression. Having two parents with psychiatric disorder leads to poorer outcome in children than having only one parent with a psychiatric disorder (Weissman et al., 1984; Beardslee et al., 1985). In a series of studies, Merikangas and associates have shown that the presence of the same diagnosis in both parents leads to a much greater likelihood that that disorder will occur in the children. This was found true for conduct disorder, alcoholism, and affective illness (Merikangas, Weissman, & Prusoff, 1990).

This review of parental diagnoses reflects the heterogeneity found in families identified because at least one parent had experienced affective disorder. When a family is selected because one parent has a clear-cut affective disorder, there are likely to be other disorders that will have an impact on the child and on family functioning. From the point of view of intervention, whether clinical or preventive, the diagnostic heterogeneity must be recognized. It implies that once an individual is identified with affective illness, there is a likelihood of comorbid disorders, of marital disharmony, and possibly of disorder in the spouse as well. If several disorders are present in one individual, careful assessment and treatment of each disorder are needed.

Parenting and Martial Discord

Poor parenting practices and marital discord and breakup are consistently described as central factors in poor child outcome (Downey & Coyne, 1990; Keitner & Miller, 1990; Rutter, 1990). Both Downey and Coyne (1990) and Rutter (1990) conclude that there is evidence that both are frequently present in children of parents with affective disorders. Because they are so often associated, it is impossible to separate the effects of parental psychiatric disorder, marital discord, and poor parenting. Sometimes one alone may be present and cause disorder. In families with affective disorder, all three are present so often that it has not been possible to disentangle the effects. All three often contribute to the transmission of disorder from parent to child.

There is considerable evidence that poor parenting practices contribute to difficulties in children (Powers, Hauser, & Kilner, 1989). In particular, depressed mothers tend to show more sustained negative affect with their babies than do nondepressed mothers (Field et al., 1985; Cohn, Campbell, Matias, & Hopkins, 1990; Field, Healy, Goldstein, & Gutherz, 1990). Depressed mothers also tend to be less responsive (Bettes, 1988) and less likely to resolve conflicts with their young children in a constructive, compromising manner (Kochanska, Kuczynski, Radke-Yarrow, & Welsh, 1987). Depressed mothers may be less effective than nondepressed mothers at disciplining and setting limits with their children. The depressed mothers studied by Kochanska and associates tended to use less effortful means to control their children and were more likely than nondepressed women to avoid confronting their children when met with resistance.

Depressed mothers of preschool children have exhibited similar parenting behaviors. Depressed women are reported to be less responsive with their young children than nondepressed women (Cox et al., 1987; Goodman & Brumley, 1990). Low response may manifest itself both behaviorally and emotionally. Depressed mothers speak less to their young children than nondepressed mothers (Cox et al., 1987) and use less structure and discipline in their parenting strategies (Goodman & Brumley, 1990). Radke-Yarrow, Cummings, Kuczynski, and Chapman (1985) report that children of parents with affective illness, particularly those whose parents have bipolar depression, are more likely to have insecure attachments to their mothers than children of well mothers and that this poor attachment may be a result of the depressed mother's inability to relate positively to her child.

Breznitz and Sherman (1987) compared interactions between depressed and non-depressed mothers and their 2½- to 3½-year-old children. The authors report that depressed women generally vocalized less with their children than nondepressed women, although they spoke more as the emotionality of the situation increased. Breznitz and Sherman hypothesize that the lack of welcome and reinforcement that mothers exhibit in response to their children's overtures may encourage their children to limit or avoid social interactions. Furthermore, the heightened emotionality of mothers in the face of stressful events may teach children to overreact to even mildly stressful events.

A study by Gordon et al. (1989) that focused on mothers of children aged 8–16 suggests that maladaptive interpersonal patterns also exist between mothers and older children. These authors found that currently depressed women were more critical and negative toward their children and that they spoke less in the presence of their children than did nondepressed mothers.

The finding that depressed mothers often use higher levels of criticism and negative verbal behavior with their children (Gordon et al., 1989; Cohn et al., 1990) indicates that depressed mothers may not be able to face the stresses of parenting as adaptively as well mothers. Zuravin (1989) has suggested that depressed mothers may be more likely than nondepressed mothers to use physical aggression with their children. In a study of single-parent mothers, Zuravin reports that moderate depression is related to an increase in maternal physical aggression. Furthermore, while severely depressed women are less likely to use increased levels of physical aggression (possibly due to anergy or emotional withdrawal), they, like moderately depressed women, are at increased risk for exhibiting greater levels of verbal or symbolic aggression. Zuravin hypothesizes that depression may lower a mother's tolerance of aversive behavior and act as a "disinhibitor." Parenting is significantly impaired through the mechanism of decreased attention, and less intensity of interaction, as well as through the inability to focus on the child (Beardslee, 1990; Downey & Coyne, 1990).

Chronic family discord is associated with child psychiatric disorders (Emery, 1982; Rutter, 1990). There is also evidence of frequent discord and disharmony in couples with a depressed partner (Rounsaville, Prusoff, & Weissman, 1980) and a higher rate of divorce (Merikangas, 1984). As mentioned above, marital dysfunction and divorce are associated with poorer child outcome in children of depressed parents (Keller et al., 1986).

In addition to the evidence presented about marital discord, it is important to note that marriages in which there is an appreciable degree of martial satisfaction and adjustment are also affected by depression (Coleman & Miller, 1975; Waring & Patton, 1984; Crowther, 1985; Merikangas, Prusoff, Kupfer, & Frank, 1985; Bouras, Vanger, & Bridges, 1986). Communication in families with affective disorder is also profoundly affected (Hinchliffe, Hooper, Roberts, & Vaughan, 1975; Ruscher & Gotlib, 1988). Bouras et al. (1986) examined the martial problems of three groups of couples: 12 with a depressed spouse, 12 with a spouse suffering from rheumatoid arthritis, and 12 with a spouse who was a cardiac patient. The depressed couples reported the highest level of marital disturbance. Of the three groups, depressed individuals and their spouses reported the highest level of dissatisfaction in three areas of their marital life: marital relationship, sexual relationship, and work and social activities. Other studies have found similar relationships between depression and marital maladjustment (Coleman & Miller, 1975; Waring & Patton, 1984; Crowther, 1985). For example, Targum, Dibble, Davenport, and Gersuon (1981), Coyne et al. (1987), and Fadden, Bebbington, and Kuipers (1987) have examined the difficulties faced by partners of depressed patients. Targum et al. (1981) described a number of difficulties in bipolar patients and their spouses. Well spouses of patients appeared to be quite distressed about their partners' illness. They expressed concern about the effects on the children.

Coyne et al. (1987) compared the experiences of 42 adults living with a currently depressed patient to 23 living with someone who had been an inpatient or outpatient but who was not currently in a depressive episode. Coyne and colleagues found that spouses of currently depressed patients felt burdened in various ways, especially by their partners' depressive symptoms, such as fatigue, hopelessness, rumination, and lack of interest in social activities. Of the relatives of patients in a current depressive episode, 40% needed psychological intervention. Coyne's analyses indicate that the differences in burden accounted almost entirely for this increased psychological distress.

Fadden et al. (1987) reported difficulties with finances, work situations, and social life. Many individuals reported a sense of having lost the husband or wife, and grief, sorrow and guilt were common. The authors also reported that many people interviewed were ignorant about their spouse's depression, and one third had no idea what caused the spouse's difficulties. A follow-up study by Krantz and Moos (1987) compared remitted, partially remitted, and nonremitted patients and their spouses. The study found that spouses of nonremitted patients had more problems than either of the other two groups, though the remitted patients still experienced difficulty. Fadden et al. (1987) suggest that practitioners should involve relatives of depressed patients in treatment plans. Fortunately, a number of therapeutic approaches are being developed that specifically target the spouses of depressed patients (Coyne, 1988; Coffman & Jacobson, 1990).

In a variety of cross-sectional and longitudinal studies of psychiatrically ill patients, Keitner and colleagues have demonstrated that family functioning is disturbed (Keitner & Miller, 1990). Significant dysfunction, with particular difficulties in the areas of communication, role allocation, affective development, and problem-solving, is evident. There is also a general lack of focus on the child in such families (Beardslee, 1990). Using the index of expressed emotion of Vaughn and Leff (1976), Hooley, Orley, and Teasdale (1986) found a strong association between levels of spouse criticism and relapse of depressed parents. Miklowitz, Goldstein, Nuechterlein, Snyder, and Mintz (1988) reported similar results in a study of key relatives of 23 hospitalized bipolar patients. Schwartz et al. (1990) demonstrated that hostility and criticism by the mother toward the child had an effect beyond the negative effect of the parental depression on child outcome.

In summary, empirical literature reveals that children whose parents experience serious affective disorders are at high risk for the development of psychopathology, especially depression, as well as impairment in overall functioning. Studies of the transmission of the disorder from parent to child are not definitive as to the relative weight of genetic and psychosocial influences. The studies reviewed above indicate the importance of both. Of particular importance, apart from genetics, are chronicity and severity of diagnosis, poor parenting practices, a lack of focus on the child, and marital discord.

Affective illness in parents should always be viewed in three fundamental, overlapping contexts: (1) Affective disorder is a *biological* disorder. (2) Affective disorder inherently involves a profound impairment in interpersonal functioning and hence is an *interpersonal* illness. (3) Affective disorder in an individual is a disorder in which the family is deeply involved; in this sense, it is a *family* disorder. These three overlapping domains of influence combine to lead to poor outcome in children.

Thus, parental affective disorder should be viewed as a factor that greatly heightens the *likelihood* of poor outcome in children. It should not be viewed as the definitive primary causal mechanism of poor outcome, because many other factors are associated with it. In this sense, the models of combining risk factors developed by Rutter (1986) and Sameroff et al. (1987) are relevant. Families in which parents have experienced affective disorders associated with a number of other risk factors—i.e., affective disorders combined with other diagnoses, particularly severe and chronic affective diagnoses; presence of divorce and separation, and difficult economic circumstances—are the families most likely to develop illness. Thus, the associated risk factors beyond the presence of affective disorder need to be fully assessed and included in understanding the connecting between parental affective disorder and poor child outcome and in working with these families clinically. These factors should be of grave concern for clinicians who treat adults with affective disorders.

Largely absent from the literature on children of parents with affective disorder is any focus on the prevention of disorder in these youngsters. The evidence is sufficient to say that these youngsters are at high risk. The major domains of influence for this risk have been identified, i.e., genetic pathways, interferences with parenting, marital discord, and divorce. A number of experts have called for nationally heightened attention to prevention and have indicated that depression is an area in which prevention efforts can be directed.

One approach is to focus on the family as a unit and the enhancement of resiliency. On the basis of these empirical findings, a preventive intervention for families with serious affective disorders has recently been developed in an attempt to incorporate findings about risk and resiliency in a family-based format that could be widely used by practitioners. Core elements of the intervention include assessment of all family members, cognitive teaching about risks, resiliency, and depression, the link of this experience to the life experience of the family, and the provision of concrete plans for the future of the child. The format consists of individual sessions with the parents, an individual session with each child in the family, and finally family meetings to work through and explain the experience of parental illness in company with the children. This approach, based on the empirical findings of risk and resiliency, offers considerable promise. A recent study demonstrated the safety and feasibility of the approach and also that families were quite pleased with the intervention (Beardslee et al., 1992). Essential components of this intervention include a recognition of the heterogeneity or differences among families with affective illness and an attempt to focus and tailor the intervention to the child's individual experiences. It also requires that the clinician be willing to engage in primary, secondary, and tertiary prevention within the same family if needed. This approach is necessary because, in families with serious affective illness, there may be high rates of untreated disorder that will need attention (tertiary prevention); there may be individuals who are manifesting signs but are not yet ill (secondary prevention); and there may be individuals who are not ill at the time of assessment but who may become ill (primary prevention). Finally, the design of this intervention was such that it could be employed by practitioners from a wide range of disciplines.

An initial study, using random assignment and blind assessment, compared families receiving this clinician-based intervention to families receiving the same information through a lecture format. Both groups report some satisfaction, but the families receiving the clinician-based intervention report significantly more behavior and attitude changes toward their children and their illnesses. These findings strongly suggest the need for the linking of cognitive information to individual life experience and the value of therapeutic focus on the children in helping parents with affective disorder (Beardslee et al., 1993b).

While the long-term effectiveness of this particular intervention remains to be established, the core principles—family involvement, incorporation of information on risk and resiliency, empirical measurement of outcomes, recognition of the heterogeneity of parental disorder and of the need to use different strategies depending on whether individuals are acutely ill or not—are elements that need attention in broad-scale preventive-intervention efforts. Beyond this particular study, however, this broad review of the children of parents with affective disorder strongly suggests that such children are at high risk for the development of disorder and are worthy subjects for the development of preventive-intervention strategies.

ACKNOWLEDGEMENTS.   This study has been conducted with the support of the William T. Grant Foundation, the Harris Trust through Harvard University, the Overseas Shipholding Group, the George P. Harrington Trust, and a Faculty Scholar Award of the William T. Grant Foundation to Dr. Beardslee.

References

Allen, M. G. (1976). Twin studies of affective illness. *Archives of General Psychiatry, 33,* 1476–1478.

Beardslee, W. R. (1981). Self-understanding and coping with cancer. In G. P. Koocher & J. E. O'Malley (Eds.), *The Damocles syndrome: Psychosocial consequences of surviving childhood cancer* (pp. 144–163). New York: McGraw-Hill.

Beardslee, W. R. (1983). *The way out must lead in: Life histories in the civil rights movement.* 2nd ed. Westport, CT: Lawrence Hill.

Beardslee, W. R. (1989). The role of self-understanding in resilient individuals: The development of a perspective. *American Journal of Orthopsychiatry, 59,* 266–278.

Beardslee, W. R. (1990). Development of a clinician-based preventive intervention for families with affective disorders. *Journal of Preventive Psychiatry and Allied Disciplines, 4,* 39–61.

Beardslee, W. R., Bemporad, J., Keller, M. B., & Klerman, G. L. (1983). Children of parents with affective disorder: A review. *American Journal of Psychiatry, 140,* 825–832.

Beardslee, W. R. Hoke, L., Wheelock, I., Rothberg, P., van de Velde, P., & Swatling, S. (1992). Preventive intervention for families with parental affective disorders: An initial study. *American Journal of Psychiatry, 149,* 1335–1340.

Beardslee, W. R., Keller, M. B., & Klerman, G. L. (1985). Children of parents with affective disorder. *International Journal of Family Psychiatry, 6,* 283–299.

Beardslee, W. R., Keller, M. B., Lavori, P. W., Klerman, G. L., Dorer, D. J., & Samuelson, H. (1988). Psychiatric disorder in adolescent offspring of parents with affective disorders in a non-referred sample. *Journal of Affective Disorders, 15,* 313–322.

Beardslee, W. R., Keller, M. B., Lavori, P. W., Stanley, J., & Sacks, N. (1993a). The impact of parental affective disorder on depression in offspring: A longitudinal follow-up in a nonreferred sample. *Journal of the American Academy of Child and Adolescent Psychiatry, 32,* 723–730.

Beardslee, W. R., & Podorefsky, D. (1988). Resilient adolescents whose parents have serious affective and other psychiatric disorder: The importance of self-understanding and relationships. *American Journal of Psychiatry, 145,* 63–69.

Beardslee, W. R., Salt, P., Porterfield, K., Rothberg, P. C., van de Velde, P., Swatling, S., Hoke, L., Mollanen, D. L., & Wheelock, I. (1993b). Comparison of preventive interventions for families with parental affective disorder. *Journal of the American Academy of Child and Adolescent Psychiatry, 32,* 254–263.

Beardslee, W. R., Schultz, L. H., & Selman, R. L. (1987). Level of social–cognitive development, adaptive functioning, and DSM-III diagnosis in adolescent offspring of parents with affective disorders: Implications of the development of the capacity for mutuality. *Developmental Psychology, 23,* 807–815.

Bettes, B. A. (1988). Maternal depression and motherese: Temporal and intonational features. *Child Development, 59,* 1089–1096.

Billings, A. G., & Moos, R. H. (1983). Comparisons of children of depressed and nondepressed parents: A social–environmental perspective. *Journal of Abnormal Child Psychology, 11,* 463–486.

Billings, A. G., & Moos, R. H. (1985). Children of parents with unipolar depression: A controlled 1-year follow-up. *Journal of Abnormal Child Psychology, 14,* 149–166.

Bouras, N., Vanger, P., & Bridges, P. K. (1986). Marital problems in chronically depressed and physically ill patients and their spouses. *Comprehensive Psychiatry, 27,* 127–130.

Breznitz, A., & Sherman, T. (1987). Speech patterning of natural discourse of well and depressed mothers and their young children. *Child Development, 58,* 395–400.

Brown, G. W., Bifulco, A., Harris, T. O., & Bridge, L. (1986). Life stress, chronic psychiatric symptoms and vulnerability to clinical depression. *Journal of Affective Disorders, 11,* 1–19.

Brown, G. W., & Davidson, S. (1978). Social class, psychiatric disorder of mothers and accidents to children. *Lancet, 1,* 378.

Buck, C., & Laughton, K. (1959). Family patterns of illness. *Acta Psychiatrica et Neurologica Scandinavica, 39,* 165–175.

Cadoret, R. J., O'Gorman, T. W., Heywood, E., & Troughton, E. (1985). Genetic and environmental factors in major depression. *Journal of Affective Disorders, 9,* 155–164.

Coffman, S. J., & Jacobson, N. S. (1990). Social learning–based marital therapy and cognitive therapy as a combined treatment for depression. In G. I. Keitner (Ed.), *Depression and families: Recent advances* (pp. 139–155). Washington, DC: American Psychiatric Press.

Cohn, J. F., Campbell, S. B., Matias, R., & Hopkins, J. (1990). Face-to-face interactions of post-partum depressed and nondepressed mother–infant pairs at 2 months. *Developmental Psychology, 26,* 15–23.

Coleman, R. E., & Miller, A. G. (1975). The relationship between depression and marital maladjustment in a clinic population: A multitrait–multimethod study. *Journal of Consulting and Clinical Psychology*, *43*, 647–651.

Costello, E. J., Costello, A. J., Edelbrock, C., Burns, B. J., Dulcan, M. K., Brent, D., & Janiszewski, S. (1988). Psychiatric disorders in pediatric primary care: Prevalence and risk factors. *Archives of General Psychiatry*, *45*, 1107–1116.

Cox, A. D., Puckering, C., Pound, A., & Mills, M. (1987). The impact of maternal depression in young children. *Journal of Child Psychology and Psychiatry*, *28*, 917–928.

Coyne, J. C. (1988). Strategic therapy with couples having a depressed spouse. In G. Haas, I. Glick, & J. Clarkin (Eds.), *Family intervention in affective illness* (pp. 89–113). New York: Guilford Press.

Coyne, J. C., Kessler, R. C., Tal, M., Turnbull, J., Wortman, C. B., & Greden, J. F. (1987). Living with a depressed person. *Journal of Consulting and Clinical Psychology*, *55*, 347–352.

Crowther, J. H. (1985). The relationship between depression and marital maladjustment: A descriptive study. *Journal of Nervous and Mental Disease*, *173*, 227–231.

Decina, P., Kestenbaum, C. J., Farber, S., Kron, L., Gargan, M., Sackeim, H. A., & Fieve, R. (1983). *American Journal of Psychiatry*, *140*, 548–553.

Downey, G., & Coyne, J. C. (1990). Children of depressed parents: An integrative review. *Psychological Bulletin*, *108*, 50–76.

Eisenberg, L. (1979). A friend, not an apple, a day will help keep the doctor away. *American Journal of Medicine*, *66*, 551–553.

Ekdahl, M. C., Rice, E. P., & Schmidt, W. M. (1962). Children of parents hospitalized for mental illness. *American Journal of Public Health*, *52*, 428–435.

Emery, R. (1982). Interpersonal conflict and the children of discord and divorce. *Psychological Bulletin*, *92*, 310–330.

Endicott, J., & Spitzer, R. L. (1978). A diagnostic interview: The Schedule for Affective Disorders and Schizophrenia. *Archives of General Psychiatry*, *35*, 837–844.

Fadden, G., Bebbington, P., & Kuipers, L. (1987). Caring and its burdens: A study of the spouses of depressed patients. *British Journal of Psychiatry*, *151*, 660–667.

Field, T., Healy, B., Goldstein, S., & Gutherz, M. (1990). Behavior–state matching and synchrony in mother–infant interactions of nondepressed versus depressed dyads. *Developmental Psychology*, *26*, 7–14.

Field, T., Sandberg, D., Carcia, R., Vega-Lahr, N., Goldstein, S., & Guy, L. (1985). Pregnancy problems, postpartum depression, and early mother–infant interactions. *Developmental Psychology*, *21*, 1152–1156.

Forehand, R., & McCombs, A. (1988). Unraveling the antecedent–consequence conditions in maternal depression and adolescent functioning. *Behavioral Research and Therapy*, *26*, 399–405.

Frank, E., Kupfer, D. J., Perel, J. M., Cornes, C., Jarrett, D. B., Mallinger, A. G., Thase, M. E., McEachran, A. B., & Grochocinski, V. J. (1990). Three-year outcomes for maintenance therapies in recurrent depression. *Archives of General Psychiatry*, *47*, 1093–1099.

Gaensbauer, T. J., Harmon, R. J., Cytryn, L., & McKnew, D. H. (1984). Social and affective development in infants with a manic–depressive parent. *American Journal of Psychiatry*, *141*, 223–229.

Garmezy, N. (1987). Stress, competence, and development: Continuities in the study of schizophrenic adults, children vulnerable to psychopathology, and the search for stress-resistant children. *American Journal of Orthopsychiatry*, *57*, 159–174.

Gershon, E. S., Hamovit, J., Guroff, J. J., Dibble, E., Leckman, J. F., Sceery, W., Targum, S. D., Nurnberger, J. I., Goldin, L. R., & Bunney, W. E. (1982). A family study of schizoaffective, bipolar I, bipolar II, unipolar, and normal control probands. *Archives of General Psychiatry*, *39*, 1157–1167.

Gershon, E. S., McKnew, D., Cytryn, L., Hamovit, J., Schreiber, J., Hibbs, E., & Pellegrini, D. (1985). Diagnoses in school-age children of bipolar affective disorder patients and normal controls. *Journal of Affective Disorders*, *8*, 283–291.

Goodman, S. H., & Brumley, H. E. (1990). Schizophrenic and depressed mothers: Relational deficits in parents. *Developmental Psychology*, *26*, 31–39.

Gordon, D., Burge, D., Hammen, C., Adrian, C., Jaenicke, C., & Hiroto, D. (1989). Observations of interactions of depressed women with their children. *American Journal of Psychiatry*, *146*, 50–55.

Hammen, C. (1988). Self-cognitions, stressful events, and the prediction of depression in children of depressed mothers. *Journal of Abnormal Child Psychology*, *16*, 347–360.

Hammen, C., Burge, D., Burney, E., & Adrian, C. (1990). Longitudinal study of diagnoses in children of women with unipolar and bipolar affective disorder. *Archives of General Psychiatry*, *47*, 1112–1117.

Hinchliffe, M., Hooper, D., Roberts, F. J., & Vaughan, P. W. (1975). A study of the interaction between depressed patients and their spouses. *British Journal of Psychiatry*, *126*, 164–172.

Hirsch, B. J., Moos, R. H., & Reischl, T. M. (1985). Psychosocial adjustment of adolescent children of a depressed, arthritic, or normal parent. *Journal of Abnormal Psychology*, *94*, 154–164.

Hooley, J. M., Orley, J., & Teasdale, J. D. (1986). Levels of expressed emotion and relapse in depressed patients. *British Journal of Psychiatry, 148,* 642–647.

Jaenicke, C., Hammen, C., Zupan, B., Hiroto, D., Gordon, D., Adrian, C., & Burge, D. (1987). Cognitive vulnerability in children at risk for depression. *Journal of Abnormal Child Psychology, 15,* 559–572.

Keitner, G. I., & Miller, I. W. (1990). Family functioning and major depression: An overview. *American Journal of Psychiatry, 147,* 1128–1137.

Keller, M. B., Beardslee, W. R., Dorer, D., Lavori, P. W., Samuelson, H., & Klerman, G. L. (1986). Impact of severity and chronicity of parental affective illness in adaptive functioning and psychopathology in children. *Archives of General Psychiatry, 43,* 930–937.

Keller, M. B., Beardslee, W. R., Lavori, P., Wunder, J., Dils, D. L., & Samuelson, H. A. (1988). Course of major depression in non-referred adolescents: A retrospective study. *Journal of Affective Disorders, 15,* 235–243.

Keller, M. B., Klerman, G. L., Lavori, P. W., Fawcett, J. A., Coryell, W., & Endicott, J. (1982). Treatment received by depressed patients. *Journal of the American Medical Association, 16,* 119–240.

Keller, M. B., Lavori, P. W., Beardslee, W. R., Wunder, J., & Ryan, N. (1991). Depression in children and adolescents: New data on "undertreatment" and a literature review on the efficacy of available treatments. *Journal of Affective Disorders, 21,* 163–171.

Kessler, R. C., Turner, J. B., & House, J. S. (1987). The effects of unemployment on health in a community survey: Main, modifying, and mediating effects. In R. Catalno & D. Dooley (Eds.), Social costs of economic stress, *Journal of Social Issues.*

Kelin, D. N., Clark, D. C., Dansky, L., & Margolis, E. T. (1988). Dysthymia in the offspring of parents with primary unipolar affective disorder. *Journal of Abnormal Psychology, 97,* 265–274.

Kochanska, G., Kuczynski, L., Radke-Yarrow, M., & Welsh, J. D. (1987). Resolutions of control episodes between well and affectively ill mothers and their young children. *Journal of Abnormal Child Psychology, 15,* 441–456.

Krantz, S. E., & Moos, R. H. (1987). Functioning and life context among spouses of remitted and nonremitted depressed patients. *Journal of Consulting and Clinical Psychology, 55,* 353–360.

Kupfer, D. J., Frank, E., & Perel, J. M. (1989). The advantage of early treatment intervention in recurrent depression. *Archives of General Psychiatry, 46,* 771–775.

Landau, R., Harth, P., & Othnay, N. (1972). The influence of psychotic parents on their children's development. *American Journal of Psychiatry, 129,* 38–43.

Lee, C. M., & Gotlib, I. H. (1989). Clinical status and emotional adjustment of children of depressed mothers. *American Journal of Psychiatry, 146,* 478–483.

McKnew, D. H., Cytryn, L., Efron, A. M., Gershon, E. S., & Bunney, W. E. (1979). Offspring of patients with affective disorders. *British Journal of Psychiatry, 134,* 148–152.

Merikangas, K. R. (1984). Divorce and assortative mating among depressed patients. *American Journal of Psychiatry, 141,* 74–76.

Merikangas, K. R., Prusoff, B. A., Kupfer, D. J., & Frank, E. (1985). Marital adjustment in major depression. *Journal of Affective Disorders, 9,* 5–11.

Marikangas, K. R., Prusoff, B. A., & Weissman, M. M. (1988). Parental concordance for affective disorders: Psychopathology in offspring. *Journal of Affective Disorders, 15,* 279–290.

Merikangas, K. R., Weissman, M. M., & Prusoff, B. A. (1990). Psychopathology in offspring of parents with affective disorders. In G. I. Keitner (Ed.), *Depression and families: Recent advances* (pp. 87–100). Washington, DC: American Psychiatric Press.

Miklowtiz, D. J., Goldstein, D. J., Nuechterlein, K. H., Snyder, K. S., & Mintz, J. (1988). Family factors and the course of bipolar affective disorder. *Archives of General Psychiatry, 45,* 225–231.

Nurnberger, J. I., & Gershon, E. S. (1982). Genetics of affective disorder. In E. S. Paykel (Ed.), *Handbook of affective disorders* (pp. 126–145). New York: Guilford Press.

Offord, D. R., Boyle, M. H., Szatmari, P., Rae-Grant, N. I., Links, P. S., Cadman, D. T., Byles, J. A., Crawford, J. W., Blum, H. M., Byrne, C., Thomase, H., & Woodward, C. A. (1987). Ontario Child Health Study. II. Six-month prevalence of disorder and rates of service utilization. *Archives of General Psychiatry, 44,* 832–836.

O'Hara, M. (1986). Social support, life events, and depression during pregnancy and the puerperium. *Archives of General Psychiatry, 43,* 569–573.

Orvaschel, H., Walsh-Allis, G., & Ye, W. (1988). Psychopathology in children of parents with recurrent depression. *Journal of Abnormal Child Psychology, 16,* 17–28.

Pellegrini, D., Kosisky, S., Nackman, D., Cytryn, L., McKnew, D., Gershon, E., Hamovit, J., & Cammuso, K. (1986). Personal and social resources in children of patients with bipolar affective disorder and children of normal control subjects. *American Journal of Psychiatry, 143,* 856–861.

Powers, S., Hauser, S., & Kilner, L. (1989). Adolescent mental health. *American Psychologist, 44,* 200–208.

Radke-Yarrow, M., Cummings, E. M., Kuczynski, L., & Chapman, M. (1985). Patterns of attachment in two- and three-year-olds in normal families and families with parental depression. *Child Development, 56,* 884–893.

Radke-Yarrow, M., & Sherman, T. (1990). Hard growing: Children who survive. In J. Rolf, A. Masten, D. Cicchetti, K. Neuchterlein, & S. Weintraub (Eds.), *Risk and protective factors in the development of psychopathology* (pp. 97–119). Cambridge, England: Cambridge University Press.

Regier, D. A., Farmer, M. E., Rae, D. S., Locke, B. Z., Keith, S. L., Judd, L. L., & Goodwin, F. K. (1990). Comorbidity of mental disorders with alcohol and other drug abuse. *Journal of the American Medical Association, 264,* 2511–2518.

Richman, N., Stevenson, J., & Graham, P. J. (1982). *Preschool to school: A behavioral study.* New York: Academic Press.

Richmond, J. B., & Beardslee, W. R. (1988). Resiliency: Research and practical implications for pediatricians. *Journal of Developmental and Behavioral Pediatrics, 9(3),* 157–163.

Robins, L. N., & Regier, D. A. (1991). *Psychiatric disorders in America: The Epidemiologic Catchment Area study.* New York: Free Press.

Rounsaville, B. J., Prusoff, B. A., & Weissman, M. M. (1980). The course of marital disputes in depressed women: A 48-month follow-up study. *Comprehensive Psychiatry, 21,* 111–117.

Ruscher, S. M., & Gotlib, I. H. (1988). Marital interaction patterns of couples with and without a depressed partner. *Behavior Therapy, 19,* 455–470.

Rutter, M. (1966). *Children of sick parents: An environmental and psychiatry study.* Institute of Psychiatry Maudsley Monograph No. 16. London: Oxford University Press.

Rutter, M. (1986). Meyerian psychobiology, personality development, and the role of life experiences. *American Journal of Psychiatry, 143,* 1077–1087.

Rutter, M. (1987). Psychosocial resilience and protective mechanisms. *American Journal of Orthopsychiatry, 57,* 316–331.

Rutter, M. (1990). Commentary: Some focus and process considerations regarding effects of parental depression on children. *Developmental Psychology, 26,* 60–67.

Sameroff, A. J., & Chandler, M. J. (1975). Reproductive risk and the continuum of caretaking casualty. In F. D. Horowitz (Ed.), *Review of child development research,* Vol. 4 (pp. 187–244).

Sameroff, A. J., Seifer, R., & Zax, M. (1982). Early development of children at risk for emotional disorder. *Monographs of the Society for Research in Child Development, 47(7),* Serial No. 199.

Sameroff, A. J., Seifer, R., Zax, M., & Barocas, R. (1987). Early indicators of developmental risk: Rochester longitudinal study. *Schizophrenia Bulletin, 13,* 383–394.

Schwartz, C. E., Dorer, D. J., Beardslee, W. R., Lavori, P. W., & Keller, M. B. (1990). Maternal expressed emotion and parental affective disorder: Risk for childhood depressive disorder, substance abuse, or conduct disorder. *Journal of Psychiatric Research, 24,* 231–250.

Strober, M., Morrell, W., Burroughs, J., Lampert, C., Danforth, H., & Freeman, R. (1988). A family study of bipolar I disorder in adolescence—early onset of symptoms linked to increased familial loading and lithium resistance. *Journal of Affective Disorders, 15,* 255–268.

Targum, S. D., Dibble, E. D., Davenport, Y. B., & Gershon, E. S. (1981). The family attitudes questionnaire: Patients' and spouses' views of bipolar illness. *Archives of General Psychiatry, 38,* 562–568.

Vaughn, C. E., & Leff, J. P. (1976). The measurement of expressed emotion in the families of psychiatric patients. *British Journal of Social and Clinical Psychology, 15,* 157–165.

Von Knorring, A.-L., Cloninger, R., Bohman, M., & Sigvardsson, S. (1983). An adoption study of depressive disorders and substance abuse. *Archives of General Psychiatry, 40,* 943–950.

Waring, E. M., & Patton, D. (1984). Marital intimacy and depression. *British Journal of Psychiatry, 145,* 641–644.

Waters, B. G. (1987). Psychiatric disorders in the offspring of parents with affective disorder: A review. *Journal of Preventive Psychiatry, 3,* 191–206.

Weissman, M. M., Gammon, G. D., John, K., Merikangas, K. R., Warner, V., Prusoff, B. A., & Sholomskas, D. (1987a). Children of depressed parents: Increased psychopathology and early onset of major depression. *Archives of General Psychiatry, 44,* 847–853.

Weissman, M. M., John, K., Merikangas, K. R., Prusoff, B. A., Wickramaratne, P. I., Gammon, G. D., Angold, A., & Warner, V. (1986). Depressed parents and their children: General health, social, and psychiatric problems. *American Journal of Diseases of Children, 140,* 801–805.

Weissman, M. M., Leaf, P., & Bruce, M. L. (1987b). Single parent women. *Social Psychiatry, 22,* 29–36.

Weissman, M. M., Paykel, E. S., & Klerman, G. L. (1972). The depressed woman as a mother. *Social Psychiatry, 7,* 98–108.

Weissman, M. M., Prusoff, B. A., Gammon, G. D., Merikangas, K. R., Leckman, J. F., & Kidd, K. K. (1984). Psychopathology of children (ages 6–18) of depressed and normal parents. *Journal of the American Academy of Child Psychiatry, 23*, 78–84.

Weissman, M. M., Warner, V., Wickramaratne, P., & Prusoff, B. A. (1988). Early-onset major depression in parents and their children. *Journal of Affective Disorders, 15*, 269–277.

Welner, Z., & Rice, J. (1988). School-aged children of depressed parents: A blind and controlled study. *Journal of Affective Disorders, 15*, 291–302.

Welner, Z., Welner, A., McCrary, M. D., & Leonard, M. A. (1977). Psychopathology in children of inpatients with depression: A controlled study. *Journal of Nervous and Mental Disease, 164*, 408–413.

Whiffen, V. E., & Gotlib, I. H. (1989). Infants of postpartum depressed mothers: Temperament and cognitive status. *Journal of Abnormal Psychology, 98*, 274–279.

Zahn-Waxler, C., Kochanska, G., Krupnick, J., & McKnew, D. H. (1990). Patterns of guilt in children of depressed and well mothers. *Developmental Psychology, 26*, 51–59.

Zahn-Waxler, C., Mayfield, A., Radke-Yarrow, M., McKnew, D. H., Cytryn, L., & Davenport, Y. B. (1988). A follow-up investigation of offspring of parents with bipolar disorder. *American Journal of Psychiatry, 145*, 506–509.

Zahn-Waxler, C., McKnew, D. H., Cummings, E. M., Davenport, Y. B., & Radke-Yarrow, M. (1984). Problem behaviors and peer interactions of young children with a manic–depressive parent. *American Journal of Psychiatry, 141*, 236–240.

Zuckerman, B., & Beardslee, W. R. (1987). Maternal depression: A concern for pediatricians. *Pediatrics, 79*, 110–117.

Zuckerman, B., Stevenson, J., & Bailey, V. (1987). Stomachaches and headaches in a community sample of preschool children. *Pediatrics, 79*, 677–682.

Zuravin, S. J. (1989). Severity of maternal depression and three types of mother-to-child aggression. *American Journal of Orthopsychiatry, 59*, 377–389.

22

Maltreatment and Childhood Depression

Geraldine Downey, Scott Feldman, Jananne Khuri, and Sarah Friedman

According to the American Psychological Association's National Task Force on Women and Depression (McGrath, Keita, Strickland, & Russo, 1990, p. 30), "Victims of interpersonal violence share many of the symptoms of persons with a primary diagnosis of depression: hopelessness, helplessness, negative self-esteem, a restricted range of affects, high-levels of self-criticism, self-defeating interpersonal strategies, and difficulties in forming and retaining intimate relationships." Studies of the sequelae of childhood victimization usually neglect these symptoms, focusing instead on documenting intergenerational continuity in violence and aggression. Yet, in her review of support for the proposition that violence begets violence, Widom (1989a, p. 24) notes, "Evidence that is often overlooked suggests that abuse and neglect in early childhood leads not only to further aggressive behavior but also to depression, withdrawal, and self-destructive behavior."

The relative inattention to depression in maltreated children is hardly surprising given that, until recently, evidence for the existence of childhood depression was thought to be "insufficient and unsubstantial" (Lefkowitz & Burton, 1978). It is now clear that even preschool children can be clinically depressed, although the disorder is extremely rare in this age group (Kashani & Carlson, 1987). The prevalence of major depressive disorder in unselected school-age children is estimated to be 2–3%, with higher rates among adolescents (Fleming & Offord, 1990). In all age groups, minor depression and dysthymia are much more prevalent than major depression. Although most depressed children recover, clinical depression can have serious developmental consequences. Childhood depression carries a specific risk for adult depression (Harrington, Fudge, Rutter, Pickles, & Hill, 1990) and portends more frequent and more severe depressive episodes over the life course. Depression impedes educational progress and is linked with poor social competence and difficulties in social relationships (Altmann & Gotlib, 1988; Goodyer,

---

Geraldine Downey, Scott Feldman, Jananne Khuri, and Sarah Friedman • Department of Psychology, Columbia University, New York, New York 10027.

Handbook of Depression in Children and Adolescents, edited by William M. Reynolds and Hugh F. Johnston. Plenum Press, New York, 1994.

Wright, & Altham, 1989; Kennedy, Spence, & Henaley, 1989; Mullins, Peterson, Wonderlich, & Reaven, 1986).

Although knowledge concerning the cause of childhood depression is still limited, there is evidence that it arises in the context of troubled family relationships (Coyne, Downey, & Boergers, 1992). The key role of the family environment in fostering and maintaining childhood depression is illustrated by the finding that many depressed children show prompt recovery when hospitalized without further specific therapeutic intervention (Kashani et al., 1987a; Puig-Antich et al., 1987). In this chapter, we consider the role that interpersonal victimization within the family—i.e., child maltreatment— plays in childhood and adult depression.

The first goal of this chapter is to review the evidence linking interpersonal victimization with depression. Toward this end, we examine the limited literature on depression and maltreatment in children. For broader evidence of a connection between victimization and depression, we draw on research on battered women and adult survivors of incest, groups in which the victimization–psychopathology association has been extensively evaluated.

The chapter also considers some possible explanations for the link between family violence and adversity and child depression. The dominant explanation for the intergenerational transmission of violence is that children learn aggression directly from abusive parents (e.g., Patterson, 1982). Similarly, the high levels of depression in the offspring of depressed persons have been attributed to the depressed persons' parenting (for a review, see Downey & Coyne, 1990). However, in addition to being prone to depression, children of depressed parents are often aggressive (Downey & Coyne, 1990). As we shall see, children from maltreating families are also at risk for both types of maladjustment. There is some suggestion that, paralleling normative gender differences in the expression of psychopathology, abused boys' distress may be more evident in aggression and disruptive disorders, whereas abused girls' distress may be more evident in depression.

Several theories have been proposed to account for the association between victimization and depression, including attribution theory (Abramson, Seligman, & Teasdale, 1978) and attachment theory (Cummings & Cicchetti, 1990). We discuss these and other theories and evaluate their potential for explaining such seeming anomalies as the frequent concurrence of depression and aggression in maltreated children and their parents and the fact that maltreatment elicits aggression at times and depression at other times. Hence, this chapter's third and final goal is to present a model that attempts to account for these and other unresolved issues in the area of victimization and depression.

Our chapter focuses on four types of child maltreatment: sexual abuse, physical abuse, emotional abuse, and neglect. We consider maltreatment to be a critical childhood stressor for three reasons. First, child maltreatment fits the profile of traumatic experiences most likely to have adverse effects on adjustment in that it is inflicted by another person and is usually repetitive (American Psychiatric Association, 1987; Terr, 1990).

Second, maltreatment may be particularly traumatic because it is perpetrated by the very people whom children expect to buffer them against the adverse impact of traumatic events. There is increasing evidence that children's adjustment following a traumatic experience depends strongly on their parents' response. This dependence is true of natural disasters (McFarlane, 1987), wars (Ziv & Israeli, 1973), kidnapping (Terr, 1983), and loss of a parent during childhood (Breier et al., 1988; Harris, Brown, & Bifulco, 1990).

Finally, victimization by family members requires attention because it is probably the most prevalent form of childhood trauma. On the basis of official reports, it is estimated that approximately 1 million children experience maltreatment each year, and the perpetrators are typically parents (American Humane Association, 1988; Westat Associates, 1987). Self-report surveys suggest that maltreatment reaching public attention forms only the tip of the iceberg (Gelles & Straus, 1988). Although official reports of sexual abuse (16% of all reports) are numerically low relative to physical abuse (28% of all reports) and neglect (52% of all reports), reports of sexual abuse have grown dramatically over the past decade. This increase parallels a burgeoning awareness of the long-term negative consequences of sexual abuse and confirms retrospective accounts of adults suggesting high rates of childhood sexual abuse (Koss, 1990).

Interpersonal Victimization and Depression

Our discussion of the research connecting victimization and depression is organized around two distinctions. We differentiate studies of the adjustment of adult victims from those of child victims. Within the adult and child literatures, we distinguish studies of sexual abuse from studies of physical abuse or neglect.

Victimization and Adult Psychopathology Research

Sexual Abuse. Research on victimization and on adult psychopathology have tended to progress independently. Awareness of the connection between victimization and adult psychopathology stemmed originally from studies of the mental health consequences of interpersonal violence, especially sexual assault and childhood history of sexual abuse. In community samples, women who were sexually abused in childhood show elevated levels of depressive symptomatology (Bagley & Ramsey, 1986; Browne & Finkelhor, 1986; Briere & Runtz, 1988) and clinical depression (Bifulco, Brown & Adler, 1991; Stein, Golding, Siegel, Burnam, & Sorenson, 1988). Other symptomatology reported by abuse victims includes dissociation, anxiety, and somaticization (Briere & Runtz, 1988; Chu & Dill, 1990; Morrison, 1989; Sanders & Giolas, 1990). This increased risk of depression associated with sexual abuse does not appear to be attributable to other adversities, such as neglect, physical abuse, and institutionalization, that are often experienced by sexually abused children (Bifulco et al., 1991). Depression is most severe following abuse that was repetitive and involved multiple perpetrators, incest, completed intercourse, and force (Briere & Runtz, 1988; Friber & Dinwiddie, 1992).

There has been little attention to male victims of childhood sexual abuse. In a notable exception, Stein et al. (1988) linked childhood sexual abuse with clinical depression in men as well as in women, although the association was stronger in women (22% in abused women vs. 14% in abused men, contrasted with 6% in nonabused women and 4% in nonabused men).

Psychopathology researchers have just begun to investigate the victimization histories of psychiatric patients, focusing particularly on female patients. Among studies that used direct interviews with female patients, the average rate of sexual abuse was 44% (Bryer, Nelson, Miller, & Krol, 1987; Briere & Zaidi, 1989; Jacobson & Richardson, 1987; Chu & Dill, 1990) and ranged from 22% (Jacobson & Richardson, 1987) to 70% (Briere & Zaidi, 1989). Consistent with findings from community studies of victimization, the few studies that included male as well as female patients have found that males were less likely than females to report sexual victimization (Jacobson & Richardson, 1987; G. R. Brown & Anderson, 1991).

Much of the work on clinical samples has sought to identify which types of diagnoses are linked with victimization history. There has been particular interest in establishing links between victimization and diagnoses theorized to result from traumatic experiences, including multiple personality disorder (MPD), borderline personality disorder (BPD), and posttraumatic stress disorder (PTSD). Indeed, there is now considerable evidence that childhood histories of abuse and victimization are common in persons with any of these disorders. Putnam (1989) reported that 97% of the MPD patients in his sample were abused as children. On the basis of averaging across studies, about half of BPD patients report histories of sexual abuse and half report histories of physical abuse (Shearer, Peters, Quaytman, & Ogden, 1990; Herman, Perry, & Van der Kolk, 1989; Ludolph et al., 1990). These rates are about twice as high as those found in psychiatric control groups with nonborderline diagnoses (Ludolph et al., 1990).

Evidence linking childhood victimization with depressive diagnoses in clinical samples is considerably more sparse, but it is unclear whether this sparsity reflects the weakness of the link or the inattention of researchers to the topic. However, there are several reasons to believe that persons with MPD, BPD, or PTSD have high levels of depressive symptomatology, if not clinical levels of depression. In fact, almost all MPD patients initially seek treatment because they feel depressed (Putnam, 1989). Furthermore, there is a strong overlap between the diagnostic criteria for affective disorders and for both BPD and PTSD. Loss of interest, a sense of a foreshortened future, impaired social relationships, and sleep problems are symptomatic of both depression and PTSD. Similarly, many of the diagnostic features of BPD involve the dysregulation of affect (Wideger & Shea, 1991). These features include emotional instability, self-destructive acts, feeling empty, and impaired social relationships. The overlap between BPD and affective disorders has prompted suggestions that borderline personality may be a characterological variant of affective disturbance (David & Akiskal, 1986).

To summarize, current research findings suggest an association between depressive symptoms and a history of sexual abuse in both clinical and nonclinical adult populations. Although there is some indication of higher rates of clinical depression in adults who were sexually abused as children, evidence linking victimization histories with clinical depression in clinical populations is still sparse.

Physical Abuse.   Studies of battered women provide the strongest evidence of a link between physical abuse and adult depression. Violence between spouses occurs in about 25% of marriages and is particularly severe in 12% of marriages (Andrews & Brown, 1988; Gelles & Straus, 1988; Jones, McLean, & Young, 1986; Hammer & Saunders, 1984). Findings from a national survey led Gelles and Straus (1988) to conclude that "women who live in the midst of violence are compromised in nearly every area of their physical and mental health." Psychological problems reported by the battered women surveyed included depression, demoralization, despondency, and despair; somatic complaints included backache, headaches, gastrointestinal problems, fatigue, restlessness, loss of appetite, and sleep difficulties. More than a third frequently felt sad or depressed, 20% felt worthless and hopeless, and suicide had been considered by many more battered women than by controls. Interviews with battered women led Walker (1979) to conclude that living in an atmosphere of constant criticism produced low self-esteem, guilt, physiological complaints, anxiety, and general suspiciousness.

The only study to examine the link between marital violence and clinical depression in a large community sample found that 45% of women who had been in a violent marital relationship were clinically depressed compared to a sample base rate of 25% (Andrews & Brown, 1988). This study echoes the conclusion of Hilberman and Munson (1978) that the most common diagnosis among battered women is depression.

Summary.   Abusive relationships seem to contribute substantially to depression, at least in women (McGrath et al., 1990). Because the connection between victimization and depression in men has not received equivalent attention, we cannot draw any conclusions about this association. However, depression was more prevalent in females than in males in the few studies of survivors of childhood sexual abuse that included males.

Evidence of a link between depression and child maltreatment comes from studies of depression in maltreated children and from studies of the family histories of depressed children.

Sexual Abuse.   Echoing the interest in the connection between childhood sexual abuse and adult depression, several studies have investigated depression in sexually abused children (for a review, see Beitchman, Zucker, Hood, DaCosta, & Ackman, 1991). Following sexual abuse, preschool (Fagot, Hagan, Youngblade, & Potter, 1989), school-age (Goldston, Turnquist, & Knutson, 1989; Kolko, Maser, & Weldy, 1988), and adolescent children show heightened levels of depression, withdrawal, and self-destructive or suicidal behavior. Such internalized responses appear more characteristic of victims of sexual abuse than does aggressive, disruptive behavior, but caution is warranted in interpreting this conclusion. Females predominate in samples of sexually abused children, reflecting their greater likelihood of being identified as victims of sexual abuse (American Humane Association, 1988). Consequently, it is not possible to determine whether the high level of depressive symptomatology in these samples reflects typically female responses to stress or specific consequences of sexual abuse. However, there is some suggestion that the former may be the case. For example, when Livingston (1987) examined depression and conduct disorders in sexually abused children, he found that, relative to their population prevalence, girls were overrepresented among abuse victims with depressive disorders (67%) and underrepresented among abuse victims with conduct disorders (13%).

There is suggestive evidence that the intensity of self-destructive, depressive responses increases with the age of the abused child, with adolescents showing the most pronounced responses, including suicide attempts and substance abuse. These behaviors often occurred in conjunction with disruptive behavior (Beitchman et al., 1991).

In summary, studies suggest that depression and internalizing symptoms may be particularly characteristic of children who have experienced sexual abuse. Unfortunately, studies have tended to use inadequate or no controls. It is noteworthy that one of the few carefully controlled studies of sexually abused children from a nonclinical population found that their depression scores did not significantly distinguish them from controls (Elliott & Tarnowski, 1990).

Physical Abuse or Neglect and Depression.   Clinical observations and controlled studies suggest that abused and neglected children are at risk for depression and low self-esteem (for a review, see Ammerman, Cassisi, Hersen, & Van Hesselt, 1986). For example, Downey and Walker (1992) found that school-age and adolescent maltreated children showed heightened levels of mother-reported depression compared with non-maltreated controls. Similar results are reported by Aber, Allen, Carlson, and Cicchetti (1989) and Toth, Manly, and Cicchetti (1992). Downey and Walker (1992) found, in addition, that a history of maltreatment also predicted a significant increase in depression over a 1-year period.

There is additional evidence that physical abuse is associated with children's self-reports of depression. In both clinical and nonclinical samples, physically abused children showed more depressive symptoms, heightened externality, lower self-esteem, and greater hopelessness about the future than controls (Allen & Tarnowski, 1989; Kazdin, Moser, Colbus, & Bell, 1985). These differences were not attributable to group differences in intelligence, gender, age, or socioeconomic status. There is also an association between parental use of physical punishment and depression in teenagers (Straus, 1992).

Only one study has reported on rates of clinical depression in maltreated children (Kaufman, 1991). Of these children, 18% had major depression (compared with population base rates of 2–3%) and 25% had dysthymia. Compared to the nondepressed children, the depressed children were more likely to have suffered severe injuries over an extended time period, to have parents who were drug-dependent, rejecting, and psychologically unavailable, and to have experienced multiple placements outside their home. Although this study is limited by its lack of a control group of nonabused children, it clearly demonstrates that clinical depression is associated with severe, repeated, and prolonged maltreatment.

As with studies of sexual abuse, the issue of gender differences in the consequences of abuse is usually not addressed. Typically, researchers commingle male and female subjects. In doing so, they cite nonsignificant differences as a rationale, but the small samples on which many of these studies are based do not provide the statistical power to detect significant sex differences. A close examination of the data suggests that females usually surpass males in depressive symptomatology and males surpass females in aggressive symptomatology. For example, the particular vulnerability of maltreated females to depression is illustrated in the finding by Dodge, Bates, and Pettit (1990) of an 86% increase in depression over base rates among physically harmed girls compared with a 19% increase among physically harmed boys.

Family History of Depressed Persons

Depressed adults describe their parents as emotionally distant, critical, punitive, authoritarian, and either rejecting or overprotective (see Burbach & Borduin, 1986). Findings from the few studies of the families of children with either clinical depression or high levels of depressive symptomatology confirm this profile. Parents of both these groups of children are characterized as emotionally distant, lacking in warmth, poor in emotion regulation and conflict resolution, inconsistent, and controlling (Amanat & Butler, 1984; Asarnow, Carlson, & Guthrie, 1987; Cole & Rehm, 1986; Kaslow, Rehm, & Siegel, 1984; Poznanski & Zrull, 1970; Puig-Antich et al., 1985a,b). Some of these studies also note abuse and neglect in the backgrounds of their subjects. For example Puig-Antich et al. (1985a,b) stated that parents of depressed children tended to be cruel and abusive. Maltreatment appears to be particularly common in the histories of depressed or suicidal preschoolers (Kashani & Carlson, 1987; Pfeffer & Trad, 1988). All the preschoolers with major depression in a large sample studied by Kashani and Carlson (1987) had been seriously physically abused or neglected.

Evidence of an association between negative, hostile, abusive parenting and child depression also comes from research on psychopathology in the offspring of depressed parents. Retrospective accounts of harsh, unfair disciplinary practices during childhood explained the relation between child abuse and depression in the adult children of depressed parents (Holmes & Robins, 1988). Child abuse is also more prognostic than parental depression of the development of child psychopathology (Kashani, Shekim, Burk, & Beck, 1987b). Downey and Walker (1992) found that parental psychopathology was associated with heightened levels and subsequent significant increases in children's depressive symptomatology only when the family was also maltreating. This portrayal of families in which depression emerges closely resembles the portrayal of families in which disruptive disorders emerge (Patterson, 1982).

Summary

Although research on the link between maltreatment and depression is still limited, convergent evidence from three sources indicates that depression is common among maltreatment victims. First, both maltreated children and adults maltreated as children show elevated levels of depressive symptomatology. Second, histories of abuse are common among women with borderline personality disorder (BPD), posttraumatic stress disorder (PTSD), and multiple personality disorder (MPD) syndromes, in all of which there is a significant symptom overlap with depression. Finally, studies of the families of depressed children and the retrospective reports of depressed adults about their parents suggest that an abusive upbringing fosters vulnerability for depression.

There are several more specific trends in the field. Notably, each type of maltreatment appears to be related with depression. When considered together with findings from research on other family stressors, this relationship suggests that depression, like aggression, may be a nonspecific response to stressors rather than a specific response to particular stressors. In addition, severity of depression is proportionate to severity of abuse. Finally, there is some suggestion that abused females may be especially vulnerable to depression, whereas abused males may be more vulnerable to aggressive problems. In evaluating these tentative conclusions, it is important to remember that this literature is plagued by the methodological difficulties identified by Widom (1989a) in studies of the "violence begets violence" hypothesis. There is a heavy reliance on retrospection, and control groups are often absent or inadequate.

Two additional factors further complicate the interpretation of findings about the maltreatment–depression association. These factors are particularly pertinent to understanding gender differences in the consequences of maltreatment. First until relatively recently, the existence of childhood depression was debatable, whereas the existence of disruptive disorders was not. Thus, when research on the consequences of maltreatment began, the focus was on aggressive, disruptive outcomes, and research on these outcomes continues to predominate. The emphasis on aggressive outcomes is not limited to maltreatment. Rather, until recently aggression has been the primary outcome studied across a variety of childhood stressors from divorce (Hetherington, Cox, & Cox, 1978) to income loss (Elder, Caspi, & Downey, 1986). This focus on aggressive outcomes has led to conclusions that preadolescent boys are more susceptible than girls to family stressors such as divorce (Hetherington et al., 1978; Elder & Caspi, 1989). However, recent research that has examined both internalizing and externalizing outcomes suggests that girls may be as vulnerable to family stress as boys, although their vulnerability may emerge in internalizing problems rather than in externalizing problems. Illustrating this point in a well-controlled study, Allison and Furstenberg (1989) found that divorce affected girls more strongly than boys. Whereas boys' difficulties were most pronounced in the behavioral domain, girls' problems emerged in academic difficulty, distress, and dissatisfaction.

A second related complication concerns distinctions between the outcomes investigated in child and adult studies. Studies of children have usually focused on aggressive outcomes in males, whereas studies of adult survivors have focused on depressive symptomatology or disorders with a strong depressive component in adult women. Thus, it may appear that males are more vulnerable to the short-term sequelae of maltreatment, as evidenced in their heightened aggressiveness in childhood, whereas females are more vulnerable to the long-term effects, as evidenced by their heightened vulnerability to depression in adulthood. Before claiming that the sequelae of maltreatment manifest themselves primarily as depression in female adults and aggression in male children, it is important to consider whether confounds in studies between life stage, gender, and measure of adjustment give rise to this pattern. Differences in the selection of child and adult samples may also contribute to these findings. The typical adult study is based on self-reports of victimization, whereas the typical child study is based on official reports of maltreatment. Because reports from adults depend on retrospective memories of childhood, they may be influenced by current mental health. Because depression facilitates memory of negative events, it may lead depressed people, who are disproportionately female, to report abusive experiences more readily than nondepressed people. Therefore, estimates of the association between victimization and depression based on retrospective self-reports may be inflated.

Studies based on official reports of child maltreatment will reflect biases inherent to the reporting process. An important point is that children's abuse is often uncovered as a consequence of disruptive behavior, which is more common in males. Other aspects of sample selection that may also affect the findings include the emphasis on female adult survivors of sexual trauma. This emphasis may have resulted in the disproportionately high representation of females in the research on adult survivors of victimization, in which men are represented in very low proportion. Males who disclose sexual abuse histories when participating in community studies of victimization may be unrepresentative of the general population of men. At the more disturbed end of the clinical spectrum, it might be found that the male equivalents of female BPDs and MPDs are more likely to populate prisons or jails than psychiatric hospitals or clinics.

These limitations aside, there is now evidence that abuse survivors are prone to depression as well as to aggression. It is now time for researchers to move beyond asking simply whether maltreatment is linked with these outcomes. Progress depends on asking more refined questions designed to elucidate the circumstances and processes that link abuse with the development of depression or aggression and to explain the link between aggression and depression. Clearly, not everyone who experiences abuse becomes depressed. Although the finding that abused children are at heightened risk for being abusive is robust, intergenerational continuity in aggression is also the exception rather than the expectation. About 30% of abused children become abusive parents (Widom, 1989a), and a similar proportion acquire a criminal record (Widom, 1989b). We know that negative outcomes, whether along the depressive or the aggressive spectrum, are linked with severity of abuse (Widom, 1989a). We also know that aggression and depression frequently co-occur, and there is the suggestion that gender differences in the consequences of abuse may parallel gender differences in the expression of psychopathology in the population.

Developing a greater understanding of the links between maltreatment and depression or aggression requires attention to (1) the broader social context of maltreatment and (2) the processes that may mediate the link between childhood abuse and subsequent depression. Specifically, researchers need to address the following issues:

1. Broader social context in which abuse emerges. As we will see, there are clear parallels among family environments in which depression, antisocial behavior, and maltreatment emerge. These parallels suggest the need to identify similarities in interactional processes in families with different presenting pathologies. A second important reason for examining the broader social context of abuse is the emerging evidence across a variety of stressors that the long-term impact of trauma on the child depends strongly on the family's reaction to it (Elder & Caspi, 1988; Briere et al., 1988; Harris et al., 1990; Terr, 1983). For example, in her pioneering work on childhood trauma, Terr (1983) found that preexisting family pathology contributed to individual differences in the long-term adjustment of a busload of children kidnapped and held for 48 hours in a subterranean hideout. At 4 years after the kidnapping, children from troubled families were more maladjusted than children from healthier families. These findings suggest that certain family environments are conducive to self-healing following trauma, whereas others are not. To fully understand the question of why some children who have encountered traumatic adversity remain resilient, we need to develop an understanding of how some families facilitate the healing process whereas others exacerbate the vulnerability. As with studies of depressed mothers (Downey & Coyne, 1990), researchers have neglected the strengths of maltreating families that may facilitate the healing process. In fact, in reviewing evidence of factors that prompt resilience in high-risk children, Garmezy (1983) identified the presence of a supportive family member as one of three recurring themes in the lives of children who transcend adversity. It is interesting that the Lynch and Roberts (1982) follow-up study of maltreated children showed that children who recovered from the maltreatment also had the support of an adult.

2. Gender differences in abuse outcomes. A crucial issue for further investigation is the influence of victim gender on maltreatment outcomes. In particular, it will be important to establish whether differential outcomes reflect gender differences in response to similar types of abuse or to different abuse experiences, as Cutler and Nolen-Hoeksema (1990) have suggested. Specifically, they propose that girls' higher rates of depression reflect their greater likelihood than boys to experience sexual abuse and the greater severity of the sexual abuse they experience. Answering these questions adequately requires the inclusion of random samples of males and females in victimization studies, the development of measures that are equally valid for males and females, and the assessment of both internalizing and externalizing symptoms.

3. Connection between childhood abusive experiences, childhood adjustment problems, and the adult consequences of abuse. We need to explain the connection between child abuse and adult psychopathology. We must also consider whether models that explain depressive symptomatology can also account for more severe disorders such as BPD, MPD, or antisocial personality disorder. Possible explanations for the link between child abuse, child maladjustment, and adult psychopathology include the following: First, depressive or aggressive reactions to childhood abuse may precipitate environmental processes that maintain the child's depression or aggression. In interviews we conducted with caretakers of children with mothers in prison, Jose and Downey (1992) found that children's reactions to their mother's imprisonment were often revealed in aggression in school and academic failure. These reactions sometimes resulted in children's being restricted to tracks for the academically limited and to delinquent peer groups. Alternatively, the children's aggressive or depressive reactions to abuse may place them directly at risk for later depression or aggression. Finally, children may develop a stormy interpersonal style (Akiskal, 1991) that puts them at risk for depressogenic experiences later in life, in that their reactions to real or imagined criticism from others may ensure rejection and other life crises that are considered depressogenic. All three processes probably operate and need to be examined.

4. Link between aggression and depression. Depression and aggression are both outcomes of maltreatment as well as of other family stressors. Depressive and aggressive symptomatologies co-occur within people (Quiggle, Garber, Panak, & Dodge, 1991; Renouf & Harter, 1990) and within families (Downey & Coyne, 1990). However, we do not yet understand how or why these different expressions of distress are related. Downey and Coyne (1990) suggested that they might co-occur among children of depressed parents because these children are exposed to both depression and conflict in the family environment.

Other possible explanations are that they are different behavioral manifestations of the same underlying distress or negative affect. The argument that aggression and depression may be different expressions of the same underlying distress, reflecting different strategies for self-regulation in the face of perceived rejection, is currently receiving some support from emotion theorists who argue that, at a biological level, there is undifferentiated negative affect that becomes socialized in its expression. How affect gets expressed may depend on the impact of the behavioral expression of affect on the environment. As we shall see, normative sex-role expectations may ensure that depressive strategies for expressing distress may be more effective for girls and aggressive strategies may be more effective for boys.

Progress in addressing the issues we have highlighted will depend on avoiding the methodological confounds we have detailed. However, to provide theoretical direction for future research, a framework that can integrate the distinct literatures on the outcomes of abuse is needed. In the next section, we consider some potential integrative frameworks.

Explaining the Link between Maltreatment and Depression

In the introduction, we noted that the dominant explanation for the intergenerational continuity of abusive behavior was that children learn such behavior directly from their parents. This learning is thought to occur through modeling and the selective reinforcement of coercive, abusive behavior (Patterson, 1982). The connection between maltreatment and depression does not evoke such a direct explanation. Therefore, we need to begin by considering what an adequate theory of the association between maltreatment and depression must explain.

First, it must provide an account of what it is about maltreatment that puts children at risk for subsequent depression. Because depressive symptomatology in victims of abuse often emerges later in life, an adequate account must describe the intervening psychological processes that children carry with them into new situations and relationships that may foster depression.

Second, the theory must account for the co-occurrence of anger and depression in maltreated children, while simultaneously accounting for the gender-differentiated expression of adult psychopathology. Specifically, from adolescence onward, women show considerably higher rates of depression than men and men show higher rates of disruptive disorders and aggressive behavior than women. These differences are found in both the general population (American Psychiatric Association, 1994) and in adults abused as children (Carmen, Rieker, & Mills, 1984).

As we turn to a discussion of efforts to explain depression in victims of maltreatment, we note that these efforts have been quite limited, and much of the evidence we review is indirect. Relevant research, to date, has focused primarily on establishing that maltreatment fosters psychological processes or states thought to play a causal role in the development of depression. The interactional processes within maltreating families that give rise to the psychological underpinnings of depression has not yet been studied. The cause of gender differences in response to abuse and victimization has received little attention from researchers.

Psychological Mediators of the Depression–Maltreatment Association

One approach to explaining the depression–maltreatment association has been to investigate the relation between maltreatment and cognitions. Self-cognitions have been the focus of considerable attention, especially self-esteem and self-blame.

Self-Esteem. In recognition of the self-deprecatory stance of depressed persons, psychoanalytical (Freud, 1968), cognitive (Abramson et al., 1978), and interactional (Coyne, 1976) perspectives all accord self-esteem a role in depression. The current cognitive emphasis in psychology has helped promote the view that negative self-cognitions play a causal role in depression.

There is much evidence that maltreated children suffer substantial impairment of their self-systems compared with children from healthier backgrounds. Low self-esteem and negative self-evaluations are common themes in the clinical literature on victims of abuse. Evidence from controlled studies using standardized measures also reports lower self-esteem in victims of maltreatment. This is true of school-age children and adolescents (Kaufman & Cicchetti, 1989; Wodarski, Kurtz, Gavdin, & Howing, 1990; Allen & Tarnowski, 1989; Kazdin et al., 1985; Oates, Forrest & Peacock, 1985; Dadds, Smith, Webber, & Robinson, 1991; Tong, Oates, & McDowell, 1987) as well as of adults who were victimized as children (Carmen et al., 1984; Gold, 1986; Hunter, 1991). The degree of impairment is proportional to the severity of maltreatment experienced (Kaufman & Cicchetti, 1989).

Although lowered self-esteem is found in victims of all forms of maltreatment, there is some suggestion that it may be a consequence of the emotional abuse that commonly accompanies neglect, physical abuse, and sexual abuse (Briere & Runtz, 1990).

Whereas many of the studies that find lowered self-esteem in victims of maltreatment also report heightened depression, the magnitude and nature of the relation between self-esteem and depression are not explored. Specifically, no study to date has demonstrated that self-esteem mediates the relation between maltreatment and depression. Moreover, no study has demonstrated that self-esteem plays a causal role in depression following maltreatment.

In fact, questions of causality are still unresolved in the literature on self-esteem and depression (e.g., Renouf & Harter, 1990) and the broader literature on cognition and affect (for contrasting views, see Lazarus, 1984; Zajonc, 1984). The cross-sectional evidence linking self-esteem with depression does not satisfactorily establish whether self-esteem is a cause, a symptom, or a consequence of depression. Researchers have rarely undertaken the longitudinal studies needed to determine whether self-esteem predicts subsequent changes in depression, a prerequisite for claiming that self-esteem plays a causal role in depression.

To address these issues, we used data from the Cornell High-Risk Study of 144 children aged 6–14 years with a maltreating or psychiatrically disturbed parent (for a general description of the study, see Downey & Walker, 1989, 1992). Whereas self-esteem, measured using the Rosenberg Self-Esteem Scale (Rosenberg, 1979), was associated cross-sectionally with mothers' reports of child depression, assessed using the Child Behavior Checklist (Achenbach, 1979), self-esteem did not explain the cross-sectional association between maltreatment and depression, nor was it associated with a change in depression over a 1-year period. Thus, our data do not support the claim that self-esteem mediates the association between maltreatment and depression.

Rather, our findings suggest that self-esteem may be a symptom rather than a precursor of depression. This view is consistent with that of Poznanski (1982) and others who have argued that self-deprecatory ideation should be a defining feature of childhood depression. In further support of this view, Renouf and Harter (1990) provide evidence that among adolescents, self-worth and depressed affect correlate at 0.81, load on the same factor, and covary over a 1-year period. Thus, it may not be fruitful to conceptualize low self-esteem as a precursor of depression in maltreated children. Rather, a better approach may be to look prior to the point at which self-esteem fails. Specifically, it may be useful to search for precursors of depression in maltreated children's attempts to maintain self-esteem under threat.

Attributing Blame.   One effort to investigate precursors of low self-worth has involved examining the role of attributions of blame in mediating the impact of negative events on self-esteem and adjustment. Accepting the assumption that negative events prompt attributional concern, attributional theories of adjustment have concentrated on the implications of particular attributions for the maintenance of self-esteem following trauma (Abramson et al., 1978; Janoff-Bulman, 1979; Wortman, 1976). Specifically, much work has concentrated on the costs and benefits of self-blame. One tradition argues that self-blame is maladaptive because it undermines self-esteem and engenders feelings of helplessness, thereby increasing risk for depression (Abramson et al., 1978). A second tradition argues that self-blame can be adaptive because it defends against the conclusion that one is helpless, thus enabling self-esteem to be maintained (Bulman & Wortman, 1977). Empirical support for either tradition has been equivocal (Downey, Silver, & Wortman, 1990).

The clinical and empirical literatures on victims of abuse reflect the interest of attribution theorists in establishing the role of self-blame in adjustment to victimization.

Studies of adult and adolescent incest and rape victims have tended to find that victims who engage in self-blame have lower self-esteem and are more depressed (Wyatt & Newcomb, 1990; Hoagwood, 1990; Meyer & Taylor, 1986; Frazier, 1991). Self-blame is intensified when the abuse is persistent or severe (Hoagwood, 1990; Brent, 1991).

Although these findings are consistent with the view that self-blame is maladaptive and inconsistent with the proposal that it is adaptive, the cross-sectional nature of the data precludes drawing any causal conclusions. In fact, evidence from recent longitudinal research on the self-blame–depression association following significant negative events such as the unexpected death of one's infant (Downey et al., 1990), an unwanted pregnancy (Major, Mueller, & Hildebrandt, 1985), and perinatal complications (Affleck, McGrade, Allen, & McQueeney, 1985) finds no support for the claim that self-blame plays a significant causal role in depression. Instead, self-blame appears to be symptomatic of distress (Downey et al., 1990).

Discouraged by continued uncertainty about the causal role of self-blame in distress, some investigators have suggested that the significant factor in adjustment to trauma is not the specific attributions people make but, rather, the extent of their preoccupation with attributing blame for the event. Among parents who lost a child to sudden infant death syndrome, Downey et al. (1990) found that those who were invested in attributing responsibility for the death were more likely to engage in blaming themselves or someone else. Future efforts to understand the connection between attributional issues following maltreatment may be more fruitful if they focus on distinguishing people who respond to negative events by attributing blame from those who do not. However, it is important to note that it has not yet been established that preoccupation with blaming per se is a distress-enhancing strategy rather than a distress-management strategy.

Summary. We began this section by considering what might be a precursor of low self-esteem. We reviewed research investigating whether self-blame might mediate the connection between negative events and self-esteem. Longitudinal studies indicate that self-blame is not causally related to self-esteem or adjustment. Instead, self-blame, like self-esteem, may be symptomatic of distress. This possibility suggests the need for a shift in focus away from self-blame as a potential mediator of the maltreatment–adjustment relation. It may be more relevant to ask which children are oriented to engage in blame following threats to self-esteem and whether they engage in self- or other-blame. This question also implies the need to focus attention on individual differences in what children identify as threats to self-esteem and on the origins of these differences.

Attachment Theory

Attachment theory has the potential to account for individual differences in self-blame and their origins (Bowlby, 1958; Ainsworth, 1973). This theory is currently of considerable interest to investigators studying the maltreatment–maladjustment association [Cicchetti, 1987; Cummings & Cicchetti, 1990; Crittenden & Ainsworth, 1989; Egeland & Sroufe, 1981; Toth et al., 1992; Cicchetti, Rogosch, & Toth (Chapter 7)]. It provides a general account of why maltreatment puts children at risk for developing psychological processes that may foster psychopathology. The core assumption of attachment theory is that human infants are innately motivated to become emotionally attached to their primary caregivers in order to feel secure. A further assumption is that children develop an internal working model that reflects the quality of their relationship with their primary caretaker. This model provides continuity between one's primary relationship and subsequent relationships.

According to attachment theory, children become securely attached to caretakers who respond sensitively to their needs. They feel confident that they are lovable, competent, and worthy and that their social environment will be supportive, should the need arise. The internal working model that embodies these beliefs mediates securely attached children's transactions with the broader world as well as with family members.

By contrast, children whose primary caretakers meet their attachment needs with intermittent or consistent rejection develop considerable anxiety about the availability of their caretaker. Consequently, the internal working model that they develop embodies doubts about the supportiveness of their broader social environment and about their self-worth. They use one of two general strategies to defend against these doubts and anxieties. Children who develop the anxious/avoidant strategy actively avoid contact with the caretakers and show hesitance about seeking support from their social environment. Their internal working model embodies the belief that the world is a threatening place and that social interactions are potential affirmations of their blameworthiness and worthlessness. Such an orientation is thought to result from parenting characterized by rejection of quests for solace or assistance.

The anxious/ambivalent defense strategy involves interspersing frequent demands for reassurance from the caretaker with displays of hostility. The internal working model of persons with this attachment style embodies the view that the supportiveness of their environment is questionable and its evaluation of their worth is subject to fluctuation. Reflecting this belief, they constantly monitor the environment's supportiveness and evaluate their self-worth by seeking expressions of support and affirmations of their worth. Such an attachment style is thought to result from caretaking marked by an unpredictable mixture of rejection and indulgence.

In sum, attachment theory is about one's sense of security and the pathologies that can arise from efforts to defend against anxiety generated by feeling insecure. Attachment theorists posit that maltreatment puts children at risk for psychopathology because the insensitive, unresponsive parenting it implies leads to the development of insecure parent–child attachments. These insecurities are mirrored in the negative internal working models that embody the child's conception of self and others and that are evoked in new situations and relationships.

Cummings and Cicchetti (1990) propose that depression is one of the pathologies that can result from a disturbed attachment relationship. Specifically, they propose that "the negative internal working model of the self that develops in the context of an insecure parent–child attachment relationship could be a major contributor to the development of depressive cognitions and symptomatology." Negative internal working models also foster depression through influencing people's perception of the supportiveness of their social environment. Persons with a negative model should be biased toward perceiving their environment as unsupportive, and the resulting feeling of rejection would promote depression.

Consistent with the view that insecure attachment may mediate the link between maltreatment and depression, there is considerable evidence that maltreated children form insecure attachments with their parents as measured by the insecure attachment paradigm (Ainsworth, 1973). Summing across studies, approximately two thirds of maltreated children are insecurely attached compared with one third of the controls (Carlson, Cicchetti, Barnett, & Braunwald, 1989; Egeland & Sroufe, 1981; Lyons-Ruth, Connell, Zoll, & Stall, 1987; Schneider-Rosen, Braunwald, Carlson, & Cicchetti, 1985). The majority of insecurely attached maltreated children are anxious/avoidant whether they are physically or emotionally abused or neglected. Rates of insecure attachment appear to be relatively stable across maltreated children from the age of 12 months to 4 years (Cicchetti & Barnett, 1992). It has recently been suggested that the traditional forced categorization of attachment styles fails to capture the full range of disturbance in relationships of children and their abusive parents in two respects: First, the parent–child relations of maltreated children classified as securely attached are more disturbed than those of securely attached nonmaltreated children (Lyons-Ruth et al., 1987). Second, there is evidence that a high proportion of maltreated children fall into a fourth attachment category, which captures very seriously disorganized parent–child relations (for a reanalysis of existing data, see Carlson et al., 1989).

Overall, attachment theory provides an integrative framework for understanding the link between maltreatment and family adversity and an interrelated set of child incompetencies, including aggression and depression. The framework identifies two key mediators of the maltreatment–child maladjustment relation. At the level of the family environment, the theory emphasizes the availability of sensitive, responsive parenting. Insecure attachments develop when it is unavailable. At the level of the child, the theory identifies internal working models acting as a lens for interpreting information relevant to one's self and one's relationships and generating behavioral responses. Children who develop a negative working model will interpret and respond to information from their social environment in ways that foster pathology.

Although this framework provides an elegantly parsimonious model of continuity between pathological parenting and pathological development, we need to consider the limitations of its current state of articulation. As Cummings and Cicchetti (1990) note, the attachment history is probably only one of many mechanisms that operate in the development of depression. Therefore, it may be useful to view the insensitive, unresponsive parenting that promotes the development of insecure attachment as a marker of risk for compromised self and social development and to consider how family environments that undermine sensitive, responsive parenting may directly influence the child's development.

The concept of internal working models is also problematic. Although the concept is theoretically distinct from that of the attachment relationship, the distinction is not yet well documented. In fact, the existence of internal working models is usually inferred from attachment behavior in children or from adults' conceptualizations of their relationships with their parents. Second, internal working models are thought to mediate the relationship between problem parenting and child incompetencies, including depression, aggression, low self-esteem, academic failure, and peer rejection. While, as a group, maltreated children show elevated rates of these incompetencies, they are not necessarily clustered in individual children. For example, abused girls appear to be more depressed than abused boys, and abused boys appear to be more aggressive than abused girls. In their present state of theoretical development, internal working models are too global to account for the development of one form of psychopathology rather than another. Finally, they do not provide an adequate account of how children will behave in the particular situations they encounter in daily life. The merit of attachment theory is in orienting us to the need to delineate the psychological consequences of maltreatment and to consider how these consequences may account for psychopathology. In sum, it is a theory of the general rather than the particular. The operation of children's internal working models in specific social interactions has not been detailed, although investigators are now beginning to undertake this task (e.g., Westen, 1991).

Summary

We have focused on two basic approaches with potential for explaining the maltreatment–depression relation. One approach focuses on what some have argued are cognitive precursors of depression: self-concept and self-blame. While child and adult victims of maltreatment who show low self-esteem and engage in self-blame tend to be depressed, current evidence suggests that these cognitions may be symptoms rather than precursors of depression. Thus, in studying self-esteem and self-blame, we may be studying depression.

Whereas attachment theory offers a broader theoretical perspective on how maltreatment may be linked with depression, all that has been established empirically is that the maltreating parent–child relationship is commonly characterized by a behavioral pattern described as insecure attachment. While attachment theorists have posited that children internalize insecure attachments as working models of relationships, evidence to support the claim is not yet available. Thus, we are left with evidence of troubled relations between maltreating parents and their children and depression accompanied by self-blame and low self-esteem. Left unexplicated are the psychological processes that are activated in children's daily activities, processes that may bridge coming from an abusive family with becoming depressed. Also, the theory does not adequately account for gender differences in psychopathology or explain why anger and depression are often combined. Finally, although attachment theory directs our attention to troubled parent–child relations—rather than specific instances of abuse—exclusive focus on this relation may be shortsighted in that it neglects the broader social context in which maltreatment is embedded.

We begin by providing a portrait of the social context of maltreatment and then turn to the model we are developing.

Maltreating Families as a Context for Development

Initially, child maltreatment became a focus of public concern because of its potential for damaging children physically. Over time, concern shifted to its impact on children's emotional development. However, there is not yet a well-articulated theory of why maltreatment compromises children's emotional development. Although efforts to date have focused on the global quality of parent–child transactions, it is becoming clear that an adequate understanding of the emotional development of maltreated children also requires attention to the broader social context in which maltreatment is embedded, as well as to the specific qualities of parent–child interaction that give rise to insecure attachment.

Parent–Child Dyad

Reflecting the roots of attachment theory in Bowlby's observations of children's response to physical separation from their mothers, some theorists argue that parental psychological unavailability is key to the development of insecure attachment and is the most harmful aspect of abuse. Support for this claim comes from a study by Egeland and Sroufe (1981) in which the attachment styles of 18-month-old children with different physical and emotional maltreatment histories are compared with those of control children. Insecure attachment was most prevalent among children of psychologically unavailable mothers, who were characterized by such behaviors as ignoring their young child's requests for comfort or assistance. Nonetheless, other forms of maltreatment were also associated with high rates of insecure attachment, and differences across maltreatment groups were not appreciable. Moreover, emotional unavailability was usually accompanied by other forms of maltreatment, obscuring the unique effects of any specific form of maltreatment. More generally, empirical efforts to link types of maltreatment with types of attachment have been unsuccessful.

These methodological difficulties aside, attachment theory reflects a much-needed shift in perspective, from viewing maltreatment as a status or an event that compromises the child's physical integrity to viewing it as a communication process that compromises psychological development. Other investigators, notably Garbarino and Gilliam (1980), echo attachment theorists' claim that emotional maltreatment is the core problem of maltreatment. Yet, instead of emphasizing emotional neglect as embodied in the concept of emotional unavailability, they emphasize the role of emotional abuse, especially overt rejection, in harming children psychologically. This perspective provides a bridge with family-systems approaches to depression (Coyne et al., 1992; Downey & Coyne, 1990; Hahlwag & Goldstein, 1987).

A major focus of research on the links between family processes and both child and adult psychopathology has centered on how families manage negative emotions. In particular, evidence is accumulating that criticism from family members may play a key role in fostering depression (Hooley & Teasdale, 1989). For example, depressed patients with spouses who are critical of the patients' characters and prior behavior are at heightened risk for relapse (Hooley, Orley, & Teasdale, 1986; Leff & Vaughn, 1985; Miklowtiz, Goldstein, Nuechterlein, & Snyder, 1988; G. W. Brown, Bifulco, & Andrews, 1990). Criticism is a stronger predictor of relapse than hostility, lack of warmth, or overinvolvement (Hooley & Teasdale, 1989). Among children at risk for depression, self-criticism is most common in children who are the direct recipients of their mother's criticism.

Thus, child-directed criticism, alone or offered as a rationale for physical maltreatment, may be an important way in which maltreating parents foster psychological vulnerability to depression in children. To summarize the effects of emotional maltreatment, both neglect and abuse appear to be crucial ways in which maltreatment affects children's psychological development.

Broader Social Context of Maltreatment

Attention to the social environment beyond the parent–child dyad is needed for two reasons: First, the environment may directly affect the quality of the parent–child relation, as when marital conflict and the ensuing depression distract mothers from effortful parenting (Downey & Coyne, 1990; Coyne et al., 1992). Second, properties of the broader family system may directly impinge on the developing child. Thus, it may be fruitful to view maltreatment as symptomatic of a troubled family environment. Viewed this way, similarities with families that include a depressed person become evident. These similarities include high levels of poverty, stress, and conflicted and violent marriages (Downey & Coyne, 1990; Gelles & Straus, 1988).

We have previously identified several system-level properties of troubled family systems that may give rise to depression (Coyne et al., 1992). Similarities between families of depressed persons and those of maltreating persons suggest that the same properties may operate in maltreating families. These properties include the absence of a sense of family coherence, that is, a sense of engagement in a common enterprise, with the attendant assumptions about security and predictability. When such a sense is absent, as it is in many abusive families, personal control is emphasized over interdependency, and individual short-term goals preempt a collective long-term agenda. Other family members are viewed as undependable, and disagreements are not easily resolved.

A sense of agency is also lost in troubled families in that, without the ability to rely on other people and routines, the scaffolding to pursue one's agenda is missing. In the absence of the mundane daily routines and rituals that lend a sense of coherence to life as a shared family venture, children have few opportunities for building competencies. As one child in our study of children of incarcerated mothers remarked, it was difficult for her to focus on schoolwork when she was constantly worried about when someone would next shoot at her home in an attempt to harm a drug-dealing family member (Jose & Downey, 1992).

Maltreating families can also be viewed as emotionally dysregulated in that negative interactions and disagreements are not resolved. Instead, they have a certain breeding quality such that they permeate the entire family system, fostering blaming and side-taking. Negative affect becomes contagious, and there is little chance that it will be transformed into positive. Small stressors are catastrophized and minor slights derail relationships.

Finally, because routine obligations, such as paying the rent, are less likely to be met, major negative life events, such as eviction, are more likely to occur. In focus groups with children of imprisoned mothers, it became obvious that children had difficulty committing themselves to current life tasks, such as paying attention to the teacher at school, when they were preoccupied with the safety of their current caretaker and with the uncertainty about whether she would still be there when they returned from school (Jose & Downey, 1992).

A Model Linking Maltreatment and Depression

Depression typically arises in the context of conflicted relationships and severe stress (Coyne et al., 1994). Families in which maltreatment occurs are characterized by these qualities (Gelles & Straus, 1988). However, an adequate explanation of the link between maltreatment and depression must also explain why children who have been maltreated early in life show heightened depression in adolescence and adulthood. We propose that being raised in a maltreating family shapes the development of key psychological processes involved in the regulation of children's social interactions. In this way, abuse fosters an orientation to social interaction that facilitates the development of psychopathology.

Specifically, we propose a model of the psychological processes involved in the regulation of children's social interactions, of the impact of maltreatment on the development of these processes, and of their relation with depression and disruptive disorders.

Rejection Sensitivity and the Regulation of Social Interaction

Our framework for explaining aggressive and depressive outcomes in abused children integrates self-esteem, attributions of blame, and children's orientation to interpersonal rejection. We define rejection sensitivity as the disposition to anxiously expect, readily perceive, and overreact to rejection in a wide variety of situations.

Specifically, we propose that sensitivity to rejection by others is a common pathway in the development of either disruptive or depressive disorders in abused children. Research on troubled families in which maltreatment, conduct disorders, and depression emerge reveals an orientation to respond to conflict with criticism, hostility, and resentful, indignant withdrawal. Verbal conflict and hostility are often precursors of physical abuse. These families provide poor models of conflict resolution and interpersonal problem-solving. Such a socialization environment is likely to foster in children (1) a tendency to associate conflict with rejection and physical danger, (2) a tendency to expect and be concerned about the possibility of rejection in all interpersonal situations, and (3) a readiness to perceive rejection in interpersonal situations. Thus, compared with non-abused children, abused children will view a wider range of situations as being suffused with threats of rejection. Perceived conflict, or even helpful suggestions, will pose a greater threat to them because they have developed no competencies for negotiating interpersonal relations and because mild conflict or criticism was frequently a precursor of overwhelming terror. Nonabused children, by contrast, are likely to view a wider, but restricted, range of situations as benign and to approach conflict situations with a problem-solving orientation. In their families, conflict was something to be resolved, and one form of resolution could be termination of the relationship when the other person's behavior was deemed grossly inappropriate. Conflict was not a prelude to inevitable terror or cruel rejection.

What happens when rejection-sensitive children perceive rejection? We argue that they become extremely distressed because their sense of self-esteem is threatened. Our discussion of self-esteem ended with the suggestion that operationalizing it as a static, traitlike cognition that operates on the affective domain does not adequately capture its role in depression. In our model, we view the fragility of self-esteem, not its level, as the risk factor. Thus, we propose that when rejection-sensitive children identify social behavior as potentially threatening to self-esteem, they attempt to regulate the ensuing negative affect by engaging in blame in lieu of problem-solving.

The socialization experiences of children from maltreating families appear particularly likely to promote blaming. First, more of the type of intractable events that are most likely to provoke an attributional search happen to them (Weiner, 1985). Because abusive families do a poor job of regulating negative emotion, mild misunderstandings are magnified and minor problems and conflicts are transformed into major, unresolvable events a disproportionate amount of the time. Moreover, role reversal is common in abusive families in that children often bear an unrealistic level of responsibility for resolving family problems (Dean, Malik, Richards, & Stringer, 1986). Evidence of the ineptness of their efforts to resolve insurmountable difficulties may prompt them to resort to blaming. Second, the criticism and verbal hostility that substitute for problem-solving in abusive households are likely to socialize children into being self-critical and blaming others when things go wrong. Thus, in abusive households, children may not learn to solve problems or even realize that problems can be solved, yet they may be given responsibility for solving family problems. The combination of deficient problem-solving skills and frequent exposure to insoluble problems may prompt them to blame someone when faced with perceived interpersonal adversity. A plummeting of self-esteem and ensuing helplessness, hopelessness, and depression may occur if children blame themselves for the event.

To forestall a plummeting of their fragile sense of self-esteem, we argue, they will directly attribute the blame to others or engage in strategies that deflect blame onto others. Examples of deflecting strategies include storming away indignantly, thus evoking apologetic, reconciliatory behavior by the perceived adversary, or engaging in overdone assuaging, ingratiating behavior, with the goal of appeasing the adversary and persuading him or her and the broader social environment that the rejection was undeserved.

Whether they deal with threats to self-esteem by attributing blame to others directly or indirectly will influence the form that their distress takes. Those who directly blame the other person will experience aggression, and their behavioral response will be aggressive. Those who are ambivalent about directly according blame will experience a mixture of resentment and sadness at the other person's behavior. Their behavioral response will involve a reciprocation of the perceived rejection in the form of withdrawal from the situation or immoderate acts of appeasement.

Sex Differences in Response to Threats to Self-Esteem

We believe that children's attributional and behavioral responses to threats to self-esteem will depend on their beliefs about what being a worthy person means. Given the prevailing sex-role stereotypes, these beliefs are likely to differ for boys and girls in ways that influence their reactions to threats to self-esteem. Stereotyped expectancies for males are that they be dominant and oriented toward justice. Expectancies for females emphasize the centrality of relationships and the importance of their preservation (Gilligan, 1982). These normative sex-role expectations are reflected in the typical socialization experiences of boys and girls. Although boys and girls in both normal (Fagot, 1984) and troubled families (Sroufe & Jacovitz, 1989) show equivalent levels of aggression early in life, aggressive behavior in girls declines between the ages of 2 and 4. A plausible explanation for this drop is that aggression is a less effective coercive strategy for girls than it is for boys. Boys' aggression elicits positive and negative responses in peers, teachers, and parents, whereas girls' aggression is more often ignored (Fagot, 1984; Fagot & Hagan, 1985, 1991;

Fagot, Hagan, Leinbach, & Kronsberg, 1985). By contrast, dependency behavior in girls is more stable between 2 and 4 years, and others respond more positively to it (Fagot, 1984; Fagot & Hagan, 1985, 1991; Fagot et al., 1985). Furthermore, girls' attempts at communication and conversation receive more encouragement than do boys' attempts. Therefore, females may find that outraged withdrawal from communication is more effective in eliciting an apology from their perceived adversary than is aggressive behavior. They may also find that appeasing behavior is more successful in "winning over" their adversary than aggression. Consequently, threats of rejection may elicit ingratiating behavior. When resentful withdrawal from the relationship and conciliatory appeasement fail, girls may be unable to avoid self-blame. Depression mixed with anger will follow.

Individual Differences in Sex-Typed Behavior and Their Origins

On the basis of findings from the adult literature showing that sex-typed people are more poorly adjusted than others (Bem, 1984), it appears reasonable to propose that children who are more sex-typed than others may show more adjustment problems and that these problems will emerge in gender-typical ways. Consistent with this argument, a study of preschool children by Sprafkin, Serbin, and Elman (1982) found that compared with children who played with both boys' and girls' toys, boys who played exclusively with male-typed toys were more defiant and aggressive and girls who played only with girls' toys were more apathetic and withdrawn. In addition, Orlofsky (1979) found that non-sex-typed adolescents had parents who were less sex-typed.

Consequently, in families with traditional sex-role beliefs, the self-esteem investment of boys and girls will probably be even more pronounced along sex-typed lines than is typical. Central to our model is the belief that normative gender differences in child socialization are more pronounced in maltreating families. Thus, we expect the patterns we now describe to emerge in male and female maltreated children.

In maltreating families where males are expected to be dominant, boys will be strongly invested in being tough, powerful, and dominant. When their esteem is threatened in social situations, efforts to regulate their distress will prompt them to engage in blaming their perceived adversary. Their sensitivity to the possibility that rejecting intent underlies negative verbal or physical interaction will result in aggressive and coercive responses. Although this esteem-maintenance behavior may be tolerated and reinforced within abusive families, such children are likely to be labeled as aggressive bullies outside the family. Consequently, their behavior will lead to recurrent social rejection, which may induce feelings of sadness and dejection (Capaldi, 1992).

By contrast, girls will be invested in maintaining and managing relationships, and dependency will be fostered. Because maintaining relationships is of primary importance, they may be more reluctant than boys to directly blame their adversary. We argue that they seek indirect ways of attributing blame to their adversary, instead. For example, they may engage in indignant withdrawal with the implicit goal of evoking an apology.

Alternatively, sensitivity to rejection in females may lead to an exaggerated tolerance of negative verbal and physical encounters with others and, more generally, to the subversion of their other needs in the service of maintaining and controlling relationships. This proposal is compatible with the fact that in this society, subordinating one's own well-being to the well-being of relationships is seen as a desirable goal for females (Belle, 1982; Goldner, Penn, Sheinberg, & Walker, 1990). Rather than view low levels of abuse and neglect as unacceptable, maltreated girls may derive esteem from their ability to tolerate and manage this behavior, and small indications of positivity may be inappropriately gratifying. This behavioral pattern may put them at risk for becoming or remaining invested in relationships with adults, peers—and, later, romantic partners—that could become seriously abusive. Consistent with this suggestion, Boeke and Markman (1992) found that marital relationships in which the woman had responded to her partner's negative, coercive behavior with positive, soothing behavior premaritally were at heightened risk for becoming violent following the marriage. Such relationships are likely to promote depression through engendering feelings of helplessness and hopelessness that eventually erode any sense of esteem or control derived from commitment to being a caring person. Thus, unlike boys who are invested in being in control, girls who are invested in relationships may be prompted into relationship-preserving behavior at any hint of adversity in the relationship. When their efforts to preserve the relationship fail, they may respond with exaggerated self-blame and resentful anger. As a result, they interpret the distress resulting from their failure in self-esteem as sadness. An alternative female strategy may involve angry, outraged, hostile withdrawal at the slightest hint of conflict. When these strategies fail to evoke an apology, self-blame, loss of self-esteem, and depression may follow.

We have argued above that parents' responses to children's expressions of distress will depend on the child's gender. Over the course of their children's development, parents may become less tolerant of sadness and vulnerability in boys and of anger in girls. Thus, parents' responses to children's expressions of distress may work to differentiate children's characteristic styles of responding to negative social interactions.

Children from abusive families are likely to develop an exaggerated tendency to show distress in sex-typed ways. First, they will display more distress, more often. In this way, they will evoke gender-differentiated responses from their parents more frequently than typical children. Second, they will have parents who are more reactive to expressions of vulnerability in boys and anger in girls. Third, they will have stronger models in their distressed parents for sex-typed expressions of distress in that mothers in maltreating families are often depressed and fathers are likely to provide models of aggressive behavior.

There is suggestive evidence that sex-typed socialization is more pronounced in maltreating families. Both Goldner et al. (1990) and Walker (1979) claim that gender-stereotyped child-rearing styles are experienced by spouses in abusive marital relationships. They posit that women in abusive relationships often come from families that foster a dependence on interpersonal relationships. They were made to feel that "they did not count unless they were tending to the needs of others" and that "being loved was contingent upon some kind of self-abnegation." By contrast, Goldner et al. (1990) and Walker (1979) portray violent men as socialized in a culture in which male violence was normative. Goldner and colleagues proposed that violent men are excessively fearful of feeling vulnerable, which they equate with being a wimp. They overcompensate for these feelings with violence. Such feelings of vulnerability are activated especially by feeling dependent on a woman. These sentiments were voiced as follows by one batterer participating in the Goldner et al. (1990) study: "I must never feel fear, know, need, respect a woman's point of view."

Although neither Goldner et al. (1990) nor Walker (1979) directly studied child-abusive families, there is evidence of a strong overlap between maritally violent and child-abusive families. Straus, Gelles, & Steinmetz (1977) reported that in a national sample, a third of battered women and a third of battering husbands abused their children. Steinmetz (1977) found a correlation of 0.50 between the use of physical force to resolve marital arguments and parent–child disputes. Herrenkohl and Herrenkohl (1981) observed that violence between adult family members had occurred in the previous year in 44% of the child-abusive families they studied. Finally, in the Straus et al. (1980) national sample, traditional sex-typed marital relationships in which husbands are dominant and wives are submissive are predictive of all types of family violence. Although no one has yet directly investigated the traditionality of male–female expectations in child-abusive families, it appears reasonable to predict that gender-differentiated behavior and expectations are exaggerated in these families. This view resonates with findings from the clinical literature documenting patterns of dominance and submissive parenting in clinical samples (Terr, 1970). In fact, there is suggestive evidence that abused children are more sex-typed that nonabused children (August & Forman, 1989).

We have argued that sex-typed socialization that fosters dominance in males and dependency in females may be exaggerated in troubled families. We believe that the gender-differentiated emphasis on dominance vs. dependency is the essential feature of sex-typed behavior that facilitates the victimization process and underlies the gender-differentiated expression of distress. If this is true, then the pattern of aggression and dependency that we believe emerges in relations between males and females from troubled families should also emerge in same-sex dyads in which one member is dominant and the other is submissive. That this may be the case at least for victimization is illustrated by the work of Troy and Sroufe (1986) with same-sex dyads in which the victimizer–victim pattern emerges. Working from an attachment perspective, they observed the interactions of same-sex dyads in which neither child, one child, or both children had an insecure attachment relationship with the mother. Victim–victimizer relationships emerged only in the interactions of two insecurely attached children. Qualitative analyses of the dyadic interactions revealed transactions that maintained the victimization relationship, in that victims often sought continuation of the relationship through unreciprocated positive overtures. For example, in one dyad the victimizer made only 2 positive overtures to the victim. By contrast, the victim made 119 attempts to initiate friendly activity, all but 6 of which were rejected. The friendly initiatives in a matched nonvictimizing dyad were balanced. It appeared that maintaining the relationship was essential to the victimized child, and rejection activated solicitous behavior rather than breaking away from the relationship.

Gender Differences in the Attributions and Adjustment of Children from Troubled Families

We review some indirect evidence for our proposal that males and females from troubled homes should show exaggerated differences in attributional and behavioral responses to perceived threats of rejection.

The work of Dodge and his colleagues provides some evidence of the model for boys. Specifically, in a series of studies, they find, first, that when expectations of rejection are activated, hostile attributional biases about peers' behaviors are activated in aggressive boys (Dodge & Somberg, 1987). Furthermore, such biases are found to mediate the association between the use of harmful physical punishment by parents and aggression in boys (Dodge et al., 1990). However, this model does not appear to hold as well for girls as for boys, in the girls did not have as strong a tendency to engage in blaming someone else when they experienced something negative. Moreover, physically harmed girls show higher levels of depressive symptomatology than physically harmed boys, and hostile attributional biases do not mediate depressive symptomatology (Dodge et al., 1990). Thus, it appears that girls' reactions to negative interpersonal events are less clearly evident in other-blame than are boys' reactions.

There is also evidence that troubled family relationships, indexed by insecure parent–child attachment relations, are linked with gender-differentiated maladaptive behavior patterns in children. Lewis, Feiring, McGuffog, and Jaskir (1984) found higher rates of internalizing problems in insecurely attached girls and heightened rates of externalizing problems in insecurely attached boys. Focusing on the social interactions of preschool children, Turner (1991) found that whereas securely attached boys and girls were moderately aggressive, assertive, and controlling, insecurely attached boys showed more aggressive, disruptive, assertive, controlling, and attention-seeking behavior than secure children. By contrast, insecurely attached girls showed more dependent behavior, positive expressive behavior, such as smiling, and more compliance than did securely attached children. These girls were also less assertive and controlling than their securely attached counterparts. Their strategy with peers appeared to be one of avoiding active participation or conflict, of being followers rather than leaders.

Although insecure attachment does not necessarily imply that a child has experienced abusive parenting, there is considerable evidence linking it with troubled parent–child interactions in the early years.

Conclusions

This chapter examined the claim that children who experience interpersonal victimization are at risk for depression in addition to aggression. Our review of the relevant literatures supports this claim. We also sought to explain why maltreated children were at heightened risk for both forms of maladjustment. We drew on existing research sources for indirect support for our model. Our general hypothesis is that rejection sensitivity—i.e., a disposition to anxiously evaluate social interactions for evidence of rejection—is common to abused children with either disruptive disorders or depression. We expect rejection sensitivity to develop in children from families that respond to conflict with criticism rather than problem-solving; because they lack the skills or orientation to resolve interpersonal problems, these children may resort to blaming when they perceive rejection.

To protect themselves from the loss of self-esteem and depression that accompany self-blame, we propose that rejection-sensitive children will engage in other-blame. Because violent families often hold traditional sex-role stereotypes (Goldner et al., 1990), abusive parents will probably emphasize a self-protective orientation in boys and a relationship-protective orientation in girls (Gilligan, 1982). Consequently, to protect themselves, rejection-sensitive boys may resort to other-blame; to protect their relationship with their adversary, rejection-sensitive girls may use more indirect means of displacing blame onto their adversary, such as storming away in the hope of obtaining an apology or engaging in appeasing behavior in the hope of changing their adversary's evaluation of their worth. Because these indirect strategies may be less successful in protecting against self-blame than direct strategies, the children may be more likely to revert to self-blame, with an accompanying loss in self-esteem and depressive affect.

More generally, we argue that progress in understanding the impact of maltreatment on children requires moving beyond simple main-effects models, in which researchers assume a direct effect of maltreatment on child outcomes. Instead, researchers need to develop models that permit the adverse effects of maltreatment to be revealed in different ways for different children. In this chapter, we have focused on the possibility that the effects of maltreatment are expressed differently in boys and girls. We have further proposed that this difference is true for the following reasons: (1) The socialization context of abusive homes affords different possibilities for the expression of distress by males and females. (2) Because of sex-typed socialization, boys and girls bring different motivational frameworks to bear on their appraisal of distressing situations. (3) Because of differential socialization in managing conflict, children from abusive families have different problem-solving competencies than children from nonabusive families.

At a broader level, we propose that understanding the impact of family stress on child development requires attention to competencies, motives, socialization goals, and contextual affordances. Thus, to facilitate progress, research on family stressors, including maltreatment, must move beyond single stressor–single outcome models.

Aber, J. L., Allen, J. P., Carlson, V., & Cicchetti, D. (1989). The effects of maltreatment on development during early childhood: Recent studies and their theoretical, clinical, and policy implications. In D. Cicchetti & V. Carlson (Eds.), *Child maltreatment* (pp. 579–619). New York: Cambridge University Press.

Abramson, L. Y., Seligman, M. E. P., & Teasdale, J. D. (1978). Learned helplessness in humans: Critique and reformulation. *Journal of Abnormal Psychology, 87*, 49–74.

Achenbach, T. M. (1979). The child behavior profile. An empirically based system for assessing children's behavioral problems and competencies. *International Journal of Mental Health, 2*, 22–42.

Affleck, G., McGrade, B. J., Allen, D., & McQueeney, M. (1985). Mothers' beliefs about behavioral causes for their developmentally disabled infant's condition: What do they signify? *Journal of Pediatric Psychology, 10*, 293–303.

Ainsworth, M. D. S. (1973). The development of infant–mother attachment. In B. M. Caldwell & H. N. Ricciuti (Eds.), *Review of child development research*, Vol. 3 (pp. 1–94). Chicago: University of Chicago Press.

Akiskal, H. S. (1991). An integrating perspective on recurrent mood disorders: The mediating role of personality. In J. Becker & A. Kleinman (Eds.), *Psychosocial aspects of depression* (pp. 215–236). Hillsdale, NJ: Erlbaum Associates.

Allen, D., & Tarnowski, K. (1989). Depressive characteristics of physically abused children. *Journal of Abnormal Child Psychology, 17*, 1–11.

Allison, P. D., & Furstenberg, F. F. (1989). How marital dissolution affects children: Variations by age and sex. *Developmental Psychology, 25*, 540–549.

Almann, E. O., & Gotlib, I. H. (1988). The social behavior of depressed children: An observational study. *Journal of Abnormal Child Psychology, 16*, 29–44.

Amanat, E., & Butler, C. (1984). Oppressive behaviors in the families of depressed children. *Family Therapy, 11*, 67–77.

American Humane Association (1988). *Highlights of official child neglect and abuse reporting*. Denver: Author.

American Psychiatric Association (1994). *Diagnostic and statistical manual of mental disorders*, 4th ed. Washington, DC: Author.

Ammerman, R., Cassisi, J., Hersen, M., & Van Hasselt, V. (1986). Consequences of physical abuse and neglect in children. *Clinical Psychology Review, 6*, 291–310.

Andrews, B., & Brown, G. W. (1988). Marital violence in the community: A biographical approach. *British Journal of Psychiatry, 153*, 305–312.

Asarnow, J. R., Carlson, G. A., & Guthrie, D. (1987). Coping strategies, self-perceptions, hopelessness, and perceived family environments in depressed and suicidal children. *Journal of Consulting and Clinical Psychology, 55*, 361–366.

August, R. L., & Forman, B. D. (1989). A comparison of sexually abused and non-sexually abused children's behavioral responses to anatomically correct dolls. *Child Psychiatry and Human Development, 20*, 39–47.

Bagley, C., & Ramsey, R. (1985). Psychosocial correlates of suicidal behavior in an urban population. *Crisis, 6*, 63–77.

Beitchman, J., Zucker, K., Hood, J., & DeCosta, G. (1991). A review of the short-term effects of child sexual abuse. *Child Abuse and Neglect, 15*, 537–556.

Belle, D. (1982). *Lives in stress: Women and depression*. Beverly Hills: Sage Publications.

Bem, S. L. (1984). Androgyny and gender schema theory: A conceptual and empirical integration. *Nebraska Symposium on Motivation, 32*, 179–226.

Bifulco, A., Brown, G., & Adler, Z. (1991). Early sexual abuse and clinical victimization in adult life. *British Journal of Psychiatry, 159*, 115–122.

Boeke, K., & Markman, H. J. (1992). Relationship violence: From premarriage to the seven year itch. Paper presented at the Life History Conference and Psychopathology Conference, Philadelphia.

Bowlby, J. (1958). The nature of the child's tie to his mother. *International Journal of Psychoanalysis, 39*, 350–373.

Breier, A., Kelsoe, J. R., Jr., Kirwin, P. D., Beller, S. A., Wolkowitz, O. M., & Pickar, D. (1988). Early parental loss and development of adult psychopathology. *Archives of General Psychiatry, 45*, 987–993.

Brent, M. K. (1991). Attributions of female adolescent incest victims regarding their molestation. *Child Abuse and Neglect, 15*, 477–483.

Briere, J., & Runtz, M. (1988). Symptomatology associated with childhood sexual victimization in a nonclinical adult sample. *Child Abuse and Neglect, 12*, 51–59.

Briere, J., & Runtz, M. (1990). Differential adult symptomatology associated with three types of child abuse histories. *Child Abuse and Neglect, 14*, 357–364.

Briere, J., & Zaidi, L. Y. (1989). Sexual abuse histories and sequelae in female psychiatric emergency room patients. *American Journal of Psychiatry, 146*, 1602–1606.

Brown, G. W., & Anderson, B. (1991). Psychiatric morbidity in adult inpatients with childhood histories of sexual and physical abuse. *American Journal of Psychiatry, 148*, 55–61.

Brown, G. W., Bifulco, A., & Andrews, B. (1990). Self-esteem and depression: Aetiological issues. *Social Psychiatry and Psychiatric Epidemiology, 25*, 235–243.

Browne, A., & Finkelhor, D. (1986). Impact of child sexual abuse: A review of the research. *Psychological Bulletin, 99*, 66–77.

Bryer, J. B., Nelson, B. A., Miler, J. B., & Krol, P. A. (1987). Childhood sexual and physical abuse as factors in adult psychiatric illness. *American Journal of Psychiatry, 144*, 1426–1430.

Bulman, R. J., & Wortman, C. B. (1977). Attributions of blame and coping in the "real world": Severe accident victims react to their lot. *Journal of Personality and Social Psychology, 35*, 351–363.

Burbach, D. J., & Borduin, C. M. (1986). Parent–child relations and the etiology of depression: A review of methods and findings. *Clinical Psychology Review, 6*, 133–153.

Capaldi, D. M. (1992). Co-occurrence of conduct problems and depressive symptoms in early adolescent boys. II. A 2-year follow-up of grade 8. *Development and Psychopathology, 4*, 125–144.

Carlson, V., Cicchetti, D., Barnett, D., & Braunwald, K. (1989). Disorganized/disoriented attachment relationships in maltreated infants. *Developmental Psychology, 25*, 525–531.

Carmen, E. H., Rieker, P. P., & Mills, T. (1984). Victims of violence and psychiatric illness. *American Journal of Psychiatry, 14*, 378–383.

Chu, J. A., & Dill, D. L. (1990). Dissociative symptoms in relation to childhood physical and sexual abuse. *American Journal of Psychiatry, 147*, 887–892.

Cicchetti, D. (1987). Development psychopathology in infancy: Illustration from the study of maltreated youngsters. *Journal of Consulting and Clinical Psychology, 55*, 837–845.

Cicchetti, D., & Barnett, D. (1992). Attachment organization in maltreated preschoolers. In D. Cicchetti & B. Nurcombe (Eds.), *Development and psychopathology* (pp. 397–411). New York: Cambridge University Press.

Cole, D. A., & Rehm, L. P. (1986). Family interaction patterns and childhood depression. *Journal of Abnormal Psychology, 14*, 297–314.

Coyne, J. C. (1976). Depression and the response of others. *Journal of Abnormal Psychology, 85*, 186–193.

Coyne, J. C., Downey, G., & Boergers, J. (1992). Depression in families: A systems perspective. In D. Cicchetti & S. Toth (Eds.), *Developmental approaches to the affective disorders: Rochester symposium on developmental psychopathology*, Vol. 4. (pp. 211–250). Rochester, NY: University of Rochester Press.

Crittenden, P. M., & Ainsworth, M. D. S. (1989). Attachment and child abuse. In D. Cicchetti & V. Carlson (Eds.), *Child maltreatment: Theory and research on the causes and consequences of child abuse and neglect* (pp. 432–463). New York: Cambridge University Press.

Cummings, E. M., & Cicchetti, D. (1990). Attachment, depression, and the transmission of depression. In M. T. Greenberg, D. Cicchetti, & E. M. Cummings (Eds.), *Attachment in the preschool years: Theory, research, and intervention* (pp. 339–374). Chicago: University of Chicago Press.

Cutler, S. E., & Nolen-Hoeksema, S. (1990). Accounting for sex differences in depression through female victimization: Childhood sexual abuse. *Sex Roles, 24*, 425–438.

Dadds, M. R., Smith, M., Webber, Y., & Robinson, A. (1991). An exploration of family and individual profiles following father–daughter incest. *Child Abuse and Neglect, 4*, 575–586.

David, G. C., & Akiskal, H. (1986). Descriptive biological, theoretical aspects of borderline personality disorder. *Hospital and Community Psychiatry, 37*, 685–692.

Dean, A., Malik, M., Richards, W., & Stringer, S. (1986). Effects of parental maltreatment on children's conceptions of interpersonal relationships. *Developmental Psychology, 22*, 617–626.

Dodge, K. A., Bates, J. E., & Pettit, G. S. (1990). Mechanisms in the cycle of violence. *Science, 250*, 1678–1683.

Dodge, K. A., & Somberg, D. R. (1987). Hostile attributional biases among aggressive boys are exacerbated under conditions of threats to the self. *Child Development, 58*, 213–224.

Downey, G., & Coyne, J. C. (1990). Children of depressed parents: An integrative review. *Psychological Bulletin, 108*, 50–76.

Downey, G., Silver, R. C., & Wortman, C. (1990). Reconsidering the attribution–adjustment relation following a major negative event: Coping with the loss of a child. *Journal of Personality and Social Psychology, 59*, 925–940.

Downey, G., & Walker, E. F. (1989). Social cognition and adjustment in children at risk for psychopathology. *Developmental Psychology, 25,* 835–845.

Downey, G., & Walker, E. (1992). Distinguishing family-level and child-level influences on the development of depression and aggression. *Development and Psychopathology, 4,* 81–86.

Egeland, B., & Sroufe, L. A. (1981). Attachment and early maltreatment. *Child Development, 52,* 44–52.

Elder, G. H. J., & Caspi, A. (1988). Human development and social change: An emerging perspective on the life course. In N. Bolger, A. Caspi, G. Downey, & M. Moorhouse (Eds.), *Persons in context: Developmental processes.* New York: Cambridge University Press.

Elder, G. H., Jr., Caspi, A., & Downey, G. (1986). Problem behavior and family relationships: Life course and intergenerational themes. In A. Sorenson, F. Weinert, & L. Sherrod (Eds.), *Human development and the life course: Multidisciplinary perspectives.* Hillsdale, NJ: Erlbaum Associates.

Elliot, D. J., & Tarnowski, K. (1990). Depressive characteristics of sexually abused children. *Child Psychiatry and Human Development, 21,* 37–48.

Fagot, B. I. (1984). The consequents of problem behavior in toddler children. *Journal of Abnormal Child Psychology, 12,* 385–396.

Fagot, B. I., & Hagan, R. (1985). Aggression in toddlers: Responses to the assertive acts of boys and girls. *Sex Roles, 12,* 341–351.

Fagot, B. I., Hagan, R., & Leinbach, M. D. (1985). Differential reactions to assertive and communicative acts of toddler boys and girls. *Child Development, 56,* 1499–1505.

Fagot, B. I., & Hagan, R. (1991). Observations of parent reactions to sex-stereotyped behaviors: Age and sex effects. *Child Development, 62,* 617–628.

Fleming, J. E., & Offord, D. R. (1990). Epidemiology of childhood depressive disorders. *Journal of the American Academy of Child and Adolescent Psychiatry, 29,* 571–580.

Frazier, P. A. (1991). Self-blame as a mediator of post-rape depressive symptoms. *Journal of Social and Clinical Psychology, 10,* 47–57.

Freud, S. (1968). Mourning and melancholia. In J. Strachey (Ed.), *Standard edition of the complete works of Sigmund Freud,* Vol. 14. London: Hogarth Press (original published in 1917).

Friber, E. F., & Dinwiddie, S. H. (1992). Psychiatric correlates of incest in childhood. *American Journal of Psychiatry, 149,* 52–56.

Garbarino, J., & Gilliam, G. (1980). *Understanding abusive families.* Lexington, MA: Lexington Books.

Garber, J., Quiggle, N. C., Panak, W. F., & Dodge, K. A. (1992). Social information processing in aggressive and depressed children. *Child Development, 63,* 1305–1320.

Garmezy, N. (1983). Stressors of childhood. In N. Garmezy & M. Rutter (Eds.), *Stress, coping and development in children* (pp. 43–84). New York: McGraw-Hill.

Gelles, R., & Straus, M. A. (1988). *Intimate violence.* New York: Touchstone.

Gilligan, C. (1982). *In a different voice.* Cambridge, MA: Harvard University Press.

Gold, E. R. (1986). Long-term effects of sexual victimization in childhood: An attributional approach. *Journal of Consulting and Clinical Psychology, 54,* 471–475.

Goldner, V., Penn, P., Sheinberg, M., & Walker, G. (1990). Love and violence: Gender paradoxes in volatile attachments. *Family Process, 29,* 343–364.

Goodyer, I. M., Wright, C., & Altham, P. M. (1989). Recent friendships in anxious and depressed school age children. *Psychological Medicine, 19,* 165–174.

Hahlwag, K., & Goldstein, M. J. (Eds.) (1987). *Understanding major mental disorder: The contribution of family interaction research.* New York: Family Process Press.

Harrington, R., Fudge, H., Rutter, M., Pickles, A., & Hill, J. (1990). Adult outcomes of childhood and adolescent depression. *Archives of General Psychiatry, 47,* 465–473.

Harris, T., Brown, G. W., & Bifulco, A. (1990). Loss of parent in childhood and adult psychiatric disorder: A tentative overall model. *Development and Psychopathology, 2,* 311–328.

Herman, J. L., Perry, C., & Van der Kolk, B. A. (1989). Childhood trauma in borderline personality disorder. *American Journal of Psychiatry, 146,* 490–495.

Herrenkohl, R. C., & Herrenkohl, E. C. (1981). Some antecedents and developmental consequences of child maltreatment. In R. Rizley & D. Cicchetti (Eds.), *New directions for child development,* Vol. 11 (pp. 57–76). San Francisco: Jossey-Bass.

Hetherington, E. M., Cox, M., & Cox, R. (1982). Effects of divorce on parents and children. In M. Lamb (Ed.), *Nontraditional families* (pp. 233–288). Hillsdale, NJ: Erlbaum Associates.

Hilberman, E., & Munson, K. (1978). Sixty battered women. *Victimology, 2,* 460–470.

Hoagwood, K. (1990). Blame and adjustment among women sexually abused as children. *Women and Therapy, 9,* 89–110.

Holmes, S. J., & Robins, L. N. (1988). The role of parental disciplinary practices in the development of depression and alcoholism. *Psychiatry, 51*, 642–647.

Hooley, J. M., Orley, J., & Teasdale, J. D. (1986). Levels of expressed emotion and relapse in depressed patients. *British Journal of Psychiatry, 148*, 642–647.

Hooley, J. M., & Teasdale, J. D. (1989). Predictors of relapse in unipolar depressives: Expressed emotion, marital distress, and perceived criticism. *Journal of Abnormal Psychology, 98*, 229–235.

Hunter, J. A. (1991). A comparison of the psychosocial maladjustment of adult males and females sexually molested as children. *Journal of Interpersonal Violence, 6*, 205–217.

Jacobson, A., & Richardson, B. (1987). Assault experiences of 100 psychiatric inpatients: Evidence of the need for routine inquiry. *American Journal of Psychiatry, 144*, 908–913.

Janoff-Bulman, R. (1979). Characterological versus behavioral self-blame: Inquiries into depression and rape. *Journal of Personality and Social Psychology, 37*, 1798–1809.

Jones, T., McClean, B., & Young, J. (1986). *The Islington crime survey*. Aldershot, England: Gower.

Jose, M. C., & Downey, G. (1992). Children with incarcerated mothers. University of Michigan.

Kashani, J. H., & Carlson, G. (1987). Seriously depressed preschoolers. *American Journal of Psychiatry, 144*, 348–350.

Kashani, J. H., Carlson, G., Beck, N. C., Hoeper, E. W., Corcoran, G. M., McAllister, J. A., Fallahi, C., Rosenberg, T. K., & Reid, J. C. (1987a). Depression, depressive symptoms, and depressed mood among a community sample of adolescents. *American Journal of Psychiatry, 144*, 931–934.

Kashani, J. H., Shekim, W. O., Burk, J. P., & Beck, N. C. (1987b). Abuse as a predictor of psychopathology in children and adolescents. *Journal of Clinical Child Psychology, 16*, 43–50.

Kaslow, N. J., Rehm, L. P., & Siegel, A. W. (1984). Social cognition and cognitive correlates of depression in children. *Journal of Abnormal Child Psychology, 12*, 605–620.

Kaufman, J. (1991). Depressive disorders in maltreated children. *Journal of the American Academy of Child and Adolescent Psychiatry, 30*, 257–265.

Kaufman, J., & Cicchetti, D. (1989). Effects of maltreatment on school-age children's socioemotional development: Assessments in a day-camp setting. *Developmental Psychology, 25*, 516–524.

Kazdin, A., Moser, J., Colbus, D., & Bell, R. (1985). Depressive symptoms among physically abused and psychiatrically disturbed children. *Journal of Abnormal Psychology, 94*, 298–307.

Kennedy, E., Spence, S. H., & Henaley, R. (1989). An examination of the relationship between childhood depression and social competence among primary school children. *Journal of Child Psychology, Psychiatry, and Allied Disciplines, 4*, 561–573.

Koss, M. (1990). The women's mental health research agenda: Violence against women. *American Psychologist, 45*, 374–380.

Lazarus, R. F. (1984). On the primacy of cognition. *American Psychologist, 39*, 124–129.

Leff, J., & Vaughn, C. E. (1985). *Expressed emotion in families: Its significance for mental illness*. New York: Guilford Press.

Lefkowitz, M. M., & Burton, N. (1978). Childhood depression: A critique of the concept. *Psychological Bulletin, 85*, 716–726.

Lewis, M., Feiring, C., McGuffog, C., & Jaskir, J. (1984). Predicting psychopathology in six-year-olds from early social relations. *Child Development, 55*, 123–136.

Livingston, R. (1987). Sexually and physically abused children. *Journal of the American Academy of Child and Adolescent Psychiatry, 26*, 413–415.

Ludolph, P. S., Westen, D., Misle, B., Jackson, A., Wixom, & Weiss, F. C. (1990). The borderline diagnosis in adolescents: Symptoms and development history. *American Journal of Psychiatry, 147*, 470–476.

Lynch, M. A., & Roberts, J. (1982). *Consequences of child abuse*. London: Academic Press.

Lyons-Ruth, K., Connell, D. B., Zoll, D., & Stahl, J. (1987). Infants at social risk: Relations among infant maltreatment, maternal behavior, and infant attachment behavior. *Developmental Psychology, 23*, 223–232.

Major, B., Mueller, P., & Hildebrandt, K. (1985). Attributions, expectations, and coping with abortion, *Journal of Personality and Social Psychology, 48*, 585–599.

McFarlane, A. C. (1987). Posttraumatic phenomena in a longitudinal study of children following a natural disaster. *Journal of the American Academy of Child and Adolescent Psychiatry, 26*, 764–769.

McGrath, E., Keita, G. P., Strickland, B. R., & Russo, N. F. (1990). *Women and depression: Risk factors and treatment issues*. Washington, DC: American Psychological Association.

Meyer, C., & Taylor, S. E. (1986). Adjustment to rape. *Journal of Personality and Social Psychology, 50*, 1226–1234.

Miklowitz, D., Goldstein, M., Nuechterlein, K., & Snyder, K. (1988). Family factors and the course of bipolar affective disorder. *Archives of General Psychiatry, 45*, 225–231.

Morrison, J. (1984). Childhood molestation reported by women with somatization disorder. *Annals of Clinical Psychiatry, 1,* 25–32.

Mullins, L. L., Peterson, L., Wonderlich, S., & Reaven, N. M. (1986). The influence of depressive symptomatology in children on the social responses and perceptions of adults. *Journal of Clinical Child Psychology, 15,* 233–240.

Oates, R. K., Forrest, D., & Peacock, A. (1985). Self-esteem of abused children. *Child Abuse and Neglect, 9,* 159–163.

Orlofsky, J. L. (1979). Parental antecedents of sex-role orientation in college men and women. *Sex Roles, 5,* 495–512.

Patterson, G. R. (1982). *Coercive family process.* Eugene, OR: Castilia Press.

Pfeffer, C., & Trad, P. (1988). Sadness and suicidal tendencies in preschool children. *Journal of Developmental and Behavioral Pediatrics, 9,* 86–88.

Poznanski, E. O. (1982). The clinical phenomenology of childhood depression. *American Journal of Orthopsychiatry, 52,* 308–313.

Poznanski, E., & Zrull, J. P. (1970). Childhood depression. *Archives of General Psychiatry, 23,* 8–15.

Puig-Antich, J., Lukens, E., Davies, M., Goetz, D., Quattrock, J. B., & Todak, G. (1985a). Psychosocial functioning in prepubertal major depressive disorders. *Archives of General Psychiatry, 42,* 500–507.

Puig-Antich, J., Lukens, E., Davies, M., Goetz, D., Quattrock, J. B, & Todak, G. (1985b). Controlled studies of psychosocial functioning in prepubertal major depressive disorders. II. Interpersonal relationships after sustained recovery from the affective episode. *Archives of General Psychiatry, 42,* 511–517.

Puig-Antich, J., Peral, J. M., Lupatkin, W., Chambers, W. J., Tabrizi, M. A., King, J., Goetz, R., Davies, M., & Stiller, R. L. (1987). Imipramine in prepubertal major depressive disorders. *Archives of General Psychiatry, 44,* 81–89.

Putnam, F. W. (1989). *Diagnosis and treatment of multiple personality disorder.* New York: Guilford Press.

Renouf, A. J., & Harter, S. (1990). Low self-worth and anger as components of the depressive experience in young adolescents. *Development and Psychopathology, 2,* 293–310.

Rosenberg, M. (1979). *Conceiving the self.* New York: Basic Books.

Sanders, B., & Giolas, M. H. (1991). Dissociation and childhood trauma in psychologically disturbed adolescents. *American Journal of Psychiatry, 148,* 50–54.

Schneider-Rosen, K., Braunwald, K. G., Carlson, V., & Cicchetti, D. (1985). Current perspectives in attachment theory: Illustrations from the study of maltreated infants. *Monographs of the Society for Research in Child Development, 50,* 194–210.

Shearer, S. L., Peters, C. P., Quaytman, M. S., & Ogden, R. L. (1990). Frequency and correlates of childhood sexual and physical abuse histories in adult female borderline patients. *American Journal of Psychiatry, 147,* 214–216.

Sprafkin, C., Serbin, L. A., & Elman, M. (1982). Sex typing of play and psychological adjustment in young children: An empirical investigation. *Journal of Abnormal Child Psychology, 10,* 559–568.

Sroufe, L. A., & Jacovitz, D. (1989). Diverging pathways, development transformations, multiple etiologies and the problem of continuity in child development. *Human Development, 32,* 196–203.

Stein, J. A., Golding, J. M., Siegel, J. M., Burnam, M. A., & Sorenson, S. B. (1988). Long-term psychological sequelae of child sexual abuse: The Los Angeles Epidemiological Catchment Area Study. In G. E. Wyatt & G. J. Powell (Eds.), *Lasting effects of child sexual abuse.* Newbury Park, CA: Sage Publications.

Steinmetz, S. (1977). *The cycle of violence.* New York: Praeger Publishers.

Straus, M., Gelles, R., & Steinmetz, S. (1980). *Behind closed doors: Violence in the American family.* New York: Anchor.

Straus, M. A. (1992). Corporal punishment of children and depression and suicide in adulthood. Paper presented at the annual meeting of the Society for Life History Research, Philadelphia.

Terr, L. A. (1970). A family study of child abuse. *American Journal of Psychiatry, 127,* 665–671.

Terr, L. A. (1983). Chowchilla revisited: The effects of psychic trauma four years after a school-bus kidnapping. *American Journal of Psychiatry, 140,* 1543–1550.

Terr, L. A. (1990). *Too scared to cry.* New York: Harper & Row.

Tong, L., Oates, K., & McDowell, M. (1987). Personality development following sexual abuse. *Child Abuse and Neglect, 11,* 371–383.

Toth, S. L., Manly, J. T., & Cicchetti, D. (1992). Child maltreatment and vulnerability to depression. *Development and Psychopathology, 4,* 97–112.

Troy, M., & Sroufe, L. A. (1986). Victimization among preschoolers: The role of attachment relationship history. *Journal of the American Academy of Child Psychiatry, 26,* 166–172.

Turner, P. J. (1991). Relationships between attachment, gender, and behavior with peers in pre-school. *Child Development, 62,* 1475–1488.

Walker, L. E. (1979). *The battered woman*. New York: Harper & Row.

Weiner, B. (1985). "Spontaneous" causal thinking. *Psychological Bulletin, 97*, 74–84.

Westat Associates (1987). *Study of National Incidence and Prevalence of Child Abuse and Neglect: Final Report*. Washington, DC: National Center on Child Abuse and Neglect, U.S. Department of Health and Human Services.

Westen, D. (1991). Social cognition and object relations. *Psychological Bulletin, 109*, 429–455.

Wideger, T. A., & Shea, T. (1991). Differentiation of Axis I and Axis II disorders. *Journal of Abnormal Psychology, 100*, 394–406.

Widom, C. (1989a). Does violence beget violence? A critical examination of the literature. *Psychological Bulletin, 106*, 3–28.

Widom, C. (1989b). The cycle of violence. *Science, 244*, 515–521.

Wodarski, J. S., Kurtz, P. D., Gaudin, J. M., & Howing, P. T. (1990). Maltreatment and the school-age child: Major academic, socioemotional, and adaptive outcomes. *Social Work, 35*, 506–513.

Wortman, C. B. (1976). Causal attributions and personal control. In J. H. Harvey, W. J. Ickes, & R. F. Kidd (Eds.), *New directions in attribution research* (pp. 23–51). Hillsdale, NJ: Erlbaum.

Wyatt, G. E., & Newcomb, M. D. (1990). Internal and external mediators of women's sexual abuse in childhood. *Journal of Consulting and Clinical Psychology, 58*, 758–767.

Zajonc, R. B. (1984). On the primacy of affect. *American Psychologist, 39*, 117–123.

Ziv, D., & Israeli, R. (1973). Effects of bombardment on the manifest anxiety level of children living in kibbutzim. *Journal of Consulting and Clinical Psychology, 40*, 287–291.

23

Psychosocial Stress and Child and Adolescent Depression

Can We Be More Specific?

Bruce E. Compas, Kathryn E. Grant, and Sydney Ey

The development of depressed mood, syndromes, and disorders during childhood and adolescence is the consequence of a complex array of personal and social factors. Evidence has been garnered to support the role of biological, psychological, familial, peer, and broader social influences. Researchers are now faced with the formidable task of integrating the contributions of these factors to the development and maintenance of depressive phenomena in young people. It is likely that the strongest explanation will reflect a broad biopsychosocial model of the etiology and course of depressive experiences (Petersen, Compas, Brooks-Gunn, Stemmler, Ey, & Grant, 1993). Our concern here is with one component of a biopsychosocial model: stressful events and processes.

Psychosocial stress plays a prominent role in most models of depression throughout the life span. Research on the relation between stress and depression in adults has provided rich information on the link between a variety of different types of stressful experiences and depressive symptoms and disorders (e.g., Brown & Harris, 1989). Theoretical perspectives on the role of stress in adult depression have typically considered the interaction of psychosocial stress with a personal vulnerability or predisposition on the part of the affected individual within the perspective of diathesis–stress models of depressive disorders (e.g., Monroe & Simons, 1991).

Research on the role of stress in depressive phenomena during childhood and adolescence has lagged behind similar research with adults. This delay is the result of several factors, including disagreement about the conceptualization of depressive phenomena in children and youth, the absence of a theoretical framework to guide research on

NOTE: This chapter was originally written in early 1992 and reflects the literature up to that point.

Bruce E. Compas • Department of Psychology, University of Vermont, Burlington, Vermont 05405-0134. **Kathryn E. Grant** • Cook County Medical Center, Chiago, Illinois 60626. **Sydney Ey** • Medical College of South Carolina, Charleston, South Carolina 29425.

Handbook of Depression in Children and Adolescents, edited by William M. Reynolds and Hugh F. Johnston. Plenum Press, New York, 1994.

stress in these age groups, and the lack of adequate measures to assess both stress and depression in young people. As we will show in this chapter, however, recent evidence has accumulated to document a clear relation between stressful experiences and depressive phenomena in children and adolescents.

In examining research on stress and depression, it is important to attend to issues of specificity in the stress–depression relation (e.g., Monroe, 1990). A primary concern is establishing whether and to what degree stress is associated with depressive phenomena. A second question, however, is concerned with the degree to which any associations that are observed between stress and depression are unique to depression as opposed to reflecting a more general association between stress and psychopathology. As we discuss below, the high degree of covariation and comorbidity of depressive symptoms and disorders with other types of symptoms and disorders presents a challenge to researchers in determining the degree of specificity in this relation.

Defining Child and Adolescent Depression and Stress

Child and Adolescent Depression

Empirical studies have established that depressed mood, depressive syndromes, and depressive disorders are related but distinct manifestations of depression (Cantwell & Baker, 1991; Compas, Ey, & Grant, 1993; Kovacs, 1989; Petersen, Kennedy, & Sullivan, 1991a). It is important to recognize these three constructs as unique representations of depressive phenomena in considering research on stress and depression. The first approach is concerned with *depressed mood* and affect (e.g., Petersen et al., 1991a; Kandel & Davies, 1982). The study of depressed mood is concerned with depression as a symptom and refers to the presence of sadness, unhappiness, or blue feelings for an unspecified period of time. The second approach is concerned with syndromes of behaviors and emotions that reflect depression; *depressive syndromes* are identified empirically through the reports of adolescents and other important informants (e.g., parents, teachers) (Achenbach, 1985, 1991). The concept of a depressive syndrome refers to a set of emotions and behaviors that have been found statistically to occur together in an identifiable pattern at a rate that exceeds chance, without implying any particular model for the nature or causes of these associated symptoms. The third approach is based on assumptions of a disease or disorder model of psychopathology and is currently reflected in the *categorical diagnostic* system of the *Diagnostic and Statistical Manual of Mental Disorders*, Fourth Edition (DSM-4), of the American Psychiatric Association (1994) and the *International Classification of Diseases, Injuries, and Causes of Death*, tenth edition (ICD-10), of the World Health Organization (1990).

It is also acknowledged in all three of these approaches that there is a high degree of covariation and comorbidity of depressive phenomena with other symptoms and disorders (e.g., Compas & Hammen, 1994). It is safe to say that with regard to all three manifestations of depressive phenomena, covariation/comorbidity is the rule rather than the exception during childhood and adolescence. Although covariation/comorbidity with anxiety symptoms and disorders is most common, depressive phenomena co-occur with a variety of other symptoms and disorders, including conduct disorders, eating disorders, and substance abuse.

The implications of these various conceptualizations for research concerned with stress and child and adolescent depression are twofold. First, it is important to specify which level of depressive phenomena has been the focus of any given piece of research, as findings that are reflective of one level of depressive phenomena may or may not hold for the other levels. Second, in light of patterns of covariation and comorbidity of depressive phenomena, attention must be given to other forms of symptoms and disorders to determine whether the findings are unique to depression as opposed to other forms of psychopathology.

511

Psychosocial Stress
and Depression

Child and Adolescent Stress

Few constructs in research on mental health and psychopathology have been as important but at the same time as difficult to define as the concept of "stress." Numerous definitions have emerged over the years, some of which have been so broad or difficult to operationalize as to render them useless for the purpose of scientific inquiry. That stress continues to play a major role despite these substantial problems in conceptualization and measurement is testimony to the centrality of this concept to most models of psychopathology.

As a result of confusion surrounding the definition of stress, several different approaches to measuring child and adolescent stressful experiences have been used. One approach has focused on stress as manifested in discrete environmental events (e.g., loss of a loved one, natural disaster, sudden economic change) that represent measurable changes in individuals' environmental conditions (e.g., Holmes & Rahe, 1967). An alternative approach is reflected in transactional models that view stress as a consequence of environmental events and circumstances as they are perceived or appraised by the individual (e.g., Lazarus & Folkman, 1984). Conceptualizations of stress have also differed in their emphasis on the occurrence of major changes in the individual's life situation that involve significant levels of social readjustment as opposed to ongoing daily transactions with the environment, as reflected in daily hassles, chronic strains, or small events. Discussion of the merits of these different approaches is beyond the scope of this chapter; we have simply included research on child and adolescent stress that reflects each of these positions.

Issues in Research Design and Measurement

Confounding of Stress and Depression. An ongoing methodological concern for stress researchers involves the possibility that measures of stress and psychopathology may be confounded, with similar items appearing on measures of both constructs (Dohrenwend & Shrout, 1985). For example, fights or conflicts with others and worries or concerns about one's life situation have been included in some indices of stress, but are also symptoms of several forms of psychopathology. Further, measures of stress and psychopathology may be confounded by response biases. An individual's appraisal of the degree of stress and his or her self-report of psychopathology may both be the consequence of a third variable (e.g., negative affectivity) that influences her or his style of responding to self-report measures of both stress and psychopathology (Watson & Pennebaker, 1989).

Concerns with possible confounding are balanced by concerns with theory. For example, models of stress and psychopathology that emphasize the role of cognitive appraisals of the self and the environment must measure stress in ways that reflect appraisal processes. To eliminate appraisals and perceptions of stress in an attempt to achieve a more "objective" index of stress would omit the core element of the stress process as conceptualized by transactional models (Lazarus, DeLongis, Folkman, & Gruen, 1985). Therefore, some researchers have chosen to include cognitive appraisals as part of the stress construct and to contend with the resulting methodological problems. Moreover, much of the research on child and adolescent stress and depression has not been guided by an explicit theoretical model. In consequence, it cannot be determined in many cases whether the measures used were consistent with any model.

Determining Specificity. It is a laudable goal for depression researchers to attempt to determine whether certain types of stress are uniquely related to depressive symptoms, syndromes, and disorders as opposed to other forms of psychopathology. Predictors of depressive outcomes, as opposed to psychopathology in general, may be especially informative about the mechanisms that underlie the effects of stress and for the development of interventions. Despite the importance of this goal, the requirements for a research design to test the specificity of stress as a predictor of depression are rarely met. That they are not is partly a function of the necessary ingredients of the design of a study to test for specificity in relation to any form of psychopathology (Garber & Hollon, 1991). This problem is further compounded by the high rates of covariation and comorbidity of depressive phenomena with other manifestations of psychopathology.

Cross-Sectional versus Longitudinal Designs. The goal of most researchers in this area has been to determine the degree to which stress functions as a cause, correlate, or consequence of depression. Cross-sectional studies are useful in establishing that there is an association between stress and depression that is worthwhile to pursue in more costly longitudinal investigations. However, cross-sectional designs cannot address temporal relations between stress and depressive phenomena. Prospective designs are essential to examine the direction of the stress–depression association—whether stress predicts increases in depressive symptoms and whether depression predicts increases in stress. Despite the hope that prospective designs could allow for the inference of causality in these associations, it is important to remember that even prospective designs fail to control for "third variables" that could be influencing both stress and depression. Causal inferences are limited to the interpretation that data may be consistent with a hypothesized model but not provide definitive proof of the causal relationships within the model.

Stress and Depression: Empirical Studies of Children and Adolescents

Studies have examined a wide range of different types of stressful experiences in relation to depressed mood, depressive syndromes, and depressive disorders using both cross-sectional and prospective designs. Findings will be summarized in response to five pertinent questions: (1) Are stressful experiences correlated with higher levels of depressive phenomena? (2) Are stressful experiences predictive of subsequent increases in depressive phenomena? (3) What types of stress are related to depressive phenomena? (4) Is stress related specifically to depression, or is stress a general risk factor for psychopathology? (5) Are there developmental differences in the stress–depression relationship? In answering each of these questions, we will consider data from studies of discrete events that are traumatic in magnitude and studies of the accumulation of major life events, daily hassles, and chronic stressful conditions. Further, we will include studies that have measured depressed mood, depressive syndromes, or depressive disorders.

Are Stressful Experiences Correlated with Higher Levels of Depressive Phenomena?

Single Events. Depressed mood, syndromes, and disorders have been examined in association with a variety of discrete events, including natural disasters (e.g., McFarlane, 1987), human-made disasters (e.g., Cornely & Bromet, 1986), childhood illness and hospitalization (e.g., Kaplan, Busner, Weinhold, & Lenon, 1987), illness or hospitalization of a parent (e.g., Compas et al., in press), and parental victimization, death, or injury (e.g., Malmquist, 1986; Payton & Krocker-Tuskan, 1988). These studies have typically used cross-sectional designs to examine self-reports and parental reports of a variety of symptoms, including depressed mood, in children and adolescents near the time of their exposure to a traumatic event. Responses of children and parents on depressive symptom scales are then compared to normative data on these scales or, more rarely, to a comparison or control sample who had not experienced the trauma.

Mixed support has been found for an association between these types of discrete events and all three levels of depressive phenomena. For example, self-reports of depressed mood and symptoms were related to the experiences of children and adolescents diagnosed with cancer (Kaplan et al., 1987). Depressive symptoms of adolescent oncology patients were related to increased negative life events; for child oncology patients, depressive symptoms were related to the total number of hospitalizations they experienced (Kaplan et al., 1987). In contrast, the relationship between the stress of losing a parent and depressive symptoms was only indirect in a sample of adolescents (Gray, 1987). Depressive syndrome scores for children and adolescents whose parents have been diagnosed with cancer were quite varied, differing as a function of the age and gender of the child and whether it was the mother or the father who had cancer (Compas et al., in press).

Several studies have examined the effects of exposure to the Three Mile Island nuclear power plant disaster in which radioactive gases were released and a meltdown almost occurred. Hanford et al. (1986) found that a majority of children (mean age 13 years) reported residual levels of anxiety 1½ years after the event even though their parents described them as anxiety-free. Actual diagnoses of anxiety or depressive disorders, however, were within the percentage expected in a general population (Hanford et al., 1986). Cornely and Bromet (1986) also fund no significant psychological effects on preschool-age children in the Three Mile Island area.

Cumulative Life Events, Hassles, and Chronic Stress. Over 40 recent studies have established that there is a cross-sectional association between stressful events and depressed mood (Adams & Adams, 1991; Allgood-Merten, Lewinsohn, & Hops, 1990; Banez & Compas, 1990; Beck & Rosenberg, 1986; L. H. Cohen, Burt, & Bjork, 1987; Garrison, Jackson, Marsteller, McKeown, & Addy, 1990; Glyshaw, Cohen, & Towbes, 1989; Ham & Larson, 1990; Hops, Lewinsohn, Andrews, & Roberts, 1990; Kanner & Feldman, 1991; Luthar, 1991; Petersen, Sarigiani, & Kennedy, 1991b; Roosa, Beals, Sandler, & Pillow, 1990; Rowlison & Felner, 1988; Siegel & Brown, 1988; Towbes, Cohen, & Glyshaw, 1989; Varni, Rubenfeld, Talbot, & Setoguchi, 1989; Vernberg, 1990; Wagner & Compas, 1990; Wagner, Compas, & Howell, 1988; Walker & Greene, 1991), depressive syndromes (Brooks-Gunn & Warren, 1989; Compas, Howell, Phares, Williams, & Giunta, 1989a; Stanger, McConaughy, & Achenbach, 1992), and depressive disorders (Costello, 1989; Hammen, 1988; Hammen, Burge, & Adrian, 1991; Velez, Johnson, & Cohen, 1989; West, Sandler, Pillow, Baca, & Gersten, 1991). This relationship has been found when stress has been measured as the accumulation of major life events (e.g., L. H. Cohen et al., 1987) as well as daily events or hassles (e.g., Banez & Compas, 1990; Kanner & Feldman, 1991; Rowlison & Felner, 1988). These correlations have ranged from modest to moderate in magnitude, with correlations for major life events typically lower than those for minor events or hassles.

Exposure of children and adolescents to chronic stressful conditions has been examined most frequently in the context of the family. Chronic stress associated with parental psychopathology (for reviews, see Downey & Coyne, 1990; Hammen, 1991), economic hardship (e.g., Conger et al., 1992; Lempers, Clark-Lempers, & Simons, 1989), single-parent status (e.g., Compas & Williams, 1990), and marital conflict and discord (for a review, see Cummings & Davies, 1994) has received the greatest attention. Depressive phenomena are typically measured through scales of depressed mood and symptoms, and frequently these symptoms are aggregated with other symptoms and reported as part of an index of overall distress. Some forms of chronic stress are associated with depressive symptoms; however, this association is rarely direct. For example, it appears that depressed mood in children is related to parental economic hardship indirectly as a result of parental psychological symptoms and disrupted parent–child relationships (e.g., Conger et al., 1992).

Are Stressful Experiences Predictive of Subsequent Increases in Depressive Phenomena?

Single Events. Few studies of traumatic events have used prospective designs, making it difficult to determine the contribution of these events to depressive phenomena over time. Prospective data are essential, however, to determine the degree to which depressive reactions to traumatic events may be short-lived, endure over time, or increase with the passage of time.

Studies that have used prospective designs have found that the effects of traumatic events endure, at least over short periods of time. For example, the McFarlane (1987) study of preschool-age children exposed to an Australian bush fire found that parental reports of children's "stress" immediately after the fire (i.e., how much they talked about the fire and worried about fires in general) were related to children's emotional and behavioral problems 18 months later. Depressive symptoms were not measured separately in this study, however. We have used a prospective design to examine the effects of the diagnosis and treatment of parental cancer on child and adolescent adjustment at the time of the parent's diagnosis and 4 months later (Compas et al., in press; Grant et al., 1992). After controlling for overall gender differences in symptom reporting, we found that adolescent girls reported significantly greater depressive syndrome scores than adolescent boys at the time of diagnosis, but adolescent girls and boys did not differ 4 months later. Preadolescent boys and girls did not differ at the time of their parent's diagnosis or at 4-month follow-up.

Cumulative Life Events, Hassles, and Chronic Stress. Fourteen recent studies have used prospective designs to examine the association between stressful events and depressed mood (Allgood-Merten et al., 1990; L. H. Cohen et al. 1987; Garrison et al., 1990; Glyshaw et al., 1989; Hops et al., 1990; Petersen et al., 1991b; Roosa et al., 1990; Siegel & Brown, 1988; Wagner et al., 1988; Walker & Greene, 1991); depressive syndromes (Compas, Howell, Phares, Williams, & Giunta, 1989a; Stanger et al., 1992), and depressive disorders (Hammen, 1988; Hammen et al., 1991; Velez et al., 1989). The time period between data collections has varied from very brief intervals [e.g., 3 months (Wagner et al. 1988)] to relatively long periods [e.g., 8 years (Velez et al., 1989)].

An association has been found between stress and depressive phenomena at follow-up, even after controlling for initial depression. In other words, concurrent stress predicted an increase in depressive symptoms, syndromes, and disorders over the time between the two data collections (e.g., Allgood-Merten et al., 1990; L. H. Cohen et al. 1987; Compas et al., 1989a; Hammen et al., 1991; Petersen et al., 1991b; Stanger et al., 1992). Thus, recent stressful events are associated with observable increases in depressive phenomena over and above the initial levels of depression reported by children and adolescents.

Support has been more mixed for a longitudinal relation in which stress at the first data collection was used to predict depression at follow-up after controlling for initial levels of depression. Several studies examined this relation and failed to find a significant association between initial stress and subsequent depressed mood once initial depressed mood was controlled (L. H. Cohen et al., 1987; Glyshaw et al., 1989; Roosa et al., 1990). The two studies that examined depressive syndromes as dependent variables found a significant longitudinal relation between initial stress and subsequent depressive syndrome scores after controlling for initial depression (Compas et al. 1989a; Stanger et al., 1992).

Similarly, Hammen and colleagues found that initial stress predicted subsequent episodes of depressive diagnoses (Hammen, 1988; Hammen et al., 1991).

These studies have provided mixed support for the utility of initial levels of stress as a predictor of increases or decreases in depressive outcomes. Evidence has generally been stronger for the prediction of depressive syndromes and disorders than for depressed mood, a surprising finding in light of the greater severity of syndromes and disorders as compared with depressed mood. Further, more attention to the impact of informant effects on reports of stress and depression is needed, as both Compas et al. (1989a) and Stanger et al. (1992) found that children's self-reports of stress predicted their own self-reports of depressive syndromes but not their parents' reports of the children's depression.

The possibility that depressive symptoms may lead to increased stressful events has also been investigated in research on cumulative events. Several studies have shown that initial levels of depressed mood and syndromes are predictive of increased stress at a later time, after controlling for initial levels of stress (L. H. Cohen et al., 1987; Compas et al., 1989a; Roosa et al., 1990; Wagner et al., 1988; Walker & Greene, 1991). When considered along with the finding that initial stress predicts subsequent depression, these results suggest that stress and depression are reciprocally related, each contributing to increases in the other in a cyclical manner. Whether depressive symptoms may contribute to the occurrence of acute traumatic events or ongoing chronic stress warrants attention.

What Types of Stress Are Related to Depressive Phenomena?

Single Events. In reviewing the literature on children's exposure to traumatic events, Garmezy (1986), Anthony (1986), and Ferholt, Hoffnung, Hunter, and Leventhal (1986) identified the need to consider the "subjective" nature of stress as well as more quantifiable aspects of the experiences (e.g., number of hospitalizations, amount of physical damage, separation from family). Furthermore, stress may be differentiated in terms of the life domain of the child who has been affected. Events involving loss of a parent are hypothesized to have a more powerful effect on depressive phenomena than are other types of traumatic events.

In brief, depressive phenomena appear to be related to stressful events involving the loss of, harm to, or absence of a parent (e.g., Gray, 1987; Malmquist, 1986; Payton & Krocker-Tuskan, 1988; Pynoos and Nader, 1988; Skinner & Swartz, 1989). Stress from natural disasters such as floods and bush fires appears to be related to posttraumatic phenomena and some generalized distress; however, depression appears less prevalent in association with these events (Burke, Moccia, Borus, & Burns, 1989; McFarlane, 1987). Stress from a long-term illness such as cancer or from physical abuse is also related to depressive symptoms (Kaplan et al., 1987; Allen & Tarnowski, 1989). The stressful experiences of Cambodian refugees, which often involved psychological and physical abuse and the loss of their family members, were also related to depressive and posttraumatic symptoms (Kinzie, Sack, Angell, Manson, & Rath, 1986).

Cumulative Life Events, Hassles, and Chronic Stress. Subtypes of stress have been examined in studies of cumulative stress in three ways. First, as noted above, the relation of depression with major life events as opposed to daily stressors has been compared. Second, stressful events representing different life domains (e.g., family, peer relationships, academic achievement) have been compared in their association with depressive phenomena. Third, stressors have been distinguished on the basis of various objective and subjective dimensions, including controllability, predictability, and valence (positive vs. negative).

In those studies in which major and daily stressors have been compared, daily stressors have been found to be more strongly related to depressive phenomena than are major events (Compas et al., 1989a; Rowlison & Felner, 1988). Further, support has been found for an integrative model in which major life events lead to increases in daily stressors, which in turn lead to depressive outcomes (Compas, Howell, Phares, Williams, & Ledoux, 1989b; Wagner et al., 1988). Thus, certain major life events such as parental divorce, moving to a new home, or a serious illness in the family may contribute to depressive phenomena through the ongoing minor stresses and strains that such events produce.

Studies examining the relation of depressive phenomena with stress in different life domains have been relatively rare. This rarity may be partly the result of the use of measures of stressful events that have not contained a sufficiently large sample of different types of stressors to make comparisons across different domains. There is some evidence that stress in different life domains is experienced at different frequencies as a function of the age and gender of children and adolescents. For example, Wagner and Compas (1990) found that adolescent boys and girls differed in their reports of the frequency and perceived stressfulness of several types of interpersonal stress. However, there is no evidence to date to suggest that events in certain life domains are more closely related to depressive phenomena than are events in other domains.

A third approach to examining subtypes of stress has been to distinguish events on the basis of their controllability, predictability, or valence. For example, L. H. Cohen et al. (1987) found that depressed mood was related to both controllable and uncontrollable events. Data on depression and predictable vs. unpredictable events have been mixed. Ham and Larson (1990) found that expected events elicited more positive affect than unexpected events, but that expected negative events that were experienced frequently were more upsetting than unexpected events. Finally, evidence is clear that depressive phenomena are associated with the accumulation of negative but not positive events (e.g., Siegel & Brown, 1988).

Is Stress Related Specifically to Depression, or Is Stress a General Risk Factor for Psychopathology?

Single Events. The majority of the studies of traumatic events have focused on identifying "posttraumatic phenomena," typically measured as symptoms of posttraumatic stress syndrome (for a review see Anthony, 1986). The impact of natural disasters such as fires, floods, and earthquakes has been found to be related to greater preoccupations with the future, nightmares, greater general distress, and avoidance of disaster-related stimuli (e.g., Burke et al., 1986; McFarlane, 1987). Many researchers have investigated posttraumatic symptoms or depressive symptoms and failed to conduct a comprehensive assessment of other types of pathology. As an example, when broader measures of psychopathology were used [e.g., clinical interviews (Kinzie et al., 1986)], depression, anxiety, and posttraumatic disorders were found to be present in a significant number of Cambodian adolescents.

Cumulative Life Events, Hassles, and Chronic Stress. Findings from studies of cumulative events and hassles suggest that stress is a nonspecific risk factor for a wide range of internalizing and externalizing symptoms, syndromes, and disorders. That is, no evidence has been reported to suggest that cumulative stress is a specific predictor of depressive phenomena. Other types of problems that have been found to be related to cumulative major and daily stress include anxiety symptoms (Banez & Compas, 1990; L. H. Cohen et al., 1987; Compas et al., 1989a; Costello, 1989; Glyshaw et al., 1989; Roosa et al., 1990; Rowlison & Felner, 1988; Velez et al., 1989; Wagner & Compas, 1990; Wagner et al., 1988), externalizing behavior problems (Beck & Rosenberg, 1986; Brooks-Gunn & Warren, 1989; Compas et al., 1989a; Stanger et al., 1992; Velez et al., 1989), lower self-esteem

(L. H. Cohen et al., 1987; Rowlison & Felner, 1988), physical health problems (Rowlison & Felner, 1988; Siegel & Brown, 1988), and poor academic performance (Luthar, 1991).

Direct comparison of the association of stress with depression as opposed to other symptoms has not been reported. For example, in a comparison of broad-band categories of symptoms, Compas et al. (1989a) found that the prospective association, after controlling for initial symptoms, of major and daily stress was greater with internalizing problems ($sr2 = 0.11$) than with externalizing problems ($sr2 = 0.05$). Although these data suggest that stressful events are more strongly related to internalizing problems, the regression coefficients were not compared statistically, nor were separate analyses conducted of depressive symptoms compared with other internalizing symptoms.

The apparent lack of specificity in the association between cumulative life stress and depressive phenomena is not surprising, for two reasons. First, research has typically not been designed to examine the association between subtypes of stress and different manifestations of psychological distress and psychopathology. Thus, these studies may have been insensitive to possible patterns of specificity. Second, in light of the high degree of covariation/comorbidity of depressive phenomena, factors that are associated with increases in depression are likely to be associated with increases in other symptoms as well.

Are There Developmental Differences in the Stress–Depression Relationship?

In research on stress and depression, little attention has been given to the role of developmental differences and processes. This appears to be a major omission, especially in light of important developmental changes in the rates of depressive phenomena from childhood to adolescence (Petersen et al., 1993). It will be important to understand whether developmental changes in exposure to stress that attend adolescence are associated with increases in depressed mood and disorders. Further, developmental changes in the responses of children and adolescents to the same stressful experiences need to be considered. Recent research has provided examples of each of these types of developmental processes.

It appears that there are significant changes in the types of stress that are experienced in adolescence as compared to childhood and that these changes are also related to depressive phenomena. For example, in a longitudinal study of adolescents, Petersen and colleagues (e.g., Petersen et al., 1991b) found that adolescent girls experienced more challenging and stressful circumstances than adolescent boys, and these differences accounted for gender differences in depressed mood. Using a cross-sectional design, Wagner and Compas (1990) also found developmental differences in the relation between subtypes of stress and negative affect. Further, negative affect was predicted only by family events in young adolescents, peer events in middle adolescents, and academic events in a sample of older adolescents attending college (Wagner & Compas, 1990).

Recent evidence also suggests that there are developmental and gender differences in depressive responses to similar stressful circumstances. In our ongoing study of the stress associated with the diagnosis and treatment of cancer in a parent, we have found that adolescents, and especially adolescent girls whose mothers are ill, reported more symptoms of depression and anxiety at the time of their parent's diagnosis and 4 months after the diagnosis than did younger children (Compas et al., in press).

Summary

It is clear that a wide range of stressful experiences and processes are associated with depressive phenomena in children and adolescents. Natural and man-made disasters, chronic adversity, and the accumulation of major and daily stressful events are all associated with depressive outcomes. Further, although a number of methodological problems remain unresolved, longitudinal studies have indicated that the association between stress and depression is not simply an artifact of self-reports of these two variables obtained at the same point in time; that is, stressful events predict meaningful increases in depression over time. Differences in this association as a function of types of stress, types of co-occurring symptoms and disorders, and developmental level are less well understood.

Where Are We and Where Do We Go From Here?

Despite the substantial contributions made by recent studies, research on the role of stress in child and adolescent depressive phenomena is in its early stages. We believe that three issues are of highest priority for future research.

Clarification of Stressful Events and Processes That Are Specific to Depressive Phenomena as Opposed to Other Manifestations of Psychopathology

As we have highlighted throughout this chapter, the answer to the question of whether stress is related to child and adolescent depression depends in part on research indicating that stress is unique to depression as opposed to other forms of psychopathology. Pursuit of the answer to this question will require increased sensitivity in the measurement of both stress and psychopathology.

First, there must be greater attention to differences in both the objective and the subjective characteristics of stressful experiences. Among the objective features of stress is the classification of events involving loss as opposed to nonloss events. Although there is evidence of a link between loss events and depressive reactions, it is important to recognize that individuals exposed to loss events are also likely to experience other types of stress, including events that involve threats to their well-being. To the extent that threatening events are likely to invoke anxiety, individuals are likely to report both depressive and anxious emotions as a result of their exposure to both threat- and loss-related events in a given time period.

Second, researchers need to cast a wide net in attempting to sample the emotions, syndromes, and disorders that individuals experience in association with stressful events. An illusion of specificity can be obtained by limiting one's focus to only one form of distress, such as depressive symptoms. The findings that we have reviewed underscore the need to examine a range of both internalizing and externalizing symptoms and disorders, as both of these broad categories of distress have been found to be related to stress.

Tests of specificity can be achieved using two very different methods. The first approach involves measuring the cumulative effects of a wide range of stressors and then categorizing them into subtypes. These subtypes can be identified on the basis of objective features of events (e.g., family, peer, school achievement) or subjective features (e.g., perceived controllability). Alternatively, researchers can focus on a single event and examine individual differences in response to such an event. Individual differences in cognitive appraisals, coping resources, coping responses, or personality characteristics may predispose some individuals to respond with depressive symptoms, whereas others do not. In either case, it is important to measure symptoms of disorders other than depression along with depressive phenomena.

Identification of Developmental Stabilities and Changes in the Relation between Stress and Depressive Phenomena

Although stress is ubiquitous throughout development, changes in individuals' appraisals and coping, as well as changes in the types of stress to which individuals are exposed, change with development. Thus, some points in development may present higher periods of risk for depressive responses to stress than others. For example, adolescence is associated with higher rates of stressful events and depressive symptoms for adolescent girls as compared with adolescent boys or preadolescent boys and girls (Petersen et al., 1991b). Further research is needed to clarify whether adolescent girls and boys experience increases in other symptoms in association with stress during adolescence. These findings indicate the need to attend to changing patterns in both stress and depression throughout childhood and adolescence.

An alternative design to examine developmental differences involves the assessment of depressive phenomena in children and adolescents of a wide age range who have been exposed to a common stressor. For example, our observations of developmental differences in depressive syndrome scores of children whose parents have cancer (Compas et al., in press) suggest that the same stressor may hold different significance for children and adolescents as a function of their developmental level. Similar research on other stressors is needed to clarify developmental patterns of response to stress.

Clarification of the Mechanisms That Underlie the Association between Stress and Depression

How do stressful events and processes contribute to depressive reactions? The mechanisms that underlie depressive responses to stress remain the most poorly understood aspect of the association between stress and depression in young people.

There has been little discussion in the literature on traumatic events of the underlying mechanisms by which stress is related to psychological distress. An exception is McFarlane (1987), who suggested that the reaction of parents to a traumatic event, not the child's reaction or the actual effects of a disaster, is the key factor by which trauma is translated to the child. Parental attitudes about traumatic events are believed to be translated to the child through the parents' subsequent overprotectiveness and irritability. In the research of McFarlane (1987), parental posttraumatic symptoms were more predictive of the child's adjustment over time than the child's initial response to a massive bush fire. It is suggested that the parental pattern of overprotectiveness may then make the child feel more vulnerable and unable to handle anxious and depressive emotions. McFarlane (1987) also offers another hypothesis: that anxiety at the time of the disaster may lead to "imprinting of memories of the event (which) maintains future (psychological) disorders" (p. 768).

Anthony (1986) offers several other explanations of how trauma may be translated into distress: (1) Some individuals are vulnerable to a sense of helplessness or hopelessness or both in the face of many stressors. (2) Individuals are more vulnerable to stress as a result of their locus of control beliefs and coping efforts. (3) Individuals differ in how physiologically alert they are to stressful stimuli, which may affect their ability to repress or minimize the impact of an event. (4) Individuals' responses to stress may be moderated by the family, work, and community context in which they occur. Anthony (1986) noted that the impact of traumatic events has not been considered in a developmental context, and he speculated that early experiences with stress "inoculate" or render them more vulnerable.

Similarly, disappointingly little attention has been given to the mechanisms through which cumulative life stress is associated with depression or other forms of distress and psychopathology. One exception is the work of Sandler, Pillow, and colleagues on the development of models for children exposed to the stress of bereavement and parental alcohol abuse (Roosa et al., 1990; West et al., 1991). These authors found that family environment variables and processes, as well as ongoing negative and positive events, mediated the relation between parental loss and parental alcohol abuse and children's depressive symptoms. Similarly, we have found that major life events are associated with depressed mood and negative affect, at least in part, through increases in daily stress (Compas et al., 1989b; Wagner et al., 1989), and that stressful events in the lives of parents are related to children's symptoms as a result of parental symptoms (Compas et al., 1989b). No research to date has examined the mechanisms of cognitive appraisals that may account for the association of life stress and depressive phenomena.

Researchers concerned with chronic stress have also focused on parental functioning and parent–child relationships as the key mechanisms through which chronic family stress affects children. For example, research indicates that chronic economic adversity affects children indirectly through increased depressive symptoms in parents, leading to disrupted parent–child relationships, which lead to emotional and behavioral difficulties in children (Conger et al., 1992). No attempt has been made, however, to identify mechanisms through which chronic stress may lead specifically to depressive outcomes.

Summary

Research on stress and child and adolescent depression has now passed through its early stages. It has been established in both cross-sectional and longitudinal research that stressful experiences are related to depressive phenomena. The challenges now facing researchers involve the careful investigation of individual differences in depressive responses to stress, the degree of specificity in this relation, and the mechanisms that underlie this association. Addressing these issues will move the field toward consideration of interventions to prevent and remediate the contribution of stress to depression and other disorders in children and adolescents.

ACKNOWLEDGMENT.   Preparation of this chapter was supported in part by National Institute of Mental Health Grant 43819.

References

Achenbach, T. M. (1985). *Assessment and taxonomy of child and adolescent psychopathology*. Newbury Park, CA: Sage.

Achenbach, T. M. (1991). The derivation of taxonomic constructs: A necessary stage in the development of psychopathology. In D. Cicchetti (Ed.), *Rochester symposium on developmental psychopathology*, Vol. 3, Hillsdale, NJ: Erlbaum.

Adams, M., & Adams, J. (1991). Life events, depression, and perceived problem-solving alternatives in adolescents. *Journal of Child Psychology and Psychiatry*, *32*, 811–820.

Allen, D. M., & Tarnowski, K. J. (1989). Depressive characteristics of physically abused children. *Journal of Abnormal Child Psychology*, *17*, 1–11.

Allgood-Merten, B., Lewinsohn, P. M., & Hops, H. (1990). Sex differences and adolescent depression. *Journal of Abnormal Psychology*, *99*, 55–63.

American Psychiatric Association (1994). *Diagnostic and statistical manual of mental disorders*, 4th ed. Washington, DC: Author.

Anthony, E. J. (1986). Children's reactions to severe stress: The response to overwhelming stress: Some introductory comments. *American Academy of Child Psychiatry*, *25*, 299–305.

Banez, G. A., & Compas, B. E. (1990). Children's and parents' daily stressful events and psychological symptoms. *Journal of Abnormal Child Psychology*, *18*, 591–605.

Beck, S., & Rosenberg, R. (1986). Frequency, quality, and impact of life events in self-rated depressed, behavioral-problem, and normal children. *Journal of Consulting and Clinical Psychology, 54*, 863–864.

Brooks-Gunn, J., & Warren, M. P. (1989). Biological and social contributions to negative affect in young adolescent girls. *Child Development, 60*, 40–55.

Brown, G. W., & Harris, T. O. (1989). Depression. In G. W. Brown & T. O. Harris (Eds.), *Life events and illness* (pp. 49–93). New York: Guilford.

Burke, J. D., Moccia, P., Borus, J. F., & Burns, B. J. (1986). Emotional distress in fifth-grade children ten months after a natural disaster. *Journal of the American Academy of Child Psychiatry, 25*, 536–541.

Cantwell, D. P., & Baker, L. (1991). Manifestations of depressive affect in adolescence. *Journal of Youth and Adolescence, 20*, 121–133.

Cohen, L. H., Burt, C. E., & Bjork, J. P. (1987). Life stress and adjustment: Effects of life events experienced by young adolescents and their parents. *Developmental Psychology, 23*, 583–592.

Compas, B. E., Ey, S., & Grant, K. E. (1993). Taxonomy, assessment, and diagnosis of depression during adolescence. *Psychological Bulletin, 114*, 373–344.

Compas, B. E., and Hammen, C. L. (1994). Child and adolescent depression: Covariation and comorbidity in development. In R. J. Haggerty, N. Garmezy, M. Rutter, & L. Sherrod (Eds.), *Risk and resilience in children: Developmental approaches* (pp. 225–267). New York: Cambridge University Press.

Compas, B. E., Howell, D. C., Phares, V., Williams, R. A., & Giunta, C. T. (1989a). Risk factors for emotional/behavioral problems in young adolescents: A prospective analysis of parent and adolescent stress and symptoms. *Journal of Consulting and Clinical Psychology, 57*, 732–740.

Compas, B. E., Howell, D. C., Phares, V., Williams, R. A., & Ledoux. (1989b). Parent and child stress and symptoms: An integrative analysis. *Developmental Psychology, 25*, 550–559.

Compas, B. E., & Williams, R. A. (1990). Stress, coping, and adjustment in mothers and young adolescents in single- and two-parent families. *American Journal of Community Psychology, 18*, 525–545.

Compas, B. E., Worsham, N., Epping, J. E., Grant, K. E., Mireault, G., Howell, D. C., & Malcarne, V. (in press). When mom or dad has cancer. Markers of psychological distress in cancer patients, spouses, and children. *Health Psychology*.

Conger, R. D., Conger, K. J., Elder, G. H., Lorenz, F. O., Simons, R. L., & Whitbeck, L. B. (1992). A family process model of economic hardship and adjustment in early adolescent boys. *Child Development, 63*, 526–541.

Cornely, P., & Bromet, E. (1986). Prevalence of behavior problems in three-year-old children living near Three Mile Island: A comparative analysis. *Journal of Child Psychology and Psychiatry, 27*, 489–498.

Costello, E. (1989). Child psychiatric disorders and their correlates: A primary care pediatric sample. *Journal of the American Academy of Child and Adolescent Psychiatry, 28*, 851–855.

Cummings, E. M., & Davies, P. T. (1994). Maternal depression and child development. *Journal of Child Psychology and Psychiatry, 35*, 73–112.

Dohrenwend, B. P., & Shrout, P. E. (1985). "Hassles" in the conceptualization of and measurement of life stress variables. *American Psychologist, 40*, 780–785.

Downey, G., & Coyne, J. C. (1990). Children of depressed parents: An integrative review. *Psychological Bulletin, 108*, 50–76.

Ferholt, J. B., Hoffnung, R. J., Hunter, D. E. K., & Leventhal, J. M. (1986). Clinical investigators under stress: A critique of Garmezy's commentary. *American Academy of Child Psychiatry, 25*, 724–727.

Garber, J., & Hollon, S. D. (1991). What can specificity designs say about causality in psychopathology research? *Psychological Bulletin, 110*, 129–136.

Garmezy, N. (1986). On measures, methods and models. *Journal of the American Academy of Child Psychiatry, 25*, 727–729.

Garrison, C. Z., Jackson, K. L., Marsteller, F., McKeown, R., & Addy, C. (1990). A longitudinal study of depressive symptomatology in young adolescents. *Journal of the American Academy of Child and Adolescent Psychiatry, 29*, 581–585.

Glyshaw, K., Cohen, L. H. & Towbes, L. C. (1989). Coping strategies and psychological distress: Prospective analyses of early and middle adolescents. *American Journal of Community Psychology, 17*, 607–623.

Grant, K. E., Ey, S., & Compas, B. E. (1992). Reactions to acute family stress: Depressive symptoms in adolescents whose parents have cancer. Paper presented at the meeting of the Society for Research on Adolescence, Washington, DC, March, 1992.

Gray, R. E. (1987). Adolescent response to the death of a parent. *Journal of Youth and Adolescence, 16*, 511–525.

Ham, M., & Larson, R. (1990). The cognitive mediation of daily stress in early adolescence. *American Journal of Community Psychology, 18*, 567–585.

Hammen, C. (1988). Self-cognitions, stressful events, and the prediction of depression in children of depressed mothers. *Journal of Abnormal Child Psychology, 16*, 347–360.

Hammen, C. (1991). *Depression in the family context.* New York: Springer-Verlag.

Hammen, C., Burge, D., & Adrian, C. (1991). Timing of mother and child depression in a longitudinal study of children at risk. *Journal of Consulting and Clinical Psychology, 59,* 341–345.

Hanford, H. A., Mayes, S. D., Mattison, R. E., Humphrey, F. J., II, Bagnato, S., Bixler, E. O., & Kales, J. D. (1986). Child and parent reaction to the Three Mile Island nuclear accident. *Journal of the American Academy of Child Psychiatry, 25,* 346–356.

Holmes, T. H., & Rahe, R. H. (1967). The Social Readjustment Rating Scale. *Journal of Psychosomatic Research, 11,* 213–218.7.

Hops, H., Lewinsohn, P. M., Andrews, J. A., & Roberts, R. E. (1990). Psychological correlates of depressive symptomatology among high school students. *Journal of Clinical Child Psychology, 19,* 211–220.

Kandel, D. B., & Davies, M. (1982). Epidemiology of depressive mood in adolescents. *Archives of General Psychiatry, 39,* 1205–1212.

Kanner, A. D., & Feldman, S. S. (1991). Control over uplifts and hassles and its relationship to adaptational outcomes. *Journal of Behavioral Medicine, 14,* 187–201.

Kaplan, S. L., Busner, J., Weinhold, C., & Lenon, P. (1987). Depressive symptoms in children and adolescents with cancer: A longitudinal study. *Journal of the American Academy of Child and Adolescent Psychiatry, 26,* 782–787.

Kinzie, J. D., Sack, W. H., Angell, R. H., Manson, S., & Rath, B. (1986). The psychiatric effects of massive trauma on Cambodian children. I. The children. *Journal of the American Academy of Child Psychiatry, 25,* 370–376.

Kovacs, M. (1989). Affective disorders in children and adolescents. *American Psychologist, 44,* 209–215.

Lazarus, R. S., DeLongis, A., Folkman, S., & Gruen, R. (1985). Stress and adaptational outcomes: The problem of confounded measures. *American Psychologist, 40,* 770–779.

Lazarus, R. S., & Folkman, S. (1984). *Stress, appraisal, and coping.* New York: Springer.

Lempers, J., Clark-Lempers, D., & Simons, R. (1989). Economic hardship, parenting practices, and adolescent distress. *Child Development, 60,* 25–39.

Luthar, L. (1991). Vulnerability and resilience: A study of high-risk adolescents. *Child Development, 62,* 600–616.

Malmquist, C. P. (1986). Children who witness parental murder: Posttraumatic aspects. *Journal of the American Academy of Child Psychiatry, 25,* 320–325.

McFarlane, A. C. (1987). Posttraumatic phenomena in a longitudinal study of children following a natural disaster. *Journal of the American Academy of Child and Adolescent Psychiatry, 26,* 764–769.

Monroe, S. M. (1990). Psychosocial factors in anxiety and depression. In J. D. Maser & C. R. Cloninger (Eds.), *Comorbidity of mood and anxiety disorders* (pp. 461–497). Washington, DC: American Psychiatric Press.

Monroe, S. M., & Simons, A. D. (1991). Diathesis–stress theories in the context of life stress research: Implications for depressive disorders. *Psychological Bulletin, 110,* 406–425.

Payton, J. B., & Krocker-Tuskan, M. (1988). Children's reactions to loss of parent through violence. *Journal of the American Academy of Child and Adolescent Psychiatry, 27,* 563–566.

Petersen, A. C., Compas, B. E., Brooks-Gunn, J., Stemmler, M., Ey, S., & Grant, K. E. (1993). Depression in adolescence. *American Psychologist, 48,* 155–168.

Petersen, A. C., Kennedy, R. E., & Sullivan, P. (1991a). Coping with adolescence. In M. E. Colton & S. Gore (Eds.), *Adolescent stress: Causes and consequences* (pp. 93–110). New York: Aldine de Gruyter.

Petersen, A. C., Sarigiani, P. A., & Kennedy, R. E. (1991b). Adolescent depression: Why more girls? *Journal of Youth and Adolescence, 20,* 247–271.

Pynoos, R. S., & Nader, K. (1988). Children who witness the sexual assaults on their mothers. *Journal of the American Academy of Child and Adolescent Psychiatry, 27,* 567–572.

Roosa, M. W., Beals, J., Sandler, I. N., & Pillow, D. R. (1990). The role of risk and protective factors in predicting symptomatology in adolescent self-identified children of alcoholic parents. *American Journal of Community Psychology, 18,* 725–741.

Rowlison, R. T., & Felner, R. D. (1988). Major life events, hassles, and adaptation in adolescence: Confounding in the conceptualization and measurement of life stress and adjustment revisited. *Journal of Personality and Social Psychology, 55,* 432–444.

Siegel, J. M., & Brown, J. D. (1988). A prospective study of stressful circumstances, illness symptoms, and depressed mood among adolescents. *Developmental Psychology, 24,* 715–721.

Skinner, D., & Swartz, L. (1989). The consequences for preschool children of a parent's detention: A preliminary south African clinical study of caregivers' reports. *Journal of Child Psychology and Psychiatry, 30,* 243–259.

Stanger, C., McConaughy, S. H., & Achenbach, T. M. (1992). Three-year course of behavioral/emotional problems in a national sample of 4- to 16-year-olds. II. Predictors of syndromes. *Journal of the American Academy of Child and Adolescent Psychiatry, 31,* 941–950.

Towbes, L. C., Cohen, L. H., & Glyshaw, K. (1989). Instrumentality as a life-stress moderator for early versus middle adolescents. *Journal of Personality and Social Psychology, 57,* 109–119.

Varni, J. W., Rubenfeld, L. A., Talbot, D., & Setoguchi, Y. (1989). Stress, social support, and depressive symptomatology in children with congenital/acquired limb deficiencies. *Journal of Pediatric Psychology, 14,* 515–530.

Velez, C. N., Johnson, J., & Cohen, P. (1989). A longitudinal analysis of selected risk factors for childhood psychopathology. *Journal of the American Academy of Child and Adolescent Psychiatry, 28,* 861–864.

Vernberg, E. M. (1990). Psychological adjustment and experiences with peers during early adolescence: Reciprocal, incidental, or unidirectional relationships. *Journal of Abnormal Child Psychology, 18,* 187–198.

Wagner, B. M., & Compas, B. E. (1990). Gender, instrumentality, and expressivity: Moderators of the relation between stress and psychological symptoms during adolescence. *American Journal of Community Psychology, 18,* 383–406.

Wagner, B. M., Compas, B. E., & Howell, D. C. (1988). Daily and major life events: A test of an integrative model of psychosocial stress. *American Journal of Community Psychology, 16,* 189–205.

Walker, L. S., & Greene, J. W. (1991). Negative life events and symptom resolution in pediatric abdominal pain patients. *Journal of Pediatric Psychology, 16,* 341–360.

Watson, D., & Pennebaker, J. W. (1989). Health complaints, stress, and distress: Exploring the central role of negative affectivity. *Psychological Review, 96,* 234–254.

West, S. G., Sandler, I. N., Pillow, D. R., Baca, L., & Gersten, J. C. (1991). The use of structural equation modeling in generative research: Toward the design of a preventive intervention for bereaved children. *American Journal of Community Psychology, 19,* 459–480.

World Health Organization (1990). *International classification of diseases, injuries, and causes of death,* 10th ed. Geneva: Author.

24

Suicide and Suicidal Behaviors in Children and Adolescents

William M. Reynolds and James J. Mazza

Introduction

Suicide and suicidal behavior have been described for nearly all of recorded history (Rosen, 1971). Historically, societal and professional perspectives on suicide have gone through continual periods of acceptance, rejection, ambivalence, and philosophical debate for millennia. Even today, the view of suicide as a pathological behavior or mental health problem to be prevented has been questioned by some (e.g., Szasz, 1986). The existential debate as to the legitimacy or normality of suicide is enervated when we consider suicidal behavior in children and adolescents.

Children and adolescents differ significantly from adults in their ability to cope with stressors and engage in problem-solving, in their perception and perspective of the future, and in their knowledge and understanding that undesirable events or situations can and often do change. These and other characteristics, such as potential deficiencies in self-regulation, contribute to a vulnerability in young people that is uncommon in mature adults. We also find many vulnerable youngsters who are exposed to situations and forces at home and elsewhere that they perceive as uncontrollable. Because of a limited repertoire of adaptive and coping skills, stresses and risk factors for suicidal behavior may be exacerbated in young people by their belief that they have little agency for control or ability to change undesirable environments and forces. We also find mental health problems such as depression among youngsters at risk for suicidal behaviors. However, our research shows that a significant number of young people who demonstrate suicidal behaviors do not manifest concomitant clinical levels of depressive symptomatology (Reynolds & Mazza, 1990).

In recent years, the news media have focused attention on suicidal behaviors among

William M. Reynolds • Psychoeducational Research and Training Centre, University of British Columbia, Vancouver, British Columbia V6T 1Z4, Canada.   **James J. Mazza** • Department of Psychology, St. John's University, Jamaica, New York 11439.

Handbook of Depression in Children and Adolescents, edited by William M. Reynolds and Hugh F. Johnston. Plenum Press, New York, 1994.

children and adolescents. This focus has increased public awareness of this problem, although public understanding still remains low, and anecdotal reports suggest that many myths and misconceptions regarding suicide continue to persevere. However, there has been a tremendous increase in the research on these problem areas in the past decade. This rapid accumulation of knowledge has occurred across many domains of study, including psychological, psychiatric, medical, and educational.

As this chapter illustrates, suicidal behavior in children and adolescents is one of the most significant mental health problems among the youth of today. Official statistics on the epidemiology of suicide indicate that the base rate for completed suicide is relatively low in comparison to formal diagnosed psychiatric disorders, such as major depression. However, research on the spectrum of suicidal behaviors, which includes suicide attempts and suicidal ideation, suggests that suicidal behaviors as a class of psychopathology are a prevalent problem among adolescents and to a somewhat lesser extent in children. In addition to the issues and warnings raised by mental health professionals, concern about adolescent suicide has also been shown by members of the United States Congress. Recently, United States Representative Gary L. Ackerman (1993), citing a Gallup Organization survey of adolescent suicidal behavior, reported that 60% of teens surveyed personally knew another teen who had attempted suicide.

The recognition of suicidal behavior as a growing and prevalent problem among children and adolescents is not new, nor are the concerns that many professionals in school and clinical settings are not providing adequate attention to this problem. Nearly 20 years ago, Toolan (1975) noted that suicidal behaviors were increasing among children and adolescents. Providing observations on a sample of approximately 900 admissions in 1960 to the child and adolescent units of Bellevue Hospital in New York City, Toolan found that 102 youngsters, including 18 children between the ages of 5 and 12 years, were seen for suicide attempts and threats. Toolan's description of youngsters and his general suggestions for treatment (Toolan, 1975) are similar to those found in contemporary reports. Thus, although our literature base on suicidal behavior in youngsters has increased exponentially over the past 20 years, our knowledge base specific to some salient issues such as treatment has shown small gains.

Suicidal Behavior as a Distinct Form of Psychopathology

For many years, suicidal behavior has been considered as a symptom component of several psychiatric disorders, such as major depression and borderline personality disorders (American Psychiatric Association, 1980, 1987, 1994). However, suicidal behavior does occur in the absence of formal psychiatric disorders (e.g., Brent, Perper, Moritz, Baugher, & Allman, 1993e). In some cases, this circumstance may obviate the provision of services or lessen the clinical significance of suicidal behaviors as a form of pathology. Irrespective of other psychopathology, however, suicidal behavior represents a significant target for intervention (Reynolds, 1988).

The need to formalize as a diagnostic category suicidal behavior or suicidality—defined to include suicidal ideation and behaviors that are deliberately self-injurious—has been presented by R. A. King, Pfeffer, Gammon, and Cohen (1992). R. A. King et al. (1992) called for the inclusion of suicidality as a diagnostic category in the then-upcoming DSM-IV, noting the inadequacies of DSM-III-R in its consideration of suicidal behavior. R. A. King et al. (1992) proposed a category of suicidal disorder of childhood and adolescence that included two subtypes, suicidal ideation and suicidal behavior, with the latter specific to suicide attempts and serious self-injurious behavior. Relatedly, Kahan and Pattison (1984) proposed the consideration of the "Deliberate Self-Harm Syndrome" (DSH) as a variant of nonlethal suicidal behavior that typically emerges during late adolescence. These authors also suggested the consideration of DSH as an Axis I disorder in DSM-IV.

The 1991 DSM-IV *Options Book* (American Psychiatric Association, 1991), which was an initial draft of proposed DSM-IV categories, included the suggested problem of suicide attempts, noting the particular relevance for adolescents who do not meet criteria for other disorders. In addition, a new option of "With Suicidal Behavior" was suggested as a subtype of Adjustment Disorder if criteria for other subtypes of Adjustment Disorder (e.g., With Depressed Mood, With Disturbance of Conduct) were not met. However, neither of these options/recommendations was included in DSM-IV (American Psychiatric Association, 1994).

With the emergence of systematic studies of suicidal behaviors in children and adolescents, and the growing awareness that such behaviors may occur without the presence of formal mental disorders, there is a need to recognize suicidal behavior in youngsters (as well as adults) as a distinct form of psychopathology with diverse presenting characteristics and biopsychosocial etiologies, if not within the context of a formal diagnostic system, then by professional acceptance of suicidal behaviors as a significant psychological disturbance irrespective of the existence of clinical or personality disorder.

The Problem of Suicidal Behavior among Children and Adolescents

It cannot be overstated that suicidal behavior is a serious and often overlooked problem among children and adolescents. Suicidal behavior has been reported as one of the most frequent psychiatric emergencies among children and adolescents (Robinson, 1986), with suicidal behaviors as one of the strongest predictors of psychiatric hospital admissions among adolescents (Hillard, Slomowitz, & Deddens, 1988). Recent surveys and government statistics suggest that suicide is the second leading cause of death among adolescents 15–19 years of age [National Institute of Mental Health (NIMH), 1992]. Although suicide is less prevalent among young children, children as young as preschool age do make suicide attempts and exhibit suicide-like behaviors (Pfeffer & Trad, 1988; Rosenthal & Rosenthal, 1984; Rosenthal, Rosenthal, Doherty, & Santora, 1986; Trad, 1990). Statistics suggest that there are over 2000 suicides by 15- to 19-year-olds each year in the United States. Most professionals view the number of suicides reported as an underestimate of the number of youngsters who purposefully take their own lives each year. As we shall show, it may be estimated that there are over 1 million additional youths who attempt suicide each year but survive. It may be inferred by rates of hospitalization that many of these attempts are of limited lethality, and many others may be considered gestures rather than true attempts. However, a significant number of youngsters who attempt suicide injure themselves physically or mentally.

Research also indicates that most parents are unaware of their youngsters' suicidal behaviors (Joffe, Offord, & Boyle, 1988; Rey & Bird, 1991; Walker, Moreau, & Weissman, 1990; Velez & Cohen, 1988; Zimmerman & Asnis, 1991a,b), and data suggest that most adolescent suicide attempters do not tell others prior to their attempt. In a sample of 59 adolescents with a history of suicide attempts whose parents sought psychiatric help for their youngsters, Zimmerman and Asnis (1991b) found that 61% of parents were unaware of their youngsters' suicide attempt. Similar findings were reported in a study of suicidal children and adolescents conducted by Kashani, Goddard, and Reid (1989), who found that 86% of parents were not aware of their youngsters' suicidal behavior. Velez and Cohen (1988), in a large community sample study of mothers' and children's reports of suicidal behavior, found little concordance between child reports of suicide attempts and suicidal ideation and mothers' reports. For instance, Velez and Cohen found a correlation of $r = 0.16$ between mother and child report of suicidal ideation, with youngsters reporting greater ideation than mothers. Of the 25 children and adolescents who reported having made one or more suicide attempts, only 2 mothers indicated an awareness of these attempts.

William M.
Reynolds and James
J. Mazza

It is important for the study and understanding of suicidal behavior in youngsters to explicate the variety and nature of clinical phenomena associated with this domain of behavioral pathology. There have been numerous perspectives taken to delineate types of suicidal behavior as well as types of suicide completion (e.g., Pokorny, 1974; Zilboorg, 1936; Zubin, 1974). Presented here is a severity perspective that delineates degrees of suicidal behavior and cognitions within a hierarchical framework. This model is viewed as providing a basis for distinguishing forms of suicidal behavior for purposes of clinical work as well as research. All too often, we create very simple constructs such as "thoughts of suicide," "suicide attempt," and so forth without considering the potentially complex and diverse nature of each domain of suicidal behaviors/cognitions. In order to gain a better understanding of how to prevent suicide, we must first recognize and understand the variety and complex nature of suicidal behavior, especially as it relates to children and adolescents.

The terminology specific to the description of suicidal behavior has varied over time, but in general three broad categories have been delineated: suicidal ideation, suicide attempts, and suicide completion. In addition, suicidal gestures or threats may also be considered as aspects of suicidal behavior. Other descriptions such as parasuicide have been used in the literature, with slight differences in definition of suicidal behavior. For this chapter, the former nomenclature will be used. This classification is consistent with that of the Center of Studies of Suicide Prevention and the National Institute of Mental Health (Ellis, 1988).

Operationally, the categories of suicide and suicidal behavior are defined as follows: Suicide is an act of intentional self-injury that was fatal to the individual. A suicide attempt represents a broad domain of self-injurious behavior that involved some degree of intentionality. A number of authors prefer to use the term "parasuicide" to describe suicide attempts and other forms of intentional self-injury, although this term is often used without implying motivation or severity of outcome (Fremouw, de Perczel, & Ellis, 1990; Kreitman, 1977; Linehan, 1981; Linehan & Nielsen, 1981; Shneidman, 1985). Although we agree that the term parasuicide is a preferred descriptor, we will use the more common term "suicide attempt" in this chapter. Moreover, as we will note, there are significant problems in the application and utility of the term suicide attempt to define a broad class of suicidal behaviors. "Suicidal ideation" as defined by Reynolds (1988, p. 4) "is the domain of thought and ideas about death, suicide, and serious self-injurious behavior, including thoughts related to the planning, conduct, and outcome of suicidal behavior." Thus, suicidal behavior is broadly described in this chapter to include the domains of suicide, suicide attempts, overt and covert threats or gestures, and suicidal ideation.

Suicide Completion

Suicide completion is only one behavior among many along the suicidal-behavior continuum. Ladame and Jeanneret (1982) describe suicide as only the tip of the iceberg of suicidal behaviors. The research and information gathered on adolescent suicide have been obtained by two primary methods. One common method of evaluation is by psychological autopsy, in which information is gathered from the family, relatives, and peers of the deceased (Phillips, 1989; Runeson, 1989; Shafii, Carrigan, Whittinghill, & Derrick, 1985). Psychological autopsies attempt to reconstruct, understand, and determine what was happening in the victim's life preceding the suicide. Premorbid status, and in particular psychiatric diagnoses, made using psychological autopsy procedures have been viewed as reasonably valid (e.g., Brent et al., 1993d). In addition to relatively in-depth psychological autopsies, a second method has been to review the medical charts and medical examiners' records of the victims (Garfinkel, Froese, & Hood, 1982; Hoberman & Garfinkel, 1988a,b; Kienhorst, Wolters, Diekstra, & Otte, 1987; Shafii, 1989).

529

**Suicide and
Suicidal Behaviors**

Methods of Suicide Completion.   The methods used for suicide completion by adolescents are quite diverse, with research suggesting that methods vary by country. This outcome is reasonable, as there are differences in the availability of means, such as firearms, between countries. In the United States, firearms are the most popular method for males and females (Jobes, 1992; Rosenberg, Smith, Davidson, & Conn, 1987). In contrast, the most widely used methods in England are suffocation, strangulation, and hanging (Hawton, 1986). In the United States, suicide by firearms in adolescents increased by 45% from the 1950s to the 1970s, while the rate for most other methods stayed fairly constant (Boyd, 1983). Hoberman and Garfinkel (1988a) found differences in methods used between males and females and between younger and older youngsters. Males and older adolescents were more likely to use firearms as a method for suicide, while females were more likely to use ingestion or carbon monoxide poisoning. Children and younger adolescents were most likely to commit suicide by hanging.

Psychopathology.   Much of our knowledge base specific to the premorbid psychological status of adolescent suicide completers has been obtained through the use of psychological autopsies (e.g., Runeson, 1989; Shafii et al., 1985; Shafii, Steltz-Lenarsky, Derrick, Beckner, & Whittinghill, 1988). On the basis of psychological autopsies, DSM-III clinical disorders found among adolescent suicide completers included mood disorders, conduct disorder, and substance abuse (Runeson, 1989; Shafii et al., 1985, 1988). In the Shafii et al. (1988) study, 95% of the suicide completers met the criteria for one or more DSM-III Axis I clinical disorders. DSM-III personality disorders such as borderline, antisocial, and avoidant were also found in 29% of the suicide completers (Shafii et al., 1988). Psychopathology and suicidal behavior will be described in more detail later in this chapter.

Individual Differences in Mortality.   Among adolescents as well as adults, more males than females complete suicide (Carlson & Cantwell, 1982; Eisenberg, 1984; Ladame & Jeanneret, 1982; Weissman, 1974). It has been suggested that males are more likely to die from their suicide attempts than females because males use more violent means (Eisenberg, 1984; Hawton, 1986; Jacobziner, 1965; Weissman, 1974). Eisenberg (1984) reported that an increase in late adolescent and young adult mortality (ages 15–24) was strongly correlated with the increase of suicides by violent means. Most countries reported males outnumbering females in their respective suicide completion rates (e.g., Kosky, 1987). In the 60 suicide cases investigated by Shafii (1989), males committed suicide 5:1 over females. However, in Asian countries, the ratio of males to females is nearly equal, 1.4:1 (Eisenberg, 1984).

The literature on suicide for children and adolescents has shown consistent racial differences in suicide completers. Caucasian adolescents commit suicide 2:1 over non-Caucasian (Shaffer & Fisher, 1981). Native American adolescents are considered the highest at-risk group for suicide, yet studies involving this population are few (Hawton, 1986; Reynolds & Mazza, 1992a). According to the National Center for Health Statistics, Native American adolescents who live on reservations commit suicide 5 times more often than Caucasian adolescents (Hawton, 1986).

Suicide Notes.   The notion that most suicidal adolescents leave a suicide note before their suicide attempt has been dispelled as a myth. Of the 505 children and adolescents seen in the hospital, only 5.3% of the attempts were accompanied by a suicide note (Garfinkel et al., 1982). Similar results regarding suicide notes were found among adolescent attempters in the general population (Reynolds & Mazza, 1993c). On the basis of clinical interviews with adolescents who had attempted suicide, only 9% left a suicide note. Suicide notes are sometimes left and can provide substantial information, but they are not as common as once thought (Leenaars, 1992).

Suicide Attempts

Suicide attempts among young people represent serious pathological behavior. Crumley (1982) suggests that suicide attempts by adolescents be considered a primary symptom of a serious psychiatric disorder. The consequences of an attempt can be devastating, both mentally and physically. Before we describe data on the epidemiology and characteristics of suicide attempts, it is important to consider the utility of this term and the domain of behavior it represents. The term *suicide attempt* encompasses such a vast array of behaviors, actions, intentions, and outcomes as to make it minimally useful in research or clinical applications for describing a class of suicidal behavior. The wide range of behaviors included in this domain is a distinct problem in the interpretation of research and in making comparisons between groups of attempters, nonattempters, and other suicidal behaviors.

Suicide attempts often have debilitating lifetime outcomes. Although data suggest that the majority of suicide attempts by young people are of limited lethality (Reynolds & Mazza, 1993a), not all adolescents who attempt suicide go back to school the next day or the next week. Some youngsters end up disfigured, scarred, or paralyzed for the rest of their lives, as was the outcome for a 16-year-old girl who attempted suicide by shooting herself in the head with a handgun. Some suicide attempts result in broken bones, such as for a 9-year-old girl who attempted suicide by running in front of a car, or a 13-year-old boy who jumped from the second story window of his home. Suicide attempts are thus quite serious and need to be viewed as indicative of severe psychological disturbance. In many cases, there is only a fine line between suicide and parasuicide, determined by the minutes saved by paramedics in the rush to the hospital or the motorist who swerves to avoid the child who purposefully runs into the street.

Because of the extreme variability in actual behaviors that constitute what is generically referred to as a suicide attempt, research that examines differences between youngsters who have made a suicide attempt and those without such a history is limited in generalizability. The basic problem, as will be elucidated in greater detail at the end of this chapter, is that the attempt group includes youngsters who have made serious and potentially life-threatening or fatal attempts, such as gunshot wounds to the head, as well as youngsters who have made attempts that are very mild or of limited lethality potential, such as taking 5 or 6 acetaminophen tablets. Grouping these youngsters together as "suicide attempters" suggests a homogeneous group that has little empirical or rational support.

Gender differences among rates of suicide attempts in the United States and most other countries show that females make more attempts than males (Diekstra, 1993; Jobes, 1992). Eisenberg (1984) reviewed epidemiological studies and estimated that among adolescent attempters, the female/male ratio is approximately 3:1. Garfinkel et al. (1982) also found a female/male attempt ratio of 3:1. In their school-based study of 469 adolescents who indicated a history of suicide attempts, Reynolds and Mazza (1992a) found a female/male ratio of 2:1 for attempters. A similar ratio was reported by Swedo (1989) in a study of 80 adolescent suicide attempters who were hospitalized for their attempts. The increased lethality of adolescent attempts is suggested in the Swedo study, as she found that significantly more males (46% vs. 19%) than females required extended inpatient therapy. Most of the research cited above has been conducted with adolescents, although some studies such as that by Swedo (1989) also included older children (i.e., ages 10 and older). Garfinkel et al. (1982) found that the ratio of males to females was approximately equal for children under the age of 13.5 years who attempted suicide.

Suicide attempts are also a primary marker for continued suicidal behavior and, in some cases, future completion. Diekstra (1993), in a review of trends in suicidal behavior in Europe and North America, notes that suicide attempts may be "the most important precursor of suicide." In a study conducted in Finland, Kotila (1992) reported that of 362 adolescent suicide attempters who were seen in a hospital emergency ward and followed up after an average of 5 years, 8.7% of males and 1.2% of females completed suicide or died violent deaths (e.g., drowning). The overall proportion of 3.6% was 20 times higher than the average mortality for suicide and violent deaths in this age group in Finland during the period of the study. Approximately 75% of the suicides occurred within 1 year of being seen in the hospital setting.

In young people, the methods used for suicide or suicide attempts are diverse and vary for male and female adolescents. Data on methods of attempts also vary by country, in part as a function of different cultures and laws, the latter of primary importance to the availability of firearms. Much of the literature reported from hospital and clinical settings indicates that overdose (drugs and alcohol) accounts for 70–90% of the suicide attempts made by adolescents (Barter, Swaback, & Todd, 1968; Crumley, 1979; Garfinkel et al., 1982; Litt, Cuskey, & Rudd, 1983; Pfeffer, Newcorn, Kaplan, Mizruchi, & Plutchik, 1988; Robbins & Alessi, 1985; Spirito et al., 1992; Spirito, Stark, Fristad, Hart, & Owens-Stively, 1987; Weissman, 1974). Females, who make significantly more suicide attempts than males, frequently use drugs as a means of attempting suicide. Litt et al. (1983), who studied 27 adolescent attempters, 21 of whom were females, found that 78% of the attempts were by drug overdose. A study conducted by Spirito et al. (1987) examining 71 adolescent suicide attempters, 55 of whom were female, found that 82% of the attempts were by drug overdose. Males, on the other hand, use more violent methods to attempt suicide, such as jumping, hanging, and guns (Eisenberg, 1984; Hawton, 1986; Mehr, Zeltzer, & Robinson, 1981).

Table 1 shows the suicide-attempt methods of 469 adolescents who reported one or more attempts from a study of over 3400 school-based adolescents conducted by Reynolds and Mazza (1993a), who found that females used pills and cutting the wrist to a greater extent than did males, with males more frequently attempting suicide by means of hanging and guns. Overall, there was a significant difference in the methods used in suicide attempts between males and females, $\chi^2(5) = 63.58$, $p < 0.0001$. A history of multiple attempts was more prevalent among females (35%) than males (22%) in the sample of attempters, $\chi^2(1) = 7.52$, $p < 0.01$. It is of interest that the difference between males and

TABLE 1. Suicide-Attempt Characteristics of Male and Female Adolescents[a]

Suicide method	Male (%)	Female (%)	Total[b]
Pills	22.5	45.1	37.7
Cut wrist	18.6	30.4	26.6
Stab self	7.0	6.6	6.9
Gun	12.4	.4	4.2
Hang/drown	7.8	3.3	4.7
Other	31.8	14.3	19.8

[a]Adapted from Reynolds and Mazza (1993a).
[b]Total sample includes a small proportion of subjects who did not report sex.

females in their reported rate of hospitalization for their attempts was not significant [males = 20.4%, females = 21.4%, χ^2 (1) = 0.05, p = ns].

Garfinkel et al. (1982) examined the methods of suicide attempts among 505 children and adolescents who appeared in a hospital emergency room in Ontario. Information was obtained by reviewing the medical charts of these youngsters. They found that children under the age of 13.5 years were significantly more likely to attempt suicide by hanging than older adolescents, χ^2 (4) = 45.16, p < 0.01. Garfinkel et al. (1982) also found that most children and adolescents used methods of low lethality and high likelihood of being rescued from their suicide attempts. Their results suggest that child and adolescent attempters may be ambivalent in the attempt to take their own lives. From the medical charts, 78% of the suicide attempts were of low lethality, 21% were of moderate lethality, and only 1% were of high lethality (Garfinkel et al., 1982). More than half (51%) of the attempters were judged as having a high likelihood of being rescued and only 3.4% were judged as low. Garfinkel et al. (1982) used the Risk–Rescue Rating Scale (Weisman & Worden, 1972) to assess lethality and the likelihood of being rescued. Attempts of low lethality and high likelihood of being rescued are more associated with communicating despair and reaching out for help, according to Weisman and Worden (1972). However, questions as to the reliability of using the Risk–Rescue Rating Scale with adolescents have been raised by Spirito, Brown, Overholser, Fritz, and Bond (1991). Smith and Crawford (1986) suggest that the low-lethality attempts by adolescents may be more of a means for communicating the chaos in their lives than a wish to die.

Many adolescents who attempt suicide are ambivalent about their intent to die, and unfortunately for some the attempt is fatal because they underestimated the lethality of the means employed (Eisenberg, 1984). The use of medical lethality as a measurement of suicidal risk, however, needs to be viewed with caution. Rotheram (1987) suggests that medical lethality is unrelated to the intention and desire of the individual to die. She states that it is the perception of the individual that is important. For example, an individual who takes 6 diet pills may have the same desire and intention to die as someone who ingests 50 aspirin (Rotheram, 1987). Relating lethality of means to intention is a tenuous undertaking. A study by Myers, Otto, Harris, Diaco, and Moreno (1992) suggests that at least in the case of acetaminophen overdose, adolescents have limited knowledge of drug toxicity.

Robbins and Alessi (1985) conducted a study that examined the communication aspects of adolescents who attempted suicide. Their study examined 64 adolescent attempters, ages 13–18, consecutively hospitalized in the adolescent psychiatric ward at the University of Michigan Hospital. Robbins and Alessi (1985) focused on two communication aspects: whether adolescents who make nonlethal attempts go on to make more dangerous attempts and whether adolescent statements about their seriousness of intent to die are accurate indicators of the lethality of their actual attempts.

Subjects were evaluated by two child psychiatrists in a structured interview that followed the Schedule for Affective Disorders and Schizophrenia (SADS) (Endicott & Spitzer, 1978). The results showed that 33 of the 64 patients had made at least one prior suicide attempt and 15 had made two or more attempts. Of the 64 patients, 6 (9.3%) had made a suicide attempt that was rated as medically dangerous, according to the SADS. Medically dangerous is defined on the SADS as "medical lethality of 4 (brief unconsciousness) to 6 (respiratory arrest)." The results showed that more females (22 of 37) (59%) than males (11 of 27) (41%) made multiple attempts. However, more males (N = 4) (36%) than females (N = 2) (9%) made medically dangerous attempts. All the adolescents who had made medically dangerous attempts had previously made nonlethal attempts. Robbins and Alessi (1985) concluded that those who make nonlethal attempts may be at higher risk for making more lethal and medically dangerous attempts than those who have not made a previous suicide attempt.

The results of the Robbins and Alessi (1985) study found that adolescent statements regarding their suicidal intent were highly correlated with their suicidal behaviors, $r = 0.67$. The correlation between the statement of intent and medical lethality was also high, $r = 0.87$. A similar correlation was reported between statement of intent and the number of suicide gestures, $r = 0.71$. Robbins and Alessi (1985) concluded that adolescents report their suicidal feelings honestly and reliably when being interviewed by someone with whom they have established rapport.

Smith and Crawford (1986) investigated the number of adolescents who received medical attention after their suicide attempt. They found that only 12% of the suicide attempters received medical attention following their attempt. Similar results were reported by Reynolds and Mazza (1992a), who examined a national sample of 3437 adolescents. They found that approximately 20% of adolescent attempters received hospital attention following their attempt. These findings also underscore the danger in generalizing the results of studies conducted in clinical settings to the general adolescent population. These results also indicate that using the medical contact process to estimate the suicide rate for adolescents is not accurate, missing approximately 80–90% of those adolescents who make suicide attempts (Reynolds & Mazza, 1992a; Smith & Crawford, 1986).

Suicidal Ideation

Suicidal ideation is an important aspect of suicidal behavior that is of great relevance for the identification of children and adolescents. Although non-self-injurious, suicidal ideation represents a common denominator of suicide-risk behavior and has the potential for being the earliest warning of a youngster at risk for more overt suicidal behaviors. Suicidal ideation may be viewed as a primary marker for more serious suicidal behavior (Bonner & Rich, 1987; Linehan, 1981) and a basic component in the classification of suicidal behaviors (Pfeffer, 1986; Pokorny, 1974; Zubin, 1974). Research on suicidal behavior in young people suggests that suicide attempts are in many cases preceded by thoughts and cognitions (ideation) of killing oneself (Andrews & Lewinsohn, 1992; Brent, 1989; Garrison, 1989; C. A. King, Raskin, Gdowski, Butkus, & Opipari, 1990; Pfeffer, Zuckerman, Plutchik, & Mizruchi, 1984; Rotheram-Borus & Trautman, 1988; Stiffman, 1989). Suicidal ideation encompasses a range of thoughts, from general cognitions about death and wishes about not being alive to more serious and specific thoughts about killing oneself, including the how, when, and where (Reynolds, 1988). Research involving suicidal behavior has shown that suicidal ideation is often a precursor to more serious suicidal behavior (Shafii et al., 1985, 1988). Thus, suicidal ideation may be viewed as the initial stage of suicidal behavior (Brent, 1989; Ellis, 1988; Ladame & Jeanneret, 1982; Pfeffer et al., 1984; Reynolds, 1988; Rudd, 1989; Shafii et al., 1985; Smith & Crawford, 1986).

The utility of suicidal ideation for the identification of suicidal youth will be described later in this chapter. It is important to note that suicidal ideation as a component of suicidal behavior needs to be viewed as a multifaceted construct and as much more than a simple question as to whether or not a youngster has thought about killing himself or herself. Research on suicidal ideation or group assignment predicated on one or two questions regarding having thoughts of suicide lacks sufficient specificity for defining this domain of suicidality and obscures the relative importance of suicidal ideation as a component of suicide risk in youth.

Suicidal ideation may be defined as thoughts and cognitions about taking one's life as well as thoughts specific to the act of suicide. Reynolds (1988) has operationalized suicidal ideation as a specific construct, delineated as a quasi-hierarchical continuum. In this continuum, suicidal ideation is characterized as ranging from low-severity general thoughts about death (morbid ideation) to general wishes that one were never born or specific wishes that one were dead to much more serious ideation about specific means of committing suicide. Included within the domain of suicidal ideation are also thoughts about suicide and the response of others and about the impact on others.

An examination of the research suggests that suicidal ideation has not, until recently, been well defined or measured as a psychological construct. Suicidal ideation, as a domain of suicidal behavior, has been studied in children and adolescents, although, as will be noted later in this chapter, there is a great deal of variability in the measurement and conceptualization of suicidal ideation in young people. However, most research suggests that suicidal ideation is a critical aspect of suicidal behavior. Pfeffer (1986), describing the results of a study of suicidal behavior in children, noted that inpatient children with suicidal ideas were considered at risk for serious suicidal behaviors. Kosky, Sliburn, and Zubrick (1986), in a sample of 628 depressed children seen in a psychiatric facility, reported that 13% indicated significant suicidal ideation, and over one third of these children had made a prior suicide attempt. Kosky et al. (1986) also noted a rapid increase in suicidal ideation after age 12, with females showing greater suicidal ideation than males.

In research using the method of "psychological autopsies" to evaluate the premorbid status of adolescents who had committed suicide, Shafii et al. (1985) found that suicidal ideation was a precursor to most adolescent suicides. They stated (p. 1064): "We believe that the suicidal ideation of yesterday is highly likely to become the suicide threat or attempt of today or the completed suicide of tomorrow." In this manner, suicidal ideation is highlighted as an important characteristic of suicidality in at-risk groups of youngsters.

Studies have also noted levels of suicidal ideation that may be considered "clinically relevant" in other populations of children and adolescents. In a study of 101 randomly selected preadolescent children from a public school setting, Pfeffer et al. (1984) found that 11.9% of the subjects demonstrated suicidal behaviors, with suicidal ideation present in 8.9% of the total sample. Pfeffer (1985) later suggested that this figure is probably an underestimate because a number of ideating children may have been reluctant to discuss these thoughts. Reynolds (1988, 1992a), using the Suicidal Ideation Questionnaire (Reynolds, 1987), reported finding clinically significant level of suicidal ideation in 9–12% of school-based adolescents with sample sizes ranging from 890 to 2139 adolescents ages 13–19. Similar results were found by Wright (1985) in a study of 207 high school seniors, 10.6% of whom indicated having suicidal thoughts. In a study of 4657 adolescents that included 101 youngsters with a history of suicide attempts, Kienhorst, De Wilde, Van den Bout, Diekstra, and Wolters (1990) examined a range of psychosocial and demographic variables and found that suicidal ideation was the most powerful predictor of a suicide attempt in this group of youngsters. Andrews and Lewinsohn (1992) found a very strong relationship between suicidal ideation and suicide attempts in a large sample of school-based adolescents, with approximately 87% of suicide attempters reporting suicidal ideation compared to approximately 1% of youngsters who had not attempted suicide. Andrews and Lewinsohn (1992) also found suicidal ideation to be a significant predictor of subsequent suicide attempts.

Epidemiology of Suicidal Behavior

The examination of the epidemiology of suicidal behavior is important for understanding the extensive and pervasive nature of suicidality among children and adolescents. To a large extent, much of the literature on the epidemiology of suicide among youngsters is specific to adolescents. As we noted, suicidal behavior has been described in young children, but there are few epidemiological studies of suicidal behavior in children. The latter circumstance may be a function of its lower incidence, as well as a natural disinclination for school personnel to permit researchers to evaluate suicidal behavior in school-based samples of children.

In our description of the epidemiology of suicidal behavior, a distinction must also be made regarding the time frame of the behavior. Suicide-completion data by their nature represent an incidence rate and are thus presented as new cases in a 12-month (typically calendar-year) period or as an average per year across a period of several years. Suicide attempts may be studied from an incidence perspective (an attempt in the 12 months preceding the data collection) or as a prevalence rate. The latter examines the extent to which a youngster has ever made a suicide attempt and is thus a lifetime occurrence. Prevalence of suicide-attempt data also depends on the respondent's age, given that older youngsters have greater potential for ever engaging in suicidal behavior, as well as potential age-cohort effects. Suicidal ideation has been reported in a number of ways from current ideation to ideation in the past week to ideation over the past 12 months to lifetime occurrence.

Suicide Completion

Attention to suicide has increased in the United States as well as in other countries over the past decade. Most countries, including the United States and Canada, have reported marked increases in the number of adolescents and young adults committing suicide (Berman, 1986; Brent, 1989; Dyck, Newman, & Thompson, 1988; Goldney & Katsikitis, 1983; Hawton, 1986; Lester, 1991; Shaffer & Fisher, 1981). Shafii et al. (1985) cited an increase of more than 80% in children (ages 10–14) and more than 100% in adolescents (ages 15–19) who committed suicide from 1976 to 1980. There are obvious questions as to the reliability of official statistics for mortality due to suicide in children and adolescents (Hoberman & Garfinkel, 1988a; Jobes, Berman, & Josselson, 1987). D. Miller (1981) suggests that there may be as many as 5 suicides for every 1 that is officially reported.

Suicide rates among children and adolescents tend to show a linear increase by age (McIntosh, 1992). Reported rates of suicide are often differentiated by age groups, e.g., 15–19 years, or 15–24 years, and so forth. These groupings often cloud our understanding of suicide-completion rates for developmental groups. For instance, McIntosh (1992) notes that the grouping of 15- to 19-year-olds masks relatively lower rates found in 13- and 14-year-olds and may therefore overestimate suicide completion during adolescence.

Reviews of the epidemiology of suicide among youth are quite widespread (e.g., Berman, 1986; Blumenthal, 1990a; Garrison, 1992; Holinger, 1989; Rosenberg, Smith, Davidson, & Conn, 1987; Shaffer, 1988), and the reader is referred to these and other studies for more in-depth examination of individual differences in the epidemiology of suicide in children and adolescents. A rough approximation is that the incidence of suicide in 15- to 19-year-olds is 11/100,000 [1989 United States data reported by the NIMH (1992)]. Significantly lower rates of suicide completion are found for younger adolescents and children, with highest rates during adolescence found among males, and in particular white males (Holinger, 1989). In 1989, over 2000 adolescents 15–19 years of age committed suicide, with a 4:1 male/female ratio of completers (NIMH, 1992).

Suicide Attempts

The rate of suicide attempts in children and adolescents varies as a function of study and sample characteristics, as well as the time frame. The latter is important in distinguishing between incidence and prevalence data. Incidence data typically report on the occurrence of a suicide attempt within the past year, and prevalence is the occurrence of a suicide attempt in the past. In this respect, prevalence is similar to evaluation of lifetime occurrence of suicide attempts. We will discuss some of the methodological issues related to potential difficulties in interpretation of research on suicide attempts in young people later in the chapter. However, it is important to note that estimates of prevalence and incidence are most useful for understanding suicide attempts in children and adolescents from the general population. This group also includes a great many youngsters who may demonstrate psychopathology but not be seen by a mental health professional or in a treatment setting. Thus, the general population is not synonymous with youngsters free from psychopathology. Similarly, individual differences (e.g., gender, race, age) for which differences in suicidal behavior have been found will affect base rates to the extent that samples vary on these variables.

Incidence of Suicide Attempts.   It was previously thought that the incidence of suicide attempts in adolescents was approximately 1/1000 (Seiden, 1969). Most epidemiological reports of suicide and suicidal behaviors among adolescents indicate that these behaviors have increased dramatically in the past 25 years. The problem of suicidality among young people may be even greater, given recent research that suggests that the actual number of adolescents from the general population who attempt suicide each year is many times more than previously thought. The studies described below are based on samples of adolescents from school-based settings and as such do not include adolescents in inpatient, correctional, or other mental health settings. Thus, if we anticipate that the many youngsters who are out of school because they have run away from home or been incarcerated for delinquent acts or are in mental health settings have a higher rate of suicidal behavior (e.g., Reynolds & Mazza, 1993b; Rotheram-Borus, 1993), the findings below are underestimates of the true proportion of adolescents who attempt suicide each year. Even as an underestimate, however, these data suggest that the number of youngsters who make a suicide attempt may be considered to be of epidemic proportion.

An incidence study of suicidal behavior in a sample of 1384 adolescents from grades 7–12 in a semirural community was reported by Dubow, Kausch, Blum, Reed, and Bush (1989), who found that 7% of their sample reported having made a suicide attempt in the past year. In a noteworthy study of 3764 adolescents from grades 9–12 in South Carolina, Garrison, McKeown, Valois, and Vincent (1993) found that 7.5% of their sample reported having made a suicide attempt in the past year. Garrison et al. (1993) reported that approximately 21% of the suicide attempters (1.6% of the total sample) reported needing medical treatment for their attempt. In a community-based study in Ontario, Canada, Joffe et al. (1988) reported 6-month incidence data on suicide attempts among a sample of 1256 children ages 12–16 years. They found that among 12- to 13-year-olds, 3.8% of females and 3.5% of males reported suicide attempts, and among 14- to 16-year-olds, 7.1% of females and 2.4% of males reported a suicide attempt in the previous 6 months.

Felts, Chenier, and Barnes (1992) surveyed 3064 adolescents from North Carolina in grades 9–12 for substance use and suicidal behavior. They found that approximately 25% of youngsters in their sample reported serious suicidal ideation during the past 12 months, and that 14.4% of the total sample had made a specific suicide-attempt plan during this time period. The authors reported that 4.5% of their sample indicated a suicide attempt in the past year. They found that 2.1% of the total sample were treated by a doctor or nurse for injuries due to their suicide attempt, suggesting that nearly half the adolescents who made an attempt in the past year required some level of medical intervention for their injuries.

In what is likely one of the most robust samples of school-based youngsters, the Centers for Disease Control (CDC, 1991) reported on the Youth Risk Behavior Survey data on adolescent suicidal behavior. The CDC report notes that among a sample of 11,631 students from all 50 states, 8.3% indicated having made a suicide attempt in the past year, including 10.3% of females and 6.2% of males. The CDC found that 2.1% of all adolescents were seen in medical settings for their suicide attempt.

Results of the CDC (1990), Dubow et al. (1989), and Garrison et al. (1993) studies are remarkably similar and suggest relatively robust statistics on the percentage of youngsters who attempt suicide each year. The base rate of 7–8% is high for a serious behavior such as suicide attempts and suggests that rather than 1/1000, as many as 1 of every 13 adolescents make a suicide attempt each year. It is also important to note that most of the studies cited above report that approximately 2% of all adolescents made an attempt of severity sufficient to require medical attention.

Prevalence of Adolescent Suicide Attempters. The prevalence of suicide attempters refers to the proportion of persons who have made one or more suicide attempts during their life. By this measure, we might expect to find a higher proportion of youngsters who have made an attempt among older adolescents, given that they have had a longer time to have engaged in suicidal behavior. However, this expectation may be mediated by cohort trends for the expression of suicidal behavior in younger adolescents. Likewise, findings based on school samples of older youngsters are biased by substantial high school dropout rates and the location of some adolescents in mental health and other placements who are not sampled. Our discussion here focuses on suicide attempts among adolescents from the general population, although there are studies that have reported on suicide attempts among psychiatric inpatient, outpatient, and other mental health or specialized treatment settings (e.g., Borst & Noam, 1989; Pfeffer et al. 1988).

Several studies of adolescents have been reported that relied on relatively modest-size samples from a single school or location. J. M. H. Friedman, Asnis, Boeck, and DiFiore (1987) reported on a sample of 380 adolescents from an academically select high school in New York, finding that 8.7% had a history of one or more suicide attempts. Smith and Crawford (1986) conducted a study assessing suicidal ideation in high school students, 237 from a public high school and 76 females from a private high school. They reported that 8.4% indicated that they had made at least one suicide attempt. In discussing their results and those of other investigators, Smith and Crawford (1986) suggested that there are over 1.5 million American youngsters between the ages of 15 and 19 who have attempted suicide at least once.

In a survey of 635 adolescents in Rhode Island, Riggs and Cheng (1988) found that 11.8% reported a history of a suicide attempt. This sample was ethnically diverse, with whites making up a minority (14.9%) of the sample. Although proportions were not reported, the authors indicated that significantly more females than males indicated a past suicide attempt. Kandel, Raveis, and Davies (1991), with a sample of 597 9th and 11th grade youngsters, reported that 12% of females and 6% of males indicated a history of a suicide attempt.

In a sample of 1048 9th grade students who responded to the item "Have you ever tried to kill yourself?," Shaffer et al. (1990) found that 97 (9.26%) responded "Yes." These youngsters were participants in a study examining effects of a suicide prevention program using a pretest–posttest design. As a function of this design, the authors were able to reassess youngsters' reports of previous suicide attempts. Shaffer et al. (1990) found that 34 youngsters who initially reported an attempt said "No" to the attempt question at the retesting and 41 youngsters who reported "No" at time one said "Yes" to an attempt history at time two. The authors suggest several reasons for this discrepancy, although the absolute rate of suicide attempts at each assessment was similar (e.g., 9% and 10%, respectively).

An investigation of adolescent health behavior conducted by Adcock, Nagy, and Simpson (1991) surveyed 3803 8th and 10th grade students in Alabama. The sample was 62% white, 35% African-American, and 3% of other ethnic origin. It was found that approximately 16% of the sample reported a past suicide attempt. By gender, 19% of female and 12% of male adolescents reported having made a suicide attempt. Windle, Miller-Tutzauer, and Domenico (1992) reported on data on suicidal behavior gathered from the 1987 National Adolescent Student Health Survey of over 11,000 early (8th grade) and midadolescents (10th grade) from a representative sample of 224 schools, along with data on alcohol use. Windle et al. (1992) found that 13.3% of white, 12.7% of African-American, and 16.8% of Hispanic youngsters indicated that they had made a suicide attempt.

In a study of suicidal behavior in a sample of 3437 adolescents drawn from 11 junior and senior high schools in 8 states across the United States, Reynolds and Mazza (1992a) examined the prevalence and characteristics of adolescent suicide attempts. Participants were in grades 7–12, with a mean age of 15.46 years and an approximately equal number of males (50.2%) and females (49.8%). Racially, the sample was heterogeneous, with a significant proportion (28.6%) of minority group participants. Our findings indicate a high prevalence of suicide attempts reported by this sample of adolescents. There were 469 (13.65%) adolescents who reported one or more suicide attempts. Significantly more females (17.9%) than males (9.5%), $\chi^2(1) = 51.30$, $p < 0.0001$, indicated a history of one or more suicide attempts. The highest rate of suicide history was found among Native American adolescents (25.5%), and the lowest was among African-American youngsters (10.6%). Suicide attempts were also reported by a large proportion (16.3%) of Hispanic youngsters.

Approximately two thirds of these youngsters who had made an attempt indicated that their attempt had been made within the past year. Of the adolescents who indicated a history of a suicide attempt, 20.9% reported that they were hospitalized for their attempt. The difference in the proportions of males and females hospitalized for their attempt was not significant. Nearly 30% of youngsters reported more than one attempt, with the difference between males and females in the mean number of attempts reported being nonsignificant.

Our investigation found that nearly 1 of 7 adolescents in a large, ethnically stratified sample reported having attempted suicide. These data are very similar to those found by Windle et al. (1992) in their examination of the National Adolescent Student Health Survey. We (Reynolds & Mazza, 1992a) also asked youngsters how long it had been since their last attempt. Although it is difficult to extrapolate from these data, a rough approximation based on the number of youngsters who made an attempt in the past 12 months suggests an incidence rate of approximately 8% that is consistent with other incidence studies (e.g., CDC, 1991; Garrison et al., 1993). We found that approximately 1 in 5 adolescents who reported a suicide attempt were hospitalized for their attempt, a proportion higher than that found by other investigators (e.g., Smith & Crawford, 1986), but consistent with findings of Garrison et al. (1993).

Suicidal Ideation

A number of studies have examined suicidal ideation in children. As noted earlier, Pfeffer et al. (1984) found suicidal ideas in 8.9% of a sample of 101 schoolchildren between the ages of 6 and 12 years who were interviewed. They also found that suicide threats were reported in 2% of their sample. Sack, Beiser, Phillips, and Baker-Brown (1993), in a study of 907 Native American and non-Native American children, ages 7–10 years, found relatively high rates of suicidal ideation (response of "A lot of the time" to the question "Have you thought of killing yourself?"), particularly among children with depressive symptoms (13.4%), conduct problems (12.1%), and comorbid conduct and depression (15.9%). Among nondepressed, non-conduct-problem children, the rate was 4.7%.

In a survey of adolescent behavior and problems conducted by the Dane County, Wisconsin, Youth Commission in 1990 (Biendseil, 1991), a stratified sample of 2215 adolescents from grades 7–12 completed a questionnaire regarding suicidal behavior and other health and mental health concerns. To the item specific to considering suicide, 22% of females and 11% of males indicated that doing so was a moderate concern, and

8% of females and 5% of males reported it to be a serious problem. Joffe et al. (1988), in their study of 1256 youngsters, reported that among 12- to 13-year-olds, 7.5% of females and 6.7% of males reported suicidal ideation in the previous 6 months, with suicidal ideation reported by 14.5% of the females and 3.3% of the males aged 14–16 years.

In a study examining suicidal ideation in 1542 younger adolescents of ages 12–14 years, Garrison, Jackson, Addy, McKeown, and Waller (1991b) found that approximately 21% of the sample reported mild suicidal ideation during the previous week, while 10% demonstrated moderate to severe levels of suicidal ideation. Females manifested higher levels of suicidal ideation than did males. In a subsample of youngsters who were interviewed with a diagnostic interview along with their parents, Garrison et al. (1991b) found that most suicidal behaviors (ideation and attempts) reported by the adolescents were not reported by their parents. In a 3-year longitudinal study of suicidal ideation in 1073 adolescents, Garrison, Addy, Jackson, McKeown, & Waller (1991a) found that approximately 8–10% of their sample manifested moderate to high levels of suicidal ideation each year, although there were few adolescents who maintained high levels across the 3 years of the study. In their study of 3764 high school students surveyed as to their suicidal behavior over the past 12 months, Garrison et al. (1993) found that 11% of youngsters reported having serious suicidal thoughts, with 6.4% having made a specific suicide plan.

As noted, Reynolds (1988) reported significant levels of suicidal ideation over the past month as measured by the Suicidal Ideation Questionnaire (SIQ) in 10% of a sample of 890 adolescents in grades 10–12, with 12% of females and 8% of males reporting significant levels of suicidal ideation. Using the SIQ—Junior High Version (SIQ-JR) with a sample of 1280 adolescents in grades 7–9, Reynolds (1988) reported significant levels of suicidal ideation in 11% of the total sample, with clinical levels found in 9% of male and 13% of female adolescents. Lamb and Pusker (1991), using the SIQ with a school-based sample of 69 adolescents, found that 16% demonstrated clinical levels of suicidal ideation. Kandel et al. (1991), with a sample of 597 9th and 11th grade youngsters, reported that over the previous few weeks, 22% of females and 11% of males reported thinking of ways to kill themselves and that 32% of females and 16% of males reported suicidal thoughts.

In the previously mentioned survey conducted by the CDC (1991) with a sample of 11,631 adolescents in grades 9–12 drawn from all 50 states, 27.3% of all students reported having thought seriously about attempting suicide in the past 12 months. In this study, 16.3% of school-based youngsters indicated that they had made specific suicide plans during the preceding 12 months. Females reported higher rates of suicidal ideation (33.9%) and plans (20.2%) than did males (20.5% and 12.3%, respectively).

The aforecited studies specific to suicidal ideation vary in the time frame as well as the procedures used to operationalize and assess suicidal ideation. A reasonable estimate is that suicidal ideation is manifested by approximately 10–15% of children and adolescents at any one time. As with other suicidal behaviors, such as attempts, significantly more adolescent females manifest suicidal ideation than do adolescent males. In children and younger adolescents, gender difference in suicidal ideation is typically not evident. Data on suicidal ideation experienced over a 1-year period suggest that serious suicidal ideation is experienced by a significant proportion of the general adolescent population.

Evaluation of Suicidal Behavior in Young People

The identification of youngsters who are at high risk for suicidal behaviors is a major step in the intervention in and prevention of these behaviors. Identification of high-risk youngsters has been seen as a significant procedure for effective intervention (e.g., Eddy, Wolpert, & Rosenberg, 1987). Due to parents' general lack of awareness of youngsters' suicidal behavior (e.g., Joffe et al., 1988; Zimmerman & Asnis, 1991b), the most suitable method for the evaluation of suicidal behavior in adolescents is by questioning the youngster directly. It has been our clinical experience in conducting hundreds of interviews with children and adolescents that youngsters are reliable reporters of their suicidal behaviors and that in many instances suicidal behaviors are not reported to parents or peers. This experience is consistent with the finding reported by Robbins and Alessi (1985).

It has been the perspective of the first author that a proactive procedure for the identification and clinical evaluation of suicidality in young persons be conducted by direct evaluation: by either self-report, clinical interview, or a combination of these approaches (Reynolds, 1988, 1991d). With younger children, parent interviews are an important part of the evaluation procedure, although in one-on-one interviews with children, we do find youngsters reporting suicide attempts that their parents thought were accidents. It should be recognized that there have been few measures developed specifically to evaluate suicidal behavior in young people that have been sufficiently tested to ascertain their psychometric quality—in particular their reliability and validity. For the most part, those measures that are available target adolescents, with few measures available for the systematic evaluation of suicidality in children.

Overt Signs of Suicidal Behavior in Youngsters

There are a number of observable behaviors that may occur and should alert one to the possibility that an adolescent is at risk for suicide. These behaviors include having frequent accidents, engaging in dangerous or risky behavior, talking about death or morbid themes, and such actions as giving away meaningful possessions. It is important to be vigilant for these indicators and treat them as signs of suicide potential. It is equally important to know that *not all suicidal youngsters* will provide such signs and symptoms of their intent, nor are all youngsters who demonstrate the behaviors listed above suicidal. Thus, it should be realized that the occurrence of these behaviors in a child or adolescent does not necessarily lead to or indicate that the youngster is at risk for suicidal behaviors. However, the behaviors noted should not be ignored.

The identification of suicidal behavior in adolescents and young adults is a difficult task. There is an obvious hesitation by some adolescents to inform others that they are thinking of taking their own life or that they are preoccupied with thoughts of death. The potential for ridicule from peers and parents often precludes the acceptability of telling others of suicidal ideation or intent. Although some adolescents will voluntarily inform professionals or parents of their problems, and some will confide in peers who may let others know, those who will do so appear to be at best a small proportion of the large number of distressed youngsters who are in need of assistance. Furthermore, it is sometimes difficult to perceive the behavior at the time of their occurrence as indicative of suicidality. Much of what we know regarding overt indicators or precursors of suicidal behavior is based on hindsight or retrospective recollection of events, behaviors, or changes in behaviors that at the time appeared relatively benign or within a normal range of functioning. It is often only after an attempt or completion that the previous behaviors take on significant meaning.

Direct Assessment of Suicidal Behaviors in Young People

After more than a decade of research on suicidal behavior involving well over 15,000 children and adolescents, the first author has noted that youngsters generally do not refer themselves for psychological help. Many of the youngsters identified through school-based screening procedures (e.g., Reynolds, 1986a, 1991d) as depressed or manifesting serious levels of suicidal ideation have indicated that they had not communicated their distress to a professional, parents, or even friends or peers. In some cases, adolescents who on being questioned have endorsed serious suicidal thoughts have also indicated that they had no intention of telling anyone. As an example of this attitude, Fig. 1 presents the responses of a 13-year-old boy on the SIQ-JR (Reynolds, 1987). This assessment was part of an annual school-based screening using the two-stage model described below. What is of interest here is the significant and frequent specific thoughts of suicide. Less frequent was mild ideation such as wishes he were dead or had never been born. Also significant is the response to item 9 on the SIQ-JR, in which the youngster, although actively thinking of killing himself, indicated that he had no thoughts of telling others he planned to kill himself. What we have inferred from this and other similar cases is that unless we ask youngsters directly, it is extremely difficult to know the extent of their suicidality.

From our work with depressed and suicidal youngsters, it is evident these are real and significant mental health problems that are demonstrated by many youngsters in school, as well as in clinical settings. This being so, there is a great need for reliable and valid assessment measures for suicidal behavior in young people. We have come to the general conclusion that the most effective method for identification of suicidal children and adolescents is by direct questioning, rather than relying on self- or peer referral or observations of others. For the most part, the latter procedures, while they may identify a small proportion of suicidal youngsters, will result in a large number of false-negatives. Given the decision-making utilities related to the identification of suicidal adolescents, to err in the direction of false-negatives, that is, to perceive a youngster as not at risk when the youth is suicidal, is highly undesirable as an outcome. Likewise, when we use psychological measures for the evaluation and identification of suicidal behavior in youngsters, we should have some information and understanding as to the anticipated proportion of false-positives and false-negatives that may occur in using a particular measure or cutoff score.

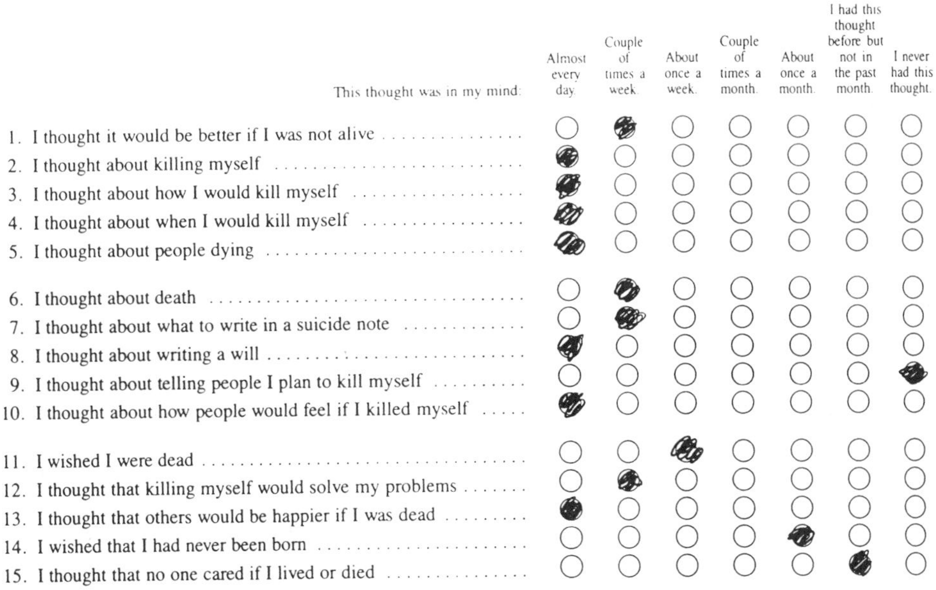

This thought was in my mind:	Almost every day	Couple of times a week	About once a week	Couple of times a month	About once a month	I had this thought before but not in the past month	I never had this thought
1. I thought it would be better if I was not alive	○	●	○	○	○	○	○
2. I thought about killing myself	●	○	○	○	○	○	○
3. I thought about how I would kill myself	●	○	○	○	○	○	○
4. I thought about when I would kill myself	●	○	○	○	○	○	○
5. I thought about people dying	●	○	○	○	○	○	○
6. I thought about death	○	●	○	○	○	○	○
7. I thought about what to write in a suicide note	○	●	○	○	○	○	○
8. I thought about writing a will	●	○	○	○	○	○	○
9. I thought about telling people I plan to kill myself	○	○	○	○	○	○	●
10. I thought about how people would feel if I killed myself	●	○	○	○	○	○	○
11. I wished I were dead	○	○	●	○	○	○	○
12. I thought that killing myself would solve my problems	○	●	○	○	○	○	○
13. I thought that others would be happier if I was dead	●	○	○	○	○	○	○
14. I wished that I had never been born	○	○	○	○	●	○	○
15. I thought that no one cared if I lived or died	○	○	○	○	○	●	○

Figure 1. Responses to the SIQ-JR by a 13-year-old boy. Adapted and reproduced by special permission of the publisher, Psychological Assessment Resources, Inc., 16204 North Florida Avenue, Lutz, FL 33549, from the Suicidal Ideation Questionnaire by William M. Reynolds, Ph.D. Copyright 1987 by Psychological Assessment Resources, Inc. Further reproduction is prohibited without permission from PAR, Inc.

Without such information, we have minimal evidence to support the use of a particular measure for the identification of at-risk children and adolescents.

Over the past decade, a number of measures have been developed that evaluate aspects of suicidal behavior in young people. These measures include paper-and-pencil self-report instruments and semistructured clinical interviews. Presented below are descriptions of a number of measures of suicidal behavior, the majority of which have been developed for use with adolescents.

Suicidal Ideation Questionnaire. Toward the goal of identification of suicidal youth, Reynolds (1987, 1988, 1989, 1991a) has developed the SIQ, a self-report measure of suicidal ideation in youngsters ages 13–19 years. A 25-item version of the SIQ, the Adult SIQ (Reynolds, 1991b), was developed for use with adults and has demonstrated high reliability with samples of college students, community adults, and psychiatric outpatients (Reynolds, 1991c; Reynolds, Kobak, & Greist, 1992, 1994) as well as sensitivity to pharmacotherapy in adult outpatients with major depressive disorder (Reynolds, Kobak, Greist, Jefferson, & Tollefson, 1993).

The SIQ was developed as a measure of adolescents' current level of suicidal ideation and is based on a model of suicidal ideation delineated by Reynolds (1988). The SIQ does not provide a probability estimate of risk for completed suicide or suicide attempt. According to the author, variability in individual characteristics such as personality, mental health status, self-regulation, motivation, psychosocial stressors, and family and social support structure does not support the assignment of a numerical probability for suicide. The SIQ does provide a measure of the seriousness of suicidal thoughts in adolescents.

There are two forms of the SIQ. The SIQ consists of 30 items and is designed for senior high school students; the SIQ-JR includes 15 items and is designed for junior high school students, but may also be used with older adolescents (e.g., C. A. King et al., 1990). On both versions, the youngster rates each item on a 7-point scale that assesses the frequency with which the cognition occurred over the past month. Included in the response format is a category indicating that the thought/cognition has never occurred, as well as a response option that indicates that the thought had previously occurred, although not in the past month. Items are scored from 0 to 6, such that a high score is indicative of numerous suicidal cognitions occurring with significant regularity over the past month. The SIQ-JR is illustrated in Fig. 1. Cutoff scores on the SIQ and SIQ-JR have been developed to define levels of suicidal ideation considered to be clinically relevant and to indicate the need for further evaluation.

The internal consistency reliabilities using the Cronbach (1951) coefficient alpha (r_α) of the SIQ and SIQ-JR reported by Reynolds (1988) for various samples and by age and sex were uniformly high and ranged from 0.93 to 0.94, with a total sample reliability coefficient of 0.94 on the SIQ-JR and a total sample reliability coefficient of 0.97 for the SIQ. The test–retest reliability of the SIQ was examined in a large sample of 801 youngsters who were retested on the SIQ approximately 4 weeks after the initial assessment. On the initial assessment, a mean of 17.76 (SD = 20.76) was obtained; 4 weeks later, a mean SIQ score of 17.49 was found (SD = 23.82), with a test–retest reliability coefficient of 0.72. This value is moderately high and consistent with the state–construct nature of suicidal ideation. There was a nonsignificant difference between mean scores between the two testings ($t = 0.45$, $p = $ ns), suggesting relative stability of raw scores.

The validity of the SIQ has been demonstrated by correlations with measures of related constructs. Correlational studies with measures of depression, hopelessness, anxiety, self-esteem, history of suicide, and other related variable have been reported in detail by Reynolds (1988, 1989, 1992a). Reynolds (1990) reported a correlation of 0.68 ($p < 0.001$) between the SIQ-JR and the Suicidal Behavior Interview (SBI) (Reynolds, in press b) and a correlation of 0.63 ($p < 0.001$) between the SIQ and the SBI. Using the SBI as criterion measure for differentiating youngsters at risk for suicidal behaviors, Reynolds (1991d) reported significant differences in SIQ scores between at-risk ($M = 77.22$) and not-at-risk ($M = 35.17$) adolescents. The clinical efficacy of SIQ and SIQ-JR cutoff scores has been described by Reynolds (1991d, 1992a) using the SBI as criterion measure.

A number of investigators have used the SIQ with clinical samples. Ritter (1990), with a sample of 28 adolescent suicide attempters evaluated with the SIQ within 24 hours of their attempt, reported a mean score of 108.6, with a range of 52–152, all scores well above the clinical cutoff of 41. Spirito et al. (1987) found a significant difference in SIQ scores between adolescent suicide attempters who were characterized as having a past history of acute (SIQ mean = 109.1) as compared to chronic (SIQ mean = 53.5) psychiatric problems. In a sample of adolescent female suicide attempters and a demographically matched sample of nonattempters, C. A. King et al. (1990) found significant differences in SIQ-JR scores between attempters ($M = 57.8$) and nonattempters ($M = 17.0$). C. A. King, Hill, Naylor, Evans, and Shain (1993) found a significant relationship between the SIQ-JR and family dysfunction ($r = 0.54$, $p < 0.001$), depression ($r = 0.53$, $p < 0.001$), and lifetime severity of suicidal behavior ($r = 0.55$, $p < 0.001$) in a sample of 54 adolescent inpatient females. In a sample of adolescents hospitalized for a suicide attempt ($N = 27$) or whose hospitalization included suicidal ideation ($N = 51$) and a nonsuicidal control group ($N = 38$), Shaunesey, Cohen, Plummer, and Berman (1993) found significantly higher SIQ scores for suicide attempters ($M = 85.70$) and suicidal ideators ($M = 73.86$) than nonsuicidal controls ($M = 26.55$), $F = 15.19$, $p < 0.01$.

The SIQ is useful both in the initial evaluation of adolescents who are potentially at risk for suicide and self-destructive behaviors and in the evaluation of youngsters who have made suicide attempts. In the latter application, the SIQ can serve as a measure for the follow-up evaluation of adolescents at continued risk. In schools and clinical settings, the SIQ provides an efficient and economical method of screening for suicidal thoughts and intent in adolescents. The SIQ may also be used for the evaluation of large-scale intervention and prevention programs, particularly those implemented in school settings. Schools that recognize mental health problems among adolescents and engage in preventative and intervention programs for suicide or other mental health problems can use the SIQ as a measure for program efficacy.

Life Orientation Inventory.   The Life Orientation Inventory (LOI) (Kowalchuk & King, 1988) is a paper-and-pencil measure of suicidal orientation, or the resolution that people have once they encompass the belief of suicide as a personal option or choice. The LOI consists of six subscales that vary in length from 16 to 24 items. These scales include: Self-Esteem Vulnerability, Overinvestment (a supplementary scale most applicable to persons who have experienced loss), Overdetermined Misery, Affective Domination, Alienation, and Suicide Tenability. The total LOI consists of 113 items. There is also a 30-item screener, although only 4 items on this scale deal specifically with suicide. The LOI item-response format is a 4-point scale from "I Am Sure I Disagree" to "I Am Sure I Agree." The LOI protocol form uses different titles for the subscales, such as "Love, Work, and What is Important to Me" for the Overinvestment subscale and "Reasons for Living or Dying" for the Suicide Tenability subscale. The authors of the LOI suggest that the scale requires 30–60 minutes to complete. Because of the linguistic complexity of some of the items, we suggest that most adolescents will require 45–60 minutes.

The LOI was developed with adolescents and adults, and the authors suggest that a 6th grade reading level is required to respond to the scale. Norms (T-scores and percentiles) are provided for youngsters 18 years and younger and for adults. There were 907 youngsters in the adolescent norms, which is a reasonably large sample. Unfortunately, there was a preponderance of Native American youngsters (approximately 16%) in the standardization sample (compared to approximately 1% in the general population). Given the relatively high rate of suicidal behavior among Native American adolescents (Berlin, 1987; Gartrell, Jarvis, & Derksen, 1993; Grossman, Milligan, & Deyo, 1991; Reynolds & Mazza, 1993a), this disproportionate representation may attenuate the utility and meaningfulness of the norms, as the norms are presented for the total sample and are not differentiated by gender or ethnic background. The authors do not discuss the potential bias in norms as a function of the relative unrepresentativeness of the sample.

The reliability of the subscales is variable, with internal consistency reliability ranging from 0.53 to 0.82 for youngsters 13–16 years and from 0.51 to 0.84 for ages 17–19 years. Test–retest reliability was not reported for adolescents, although a sample of college students were tested twice, with subscale test–retest coefficients ranging from 0.62 to 0.83. Validity data are sparse for adolescents. These data consist of correlations between the LOI subscales and two hopelessness measures for two groups of 40 youngsters who are not adequately described. Only significant correlations are reported, and they are adjusted for restriction of range. Overall, the LOI is an interesting measure, although at this time there are insufficient data to support its clinical use. Further reliability, validity, and normative data need to be established with the general adolescent population.

Reasons for Living Inventory. The Reasons for Living Inventory (RFL) was developed for adults by Linehan, Goodstein, Nielsen, and Chiles (1983) as a self-report measure of persons' beliefs related to reasons for not committing suicide. The RFL consists of 48 items that provide scores on 6 factors: Survival and Coping Beliefs, Responsibility to Family, Child-Related Concerns, Fear of Suicide, Fear of Social Disapproval, and Moral Objections. Although the RFL has been used in several research studies with adolescents (e.g., Cole, 1989a; Fremouw, Callahan, & Kashden, 1993), data suggest that additional research is needed with youngsters. In a study reported by Fremouw et al. (1993), the RFL did not differentiate between suicidal and nonsuicidal hospitalized adolescents, although a significant difference was found between suicidal inpatients and normal controls. Cole (1989a) found mixed results in groups of normal and delinquent adolescents, reporting some evidence of discrimination between groups of adolescents based on suicidal status, but relatively low correlations with related measured.

Adolescent Psychopathology Scale: Suicide Scale. The Adolescent Psychopathology Scale (APS) (Reynolds, in press a) is a multidimensional self-report measure of psychopathology in adolescents. The APS consists of 20 scales that evaluate DSM-IV Axis I domains, 5 personality disorder scales, and 11 content scales (e.g., self-concept, alienation, disorientation). The Suicide Scale of the APS is one of the content scales and consists of 8 items that reflect aspects of suicidal behaviors, e.g., suicidal ideation, attempts, intent. Norms for the APS are provided for a national sample of over 1800 adolescents, with data also presented for a clinical sample of 506 youngsters drawn from 21 states. Reynolds (in press a) reports an internal consistency reliability of 0.88 for the standardization sample of school-based adolescents and 0.92 for a clinical sample drawn from mental health settings. As a component of a broad-based measure of adolescent psychopathology, the Suicide Scale of the APS allows for the examination of suicidality in conjunction with psychopathology and other problems in adolescents.

Suicidal Behaviors Interview. The SBI (Reynolds, 1990, in press b) is a semistructured clinical interview developed for the clinical evaluation of suicidal behavior in adolescents. There are 20 questions on the SBI, 18 of which are scored on either a 0–2 or a 0–4 point scale. Two questions specific to attempted suicide are not scored—i.e., length of time the youngster thought about the attempt before acting and what precipitated the attempt—but are included in the interview to gain further clinical insight into components of a youngster's suicidal behavior.

The SBI consists of two parts, the first of which includes four sets of questions that have been shown to be related to suicidal behaviors in adolescents and important aspects to examine in the evaluation of suicidal youngsters (Brent et al., 1988; Garfinkel & Golombek, 1983; Hawton, 1986; Reynolds, 1988). These questions evaluate generalized levels of psychological distress (including anxiety, depression, and hopelessness), the severity of daily hassles, general level of social support from family, friends, school, work, and other factors (reverse scored), and evaluation of recent major negative life events. Each set of questions is scored using a global rating (0–4), with a high score indicative of severe problems in each domain.

The second section consists of questions specific to suicidal behavior and related risk factors. Questions in this section follow the hierarchy of suicidal cognitions and behaviors described by Reynolds (1988). Thus, the first items in this section focus on mild suicidal ideation, followed by items dealing with specific thoughts of how, when, and where the youngster has contemplated suicide. Overt suicide-related behaviors, such as writing a will, leaving a suicide note, and giving away possessions, are then evaluated, followed by questions about prior suicide attempt(s). The latter focus on these specifics: length of time since the most recent attempt, the youngster's perception at the time that the attempt would be successful, and information about the method used and circumstances of the attempt (i.e., location of significant others who might intervene or probability of rescue).

Items are scored by the interviewer, with higher scores indicative of greater severity of suicidal behavior. Each item has descriptors associated with specific points on the rating scale. Descriptors vary across items and are specific to the suicidal behavior delineated by the item. For instance, item 6, which deals with general thoughts of killing oneself, is scored on the basis of frequency from absent (0) or infrequently (1) to most of the time (4). Item 7, which is specific to thoughts of how the youngster might kill himself or herself, is scored on the basis of how well formulated the plan is, with possible scores ranging from absent (0) or vague plan (1) to detailed plan (4). As a semistructured clinical interview, SBI items are presented and scored in a reasonably objective format, with operational anchors associated with score points on each item.

In the original development study (Reynolds, 1990), the reliability of the SBI was examined from the perspective of internal consistency reliability and interrater reliability. The sample consisted of 352 subjects, ages 12–19 years. Racially, one third of the sample were nonwhite. Subjects were individually interviewed by one of seven trained interviewers using the SBI. For a subsample of 36 youngsters, a second interviewer was present and independently scored the SBI to establish interrater reliability. The coefficient alpha reliability (r_α) was 0.92 for the 18-item (scored portion) SBI. Internal consistency reliability coefficients were somewhat higher for females ($r_\alpha = 0.93$) as compared to males ($r_\alpha = 0.89$). For a group of 62 youngsters who reported a history of one or more suicide attempts, a coefficient alpha reliability of 0.88 was found. Interrater reliability coefficients were high, with a zero-order correlation of 0.97 and an intraclass correlation coefficient (r_{icc}) of 0.99 between the sets of interviewers. This high reliability between raters is consistent with that achieved during the training.

A factor analysis of SBI items produced three factors that the author delineated as specific to: (1) covert and overt suicidal behaviors, (2) psychological distress and stress, and (3) history of suicide attempt. Scores on these subscales were moderately related to each other and demonstrated moderate to high reliability ($r_\alpha = 0.83$–0.90). Further evidence of validity was presented in the form of correlations between the SBI total scale and subscales and the SIQ, Reynolds Adolescent Depression Scale (RADS) (Reynolds, 1986b), and history of previous suicide attempt. Moderate to high correlations were reported between the SBI and related measures. A series of multiple regression analyses with the SBI as dependent variable and related measures, age, and sex as independent variables produced a multiple correlation of 0.82 for the junior high school subjects and 0.79 for the senior high school subjects.

Reynolds and Mazza (1993c) examined the reliability of the SBI, using a different sample of 486 adolescents (M age = 14.57 years) including 191 males and 295 females from grades 7–12 in three schools. Adolescents were interviewed with the SBI as part of a two-stage school-based procedure for the identification of suicidal youngsters. This procedure is described in more detail below. Interviewers were eight graduate students who received extensive training on the administration and scoring of the SBI by the author. For a subsample of 47 adolescents, a second interviewer was present and scored the SBI as it was administered to establish interrater reliability. The reliability of the SBI was examined from the perspective of internal consistency reliability using the coefficient alpha of Cronbach (1951) and interrater reliability. The coefficient alpha was 0.90 for the total 18-item interview. The interrater reliability was high, with a zero-order correlation of 0.95. In addition, a dependent sample t-test between SBI scores for the pairs of raters was nonsignificant ($t = 0.52, p$ = ns). The mean difference between raters was less than 1 point. These results support the high internal consistency and interrater reliability of the SBI with adolescents. Given the seriousness of the behavior assessed, high reliability is a prerequisite for a measure of suicidal behavior.

Suicidal Behavior History Form. The Suicidal Behavior History Form (SBHF) (Reynolds & Mazza, 1992c) is a formal guide for the evaluation of a youngster's past history of suicidal behavior, in particular suicide attempt(s). The SBHF is a four-page form and a detailed Clinicians Guide that describes the administration, interpretation, and rationale for the SBHF. Page 1 of the SBHF provides for the documentation of client information, including psychosocial risk factors, health considerations, family factors, major life events, drug and alcohol use, current and past mental health diagnoses, current prescription medications, social supports, previous hospitalization, significant others/contact persons, interviewer information, and circumstances of the interview. Pages 2–4 of the SBHF focus on questions specific to recent and past suicide attempts, with questions including method, place, and circumstances of attempt, planning of attempt, intention to complete suicide, availability of rescue, reasons for attempt, outcome immediately following attempt, communication with others, specifics of suicide note, writing of a will, giving away possessions, medical and psychiatric attention for attempt, current status, availability of guns, pills, family history of suicidal behavior, and other questions including current level of suicidal intent.

Although not a formal assessment measure, the SBHF allows for the systematic evaluation of past and present suicidal behavior in adolescents and adults. In this manner, the SBHF provides the clinician with a formal documented history of an individual's suicidal behavior and allows for the integration of this information along with test data, clinical observations, and other information for the evaluation of suicide risk and the development of an intervention program or plan. The SBHF may also be used in conjunction with formal measures of suicidal behavior for providing documentation of evaluation of suicidality, an important consideration when working with suicidal individuals (Berman, 1990; Jobes & Berman, 1993).

Summary

The measures described above represent a majority of measures developed for use with youngsters and, with the exception of the SBHF, have demonstrated psychometric characteristics that allow for their evaluation for research and clinical applications. Space limitations preclude a comprehensive review of all measures of suicidality used in research with young people. For example, our review did not include the Pfeffer (1986) Spectrum of Suicidal Behaviors (SBS) scale, a 5-point scale that classifies behavior as (1) nonsuicidal, (2) suicidal ideation, (3) suicidal threats, (4) mild suicide attempt, or (5) serious suicide attempt. The SBS has been used in numerous studies of child and adolescent suicide as a descriptive measure for categorizing groups as to levels of suicidality. A number of other measures, some of which were developed for adults, have also bee used with children or adolescents. Rich, Kirkpatrick-Smith, Bonner, and Jans (1992) used an adapted version of the Scale for Suicidal Ideation (SSI) (Beck, Kovacs, & Weissman, 1979) with a sample of high school students, although these authors did not report on the psychometric characteristics of the SSI with high school students. Brent et al. (1993d) used the Beck Suicide Intent Scale (BSIS) (Beck, Schuyler, & Herman, 1974), a 16-item clinical interview with an inpatient sample of adolescents, and while reliability estimates were ascertained for other interview and self-report measures in their study, no psychometric data were reported for the BSIS. In addition, the Suicide Probability Scale (Cull & Gill, 1982) was not reviewed, and although Cull and Gill included a limited number of adolescents in their normative sample, research (Tatman, Greene, & Karr, 1993) has raised questions as to the utility of this measure with adolescents.

We also did not review measures such as the Death/Suicide Interview used in research by Carlson, Asarnow, and Orbach (1987), for which no psychometric information was reported. Orbach, Feshbach, Carlson, Blaugman, and Gross (1983) reported on the Suicidal Tendencies Test, designed to measure four attitudes toward death and suicide (attraction to life, repulsion by life, attraction to death, and repulsion by death) using fairy tales that require resolution to a story. Orbach et al. (1983) found low test–retest reliability coefficient for scores on this interview measure with a sample of suicidal and nonsuicidal children. A self-report form, the Multi-Attitude Suicide Tendency Scale (Orbach et al., 1991), was developed for use with adolescents and shows moderate levels of reliability and validity. Rudd (1989, 1990) reported on the 10-item Suicidal Ideation Scale that he developed for use with college students, including older adolescents. Rudd (1989) reports adequate internal consistency reliability ($r_\alpha = 0.86$) and correlations with related constructs as validity evidence. Using a structured diagnostic interview, Velez and Cohen (1988) constructed a 6-item measure of suicidal ideation and reported an internal consistency reliability coefficient of 0.73 for this scale, minimally adequate for use in research.

Identifying Youngsters at Risk for Suicidal Behaviors: A Two-Stage School-Based Screening Procedure

We have noted that schools represent one of the few settings that allow for the potential identification of the significant numbers of youngsters who demonstrate or are potentially at risk for suicidal behaviors. For the most part, schools have not engaged in proactive approaches for the identification of suicidal youth. Although schools are beginning to recognize this need, most schools are ill-equipped or relatively unsophisticated in procedures and methods for identifying affected youngsters. On the basis of over a decade of research and applications, the first author has developed and tested procedures for the school-based identification of youngsters who demonstrate significant suicidal ideation and who report an intent or propensity for self-injurious behavior.

School-based screening for at-risk youngsters is a cost-effective means of identifying and directing intervention services to high-risk youngsters. As Shaffer, Garland, Gould, Fisher, and Trautman (1988) point out, even with a high rate of success, school-based prevention programs that utilize educational approaches would prevent fewer than 1% of adolescent suicides. They note that a better strategy is to provide services to those youngsters who are at greatest risk. It is our conclusion that by identifying these youngsters via school-based screening procedures, we are best able to target those youngsters who might be in greatest need of intervention, as well as tailor interventions to individual needs. Shaffer et al. (1988) and Garfinkel (1986) view procedures that assist in the early identification of suicidal youth as preventative approaches to youth suicide.

The identification of adolescents' severity of suicidal ideation serves as a viable proactive approach for the identification of youths at risk for suicide. Although it is not suggested that all adolescents who manifest suicidal ideation will attempt suicide, suicidal ideation appears to be a precursor for the vast majority who do attempt suicide and many who commit suicide (e.g., Shafii et al., 1988). Andrews and Lewinsohn (1992), in a longitudinal study of school-based adolescents, found that suicidal ideation was a significant predictor of future suicide attempts, even when controlling for previous suicide attempts. In addition, suicidal ideation represents a domain of maladaptive cognitions that are worthy of treatment consideration.

The procedure described below may be viewed as a multiple-gate or multiple-stage screening procedure. Multiple-stage screening methods have been proposed and found useful for the identification of mental health problems in children and adolescents in school settings (Reynolds, 1986a). School-based screening procedures are a viable strategy for the identification of youngsters who are thinking about suicide and other self-destructive behaviors. For professionals in school settings, the importance of screening for suicidal behaviors can be readily appreciated if one considers the thousands of adolescents who kill themselves each year and the estimated 1–2 million youngsters who make suicide attempts. As noted, studies suggest that approximately 9–12% of adolescents endorse significant levels of suicidal thoughts, making the identification of youngsters who are actively thinking about suicide an important quest.

A major problem in the identification of suicidal adolescents is the lack of self-referral by suicidal youngsters. Many youngsters do not communicate suicidal thoughts to others, which makes the identification of suicidal adolescents by peers, teachers, or others a difficult undertaking. Reliance on teachers for the identification of suicidal youngsters is a misguided expectation, given that high school teachers have limited contact with 100–200 students per day. It is unrealistic to expect the average teacher, even with training, to have complete insight into the problems of students. Likewise, the psychoeducational approaches that suggest that teachers and other professionals be vigilant for signs of depression are based in part on the false assumptions that professionals are reliable in their identification of depressed youngsters and that suicidal youngsters are also depressed. In a study of over 1400 adolescents who were screened with the SIQ and RADS, 330 of whom were interviewed with the SBI, Reynolds and Mazza (1990) found 39 youngsters who were at risk for suicidal behaviors. Of these, 13 (33%) did not evidence a clinical level of depressive symptomatology on the RADS. The authors also found a higher rate of past history of attempts among the suicidal nondepressed adolescents (92.3%) compared to the suicidal depressed youngsters (76.9%). On the basis of clinical interviews with a sample of 2787 adolescents seen in community mental and health care clinics, Stiffman, Earls, Robins, and Jung (1988) found that only 18% of 677 youngsters who reported suicidal ideation and suicidal behavior met criteria for major depression. Thus, depression, although a related clinical problem, is not always found in suicidal adolescents.

The screening procedure delineated below uses a two-stage assessment approach for the identification of youngsters who may be characterized as demonstrating clinically significant levels of suicidal thoughts. This procedure includes the group administration of the SIQ within classrooms as the initial screen. Following collection and scoring of the SIQ, those youngsters who score at or above the cutoff score are interviewed by a trained professional for more specific suicidal behaviors. In our research and clinical practice, we have used the SBI as the clinical interview for youngsters identified in the initial stage of the screening. Detailed descriptions and efficacy of the screening procedure described below can be found in Reynolds (1991a,d).

The first stage is the group screening of a school or of specific grade levels in a school with the SIQ or similar measure. In practice, this screening has been accomplished by teachers, who, after receiving a brief in-service training session, administer the SIQ to students in their classrooms. This assessment, including administration, directions, and distribution of the SIQ, can be conducted in less than 20 minutes. We have found it best to administer the screening at the same time for all students, preferably in the morning (second or third period). Once teachers have administered the SIQ, the questionnaires are collected and scored (a same-day mail-in scoring service is available for the SIQ).

At this first screening stage, we have typically found between 9% and 12% of youngsters to score at or above the cutoff score on the SIQ. The basic strategy is to identify students who report significant levels of suicidal thoughts at the initial screening. These youngsters are then evaluated by qualified school professionals with a semistructured clinical interview or other similar measures to determine specific suicide risk and decide on intervention/referral procedures. The sensitivity of the initial-stage selection procedure is a function of the cutoff score used to identify youngsters who demonstrate significant suicidal ideation. By selecting a somewhat more conservative (lower) cutoff score on the SIQ and SIQ-JR, Reynolds (1991a) reported a 100% sensitivity for the identification of youngsters who were considered to be at-risk for more severe suicidal behaviors on the basis of clinical interviews using the SBI.

Stage 2

The second stage of the screening process involves a comprehensive interview with those youngsters who report significant suicidal thoughts on the initial assessment measure. In our experience, this interview can be conducted by school psychologists, counselors, and other health professionals who are knowledgeable about psychological disorders in adolescents and have had training on the interview procedures. This interview should include a detailed assessment of suicidal behaviors, evaluate the possibility of diagnosable disorders (e.g., depression), and establish a plan for follow-up and, if necessary, protection of the adolescent against self-destructive behaviors.

In our research with this identification procedure, we have used the SBI as the primary assessment measure for Stage 2, along with the SBHF for obtaining greater detailed information from youngsters who have reported a history of one or more suicide attempts. As noted above, youngsters identified as demonstrating a clinical level of suicidal ideation at the initial screening are then interviewed. We have found it useful to begin interviews with those youngsters who score highest on the SIQ or SIQ-JR as soon as possible after the screening. In some cases in which the school has observed very high scores on the SIQ after the screening, youngsters were seen that day, and in some cases referred for services.

Summary

The procedures outlined here for the identification of youngsters thinking about suicide are effective in targeting students who are actively thinking of suicide and in need of intervention. This procedure results in the identification of numerous school-based adolescents who are seriously thinking of killing themselves. The school-based screening for suicidal behavior also fits into multicomponent intervention programs, such as those suggested by Blumenthal and Kupfer (1988) and Garfinkel (1989). It should also be noted that there is a need for formal evaluation of suicidality in youngsters seen in mental health and other treatment facilities. Pfeffer (1981a) notes the importance for all children seen for a psychiatric evaluation to also be assessed for signs of suicidality.

Suicidal Behavior and Psychopathology in Adolescents

William M.
Reynolds and James
J. Mazza

Studies investigating suicidal behavior and psychopathology in adolescents have been for the most part conducted in hospital and clinical settings (e.g., Asarnow & Guthrie, 1989; Brent, 1987; Brent et al., 1993a,b; Christoffel, Marcus, Sagerman, & Bennett, 1988; R. C. Friedman et al., 1984b; Garfinkel et al., 1982; Pfeffer et al., 1988; Robbins & Alessi, 1985; Rotheram-Borus & Trautman, 1988). Most of these studies have examined the relationship of formal psychiatric disorders (DSM-III/DSM-III-R Axis I and Axis II disorders) and suicidal behavior in children and adolescents. Research investigating formal DSM-III Axis I clinical disorders in suicidal children and adolescents has found psychiatric disorders of depression, substance abuse, schizophrenia, eating disorders, and conduct disorder in completers and attempters (Apter, Bleich, Plutchik, Mendelsohn, & Tyano, 1988; Brent, 1987; R. C. Friedman et al., 1984b; Kosky, Silburn, & Zubrick, 1990; Kovacs & Puig-Antich, 1989; Pfeffer et al., 1988; Schreiber & Johnson, 1986; Shafii et al., 1985, 1988; Weiner & Pfeffer, 1986).

The most common DSM-III/DSM-III-R clinical disorder diagnosis reported among suicidal children and adolescents is depression (Brent et al., 1988, 1993a,b; R. C. Friedman et al., 1984b; Kosky et al., 1990; Lewinsohn, Rohde, & Seeley, 1993; Myers, Burke, & McCauley, 1985; Pfeffer et al., 1988; Robbins & Alessi, 1985). Brent et al. (1993a) found an affective disorder in 86.5% of a sample of 37 inpatient adolescent suicide attempters. In a study conducted by Shafii et al. (1988) examining the diagnoses of 21 adolescent suicide completers via psychological autopsies, depression was diagnosed in 76% (16) of the suicide completers as either a primary or a secondary psychiatric disorder. Similar results were reported in a study conducted by Robbins and Alessi (1985), who studied 64 adolescent attempters hospitalized in a psychiatric unit and found that 76.6% (49) were diagnosed with depression. In a study of 231 children and adolescents of ages 6–18 years, Brent et al. (1986) found a high rate of dysthymic disorder (DSM-III criteria) among youngsters who had made one or more suicide attempts. Depression has also been noted in very young children who attempt suicide. Rosenthal and Rosenthal (1984), using modified Weinberg criteria, found that 56% of 16 preschool children who made one or more suicide attempts were depressed.

Depressive disorders are also frequent in adolescent suicide attempters found in school-based samples. Andrews and Lewinsohn (1992), in an epidemiological study of 1710 older adolescents, found that approximately 80% of 121 youngsters who had attempted suicide prior to the evaluation also met criteria for a depressive disorder during this time period. Alcohol and drug abuse were also relatively common diagnoses in this group of attempters. In a community study of suicidal behavior in a sample of children and adolescents from 752 families, Velez and Cohen (1988) found major depressive disorder (MDD) present in 19% of suicide attempters compared to 1.1% of nonattempters and a past episode of MDD in 35% of attempters compared to 4.5% of nonattempters.

Substance abuse is also a common DSM-III Axis I diagnosis among completers and attempters (Brent et al., 1986, 1988, 1993a; Kotila & Lonnqvist, 1988; Levy & Deykin, 1989; Lewinsohn et al., 1993; Pfeffer et al., 1988; Robbins & Alessi, 1985; Schreiber & Johnson, 1986; Schuckit & Schuckit, 1989; Shafii et al., 1988). In the Shafii et al. (1988) study, substance abuse was a primary or secondary diagnosis in 62% of the adolescent suicide completers. Kandel et al. (1991) found drug use highly related to suicide attempts in adolescents, particularly females. In a study of 424 older adolescents, Levy and Deykin (1989) found substance-abuse disorder as a risk factor for suicide attempts and ideation, with somewhat greater effects found for males. In older adolescents, there also appears to be an increased frequency of comorbidity of substance-abuse and depressive disorders (Carlson, Rich, Grayson, & Fowler, 1991) and substance-abuse and borderline personality disorder (Runeson & Beskow, 1991) among suicide completers.

Although formal psychiatric diagnoses were not reported by Kotila and Lonnqvist (1988), who described the characteristics of 422 adolescent suicide attempters, they did find that 53% of males and 40% of females had consumed alcohol when making their suicide attempt. Kotila and Lonnqvist (1988) also found that males (15%) were significantly more likely to report that their attempt was influenced by alcohol than females (5%), $\chi^2 = 17.5, p < 0.001$. Berman and Schwartz (1990) reported on suicidal behavior among adolescent drug users seen in four outpatient drug treatment facilities. Of 298 drug users surveyed, 29.9% reported a history of one or more suicide attempts. Although substance abuse is relatively prevalent among youngsters who attempt suicide, the rate is not necessarily higher than rates found in nonattempter psychiatric samples.

Research investigating formal clinical disorders has found that the diagnosis of conduct disorder is not uncommon among male and female adolescent suicide attempters (Schreiber & Johnson, 1986; Taylor & Stanfeld, 1984). Taylor and Stansfeld (1984) reported that in a sample of 50 youngsters ranging in age from 8 to 17 years who attempted suicide by poison, approximately 20% had a diagnosis of conduct disorder. However, a similar rate was found in a matched sample of nonsuicidal psychiatric controls. In a report by Borst and Noam (1989), the diagnosis of conduct disorders was also found to be the most frequent diagnosis (44.5%) in a sample of 36 suicide attempters (both children and adolescents) who were inpatients in a psychiatric hospital. It should also be noted that a similar rate of conduct disorders (51%) was found among nonsuicidal youngsters in the hospital sample.

There have been few research studies examining adjustment disorder among adolescents in relation to suicidal behavior (e.g., C. A. King et al., 1990; Pfeffer et al., 1988). In the Pfeffer et al. (1988) study, adjustment disorder was diagnosed in 7.4% ($N = 6$) of males and 9.2% ($N = 11$) of females. The results of the Pfeffer et al. (1988) study must be interpreted cautiously because adolescents could receive multiple diagnoses. C. A. King et al. (1990) compared 19 female adolescent attempters to 21 "normal" adolescent females. Adjustment disorder was measured by the Personality Inventory for Children (Lachar, 1982). The results of this study showed that female attempters had significantly higher adjustment disorder scores than "normal" adolescents. Reynolds and Mazza (1992b), in their school-based study of 378 suicide attempters and 2419 nonattempters, also found significantly higher scores on the APS Adjustment disorder scale ($F = 382.02, p < 0.0001$) in adolescents who had a history of attempted suicide than in those without a suicide-attempt history. The results of these studies suggest the need to examine adjustment disorder in relation to suicidal behavior in adolescents. These results are also limited by the use of severity measures, rather than formal diagnosis, by C. A. King et al. (1990) and Reynolds and Mazza (1992b).

Another clinical disorder that needs to be further examined in relation to suicidal behavior is schizophrenia. The research on schizophrenia in relation to suicidal adolescents has been minimal. In the Pfeffer et al. (1988) study, schizophrenia was diagnosed significantly more often in males, 22.2% (18), than in females, 6.7% (8), ($\chi^2 = 8.8$, $p < 0.003$). It appears from this study that schizophrenia may be more related to suicidal behavior in adolescents than has been thought in the past, especially for males.

Personality disorders have also been found to be prevalent in youngsters who demonstrate suicidal behaviors. Brent et al. (1993a), in a study of 37 inpatient adolescent suicide attempters, found that 81% manifested a DSM-III-R personality disorder or trait as assessed by the Structured Clinical Interview for the DSM-III-R for personality disorders (Spitzer, Williams, Gibbon, & First, 1989).

Coexisting Clinical and Personality Disorders

Studies examining formal DSM-III or DSM-III-R clinical and personality disorders in suicide completers and suicide attempters have begun to focus on coexisting disorders.

Shafii et al. (1988) found that 81% of completers fulfilled the DSM-III criteria for more than one mental disorder at the time of their death. Similar results were reported in the R. C. Friedman et al. (1984b) study; 60% of attempters with an Axis I disorder also met the criteria for a formal Axis II personality disorder. Results from other studies suggest that adolescents with concurrent coexisting mental disorders, DSM Axis I or Axis II or both, are more at risk for suicidal behavior than those with only one mental disorder (Alessi, McManus, & Brickman, 1984; Brent, Kolko, Allan, & Brown, 1990; Clarkin, Friedman, Hurt, Corn, & Aronoff, 1984; R. C. Friedman et al., 1982; R. C. Friedman, Aronoff, Clarkin, Corn, & Hurt, 1983; Shafii et al., 1988).

Research findings suggest that a coexisting personality disorder with certain Axis I clinical disorders may increase the risk of suicidal behavior in adolescents (Alessi et al., 1984; R. C. Friedman et al., 1983; Fyer, Frances, & Sullivan, 1988). The combination or "comorbidity" of antisocial personality and depressive symptoms has been found to be particularly lethal in adolescents and young adults (Blumenthal & Kupfer, 1986, 1988). Fyer et al. (1988) examined 180 patients who were diagnosed with borderline personality disorder. Among the 180 patients, Fyer et al. (1988) reported that those with coexisting borderline and an affective disorder engaged in more suicidal behavior than those with only a borderline personality disorder.

Reynolds and Mazza (1992d) examined clinical levels of comorbidity in 306 school-based adolescents who had a history of one or more suicide attempts using six scales on the APS: depression, adjustment disorder, conduct disorder, substance abuse, borderline personality disorder, and anger. They reported that 13.4% of the attempters had two or more APS scale T-scores at or above 70 (Reynolds & Mazza, 1992b). The two scales showing the highest proportions above a T-score of 70 were borderline personality disorder and depression, 20.4% and 18.3%, respectively. Because of the reliance on the APS, a severity measure, rather than formal diagnoses, caution must be taken in interpreting this study.

The investigation of specific combinations of disorders or patterns of comorbidity and suicidal behavior has received little attention in clinical studies (Blumenthal & Kupfer, 1986, 1988). Research needs to be conducted that examines patterns of comorbidity that occur most frequently in completers, attempters, and school-based populations.

Relationship with Depression

Of special note is the relationship between depression and suicidal behavior. Depression is diagnostically and phenomenologically linked to suicide and suicidal behavior (Reynolds, 1992b, 1994). Of persons who commit suicide, approximately half have a diagnosis of depression (Goodwin & Runck, 1992). Depression in children and adolescents is a serious clinical problem involving cognitive (disturbances in thinking), affective, motivational, somatic (physical complaints), and vegetative symptoms (eating and sleeping problems), as well as the emotional symptom of sadness. Myers et al. (1991) suggest that suicidal youngsters with major depression may constitute a distinct group of youngsters with depressive disorders. In the past 15 years, a great deal has been learned regarding depression in children and adolescents. Most of this research is descriptive, focusing on correlates of depression in youngsters. There has also been significant research on the psychobiology of childhood depression, with researchers examining biological and neuroendocrine correlates as well as genetic factors [Emslie, Weinberg, Kennard, and Kowatch (Chapter 8); Puig-Antich, 1987]. Biological markers have also been examined for suicidal behavior (Cohen, Winchel, & Stanley, 1988; Ryan et al., 1988; van Praag, 1982, 1986). In addition, advances in the development of methodologies for the identification and assessment of depression [Hodges (Chapter 10); Reynolds (Chapter 11)], as well as research on treatment strategies for the amelioration of depressive symptomatology in youngsters

[Stark, Rouse, and Kurowski (Chapter 14); Lewinsohn, Clarke, and Rohde (Chapter 15)], have greatly enhanced our understanding of and ability to deal with this disorder.

Youngsters with depressive disorders (e.g., major depression, dysthymia) appear to be at greater risk for suicidal behavior than those with other psychiatric disorders. Kovacs, Goldston, and Gatsonis (1993), in a longitudinal study of suicidal behavior in children with depressive disorders and other psychiatric disorders, found a significantly greater proportion of youngsters with depression who attempted suicide compared to nondepressed psychiatric controls. The highest rate of attempts found at follow-up (late teens) was 37% for youngsters with major depression as their study index diagnosis. In a longitudinal study, Rao, Weissman, Martin, and Hammond (1993) found 7 suicides among a subsample of 159 individuals who as children or adolescents had an initial diagnosis of major depression. On the basis of psychological autopsies, 5 of these 7 cases had a diagnosis of major depression at the time of their suicide.

The relationship between suicidal behavior and depression is by no means clear. Sample characteristics, as well as aspects of suicidality, appear related to depression. In a study of adolescent suicide attempters hospitalized in a pediatric unit and differentiated as impulsive or nonimpulsive on the basis of their premeditation, Brown, Overholser, Spirito, and Fritz (1991) found nonimpulsive suicide attempters to be significantly more depressed than impulsive suicide attempters. Nonimpulsive attempters also demonstrated a high level of suicidal ideation on the SIQ ($M = 75.6$) that approached statistical significance ($p < 0.06$) compared to SIQ scores of the impulsive suicide attempters ($M = 53.3$).

Personality and Psychosocial Characteristics and Suicidal Behavior

There are some limitations to the heavy reliance on the use of formal DSM-III (American Psychiatric Association, 1980) or DSM-III-R (American Psychiatric Association, 1987) diagnoses in the study of suicidal behavior in children and adolescents. Although formal diagnoses are useful for description and in making group comparisons, such as completers vs. attempters, they also produce a rigid structure for labeling individuals. The diagnosis itself may overshadow specific symptom(s) or trait(s) that are precipitating or play a more causal role in the suicidal behavior. Goldsmith, Fryer, and Frances (1990) suggest that personality traits such as impulsivity may be better predictors of suicidal behaviors than are personality disorders. Several studies have focused on specific symptoms or traits within clinical and personality disorders that may be related to adolescent suicidal behavior (e.g., Blumenthal & Kupfer, 1988; Brent & Kolko, 1990). For example, personality characteristics of impulsivity and aggression have been found to be important potential precursors of adolescent suicidal behavior (Cairns, Peterson, & Neckerman, 1988; Cantor, 1976; Gispert, Wheeler, Marsh, & Davis, 1985; Patsiokas, Clum, & Luscomb, 1979; Pfeffer et al., 1988) and to be related to neurobiological correlates of suicide (Goodwin & Brown, 1989; Plutchik & van Pragg, 1989). Impulsivity and aggression, as personality characteristics, have been reported more frequently in hospitalized female attempters than in female psychiatric controls and male attempters (Cantor, 1976; Gispert et al., 1985). Kashden, Fremouw, Callahan, and Franzen (1993) found that adolescent suicidal inpatients demonstrated greater impulsivity than nonsuicidal inpatients or a high school control group. Pfeffer et al. (1988) found that aggressive behavior was a significant predictor for suicidal risk in females, but not for males. The importance of anger, aggression, and hopelessness as characteristics for understanding suicidal behavior is not new (e.g., Shaw & Schelkun, 1965) and has also been raised in the psychodynamic literature (e.g., Hendin, 1991).

A number of psychosocial characteristics have been studied in various samples of children and adolescents. Foremost among these variables have been hopelessness and depression along with environmental variables of social support and major and minor negative events, the latter often conceptualized as chronic strains or hassles. These studies have been conducted with clinical and nonclinical samples of children and adolescents (e.g., Asarnow & Guthrie, 1989; Asarnow, Carlson, & Guthrie, 1987; Cole, 1989b; Kazdin, French, Unis, Esveldt-Dawson, & Sherick, 1983; Mazza & Reynolds, 1991, 1993; Reynolds, 1988; Reynolds & Waltz, 1986; Rich et al., 1992) and constitute an extensive literature base. In general, depression and hopelessness have shown strong relationships to suicidal behavior, the latter typically operationalized as suicide attempts or suicidal ideation or both. However, many studies have found gender differences in the relationship of psychosocial variables to suicidal behavior, particularly in adolescents (e.g., Cole, 1989b; Mazza & Reynolds, 1991).

Family Dysfunction and Abuse

Family problems or difficult child–parent relationships or both are frequent issues among suicidal children and adolescents (Asarnow et al., 1987; Brent et al., 1993f; Carlson, 1983; Hawton, 1987; Kerfoot, 1987; Orbach, 1988; Pfeffer, 1981b, 1986, 1989a; Sabbath, 1969; Schrut & Michels, 1969; Taylor & Stansfeld, 1984). In a study of adolescent suicidal inpatients, nonsuicidal inpatients, and a normal adolescent control group, C. A. King, Segal, Naylor, and Evans (1993) found that fathers of suicidal adolescents reported greater depression and family problems than fathers of the other two groups. Suicidal inpatients reported greater problems with fathers in a number of relationship domains. Adolescents' relationship with their mothers was not significantly different between groups. C. A. King et al. (1993) suggest the need to engage parents, and in particular fathers, in treatment.

Family problems are prevalent among children who attempt suicide (Asarnow & Carlson, 1988; Kienhorst et al., 1987; Kosky, 1983; Orbach, Gross, & Glaubman, 1981). An impaired or dysfunctional parent–child relationship may play an important role as a precipitating factor in child and adolescent suicidal behavior. Kerfoot (1988), in a sample of 100 child and young adolescent suicide attempters, found that a serious disagreement with parents was the most frequent reason given for youngsters' suicide attempts. Kienhorst et al. (1987) examined motives for suicide attempts in a sample of 40 children, finding family problems the most frequent reason. Similar findings were reported by Paulson, Stone, and Sposto (1978), who found that reasons for suicide attempts in young children included escape from traumatic home situation and perceived abandonment or rejection by parents. Asarnow and Carlson (1988) found that family support in comparison to depression and hopelessness was a major discriminator between child psychiatric inpatients who attempted suicide and those who had not, with suicide attempters reporting lower perceived family support. In a sample of adolescent psychiatric inpatients, C. A. King, Naylor, Evans, and Segal (1991) found moderate and significant correlations between suicidal ideation as measured by the SIQ-JR and youngsters' reports of family problems.

Suicidal behavior in children and adolescents has also been associated with parental abuse and neglect, as well as physical and sexual abuse in general (Deykin, Alpert, & McNamarra, 1985; Garnefski, Diekstra, & de Heus, 1992; Green, 1978; Hibbard, Brack, Rauch, & Orr, 1988; Livingston, Lawson, & Jones, 1993; Stone, 1993). Hibbard et al. (1988) conducted a community-based study of 706 junior high school students who completed a questionnaire on physical and sexual abuse and mental health problems, 130 (18.4%) of whom indicated some form of abuse. Approximately 30% of youngsters who experienced abuse also noted a history of suicide attempts compared with 11.6% of adolescents who reported no abuse. De Wilde, Kienhorst, Diekstra, and Wolters (1992), in a community sample study of adolescents, found that adolescents who attempted suicide reported significantly more physical and sexual abuse during adolescence than nonattempters, and significantly more physical abuse during childhood. In a school-based study comparing male and female suicide attempters with a matched sample of nonattempters, Shaunesey et al. (1993) found a higher frequency of suicide attempts among a sample of adolescent psychiatric inpatients who had been abused physically or sexually or both ($N = 55$) than among those with no history of abuse ($N = 65$). Youngsters who were hospitalized for a suicide attempt and had been abused also demonstrated significantly higher levels of suicidal ideation on the SIQ ($M = 107.60$) than attempters without a history of abuse ($M = 58.33$). Shaunesey et al. (1993) also found significant differences in SIQ scores between groups of youngsters who had experienced frequent physical abuse ($M = 85.63$) or infrequent physical abuse ($M = 62.67$) and those who had not been physically abused ($M = 53.95$). Garnefski et al. (1992) found that female adolescents who had attempted suicide vs. female nonattempters reported greater physical abuse (51% vs. 24%; $\chi^2 = 26.4$, $p < 0.001$) and sexual abuse (32% vs. 7%; $\chi^2 = 32.3$, $p < 0.001$). Male suicide attempters reported significantly more sexual abuse than did nonattempters ($\chi^2 = 16.7$, $p < 0.001$), but these two groups did not differ in rates of reported physical abuse. Suicide attempts and behavior have also been noted to a significant extent in physically and sexually abused youngsters seen in inpatient settings (Sansonnet-Hayden, Haley, Marriage, & Fine, 1987) and in pregnant adolescents (Bayatpour, Wells, & Holford, 1992), although abused youngsters are victimized by others as well as parents.

It is important to note the potential for suicidal behavior among parents, particularly as this may be a risk factor for suicidal behavior in some youngsters (Pfeffer, 1981c; Roy, 1989). Kerfoot (1988), in his study of deliberate self-poisoning in 100 children and young adolescents, found similar suicidal behavior in 30% of the first-degree relatives, primarily mothers, compared to 4% in a psychiatric control sample. Similar findings were reported by Myers et al. (1985), who found suicidal behaviors in 25% of families of suicidal children compared to 6% of a matched group of controls. In a descriptive study of 11 children who manifested suicidal behaviors, Orbach et al. (1981) found a suicidal parent in the majority of cases. Orbach et al. (1981) also found that all but one of the families of these children were experiencing a major family crisis. Related to suicidal behavior in parents is the significant issue of parental depression and other forms of psychopathology that may interfere with effective parenting and relate to child and adolescent psychopathology [Cicchetti, Rogosch, and Toth (Chapter 7); Downey, Feldman, Khuri, and Friedman (Chapter 22)].

Family problems and discord are significant but by no means singular in their contribution to the etiology and development of suicidal behaviors in young persons. Other externalizing as well as internalizing problems can be viewed as precursors or augmenters of suicide risk (Hoberman, 1989). Although not all suicidal youngsters have families that manifest disturbed relations or are a source of abuse or stress, parental and family dysfunction appears to be the single most prevalent problem domain among suicidal children and adolescents.

Interventions for Suicidal Behavior in Young People

Introduction

Intervention, as compared to prevention, is aimed at the active treatment of youngsters who demonstrate suicidal behaviors. It is evident that many youngsters do receive treatment for suicidal behavior, given the large number of suicide attempts that result in medical or psychiatric hospitalization. Furthermore, the number of youngsters seen in treatment settings for psychiatric disorders such as depression, borderline personality disorder, and other psychopathology includes significant numbers of youngsters who are also at-risk for suicidal behavior (Reynolds & Mazza, 1993b). Thus, it can be inferred that there are many different treatment strategies that have been implemented with suicidal youngsters. Less evident is the efficacy of these procedures. From follow-up studies of previously hospitalized youngsters, it appears that many youngsters treated for suicidal behavior go on to complete suicide (Shaffer et al., 1988) or repeat an attempt (Spirito et al., 1992). Likewise, adolescent suicide attempters tend to be relatively noncompliant with regard to outpatient care (Spirito et al., 1992; Trautman, Stewart, & Morishima, 1993).

Our review of treatment studies includes several with adults that may prove applicable to adolescents as well as several studies that target adolescents. We also limit our discussion to psychological treatments, although pharmacological interventions with depressed suicidal youngsters are viable, particularly when presented along with psychotherapy. However, pharmacotherapy of suicidal youngsters with antidepressants needs to be a cautious undertaking, given the high level of toxicity of most tricyclic antidepressants (Kragh-Sorensen, 1993) and a noted increase in antidepressant overdose as a method for suicide (Retterstol, 1993). With reference to antidepressants, we anticipate that some of the newer selective serotonin reuptake inhibitors (SSRIs) such as fluoxetine may prove effective with suicidal youngsters, as they have shown efficacy in reducing suicidal ideation in adults (Reynolds et al., 1993). Furthermore, SSRIs have fewer side effects and are safer when taken in large doses then other antidepressant medications [Johnston & Freuhling (Chapter 17)]. It is also important to note that suicidal youngsters may demonstrate other forms of psychopathology and may benefit from other medications that are more specific to their psychiatric disorder (Pfeffer, 1984).

Most of the empirical psychological treatment literature has focused on behavioral and cognitive–behavioral interventions, with a strong emphasis on problem-solving strategies. A number of professionals have advocated the use of cognitive and problem-solving therapies for the treatment of suicidal behaviors (e.g., Brent & Kolko, 1990; Ellis, 1986; Weishaar & Beck, 1990), and research has shown deficits in these domains among suicidal youngsters (e.g., Asarnow et al., 1987; Rotheram-Borus, Trautman, Dopkins, & Shrout, 1990; Sadowski & Kelly, 1993). Treatment-outcome research on suicidal youngsters is virtually nonexistent and is likewise sparse with adults. A review of the literature on the treatment of suicidal behavior in children and adolescents indicates a primary focus on articles that suggest treatments rather than testing the efficacy of treatments or reports of case studies or case examples. Thus, the professional is faced with accepting treatment prescriptions that have no proven efficacy. As will be noted later, the same conditions exist with regard to many school-based prevention programs.

Interventions for suicidal youngsters vary, in part, as a function of the nature of the suicidal behavior, as well as the youngster's psychological or diagnostic status. Blumenthal (1990a) delineates four components in the treatment of suicidal youths: psychological interventions; medications targeted to existing mental health problems, if necessary; use of psychiatric consultation and, if needed, hospitalization; and changes directed at the youngster's environment and social support system. Similarly, Pfeffer (1990) suggests and describes three intervention formats: a psychotherapeutic–cognitive approach, pharmacotherapy, and interventions that focus on stabilizing the environment, including major life stressors and family therapy and involvement. Pfeffer (1990) considers these interventions most useful when used together to decrease or alleviate suicidal behavior. Pfeffer (1977, 1990) also describes psychiatric hospitalization as a strategy for preventing self-harm to actively suicidal youngsters and notes the importance of involving the family in the treatment of suicidal children (Pfeffer, 1977, 1982).

Likewise, the mental state of the youngster when presenting for treatment can vary greatly. In many cases, the child or adolescent may have an acute suicidal episode or crisis in which a host of environmental, interpersonal, and internal problems and stressors combine to create a confused and intensely distressed youngster. Jobes and Berman (Jobes

& Berman, 1991; Berman & Jobes, 1991) have developed a crisis intervention model for the treatment of suicidal youngsters that appears to have a great deal of promise.

Research on the treatment of suicidal behavior presents a host of formidable difficulties if experimental designs are to be implemented. Foremost is the ethical consideration that precludes the use of most control-group designs. The utilization of wait-list or placebo conditions places suicidal subjects at potentially grave risk, given that such procedures will knowingly endanger subjects. Likewise, engaging subjects in treatment for suicidal behavior introduces the possibility that if an experimental procedure is not 100% effective, subject mortality may result. Further complications are specific to the nature of the behavior pathology, in that many suicidal individuals, because of their desire to end their life, are noncompliant or reject treatment. Characteristics of the therapist and the development of a therapeutic relationship are also important aspects for effective treatment (Bongar, Peterson, Harris, & Aissis, 1989; Pfeffer, 1984).

Because of the high comorbidity of suicidal behavior and depression, treatment for suicidal behavior may in many cases be combined with therapy for depression. In this regard, there have been a few experimental treatment studies for the amelioration of depression in children and adolescents. In a number of studies reported (e.g., Kahn, Kehle, Jenson, & Clark, 1990; Reynolds & Coats, 1986; Stark, Reynolds, & Kaslow, 1987), suicidal youngsters were either excluded or not dealt with as a specific group. Likewise, Mufson, Moreau, Weissman, and Klerman (1993), in describing the application of interpersonal psychotherapy for depressed adolescents (IPT-A), indicate that youngsters who are at risk for suicidal behaviors should not be viewed as candidates for IPT-A. Thus, although literature describing the nature and efficacy of psychological treatments for depression in youngsters has appeared, youngsters included in these therapies are typically not at imminent risk for suicidal behaviors. The utility of these therapies for suicidal youngsters remains to be determined, and it will be necessary to make extensive modification and enhancement of these procedures to include a substantial focus on dealing with suicidal behaviors and risk. Research by Rotheram-Borus et al. (1990) suggests that some adult models of depression may not be appropriate in defining targets for intervention with suicidal adolescents, although their research supports the application of cognitive–behavioral treatments for suicidal youngsters.

Suicidal behavior is often found in persons with borderline personality disorder or borderline characteristics (Cohen-Sandler, Berman, & King, 1982; Mazza & Reynolds, 1993; Reynolds & Mazza, 1992b). These findings are due in part to the inclusion of suicidal behavior as a symptom within the criteria for the diagnosis of borderline personality disorder in DSM-III-R and DSM-IV (American Psychiatric Association, 1987, 1994). Linehan (1993a,b) has developed a structured therapy that integrates cognitive and behavioral components for the treatment of borderline personality disorder along with suicidal behaviors, although these procedures have not been tested with adolescents. Known as dialectical behavior therapy (DBT), this therapy was developed and tested on adults with borderline personality disorder, most of whom also demonstrated significant suicidal behaviors. A primary target of DBT is "high-risk suicidal behaviors," ". . . simply because," as Linehan (1987, p. 329) succinctly notes, "psychotherapy is not effective with dead patients." The structured nature of this therapy, along with its - skill-building, problem-solving, and behavior-change orientations and focus on suicidal behaviors, suggests that it has a great deal of potential for use with adolescents. The work of Linehan and colleagues (e.g., Linehan, 1993a; Linehan, Armstrong, Suarez, Allmon, & Heard, 1991; Linehan, Heard, & Armstrong, 1993) on the treatment of suicidal behaviors with DBT stands as an excellent model for modification and application with at-risk adolescents.

Although there is not an extensive research base on contemporary psychotherapies for suicidal behaviors in adults, there is some evidence to suggest that cognitive–

behavioral and behavioral therapies are effective for reducing suicidal behaviors (e.g., Salkovskis, Atha, & Storer, 1990). Clum, Patsiokas, and Luscomb (1979) note the potential utility of problem-solving treatment approaches, particularly for persons who have made multiple attempts and for whom attempts may in part be a response to interpersonal problems. Because of the relatively high numbers of multiple attempters found in samples of adolescent suicide attempters, interpersonal problem-solving approaches may be important for some youngsters, particularly if the purpose of suicidal behavior is to manipulate or effect change in the youngster's interpersonal relations.

An examination of treatment studies for suicidal behaviors suggests at least two primary groups for attention: treatment of individuals identified as suicide attempters and treatment of individuals who are identified as at imminent risk for suicide or an attempt. The latter group includes those individuals who contact significant others, professionals, crisis hot lines, or persons who are identified as at risk by school-based screening or by others, such as a therapist or other mental health professional.

A field-based intervention study of adolescents of ages 13–17 who had received services at one of two geographically separate hospitals in the Boston area and who demonstrated suicidal behaviors including suicide attempts, gestures, extreme risk-taking behaviors, and suicidal ideation was described by Deykin (1986) and Deykin, Hsieh, Joshi, and McNamarra (1986). The intervention was provided to youngsters seen in one of the two hospitals, with youngsters from the second hospital acting as control subjects. The intervention consisted of a brief psychoeducational mental health awareness program along with direct contact (minimum of 4 times per year) with a community outreach worker to maintain contact between the subject and the study program. Treatments were tailored to the individual needs of each subject. Outcome variables included repeated admission to area hospitals, percentage of subjects who attended follow-up visits or clinic referrals, and subject mortality. The intervention appeared to be effective in increasing the rate of compliance with medical recommendations and keeping medical appointments. However, no treatment superiority was found specific to reducing suicidal behaviors.

Cognitive–Behavioral Interventions

Several relevant studies have been conducted that used cognitive–behavioral and social problem-solving treatment components. Some of these studies have been conducted with adults or older adolescents, but are reviewed here because of their relevance and potential for use with adolescents. It should also be noted that treatment studies using experimental designs are difficult to conduct and a challenge for researchers.

In a preliminary report of a pilot study examining the efficacy of combined cognitive and interpersonal therapy for suicidality in adolescents, Kolko and Brent (1988) found that in a sample of 127 youngsters seen in a treatment program for suicidality, about 80% showed remission for suicidal behavior. Although this was an uncontrolled study and about one third of the sample also received medication for depression, this study is useful in pointing out the difficulty in treating suicidal youngsters. One potential problem noted by the authors of this study was compliance, with about half the sample completing treatment and follow-up. The authors suggested that active support is needed to enhance family involvement and assistance in therapy and communication.

In an experimental study with 24 adult suicide attempters, Liberman and Eckman (1981) compared a behavior-therapy approach with an insight-oriented therapy. The behavior therapy consisted of 17 hours of social-skills training, along with 10 hours of anxiety-management techniques (e.g., relaxation training) and 5 hours of "family negotiation and contingency contracting." The insight-oriented treatment consisted of 17 hours of individual insight psychotherapy, 10 hours of psychodrama and group psychotherapy, and 5 hours of family therapy. Therapy was quite intense, consisting of 4 hours of therapy per day, administered over an 8-day period. A noteworthy aspect of this study was the continued follow-up of subjects at six points over a 2-year period. Outcome measures included depression measures and subject reports of suicidal behavior (e.g., ideation, plans, attempts). Liberman and Eckman (1981) reported relatively positive results for both groups, although the behavior-therapy group demonstrated less frequent suicidal ideation at the long-term follow-up assessments. Specific to suicide attempts at the 2-year follow-up, results were identical for both groups, with 9 subjects in each group free from suicide attempts, 2 subjects in each group who made suicide threats or preparations, and 1 subject in each group who attempted suicide postintervention. Although the level of repeat attempts appears low, we need to consider that 8% of the sample reattempted within 2 years after treatment and an additional 17% made threats or plans to attempt in each group. Before therapeutic efficacy can be claimed, we need to know the extent to which these outcomes are superior to those expected in a similar sample without treatment. Such a study becomes a complex undertaking, however, because for ethical and moral reasons we cannot conduct or condone a treatment study that includes a placebo or wait-list control group for suicidal behaviors.

In an experimental treatment study of adult suicide attempters, Patsiokas and Clum (1985) randomly assigned 15 hospitalized suicide attempters to one of three groups: a cognitive-restructuring group based on Beck's cognitive therapy, a problem-solving group based on the procedures of D'Zurilla and Goldfried (1971), and a nondirective control group designed as an attention control. Treatments were individually administered in 10 1-hour sessions over 3 weeks. There were significant decreases in suicidal ideation and hopelessness by all groups between pretest and posttest. However, differences between experimental and control groups were nonsignificant. As one of the first controlled treatment-outcome studies, this investigation is noteworthy. Limitations in the number of subjects (5) per condition, and the fact that there was no follow-up, particularly posthospitalization, need to be noted.

In a significant study of older adolescents and young adults, Lerner and Clum (1990) examined the efficacy of a problem-solving treatment in comparison to the generalized nonspecific supportive therapy. The participants were 18 persons of ages 18–24 years with a mean age of 19.17 years, although it should be noted that these were subjects who completed the study. No data are reported for individuals who did not complete therapy. Subjects were selected on the basis of experiencing significant suicidal ideation as determined by an interview using the Modified Scale for Suicidal Ideation (MSSI) (I. W. Miller, Norman, Bishop, & Dow, 1986). There were 8 subjects in each group. Treatments were administered in 10 90-minute sessions over a 5- to 7-week period. A small-group treatment format (2–5 subjects) was used for the presentation of therapy. The active condition was a problem-solving therapy incorporating components delineated by D'Zurilla and Goldfried (1971). The supportive therapy included empathic listening, sharing of experiences, and instruction on active listening skills. Assessment with the MSSI, and measures of depression, hopelessness, loneliness, and social problem-solving, were obtained at pretest, posttest, and 3-month follow-up.

At pretest, the problem-solving group showed higher scores on measures of depression, suicidal ideation, and hopelessness. After treatment, both groups reported reductions in suicidal ideation. A significantly greater reduction in depression was found in the problem-solving group as compared to the support therapy at posttreatment. At the 3-month follow-up, the problem-solving group continued to show treatment superiority on measures of depression, hopelessness, and loneliness. Although not statistically significant, an increase in suicidal ideation was reported for the supportive therapy group at follow-up. The relatively small sample size and limitations in the power of this study are concerns in the interpretation of the data; however, the results are generally positive. Experimental studies specific to the treatment of suicidal behaviors in adolescents and adults are virtually nonexistent. Thus, the Lerner and Clum study is an important contribution to our understanding of methods for the treatment of suicidality in young people.

Role of the Family

Most of the anecdotal and clinical literature on the multimodal treatment of suicidality in young people notes that family involvement in therapy or family therapy is an important component. The inclusion of the family in the treatment of suicidal youngsters is not a new or novel perspective (e.g., Motto, 1975). As we noted above, family dysfunction and parent–child relationship problems are frequently found among suicidal children and adolescents (Asarnow et al., 1987; Carlson, 1983; Kerfoot, 1987; Orbach, 1988; Pfeffer, 1981b, 1986, 1989a; Sabbath, 1969; Schrut & Michels, 1969).

The role of the family in the treatment of suicidal behavior among children and adolescents is complex and to a large extent dependent on the existing family situation and dynamics. Treatment will vary as a function of the integrity of the family, as well as the extent to which family or parental problems may contribute to, or maintain, suicidal behavior in youngsters. A number of researchers have noted the importance and utility of integrating contemporary individual psychotherapies and family-systems approaches for the treatment of suicidal adolescents (Brent & Kolko, 1990; Cantor, 1992; Turgay, 1989; Vaz-Leal, 1989; Zimmerman & La Sorsa, 1992). The involvement of the family is particularly important when dealing with what Smith (1992) refers to as *suicidogenic family processes*, which are particularly problematic in families in which children are overtly rejected by their parents. Family members can also play a critical role in assisting in removing or securing potentially lethal methods of self-harm, such as weapons and medications (Motto, 1975). The role of parents in limiting access to handguns is particularly important and can result in a significant decrease in adolescent suicides and attempts (Cantor, 1989, 1990).

Family therapy is rarely presented as the sole treatment modality, nor is it recommended for all suicidal youngsters. Aspects to consider when evaluating the potential of family therapy have been described by Frances and Clarkin (1985). Relying to a large extent on family involvement and therapy, Gutstein and Rudd (1990) described the Systemic Crisis Intervention Program, an intervention designed for use with suicidal children and adolescents and their families. The authors present this treatment as an outpatient therapy and define some criteria for who might best be served by this intervention. Suggestions for the efficacy of this program were provided on a sample of 47 youngsters and their families and included long-term follow-up evaluations.

Efficacy of Suicide-Prevention Programs

Schools across the country are becoming increasingly aware of the possibility of student suicide. Although most evident in adolescents, suicidal behavior occurs in children and even preschool-age children. Because of the limited avenues for the identification of suicidal youngsters and the delivery of preventative and therapeutic services, schools are in a unique position to intervene with at-risk children and adolescents. After many years of unsubstantiated claims of efficacy (e.g., Ross, 1983, 1987), a number of investigators have examined the response of adolescents to school-based suicide-prevention programs and curricula. For the most part, reviewers find little empirical evidence to support claims of prevention-program efficacy (e.g., Diekstra, 1992). This is not to say that there may not be some positive results from the implementation of a school-based suicide-prevention curriculum. Spirito, Overholser, Ashworth, Morgan, and Benedict-Drew (1988) found a small increase in adolescent's knowledge of suicidal youths as a function of participation in a school-based suicide-awareness curriculum.

Unfortunately, many of the positive claims for the efficacy of school-based prevention

programs are anecdotal or based on secondary attitudes or knowledge without a determination of effects on those youngsters who are at risk or whether at-risk youngsters are
identified or referred for services. In a study of school-based suicide-prevention programs
that examined effects on adolescent attempters and nonattempters, Shaffer et al. (1990)
found that there was little positive change in adolescent suicide attempters' attitudes after
exposure to the prevention program.

It has been found that curriculum-based suicide-prevention programs generally
ignore or even downplay the role of mental health problems associated with at-risk
youngsters (Garland, Shaffer, & Whittle, 1989). This is a significant oversight, since mental
health problems are prevalent among school-based adolescent suicide attempters. In a
school-based mental health study, Andrews and Lewinsohn (1992) found that approximately 80% of adolescent suicide attempters met criteria for a psychiatric disorder, with
major depression the most frequently found mental disorder (64.5% of male attempters,
55.6% of female attempters). In their survey of school-based curriculum programs in the
United States, Garland et al. (1989) reported that fewer than 1% of adolescents are exposed
to these programs. On the basis of their review of programs and efforts by schools, Garland
et al. (1989, p. 933) concluded, "Not only is the potential impact of these programs limited
by the low risk strategy used, it has yet to be shown that the programs are either effective,
safe or necessary." Although well meant, the reality is that there is little quality research to
support the efficacy, expense, and false sense of intervention of curriculum-based suicide-
prevention programs. There is also evidence to suggest that such programs may have a
deleterious effect on some youngsters (Overholser, Hemstreet, Spirito, & Vyse, 1989).

It is important that school-based as well as other mental health professionals have a
well-grounded understanding of the nature of this problem, be aware of potential avenues
for the identification of suicidal youngsters, and be able to evaluate procedures suggested
for the prevention of suicide in children and adolescents. Toward the latter point, Streiner
and Adam (1987) have provided useful guidelines for the design and evaluation of suicide-
prevention programs.

In addition to school-based programs, suicide hot lines and community prevention
and crisis centers have also targeted adolescents as a group in need of intervention.
Although a large number of such hot lines and suicide-prevention centers exist around the
country, their effectiveness appears to be minimal (Dew, Bromet, Brent, & Greenhouse,
1987; Garland & Zigler, 1993). In a similar manner, there are few data to support the
widespread implementation of school-based postvention programs that target students in
schools following adolescent suicides. In one of the few outcome studies, Hazell and Lewin
(1993) examined levels of suicidal behavior of students who were counseled and those not
counseled after exposure to adolescent suicide, controlling for a number of salient
variables such as proximity to the completed suicide, past suicidal behavior, and subject
characteristics. Results indicated no difference in levels of suicidal ideation or related
domains of self-reported problem behaviors between students who were counseled after a
suicide completion in the school and those who did not receive counseling. It is evident
that we need to develop an adequate empirical basis and documentation of efficacy of
school-based prevention and postvention programs.

Issues and Difficulties in the Study of Suicidal Behavior

A major difficulty in studying and synthesizing existing information on adolescent
suicidal behavior is the amount of diversity in the methodologies, settings, and populations
being studied. The settings in which suicidal behavior research are conducted are quite
diverse, ranging from psychiatric hospitals (Carlson & Cantwell, 1982; Christoffel et al.,
1988; Garfinkel et al., 1982; Robbins & Alessi, 1985) to psychiatric outpatient clinics

(Bettes & Walker, 1986; Goldacre & Hawton, 1985; Hawton, O'Grady, Osborne, & Cole, 1982) and from emergency rooms (Brent, 1987; Shafii et al., 1985; Spirito, Brown, & Overholser, 1989) to junior and senior high school classrooms (Cole, 1989b; Dubow et al., 1989; J. M. H. Friedman et al., 1987; Reynolds, 1988; Reynolds & Mazza, 1990; Smith & Crawford, 1986). The methods used for collecting data also vary from study to study, including psychological autopsies, examining medical charts, clinical interviews, psychiatric evaluations, and self-report measures. The adolescent populations being investigated for suicidal behavior range from junior and senior high school students (Cole, 1989b; J. M. H. Friedman et al., 1987; Reynolds, 1989; Reynolds & Mazza, 1993a; Smith & Crawford, 1986) to adolescent attempters seen in hospital settings (R. C. Friedman et al., 1984b; C. A. King et al., 1990) to suicide completers evaluated via psychological autopsies (Runeson, 1989; Shafii et al., 1985, 1988). The numerous at-risk adolescent populations being studied, in conjunction with the diverse settings and methods for collecting data, make it difficult to combine results from one study with those from another and limit the generalizations that can be made.

The interpretation of research on clinical disorders among youngsters who demonstrate suicidal behaviors needs to consider the variability of settings. Differences in the type, nature, and severity of psychiatric disorders can be found across different settings that focus on different populations. Thus, differences in prevalence of suicidal behaviors in youngsters with psychopathology may occur as a function of inpatient vs. outpatient, psychiatric vs. general hospital, mental health setting vs. correctional setting, private vs. public facility, and other setting differentiation. Research has shown that prevalence rates for comorbidity of addictive disorders and other psychiatric diagnoses vary as a function of setting type (e.g., N. S. Miller & Fine, 1993). Likewise, it can be expected that the suicidality found among youngsters with psychiatric disorders and problems will also vary as a function of these setting variables. For instance, a youngster with an affective disorder may be more likely to be referred or receive services in a particular setting if the depressive disorder is accompanied by serious suicidal behavior.

A second major difficulty in studying suicidal behavior, particularly suicide completion, is that the event of suicide itself is rare. The suicide rate in the United States is just under 13/100,000 per year (Hawton, 1986) and somewhat lower for adolescents. Even among high-risk groups, a study would need to encompass a very large number of subjects over a long period of time to provide reliable and valid results (i.e., hundreds of thousands of subjects over a 10- to 15-year period). This type of research study is neither economical nor realistically feasible (Eisenberg, 1984). However, as we have shown, estimated base rates for suicide attempts and suicidal ideation are sufficiently high to alleviate some of the statistical problems inherent in the study of suicide completion.

A third difficulty involves assessing suicidal ideation and intent, which are considered internal cognitions. Unless specific questions are asked pertaining to suicide or thoughts of suicide, assessing suicidal ideation and intent in adolescents is extremely difficult. Most schools do not use assessment measures or interviews that ask these pertinent questions because they do not have the time or the trained personnel to do so. Even when the opportunities or resources are available, parents or school boards often reject programs that have been offered.

Sample and Design Characteristics

Unraveling the interpretability and generalizability of research findings is in large part a function of understanding the characteristics of the sample used in the research. Berman and Carroll (1984) described three major methodological flaws that are related to sample characteristics and are commonly found in suicide research: combining diverse groups to increase sample size, making inappropriate generalizations across different groups, and the lack of a control group. Combining of diverse groups is problematic, because it implies that suicidal adolescents are a homogeneous group. One example of this problem is combining youngsters who are thinking about suicide with those who have attempted suicide and characterizing them "suicidal" or "at risk." Ellis (1988) reported the necessity of defining suicidal groups and the importance of keeping these groups separate when conducting research and making generalizations. In this chapter, we have also noted the difficulty in conceptualizing suicide attempters as a homogeneous group given the variability in lethality, intentionality, and other differences in attempt characteristics. Berman and Carroll (1984) note that a distinction needs to be made between adolescents with current suicidal thoughts without a history of suicide attempts and those with a past history of suicidal behavior.

According to Ellis (1988) and Berman and Carroll (1984), there appear to be five important groups that need to be kept separate when conducting suicidal behavior research: (1) suicide completers, (2) suicide attempters who are currently thinking about suicide, (3) suicide attempters who are not currently thinking about suicide, (4) suicidal ideators (those who are currently thinking about suicide but have not made a suicide attempt), and (5) a control group (nonsuicidal adolescents, those who have not attempted suicide and are not currently thinking about suicide). A caveat regarding the creation of suicide groups, particularly nonfatal groups, is the diversity within groups (Goodwin & Runck, 1992). Issues of severity, intentionality, and other factors related to attempts, as well as the determination of what constitutes a clinical level of suicidal ideation, need to be examined in the determination of group membership and subsequent generalizability of research findings.

The implementation of a control group in suicidal-behavior research cannot be emphasized enough (Berman & Jobes, 1991; Berman & Carroll, 1984). According to Berman and Carroll, one of every two empirical research studies of suicidal behavior in youths from 1980 to 1983 did not incorporate a control or comparison group. Research results derived from groups of suicidal youngsters should be evaluated in relation to a control group to provide a meaningful comparison. Too often, results are linked to causation or given great importance without incorporating the findings from the control group (Berman & Carroll, 1984). In clinical settings, control groups are often nonsuicidal psychiatric patients, although the makeup and generalizability of this group across studies and settings are difficult. Another control group to consider is that of nonsuicidal depressed youngsters. Because of the prevalence of depression among suicidal youngsters, the differentiation of factors specific to suicidal adolescents as distinct from depression needs to be considered. The best case for making this distinction can be found in the research program of de Wilde and colleagues (de Wilde, 1992; de Wilde, Kienhorst, Diekstra, & Wolters, 1993), who found that many of the psychosocial variables that differed between adolescent suicide attempters and nonattempters did not differentiate attempters from depressed nonattempters.

Issues in the Assessment, Measurement, and Operationalization of Suicidal Behavior

Making comparisons across studies, particularly those that focus on suicidal ideation, is to some extent dependent on the manner in which the specific component of suicidal behavior is operationalized and measured. The use of single- or several-item question-naires provides little evidence of reliability and validity from a measurement perspective. For example, a number of investigators (e.g., Friedrich, Reams, & Jacobs, 1982; Kaplan, Hong, & Weinhold, 1984) evaluated suicidal ideation in young adolescents by the suicide item on the Beck Depression Inventory (Beck, Ward, Mendelson, Mock, & Erbaugh, 1961), and Domenech, Canals, and Fernandez-Ballart (1992) evaluated suicidal ideation in young adolescents with a single item from the Children's Depression Inventory (Kovacs, 1979). Simons and Murphy (1985) sought to explain the etiology of suicidal ideation in adolescents using the item "Do you ever have thoughts about possibly ending your life?" as the sole dependent variable of suicidal ideation. Without any indication of severity, time frame, or specificity of thoughts, it is difficult to consider this as an adequate assessment of youngsters' suicidal ideation.

Even a multiple-item scale may not show sufficient reliability. For example, Howard-Pitney, LaFromboise, Basil, September, and Johnson (1992) studied suicidal ideation in Zuni adolescents using an 8-item measure of suicidal ideation adapted from the Suicide Probability Scale. The authors report an internal consistency reliability of 0.69 for this measure, significantly lower than reliabilities they report for related measures of psychological distress. Numerous other studies base their evaluation of suicidality on one to four questions without the determination of reliability or validity (e.g., Rey & Bird, 1991). Particularly problematic is the classification of suicidality based on single questions from structured interviews such as the Diagnostic Interview Schedule for Children—Child Version. Recklitis, Noam, and Borst (1992) classified adolescent psychiatric patients as suicidal ideators if they responded "Yes" to the question "Have you ever thought of killing yourself?" It is difficult to conceptualize this group of adolescents as suicidal ideators given the lack of specificity, frequency, duration, or time frame inherent in the single question. Rubenstein, Heeren, Housman, Rubin, and Stechler (1989) included youngsters as "suicidal" if they answered "True" to the statement "I tried to hurt myself" over the past year. Although they also classified students as suicidal if they responded "Yes" to the statement "I tried to kill myself," only 6 of 60 students classified as suicidal responded affirmatively to the latter statement. On the basis of the group of 60 students who answered affirmative to the two questions listed above, Rubenstein et al. (1989) reported that 20% of their sample engaged in suicidal behavior in the past year. This is a tenuous assumption since 90% of the suicidal group did not report making a suicide attempt, and there is no way of knowing what an affirmative response to the question concerning the attempt to "hurt myself" means. For some youngsters, it may mean hitting their hand against a wall in anger or frustration. Unfortunately, data such as the 20% prevalence rate described by Rubenstein et al. (1989) have been used by others to characterize rates of suicide attempts among adolescents (e.g., Cantor, 1992; Diekstra, 1993; Garnefski et al., 1992).

Summary

The current literature and research findings suggest that suicidal behaviors are a prevalent problem among adolescents and, to a lesser extent, children. School and community-based studies of adolescents suggest that between 10% and 13% of adolescents in the United States have made one or more suicide attempts and that approximately 7% of adolescents make suicide attempts of varying lethality each year. Because these studies generally do not include special at-risk populations of youngsters, such as those in mental health and correctional settings, as well as runaways and dropouts, these prevalence and incidence values are most likely underestimates.

Adolescents, as well as children, find themselves under tremendous stress. Problems most often occur when stresses at home, school, with peers, and in other circumstances are concomitant with minimal social and emotional supports. As was described, a consistent finding is the role of parents and family dysfunction as reasons for suicidal behavior in children and adolescents. These problems are further exacerbated if the youngster lacks adequate coping strategies or if serious cognitive or behavioral deficits or dysfunctions exist. Our research has shown that many adolescents are at greatest risk for suicidal behaviors when they are experiencing major negative life events, having many daily hassles, and have few social supports (Reynolds & Waltz, 1986).

When considering suicidal behavior in children, it is important to view the act itself as primary and attend less to the question of whether the child understands that death is permanent. The same is true with regard to determining the seriousness of a child's suicidal behavior. As Pfeffer (1986) notes, a child's understanding of the lethality of a suicidal action is difficult to determine. It is therefore expeditious to place primary emphasis on the observable behavior and aspects of intention, rather than on the child's understanding of his or her actions, in evaluating the seriousness of the suicidal behavior.

A significant but minimally researched question is that of what predisposes youngsters to suicidal behaviors. Knowing that suicidal behavior occurs in psychiatric disorders, such as major depression or adjustment disorder, does not deal with the question of why, since many youngsters with these disorders do not engage in suicidal behavior. Likewise, environmental stressors and interpersonal difficulties or crises are experienced by many adolescents, the majority of whom do not engage in self-destructive behaviors. Smith (1992), drawing from the literature and his clinical experience, has posited an "ego vulnerability model" to explain why some youngsters are vulnerable to suicidal behavior. This interactional model incorporates a number of ego structures, including an excessively demanding or harsh conscience, and high self-expectations, along with an internalized sense of helplessness, dysfunctional impulse control (either over- or undercontrolled), and overdependence on external approval for the regulation of self-esteem.

Attempts at the clinical prediction of suicidal behavior in adolescents are generally concerned with a myriad of variables, such as demographic characteristics (e.g., age, gender, race), family structure, parental psychopathology, social class, loss, psychiatric disturbances, major and minor stressors, previous suicidal behavior, exposure to others' suicidal behavior (modeling), substance use, and other characteristics. These variables are generally described as "risk factors," although most of these variables are considered risk factors when considered in a multivariate model rather than in isolation.

For the most part, the aforementioned factors are external to the individual, although some variables such as psychiatric disorders are trait or state characteristics that may have a major impact on the increased probability of or risk for suicide. For example, in an autopsy study of 170 youngsters who completed suicide in New York, Gould, Shaffer, Fisher, Kleinman, and Morishima (1992) found that for males with an affective disorder, the risk for suicide was 60/100,000 compared to the general rate of 16/100,000 for adolescent males. The highest risk of suicide was found for males who had a history of prior suicide attempts, with an estimated incidence of 250/100,000. What is generally overlooked in the prediction of suicide and suicidal behaviors is the cognitive and intrapsychic aspects of the individual that may predispose the individual to, or interact with other factors to increase the individual's vulnerability to, suicidal behavior.

It is not surprising to find that the highest risk for suicide among the demographic and personal variables studied by Gould et al. (1992) was a history of previous suicide attempts, since such a history is probably most indicative of youngsters who manifest incompetence in cognitive and intrapsychic domains. The critical nature of a suicide attempt in adolescence can be seen in the high rates of repeat attempts. In a study of adolescent suicide attempters in the Netherlands, Kienhorst et al. (1991) found that 12.5% made a repeat attempt between an initial interview and a 1-year follow-up. Brent et al. (1993b) and Spirito et al. (1992), respectively, conducted 6- and 3-month follow-up evaluations of attempters, reporting reattempt rates of 14.6% and 10%, respectively. In a sample of children and young adolescents previously hospitalized for suicidal behavior and followed up 6–8 years later, Pfeffer et al. (1991) found that 23.2% had made at least one repeat suicide attempt vs. 6.3% in a nonpsychiatric comparison sample. In the total sample, there were 26 youngsters who had attempted suicide at the initial evaluation, 30.8% of whom subsequently reattempted during the follow-up period. From these studies, we can see that a significant number of adolescent suicide attempters, including those who receive treatment for their attempt, go on to make one or more additional attempts.

Researchers studying at-risk groups of youngsters typically find relatively high rates of suicidal behavior. In a study of 576 runaway youths in New York City, Rotheram-Borus (1993) found that 29% of males and 44% of females had a history of suicide attempts. Furthermore, 12.7% of males and 15.5% of females reported having made a suicide attempt in the past month. In a sample of 291 adolescents who were seen in a home for runaway youths, Stiffman (1989) reported that 30% of the sample had a history of suicide attempt. Approximately 19% of the suicide attempters had made their initial attempt before 12 years of age.

Concluding Thoughts

The number of adolescents who engage in suicidal behaviors may be considered to be of epidemic proportion. Although completed suicide remains a relatively rare event, other suicidal behaviors such as suicide attempts and suicidal ideation are experienced by a significant proportion of young people. It is clear from this review and others (e.g., Pfeffer, 1989b) that a multitude of factors are associated with children's and adolescents' suicidal behaviors. The number, magnitude, and complexity (e.g., interactions among factors, predisposing conditions) of these factors make it nearly impossible for any one study to adequately evaluate or explain suicidal behavior in children and adolescents. Likewise, the heterogeneity of suicidal behavior creates further complexity in attempts to study it and ascertain its etiology.

As we noted earlier, the generally accepted rate of suicide in adolescents is approximately 11/100,000. This rate may be considered a conservative underestimate that ignores suicides presented as accidents (e.g., single car fatalities, drowning, drug overdoses) and failures or errors in coroners' reports. Data from the CDC and other studies suggest that approximately 8% of school-based adolescents make a suicide attempt each year, with higher rates found in clinical and other at-risk populations. The data suggest that every year between 1 and 2 million adolescents attempt suicide in the United States and that a significant number of attempts are of severity sufficient to require medical attention.

Several responsible questions to ask are these: How do we prevent such behaviors from developing? Given the existence of these problems how do we intervene? We believe that schools can and should do more to take a proactive approach to the prevention of suicide in children and adolescents. Likewise, we feel that professionals can do more to work and provide consultation with schools in procedures and methods for the prevention of suicidal behavior in young people. Both authors have been dismayed, on numerous occasions, to find that a school or school district proudly presents its program for crisis intervention or postvention after a suicide has occurred, yet has not plans or programs for the prevention of the initial suicide. We do not wish, however, to dissuade schools from development of crisis-situation programs. Several school-based crisis-situation programs have been developed for use in schools that relate to youth suicide as well as other serious events that appear reasonable responses to such crises (e.g., Poland & Pitcher, 1990; Pitcher & Poland, 1992). Likewise, a number of authors have provided suggestions for the development of school-based postvention programs (e.g., Leenaars & Wenckstern, 1991; Wenckstern & Leenaars, 1993).

Given the general failure and often poor conceptualization of school-based psychoeducational approaches for suicide prevention, schools and society would be better served by the identification of youngsters at greatest risk and the focusing of resources and efforts on this group. Medical professionals must also take a more active role in the identification of suicidal youth (Blumenthal, 1990b). Research suggests that adolescents seen in pediatric settings are unlikely to be asked about current or previous suicidal behavior (e.g., Hodgman & Roberts, 1982; Slap, Vorters, Khalid, Margulies, & Forke, 1992). Professionals and the general public should also be aware that targeting only suicide completion as the focus of intervention ignores the vast numbers of youngsters who are at risk for other suicidal behaviors. Although many of these suicidal behaviors, such as suicidal ideation and suicide threat, may not be immediately life-threatening, they are meaningful aspects of psychopathology and frequent precursors to more serious and sometimes lethal behaviors.

The prevention of suicide in actively or potentially suicidal youngsters is an enormously involved and challenging undertaking, even for a well-trained therapist. To expect schools to be efficacious in this endeavor may be overextending the role and function of the school. However, schools can do a great deal in the active identification of at-risk youngsters who can then be referred for further evaluation and, if deemed advisable, treatment. Poland (1989) has presented a useful set of guidelines and recommendations for schools in dealing with suicidal youngsters. We anticipate that significant reductions in the incidence of suicidal behavior among children and adolescents will be realized when mental health professionals and school personnel engage in collaborative programs of active identification, treatment, and support of youngsters at risk for suicidal behaviors.

References

Ackerman, G. L. (1993). A Congressional view of youth suicide. *American Psychologist, 48,* 183–184.

Adcock, A., Nagy, S., & Simpson, J. A. (1991). Selected risk factors in adolescent suicide attempts. *Adolescence, 26,* 817–828.

Alessi, N. E., McManus, M., & Brickman, A. (1984). Suicidal behavior among serious juvenile offenders. *American Journal of Psychiatry, 141,* 286–287.

American Psychiatric Association (1980). *Diagnostic and statistical manual of mental disorders,* 3rd ed. Washington, DC: Author.

American Psychiatric Association (1987). *Diagnostic and statistical manual of mental disorders,* 3rd ed., revised. Washington, DC: Author.

American Psychiatric Association (1991). *DSM-IV options book: Work in progress.* Washington, DC: Author.

American Psychiatric Association (1994). *Diagnostic and statistical manual of mental disorders,* 4th ed. Washington, DC: Author.

Andrews, J. A., & Lewinsohn, P. M. (1992). Suicidal attempts among older adolescents: Prevalence and co-occurrence with psychiatric disorders. *Journal of the American Academy of Child and Adolescent Psychiatry, 31,* 655–662.

Apter, A., Bleich, A., Plutchik, R., Mendelsohn, S., & Tyano, S. (1988). Suicidal behavior, depression, and conduct disorder in hospitalized adolescents. *Journal of the American Academy of Child and Adolescent Psychiatry, 27,* 696–699.

Asarnow, J. R., & Carlson, G. (1988). Suicide attempts in preadolescent child psychiatry inpatients. *Suicide and Life-Threatening Behavior, 18,* 129–136.

Asarnow, J. R., Carlson, G. A., & Guthrie, D. (1987). Coping strategies, self-perceptions, hopelessness, and perceived family environments in depressed and suicidal children. *Journal of Consulting and Clinical Psychology, 55,* 361–366.

Asarnow, J. R., & Guthrie, D. (1989). Suicidal behavior, depression, and hopelessness in child psychiatric inpatients: A replication and extension. *Journal of Clinical Child Psychology, 18,* 129–136.

Barter, J. T., Swaback, D. O., & Todd, D. (1968). Adolescent suicide attempts: A follow-up study of hospitalized patients. *Archives of General Psychiatry, 26,* 523–527.

Bayatpour, M., Wells, R. D., & Holford, S. (1992). Physical and sexual abuse as predictors of substance use and suicide among pregnant teenagers. *Journal of Adolescent Health, 13,* 128–132.

Beck, A. T., Kovacs, M., & Weissman, A. (1979). Assessment of suicidal intention: The Scale for Suicidal Ideation. *Journal of Consulting and Clinical Psychology, 47,* 343–352.

Beck, A. T., Schuyler, D., & Herman, I. (1974). Development of suicidal intent scales. In A. T. Beck, H. L. P. Resnik, & D. J. Lettieri (Eds.), *The prediction of suicide* (pp. 45–56). Bowie, MD: Charles Press.

Beck, A. T., Ward, C., Mendelson, M., Mock, J., & Erbaugh, J. (1961). An inventory for measuring depression. *Archives of General Psychiatry, 4,* 561–571.

Berlin, I. N. (1987). Suicide among American Indian adolescents: An overview. *Suicide and Life-Threatening Behavior, 17,* 218–232.

Berman, A. L. (1986). Adolescent suicide: Issues and challenges. *Seminars in Adolescent Medicine*, *2*, 269–277.

Berman, A. L. (1990). Standard of care in assessment of suicidal potential. *Psychotherapy in Private Practice*, *8*, 35–41.

Berman, A. L., & Carroll, T. A. (1984). Adolescent suicide: A critical review. *Death Studies*, *8*, 53–63.

Berman, A. L., & Jobes, D. A. (1991). *Adolescent suicide: Assessment and intervention*. Washington, DC: American Psychological Press.

Berman, A. L., & Schwartz, R. H. (1990). Suicide attempts among adolescent drug users. *American Journal of Diseases of Children*, *144*, 310–314.

Bettes, B. A., & Walker, E. (1986). Symptoms associated with suicidal behavior in childhood and adolescence. *Journal of Abnormal Child Psychology*, *14*, 591–604.

Biendseil, R. E. (1991). *1990 Dane county youth survey: Characteristics, problems, needs and opinions of 7th–12th grade students*. Madison, WI: Dane County Youth Commission.

Blumenthal, S. J. (1990a). Youth suicide: Risk factors, assessment, and treatment of adolescents and young adult suicidal patients. *Psychiatric Clinics of North America*, *13*, 511–556.

Blumenthal, S. J. (1990b). Youth suicide: The physician's role in suicide prevention. *Journal of the American Medical Association*, *264*, 3194–3196.

Blumenthal, S. J., & Kupfer, D. J. (1986). Generalizable treatment strategies for suicidal behavior. *Annals of the New York Academy of Science*, *48*, 327–340.

Blumenthal, S. J., & Kupfer, D. J. (1988). Overview of early detection and treatment strategies for suicidal behavior in young people. *Journal of Youth and Adolescence*, *17*, 1–24.

Bongar, B., Peterson, L. G., Harris, E. A., & Aissis, J. (1989). Clinical and legal considerations in the management of suicidal patients: An integrative overview. *Journal of Integrative and Eclectic Psychotherapy*, *8*, 53–67.

Bonner, R. L., & Rich, A. R. (1987). Toward a predictive model of suicidal ideation and behavior: Some preliminary data in college students. *Suicide and Life-Threatening Behaviors*, *17*, 50–63.

Borst, S. R., & Noam, G. G. (1989). Suicidality and psychopathology in hospitalized children and adolescents. *Acta Paedopsychiatrica*, *52*, 165–175.

Boyd, J. H. (1983). The increasing rate of suicide by firearms. *New England Journal of Medicine*, *308*, 872–874.

Brent, D. A. (1987). Correlates of the medical lethality of suicide attempts in children and adolescents. *Journal of the American Academy of Child and Adolescent Psychiatry*, *26*, 87–89.

Brent, D. A. (1989). The psychological autopsy: Methodological considerations for the study of adolescent suicide. *Suicide and Life-Threatening Behaviors*, *19*, 43–57.

Brent, D. A., Johnson, B., Bartle, S., Bridge, J., Rather, C., Matta, J., Connolly, J., & Constantine, D. (1993a). Personality disorder, tendency to impulsive violence, and suicidal behavior in adolescents. *Journal of the American Academy of Child and Adolescent Psychiatry*, *32*, 69–75.

Brent, D. A., Kalas, R., Edelbrock, C., Costello, A. J., Dulcan, M. K., & Conover, N. (1986). Psychopathology and its relationship to suicidal ideation in childhood and adolescents. *Journal of the American Academy of Child and Adolescent Psychiatry*, *25*, 666–673.

Brent, D. A., & Kolko, D. J. (1990). The assessment and treatment of patients at risk for suicide. In S. J. Blumenthal & D. J. Kupfer (Eds.), *Suicide over the life cycle: Risk factors, assessment and treatment of suicidal patients* (pp. 253–302). Washington, DC: American Psychiatric Press.

Brent, D. A., Kolko, D. J., Allan, M. J., & Brown, R. V. (1990). Suicidality in affectively disordered adolescent inpatients. *Journal of the American Academy of Child and Adolescent Psychiatry*, *29*, 586–593.

Brent, D. A., Kolko, D. J., Wartella, M. E., Boylan, M. B., Mortiz, G., Baugher, M., & Zelenak, J. P. (1993b). Adolescent psychiatric inpatients' risk of suicide attempt at 6-month follow-up. *Journal of the American Academy of Child and Adolescent Psychiatry*, *32*, 95–105.

Brent, D. A., Perper, J. A., Goldstein, C. E., Kolko, D. J., Allan, M. J., Allman, C. J., & Zelenak, J. P. (1988). Risk factors for adolescent suicide: A comparison of adolescent victims with suicidal inpatients. *Archives of General Psychiatry*, *45*, 581–588.

Brent, D. A., Perper, J. A., Moritz, G., Allman, C. J., Roth, C., Schweers, J., & Balach, L. (1993d). The validity of diagnoses obtained through the psychological autopsy procedure in adolescent suicide victims: Use of family history. *Acta Psychiatrica Scandinavia Supplementum*, *87*, 118–122.

Brent, D. A., Perper, J. A., Mortiz, G., Baugher, M., & Allman, C. (1993e). Suicide in adolescents with no apparent psychopathology. *Journal of the American Academy of Child and Adolescent Psychiatry*, *32*, 494–500.

Brent, D. A., Perper, J. A., Moritz, G., Baugher, M., Roth, C., Balach, L., & Schweers, J. (1993f). Stressful life events, psychopathology, and adolescent suicide: A case control study. *Suicide and Life-Threatening Behaviors*, *23*, 179–187.

Brown, L. K., Overholser, J., Spirito, A., & Fritz, G. K. (1991). The correlates of planning in adolescent suicide attempts. *Journal of the American Academy of Child and Adolescent Psychiatry, 30*, 95–99.

Cairns, R. B., Peterson, G., & Neckerman, H. J. (1988). Suicidal behavior in aggressive adolescents. *Journal of Clinical Child Psychology, 17*, 298–309.

Cantor, P. C. (1976). Personality characteristics found among youthful female suicide attempters. *Journal of Abnormal Psychology, 85*, 324–329.

Cantor, P. C. (1989). Intervention strategies: Environmental risk reduction for youth suicide. *Report of the secretary's task force on youth suicide*, Vol. 3, *Prevention and interventions in youth suicide* (pp. 285–293) (DHHS Publication No. ADM-89-1623). Washington, DC: U.S. Government Printing Office.

Cantor, P. C. (1990). Symptoms, prevention, and treatment of attempted suicide. In B. Wolman & G. Stricker (Eds.), *Depressive disorders: Facts, theories, and treatment methods* (pp. 189–202). New York: John Wiley.

Cantor, P. (1992). Environmental, educational, and psychological interventions in suicidal adolescents. In D. Jacobs (Ed.), *Suicide and clinical practice* (pp. 131–146). Washington, DC: American Psychiatric Press.

Carlson, G. A. (1983). Depression and suicidal behavior in children and adolescents. In D. P. Cantwell & G. A. Carlson (Eds.), *Affective disorders in childhood and adolescence: An update* (pp. 335–352). Jamaica, NY: Spectrum Publications.

Carlson, G. A., Asarnow, J. R., & Orbach, I. (1987). Developmental aspects of suicidal behavior in children I. *Journal of the American Academy of Child and Adolescent Psychiatry, 26*, 186–192.

Carlson, G. A., & Cantwell, D. P. (1982). Suicidal behavior and depression in children and adolescents. *Journal of the American Academy of Child Psychiatry, 21*, 361–368.

Carlson, G. A., Rich, C. L., Grayson, P., & Fowler, R. (1991). Secular trends in psychiatric diagnoses of suicide victims. *Journal of Affective Disorders, 21*, 127–132.

CDC (Centers for Disease Control) (1991). Attempted suicide among high school students: United States, 1990. *Morbidity and Mortality Weekly Report, 40(37)*, 633–635.

Christoffel, K. K., Marcus, D., Sagerman, S., & Bennett, S. (1988). Adolescent suicide and suicide attempts: A population study. *Pediatric Emergency Care, 4*, 32–40.

Clum, G. A., Patsiokas, A. T., & Luscomb, R. L. (1979). Empirical based comprehensive treatment program for parasuicide. *Journal of Consulting and Clinical Psychology, 47*, 937–945.

Cohen, L. S., Winchel, R. M., & Stanley, M. (1988). Biological markers of suicide risk and adolescent suicide. *Clinical Neuropharmacology, 11*, 423–435.

Cohen-Sandler, R., Berman, A. L., & King, R. A. (1982). Life stress and symptomatology: Determinants of suicidal behavior in children. *Journal of the American Academy of Child and Adolescent Psychiatry, 21*, 178–186.

Cole, D. A. (1989a). Validation of the Reasons for Living Inventory in general and delinquent adolescent samples. *Journal of Abnormal Child Psychology, 17*, 13–27.

Cole, D. A. (1989b). Psychopathology of adolescent suicide: Hopelessness, coping beliefs, and depression. *Journal of Abnormal Psychology, 98*, 248–255.

Cronbach, L. J. (1951). Coefficient alpha and the internal structure of tests. *Psychometrika, 16*, 297–334.

Crumley, F. E. (1979). Adolescent suicide attempts. *Journal of the American Medical Association, 241*, 2404–2407.

Crumley, F. E. (1982). The adolescent suicide attempt: A cardinal symptom of a serious psychiatric disorder. *American Journal of Psychotherapy, 36*, 158–165.

Cull, J. G., & Gill, W. S. (1982). *Suicide Probability Scale*. Los Angeles: Western Psychological Services.

Dew, M. A., Bromet, E. J., Brent, D., & Greenhouse, J. B. (1987). A quantitative literature review of the effectiveness of suicide prevention centers. *Journal of Consulting and Clinical Psychology, 55*, 239–244.

de Wilde, E. J. (1992). *Specific characteristics of adolescent suicide attempters*. Utrecht, The Netherlands: Proefschrift Rijksuniversiteit Utrecht.

de Wilde, E. J., Kienhorst, I. C. W. M., Diekstra, R. F. W., & Wolters, W. H. G. (1992). The relationship between adolescent suicidal behavior and life events in childhood and adolescence. *American Journal of Psychiatry, 149*, 45–51.

de Wilde, E. J., Kienhorst, I. C. W. M., Diekstra, R. F. W., & Wolters, W. H. G. (1993). The specificity of psychological characteristics of adolescent suicide attempters. *Journal of the American Academy of Child and Adolescent Psychiatry, 32*, 51–59.

Deykin, E. Y. (1986). Adolescent suicidal and self-destructive behavior: An intervention study. In G. L. Klerman (Ed.), *Suicide and depression among adolescents and young adults* (pp. 279–297). Washington, DC: American Psychiatric Press.

Deykin, E. Y., Alpert, J. J., & McNamarra, J. J. (1985). A pilot study of the effect of exposure to child abuse or neglect on adolescent suicide. *American Journal of Psychiatry, 142,* 1299–1303.

Deykin, E. Y., Hsieh, C. C., Joshi, N., & McNamarra, J. J. (1986). Adolescent suicidal and self-destructive behavior: Results of an intervention study. *Journal of Adolescent Health Care, 7,* 88–95.

Diekstra, R. F. W. (1992). The prevention of suicidal behavior: Evidence for the efficacy of clinical and community-based programs. *International Journal of Mental Health, 21,* 69–87.

Diekstra, R. F. W. (1993). The epidemiology of suicide and parasuicide. *Acta Psychiatrica Scandinavica Supplementum, 371,* 9–20.

Domenech, E., Canals, J., & Fernandez-Ballart, J. (1992). Suicidal ideation among Spanish schoolchildren: A three-year follow-up study of a pubertal population. *Personality and Individual Differences, 13,* 1055–1057.

Dubow, E. F., Kausch, D. F., Blum, M. C., Reed, J., & Bush, E. (1989). Correlates of suicidal ideation and attempts in a community sample of junior and high school students. *Journal of Clinical Psychology, 18,* 158–166.

Dyck, R. J., Newman, S. C., & Thompson, A. H. (1988). Suicide trends in Canada, 1956–1981. *Acta Psychiatrica Scandinavica, 77,* 411–419.

D'Zurilla, T., & Goldfried, M. (1971). Problem-solving and behavior modification. *Journal of Abnormal Psychology, 78,* 107–126.

Eddy, D. M., Wolpert, R. L., & Rosenberg, M. L. (1987). Estimating the effectiveness of interventions to prevent youth suicide. *Medical Care, 25(Supplement),* S57–S65.

Eisenberg, L. (1984). The epidemiology of suicide in adolescents. *Pediatric Annals, 13,* 47–54.

Ellis, T. E. (1986). Toward a cognitive therapy for suicidal individuals. *Professional Psychology: Research and Practice, 17,* 125–130.

Ellis, T. E. (1988). Classification of suicidal behavior: A review and step toward integration. *Journal of Suicide and Life-Threatening Behavior, 18,* 358–371.

Endicott, J., & Spitzer, R. L. (1978). A diagnostic interview: The Schedule for Affective Disorders and Schizophrenia. *Archives of General Psychiatry, 35,* 837–844.

Feltz, W. M., Chenier, T., & Barnes, R. (1992). Drug use and suicide ideation and behavior among North Carolina public school students. *American Journal of Public Health, 82,* 870–872.

Frances, A., & Clarkin, J. G. (1985). Considering family versus other therapies after a teenager's suicide attempt. *Hospital and Community Psychiatry, 36,* 1041–1042, 1046.

Fremouw, W., Callahan, T., & Kashden, J. (1993). Adolescent suicidal risk: Psychological, problem solving, and environmental factors. *Journal of Suicide and Life-Threatening Behavior, 23,* 46–54.

Fremouw, W. J., de Perczel, M., & Ellis, T. E. (1990). *Suicide risk: Assessment and response guidelines.* New York: Pergamon Press.

Friedman, J. M. H., Asnis, G. M., Boeck, M., & Difiore, J. (1987). Prevalence of specific behaviors in a high school sample. *American Journal of Psychiatry, 144,* 76–79.

Friedman, R. C., Aronoff, M. S., Clarkin, J. F., Corn, R., & Hurt, S. W. (1983). History of suicidal behavior in depressed borderline inpatients. *American Journal of Psychiatry, 140,* 1023–1026.

Friedman, R. C., Clarkin, J. F., Corn, R., Aronoff, M. S., Hurt, S. W., & Murphy, M. C. (1982). DSM-III and affective pathology in hospitalized adolescents. *Journal of Nervous and Mental Disease, 170,* 511–521.

Friedman, R. C., Corn, R., Hurt, S. W., Fibel, B., Schulick, J., & Swirsky, S. (1984b). Family history of illness in the seriously suicidal adolescent: A life-cycle approach. *American Journal of Orthopsychiatry, 54,* 390–397.

Friedrich, W., Reams, R., & Jacobs, J. (1982). Depression and suicidal ideation in early adolescents. *Journal of Youth and Adolescence, 11,* 403–407.

Fyer, M. R., Frances, A. J., & Sullivan, T. (1988). Comorbidity of borderline personality disorder. *Archives of General Psychiatry, 45,* 348–352.

Garfinkel, B. D. (1986). School based prevention programs. Paper presented at the National Conference on Prevention and Intervention in Youth Suicide, Oakland, CA, June 1986.

Garfinkel, B. D. (1989). School-based prevention programs. *Report of the secretary's task force on youth suicide,* Vol. 2, *Prevention and interventions in youth suicide* (pp. 294–304) (DHHS Publication No. ADM-89-1623). Washington, DC: U.S. Government Printing Office.

Garfinkel, B. D., Froese, A., & Hood, J. (1982). Suicide attempts in children and adolescents. *American Journal of Psychiatry, 139,* 1257–1261.

Garfinkel, B. D., & Golombek, H. (1983). Suicidal behavior in adolescence. In H. Golombek & B. D. Garfinkel (Eds.), *The adolescent and mood disturbance.* New York: International Universities Press.

Garland, A., Shaffer, D., & Whittle, B. (1989). A national survey of school-based adolescent suicide prevention programs. *Journal of the American Academy of Child and Adolescent Psychiatry, 28,* 931–934.

Garland, A. F., & Zigler, E. (1993). Adolescent suicide prevention: Current research and social policy implications. *American Psychologist, 48,* 169–182.

Garnefski, N., Diekstra, R. F. W., & de Heus, P. (1992). A population-based survey of the characteristics of high school students with and without a history of suicidal behavior. *Acta Psychiatrica Scandinavica, 86,* 189–196.

Garrison, C. Z. (1989). The study of suicidal behavior in the schools. *Journal of Suicide and Life-Threatening Behavior, 19,* 120–131.

Garrison, C. Z. (1992). Demographic predictors of suicide. In R. W. Maris, A. L. Berman, J. T. Maltsberger, & R. I. Yufit (Eds.), *Assessment and prediction of suicide* (pp. 484–498). New York: Guilford Press.

Garrison, C. Z., Addy, C. L., Jackson, K. L., McKeown, R. E., & Waller, J. L. (1991a). A longitudinal study of suicidal ideation in young adolescents. *Journal of the American Academy of Child and Adolescent Psychiatry, 30,* 597–603.

Garrison, C. Z., Jackson, K. L., Addy, C. L., McKeown, R. E., & Waller, J. L. (1991b). Suicidal behaviors in young adolescents. *American Journal of Epidemiology, 133,* 1005–1014.

Garrison, C. Z., McKeown, R. E., Valois, R. F., & Vincent, M. L. (1993). Aggression, substance use, and suicidal behaviors in high school students. *American Journal of Public Health, 83,* 179–184.

Gartrell, J. W., Jarvis, G. K., & Derksen, L. (1993). Suicidality among adolescent Alberta Indians. *Journal of Suicide and Life-Threatening Behavior, 23,* 366–373.

Gispert, M., Wheeler, K., Marsh, L., & Davis, M. S. (1985). Suicidal adolescents: Factors in evaluation. *Adolescence, 20,* 753–762.

Goldacre, M., & Hawton, K. (1985). Repetition of self-poisoning and subsequent death in adolescents who take overdoses. *British Journal of Psychiatry, 146,* 395–398.

Goldney, R. D., & Katsikitis, M. (1983). Cohort analysis of suicide rates in Australia. *Archives of General Psychiatry, 40,* 71–74.

Goldsmith, S. J., Fyer, M., & Frances, A. (1990). Personality and suicide. In S. J. Blumenthal & D. J. Kupfer (Eds.), *Suicide over the life cycle: Risk factors, assessment and treatment of suicidal patients* (pp. 155–176). Washington, DC: American Psychiatric Press.

Goodwin, F. K., & Brown, G. L. (1989). Summary and overview of risk factors in suicide. *Report of the secretary's task force on youth suicide,* Vol. 2, *Prevention and interventions in youth suicide* (pp. 263–271). (DHHS Publication No. ADM-89-1622). Washington, DC: U.S. Government Printing Office.

Goodwin, F. K., & Runck, B. L. (1992). Suicide intervention: Integration of psychosocial, clinical, and biomedical traditions. In D. Jacobs (Ed.), *Suicide and clinical practice* (pp. 1–22). Washington, DC: American Psychiatric Press.

Gould, M. S., Shaffer, D., Fisher, P., Kleinman, M., & Morishima, A. (1992). The clinical prediction of adolescent suicide. In R. W. Maris, A. L. Berman, J. T. Maltsberger, & R. I. Yufit (Eds.), *Assessment and prediction of suicide* (pp. 130–143). New York: Guilford Press.

Green, A. H. (1978). Self-destructive behavior in battered children. *American Journal of Psychiatry, 135,* 579–582.

Grossman, D. C., Milligan, B. C., & Deyo, R. A. (1991). Risk factors for suicide attempts among Navajo adolescents. *American Journal of Public Health, 81,* 870–874.

Gutstein, S. E., & Rudd, M. D. (1990). An outpatient treatment alternative for suicidal youth. *Journal of Adolescence, 13,* 265–277.

Hawton, K. (1986). *Suicide and attempted suicide among children and adolescents.* Newbury Park, CA: Sage Publications.

Hawton, K. (1987). Assessment and aftercare of adolescents who take overdoses. In R. F. W. Diekstra & K. Hawton (Eds.), *Suicide in adolescence* (pp. 79–93). Dordrecht, The Netherlands: Martinus Nijhoff Publishers.

Hawton, K., O'Grady, J., Osborne, M., & Cole, D. (1982). Adolescents who take overdoses: Their characteristics, problems, and contacts with helping agencies. *British Journal of Psychiatry, 140,* 118–123.

Hazell, P., & Lewin, T. (1993). An evaluation of postvention following adolescent suicide. *Suicide and Life-Threatening Behavior, 23,* 101–109.

Hendin, H. (1991). Psychodynamics of suicide, with particular reference to the young. *American Journal of Psychiatry, 148,* 1150–1158.

Hibbard, R. A., Brack, C. J., Rauch, S., & Orr, D. P. (1988). Abuse, feelings, and health behaviors in a student population. *American Journal of Diseases of Children, 142,* 326–330.

Hillard, J. R., Slomowitz, M., & Deddens, J. (1988). Determinants of emergency psychiatric admission for adolescents and adults. *American Journal of Psychiatry, 145,* 1416–1419.

Hoberman, H. M. (1989). Completed suicide in children and adolescents: A review. *Residential Treatment for Children and Youth, 7,* 61–88.

Hoberman, H. M., & Garfinkel, B. D. (1988a). Completed suicide in children and adolescents. *Journal of the American Academy of Child and Adolescent Psychiatry, 27*, 689–695.

Hoberman, H. M., & Garfinkel, B. D. (1988b). Completed suicide in youth. *Canadian Journal of Psychiatry, 33*, 494–504.

Hodgman, C. H., & Roberts, F. N. (1982). Adolescent suicide and the pediatrician. *Journal of Pediatrics, 101*, 118–123.

Holinger, P. C. (1989). Epidemiologic issues in youth suicide. In C. R. Pfeffer (Ed.), *Suicide among youth: Perspectives on risk and prevention* (pp. 41–62). Washington, DC: American Psychiatric Press.

Howard-Pitney, B., LaFromboise, T. D., Basil, A., September, C., & Johnson, M. D. (1992). Psychological and social indicators of suicidal ideation and suicide attempts in Zuni adolescents. *Journal of Consulting and Clinical Psychology, 60*, 473–476.

Jacobziner, H. (1965). Attempted suicide in adolescence. *Journal of the American Medical Association, 191*, 101–105.

Jobes, D. (1992). Evaluation of suicide patients. Paper presented at the Annual Meeting of the American Association of Suicidology, Chicago, IL, May 1992.

Jobes, D. A., & Berman, A. L. (1991). Crisis intervention and brief treatment for suicidal youth. In A. Roberts (Ed.), *Contemporary perspectives on crisis intervention and prevention* (pp. 53–69). Englewood Cliffs, NJ: Prentice Hall.

Jobes, D. A., & Berman, A. L. (1993). Suicide and malpractice liability: Assessing and revising policies, procedures, and practice in outpatient settings. *Professional Psychology: Research and Practice, 24*, 91–99.

Jobes, D. A, Berman, A. L., & Josselson, A. R. (1987). Improving the validity and reliability of medical–legal certifications of suicide. *Suicide and Life-Threatening Behavior, 17*, 310–325.

Joffe, R. T., Offord, D. R., & Boyle, M. H. (1988). Ontario Child Health Study: Suicidal behavior in youth age 12–16 years. *American Journal of Psychiatry, 145*, 1420–1423.

Kahan, J., & Pattison, E. M. (1984). Proposal for a distinctive diagnosis: The Deliberate Self-Harm Syndrome (DSH). *Suicide and Life-Threatening Behavior, 14*, 17–35.

Kahn, J. S., Kehle, T. J., Jenson, W. R., & Clark, E. (1990). Comparison of cognitive–behavioral, relaxation, and self-modeling interventions for depression among middle-school students. *School Psychology Review, 19*, 196–211.

Kandel, D. B., Raveis, V. H., & Davies, M. (1991). Suicidal ideation in adolescence: Depression, substance use, and other risk factors. *Journal of Youth and Adolescence, 20*, 289–308.

Kaplan, S. L., Hong, G. K., & Weinhold, C. (1984). Epidemiology of depressive symptomatology in adolescents. *Journal of the American Academy of Child Psychiatry, 23*, 91–98.

Kashani, J. H., Goddard, P., & Reid, J. C. (1989). Correlates of suicidal ideation in a community sample of children and adolescents. *Journal of the American Academy of Child and Adolescent Psychiatry, 28*, 912–917.

Kashden, J., Fremouw, W. J., Callahan, T. S, & Franzen, M. D. (1993). Impulsivity in suicidal and nonsuicidal adolescents. *Journal of Abnormal Child Psychology, 21*, 339–353.

Kazdin, A. E., French, N. H., Unis, A. S., Esveldt-Dawson, K., & Sherick, R. B. (1983). Hopelessness, depression and suicidal intent among psychiatrically disturbed inpatient children. *Journal of Consulting and Clinical Psychology, 51*, 504–510.

Kerfoot, M. (1987). Family therapy and psychotherapy following suicidal behaviour by young adolescents. In R. F. W. Diekstra & K. Hawton (Eds.), *Suicide in adolescence* (pp. 95–111). Dordrecht, The Netherlands: Martinus Nijhoff Publishers.

Kerfoot, M. (1988). Deliberate self-poisoning in childhood and early adolescence. *Journal of Child Psychology and Psychiatry, 29*, 335–343.

Kienhorst, C. W. M., De Wilde, E. J., Van den Bovt, J., Diekstra, R. F. W., & Wolters, W. H. G. (1990). Characteristics of suicide attempters in a population-based sample of Dutch adolescents. *British Journal of Psychiatry, 156*, 243–248.

Keinhorst, C. W. M., De Wilde, E. J., Diekstra, R. F. W., & Wolters, W. H. G. (1991). Construction of an index for predicting suicide attempts in depressed adolescents. *British Journal of Psychiatry, 159*, 676–682.

Kienhorst, C. W. M. Wolters, W. H. G., Diekstra, R. F. W., & Otte, E. (1987). A study of the frequency of suicidal behaviour in children aged 5 to 14. *Journal of Child Psychology and Psychiatry, 28*, 153–165.

King, C. A., Hill, E. M., Naylor, M., Evans, T., & Shain, B. (1993). Alcohol consumption in relation to other predictors of suicidality among adolescent inpatient girls. *Journal of the American Academy of Child and Adolescent Psychiatry, 32*, 82–88.

King, C. A., Naylor, M. W., Evans, T., & Segal, H. (1991). Adolescents at risk for suicide: Family systems protective factors. Paper presented at the Annual Conference of the American Psychological Association, San Francisco, August 1991.

King, C. A., Raskin, A., Gdowski, C. L., Butkus, M., & Opipari, L. (1990). Psychosocial factors associated with urban adolescent female suicide attempts. *Journal of the American Academy of Child and Adolescent Psychiatry, 29*, 289–294.

King, C. A., Segal, H. G., Naylor, M., & Evans, T. (1993). Family functioning and suicidal behavior in adolescent inpatients with mood disorders. *Journal of the American Academy of Child and Adolescent Psychiatry, 32*, 1198–1206.

King, R. A., Pfeffer, C., Gammon, G. D., & Cohen, D. J. (1992). Suicidality of childhood and adolescence: Review of the literature and proposal for establishment of a DSM-IV category. In B. B. Lahey & A. E. Kazdin (Eds.), *Advances in clinical child psychology*, Vol. 14 (pp. 297–325). New York: Plenum Press.

Kolko, D. J., & Brent, D. A. (1988). Cognitive–behavioral interventions for adolescent suicide attempters: Procedures, processes, and preliminary outcomes. Paper presented at the Annual Meeting of the American Psychological Association, Atlanta, August 1988.

Kosky, R. (1983). Childhood suicidal behaviour. *Journal of Child Psychology and Psychiatry, 24*, 457–468.

Kosky, R. (1987). Is suicidal behavior increasing among Australian youth? *Medical Journal of Australia, 147(8)*, 164–166.

Kosky, R., Silburn, S., & Zubrick, S. (1986). Symptomatic depression and suicidal ideation: A comparative study with 628 children. *Journal of Nervous and Mental Disease, 174*, 523–528.

Kosky, R., Silburn, S., & Zubrick, S. R. (1990). Are children and adolescents who have suicidal thoughts different from those who attempt suicide? *Journal of Nervous and Mental Disease, 178*, 38–43.

Kotila, L. (1992). The outcome of attempted suicide in adolescence. *Journal of Adolescent Health, 13*, 415–417.

Kotila, L., & Lonnqvist, J. (1988). Adolescent suicide attempts: Sex differences predicting suicide. *Acta Psychiatrica Scandinavica, 77*, 264–270.

Kovacs, M. (1979). *Children's Depression Inventory*. Pittsburgh: University of Pittsburgh School of Medicine.

Kovacs, M., Goldston, D., & Gatsonis, C. (1993). Suicidal behaviors and childhood-onset depressive disorders: A longitudinal investigation. *Journal of the American Academy of Child and Adolescent Psychiatry, 32*, 8–20.

Kovacs, M., & Puig-Antich, J. (1989). "Major psychiatric disorders" as risk factors in youth suicide. *Report of the secretary's task force on youth suicide*, Vol. 2, *Prevention and interventions in youth suicide* (pp. 143–159) (DHHS Publication No. ADM-89-1622). Washington, DC: U.S. Government Printing Office.

Kowalchuk, B., & King, J. D. (1988). *Life Orientation Inventory: A method for assessing suicide risk*. Austin, TX: Pro-Ed.

Kragh-Sorensen, P. (1993). Pharmacotherapy of the suicidal patient. *Acta Psychiatrica Scandinavica Supplementum, 371*, 57–59.

Kreitman, N. (1977). *Parasuicide*. London: John Wiley.

Lachar, D. (1982). *Personality Inventory for Children Revised Format Manual Supplement*. Los Angeles: Western Psychological Services.

Ladame, F., & Jeanneret, O. (1982). Suicide in adolescence: Some comments on epidemiology and prevention. *Journal of Adolescence, 5*, 355–366.

Lamb, J., & Pusker, K. R. (1991). School-based adolescent mental health project survey of depression, suicidal ideation, and anger. *Journal of Child and Adolescent Psychiatric and Mental Health Nursing, 4*, 101–104.

Leenaars, A. (1992). Suicide notes and their implications for intervention. Paper presented at the Annual Convention of the American Association of Suicidology, Chicago, April 1992.

Leenaars, A. A., & Wenckstern, S. (1991). Posttraumatic stress disorder: A conceptual model for postvention. In A. A. Leenaars & S. Wenckstern (Eds.), *Suicide prevention in schools* (pp. 173–180). New York: Hemisphere Publishing.

Lerner, M. S., & Clum, G. A. (1990). Treatment of suicide ideators: A problem-solving approach. *Behavior Therapy, 21*, 403–411.

Lester, D. (1991). A cross-cultural look at the suicide rates of children and teenagers. In A. A. Leenaars & S. Wenckstern (Eds.), *Suicide prevention in schools* (pp. 17–25). New York: Hemisphere Publishing.

Levy, J. C., & Deykin, E. Y. (1989). Suicidality, depression, and substance abuse in adolescence. *American Journal of Psychiatry, 146*, 1462–1467.

Lewinsohn, P. M., Rohde, P., & Seeley, J. R. (1993). Psychosocial characteristics of adolescents with a history of suicide attempt. *Journal of the American Academy of Child and Adolescent Psychiatry, 32*, 60–68.

Liberman, R. P., & Eckman, T. (1981). Behavior therapy vs insight-oriented therapy for repeated suicide attempters. *Archives of General Psychiatry, 38*, 1126–1130.

Linehan, M. M. (1981). A social–behavioral analysis of suicide and parasuicide: Implications for clinical assessment and treatment. In J. F. Clarkin & H. Glazer (Eds.), *Depression: Behavioral and directive treatment strategies* (pp. 229–294). New York: Garland Press.

Linehan, M. M. (1987). Dialectical behavior therapy: A cognitive behavioral approach to parasuicide. *Journal of Personality Disorders, 1*, 328–333.

Linehan, M. M. (1993a). *Cognitive–behavioral treatment of borderline personality disorder.* New York: Guilford Press.

Linehan, M. M. (1993b). *Skills training manual for treating borderline personality disorder.* New York: Guilford Press.

Linehan, M. M., Armstrong, H. E., Suarez, A., Allmon, D., & Heard, H. L. (1991). Cognitive–behavioral treatment of chronically parasuicidal borderline patients. *Archives of General Psychiatry, 48*, 1060–1064.

Linehan, M. M. Goodstein, J. L., Nielsen, S. L., & Chiles, J. A. (1983). Reasons for staying alive when you're thinking of killing yourself: The Reasons for Living Inventory. *Journal of Consulting and Clinical Psychology, 51*, 276–286.

Linehan, M. M., Heard, H. L., & Armstrong, H. E. (1993). Naturalistic follow-up of a behavioral treatment for chronically parasuicidal borderline patients. *Archives of General Psychiatry, 50*, 971–974.

Linehan, M. M., & Nielsen, S. L. (1981). Assessment of suicidal ideation and parasuicide: Hopelessness and social desirability. *Journal of Consulting and Clinical Psychology, 49*, 773–775.

Litt, I. F., Cuskey, W. R., & Rudd, S. (1983). Emergency room evaluation of the adolescent who attempts suicide: Compliance with follow-up. *Journal of Adolescent Health Care, 4*, 106–108.

Livingston, R., Lawson, L., & Jones, J. G. (1993). Predictors of self-reported psychopathology in children abused repeatedly by a parent. *Journal of the American Academy of Child and Adolescent Psychiatry, 32*, 948–954.

Mazza, J. J., & Reynolds, W. M. (1991). Longitudinal investigation of psychosocial factors and suicidal ideation in adolescents. Paper presented at the Annual Convention of the American Psychological Association, San Francisco, August 1991.

Mazza, J. J., & Reynolds, W. M. (1993). Investigation of psychopathology in suicidal and nonsuicidal school-based adolescents. Unpublished manuscript.

McIntosh, J. L. (1992, April). Epidemiology of teen suicide in the United States. Paper presented at the Annual Convention of the American Association of Suicidology, Chicago.

Mehr, M., Zeltzer, L. K., & Robinson, R. (1981). Continued self-destructive behaviors in adolescent suicide attempters: Part I. *Journal of Adolescent Health Care, 1*, 269–274.

Miller, D. (1981). Adolescent suicide: Etiology and treatment. In S. C. Feinstein, J. G. Looney, A. Z. Schwartzberg, & A. D. Sorosky (Eds.), *Adolescent psychiatry*, Vol. 9, *Developmental and clinical studies* (pp. 327–342). Chicago: University of Chicago Press.

Miller, I. W., Norman, W. H., Bishop, S. B., & Dow, M. G. (1986). The Modified Scale for Suicidal Ideation: Reliability and validity. *Journal of Consulting and Clinical Psychology, 54*, 724–725.

Miller, M. L., Chiles, J. A., & Barnes, V. E. (1982). Suicide attempts within a delinquent population. *Journal of Consulting and Clinical Psychology, 50*, 491–498.

Miller, N. S., & Fine, J. (1993). Current epidemiology of comorbidity of psychiatric and additive disorders. *Psychiatric Clinics of North America, 16*, 1–10.

Motto, J. A. (1975). Treatment and management of suicidal adolescents. *Psychiatric Opinion, 12(6)*, 14–20.

Mufson, L., Moreau, D., Weissman, M. M., Klerman, G. L. (1993). *Interpersonal psychotherapy for depressed adolescents.* New York: Guilford Press.

Myers, K. M., Burke, P., & McCauley, E. (1985). Suicidal behavior by hospitalized preadolescent children on a psychiatric units. *Journal of the American Academy of Child and Adolescent Psychiatry, 24*, 474–480.

Myers, K., McCauley, E., Calderon, R., Mitchell, J., Burke, P., & Schloredt, K. (1991). Risks for suicidality in major depressive disorder. *Journal of the American Academy of Child and Adolescent Psychiatry, 30*, 86–94.

Myers, W. C., Otto, T. A., Harris, E., Diaco, D., & Moreno, A. (1992). Acetaminophen overdose as a suicide gesture: A survey of adolescents' knowledge of its potential toxicity. *Journal of the American Academy of Child and Adolescent Psychiatry, 31*, 686–690.

NIMH (National Institute of Mental Health) (1992). *Suicide facts.* Bethesda, MD: Author, March 1992.

Orbach, I. (1988). *Children who don't want to live: Understanding and treating the suicidal child.* San Francisco: Jossey-Bass.

Orbach, I., Feshbach, S., Carlson, G., Glaubman, H., & Gross, Y. (1983). Attraction and repulsion by life and death in suicidal and in normal children. *Journal of Consulting and Clinical Psychology, 51,* 661–670.

Orbach, I., Gross, Y., & Glaubman, H. (1981). Some common characteristics of latency-age suicidal children: A tentative model based on case study analyses. *Suicide and Life-Threatening Behavior, 11,* 180–190.

Orbach, I., Milstein, I., Har-Even, D., Apter, A., Tiano, S., & Elizur, A. (1991). A multi-attitude suicide tendency scale for adolescents. *Psychological Assessment, 3,* 398–404.

Overholser, J. C., Hemstreet, A. H., Spirito, A., & Vyse, S. (1989). Suicide awareness programs in the schools: Effects of gender and personal experience. *Journal of the American Academy of Child and Adolescent Psychiatry, 28,* 925–930.

Patsiokas, A. T., & Clum, G. A. (1985). Effects of psychotherapeutic strategies in the treatment of suicide attempters. *Psychotherapy, 22,* 281–290.

Patsiokas, A. T., Clum, G. A., & Luscomb, R. L. (1979). Cognitive characteristics of suicide attempters. *Journal of Consulting and Clinical Psychology, 47,* 478–484.

Paulson, M. J., Stone, D., & Sposto, R. (1978). Suicide potential and behavior in children ages 4 to 12. *Suicide and Life-Threatening Behavior, 8,* 225–242.

Pfeffer, C. R. (1977). Psychiatric hospital treatment of suicidal children. *Suicide and Life-Threatening Behavior, 8,* 150–160.

Pfeffer, C. R. (1981a). Suicidal behavior of children: A review with implications for research and practice. *American Journal of Psychiatry, 138,* 154–159.

Pfeffer, C. R. (1981b). The family system of suicidal children. *American Journal of Psychotherapy, 35,* 330–341.

Pfeffer, C. R. (1981c). Parental suicide: An organizing event in the development of latency age children. *Suicide and Life-Threatening Behavior, 11,* 43–50.

Pfeffer, C. R. (1982). Interventions for suicidal children and their parents. *Suicide and Life-Threatening Behavior, 12,* 240–248.

Pfeffer, C. R. (1984). Modalities of treatment for suicidal children: An overview of the literature on current practice. *American Journal of Psychotherapy, 38,* 364–372.

Pfeffer, C. R. (1985). Suicidal fantasies in normal children. *Journal of Nervous and Mental Disease, 173,* 78–84.

Pfeffer, C. R. (1986). *The suicidal child.* New York: Guilford Press.

Pfeffer, C. R. (1989a). Life stress and family risk factors for youth fatal and nonfatal suicidal behavior. In C. R. Pfeffer (Ed.), *Suicide among youth: Perspectives on risk and prevention* (pp. 143–164). Washington, DC: American Psychiatric Press.

Pfeffer, C. R. (1989b). Family characteristics and support systems as risk factors for youth and suicidal behavior. *Report of the secretary's task force on youth suicide,* Vol. 2, *Prevention and interventions in youth suicide* (pp. 71–87). (DHHS Publication No. ADM-89-1622). Washington, DC: U.S. Government Printing Office.

Pfeffer, C. R. (1990). Clinical perspectives on treatment of suicidal behavior among children and adolescents. *Psychiatric Annals, 20,* 143–150.

Pfeffer, C. R., Klerman, G. L., Hurt, S. W., Lesser, M., Peskin, J. R., & Siefker, C. A. (1991). Suicidal children grow up: Demographic and clinical risk factors for adolescent suicide attempts. *Journal of the American Academy of Child and Adolescent Psychiatry, 30,* 609–616.

Pfeffer, C. R., Newcorn, J., Kaplan, G., Mizruchi, M. S., & Plutchik, R. (1988). Suicidal behavior in adolescent psychiatric inpatients. *Journal of the American Academy of Child and Adolescent Psychiatry, 27,* 357–361.

Pfeffer, C. R., & Trad, P. V. (1988). Sadness and suicidal tendencies in preschool children. *Developmental and Behavioral Pediatrics, 9,* 86–88.

Pfeffer, C. R., Zuckerman, S., Plutchik, R., & Mizruchi, M. S. (1984). Suicidal behavior in normal and psychiatric inpatients. *Journal of the American Academy of Child Psychiatry, 23,* 416–423.

Phillips, D. P. (1989). Effects of mass media news stores on suicide, with new evidence on the role of story content. In C. R. Pfeffer (Ed.), *Suicide among youth: Perspectives on risk and prevention* (pp. 101–116). Washington, DC: American Psychiatric Press.

Pitcher, G. D., & Poland, S. (1992). *Crisis intervention in the schools.* New York: Guilford Press.

Plutchik, R., & van Praag, H. (1989). The measurement of suicidality, aggressivity and impulsivity. *Progress in Neuro-Psychopharmacology and Biological Psychiatry, 13,* S23–S34.

Pokorny, A. D. (1974). A scheme for classifying suicidal behaviors. In A. T. Beck, H. L. P. Resnik, & D. J. Lettieri (Eds.), *The prediction of suicide* (pp. 29–44). Bowie, MD: Charles Press.

Poland, S. (1989). *Suicide intervention in the schools.* New York: Guilford Press.

Poland, S., & Pitcher, G. (1990). Expect the unexpected. *School Safety, 14(Fall)*, 14–17.

Puig-Antich, J. (1987). Affective disorders in children and adolescents: Diagnostic validity and psychobiology. In H. Y. Meltzer (Ed.), *Psychopharmacology: The third generation of progress* (pp. 843–859). New York: Raven Press.

Rao, U., Weissman, M. M., Martin, J. A., & Hammond, R. W. (1993). Childhood depression and risk of suicide: A preliminary report of a longitudinal study. *Journal of the American Academy of Child and Adolescent Psychiatry, 32*, 21–27.

Recklitis, C. J., Noam, G. G., & Borst, S. R. (1992). Adolescent suicide and defensive style. *Suicide and Life-Threatening Behavior, 22*, 374–387.

Retterstol, N. (1993). Death due to overdose of antidepressants: Experiences from Norway. *Acta Psychiatrica Scandinavica Suppplementum, 371*, 28–32.

Rey, J. M., & Bird, K. D. (1991). Sex differences in suicidal behaviour of referred adolescents. *British Journal of Psychiatry, 158*, 776–781.

Reynolds, W. M. (1986a). A model for the screening and identification of depressed children and adolescents in school settings. *Professional School Psychology, 1*, 117–129.

Reynolds, W. M. (1986b). *Reynolds Adolescent Depression Scale.* Odessa, FL: Psychological Assessment Resources.

Reynolds, W. M. (1987). *Suicidal Ideation Questionnaire.* Odessa, FL: Psychological Assessment Resources.

Reynolds, W. M. (1988). *Suicidal Ideation Questionnaire: Professional Manual.* Odessa, FL: Psychological Assessment Resources.

Reynolds, W. M. (1989). Suicidal ideation and depression in adolescents: Assessment and research. In P. F. Lovibond & P. Wilson (Eds.), *Clinical and abnormal psychology* (pp. 125–135). Amsterdam: Elsevier.

Reynolds, W. M. (1990). Development of a semistructured clinical interview for suicidal behaviors in adolescents. *Psychological Assessment: Journal of Consulting and Clinical Psychology, 2*, 382–390.

Reynolds, W. M. (1991a). Efficacy of the SIQ for the identification of suicidal youth. Paper presented at the Annual Convention of the American Psychological Association, San Francisco, August 1991.

Reynolds, W. M. (1991b). *Adult Suicidal Ideation Questionnaire: Professional Manual.* Odessa, FL: Psychological Assessment Resources.

Reynolds, W. M. (1991c). Psychometric characteristics of the Adult Suicidal Ideation Questionnaire in college students. *Journal of Personality Assessment, 56*, 289–307.

Reynolds, W. M. (1991d). A school-based procedure for the identification of adolescents at-risk for suicidal behaviors. *Family and Community Health, 14*, 64–75.

Reynolds, W. M. (1992a). *Measurement of suicidal ideation in adolescents.* Paper presented at the Annual Convention of the American Association of Suicidology, Chicago, April 1992.

Reynolds, W. M. (1992b). Depression in children and adolescents. In W. M. Reynolds (Ed.), *Internalizing disorders in children and adolescents* (pp. 149–254). New York: John Wiley.

Reynolds, W. M. (1994). Depression in adolescents: Contemporary issues and perspectives. In T. H. Ollendick & R. J. Prinz (Eds.), *Advances in clinical child psychology*, Vol. 16 (pp. 261–316). New York: Plenum Press.

Reynolds, W. M. (in press-a). *Adolescent Psychopathology Scale.* Odessa, FL: Psychological Assessment Resources.

Reynolds, W. M. (in press-b). *Suicidal Behaviors Interview.* Odessa, FL: Psychological Assessment Resources.

Reynolds, W. M., & Coats, K. I. (1986). A comparison of cognitive–behavioral therapy and relaxation training for the treatment of depression in adolescents. *Journal of Consulting and Clinical Psychology, 54*, 653–660.

Reynolds, W. M., Kobak, K. A., & Greist, J. H. (1992). Suicidal behavior in outpatients with panic disorder, OCD, and major depression. Paper presented at the International Conference on Suicidal Behavior, Western Psychiatric Institute and Clinic, Pittsburgh, June 1992.

Reynolds, W. M., Kobak, K. A., & Greist, J. H. (1994). Measurement of suicidal ideation in psychiatric outpatients: Psychometric characteristics of the Adult Suicidal Ideation Questionnaire (submitted).

Reynolds, W. M., Kobak, K. A., Greist, J. H., Jefferson, J. W., & Tollefson, G. D. (1993). Fluoxetine versus imipramine: Changes in suicidal ideation. Paper presented at the Annual Convention of the American Psychiatric Association, San Francisco, May 1993.

Reynolds, W. M., & Mazza, J. J. (1990). Suicidal behavior and depression in adolescents. Paper presented at the Annual Meeting of the American Psychological Association, Boston.

Reynolds, W. M., & Mazza, J. J. (1992a, June). Suicidal behavior in nonreferred adolescents. Paper presented at the International Conference for Suicidal Behavior, Western Psychiatric Institute and Clinic, Pittsburgh, PA.

Reynolds, W. M., & Mazza, J. J. (1992b, June). Psychosocial characteristics of adolescent suicide attempts. Paper presented at the International Conference for Suicidal Behavior, Western Psychiatric Institute and Clinic, Pittsburgh, PA.

Reynolds, W. M., & Mazza, J. J. (1992c). *Suicide Behavior History Form*. Odessa, FL: Psychological Assessment Resources.

Reynolds, W. M., & Mazza, J. J. (1992d). Suicide attempts and psychopathology in youth. Paper presented at the Annual Conference of the American Association for Suicidology, Chicago, April 1992.

Reynolds, W. M., & Mazza, J. J. (1993a). Suicidal behavior in adolescents. I. Suicide attempts in school-based youngsters. Unpublished manuscript.

Reynolds, W. M., & Mazza, J. J. (1993b). Suicidal behavior in adolescents. II. Suicide attempts in youngsters seen in mental health facilities. Unpublished manuscript.

Reynolds, W. M., & Mazza, J. J. (1993c). Evaluation of suicidal behavior in adolescents: Reliability of the Suicidal Behaviors Interview. Unpublished manuscript.

Reynolds, W. M., & Waltz, J. (1986). Life events, social support and suicidal ideation in adolescents. Paper presented at the annual meeting of the American Psychological Association, Washington, DC, August 1986.

Rich, A. R., Kirkpatrick-Smith, J., Bonner, R. L., & Jans, F. (1992). Gender differences in the psychosocial correlates of suicidal ideation among adolescents. *Suicide and Life-Threatening Behavior, 22,* 364–373.

Riggs, S., & Cheng, T. (1988). Adolescents' willingness to use a school-based clinic in view of expressed health concerns. *Journal of Adolescent Health Care, 9,* 208–213.

Ritter, D. R. (1990). Adolescent suicide: Social competence and problem behavior of youth at high risk and low risk for suicide. *School Psychology Review, 19,* 83–95.

Robbins, D. R., & Alessi, N. E. (1985). Depressive symptoms and suicidal behavior in adolescents. *American Journal of Psychiatry, 142,* 588–592.

Robinson, J. (1986). Emergencies I. In K. S. Robson (Ed.), *Manual of clinical child psychiatry* (pp. 185–211). Washington, DC: American Psychiatric Press.

Rosen, G. (1971). History in the study of suicide. *Psychological Medicine, 1,* 267–285.

Rosenberg, M. L., Smith, J. C., Davidson, L. E., & Conn, J. M. (1987). The emergence of youth suicide: An epidemiologic analysis and public health perspective. *Annual Review of Public Health, 8,* 417–440.

Rosenthal, P. A, & Rosenthal, S. (1984). Suicidal behavior by preschool children. *American Journal of Psychiatry, 141,* 520–525.

Rosenthal, P. A, Rosenthal, S., Doherty, M. B., & Santora, D. (1986). Suicidal thoughts and behaviors in depressed hospitalized preschoolers. *American Journal of Psychotherapy, 40,* 201–212.

Ross, C. P. (1983). Teaching suicide prevention in schools. In J. P. Soubrier & J. Vedrinne (Eds.), *Depression et suicide: Aspects médicaux, psychologiques et socio-culturels* (pp. 632–637). Paris: Pergamon Press.

Ross, C. P. (1987). School and suicide: Education for life and death. In R. F. W. Diekstra & K. Hawton (Eds.), *Suicide in adolescence* (pp. 155–178). Dordrecht, The Netherlands: Martinus Nijhoff Publishers.

Rotheram, M. J. (1987). Evaluation of imminent danger for suicide among youth. *American Journal of Orthopsychiatry, 57,* 102–110.

Rotheram-Borus, M. J. (1993). Suicidal behavior and risk factors among runaway youths. *American Journal of Psychiatry, 150,* 103–107.

Rotheram-Borus, M. J., & Trautman, P. D. (1988). Hopelessness, depression, and suicide intent among adolescent suicide attempts. *Journal of the American Academy of Child and Adolescent Psychiatry, 27,* 700–704.

Rotheram-Borus, M. J., Trautman, P. D., Dopkins, S. C., & Shrout, P. E. (1990). Cognitive style and pleasant activities among female adolescent suicide attempters. *Journal of Consulting and Clinical Psychology, 58,* 554–561.

Roy, A. (1989). Genetics and suicidal behavior. *Report of the secretary's task force on youth suicide,* Vol. 2, *Prevention and interventions in youth suicide* (pp. 247–262) (DHHS Publication No. ADM-89-1622). Washington, DC: U.S. Government Printing Office.

Rubenstein, J. L., Heeren, T., Housman, D., Rubin, C., & Stechler, G. (1989). Suicidal behavior in "normal" adolescents: Risk and protective factors. *American Journal of Orthopsychiatry, 59,* 59–71.

Rudd, M. D. (1989). The prevalence of suicidal ideation among college students. *Suicide and Life-Threatening Behavior, 19,* 173–183.

Rudd, M. D. (1990). An integrative model of suicidal ideation. *Suicide and Life-Threatening Behavior, 20,* 16–30.

Runeson, B. (1989). Mental disorder in youth suicide. DSM-III-R axis I and II. *Acta Psychiatrica Scandinavica, 79,* 490–497.

Runeson, B., & Beskow, J. (1991). Borderline personality disorder in young Swedish suicides. *Journal of Nervous and Mental Disease, 179*, 153–156.

Ryan, N. D., Puig-Antich, J., Rabinovich, H., Ambrosini, P., Robinson, D., Nelson, B., & Novacenko, H. (1988). Growth hormone response to desmethylimipramine in depressed and suicidal adolescents. *Journal of Affective Disorders, 15*, 323–337.

Sabbath, J. C. (1969). The suicidal adolescent—The expendable child. *Journal of the American Academy of Child Psychiatry, 8*, 272–289.

Sack, W. H., Beiser, M., Phillips, N., & Baker-Brown, G. (1993). Co-morbid symptoms of depression and conduct disorder in First Nation children: Some findings from the Flower of Two Soils Project. *Culture, Medicine and Psychiatry, 16*, 471–786.

Sadowski, C., & Kelley, M. L. (1993). Social problem-solving in suicidal adolescents. *Journal of Consulting and Clinical Psychology, 61*, 121–127.

Salkovskis, P. M., Atha, C., & Storer, D. (1990). Cognitive–behavioural problem solving in the treatment of patients who repeatedly attempt suicide: A controlled trial. *British Journal of Psychiatry, 157*, 871–876.

Sansonnet-Hayden, H., Hayley, G., Marriage, K., & Fine, S. (1987). Sexual abuse and psychopathology in hospitalized adolescents with outpatient care. *Journal of the American Academy of Child and Adolescent Psychiatry, 26*, 753–757.

Schreiber, T. J., & Johnson, R. L. (1986). The evaluation and treatment of adolescent overdoses in an adolescent medical service. *Journal of the National Medical Association, 78*, 101–108.

Schrut, A., & Michels, T. (1969). Adolescent females who attempt suicide—Comments on treatment. *American Journal of Psychotherapy, 23*, 243–251.

Schuckit, M. A., & Schuckit, J. J. (1989). Substance use and abuse: A risk factor in youth suicide. *Report of the secretary's task force on youth suicide*, Vol. 2, *Prevention and interventions in youth suicide* (pp. 172–183) (DHHS Publication No. ADM-89-1622). Washington, DC: U.S. Government Printing Office.

Seiden, R. H. (1969). *Suicide among youth* (U.S. Public Health Service Publication 1971). Washington, DC: U.S. Government Printing Office.

Shaffer, D. (1988). The epidemiology of teen suicide: An examination of risk factors. *Journal of Clinical Psychiatry, 49(Supplement)*, 36–41.

Shaffer, D., & Fisher, P. (1981). The epidemiology of suicide in children and young adolescents. *Journal of the American Academy of Child Psychiatry, 20*, 545–565.

Shaffer, D., Garland, A., Gould, M., Fisher, P., & Trautman, P. (1988). Preventing teenage suicide: A critical review. *Journal of the American Academy of Child and Adolescent Psychiatry, 27*, 675–687.

Shaffer, D., Vieland, V., Garland, A., Rojas, M., Underwood, M., & Busner, C. (1990). Adolescent suicide attempters: Response to suicide prevention programs. *Journal of the American Medical Association, 264*, 3151–3155.

Shafii, M. (1989). Completed suicide in children and adolescents: Methods of psychological autopsy. In C. R. Pfeffer (Ed.), *Suicide among youth: Perspectives on risk and prevention* (pp. 1–19). Washington, DC: American Psychiatric Press.

Shafii, M., Carrigan, S., Whittinghill, J. R., & Derrick, A. (1985). Psychological autopsy of completed suicide in children and adolescents. *American Journal of Psychiatry, 142*, 1061–1064.

Shafii, M., Steltz-Lenarsky, J., Derrick, A. M., Beckner, C., & Whittinghill, J. R. (1988). Comorbidity of mental disorders in the post-mortem diagnosis of completed suicide in children and adolescents. *Journal of Affective Disorders, 15*, 227–233.

Shaunesey, K., Cohen, J. L., Plummer, B., & Berman, A. (1993). Suicidality in hospitalized adolescents: Relationship to prior abuse. *American Journal of Orthopsychiatry, 63*, 113–119.

Shaw, C. R., & Schelkun, R. F. (1965). Suicidal behavior in children. *Psychiatry, 28*, 157–168.

Shneidman, E. (1985). *Definition of suicide*. New York: John Wiley.

Simons, R. L., & Murphy, P. L. (1985). Sex differences in the causes of adolescent suicide ideation. *Journal of Youth and Adolescence, 14*, 423–434.

Slap, G. B., Vorters, D. F., Shalid, N., Margulies, S. R., & Forke, C. M. (1992). Adolescent suicide attempters: Do physicians recognize them? *Journal of Adolescent Health, 13*, 286–292.

Smith, K. (1992). Suicidal behavior in children and adolescents. In W. M. Reynolds (Ed.), *Internalizing disorders in children and adolescents* (pp. 255–282). New York: John Wiley.

Smith, K., & Crawford, S. (1986). Suicidal behavior among "normal" high school students. *Suicide and Life-Threatening Behavior, 16*, 313–325.

Spirito, A., Brown, L., Overholser, J., & Fritz, G. (1989). Attempted suicide in adolescence: A review and critique of the literature. *Clinical Psychology Review, 9*, 335–363.

Spirito, A., Brown, L., Overholser, J., Fritz, G., & Bond, A. (1991). Use of the Risk–Rescue Rating Scale with adolescent suicide attempters: A cautionary note. *Death Studies, 15*, 269–280.

Spirito, A., Overholser, J., Ashworth, S., Morgan, J., & Benedict-Drew, C. (1988). Evaluation of a suicide awareness curriculum for high school students. *Journal of the American Academy of Child and Adolescent Psychiatry, 27,* 705–711.

Spirito, A., Plummer, B., Gispert, M., Levy, S., Kurkjian, J., Lewander, W., Hagberg, S., & Devost, L. (1992). Adolescent suicide attempts: Outcomes at follow-up. *American Journal of Orthopsychiatry, 62,* 464–468.

Spirito, A., Stark, L., Fristad, M., Hart, K., & Owens-Stively, J. (1987). Adolescent suicide attempters hospitalized on a pediatric unit. *Journal of Pediatric Psychology, 12,* 171–190.

Spitzer, R. L., Williams, J. B., Gibbon, M., & First, M. B. (1989). *Structured Clinical Interview for DSM-III-R Personality Disorders.* New York: Biometrics Research Department, New York Psychiatric Institute.

Stark, K. D., Reynolds, W. M., & Kaslow, N. J. (1987). A comparison of the relative efficacy of self-control therapy and behavioral problem-solving therapy for depression in children. *Journal of Abnormal Child Psychology, 15,* 91–113.

Stiffman, A. R. (1989). Suicide attempts in runaway youths. *Suicide and Life-Threatening Behavior, 19,* 147–159.

Stiffman, A. R., Earls, F., Robins, L. N., & Jung, K. G. (1988). Problems and help seeking in high-risk adolescent patients in health clinics. *Journal of Adolescent Health Care, 9,* 305–309.

Stone, N. (1993). Parental abuse as a precursor to childhood onset depression and suicidality. *Suicide and Life-Threatening Behavior, 24,* 13–24.

Streiner, D. L., & Adam, K. S. (1987). Evaluation of the effectiveness of suicide prevention programs: A methodological perspective. *Suicide and Life-Threatening Behavior, 17,* 93–106.

Swedo, S. E. (1989). Postdischarge therapy of hospitalized adolescent suicide attempters. *Journal of Adolescent Health Care, 10,* 541–544.

Szasz, T. (1986). The case against suicide prevention. *American Psychologist, 41,* 806–812.

Tatman, S. M., Greene, A. L., & Karr, L. C. (1993). Use of the Suicide Probability Scale (SPS) with adolescents. *Suicide and Life-Threatening Behavior, 23,* 188–203.

Taylor, E. A., & Stansfeld, S. A. (1984). Children who poison themselves. I. A clinical comparison with psychiatric controls. *British Journal of Psychiatry, 145,* 127–135.

Toolan, J. M. (1975). Suicide in children and adolescents. *American Journal of Psychotherapy, 29,* 339–344.

Trad, P. V. (1990). *Treating suicidelike behavior in a preschooler.* Madison, CT: International Universities Press.

Trautman, P. A., Stewart, N., & Morishima, A. (1993). Are adolescent suicide attempters noncompliant with outpatient care? *Journal of the American Academy of Child and Adolescent Psychiatry, 32,* 89–94.

Turgay, A. (1989). An integrative treatment approach to child and adolescent suicidal behavior. *Psychiatric Clinics of North America, 12,* 971–983.

van Praag, H. M. (1982). Depression, suicide and the metabolism of serotonin in the brain. *Journal of Affective Disorders, 4,* 275–290.

van Praag, H. M. (1986). Biological suicide research: Outcome and limitations. *Biological Psychiatry, 21,* 1305–1323.

Vaz-Leal, F. J. (1989). Psychotherapeutic management of suicide attempts in children and early adolescents: Working with parents. *Psychotherapy and Psychosomatics, 52,* 125–132.

Velez, C. N., & Cohen, P. (1988). Suicidal behavior and ideation in a community sample of children: Maternal and youth reports. *Journal of the American Academy of Child and Adolescent Psychiatry, 27,* 349–356.

Walker, M., Moreau, D., & Weissman, M. M. (1990). Parents' awareness of children's suicide attempts. *American Journal of Psychiatry, 147,* 1364–1366.

Weiner, A. S., & Pfeffer, C. R. (1986). Suicidal status, depression, and intellectual functioning in preadolescent psychiatric inpatients. *Comprehensive Psychiatry, 27,* 372–380.

Weishaar, M. E., & Beck, A. T. (1990). Cognitive approaches to understanding and treating suicidal behavior. In S. J. Blumenthal & D. J. Kupfer (Eds.), *Suicide over the life cycle: Risk factors, assessment and treatment of suicidal patients* (pp. 469–498). Washington, DC: American Psychiatric Press.

Weisman, A. D., & Worden, J. W. (1972). Risk–rescue rating in suicide assessment. *Archives of General Psychiatry, 26,* 553–560.

Weissman, M. (1974). The epidemiology of suicide attempts, 1960 to 1971. *Archives of General Psychiatry, 30,* 737–746.

Wenckstern, S., & Leenaars, A. A. (1993). Trauma and suicide in our schools. *Death Studies, 17,* 151–171.

Windle, M., Miller-Tutzauer, C., & Domenico, D. (1992). Alcohol use, suicidal behavior, and risky activities among adolescents. *Journal of Research on Adolescence, 2,* 317–330.

Wright, L. S. (1985). Suicidal thoughts and their relationship to family stress and personal problems among high school seniors and college undergraduates. *Adolescence, 20,* 575–580.

Zilboorg, G. (1936). Differential diagnostic types of suicide. *Archives of Neurology and Psychiatry, 35,* 270–291.

Zimmerman, J. K., & Asnis, G. M. (1991a). Parents' knowledge of children's suicide attempts: Awareness or denial (letter). *American Journal of Psychiatry, 148,* 1091–1092.

Zimmerman, J. K., & Asnis, G. M. (1991b). Parents' knowledge of children's suicide attempts: Findings and implications for treatment. Paper presented at the Annual Conference of the American Psychological Association, San Francisco, August 1991.

Zimmerman, J. K., & La Sorsa, V. A. (1992). Being the family's therapist: An integrative approach. Paper presented at the Annual Conference of the American Association of Suicidology, Chicago, April 1992.

Zubin, J. (1974). Observations on nosological issues in the classification of suicidal behavior. In A. T. Beck, H. L. P. Resnik, & D. J. Lettieri (Eds.), *The prediction of suicide* (pp. 3–25). Bowie, MD: Charles Press.

25

Comorbidity of Depression in Children and Adolescents

Jessie C. Anderson and Rob McGee

Interest in the coexistence of depressive disorders with other behavioral and emotional problems in childhood and adolescence is relatively recent (Caron & Rutter, 1991; Biederman, Newcorn, & Sprich, 1991). This interest has followed the recognition of depression in young people (Carlson & Cantwell, 1980a) as a symptom and as a disorder and the availability of standardized interview schedules for affective disorders in younger subjects, in both patient and nonpatient populations (for reviews, see Angold, 1988; A. J. Costello, 1986; E. J. Costello & Angold, 1988; Edelbrock & Costello, 1988; Strober & Werry, 1987). Historically, the question of whether a syndrome similar to the affective disorders in adults also exists for children has been the subject of considerable discussion in the psychiatric literature. The major focus of this discussion has been on depressive disorders, largely major depressive disorder (MDD), rather than on dysthymic disorder, adjustment disorders, with depressed mood, or mania. There has been some inclusion of the other depressive disorders in research by Kovacs and colleagues (Kovacs, Feinberg, Crouse-Novak, Paulauskas, & Finkelstein, 1984a; Kovacs et al., 1984b), but still relatively little interest in mania.

Childhood depression has passed through several phases in its status as a syndrome. These phases have been summarized by Cantwell and Carlson (1979) and Cantwell (1982) as representing four points of view. The first view is that depression did not and could not exist in children, who did not have the emotional or cognitive maturity required to exhibit the adult form of the disorder. This view has frequently been attributed to the psychoanalytic schools of thought, as described by Kashani et al. (1981) and others (Petti, 1983; Waters & Storm, 1985) in their reviews.

Cantwell and Carlson's second stage, that of recognizing the existence of depression in children, with features unique to childhood such as enuresis, phobic behavior, or aggres-

Jessie C. Anderson • Division of Child and Adolescent Psychiatry, Children's Pavilion, Dunedin Hospital, Dunedin, New Zealand.   **Rob McGee** • Department of Preventive and Social Medicine, University of Otago Medical School, Dunedin, New Zealand.

Handbook of Depression in Children and Adolescents, edited by William M. Reynolds and Hugh F. Johnston. Plenum Press, New York, 1994.

sive, arose from the empirical observations of depressed (or miserable) children, initially appearing in individual case reports. Cantwell (1982) cites a review by Kovacs and Beck (1977) in which the proponents of the "unique features" school of thought are examined and their many "essential" symptoms listed, ranging from irritability to poor school performance, social withdrawal, suicidal thoughts, poor concentration, and aggressive behavior. The distinction between essential symptoms and associated symptoms is not clear in many cases, but the "core" disturbance in mood is described as central to the diagnosis by most authors (for a review, see Cantwell, 1982). This perspective allows for childhood depression to present with mood disorder, plus other associated symptoms that may be age-dependent and change with developing social, emotional, and cognitive skills as the child grows. There is some empirical evidence in favor of this view in the work of McConville, Boag, and Purohit (1973), who found that children presented with different types of symptoms at different ages, associated with depressed mood. These "unique features" represent the early recognition that symptoms not associated with adult depression are commonly associated with childhood affective syndromes and can be seen as the beginnings of an interest in comorbidity.

The next stage, and historically one of the most controversial, was the school of thought that proposed that depression could be diagnosed in the absence of and even with the denial of depressed mood, given certain observable behaviors. These behavioral presentations were held to be depressive "equivalents" or to "mask" the presentation of the depressive affect (Cytryn & McKnew, 1972; Glaser, 1967). Cantwell (1982) describes the problems with this concept, and its eventual decline, at least within the United States. Other reviewers take a similar stand, that "masked" depression is no longer a viable concept, particularly as careful history-taking will usually elicit the depressed mood and other symptoms of depression claimed to have been masked by a wide variety of disorders, such as aggression, inattention, hyperactivity, social withdrawal, phobias, and anxiety disorders (Cantwell & Carlson, 1979; Petti, 1983; Shaffer, 1985). Apart from the rare psychoses that occur in childhood, almost every other condition in childhood psychopathology was at some time claimed to be "masking" an underlying depression. This situation was analogous to the problems with the "minimal brain dysfunction" label described for childhood attention-deficit hyperactivity disorder (ADHD) by Rutter (1982). Carlson and Cantwell (1980b) demonstrated that "masked" depression could be "unmasked" by careful inquiry and that the depressed mood and other depressive symptoms were present alongside the so-called masking or behavioral symptoms. Cantwell (1982, p. 42), in reviewing this study, claims that "the mask may well be on the face of the clinician rather than the patient."

The fourth stage, currently the most widely accepted, is that childhood depression is similar to depression in adults and, at least in school-age children and adolescents, can be recognized if the appropriate questions are asked [although there is dissent on the status of depression as an identifiable disorder in childhood and adolescence (see Nurcombe et al., 1989; Seifer, Nurcombe, Sciolo, & Grapentine, 1989)]. The emerging consensus is to adopt DSM-III-R (American Psychiatric Association, 1987) criteria for diagnosing MDD in childhood, although other criteria have been used, as will be discussed further. The widespread adoption of DSM-III-R criteria followed the empirical demonstration that there are children whose emotional disturbance fulfills the adult criteria for major depression (e.g., Kashani et al., 1981).

As Waters and Storm (1985) point out, the high rates of associated behavior problems make childhood depression appear quite different from depression in adults. Empirical studies using DSM-III-R have uncovered the extent of the coexistence of other recognizable and diagnosable psychopathology in depressed children and adolescents. Is "comorbidity" a new name for an old problem, previously identified as "masked" depression or "depressive equivalents," or is it an artifact of recent diagnostic systems that allow for multiple concurrent diagnoses? The evidence in empirical studies for comorbidity of affective disorders with other childhood disorders can be found in older studies and in those using different systems to identify psychopathology, suggesting that the phenomenon is not merely an artifact of DSM-III (American Psychiatric Association, 1980). However, where other systems subsume emotional/mood disorders into the behavioral disorder categories when both types of disorder are present (such as in the ICD systems), comorbidity could not be recognized. Similarly, studies that looked for only one disorder or a small number of disorders were unlikely to find comorbidity, especially if diagnostic instruments designed predominantly to identify behavioral (externalizing) disorders, or to identify only depression, were used. It is not surprising, therefore, that the current interest in comorbidity can be seen as a "DSM" phenomenon when it has in fact been evident more widely for some time.

Early Studies

In one of the first major population studies of childhood psychopathology, Rutter, Tizard, and Whitmore (1970) found a sizeable group of children in the Isle of Wight sample who had "mixed" conduct and emotional disorders. Further, child reports of being miserable and unhappy were more often associated with having a behavioral or emotional disorder than having no disorder. The disorder most commonly associated with low mood was some form of conduct disorder, and children who had both emotional and conduct disorders, including depressed mood, were more like children with "pure" conduct problems than those with "pure" emotional problems when compared for sex, IQ, higher levels of learning problems, and more frequent family problems. Rutter et al. (1970) found that 42% of the preadolescent children presenting with antisocial behavior problems also had an affective disturbance, usually described as low or depressed mood. When followed up at age 14, the Isle of Wight sample reported higher rates of depression, with greater numbers of girls reporting depressive symptoms than previously and less comorbidity with externalizing conduct-type problems than were found when the children were 11 years old (Graham & Rutter, 1973), suggesting a developmental change in the patterns of comorbidity.

Dimensional Studies

Studies using dimensional systems of classification (i.e., those that regard disorders as extremes of a continuum, rather than as a categorical difference in type of behavior or emotional state) have also found affective disorders to be comorbid. Depression in children in these studies presents either as part of an anxious–withdrawn syndrome, as an anxious–depressed disorder, or linked with conduct-type symptoms for particular groups such as boys 6–11 years old (see Edelbrock & Achenbach, 1980; Achenbach & Edelbrock, 1978; Quay, 1986). These studies have identified syndromes using a variety of multivariate techniques, including factor analysis, cluster analysis, combinations of factor and cluster analysis, and samples both from the general population (McDermott, 1980) and clinical samples of boys and girls for a wide age range (Edelbrock & Achenbach, 1980; Soli, Neuchterlein, Garmezy, Devine, & Shaefer, 1981; Neuchterlein, Soli, Garmezy, Devine, & Shaefer, 1981; Lessing, Williams, & Gil, 1982). Interestingly, all the clinical studies found groups of children who were unclassifiable, because of high numbers of symptoms, across all the major disorder groups (Lessing et al., 1982; Edelbrock & Achenbach, 1980; Soli et al., 1981; Neuchterlein et al., 1981).

In a recent cooperative effort among the major researchers of dimensional systems of classification, using large clinic samples and principal-components analysis (Achenbach, Conners, Quay, Verhulst, & Howell, 1989), the DSM-III-R syndromes of overanxious disorder and dysthymia appeared in a mixed anxious–depressed syndrome, but there were no consistent syndromes similar to major depression, separation anxiety, or phobias. These results were replicated across the instruments used and the gender, age groups, and cultures of the children studied.

Categorical Systems

Recent studies using categorical diagnoses (usually DSM-III) have shown considerable comorbidity among disorders in nonclinical populations, both as double disorders and as multiple (more than two) concurrent disorders in small groups of children. Of these studies, 11 have used large databases (200 or more subjects), structured and replicable means of data collection and diagnosis, and multiple sources of information, making them the most likely to reliably represent the general population (or nonpsychiatric population) for prevalence, extent of comorbidity, and risk factors for commonly occurring disorders of behavior and emotional states among children and adolescents. The major findings of seven studies that reported rates of comorbidity have been summarized by Fleming and Offord (1990) and show levels of comorbidity for depressive disorders ranging from 33% to 100%, with the majority in the 60–80% range.

Despite differences in age and sources of information, there are considerable similarities in overall prevalence rates, but fewer similarities in prevalence for individual disorders (see E. J. Costello, 1989) for the five major studies recently conducted on nonclinical samples, with a range from 17.6% to 22% for overall disorder (Anderson, Williams, McGee, & Silva, 1987; Bird et al., 1988; Cohen, Velez, & Garcia, 1985; E. J. Costello et al., 1988; Offord et al., 1987). The comorbidity of depressive disorders with anxiety disorders, ADHD, and conduct disorders has been studied in clinic samples, but the problem of multiple comorbidity is less often described. Kovacs et al. (1984a,b) and Kovacs, Paulauskas, Gatsonis, and Richards (1988) described a clinic sample of children with different types of affective disorders who had considerable comorbidity between affective disorders, conduct disorders, ADHD, and anxiety disorders. Among children with MDD and dysthymic disorder, the rates of comorbidity at intake into Kovacs' study were 79% and 93%, respectively, with other affective disorders being the most common, followed by anxiety disorder, ADHD, and conduct disorder. A further group developed nonaffective disorders during the progress of the study.

Among the studies of "double diagnosis," Kovacs and colleagues have examined depression with anxiety (Kovacs, Gatsonis, Paulauskas, & Richards, 1989) and depression with conduct disorder (Kovacs et al., 1988), showing that the comorbidity influences both the long-term outcome and the severity of the depressive disorder, compared to "pure" depression, in their sample. The effect of comorbidity on recovery from depression depended on the type of depressive disorder and the comorbid disorder. Comorbid conduct disorder did not influence rates of recovery from depression, whereas comorbid anxiety disorder influenced recovery from MDD (by prolonging MDD) but not from dysthymia. Bernstein (1991) also found that comorbid anxiety and affective disorders were more severe than either disorder on its own, while Bernstein and Garfinkel (1986) found considerable overlap between anxiety and affective disorders in children presenting with school refusal.

In a review of patterns of comorbidity of ADHD with other disorders, including affective disorders, Biederman et al. (1991) describe the variable comorbidity of ADHD and mood disorders in both clinic and general population samples and in family studies of children with ADHD. Overall, mood disorders are more common among children with

ADHD and their relatives than expected by chance, and the combination of ADHD and mood disorders predicts a poorer outcome than for either disorder alone. Whether the combination of disorders identifies a specific subgroup of children with ADHD and depression is a matter for further research (Biederman et al., 1991). In a general population study, McGee, Anderson, Williams, and Silva (1986) found that the cognitive deficits among depressed children were due to comorbid ADHD and disappeared once the inattentiveness was controlled for. Comorbidity of depressive and conduct disorders in childhood has also been investigated by Puig-Antich (1982) and Harrington, Fudge, Rutter, Pickles, and Hill (1991), with variable conclusions. Puig-Antich considered much of the conduct disorder (CD) in his sample to be secondary to the depression and to ameliorate once the depression was treated, whereas Harrington et al. (1991) described a British clinic study of children with conduct and depressive disorders in which the comorbid group were more like the CD group in terms of both short-term and long-term outcomes for antisocial behavior and criminality. Cole and Carpentieri (1990) found that the comorbid CD and depression groups had poor social status and that the two disorders were highly correlated in a nonclinic sample of 1400 children. The social rejection described was related to having both depression and CD disorders. Other disorders that frequently co-occur with depression are learning disorders (Weinberg, Rutman, Sullivan, Pennick, & Dietz, 1973) and substance-abuse disorders (see Rutter, 1989).

The major issues raised by the widespread occurrence of comorbidity for all childhood and adolescent disorders have been clarified recently by Caron and Rutter (1991). They demonstrated that for two general population studies (Anderson et al., 1987; Kashani et al., 1987), the rates of comorbidity for all disorders were higher by a factor of 2 or more than one would expect by chance from the individual prevalence rates. While clinic samples have major problems with referral bias and the increased probability of being referred if more than one disorder is present, the general population studies may also have artifactual comorbidity for a variety of reasons. These reasons include overlapping diagnostic criteria, subdivision of syndromes into too many categories, artificial separation of early and late manifestations of the same disorder, and splitting up parts of the same disorder into separate categories. Some of these issues can be resolved by longitudinal data bases and others by looking at disorders on a dimensional basis, as well as categories of disorder, to examine the effects of time, severity, and outcomes on the comorbid disorder patterns. If true comorbidity is assumed, the major questions that arise in relation to cause are concerned with common risk factors, overlapping risk, one disorder increasing risk for the other, and the comorbid pattern representing a meaningful separate syndrome (Caron & Rutter, 1991; Biederman et al., 1991; Rutter, 1989).

This chapter will report on some of the findings of the Dunedin, New Zealand, sample, to examine the longitudinal and developmental aspects of comorbidity in more detail, in relation to some of these questions.

Dunedin Longitudinal Study

The data presented come from the Dunedin Multidisciplinary Health and Development Study, a longitudinal study of the health and development of a birth cohort of children born during the 12 months from April 1, 1972 to March 31, 1973, in one maternity hospital in Dunedin, New Zealand. The children have been assessed every 2 years from age 3 years. The history and description of the sample may be found in Silva (1990). Currently, the mental health data at the age of 15 years have been presented (McGee et al., 1990), and further phases when the subjects were aged 18 years and 21 years are being analyzed and collected, respectively. Mental health data were collected on the whole sample by structured interview, using the Diagnostic Interview Schedule for Children

(DISC) (A. Costello, Edelbrock, Kalas, Kessler, & Klaric, 1982), at age 11 years and in a modified form at ages 13 and 15 years (see Anderson et al., 1987; Frost, Moffit, & McGee, 1989; McGee et al., 1990). Parent and teacher data (including behavior problem reports) were available at ages 5–13 years, and at age 15 years parent information only, as the children had moved into the high school system, with more anonymity, and no one teacher could report details on them. Correlates and risk factors for disorder for the age groups 11, 13, and 15 years have been reported (Anderson, Williams, McGee, & Silva, 1989; Williams, Anderson, McGee, & Silva, 1990; Williams, McGee, Anderson, & Silva, 1989; McGee et al., 1990; McGee, Feehan, Williams, & Anderson, 1992; McGee et al., 1986; Frost et al., 1989).

At age 9 years, a study of depression, using a subsample of the study population, reported prevalence rates for MDD and minor depression of 1.8% and 2.5%, respectively, and past depression of 1.1%. However, the presence of other coexisting disorders was not fully assessed for that sample at age 9 years (Kashani et al., 1983). In a follow-up study of the children from age 9 to 13 years, McGee and Williams (1988) reported that depression was relatively persistent, as a symptom as well as a diagnosable disorder, and that children identified as depressed at age 9 years had high levels of disorder at age 11 years and significantly higher levels of parent- and teacher-reported behavioral problems at age 9 years.

At ages 11 and 15 years, the overall prevalence rates of disorder were 17.6% and 22%, respectively, with a male/female ratio for one or more disorders at age 11 years of 1.7:1 and a female/male ratio at age 15 years of 1.4:1. The prevalence rates for depressive disorders (combining MDD and dysthymia) were 1.8% at age 11 years and 4.2% at age 15 years.

The next section will examine changing patterns in prevalence, gender, comorbidity, stability, and severity of depressive disorders between ages 11 and 15 years and behavioral background from age 5 years. Further analyses comparing children with a lesser degree of depression (measured by depressed mood but with insufficient symptoms for a diagnosis of depression) with the depressed group will also be presented.

Categorical Diagnosis: Patterns of Comorbidity

The comorbidity of depression/dysthymia (1-year prevalence) at ages 11 and 15 years is shown in Fig. 1. At age 11 years, there were 14 children with one or more depressive disorders, 11 of whom had combinations of two or more disorders. Of these 11 children, 10 were in the multiple disorders group, with three to seven confirmed diagnoses each (or three to four diagnoses when the anxious and phobic disorders were combined into one group). All 10 children had either conduct or oppositional disorders, 8 had ADHD, and 8 had one or more anxious/phobic disorders, as well as depression/dysthymia. Of the other 4 children with depression/dysthymia, 1 had CD, and there were 3 "pure" cases of depression, comprising one child with MDD, one with dysthymia, and one with "double depression" (with MDD occurring on a background of dysthymia).

Overall, there were 13 children with dysthymia and 4 with MDD, 3 of the latter presenting with "double depression," leaving 1 child with a single diagnosis of MDD. This group can therefore be regarded as presenting almost entirely with dysthymic disorder, with or without MDD, in preadolescence. In comparison, at age 15 years, there were 26 children with MDD, 14 with Dysthymia, and 2 with "double depression."

The patterns of comorbidity are different at the two ages, with the high levels at age 11 years reducing greatly at 15 years for ADHD and less so for anxious/phobic disorders and for conduct/oppositional disorders. The proportion of cases of "pure" depression or dysthymia or both has doubled by age 15 years compared to 11 years, and comorbid ADHD has nearly disappeared by age 15.

Major Depression Compared to Dysthymia. When the two depressive disorders, MDD and dysthymic disorder, are examined separately at age 15, it is apparent that
dysthymia is the more highly comorbid disorder, with only 14% of pure cases, compared to
depression, with 50% pure cases. The two cases with "double depression" were counted
as dysthymia, as it was likely to be the more long-standing disorder. Figure 2 shows the
differences between the two depressive disorders at age 15 years. (This comparison was
not possible at age 11, as the cases of depressive disorder were almost entirely dysthymic
at that age, with one case of pure MDD and three of "double depression.")

The pattern of comorbidity for dysthymia at age 15 resembles that seen at age 11,
although to a lesser degree, and is notable for its preponderance of comorbidity with
externalizing disorders (ADHD and CD/OPP).

Gender Differences. There are also clear gender differences at ages 11 and 15
years, with a reversal of the 5:1 male predominance in preadolescent depressive disorders
to female dominance for both MDD and dysthymia by age 15 years. This shift in gender
patterns reflects the overall shift in prevalence rates of disorder from the higher male rates
at age 11 to the higher female rates at age 15 years. Table 1 shows the sex ratios for
depressive disorders at ages 11 and 15 years, with the consistently high male/female ratios
at age 11 years and the high female/male ratios at age 15 years. Comorbidity with other
disorders was consistent with sex ratios. Overall prevalence for one or more disorders at
age 11 years had a male/female sex ratio of 1.7:1 and at age 15 years a female/male sex ratio
of 1.4:1.

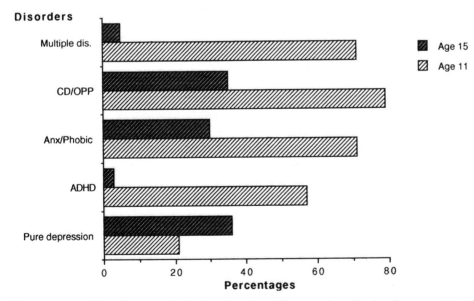

Figure 1. Comorbidity for depression/dysthymia at 11 and 15 years of age showing the percentages of
depressed groups with comorbid disorders. Key for Figs. 1 and 2: (Multiple dis.) three or more concurrent
disorders; (CD/OPP) conduct or oppositional disorder; (Anx/Phobic) one or more anxious or phobic
disorders; (ADHD) attention-deficit hyperactivity disorder; (Pure depression) no comorbid disorder. *Note:*
The groups are not mutually exclusive; the multiple disorders group includes the majority of children in the
other groups.

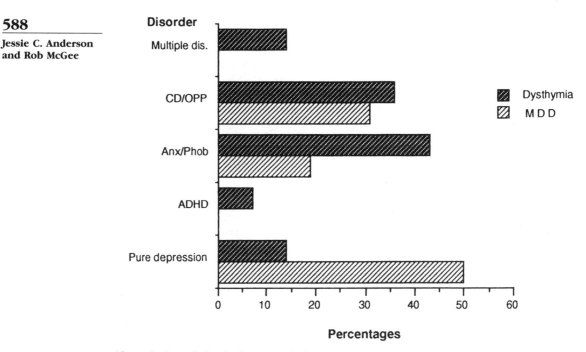

Figure 2. Comorbidity for depression/dysthymia at 15 years of age showing the percentages of depressed groups with comorbid disorders. Key: See the Fig. 1 caption.

Stability of the Disorder. The stability of both the depressive disorders and their comorbid disorders can also be examined from the child's past history and compared between ages 11 and 15 years. A previous analysis by McGee and Williams (1988) has shown depressive disorders in this sample to be stable between ages 9 and 13 years. Examination of the background reports of behavioral and emotional problems [using Parent and Teacher Rutter subscale scores (see Anderson et al., 1987)] from age 5 years onward showed that the multiple-disorders group had consistently higher scores for aggression and hyperactivity than the anxious/phobic or no-disorder groups. As the multiple-disorders group included most of the children with depression, the results indicate a high level of externalizing symptomatology over time for this group, and the

Table 1. Sex Distribution of Depression and Dysthymia at 11 and 15 Years of Age

Disorder	Boys	Girls	Total	M/F ratio
Any depression at 11 years	12	2	14	5.4:1
MDD at 11 years	4	0	4	—
Dysthymia at 11 years	11	2	13	4.9:1
Double depression[a] at 11 years	3	0	3	—
Any depression at 15 years	11	29	40	0.4:1
MDD at 15 years	8	21	29	0.4:1
Dysthymia at 15 years	4	10	14	0.4:1
Double depression[a] at 15 years	1	2	3	—

[a]Double depression indicates concurrent MDD and dysthymia.

rather later rise of emotional symptoms (between ages 9 and 11 years according to Parent and Teacher reports) suggests that the comorbid anxiety disorders and the depressive symptoms may have followed the aggressive or hyperactive problems, or both, rather than preceding them, for this group. [The mean subscale scores for the disorder groups at age 11 years can be found in Fig. 2 (Anderson et al., 1987).] Tables 2 and 3 show the persistence of disorders from ages 11 to 15 years, when all 14 children with depression/dysthymia at age 11 years were reassessed at age 15 years. It is clear from Table 2 that the comorbid disorders were more stable than the depression. Of the 3 children with "pure" depression at age 11 years, none had disorder at age 15 years, whereas of the 11 children with comorbid depression and other disorders at age 11 years, 9 continued to have disorder at age 15 years. Only 1 child with depression at age 11 years had dysthymia at age 15 years, and none had MDD at 15 years. For some children, the follow-up diagnoses changed between the broad internalizing/externalizing groups, but in general ADHD and CD/OPP were the most persistent disorders.

Follow-back of subjects diagnosed as depressed/dysthymic at age 15 years showed a lesser degree of persistence, with only 7 cases (of 40) at age 15 years having had any disorder at age 11 years (see Table 3). Those with dysthymia at age 15 years were more likely to have had disorder at age 11 years ($p = 0.03$, Fisher's exact test).

All those with disorder at age 11 years on follow-back and depression/dysthymia at age 15 years had externalizing disorders at age 11 years, being in the ADHD, CD/OPP, or multiple-disorders groups. The relatively high number of young people with depression/dysthymia at age 15 years who were not seen at age 11 years reflected the increased number of subjects seen at age 15 years compared to 11 years (792 subjects at age 11 years compared to 925 subjects at age 15 years, from the original birth cohort of 1660 subjects). It is possible that some of the 12 subjects not seen at age 11 years may have had disorders at 11 years. New cases in adolescence outnumbered persisting cases for all disorders (see McGee et al., 1990), suggesting that different mechanisms were operating for onset of disorder in adolescence compared to onset and persistence in preadolescence.

Table 2. Persistence of Disorders from 11 to 15 years of Age in Subjects with Depression/Dysthymia at 11 years of Age[a]

Case No.	Disorder(s) at 11 years				Disorder(s) at 15 years	
1	DD	Anx/Phob	CD/OPP		DD	CD/OPP
2	DD	Anx/Phob	CD/OPP	ADHD	CD/OPP	ADD
3	DD				No disorder	
4	DD	CD/OPP			Anx/Phob	
5	MDD				No disorder	
6	DD	Anx/Phob	CD/OPP	ADHD	ADD	
7	DD	Anx/Phob	CD/OPP	ADD	ADD	
8	DD	MDD	Anx/Phob	CD/OPP	CD/OPP	
9	DD	Anx/Phob	CD/OPP	ADHD	No disorder	
10	DD	Anx/Phob	CD/OPP	ADD	CD/OPP	
11	DD	MDD	CD/OPP	ADHD	ADD	CD/OPP
12	DD	Anx/Phob	CD/OPP	ADHD	ADD	
13	DD	Anx/Phob	CD/OPP	ADHD	No disorder	
14	DD	MDD			No disorder	

[a]Key: (DD) depression/dysthymia; (Anx/Phob) multiple anxious/phobic disorders; (CD/OPP) conduct or oppositional disorder; (ADD) attention-deficit disorder; (ADHD) attention-deficit hyperactivity disorder; (MDD) major depressive disorder.

Table 3. Disorders vs. No Disorders at 11 Years of Age for Depressed/Dysthymic Groups at 15 Years of Age

Group	Disorder(s) at 11	No disorder(s) at 11	Not seen at 11
MDD at 15	2	15	9
DD at 15	5	6	3
Totals:	7	21	12

Dimensional Analyses

When the relationship between comorbidity and dimensional scores is examined, the effect of severity of disorder becomes apparent and the artifacts produced by using cutoff scores to create categories are lessened. The use of the DISC at ages 11 and 15 years allowed for scales to be created on which the subjects could be rated on all dimensions of psychopathology at the same time. The interrelations of these scales at age 11 years have been reported by Williams et al. (1989), who found that all the disorders were highly intercorrelated and that even subjects with "pure" disorders on categorical diagnoses had higher symptom loadings from other disorders than those children with no disorder. This "contaminating" effect between disorders was notable for all disorders, including those not traditionally correlated, e.g., anxiety and CD symptoms, and was quite marked for depression, as would be expected from the degree of comorbidity among categorical diagnoses.

At age 15 years, the intercorrelations between dimensional scale scores were again calculated and, although less than at age 11 years, were still significant for depression and all other disorders. The patterns were rather different for boys than for girls (see Table 4), with the depression–CD correlation for girls remaining at the high levels reported at age 11 years. This pattern was not seen for boys, in whom all the disorder scales were becoming more distinguishable by age 15 years.

Table 4. Relationship between Self-Reported Depression and Other Disorders at 11 and 15 Years of Age for Boys and Girls (Intercorrelations between Scales)

Depression vs. age	ADHD	CD/OPP	Anx/Phob
		Girls	
Depression:			
At 11	0.43	0.46	0.56
At 15	0.34	0.42	0.28
		Boys	
Depression:			
At 11	0.46	0.51	0.63
At 15	0.32	0.28	0.27

Severity of the Disorder. The effects of severity on comorbidity were examined for the data at the ages of 11 years and 15 years. At age 11 years, the 14 children with a diagnosis of either depression or dysthymia or both were compared to children who had either a self-report of depressed mood for 2 or more weeks or a Parent or Teacher score of 2 for the items of being sad or miserable. The group of children with depressed mood but no diagnosis of depression/dysthymia was further divided into two subgroups: those with and those without depressive symptoms other than mood disorder, as reported by any of the three sources (self, parent, or teacher). The remainder of the sample, with no depressed mood, were the fourth group. The resulting groups were: (1) identified depression/dysthymia ($N = 14$), (2) depressed mood plus one to three depressive symptoms ($N = 34$), (3) depressed mood and no additional symptoms ($N = 36$), (4) no depressed mood ($N = 708$).

The four groups were compared for sex distribution, presence of other concurrent disorders, behavioral background, and other cognitive and family/social measures. The sex distribution was significantly different between the groups (see Table 5). The group with DSM-III depression had more boys and a much higher sex ratio of boys to girls than the other two groups with depressed mood or the group with no depressed mood.

Comparisons on background measures as recorded at age 11 years showed no significant between-group differences for IQ, but did show a significant difference for global self-esteem measured by the Rosenberg Scale (Rosenberg, 1965) and for academic self-esteem (Chapman, Silva, & Boersma, 1983), with the depressed group showing significantly lower mean scores than the other groups. Mean scores on a cumulative measure of family and social disadvantage to age 11 years (for a description of this measure, see Anderson et al., 1989) were significantly higher for the depressed group and the depressed mood plus symptoms group than for the other groups. The depressed group also had mothers with higher maternal depression scores than the other three groups and had been reported by parents or teachers or both as more consistently disliked or solitary since 5 years of age.

When compared for the presence of other concurrent disorders, the groups were significantly different, with the depressed group followed by the two depressed mood groups being significantly different from the rest of the sample, with more concurrent disorders (see Fig. 3). When the analysis was repeated on the more stringently defined pervasive-disorder groups [with disorder or symptoms identified by more than one source of information (see Anderson et al., 1987)], including the diagnosis of depression/dysthymia, the differences were even more marked. Only the depressed group was significantly different from the other three groups for extent of comorbidity with pervasive disorder, which was higher than that for all disorders.

Table 5. Sex Distribution for Depressed Mood Groups

Group	Female	Male	M/F ratio
Group 1			
Diagnosed depressed	2	12	5.4:1
Group 2			
Depressed mood + 1–3 symptoms	21	13	0.6:1
Group 3			
Depressed mood, no symptoms	22	14	0.6:1
Group 4			
No depressed mood	331	377	1.0:1
Totals:	376	416	

The four groups were also compared for their background of behavioral or emotional problems at younger ages, as measured by the Parent and Teacher reports collected at ages 5, 7, and 9 years using the Rutter Parent and Teacher Scales. The mean total scores for the groups at each age are shown in Figs. 4 and 5. Statistical analysis for between-group differences showed the groups to be significantly different for both Parent scores and Teacher scores. The depressed group had significantly higher levels of psychopathology from an early age, which were related to their higher rates of aggressive and inattentive/hyperactive symptoms (see Anderson et al., 1987).

In summary, children with DSM-III depression were much more likely to have other concurrent disorders and a history of behavioral problems, to be male, and to come from disadvantaged families compared to children who had depressed mood but fewer other symptoms of depression. The increased stringency of the "pervasive" disorder categories further discriminated DSM-III depression from lesser forms of depression, regarding the extent of comorbidity with other disorders.

The relationship between severity and comorbidity at age 15 years was examined by comparing mean scores across the depression, anxiety, and CD scales for the three "pure"

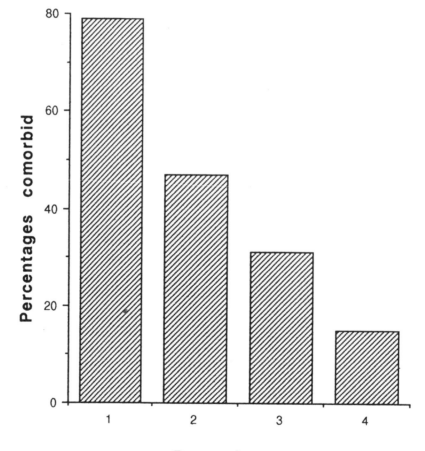

Figure 3. Comorbidity of all disorders for the depression groups at the age of 11 years. Groups: (1) DSM-III MDD/dysthymia ($N = 14$); (2) 2 weeks depressed mood and one to three symptoms ($N = 34$); (3) 2 weeks depressed mood and no symptoms ($N = 26$); (4) no depressed mood ($N = 708$).

disorder groups and the two comorbid groups. (As there was only one adolescent with comorbid ADHD and depression at age 15 years, this combination was not included.) The results are presented in Table 6.

The results for each scale are summarized below.

For Anxiety scores: Pure Anx = Depr + Anx > Pure Depr = Depr + CD > Pure CD = No disorder

For Depression scores: Depr + CD > Depr + Anx = Pure Depr > Pure Anx = Pure CD > No disorder

For Conduct Disorder scores: Depr + CD > Pure CD > Pure Depr > Depr + Anx = Pure Anx = No disorder

From these results, it can be seen that the combination of depression and CD has the most severe depression and conduct scores and an intermediate level of anxiety score. These scores are greater than for either pure component disorder and much greater than would be expected if either disorder were ameliorating the severity of the other.

Anxious and depressive disorders in combination are more like their appropriate pure disorder for each scale and do not appear to amplify each other to any great extent. The low depression + anxiety mean score on the conduct scale indicates that the traditionally low interrelationships between anxiety and aggression are holding for this sample and that the higher scores for the comorbid disorders are not simply a function of more symptoms

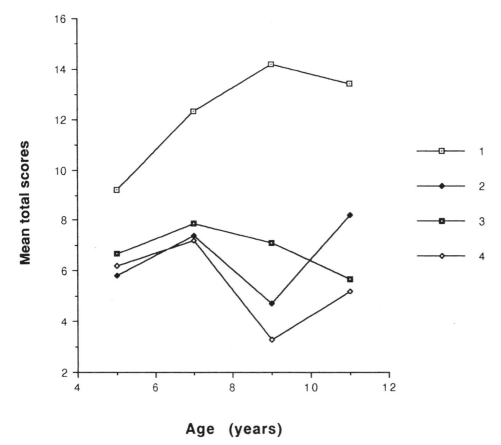

Age (years)

Figure 4. Behavioral background of the depression groups showing the mean total scores for the Parent Rutter scale. Groups: See the Fig. 3 caption.

across the board, but reflect some discrimination between disorders. The relationship of comorbidity with severity of each disorder is therefore not a simple one and depends on the disorders involved, on their likelihood of sharing symptoms in common, and on underlying mechanisms in common, such as self-esteem.

When adolescents with MDD and dysthymia at age 15 years were compared for mean scale scores on the anxiety, CD, and attention-deficit scales, there were no significant differences between the two groups (see Table 7). However, the dysthymic group had higher mean scores on every scale, reflecting the higher numbers of comorbid symptoms in this group.

Discussion

From our results, it can be seen that depression in childhood (preadolescence) is largely represented by dysthymic disorder, which is highly comorbid with both internalizing and externalizing disorders. This pattern of comorbidity is less marked for dysthymia at age 15 years and greatly reduced for MDD at age 15 years.

The prevalence of dysthymia has remained relatively constant from ages 11 to 15 years, although affecting a different group of children at each age, with only one child having the disorder at both 11 and 15 years of age. MDD appears to be newly emergent in

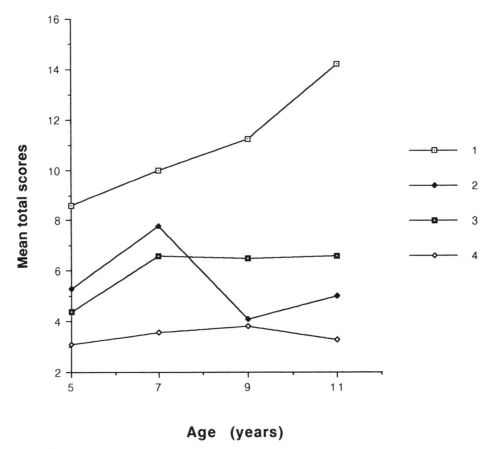

Figure 5. Behavioral background of the depression groups showing the mean total scores for the Teacher Rutter scale. Groups: See the Fig. 3 caption.

Table 6. Mean Scale Scores for Pure and Comorbid Disorders

Group	Total mean scores		
	Anxiety disorders	Depression	Conduct disorders
Pure Depr	11.3	22.3	5.3
Depr + Anx	18.0	25.3	2.8
Depr + CD	11.6	29.0	18.2
Pure Anx	18.2	5.4	3.2
Pure CD	8.3	4.4	15.1
No disorder	7.3	1.8	2.4

adolescence, with greater "purity" of diagnosis, and where comorbidity exists, it is likely to be with anxiety disorders rather than the externalizing disorders associated with dysthymia. There was also a shift in gender distribution between ages 11 and 15 years, with the predominantly male dysthymia at age 11 years being replaced by more female cases at age 15 years for both depression and dysthymia equally. These results indicate that childhood and preadolescent affective disorders may present early on as predominantly dysthymic disorder in boys, highly comorbid and associated with externalizing disorders to a greater degree than with anxiety disorders. By age 15 years, or midadolescence, the pattern has shifted to more prevalent major depression than dysthymia, presenting in girls more often than in boys and with less overall comorbidity, particularly with externalizing disorders, also described in other longitudinal studies (see Rutter, 1989). This shift from dysthymia to major depression, with a change in predominant gender from boys to girls, and less comorbidity, especially for externalizing disorders, may reflect a developmental change in the way children who are vulnerable genetically or socially or both express affective disorders. This is similar to the shift in anxiety disorders over time described by Last, Hersen, Kadzin, Finkelstein, and Strauss (1987), from early separation anxiety to later overanxious disorders, and the suggested developmental links between early oppositional disorder progressing to CD with age in vulnerable children and adolescents (Rutter, 1989).

The near-disappearance of comorbidity with ADHD at age 15 years may reflect the decline in prevalence of ADHD with age once adolescence is reached and also the lack of teacher information at age 15 years. Residual ADHD is often a problem noticed at school rather than at home, particularly as the hyperactivity lessens and leaves an inattentive but less overactive and disruptive young person in the residual state (Aman, 1984).

By age 15 years, the presentation and comorbidity patterns of depressive disorders are becoming more like those seen in adults, with higher female than male rates, less comorbidity, and less association with externalizing disorders compared to the association

Table 7. Mean Scores for Adolescents with Depression and Dysthymia on Self-Report Scales at 15 Years of Age

Group	ADD		Conduct		Anxiety		Depression	
	Mean	SD	Mean	SD	Mean	SD	Mean	SD
MDD	3.8	5.0	2.4	2.0	5.9	4.0	6.4	5.2
DD	6.3	6.1	4.1	4.5	7.5	5.9	9.0	8.5

with anxiety disorders (Rutter, 1989; Weissman & Klerman, 1977). The stable prevalence rate of dysthymia, though affecting a different group of children, is of interest and may continue into adult life, forming the basis for the adult group with "double depression," as described by Keller and Shapiro (1982). Kovacs et al. (1984a,b) describe a chronic course for dysthymia, with superimposed episodes of MDD, in their longitudinal study of a clinic sample with earlier onset of dysthymia. However, some of the children in their study with MDD did not have a preceding or underlying dysthymia and not all children with dysthymia developed MDD, suggesting that the two disorders are related but are not necessarily the early- and later-onset forms of the same illness.

In our sample, there was less evidence of chronicity of dysthymia in the 4-year interval measured. The stability of disorders in both the follow-up and the follow-back studies indicated that the comorbid disorders were more long-standing than the depression and that this persistence was especially so for externalizing disorders, including ADHD, conduct, and oppositional disorders. There were indications that these externalizing disorders had been present with a high level of symptomatology for some time in the children diagnosed as depressed at age 11 years, but that this relationship weakened with the lesser forms of depression, exemplified by the two groups with depressed mood. The long-standing nature of these parent- and teacher-reported behavior problems makes it more likely that for the diagnosed depressed group at age 11 years, the diagnosed affective disorders were secondary to the behavior disorders, and that the behavior disorders tended to remain after the affective disorders remitted in a significant number of the children.

Depressive disorders at age 15 years likewise either presented on a background of behavioral problems (especially for dysthymia) or arose in subjects with no previous disorder, suggesting a lack of continuity in affective disorders from preadolescence to midadolescence. This lack of continuity between preadolescent and adolescent disorders had also been described for the Isle of Wight sample and other longitudinal studies (Rutter, 1989; Esser, Schmidt, & Woerner, 1990; Verhulst, Berden, & Sanders-Woudstra, 1985; Verhulst, Koot, & Berden, 1990; Velez, Johnson, & Cohen, 1989), suggesting that the factors operating in early onset of disorder do not have such a strong influence on adolescent disorders, including affective disorders. McGee et al. (1992) found in the Dunedin sample that many of the early childhood factors correlated with disorder at age 11 years were not correlated with adolescent disorder, but that new sets of correlates, related to current family and social functioning, were important in adolescence.

These changes reflect developmental differences in important correlates with age for both the depressive disorders and the comorbid disorders, giving important clues to the necessary and sufficient conditions for onset and maintenance of disorder. Differences in these correlated variables between pure and comorbid disorder groups may be valuable indicators in determining why some children and not others develop particular disorders.

Examination of the relationships of disorders with particular correlates or risk factors is important in establishing the external validity of diagnostic categories. To date, the major diagnostic categories in child and adolescent psychopathology do not have strong support from external validity as independent syndromes. While many studies find differences between disorder and nondisorder groups, there is less distinction when various disorder groups are compared with each other (Werry, Elkind, & Reeves, 1988; Werry, Reeves, & Elkind, 1987; Reeves, Werry, Elkind, & Zametkin, 1987; Williams et al., 1989, 1990; Anderson et al., 1989), and this situation is compounded by the high degrees of comorbidity at both disorder and symptom level.

The dimensional analyses reported in this chapter also reinforce the strong interrelatedness of the major disorders when measured as dimensions rather than categories in preadolescence. More distinctiveness emerges in adolescence (greater for boys than for girls). It has been suggested that comorbidity may be an artifact arising either from too many categories/dimensions being imposed on symptoms or from the likelihood that more severe disorders will have a larger number of symptoms in a wider pattern and are therefore likely to cover the diagnostic criteria of more disorders (Caron & Rutter, 1991).

The data presented on the relationship between comorbidity and severity of the pure or comorbid disorders do not fit readily with either of the aforementioned hypotheses. While there may be debate on the validity of subtypes of anxiety disorders (Gould, Shaffer, Rutter, & Sturge, 1988) or conduct/oppositional disorders (Werry et al., 1987, 1988), this study used wide categories rather than narrowly defined subtypes. It would be against the weight of evidence from many nosological studies to suggest that depressive disorders and conduct disorders are subtypes of the same disorder (Quay, 1986), even if such an argument could be made for depressive and anxiety disorders (Kovacs et al., 1989; Bernstein, 1991). Further, the patterns of interrelatedness between disorders at age 11 years show broad separations between externalizing and internalizing disorders, both for correlates/risk factors and for interrelations between the disorder scales (Anderson et al., 1989; Williams et al., 1989, 1990). At age 15 years, the "pure" and comorbid disorders also show some discrimination, with the comorbid disorders having high mean scores for some scales but not others, suggesting underlying patterns to the symptoms rather than a broad scatter of symptoms increasing randomly across all categories with increasing severity of disorder.

Further evidence against the hypothesis that severity equates with more general symptomatology comes from the finding that when disorders were more stringently defined, comorbidity increased for an identified DSM-III depressed group, but fell for the group with lesser forms of depression. If comorbidity were arising either from chance association of common disorders or from the wide spread of symptoms across disorders, it would be expected to decrease with increased stringency of identification of those disorders.

For the major patterns of comorbidity in preadolescence, the comorbid groups had the risk factors present for both (or all) component disorders, including social, family, and cognitive/constitutional risks (Anderson et al., 1989; Williams et al., 1989, 1990), indicating that the comorbidity may well have arisen from the particular combinations of risks and vulnerabilities presented by the children and their families. The suggestion that comorbid disorders may represent distinct disorders or subtypes of a disorder has been raised for several commonly occurring comorbid patterns, e.g., conduct disorder plus ADHD, and ADHD plus anxiety disorders. The distinctiveness of these comorbid groups from either "parent" disorder in terms of severity, response to treatment, or outcome lends validity to seeing them as separate disorder patterns (Werry et al., 1987; Caron & Rutter, 1991; Biederman et al., 1991). The evidence for seeing comorbid depressive disorders in this way is less clear (Fleming & Offord, 1990; Rutter, 1989) and will depend on longitudinal outcome and treatment studies that focus on comorbid disorders rather than ignore or reject them.

In both preadolescent and adolescent samples, it is clear that comorbidity cannot be ignored and may have major treatment implications. If the comorbid disorder precedes the depression and influences both recovery from and relapse rates for depression, then treatment of the comorbid condition is essential in managing the depressive illness. Conversely, effective management of preadolescent depression may be important in treating externalizing disorders and anxiety disorders, as well as offering some protection from developing these disorders in adolescence (McGee et al., 1990, 1992).

The levels of comorbidity between all disorders, and especially between depression and other disorders, have implications for taxonomic systems. Changes in prevalence rates in the same sample arising from the changes between DSM-III and DSM-III-R are quite marked (Lahey et al., 1990), and planned changes in ICD-10 to incorporate mixed diagnoses such as depression and conduct disorder (Caron & Rutter, 1991) will alter reported comorbidity in future. If classifications do not take account of comorbidity, they will fail to be clinically or heuristically useful, in the same way that earlier DSMs were poorly used. Rapid changes, however, create major difficulties for just the longitudinal studies needed to investigate the causes, origins, and natural history of comorbid disorders (see Werry, 1988). Eisenberg (1986) described the way disorders change over time with new knowledge, from descriptive clinical classifications to systems based on underlying causes, genetic links, or biochemical markers. These changes may eventually exclude some of the original clinical cases (Eisenberg, 1986). Childhood depression is still firmly in the clinical descriptive stage, along with most other disorders of child and adolescent psychopathology, relying on descriptive classification systems. In the future, this classificatory scheme may well move toward etiological systems.

The importance of comorbidity lies in what it tells us about the effective treatment strategies for childhood and adolescent disorders and about the strength of and specificity of risk factors and vulnerabilities to disorder, as well as the likely outcomes for the different patterns and mixtures of disorder. Once we have this information, it will be possible to diagnose, prognose, treat, and eventually prevent the distressing, disabling, and often prolonged clinical disorders represented by these comorbid disorder groups.

ACKNOWLEDGMENTS.   The Dunedin Multidisciplinary Research and Development Unit is supported by the Medical Research Council of New Zealand and involves several departments of the University of Otago. Much of the data has been collected by voluntary workers from the local community. The authors are indebted to the many people whose valuable contributions continue to make this ongoing study possible, in particular the statistical analyses by Mrs. Sheila Williams, biostatistician. Collection of the mental health data was partially supported by U.S.P.H.S. Grants 1-23-MH42723-01 and 1-R01-MH43746 from the Antisocial and Violent Behavior Branch of the U.S. National Institutes of Mental Health.

References

Achenbach, T. M., & Edelbrock, C. S. (1978). The classification of child psychopathology: A review and analysis of empirical efforts. *Psychological Bulletin, 85,* 1275–1301.

Achenbach, T. M., Conners, K., Quay, H. C., Verhulst, F. C., & Howell, C. T. (1989). Replication of empirically derived syndromes as a basis for taxonomy of child/adolescent psychopathology. *Journal of Abnormal Child Psychology, 17,* 299–323.

Aman, M. G. (1984). Hyperactivity: Nature of the syndrome and its natural history. *Journal of Autism and Developmental Disorders, 14,* 39–55.

American Psychiatric Association (1980). *Diagnostic and statistical manual of mental disorders,* 3rd ed. Washington, DC: Author.

American Psychiatric Association (1987). *Diagnostic and statistical manual of mental disorders,* 3rd ed., revised. Washington, DC: Author.

Anderson, J. C., Williams, S. M., McGee, R., & Silva, P. (1987). DSM-III disorders in preadolescent children: Prevalence in a large sample from the general population. *Archives of General Psychiatry, 44,* 69–76.

Anderson, J. C., Williams, S. M., McGee, R., & Silva, P. (1989). Cognitive and social correlates of DSM-III disorders in preadolescent children. *Journal of the American Academy of Child and Adolescent Psychiatry, 28,* 842–846.

Angold, A. (1988). Childhood and adolescent depression. I. Epidemiological and aetiological aspects. *British Journal of Psychiatry, 152,* 601–617.

Bernstein, G. A. (1991). Comorbidity and severity of anxiety and depressive disorders in a clinic sample. *Journal of the American Academy of Child and Adolescent Psychiatry, 30,* 43–50.

Bernstein, G., & Garfinkel, B. D. (1986). School phobia: The overlap of affective and anxiety disorders. *Journal of the American Academy of Child and Adolescent Psychiatry, 25,* 235–241.

Biederman, J., Newcorn, J., & Sprich, S. (1991). Comorbidity of attention deficit hyperactivity disorder with conduct, depressive, anxiety, and other disorders. *American Journal of Psychiatry, 148,* 564–577.

Bird, H., Canino, G., Rubio-Stipec, M., Gould, M. S., Ribera, J., Sesman, M., Woodbury, M., Heurtas-Goldman, S., Pagan, A., Sanchez-Lacay, A., & Moscoso, M. (1988). Estimates of the prevalence of childhood maladjustment in a community survey in Puerto Rico: The use of combined measures. *Archives of General Psychiatry, 45*, 1120–1126.

Cantwell, D. P. (1982). Childhood depression: A review of current research. In B. B. Lahey & A. E. Kazdin (Eds.), *Advances in clinical child psychology*, Vol. 5 (pp. 39–93). New York: Plenum Press.

Cantwell, D. P., & Carlson, G. (1979). Problems and prospects in the study of childhood depression. *Journal of Nervous and Mental Disease, 167*, 522–529.

Carlson, G., & Cantwell, D. P. (1980a). A survey of depressive symptoms, syndrome and disorder in a child psychiatric population. *Journal of Child Psychology and Psychiatry, 21*, 19–25.

Carlson, G., & Cantwell, D. P. (1980b). Unmasking masked depression in children and adolescents. *American Journal of Psychiatry, 137*, 445–449.

Caron, C., & Rutter, M. (1991). Comorbidity in child psychopathology: Concepts, issues and research strategies. *Journal of Child Psychology and Psychiatry, 32*, 1063–1080.

Chapman, J. W., Silva, P. A., & Boersma, F. J. (1983). Student's perception of ability scales: Development of a short form. *Perceptual and Motor Skills, 57*, 799–802.

Cohen, P., Velez, C. N., & Garcia, M. (1985). The epidemiology of childhood depression. Paper presented at the Annual Meeting of the American Academy of Child Psychiatry, San Antonio, October 1985.

Cole, D. A., & Carpentieri, S. (1990). Social status and the comorbidity of child depression and conduct disorder. *Journal of Consulting and Clinical Psychology, 58*, 748–757.

Costello, A. J. (1986). Assessment and diagnosis of affective disorders in children. *Journal of Child Psychology and Psychiatry, 27*, 565–574.

Costello, A., Edelbrock, C., Kalas, R., Kessler, M., & Klaric, S. A. (1982). *Diagnostic Interview Schedule for Children (DISC)*. Bethesda, MD: National Institute for Mental Health (Contract No. RFP-DB-81-0027).

Costello, E. J. (1989). Developments in child psychiatric epidemiology. *Journal of the American Academy of Child and Adolescent Psychiatry, 28*, 836–841.

Costello, E. J., & Angold, A. (1988). Scales to assess child and adolescent depression: Checklists, screens and nets. *Journal of the American Academy of Child and Adolescent Psychiatry, 27*, 726–737.

Costello, E. J., Costello, A. J., Edelbrock, C. S., Burns, B. J., Dulcan, M. K., Brent, D., & Janiszewski, S. (1988). DSM-III disorders in pediatric primary care: Prevalence and risk factors. *Archives of General Psychiatry, 45*, 1107–1116.

Cytryn, L., & McKnew, D. H. (1972). Proposed classification of childhood depression. *American Journal of Psychiatry, 129*, 149–155.

Edelbrock, C., & Achenbach, T. M. (1980). A typology of child behaviour profile patterns: Distribution and correlates for disturbed children aged 6–16. *Journal of Abnormal Child Psychology, 8*, 441–470.

Edelbrock, C., & Costello, A. (1988). Structured psychiatric interviews for children. In M. Rutter, A. Tuma, & I. Lann (Eds.), *Assessment and diagnosis in child psychopathology* (pp. 87–112). London: Guilford Press.

Eisenberg, L. (1986). When is a case a case? In M. Rutter, C. Izard, & P. Read (Eds.), *Depression in young people* (pp. 469–479). New York: Guilford Press.

Esser, G., Schmidt, M. H., & Woerner, W. (1990). Epidemiology and course of psychiatric disorders in school-age children: Results of a longitudinal study. *Journal of Child Psychology and Psychiatry, 31*, 243–263.

Fleming, J. E., & Offord, D. R. (1990). Epidemiology of childhood depressive disorders: A critical review. *Journal of the American Academy of Child and Adolescent Psychiatry, 29*, 571–580.

Frost, L. A., Moffit, T. E., & McGee, R. (1989). Neuropsychological correlates of psychopathology in an unselected cohort of young adolescents. *Journal of Abnormal Psychology, 98*, 307–313.

Glaser, K. (1967). Masked depression in children and adolescents. *American Journal of Psychotherapy, 21*, 565–574.

Gould, M., Shaffer, D., Rutter, M., & Sturge, C. (1988). UK/WHO study of ICD-9. In M. Rutter, A. Tuma, & I. Lann (Eds.), *Assessment and diagnosis in child psychopathology* (pp. 37–65). London: Guilford Press.

Graham, P., & Rutter, M. (1973). Psychiatric disorder in the young adolescent: A follow-up study. *Proceedings of the Royal Society of Medicine, 66*, 1226–1229.

Harrington, R., Fudge, H., Rutter, M., Pickles, A., & Hill, J. (1991). Adult outcomes of childhood and adolescent depression. II. Links with antisocial disorders. *Journal of the American Academy of Child and Adolescent Psychiatry, 30*, 434–439.

Kashani, J. H., Beck, N. C., Hoeper, E. W., Fallahi, C., Corcoran, C. M., McAllister, J. A., Rosenberg, T. K., & Reid, J. C. (1987). Psychiatric disorders in a community sample of adolescents. *American Journal of Psychiatry, 144*, 584–589.

Kashani, J., Husain, A., Shekim, W., Hodges, K., Cytryn, L., & McKnew, D. (1981). Current perspectives on childhood depression: An overview. *American Journal of Psychiatry, 138*, 143–153.

Kashani, J., McGee, R., Clarkson, S., Anderson, J., Walton, L., Williams, S., Silva, P., Robins, A., Cytryn, M., & McKnew, D. (1983). Depression in a sample of 9 year old children: Prevalence and associated characteristics. *Archives of General Psychiatry, 40*, 1217–1223.

Keller, M. B., & Shapiro, R. W. (1982). "Double depression": Superimposition of acute depressive episodes on chronic depressive disorders. *American Journal of Psychiatry, 139*, 438–442.

Kovacs, M., & Beck, A. T. (1977). An empirical clinical approach towards a definition of childhood depression. In J. Shulterbrandt & A. Raskin (Eds.), *Depression in childhood* (pp. 1–26). New York: Raven Press.

Kovacs, M., Feinberg, T. L., Crouse-Novak, M. A., Paulauskas, S. L., & Finkelstein, R. (1984a). Depressive disorders in childhood. I. *Archives of General Psychiatry, 41*, 229–237.

Kovacs, M., Feinberg, T. L., Crouse-Novak, M. A., Paulauskas, S. L., Pollock, M., & Finkelstein, R. (1984b). Depressive disorders in childhood. II. A longitudinal study of the risk for a subsequent major depression. *Archives of General Psychiatry, 41*, 643–649.

Kovacs, M., Gatsonis, C., Paulauskas, S. L., & Richards, C. (1989). Depressive disorders in childhood. IV. A longitudinal study of comorbidity with and risk for anxiety disorders. *Archives of General Psychiatry, 46*, 776–782.

Kovacs, M., Paulauskas, S., Gatsonis, C., & Richards, C. (1988). Depressive disorders in childhood. III. A longitudinal study of comorbidity with and risk for conduct disorders. *Journal of Affective Disorders, 15*, 205–217.

Lahey, B. B., Loeber, R., Stouthamer-Loeber, M., Christ, M. G., Green, S., Russo, M. F., Frick, P. J., & Dulcan, M. (1990). Comparison of DSM-III and DSM-III-R diagnoses for prepubertal children: Changes in prevalence and validity. *Journal of the American Academy of Child and Adolescent Psychiatry, 29*, 620–626.

Last, G. C., Hersen, M., Kazdin, A. E., Finkelstein, R., & Strauss, C. C. (1987). Comparison of DSM-III separation anxiety and overanxious disorders: Demographic characteristics and patterns of comorbidity. *Journal of the American Academy of Child and Adolescent Psychiatry, 26*, 528–531.

Lessing, E. E., Williams, V., & Gil, E. (1982). A cluster-analytically derived typology: Feasible alternatives to clinical diagnostic classification of children? *Journal of Abnormal Child Psychology, 10*, 451–482.

McConville, B. J., Boag, L. C., & Purohit, A. P. (1973). Three types of childhood depression. *Canadian Psychiatric Association Journal, 18*, 133–138.

McDermott, P. A. (1980). Prevalence and constituency of behavioural disturbance taxonomies in the regular school population. *Journal of Abnormal Child Psychology, 4*, 523–536.

McGee, R., Anderson, J. C., Williams, S. M., & Silva, P. (1986). Cognitive correlates of depressive symptoms in eleven year old children. *Journal of Abnormal Child Psychology, 14*, 517–524.

McGee, R., Feehan, M., Williams, S. M., & Anderson, J. C. (1992). DSM-III disorders from age 11 to age 15 years. *Journal of the American Academy of Child and Adolescent Psychiatry, 31*, 50–59.

McGee, R., Feehan, M., Williams, S. M., Partridge, F., Silva, P. A., & Kelly, A. B. (1990). The prevalence of DSM-III disorders in a large sample of adolescents. *Journal of the American Academy of Child and Adolescent Psychiatry, 29*, 611–619.

McGee, R., & Williams, S. (1988). A longitudinal study of depression in nine-year-old children. *Journal of the American Academy of Child and Adolescent Psychiatry, 27*, 342–348.

Nuechterlein, K. H., Soli, S. D., Garmezy, N., Devine, V. T., & Shaefer, S. M. (1981). A classification system for research in childhood psychopathology: Part II. *Progress in Experimental Personality Research, 10*, 163–202.

Nurcombe, B., Seifer, R., Sciolo, A., Tramontana, M. G., Grapentine, W. L., & Beauchesne, H. C. (1989). Is major depressive disorder in adolescence a distinct diagnostic entity? *Journal of the American Academy of Child and Adolescent Psychiatry, 28*, 333–342.

Offord, D. R., Boyle, M. H., Szatmari, P., Rae-Grant, N. I., Links, P. S., Cadman, D. T., Byles, J. A., Crawford, J. W., Monroe Blum, H., Byrne, C., Thomas, H., & Woodward, C. (1987). Ontario Child Health Study. II. Six month prevalence of disorder and rates of service utilisation. *Archives of General Psychiatry, 44*, 832–836.

Petti, T. A. (1983). Depression and withdrawal in children. In T. H. Ollendick & M. Hersen (Eds.), *Handbook of child psychopathology* (pp. 293–321). New York: Plenum Press.

Puig-Antich, J. (1982). Major depression and conduct disorder in prepuberty. *Journal of the American Academy of Child Psychiatry, 21*, 118–128.

Quay, H. C. (1986). Classification. In H. C. Quay & J. S. Werry (Eds.), *Psychopathological disorders of childhood*, 3rd ed. (pp. 1–34). New York: John Wiley.

Reeves, J., Werry, J., Elkind, G., & Zametkin, A. (1987). Attention deficit, conduct, oppositional and anxiety disorders in children. II. Clinical characteristics. *Journal of the American Academy of Child Psychiatry, 26*, 144–155.

Rosenberg, M. (1965). *Society and the adolescent self-image*. Princeton, NJ: Princeton University Press.

Rutter, M. (1982). Syndromes attributed to "minimal brain dysfunction" in childhood. *American Journal of Psychiatry, 139*, 21–33.

Rutter, M. (1989). Isle of Wight revisited: Twenty-five years of child psychiatric epidemiology. *Journal of the American Academy of Child and Adolescent Psychiatry, 28*, 633–653.

Rutter, M., Tizard, J., & Whitmore, K. (1970). *Education, health, and behaviour*. London: Longmore.

Seifer, R., Nurcombe, B., Sciolo, A., & Grapentine, W. L. (1989). Is major depressive disorder in childhood a distinct diagnostic entity? *Journal of the American Academy of Child and Adolescent Psychiatry, 28*, 935–941.

Shaffer, D. (1985). Depression, mania and suicidal acts. In M. Rutter & L. Hersov (Eds.), *Child and adolescent psychiatry* (pp. 698–719). London: Blackwell.

Silva, P. A. (1990). The Dunedin multidisciplinary health and development study: A fifteen year longitudinal study. *Paediatric and Perinatal Epidemiology, 4*, 96–127.

Soli, S. D., Nuechterlein, K. H., Garmezy, N., Devine, V. T., & Shaefer, S. M. (1981). A classification system for research in childhood psychopathology: Part I. *Progress in Experimental Personality Research, 10*, 115–161.

Strober, M., & Werry, J. (1987). The assessment of depression in children and adolescents. In T. Ban & N. Sartorius (Eds.), *Assessment of depression* (pp. 324–342). Heidelberg: Springer-Verlag.

Velez, C. N., Johnson, J., & Cohen, P. (1989). A longitudinal analysis of selected risk factors for childhood psychopathology. *Journal of the American Academy of Child and Adolescent Psychiatry, 28*, 861–864.

Verhulst, F. C., Berden, G. F. M., & Sanders-Woudstra, J. A. R. (1985). Mental health in Dutch children. II. The prevalence of psychiatric disorder and relationship between measures. *Acta Psychiatrica Scandinavica Supplementum, 72*, 1–45.

Verhulst, F. C., Koot, H. M., & Berden, G. F. M. G. (1990). Four year follow-up of an epidemiological sample. *Journal of the American Academy of Child and Adolescent Psychiatry, 29*, 440–448.

Waters, B., & Storm, V. (1985). Depression in prepubertal children. *Australian and New Zealand Journal of Psychiatry, 19*, 6–17.

Weinberg, W. A., Rutman, J., Sullivan, L., Pennick, E. C., & Dietz, S. G. (1973). Depression in children referred to an educational diagnostic centre: Diagnosis and treatment. *Journal of Pediatrics, 83*, 1065–1072.

Weissman, M. M., & Klerman, G. L. (1977). Sex differences and the epidemiology of depression. *Archives of General Psychiatry, 34*, 98–111.

Werry, J. S. (1988). Letter to the editor: In memoriam—DSM-III. *Journal of the American Academy of Child and Adolescent Psychiatry, 27*, 138–139.

Werry, J., Elkind, G., & Reeves, J. (1988). Attention deficit, conduct, oppositional and anxiety disorders in children. III. Laboratory differences. *Journal of Abnormal Child Psychology, 15*, 409–428.

Werry, J., Reeves, J., & Elkind, G. (1987). Attention deficit, conduct, oppositional and anxiety disorders in children. I. A review of research on differentiating characteristics. *Journal of the American Academy of Child Psychiatry, 26*, 133–143.

Williams, S. M., Anderson, J. C., McGee, R., & Silva, P. (1990). Risk factors for behavioural and emotional disorder in preadolescent children. *Journal of the American Academy of Child and Adolescent Psychiatry, 29*, 413–419.

Williams, S. M., McGee, R., Anderson, J. C., & Silva, P. A. (1989). The structure and correlates of self-reported symptoms in 11-year old children. *Journal of Abnormal Child Psychology, 17*, 55–71.

Index

Abandonment, 72, 224, 315, 554

Abnormal development, 125

Abuse, 8, 25, 27, 31, 33, 46, 49, 50, 70, 72, 82, 86, 87, 126, 133, 155, 179, 188, 262, 310, 315, 323, 328, 329, 333, 345, 346, 366, 386, 408, 415, 418, 419, 427, 436, 470, 481–502, 481, 482, 483, 484, 485,486, 487, 488, 489, 490, 491, 493, 494, 495, 496, 497, 499, 500, 401, 502, 510, 515, 520, 529, 550, 551, 552, 555, 585

    maltreatment, 4, 8, 11, 83, 89, 92, 94, 133, 346, 482, 485, 486, 487, 488, 489, 490, 491, 492, 493, 494, 495, 496, 497, 502

Academic. See School

Accommodation, 128

Acetylcholine, 151, 152, 154, 370

ACH. See acetylcholine

Achievement, 4, 87, 90, 91, 92, 108, 109, 111, 113, 130, 133, 148, 235, 284, 347, 355, 357, 402, 515, 518

ACTH, 153, 405, 407, 408, 409, 410, 411

Acting-out, 186, 196, 213, 215, 293, 315

Adaptation, 7, 90, 127, 128, 130, 131, 132, 133, 138, 139, 222, 243, 369, 433

ADHD. See attention deficit hyperactivity disorder

Adjustment disorder, 6, 42, 66, 173, 178, 196, 199, 427, 428, 436, 527, 551, 552, 565

Admixture analysis, 65

Adolescent Psychopathology Scales, 221, 544

Aggression, 51, 52, 68, 84, 152, 252, 255, 259, 261, 267, 277, 384, 410, 472, 481, 482, 487, 488, 489, 494, 498, 501, 502, 553, 582, 588, 593

AIDS, 436

Alcohol, 27, 31, 33, 254, 313, 316, 427, 428, 436, 520, 531, 538, 546, 551

Alcohol abuse, 31, 33, 428, 436, 520

Alcoholism, 67, 70, 133, 155, 219, 348, 470

Amitriptyline, 66, 156, 370, 372, 382, 384, 388, 441

Amoxapine, 370, 371, 374

Amygdala, 145, 405

Anaclitic depression, 63, 84, 315, 414, 419, 446

Anafranil. See clomipramine

Androgen, 155

Anger, 4, 48, 51, 68, 82, 83, 128, 129, 153, 179, 185, 186, 283, 289, 290, 302, 306, 314, 348, 428, 430, 437, 490, 495, 499, 500, 552, 553, 564

Anhedonia, 68, 91, 174, 180, 188, 200, 215, 280, 355, 356, 366, 367, 391, 402

Antisocial, 47, 68, 70, 129, 193, 267, 315, 345, 387, 428, 488, 489, 552, 583, 585

Anxiety, 33, 63, 68, 69, 70, 71, 82, 91, 98, 128, 131, 152, 187, 188, 193, 201, 253, 254, 261, 262, 277, 288, 289, 290, 291, 293, 314, 316, 319, 324, 336, 345, 358, 418, 427, 430, 452, 483, 484, 493, 510, 513, 516, 517, 518, 519, 542, 545, 558, 584, 590, 592, 593, 594, 595

    anxiety disorders, 8, 31, 32, 33, 105, 126, 156, 178, 186, 195, 213, 266, 333, 346, 348, 366, 427, 428, 436, 470, 516, 582, 584, 587, 588 589, 595, 596, 597

    separation anxiety, 134, 238, 387, 584

Appetite, 5, 21, 22, 62, 68, 84, 145, 152, 174, 177, 180, 210, 244, 323, 410, 434, 445, 446, 448, 449

APS. See Adolescent Psychopathology Scales

Arecoline, 153

Arginine vasopressin, 65

Asendin. See Amoxapine

ASQ. See Attributional Style Questionnaire

ASSA. See Attributional Style Scale for Adolescents

Assessment, 7, 26, 209, 210, 220, 223, 238, 240, 241, 249, 252, 330, 331, 335, 350, 351, 519, 546, 548, 564

    diagnostic assessment, 24, 251, 311

    epidemiological assessment, 177, 192

    functional assessment, 311

    interview assessment, 48, 184, 195, 203

    neurobiological assessment, 145

    parent report, 7, 193, 196, 257, 258, 262, 266, 267

603

Assessment (*cont.*)
  peer report, 7
  self-report, 7, 24, 25, 26, 27, 28, 100, 103, 104,
      107, 111, 115, 147, 148, 183, 186, 187, 193,
      196, 197, 201, 202, 209, 210, 211, 212,
      213, 216, 217, 218, 219, 220, 221, 222,
      223, 224, 225, 226, 235, 236, 238, 239,
      245, 259, 261, 262, 284, 313, 326, 328,
      329, 335, 385, 511, 540, 542, 544, 547,
      562, 591
  validity, 210
Assimilation, 128
Assortative mating, 50
ATQ. *See* Automatic Thoughts Questionnaire
Attachment, 4, 5, 63, 71, 72, 83, 84, 98, 113, 125,
      126, 128, 130, 131, 132, 134, 135, 136, 138,
      139, 346, 348, 351, 358, 410, 411, 418,
      419, 431, 466, 471, 482, 492, 493, 494,
      495, 501, 502
  insecure attachment, 125, 348, 418, 471, 493, 495
  secure attachment, 113, 125, 128, 130, 346, 410
Attention deficit disorder, 4, 31, 32, 100, 150,
      175, 176, 200, 213, 252, 264, 266, 371,
      582, 587, 589, 594
Attention deficit hyperactivity disorder, 49, 50,
      151, 348, 371, 378, 389, 582, 584, 585,
      586, 587, 588, 589, 590, 593, 595, 596,
      597
Attributional style, 99, 100, 110, 111, 112, 113,
      114, 116, 123, 129, 133, 239, 261, 279,
      281, 317, 415, 451, 466
Attributional Style Questionnaire, 112
Attributional Style Scale for Adolescents, 112
Atypical, 43, 91, 180, 378
Autistic disorder, 151, 175, 250, 264
Automatic Thoughts Questionnaire, 103
Autonomy, 83, 89, 91, 92, 128, 134, 316, 323,
      335, 431, 438
Aventyl. *See* Nortriptyline

BDI. *See* Beck Depression Inventory
BDIS. *See* Behavior Disorders Identification Scale
Beck Depression Inventory, 27, 112, 187, 212,
      220, 265, 563
Beck Suicide Intent Scale, 547
Behavior Disorders Identification Scale, 241
Behavior Rating Profile, 241
Behavioral Evaluation Scale-2, 240
Behavioral interventions, 241, 318
Bellevue Index of Depression, 216, 218, 252,
      325, 382, 384, 432, 435
Benzodiazepines, 368, 436
Bereavement, 22, 71, 72, 85, 179, 315, 332, 436,
      469, 520
BES-2. *See* Behavioral Evaluation Scale-2
Beta endorphin, 153
Bimodality analysis, 65
Biological correlates. *See* Biological markers
Biological markers, 9, 64, 83, 171, 198, 405
  anorexia, 68, 430

Biological markers (*cont.*)
  appetite, 5, 21, 22, 62, 68, 84, 145, 152, 174,
      177, 180, 210, 244, 323, 410, 434, 445,
      446, 448, 449
  arginine vasopressin, 65
  beta-endorphin, 409
  cholinergic REM induction test, 153
  circadian rhythm, 65, 70, 404, 406
  decreased weight, 68
  dexamethasone suppression test, 9, 65, 67,
      145, 154, 155, 198, 238, 406, 407, 408, 437
  early morning awakening, 65, 156
  growth hormone, 9, 65, 67, 145, 153, 158, 408
  hypercortisolism, 64, 67
  hypersomnia, 47, 53, 68, 174, 180, 323, 367
  immune system, 10, 331, 436
      natural killer cell, 10
  insomnia, 4, 53, 68, 69, 174, 210, 331, 382
  melatonin, 67
  nightmares, 69, 70, 446
  physostigmine challenge test, 153
  prolactin response, 152
  psychomotor disturbance, 4, 21, 22, 53, 62, 68,
      85, 147, 174, 176, 177, 196, 402, 417, 434,
      445, 446
  REM latency, 65, 67, 144, 156, 157, 158
  scopolamine challenge test, 153
  sleep, 5, 10, 21, 22, 23, 32, 53, 65, 67, 84, 85,
      130, 152, 154, 156, 157, 158, 174, 198,
      215, 235, 244, 253, 366, 367, 368, 386,
      390, 391, 406, 407, 411, 417, 427, 428,
      430, 434, 446, 448, 449, 484, 552
  slow wave sleep, 67
  somatostatin, 65
  thyroid-stimulating hormone, 65, 67, 155
  thyrotropin-releasing hormone challenge test, 155
  weight gain, 44
Bipolar disorder, 6, 8, 9, 11, 17, 19, 21, 22, 23, 29,
      30, 34, 41–56, 41, 42, 43, 44, 45, 46, 48,
      50, 51, 52, 53, 54, 55, 62, 65, 150, 153,
      172, 176, 180, 208, 309, 369, 378, 384,
      435, 469
  bipolar "variant" disorder, 51
  bipolar I disorder, 6
  bipolar II disorder, 6
  cyclothymia, 22, 23, 55, 222
  family history, 44
  hypersexuality, 49
  hypomania, 6, 22, 23, 29, 44, 47, 48, 49, 50,
      51, 62, 179, 376, 384
  in mental retardation, 53
  lithium efficacy, 54
  mania, 6, 29, 41
  manic, 6, 22, 23, 29, 30, 34, 41, 42, 43, 44, 45,
      47, 48, 49, 50, 51, 52, 55, 62, 153, 170,
      179, 187, 407, 446, 464, 466, 469
  mixed manic/depressed states, 23
  onset, 42–44
  phenomenology, 46–53
      atypical, 43

Bipolar disorder (*cont.*)
  prognosis, 43, 47
  psychotic mania, 51–52
  rapid cycling, 54
  recovery, 45
  "switching", 45, 47
  treatment, 53–56
Birleson Depression Self-Rating, 188
Blood levels, 55
Body image, 105, 106, 281, 431
Bone marrow transplant, 438
Borderline personality disorder, 483, 552, 557
Brain imaging, 148–151, 148, 150, 151
Brazelton Neonatal Assessment Scale, 406
BRP. *See* Behavior Rating Profile
BSIS. *See* Beck Suicide Intent Scale
Bupropion, 378, 383
Burn injury, 438

Cancer, 331, 417, 432, 434, 436, 440, 467, 513,
  514, 515, 517, 519
Carbamazepine, 53, 54
CAS. *See* Child Assessment Schedule
CASQ. *See* Children's Attributional Style
  Questionnaire
CAT. *See* Computed axial tomography
Catatonia, 6
Catecholamine, 151, 404
CBCL. *See* Child Behavior Checklist
CBQC. *See* Cognitive Bias Questionnaire for
  Children
CDI. *See* Children's Depression Inventory
CDRS. *See* Children's Depression Rating Scale
Center for Epidemiological Studies-Depression
  Scale, 212, 221
Cerebral blood flow, 145, 146, 149, 150
Cerebral hemispheres, 145, 146, 147, 158
Cerebral lateralization, 145, 147
Cerebral palsy, 447
Cerebral spinal fluid, 152
CES-D. *See* Center for Epidemiological Studies-
  Depression Scale
CGI. *See* Clinical Global Impressions
Child Assessment Schedule, 184, 185–189, 202,
  210, 224
Child Behavior Checklist, 69, 184, 222, 237, 313
Childhood Depression Assessment Tool, 222
Children's Attributional Style Questionnaire, 110
Children's Depression Adjective Check Lists, 222
Children's Depression Inventory, 25, 69, 102,
  147, 183, 202, 212–216, 212, 236, 251,
  252, 260, 265, 326, 384, 432, 564
Children's Depression Rating Scale, 183, 201–
  202, 217, 218, 386, 387, 434
Children's Depression Scale, 212, 216, 238
Children's Negative Cognitive Error
  Questionnaire, 103
Cingulate gyrus, 145
Circadian rhythm, 65, 70, 404, 406
Circumcision, 406, 408

Classroom, 109, 113, 223, 238, 242, 243, 262,
  264, 328, 455
Clinical Global Impressions, 386
Clomipramine, 152, 370, 371, 372, 388
Clonidine, 65, 152, 154, 155
Cluster analysis, 63, 65, 68, 69
CNCEQ. *See* Children's Negative Cognitive Error
  Questionnaire
Cognition, 48, 68, 109, 129, 136, 137, 250, 255,
  263, 282, 293, 300, 449, 452, 491, 498, 542
Cognitive attributions, 261
Cognitive Bias Questionnaire for Children, 103
Cognitive deficit, 3, 147, 148, 415, 585
Cognitive development, 35, 107, 138, 148, 176,
  255, 264, 450, 452, 453, 456
Cognitive distortions, 98, 103, 104, 113, 115, 136,
  281, 354, 355, 451
Cognitive impairment, 147, 174
Cognitive Process Inventory for Children, 112
Cognitive processes, 104, 114, 250, 259, 265
Cognitive style, 87
Cognitive-behavioral therapy, 10, 97, 104, 105,
  106, 116, 276, 277, 279, 281, 285, 286,
  306, 315, 317, 319, 324, 325, 326, 328,
  329, 332, 345, 350, 351, 355, 556, 558
Comorbidity, 8, 26, 30, 31–33, 34, 50, 54, 68,
  70, 105, 129, 171, 176, 184, 196, 198, 202,
  310, 327, 331, 333, 349, 387, 389, 391,
  470, 471, 510, 512, 517, 538, 550, 552,
  557, 562, 581–598
  dysthymia, 586, 588
  prevalence, 585
  speech and language, 26–27
Computed axial tomography, 148, 149, 151
Concrete operations, 87
Conduct disorder, 4, 31, 32, 50, 67, 175, 176,
  186, 187, 193, 213, 219, 348, 366, 471,
  485, 497, 510, 529, 550, 551, 552, 583,
  584, 585, 587, 588
Confidentiality, 330, 334
Conflict, 9, 92, 133, 261, 283, 291, 300, 303, 304,
  305, 306, 311, 313, 314, 315, 321, 323,
  324, 326, 332, 334, 346, 347, 349, 355,
  357, 439, 466, 486, 489, 496, 497, 500,
  502, 513
Conscious, 55, 62, 68, 71, 86, 135, 295, 313
Construct validity, 64, 65–66, 67, 240
Contingency reinforcement, 100
Control group, 25, 50, 107, 155, 187, 196, 220,
  279, 326, 335, 408, 412, 432, 464, 486,
  543, 553, 554, 563
Convergent validity, 259
Coopersmith Self-Esteem Inventory, 104
Coping, 63, 70, 71, 72, 126, 131, 133, 287, 288,
  289, 290, 291, 294, 296, 299, 300, 302,
  306, 311, 313, 314, 336, 352, 353, 354,
  355, 356, 358, 403, 431, 438, 439, 450,
  455, 456, 467, 468, 518, 519, 525, 564
Coping skills, 294, 299, 300, 302, 306, 311, 336,
  450, 455, 456, 525

Corpus striatum, 153

Cortex, 9, 145, 150, 151, 152, 153, 405

Corticotropin-releasing factor, 405

Cortisol, 145, 153, 158, 198, 405, 406, 407, 408, 409, 410, 411
  salivary cortisol, 407

Criterion variance, 170, 183, 197

Crohn's disease, 433

Cross-sectional, 104, 180, 464, 473, 491, 492, 512, 513, 517, 520

Crying, 84, 128, 217, 237, 241, 254, 356, 403, 406, 408, 417, 430

CSEI. *See* Coopersmith Self-Esteem Inventory

CSF. *See* Cerebral spinal fluid

CT. *See* Computed axial tomography

Cycle, 43, 45, 54, 137, 151, 180, 293, 296, 302, 348, 357, 359, 419

Cyclothymia, 6, 22, 23, 55, 222

Cystic fibrosis, 188, 433, 447

DBH. *See* Dopamine beta-hydroxylase

DBT. *See* Dialectical Behavior Therapy

Death, 22, 46, 51, 94, 133, 174, 175, 200, 216, 237, 324, 332, 346, 367, 371, 378, 389, 393, 431, 437, 445, 446, 492, 510, 512, 527, 528, 533, 540, 547, 552, 565

Death/Suicide Interview, 547

Delinquency, 68, 192, 310, 324, 331, 332, 489, 536, 544

Delirium, 51, 427, 428

Delusional disorder, 179, 180

Delusions, 22, 23, 44, 47, 51, 53, 62, 195, 254, 385

Dementia, 45, 47, 62, 156, 428, 436

Demographic factors
  parental education, 28
  race, 28, 111, 214, 256, 264, 267, 433, 536, 565
  religion, 28
  socioeconomic status, 28, 111, 133, 134, 188, 217, 239, 242, 251, 256, 264, 267, 434, 485

Depression Adjective Check List, 382

Depression Self-Rating Scale, 103, 212, 217

Depression Symptom Checklist, 252

Depressive Affect Self-Report Scale, 222

Depressive equivalent, 20, 123, 401, 582

Depressive Experiences Questionnaire for Adolescents, 222

Deprivation, 82, 87, 90, 92, 94, 173, 315, 346, 355, 433, 449

DES. *See* Differential Emotions Scale—IV

Desipramine, 154, 155, 370, 371, 372, 385, 389

Desyrel. *See* Trazodone

Developmental psychophathology, 123–139

Dexamethasone suppression test, 9, 65, 67, 145, 154, 155, 198, 238, 406, 407, 408, 437

Diagnostic and Statistical Manual of Mental Disorders (American Psychiatric Association), 5, 6, 8, 21, 22, 23, 24, 25, 26, 27, 29, 34, 41, 43, 45, 46, 47, 48, 49, 52, 55, 62, 63, 85, 149, 169, 170, 171, 172, 173, 174, 175, 176, 177, 178, 179, 180,

Diagnostic and Statistical Manual of Mental Disorders (American Psychiatric Association) (*cont.*)
  183, 185, 186, 187, 189, 191, 192, 194, 197, 200, 201, 210, 213, 218, 221, 238, 239, 243, 244, 265, 277, 309, 311, 326, 328, 329, 366, 367, 387, 401, 402, 415, 417, 418, 428, 432, 433, 436, 464, 469, 510, 526, 527, 529, 544, 550, 551, 552, 553, 557, 582, 583, 584, 591, 592, 597

Diagnostic clinical interview, 183–203

Diagnostic Interview for Children and Adolescents, 27, 184, 189–191, 203, 210

Diagnostic Interview Schedule for Children, 184, 191–195, 202, 210, 585

Diagnostic validity, 61–72
  construct validity, 64, 65–66, 67, 171, 240, 245, 258, 259
  descriptive validity, 171
  external validity, 171, 172, 596
  face validity, 171
  predictive validity, 171

Dialectical behavior therapy, 557

Diathesis, 99, 113, 114, 132, 509

DICA. *See* Diagnostic Interview for Children and Adolescents

Diencephalon, 145

Differential Emotions Scale—IV, 186, 219

Direct Observation Form, 243

Disability, 4, 26, 158, 366, 367, 431, 445, 446, 447, 448, 449, 450, 452, 453, 455, 456, 457

DISC. *See* Diagnostic Interview Schedule for Children

Discipline, 283, 302, 471

Discriminant validity, 187, 189, 192, 193, 202, 218, 259, 261

Disruptive behaviors, 199, 262

Dissociation, 146, 483

Diurnal variation, 62, 68, 224, 449

Divorce, 9, 25, 133, 346, 366, 472, 473, 474, 487, 516

DOF. *See* Direct Observation Form

Dopamine, 151, 154, 370, 404, 409

Dopamine beta-hydroxylase, 152

Double depression, 22, 329, 586, 587, 588, 596

Drug abuse, 27, 31, 33, 46, 50, 70, 82, 126, 133, 179, 310, 315, 329, 345, 346, 386, 427, 436, 470, 485, 529, 550, 551, 552

DSCL. *See* Depression Symptom Checklist

DSM. *See* *Diagnostic and Statistical Manual of Mental Disorders* (American Psychiatric Association)

DSRS. *See* Depression Self-Rating Scale

Dysphoria, 5, 20, 23, 24, 25, 27, 28, 31, 46, 48, 52, 54, 68, 71, 81, 85, 86, 87, 90, 92, 93, 109, 110, 129, 136, 137, 174, 175, 177, 178, 186, 188, 200, 213, 217, 239, 240, 244, 277, 288, 313, 314, 316, 321, 323, 349, 355, 367, 382, 417, 428, 432, 435, 436, 445

Dysthymia, 21, 22, 25, 27, 31, 61, 62, 63, 64, 65, 66, 70, 71, 72, 155, 172, 175, 177, 179, 193, 199, 221, 222, 238, 277, 280, 309, 329, 407, 428, 435, 446, 470, 481, 486, 553, 584, 586, 587, 588, 589, 591, 592, 594, 595, 596

Dysthymic disorder, 6, 8, 21, 24, 25, 27, 31, 32, 67, 85, 107, 184, 190, 199, 210, 218, 221, 329, 407, 550, 581, 584, 586, 587, 589, 594, 595

Early morning awakening, 65, 156
ECT. *See* Electroconvulsive therapy
Education. See school
Education for All Handicapped Act, 241
EEG. *See* Electroencephalography
Ego, 82, 83, 90, 92, 93 123, 315, 352, 430, 565
Elavil. *See* Amitriptyline
Electroconvulsive therapy, 64, 65
Electroencephalography, 156, 157, 198, 440
EMR. *See* Educable mentally retarded
Endogenous, 9, 42, 43, 61, 62, 68, 70, 130, 153, 154, 155, 156, 157, 385, 408, 409
  endogenous depression, 62, 68, 156
Endorphin, 153, 404, 407, 409
Enuresis, 31, 254, 370, 391, 430, 581
Environmental factors, 8
Epidemiology, 4, 7, 17, 19, 23, 24, 25, 26, 29, 30, 23–30, 31, 32, 63, 83, 89, 124, 171, 177, 178, 191, 192, 194, 195, 215, 222, 310, 328, 348, 431, 447, 464, 468, 469, 526, 530, 534, 535, 550
  adolescents, 27–28
  bipolar disorder, 29
  incidence, 24, 66, 154, 328, 349, 408, 417, 427, 432, 445, 447, 464, 534, 535, 536, 538, 564, 565, 567
  pre-school children, 24–25
  prevalence, 3, 7, 10, 11, 23, 24, 25, 26, 27, 28, 29, 30, 32, 83, 87, 89, 146, 171, 175, 191, 194, 309, 310, 431, 432, 433, 447, 481, 485, 535, 537, 538, 562, 563, 564, 584, 585, 586, 587, 594, 595, 596, 597. *See* Epidemiology
  lifetime prevalence, 7, 27, 29, 310, 433
  1-year prevalence, 25
  point prevalence, 7, 25, 27
  school-age children, 25–27
  suicide, 29, 527, 534–39
Estrogen, 155
Ethnicity, 214, 218, 266, 537, 538
Ethnology, 71, 84, 85
Etiology, 5, 7, 9, 11, 35, 61, 62, 64, 71, 81, 83, 84, 126, 156, 169, 170, 171, 173, 175, 176, 178, 179, 280, 309, 314, 315, 334, 335, 345, 354, 403, 404, 415, 433, 434, 436, 445, 469, 470, 509, 555, 564, 566, 598
Existential, 90, 324, 525
Externalizing, 4, 8, 31, 48, 100, 101, 192, 253, 254, 256, 266, 267, 311, 313, 314, 330, 332, 466, 487, 489, 501, 516, 517, 518, 555, 583, 587, 588, 589, 594, 595, 596, 597

Eye contact, 88, 277, 280, 291, 303, 304, 318

Face Valid Depression Scale for Adolescents, 222
FAD. *See* Family Assessment Device
Failure to thrive, 408, 419
Family Assessment Device, 219
Family conflict, 261, 332, 346
Family history, 21, 32, 33, 44, 50, 51, 52, 67, 69, 173, 175, 176, 178, 266, 348, 354, 384, 428, 433, 435, 546
Family studies, 50, 144, 157, 171, 584
Family therapy, 277, 282, 283, 303, 306, 324, 325, 326, 330, 345, 350, 351, 352, 354, 355, 359, 438, 439, 441, 556, 558, 560
Father, 88, 114, 239, 240, 252, 253, 255, 256, 259, 267, 345, 349, 354, 500, 554
Fatigue, 4, 53, 68, 174, 179, 323, 331, 434, 473, 484
Fear, 69, 88, 89, 90, 131, 185, 236, 241, 253, 254, 261, 289, 291, 315, 316, 351, 410, 414, 439, 500
Fenfluramine, 152
5-HIAA. *See* 5-hydroxyindole acetic acid
5-HT. *See* Serotonin
5-hydroxyindoleacetic acid, 152
Fluoxetine, 11, 48, 368, 371, 376, 377, 386, 388, 441, 556
Fluvoxamine, 376
Follow-up studies, 46, 50, 53, 171, 185, 464, 556
Food and Drug Administration, 370, 390

GABA. *See* Gamma-aminobutyric acid
Games, 137, 276, 285, 287, 291, 297
Gamma-aminobutyric acid, 153, 154
Gender, 9, 32, 103, 105, 106, 108, 111, 112, 143, 188, 215, 238, 246, 310, 314, 329, 334, 335, 385, 482, 485, 486, 487, 488, 489, 490, 495, 499, 500, 501, 513, 514, 516, 517, 536, 537, 539, 544, 554, 565, 584, 586, 587, 595
  gender differences, 9, 105, 108, 112, 188, 314, 334, 335, 482, 486, 487, 488, 489, 495, 498, 499, 514, 517, 554, 587
General Behavior Inventory, 222
Genetic, 7, 9, 61, 62, 64, 65, 67, 71, 72, 83, 84, 130, 133, 139, 144, 171, 178, 198, 200, 309, 348, 428, 448, 449, 468, 469, 470, 473, 474, 552, 598
  chromosome, 64
Grandiosity, 23, 49, 53
Grief, 70, 323, 332, 358, 411, 427, 435, 436, 439, 473
Group therapy, 200, 325, 326, 330, 335, 359, 438, 440
Growth hormone, 9, 65, 67, 145, 152, 153, 154, 155, 158, 408, 409
Growth hormone releasing factor, 154
Guilt, 22, 42, 63, 68, 69, 70, 86, 90, 91, 123, 129, 173, 174, 175, 179, 186, 210, 216, 226, 236, 238, 244, 304, 315, 323, 354, 367, 417, 431, 435, 437, 446, 466, 467, 473, 484

Hallucinations, 22, 23, 44, 47, 51, 62, 177, 195, 254, 385
   auditory hallucinations, 49
HAM-D. *See* Hamilton Depression Rating Scale
Hamilton Depression Rating Scale, 201, 220, 386
Handicap, 433
Head injury, 466
Helplessness, 72, 82, 97, 99, 103, 108, 109, 110, 111, 112, 113, 114, 115, 116, 123, 128, 131, 133, 134, 135, 136, 137, 173, 241, 317, 347, 348, 351, 353, 354, 357, 410, 414, 415, 419, 428, 430, 433, 439, 449, 451, 455, 468, 481, 491, 500, 519, 565
Heritability, 61, 70, 72, 83
   pedigree, 70
HGI. *See* Hostility-Guilt Inventory
Hippocampus, 145, 151, 152
Histamine, 370
Historical perspective, 21, 41–43, 51, 62–64, 169–170, 581–583
Hopelessness, 22, 72, 82, 85, 86, 87, 94, 98, 99, 100, 107, 110, 113, 115, 128, 129, 133, 173, 179, 210, 224, 261, 265, 266, 298, 317, 352, 353, 357, 431, 449, 451, 455, 473, 481, 485, 498, 500, 519, 542, 544, 545, 553, 554, 559
Hopelessness Scale for Children, 107
Hopkins Symptom Checklist, 222, 256, 386
Hospitalization, 26, 42, 43, 44, 45, 47, 48, 52, 54, 67, 69, 71, 154, 187, 201, 252, 265, 277, 310, 323, 325, 334, 352, 353, 382, 389, 405, 415, 417, 428, 429, 430, 432, 433, 438, 466, 470, 473, 482, 512, 527, 530, 532, 538, 543, 544, 546, 550, 553, 555, 556, 559, 565. *See* Inpatient
Hostility, 42, 48, 84, 133, 186, 334, 347, 384, 450, 473, 493, 496, 497, 498
Hostility-Guilt Inventory, 260
HPA axis. *See* Hypothalamic-pituitary-adrenal axis
HSC. *See* Hopelessness Scale for Children
Hypercortisolism, 64, 67
Hypersomnia, 47, 53, 68, 174, 180, 323, 367
Hypothalamic-pituitary-adrenal axis, 153, 154, 405, 406, 407, 408
Hypothalamus, 145, 151, 152, 154, 155, 405

Id, 90
IA. *See* Interview for Aggression
IDEA. *See* Individuals with Educational Disabilities Act
Imipramine, 32, 34, 66, 277, 365, 368, 370, 371, 373, 382, 384, 385, 391, 404, 441
Immaturity, 53, 64, 86, 123, 235, 402
Immune system, 10, 331, 436
Incest, 482, 483, 492
Incidence. *See* Epidemiology
Individuals with Educational Disabilities Act, 241

Infant, 4, 5, 63, 84, 85, 92, 93, 110, 128, 134, 136, 187, 349, 401, 402, 403, 405, 406, 407, 408, 409, 410, 411, 412, 413, 414, 415, 416, 417, 418, 419, 430, 465, 467, 492
Inferiority, 104, 316
Inherit. *See* Heritability
Inpatient, 26, 28, 44, 66, 68, 69, 70, 71, 86, 100, 103, 107, 109, 111, 113, 114, 147, 148, 149, 154, 155, 157, 158, 186, 187, 188, 189, 190, 192, 198, 201, 202, 213, 217, 219, 220, 221, 236, 243, 252, 254, 259, 325, 329, 376, 386, 428, 432, 433, 438, 441, 472, 530, 534, 536, 537, 543, 544, 547, 550, 551, 553, 554, 555, 562. *See* Hospitalization
Insomnia, 4, 53, 68, 69, 174, 210, 331, 382
Instruments (rating scales, self reports, structured interviews, questionnaires etc.)
   Adolescent Psychopathology Scales, 221, 544
   Attributional Style Questionnaire, 112
   Attributional Style Scale for Adolescents, 112
   Automatic Thoughts Questionnaire, 103
   Beck Depression Inventory, 27, 112, 187, 212, 220, 265, 563
   Beck Suicide Intent Scale, 547
   Behavior Disorders Identification Scale, 241
   Behavior Rating Profile, 241
   Behavioral Evaluation Scale-2, 240
   Bellevue Index of Depression, 216, 218, 252, 260, 325, 382, 384, 432, 435
   Birleson Depression Self-Rating, 188
   Brazelton Neonatal Assessment Scale, 406
   Center for Epidemiological Studies-Depression Scale, 212, 221
   Child Assessment Schedule, 184, 185–189, 202, 210, 224
   Child Behavior Checklist, 69, 184, 222, 237, 313
   Childhood Depression Assessment Tool, 222
   Children's Attributional Style Questionnaire, 110
   Children's Depression Adjective Check Lists, 222
   Children's Depression Inventory, 25, 69, 102, 147, 183, 202, 212–216, 236, 251, 252, 265, 326, 384, 432, 564
   Children's Depression Rating Scale, 183, 201–202, 212, 217, 218, 386, 387, 434
   Children's Depression Scale, 212, 216, 238
   Children's Negative Cognitive Error Questionnaire, 103
   Clinical Global Impressions, 386
   Cognitive Bias Questionnaire for Children, 103
   Cognitive Process Inventory for Children, 112
   Coopersmith Self-Esteem Inventory, 104
   Death/Suicide Interview, 547
   Depression Adjective Check List, 382
   Depression Self-Rating Scale, 103, 212, 217
   Depression Symptom Checklist, 252

Instruments (rating scales, self reports, structured interviews, questionnaires etc.) (*cont.*)

Depressive Affect Self-Report Scale, 222

Depressive Experiences Questionnaire for Adolescents, 222

Diagnostic Interview for Children and Adolescents, 27, 184, 189–191, 203, 210

Diagnostic Interview Schedule for Children, 184, 191–195, 202, 210, 585

Differential Emotions Scale—IV, 186, 219

Direct Observation Form, 243

Face Valid Depression Scale for Adolescents, 222

Family Assessment Device, 219

General Behavior Inventory, 222

Hamilton Depression Rating Scale, 201, 220, 386

Hopelessness Scale for Children, 107

Hopkins Symptom Checklist, 222, 256, 386

Hostility-Guilt Inventory

Interview for Aggression, 260

Interview Schedule for Children, 184, 195–197, 195, 202, 311, 564

Inventory to Diagnose Depression, 222

Kiddie Global Assessment Scale, 385

Life Orientation Inventory, 543

Matching Familiar Figures Test, 104, 108

Minnesota Multiphasic Personality Inventory, 69, 211, 382

Modified Scale for Suicidal Ideation, 559

Moyal–Miezitis Stimulus Appraisal Scale, 109

Multi-Attitude Suicide Tendency Scale, 547

Multiscore Depression Inventory, 222

My Standards Questionnaire—Revised, 296

Nowicki-Strickland Children's Locus of Control Scale, 109

Offer Self-Image Questionnaire, 104

Peer Nomination Inventory of Depression, 105, 222, 239, 245

Personality Inventory for Children, 237, 551

Piers–Harris Children's Self-Concept Scale, 104

Pleasant Events Schedule, 319

Psychiatric Rating Scale, 382

Raskin Depression Scale, 386

Rating Scale of Dysphoria, 212, 222, 239

Reasons for Living Inventory, 544

Research Diagnostic Criteria, 326

Reynolds Adolescent Depression Scale, 212, 218–220, 222, 223, 325, 325, 545, 548

Reynolds Child Depression Scale, 212, 217

Scale for Suicidal Ideation, 547

Schedule for Affective Disorders and Schizophrenia, 220, 432

Schedule for Affective Disorders and Schizophrenia in School-Age Children, 197–201

Schedule for Affective Disorders and Schizophrenia in School-Age Children, 68, 155, 184, 210, 236, 311, 385, 433

Instruments (rating scales, self reports, structured interviews, questionnaires etc.) (*cont.*)

Schedule for Affective Disorders and Schizophrenia—Lifetime Version, 469

School Age Depression Listed Inventory, 384

Self-Perception Profile for Children, 104

Self-Rating Depression Scale, 222

Spectrum of Suicidal Behaviors, 547

Suicidal Behavior History Form, 546

Suicidal Behaviors Interview, 542, 543, 544, 545, 546, 548, 549

Suicidal Ideation Questionnaire, 225, 534, 539, 541, 542, 543, 545, 548, 549, 553, 554, 555

Symptom Checklist for Major Depressive Disorders, 244

Teacher Affect Rating Scale, 242

Teacher Report Form, 242

Wechsler Intelligence Scale for Children-Revised, 108,147

Weinberg Index of Depression, 384

Youth Depression Adjective Checklist, 219

Youth Self-Report, 192, 222

Intelligence, 110, 148, 249, 301, 321, 485

Internalize, 7, 42, 89, 91, 92, 129, 131, 135, 485, 565

Internalizing, 4, 8, 31, 192, 210, 225, 252, 253, 254, 257, 261, 266, 267, 311, 313, 350, 466, 487, 489, 501, 516, 517, 518, 555, 589, 597

Interpersonal therapy, 10

Intervention, 86, 106, 123, 139, 185, 217, 241, 242, 275, 276, 277, 278, 279, 280, 282, 283, 290, 293, 296, 299, 306, 310, 311, 314, 318, 319, 322, 323, 325, 326, 327, 332, 333, 335, 336, 350, 351, 352, 353, 354, 356, 357, 358, 391, 403, 428, 435, 438, 439, 440, 452, 468, 470, 471, 473, 474, 482, 526, 536, 539, 543, 546, 547, 549, 556, 557, 558, 560, 561, 566, 567

Interview Schedule for Children, 184, 195–197, 195, 311, 564

Interviewing, 24, 25, 45, 48, 63, 148, 183, 184, 185, 186, 187, 188, 189, 190, 191, 192, 193, 195, 196, 197, 198, 199, 200, 201, 202, 203, 209, 211, 217, 218, 220, 222, 224, 225, 226, 236, 253, 259, 262, 265, 266, 267, 276, 287, 290, 292, 311, 313, 326, 328, 331, 351, 384, 432, 464, 468, 532, 539, 540, 544, 545, 546, 547, 548, 549, 559, 565, 581, 585

Intraclass Correlation Coefficient, 185

Introjective depression, 315

Introversion, 52

Inventory to Diagnose Depression, 222

IPT. *See* Interpersonal psychotherapy

Irritability, 23, 44, 52, 63, 68, 130, 174, 179, 226, 314, 323, 366, 378, 391, 449, 519, 582

ISC. *See* Interview Schedule for Children
Isocarboxazid, 376, 379

Juvenile court, 188, 331

Kappa statistic, 185, 186, 187, 189, 190, 191, 192, 193, 196, 198, 199, 200, 201, 221, 251, 253, 257
KASTAN Children's Attributional Style Questionnaire. *See* Children's Attributional Style Questionnaire
K-GAS. *See* Kiddie Global Assessment Scale
Kiddie Global Assessment Scale, 385
Kindergarten, 241
Klein-Levin syndrome, 146
K-SADS. *See* Schedule for Affective Disorders and Schizophrenia in School-Age Children

Language, 10, 26, 53, 87, 131, 145, 175, 190, 209, 211, 212, 218, 219, 282, 300, 333, 402, 419, 447, 452, 453, 466
Lead exposure, 369
Learned-helplessness, 97, 99, 108, 109, 110, 111, 113, 114, 115, 123, 135, 136, 137, 317, 410, 414, 415, 419, 430
Learning disability, 4, 26, 158, 447, 448
Libido, 448
Life Orientation Inventory, 543
Limbic system, 145, 146, 152, 153, 405, 448
Lithium, 11, 33, 35, 50, 51, 53, 54, 55, 151, 369, 378, 389, 405, 449
Locus ceruleus, 151
Locus of control, 100, 103, 109, 245, 261, 519
LOI. *See* Life Orientation Inventory
Longitudinal, 21, 33, 46, 50, 66, 71, 104, 107, 113, 114, 148, 157, 193, 196, 197, 199, 239, 263, 406, 466, 473, 491, 492, 512, 514, 517, 518, 520, 539, 548, 553, 585, 595, 596, 597, 598
Loss, 5, 21, 23, 62, 63, 68, 81, 82, 83, 84, 85, 86, 87, 88, 90, 91, 92, 94, 124, 126, 128, 134, 136, 173, 174, 175, 177, 178, 179, 186, 210, 213, 226, 243, 244, 315, 324, 332, 346, 358, 367, 410, 413, 414, 428, 431, 432, 437, 445, 449, 450, 452, 469, 482, 484, 487, 500, 502, 511, 515, 518, 520, 543, 565
Love, 81, 87, 301, 315, 323, 352
Ludiomil. *See* Maprotiline
Luvox. *See* Fluvoxamine

Magnetic resonance imaging, 148, 149, 151
Magnetic resonance spectroscopy, 148, 149, 151
Major depressive disorder, 6, 8, 9, 22, 25, 27, 44, 45, 50, 61, 64, 65, 66, 67, 70, 85, 107, 146, 148, 149, 150, 153, 154, 157, 158, 178, 210, 215, 218, 219, 220, 221, 238, 277, 348, 350, 407, 409, 418, 427, 428, 429, 432, 434, 435, 464, 470, 481, 486, 526, 548, 552, 553, 561, 565, 582, 584, 595

Maltreatment, 87, 481–502, 481, 482, 485, 486, 489, 490, 491, 493, 494, 495, 497, 499, 502
Manic-depressive. *See* Bipolar disorder
MAOI. *See* Monoamine oxidase inhibitor
Maprotiline, 378, 383
Marital therapy, 299
Marplan. *See* Isocarboxazid
Masked depression, 20, 63, 401, 430, 433
Mastery, 53, 89, 90, 91, 108, 109, 110, 113, 131, 277, 282, 284, 285, 287, 298, 322, 413
Matching Familiar Figures Test, 104, 108
Maturity, 55, 82, 83, 85, 89, 90, 235, 236, 316, 368, 581
Maximum covariance analysis, 65
Medical illness, 310, 331, 427, 429, 430, 435
Medications, 44, 63, 66, 176, 323, 325, 365–393, 366, 367, 371, 378, 388, 389, 390, 391, 392
  anticonvulsants
    carbamazepine, 53, 54
    valproic acid, 53, 54
  arecoline, 153
  benzodiazepines, 368, 436
  blood level, 388
  blood levels, 34, 55, 391, 392, 440
  bupropion, 378, 383
  clonidine, 65, 152, 154, 155
  compliance, 55, 56, 289, 301, 369, 389, 392, 428, 429, 439, 456, 502, 558
  desipramine, 154, 155 372
  dexamethasone, 9, 67, 145, 154, 198, 238, 406, 407, 409, 410, 437
  dose, 34, 154, 156, 368, 382, 384, 385, 386, 391, 392, 404, 440
  drug "holidays", 55
  efficacy, 34, 382
  fenfluramine, 152
  lithium, 11, 33, 35, 50, 51, 53, 54, 55, 151, 369, 378, 389, 405, 449
  maprotiline, 378, 383
  metabolism, 368
  monoamine oxidase inhibitor, 11, 33, 83, 151, 369, 376, 440, 449
    isocarboxazid, 376
    phenelzine, 378, 380
    tranylcypromine, 378, 381
  neuroleptics, 53, 55, 389
  overdose, 370, 371, 376, 391, 392, 531, 532, 556
  phenobarbital, 368
  physostigmine, 153
  placebo, 34, 51, 53, 54, 66, 144, 369, 376, 378, 382, 384, 385, 386, 387, 388, 440, 557, 559
  plasma levels, 34, 67, 382, 384, 385, 386, 387, 388, 406, 407, 408, 409
  psycho-stimulant, 51, 440
    methylphenidate, 150, 389
  reserpine, 151, 152, 404
  scopolamine, 153

Medications (*cont.*)
  selective serotonin reuptake inhibitor, 11, 449,
    556
    fluoxetine, 11, 48, 49, 368, 371, 376, 377,
      386, 388, 441, 556
    fluvoxamine, 376
    paroxetine, 369, 376, 377
    sertraline, 369, 376, 377, 388
  serotonin reuptake inhibitor, 11, 449, 556
  side effects, 10, 35, 368, 369, 370, 371, 376,
    384, 389, 391, 392, 393, 440, 441, 449,
    556
    anticholinergic, 152, 368, 370, 392, 440
    behavioral side effects, 376
    mania, 371
    sudden death, 371, 378
    withdrawal, 371
  trazodone, 378, 383, 441
  tricyclic antidepressant, 11, 83, 146, 151, 180,
    368, 369, 405, 407, 440, 449, 556
    amitriptyline, 66, 156, 370, 372, 382, 384,
      388, 441
    amoxapine, 370, 371, 374
    clomipramine, 152, 370, 371, 372, 388
    desipramine, 370, 371, 372, 385, 389
    imipramine, 32, 34, 66, 277, 365, 368, 370,
      371, 373, 382, 384, 385, 391, 404, 441
    nortriptyline, 66, 368, 370, 371, 385, 386, 387
    protriptyline, 370, 371, 374
    trimipramine, 370, 371, 375
    zimelidine, 154
Melancholia, 6, 22, 46, 61, 62, 63, 65, 71, 72, 81,
    82, 83, 85, 154, 156, 176, 180
Melatonin, 67
Memory, 101, 102, 135, 179, 284, 412, 487
Mental retardation, 53, 54, 62, 175, 218, 219,
    250, 264, 446, 447, 456, 457
Methodology, 24, 27, 100, 102, 209, 220, 226, 331
Methylphenidate, 150, 389
MHPG. *See* 3-methoxy-4- hydroxyphenylglycol
Minnesota Multiphasic Personality Inventory, 69,
    211, 382
MMPI. *See* Minnesota Multiphasic Personality
    Inventory
Modified Scale for Suicidal Ideation, 559
Monoamine oxidase inhibitor. *See* Medications *or
    specific drug*
Mood-congruent symptoms, 45, 62, 102, 178
Mood-incongruent symptoms, 45, 54
Mother, 62, 63, 81, 84, 85, 86, 88, 91, 92, 94,
    102, 113, 114, 115, 128, 129, 130, 134, 135,
    187, 188, 199, 200, 201, 237, 239, 240,
    245, 252, 253, 256, 259, 261, 262, 266,
    267, 277, 278, 315, 321, 322, 323, 324,
    345, 346, 347, 348, 349, 354, 384, 407,
    411, 414, 418, 419, 430, 433, 465, 466,
    467, 468, 469, 471, 472, 473, 485, 488,
    489, 491, 495, 496, 497, 500, 501, 513,
    517, 527, 554, 555, 591
Mourning, 85, 90, 134, 332

Moyal–Miezitis Stimulus Appraisal Scale, 109
MRI. *See* Magnetic resonance imaging
MRS. *See* Magnetic resonance spectroscopy
MSSI. *See* Modified Scale for Suicidal Ideation
Multi-Attitude Suicide Tendency Scale, 547
Multiple sclerosis, 447
Multiscore Depression Inventory, 222
Multivariate analysis, 64, 69, 170
My Standards Questionnaire—Revised, 296

Narcissism, 82, 90, 92
Nardil. *See* Phenelzine
National Institute of Mental Health, 45, 139, 191,
    268, 309, 527, 528
Natural-killer cell, 10
Nature vs. nurture, 9
Negative life events, 99, 111, 112, 113, 123, 346,
    497, 513, 545, 564
Neglect, 17, 25, 33, 49, 72, 81, 83, 243, 244,
    290, 309, 358, 389, 408, 418, 419, 450,
    481, 482, 483, 484, 485, 486, 488, 491,
    493, 495, 496, 499, 554
Neurobiology, 9, 98, 143, 144, 145, 157, 158, 553
Neurochemistry, 143, 145, 153, 158
Neuroendocrine, 67, 70, 72, 143, 145, 152, 153,
    155, 403, 404, 405, 407, 408, 409, 411, 413
Neuroimaging, 143, 145, 151, 158. *See* Brain
    imaging
Neuroleptics, 53
Neurology, 143, 145, 158
  neurological findings, 145, 146, 158
  neurological signs (focal), 146
  neurological signs (soft), 144
Neuromodulators, 153
Neuropeptide, 151, 153
Neuropsychological testing, 144, 147, 148
Neuropsychology, 143, 144, 145, 147, 148, 158
Neurosis, 21, 62, 63, 68, 70, 88, 170, 173, 254,
    347, 446
Neurotoxicity, 369
Neurotransmitter, 83, 85, 150, 151, 152, 153, 154,
    157, 158, 369, 370, 378, 404, 410
  acetylcholine, 151, 152, 154, 370
  catecholamine, 151, 404
  dopamine, 151, 152, 154, 370, 404, 409
  histamine, 370
  neuropeptide, 151, 153
  norepinephrine, 85, 151, 152, 370, 404, 406,
    409, 410
  serotonin, 11, 151, 152, 155, 370, 376, 388,
    389, 404, 405, 407, 409, 411, 449, 556
Neuro-vegetative signs. *See* Biological markers
Nightmares, 69, 70, 446
Noncompliance, 176, 285, 389, 439
Norepinephrine, 85, 151, 152, 370, 404, 406,
    409, 410
Normative data, 143, 158, 214, 237, 245, 265,
    513, 544
Norpramin. *See* Desipramine
Nortriptyline, 66, 368, 370, 371, 385, 386, 387

Nosology, 5, 61–72, 169–180
Nowicki–Strickland Children's Locus of Control Scale, 109

Object relations, 345, 351
Obsessions, 145, 253, 254
Offer Self-Image Questionnaire, 104
Onset, 27, 29, 33, 41, 42, 43, 44, 45, 46, 47, 50, 51, 52, 54, 55, 56, 64, 98, 132, 153, 156, 175, 177, 178, 179, 180, 185, 187, 196, 197, 310, 318, 336, 347, 387, 403, 404, 415, 431, 432, 433, 435, 436, 448, 449, 457, 469, 470, 589, 596
Oppositional defiant disorder, 50, 587, 588
Organic mood disorder, 436
Organic problems, 52
OSIQ. *See* Offer Self-Image Questionnaire
Outcome, 4, 11, 43, 46, 49, 52, 55, 64, 69, 72, 99, 109, 124, 125, 126, 129, 144, 171, 184, 199, 200, 210, 211, 213, 218, 220, 222, 262, 276, 277, 282, 284, 291, 294, 295, 297, 298, 299, 310, 317, 326, 330, 333, 334, 335, 336, 359, 385, 414, 418, 451, 464, 465, 467, 468, 470, 471, 472, 473, 487, 502, 528, 529, 530, 541, 546, 556, 559, 561, 584, 585, 597

Pain, 82, 86, 89, 352, 406, 414, 438
Pamelor. *See* Nortriptyline
Parents
    father, 88, 114, 115, 135, 200, 237, 239, 240, 252, 253, 255, 256, 259, 267, 324, 332, 345, 347, 349, 354, 500, 513, 554
    mother, 62, 63, 81, 84, 85, 86, 88, 91, 92, 94, 102, 113, 114, 115, 128, 129, 130, 134, 135, 187, 188, 199, 200, 201, 237, 239, 240, 245, 252, 253, 256, 259, 261, 262, 266, 267, 277, 278, 315, 321, 322, 323, 324, 345, 346, 347, 348, 349, 354, 384, 407, 411, 414, 418, 419, 430, 433, 465, 466, 467, 468, 469, 471, 472, 473, 485, 488, 489, 491, 495, 496, 497, 500, 501, 513, 517, 527, 554, 555, 591
    parent training, 277, 282, 283, 299, 300, 303, 306
    parental depression, 417
        maternal depression, 102, 349, 471
        parents with affective disorders, 463–474
    parental education, 28
    parental psychopathology, 8, 133, 346, 418, 486, 513, 565
    parental report, 237, 239, 513, 514
    parenting, 71, 133, 256, 283, 299, 300, 302, 303, 306, 334, 349, 351, 356, 357, 471, 472, 473, 474, 482, 486, 493, 494, 496, 501, 502, 555
Parnate. *See* Tranylcypromine
Paroxetine, 369, 376, 377
Pathophysiology, 5, 64, 144, 145, 151, 156
Paxil. *See* Paroxetine
Pearson correlation, 185

Pedigree, 70
Peer Nomination Inventory of Depression, 105, 222, 239, 245
Peer relationship, 131
Peers, 4, 6, 54, 85, 87, 88, 89, 91, 92, 100, 101, 108, 112, 113, 114, 115, 129, 131, 235, 244, 245, 246, 249, 250, 251, 252, 258, 261, 263, 265, 266, 267, 278, 280, 281, 282, 283, 290, 315, 316, 321, 322, 335, 336, 351, 356, 440, 447, 448, 450, 452, 453, 455, 456, 498, 499, 501, 502, 528, 540, 541, 548, 564
Perfectionism, 70
Perseveration, 49, 53
Personality, 46, 48, 52, 53, 54, 70, 88, 94, 126, 129, 134, 137, 171, 175, 237, 239, 245, 249, 259, 263, 402, 428, 430, 435, 483, 484, 487, 489, 518, 526, 527, 529, 542, 544, 550, 551, 552, 553, 555, 557
Personality disorder, 46, 402, 483, 487, 489, 527, 544, 551, 552, 557
Personality Inventory for Children, 237, 551
Pertofrane. *See* Desipramine
PES. *See* Pleasant Events Schedule
PET. *See* Positron emission tomography
Pharmacodynamics, 367, 368
Pharmacokinetics, 367, 391
Pharmacology, 10, 11, 21, 33, 34, 70, 152, 154, 158, 176, 178, 366, 389, 436, 449, 556
Pharmacotherapy, 10, 365–393, 440
Phenelzine, 378, 380
Phenobarbital, 368
Phenocopy, 53, 67
Phenomenology, 17, 19, 20, 21, 22, 23, 24, 30, 31–35, 43, 46, 53, 63, 70. *See also specific disorder*
Phenotype, 61
Phobias, 582, 584, 587, 588
Physical abuse, 86, 87, 262, 346, 418, 482, 483, 484, 485, 491, 497, 515, 554
Physical illness, 9, 355, 391, 429, 432
Physostigmine, 153
PIC. *See* Personality Inventory for Children
Piers–Harris Children's Self-Concept Scale, 104
Placebo, 34, 51, 53, 54, 66, 144, 369, 376, 378, 382, 384, 385, 386, 387, 440, 557, 559
Placement, 9
Plasma levels. *See* Blood levels
Pleasant Events Schedule, 319
PNID. *See* Peer Nomination Inventory of Depression
Polysomnography, 65, 67, 143, 145, 156–157, 156
Positron emission tomography, 148, 149, 150
Postpartum, 6
Posttraumatic stress disorder, 410, 436, 438, 483
Premorbid, 46, 48, 49, 52, 53, 56, 90, 170, 529, 534
Prevention, 53, 123, 139, 310, 327, 328, 438, 448, 449, 450, 452, 474, 528, 537, 539, 543, 547, 555, 556, 560, 561, 566, 567
    primary prevention, 474

Prevention (*cont.*)
  secondary prevention, 327, 474
  suicide prevention, 560
  tertiary prevention, 327, 474
Primate, 85
Prodrome, 43, 50, 51
Prognosis, 43, 44, 45, 47, 55, 144, 148, 184, 429,
    433, 486
Prolactin, 152, 153, 409
Promiscuity, 315
Prophylaxis, 53, 54, 55
Prosody, 145
Protriptyline, 370, 371, 374
Prozac. *See* Fluoxetine
PRS. *See* Psychiatric Rating Scale
Psychiatric Rating Scale, 382
Psychobiology. *See* Neurobiology
Psychoimmunology, 331
Psychometric, 7, 112, 183, 184, 189, 190, 191,
    194, 195, 196, 197, 201, 202, 213, 214,
    216, 217, 237, 239, 240, 242, 335, 540,
    546, 547
Psychomotor agitation, 21, 174, 446
Psychomotor disturbance, 4, 21, 22, 53, 62, 68,
    85, 147, 174, 176, 177, 196, 402, 417, 434,
    445, 446
Psychopharmacology, 10, 371, 393. *See*
    Pharmacology
Psychosis, 29, 34, 41, 42, 43, 44, 45, 47, 48, 49,
    51, 52, 53, 55, 62, 170, 173, 178, 193, 323,
    385, 386, 389, 428, 582
Psychosocial deficits, 314
Psychosocial factors, 25, 34, 35, 72, 84, 171, 455
Psychosocial problems, 310, 313, 314
Psychosocial stress, 509–20
Psycho-stimulant. *See* Medications *or specific*
    drug
Psychotherapy, 10, 101, 322, 323, 325, 332, 334,
    384, 391, 439, 440, 557, 558
  cognitive-behavioral therapy, 10, 97, 104, 105,
    106, 116, 276, 277, 279, 281, 285, 286, 293,
    306, 315, 317, 319, 324, 325, 326, 328, 329,
    332, 345, 350, 351, 355, 439, 556, 558
    attribution retraining, 114, 278
    behavioral problem-solving therapy, 105
    relaxation training, 106, 279, 280, 288, 289,
      300, 302, 318, 319, 325, 326, 558
    self-control therapy, 105, 202, 324, 325, 336
    social-skills training, 200, 277, 280, 281,
      290, 318, 558
  dialectical behavior therapy, 557
  existential therapy, 324
  family therapy, 277, 282, 283, 303, 306, 324,
    325, 326, 330, 345–359, 345, 350, 351,
    352, 353, 354, 355, 359, 438, 439, 441,
    556, 558, 560
  group therapy, 200, 325, 326, 330, 335, 359,
    438, 440, 558
  interpersonal therapy, 10, 322, 557
  kinetic psychotherapy, 325

Psychotherapy (*cont.*)
  marital therapy, 299
  parent training, 277, 282, 283, 299, 300, 303, 306
  play therapy, 63, 439
  psychoanalysis, 20, 42, 63, 81, 83, 84, 90, 173,
    315, 316, 401, 446, 490
    countertransference, 435
    transference, 316
  psychodynamic, 3, 62, 81, 82, 83, 84, 104, 177,
    315, 316, 317, 553
  relaxation training, 106, 279, 280, 319, 558
  supportive psychotherapy, 439
PTSD. *See* Posttraumatic stress disorder
Puberty, 11, 24, 28, 29, 34, 89, 91, 131, 155, 158, 449
  prepuberty, 17,19, 21, 24, 25, 26, 28, 29, 30,
    31, 32, 34, 43, 44, 48, 50, 51, 53, 66, 67,
    68, 69, 71, 154, 155, 157, 173, 176, 371,
    385, 402, 405
Public Law 101-476, 241
Public Law 94-142, 241
Punishment, 71, 99, 115, 292, 318, 324, 419, 430,
    452, 485, 501

Questionnaires. *See* Instruments

Race, 28, 111, 214, 242, 246, 256, 264, 267, 310,
    332, 333, 433, 529, 536, 565
RADS. *See* Reynolds Adolescent Depression Scale
Raphe nuclei, 152
Raskin Depression Scale, 386
Rating scales. *See* Instruments
Rating Scale of Dysphoria, 222, 239
RDC. *See* Research Diagnostic Criteria
Reactive depression, 26, 63
Reading ability, 211, 218, 220, 235, 238, 286,
    288, 319, 543
Reasons for Living Inventory, 544
Receiver operating characteristic, 238
Receptors, 83, 150, 152, 153, 157, 158, 405
Recovery, 45, 46, 47, 86, 115, 153, 154, 155, 196,
    314, 326, 330, 335, 336, 438, 470, 482,
    584, 597
Recurrence, 32, 41, 44, 46, 47, 55, 66, 144, 335
Rejection, 72, 88, 89, 101, 180, 240, 244, 278,
    290, 315, 346, 347, 348, 417, 430, 440,
    456, 489, 493, 494, 496, 497, 498, 499,
    501, 502, 554, 585
Relapse, 53, 144, 154, 155, 276, 310, 328, 334,
    335, 473, 496, 597
Relaxation training, 106, 319, 558
Religion, 28, 49
REM latency, 65, 67, 144, 156, 157, 158
Remission, 30, 56, 101, 144, 146, 154, 156, 157,
    175, 335, 346, 347, 348, 558
Research Diagnostic Criteria, 21, 42, 178, 180,
    210, 326, 385
Reserpine, 151, 152, 404
Residential treatment, 243
Resiliency, 98, 131, 467, 468, 474
Reticular activating system, 405

Reticular system, 152
Rewards, 109, 115, 137, 284, 289, 292
Reynolds Adolescent Depression Scale, 212, 218–220, 218, 545
Reynolds Child Depression Scale, 212, 217
RFL. *See* Reasons for Living Inventory
Risk factors, 72, 133, 332, 346, 414, 415, 419, 468, 473, 525, 546, 565, 584, 585, 586, 596, 597, 598
RSD. *See* Rating Scale for Dysphoria

SADS-L. *See* Schedule for Affective Disorders and Schizophrenia—Lifetime Version
SBHF. *See* Suicidal Behavior History Form
SBI. *See* Suicidal Behaviors Interview
SBS. *See* Spectrum of Suicidal Behaviors Scale
Scale for Suicidal Ideation, 547
Scapegoating, 354
Schedule for Affective Disorders and Schizophrenia, 220, 432
Schedule for Affective Disorders and Schizophrenia in School-Age Children, 184, 197–201, 210, 236, 311, 385
Schedule for Affective Disorders and Schizophrenia—Lifetime Version, 469
Schizoaffective disorder, 33, 52, 54, 55, 179, 407
Schizoid, 68
Schizophrenia, 42, 44, 45, 46, 48, 51, 52, 55, 155, 156, 179, 180, 199, 253, 329, 334, 433, 532, 550, 551
Schizophreniform disorder, 179
School
  academic achievement, 109, 148, 515
  academic performance, 89, 106, 262, 278, 517
  education, 28, 94, 219, 282, 283, 285, 289, 291, 297, 298, 301, 302, 303, 304, 305, 354, 445, 447, 450, 452, 453, 457
    special education, 219, 445, 447, 450, 452, 453, 457
  grade point average, 262, 313, 335
  grades, 4
  high school, 104, 110, 114, 214, 219, 223, 224, 310, 323, 328, 534, 537, 539, 542, 546, 547, 548, 554, 562, 586
  school achievement, 109, 113, 518
  school psychologists, 223, 549
  school-based assessment, 214, 218, 220, 221, 222, 225, 278, 310, 326, 327, 329, 530, 531, 534, 536, 539, 540, 544, 546, 547, 548, 549, 550, 551, 552, 554, 556, 558, 560, 561, 566
  teacher, 4, 6, 24, 68, 89, 104, 105, 108, 109, 113, 115, 184, 190, 193, 199, 211, 223, 225, 235, 236, 237, 238, 240, 241, 242, 243, 244, 245, 246, 249, 250, 251, 252, 253, 254, 255, 256, 258, 259, 261, 262, 263, 264, 265, 266, 267, 282, 283, 284, 290, 294, 295, 296, 297, 310, 333, 336, 351, 390, 446, 447, 448, 450, 451, 452, 455, 456, 497, 498, 510, 548, 549, 586, 591, 595, 596

School Age Depression Listed Inventory, 384
Scopolamine, 153
Seasonal affective disorder, 6
SED. *See* Severely emotionally disturbed
Seizure, 436, 440
Selective serotonin reuptake inhibitor. *See* Medications *or specific drug*
Self-blame, 44, 490, 491, 492, 494, 495, 499, 500, 502
Self-esteem, 22, 53, 63, 82, 83, 85, 86, 87, 89, 92, 98, 99, 103, 104, 105, 106, 107, 109, 110, 115, 128, 129, 131, 133, 136, 137, 173, 174, 177, 178, 179, 215, 261, 265, 276, 279, 281, 283, 292, 300, 301, 302, 306, 311, 313, 314, 315, 318, 335, 348, 357, 410, 431, 432, 434, 437, 451, 455, 466, 467, 481, 484, 485, 490, 491, 492, 494, 495, 497, 498, 499, 500, 502, 516, 542, 565, 591, 594
Self-image, 88, 185, 241, 335, 437, 467
Self-medication, 33, 436
Self-monitoring, 99, 114, 116, 278, 279, 295, 296, 297, 324, 326
Self-Perception Profile for Children, 104
Self-pity, 44
Self-Rating Depression Scale, 222
Self report. *See* Instruments
Self-regulation, 90, 114, 115, 136, 284, 408, 419, 489, 542
Self-schema, 101, 102, 354
Separation, 5, 9, 32, 63, 84, 85, 94, 124, 128, 129, 134, 172, 237, 238, 346, 366, 387, 410, 411, 417, 418, 430, 433, 436, 473, 495, 515, 584, 595
Sequelae, 92, 124, 481, 487
Serotonin, 11, 151, 152, 155, 370, 376, 388, 404, 405, 407, 409, 411, 449, 556
Serotonin reuptake inhibitor. *See also* Medications *or specific drug*
Serotonin syndrome, 389
Sertraline, 369, 376, 377, 388
Severely emotionally disturbed, 447
Sexual abuse, 188, 483–484
Sexuality, 49, 89, 315, 323, 392, 427, 431, 472, 482, 483, 484, 485, 486, 488, 489, 491, 554, 555
  masturbation, 49
Shyness, 68, 69, 186
Siblings, 100, 115, 256, 291, 333, 351, 356, 359, 434, 437
Signal-detection theory, 238
Single-photon emission computed tomography, 148, 149, 150.
SIQ. *See* Suicidal Ideation Questionnaire
Sleep, 5, 10, 21, 22, 23, 32, 53, 65, 67, 69, 84, 85, 130, 152, 154, 156, 157, 158, 174, 177, 198, 215, 226, 235, 244, 245, 253, 366, 367, 368, 386, 390, 391, 406, 407, 411, 417, 427, 428, 430, 434, 446, 448, 484, 552

Slow wave sleep, 67
Social class, 109
Social competence, 105, 148, 262, 348, 453
Social isolation, 101, 237, 440
Social support, 9, 124, 311, 313, 314, 322, 335, 448, 450, 455, 456, 545, 554, 556
Social withdrawal, 84, 174, 179, 262, 330, 582
Social-skills deficit, 100, 277
Social-skills training, 200, 277, 280, 281, 290, 318, 558
Somatic, 5, 22, 49, 63, 68, 154, 174, 176, 177, 178, 185, 192, 210, 215, 218, 254, 277, 429, 430, 432, 434, 441, 484, 552
Somatizing, 68
Somatostatin, 65
Special education, 219, 445, 447, 450, 452, 453, 457
SPECT. *See* Single-photon emission computed tomography
Spectrum of Suicidal Behaviors, 547
Speech, 26, 47, 49, 52, 53, 114, 146, 190, 244, 277, 318, 446, 447, 452
SSRI. *See* Selective serotonin reuptake inhibitor
State variable, 144, 148
Stepfathers, 256
Stigma, 169, 390
Stressors, 8, 11, 133, 175, 322, 333, 353, 354, 366, 403, 430, 435, 436, 439, 469, 487, 488, 489, 496, 502, 515, 516, 518, 519, 525, 542, 556, 565
  abandonment, 72, 224, 315, 554
  abuse, 8, 25, 27, 31, 33, 46, 49, 50, 70, 72, 82, 86, 87, 126, 133, 155, 179, 188, 262, 310, 315, 323, 329, 333, 345, 346, 366, 386, 408, 415, 418, 419, 427, 436, 470, 481–502, 481, 482, 483, 484, 485, 486, 487, 488, 489, 490, 491, 492, 493, 494, 495, 496, 497, 499, 500, 501, 502, 510, 515, 520, 529, 550, 551, 552, 555, 585
    physical abuse, 86, 87, 262, 346, 418, 482, 483, 484, 485, 491, 497, 515, 554, 555
    sexual abuse, 188, 483–484
  bereavement, 22, 71, 72, 85, 179, 315, 332, 436, 469, 520
  deprivation, 82, 87, 90, 92, 94, 173, 315, 346, 355, 433, 449
  disasters, 482, 512, 515, 516, 517
  divorce, 9, 133, 346, 366, 472, 473, 474, 487, 516
  family conflict, 261, 332, 346
  grief, 70, 323, 332, 358, 411, 427, 435, 436, 439, 473
  helplessness, 72, 82, 97, 99, 103, 108, 109, 110, 111, 112, 113, 114, 115, 116, 123, 128, 131, 133, 134, 135, 136, 137, 173, 241, 317, 347, 348, 351, 353, 354, 357, 410, 414, 415, 419, 428, 430, 433, 439, 449, 451, 455, 468, 481, 491, 500, 519, 565
  isolation, 68, 88, 89, 101, 209, 237, 283, 417, 437, 440

Stressors (*cont.*)
  loss, 5, 21, 23, 62, 63, 68, 81, 82, 83, 84, 85, 86, 87, 88, 90, 91, 92, 94, 124, 126, 128, 134, 136, 173, 174, 175, 177, 178, 179, 186, 210, 213, 226, 243, 244, 315, 324, 332, 346, 358, 367, 410, 413, 414, 428, 431, 432, 437, 445, 449, 450, 452, 469, 482, 484, 487, 500, 502, 511, 515, 518, 520, 543, 565
  maltreatment, 87, 481, 482, 485, 486, 489, 490, 491, 493, 494, 495, 497, 499, 502
  negative life events, 99, 111, 112, 113, 123, 346, 497, 513, 545, 564
  neglect, 17, 25, 33, 49, 72, 81, 83, 243, 244, 290, 309, 358, 389, 408, 418, 419, 450, 481, 482, 483, 484, 485, 486, 488, 491, 493, 495, 496, 499, 554
    failure to thrive, 408, 419
  pain, 82, 86, 89, 352, 406, 414, 438
  psychosocial stress, 509–520
  rejection, 72, 88, 89, 101, 180, 240, 244, 278, 290, 315, 346, 347, 348, 417, 430, 440, 456, 489, 493, 494, 496, 497, 498, 499, 501, 502, 554, 585
  separation, 5, 9, 32, 63, 84, 85, 94, 124, 128, 129, 134, 237, 238, 346, 366, 387, 410, 411, 417, 418, 430, 433, 436, 473, 495, 515, 584, 595
  social class, 109
  stressful events, 313, 409, 472, 509, 513, 514, 515, 516, 517, 518, 519, 520
  war, 63
Stroke, 145, 146, 158
Structured interviews. *See* Instruments
Substance abuse, 6. *See* Drug abuse
Substance-abuse, 8, 50, 155, 333, 550, 585
Substantia nigra, 153
Subsyndromal, 51, 55
Subtypes, 8, 9, 21, 42, 147, 173, 178, 180, 196, 202, 516, 517, 518, 526, 527, 597
Suicidal Behavior History Form, 546
Suicidal Behaviors Interview, 542, 544
Suicidal Ideation Questionnaire, 225, 534, 539, 541, 542
Suicide, 3, 68, 101, 112, 154, 157, 219, 225, 238, 239, 253, 266, 327, 332, 346, 376, 382, 486, 525–567, 525, 526, 527, 529, 533, 535, 540, 541, 542, 544, 545, 546, 547, 548, 550, 551, 552, 553, 554, 555, 556, 557, 558, 560, 563, 564, 566, 567
  assessment, 225, 539–549
  attempt, 537, 545, 551, 552
  attempts, 51, 69
  epidemiology, 64, 70, 527, 534–539, 535, 537, 566
  gender differences, 530
  intervention, 326, 327, 555–561, 556, 557, 560
  method, 529, 531, 532
    lethality, 527, 530, 532, 533, 563, 564, 565

Suicidal Ideation Questionnaire (*cont.*)
method (*cont.*)
overdose, 370, 371, 376, 391, 392, 531, 532, 556
notes, 529
parasuicide, 528, 530
prevention, 537, 560, 561
psychological autopsy, 528, 529, 534, 550, 553, 562
screening, 549
suicidal behavior, 29, 107, 108, 115, 219, 225, 311, 326, 329, 331, 352, 385, 485, 525, 526, 527, 528, 529, 530, 531, 533, 534, 535, 536, 537, 538, 539, 540, 541, 542, 543, 544, 545, 546, 547, 548, 549, 550, 551, 552, 553, 554, 555, 556, 557, 558, 559, 560, 561, 562, 563, 564, 565, 566, 567
suicidal ideation, 22, 24, 44, 68, 69, 85, 86, 91, 107, 174, 175, 200, 210, 225, 236, 241, 243, 253, 254, 264, 266, 327, 353, 367, 376, 417, 427, 445, 446, 484, 526, 527, 528, 533, 534, 536, 537, 538, 539, 540, 541, 542, 543, 544, 545, 546, 547, 548, 549, 553, 554, 555, 556, 558, 559, 561, 562, 563, 564, 566, 567, 582
suicidal risk, 47, 532
suicide attempt, 29, 113, 219, 239, 261, 262, 328, 329, 367, 407, 445, 470, 485, 527, 530, 531 532, 533
suicide completion, 29, 529, 550
suicide risk, 107, 327, 348, 350, 431, 553, 557
superego, 42, 63, 81, 90, 91, 173, 401
Surmontil. *See* Trimipramine
Symptom Checklist for Major Depressive Disorders, 244

TARS. *See* Teacher Affect Rating Scale
Taxonomic. *See* Nosology
TCA. *See* Tricyclic antidepressant
Teacher Affect Rating Scale, 242
Teacher Report Form, 242
Television, 49, 244
Temperament, 4, 48, 61, 71, 100, 451, 467
Thalamus, 145
Theories, 63, 71, 81, 82, 97, 100, 104, 136, 263, 317, 404, 445, 448, 482, 491
Therapeutic alliance, 316, 317, 330, 336
Thought disorder, 22, 23, 192
Thyroid, 65, 67, 153, 155, 436
Thyroid-stimulating hormone, 65, 67, 155

Thyrotropin-releasing hormone, 65, 67, 155
Tofranil. *See* Imipramine
Trait variable, 144, 148, 154, 157
Tranylcypromine, 378. 381
Trauma, 8, 9, 11, 83, 410, 431, 437, 438, 482, 483, 488, 491, 492, 512, 513, 514, 515, 516, 519, 554
Trazodone, 378, 383, 441
TRF. *See* Teacher Report Form
TRH. *See* Thyrotropin-releasing hormone
Tricyclic antidepressant. *See* Medications *or specific drug*
Trimipramine, 370, 371, 375
Truancy, 254, 315
Tryptophan, 152, 404
Twin studies, 64, 65, 67, 70, 449, 469

Ulcerative colitis, 433
Unconscious, 62, 86, 91, 405, 532
Unipolar, 5, 21, 42, 44, 45, 47, 62, 64, 65, 150, 153, 176, 187, 199, 310, 407, 408, 464, 465, 469, 470

Validity. *See* Diagnostic validity
Valproic acid, 53, 54
Vegetative symptoms, 53, 101, 213, 402, 429, 435, 552
Vivactil. *See* Protriptylin
Vulnerability, 8, 33, 54, 67, 72, 83, 90, 94, 102, 106, 113, 126, 127, 128, 130, 131, 132, 133, 134, 157, 176, 315, 322, 332, 346, 353, 354, 368, 405, 413, 418, 431, 466, 469, 486, 487, 488, 496, 499, 500, 509, 519, 525, 565, 595

War, 63
Wechsler Intelligence Scale for Children— Revised, 108, 147
Weight gain, 44, 55
Weinberg Index of Depression, 384
Wellbutrin. *See* Bupropion
WISC-R. *See* Wechsler Intelligence Scale for Children—Revised

Y-DACL. *See* Youth Depression Adjective Checklist
Youth Depression Adjective Checklist, 219
Youth Self-Report, 192, 222

Zimelidine, 154
Zoloft. *See* sertraline